P9-BYT-329

FIFTH EDITION

PSYCHIATRIC NURSING

Holly Skodol Wilson

PhD, RN, FAAN

Carol Ren Kneisl

MS, RN, CS

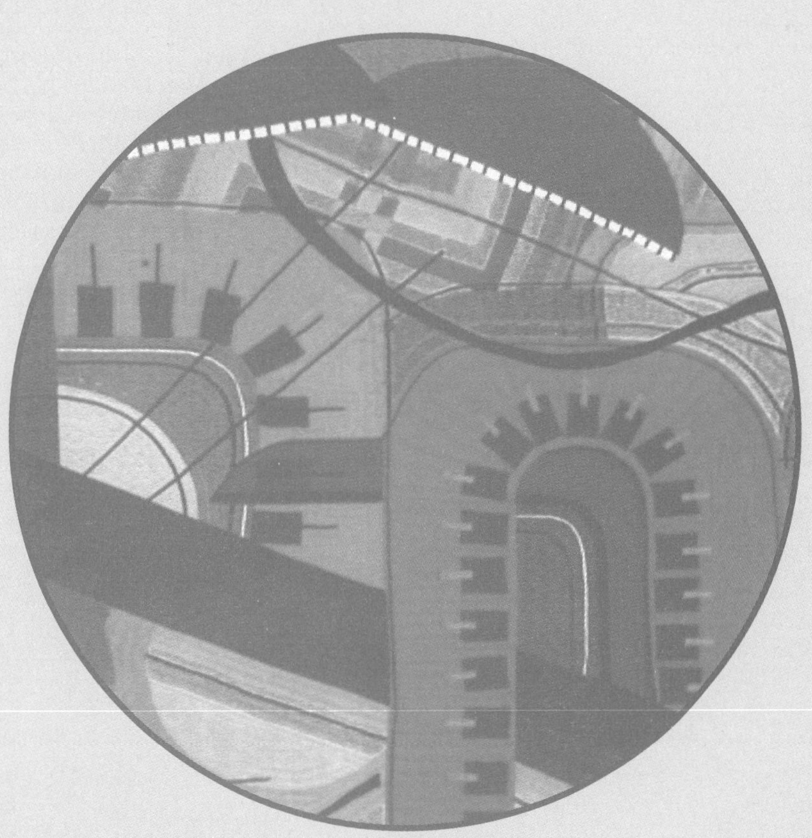

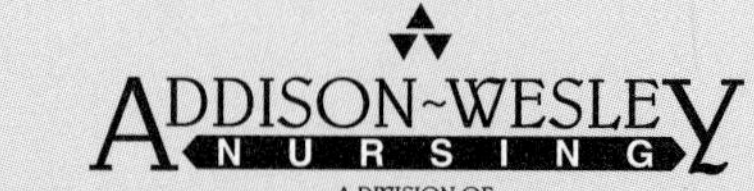

A DIVISION OF

THE BENJAMIN/CUMMINGS PUBLISHING COMPANY, INC.

Menlo Park, California • Reading, Massachusetts • New York • Don Mills, Ontario
Wokingham, U.K. • Amsterdam • Bonn • Paris • Milan • Madrid • Sydney • Singapore
Tokyo • Seoul • Taipei • Mexico City • San Juan, Puerto Rico

Executive Editor: Patricia L. Cleary
Developmental Editor: Mark J. Wales
Managing Editor: Wendy Earl
Production Supervisor: Karen Gulliver
Editorial Assistant: Marla Nowick
Text and Insert Designer: Gary Head Design
Cover Designer: Yvo Riezebos
Copy Editor: Betsy Dilernia
Proofreader: Anita Wagner
Indexer: Sylvia Coates
Composition Manager: Lillian Hom
Compositor and Prepress Supplier: GTS Graphics
Art Production: GTS Graphics
Manufacturing Coordinator: Merry Free Osborn
Text Printer and Binder: Von Hoffmann Press, Inc.
Cover Printer: Color Dot, Inc.

Credits may be found on page CR-1.

The quilt pictured on the cover, "Clamscape" was designed by Lynn Last. The image was supplied by Mitsumura Suiko Shoin Co., Ltd., Kyoto, Japan.

Library of Congress Cataloging-in-Publication Data

Wilson, Holly Skodol.
Psychiatric nursing / Holly Skodol Wilson, Carol Ren Kneisl.—5th ed.
p. cm.
Includes bibliographical references and index.
ISBN 0-8053-9408-7
1. Psychiatric nursing. I. Kneisl, Carol Ren. II. Title.
[DNLM: 1. Psychiatric Nursing. WY 160 W748p 1996]
RC440.W5 1996
610.73'68—dc20
DNLM/DLC 95-37750
for Library of Congress CIP

ISBN 0-8053-9408-7

1 2 3 4 5 6 7 8 9 10—VH—99 98 97 96 95

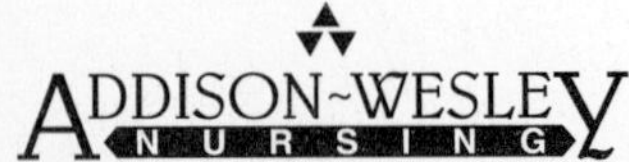

A DIVISION OF
THE BENJAMIN/CUMMINGS PUBLISHING COMPANY, INC.

2725 Sand Hill Road,
Menlo Park, California 94025

Care has been taken to confirm the accuracy of information presented in this book. The authors, editors, and the publisher, however, cannot accept any responsibility for errors or omissions or for the consequences from application of information in this book and make no warranty, express or implied, with respect to its contents.

The authors and publisher have exerted every effort to ensure that drug selections and dosages set forth in this text are in accord with current recommendations and practice at time of publication. However, in view of ongoing research, changes in government regulations, and the constant flow of information relating to drug therapy and drug reactions, the reader is urged to check the package inserts of all drugs for any change in indications of dosage and for added warnings and precautions. This is particularly important when the recommended agent is a new and/or infrequently employed drug.

AUTHORS AND CONTRIBUTORS

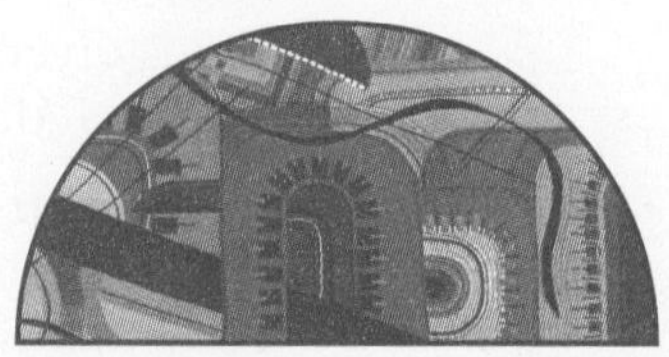

Holly Skodol Wilson, PhD, RN, FAAN, is a Professor in the Department of Mental Health, Community and Administrative Nursing, School of Nursing, University of California at San Francisco. Her clinical and research interests are in the fields of community care for the demented elderly and quality of life in advanced HIV/AIDS. She is active as an international lecturer on topics ranging from research in nursing to the future of psychiatric nursing practice, education, and science.

Carol Ren Kneisl, MS, RN, CS, is an internationally known nursing author, lecturer, and consultant, and is President and Educational Director of Nursing Transitions, Inc., a nursing continuing education company in Williamsville, New York. Actively involved in clinical practice issues, she encourages psychiatric nurses through her consultation, writing, and speaking activities to provide expert, humanistic care in psychiatric–mental health nursing and to take active leadership roles in the AIDS era.

Contributors

Judy Banks Campbell, EdD, MSN, ARNP
Professor
Palm Beach Community College
Lake Worth, Florida

Linda Chafetz, DNSc, RN
Associate Professor and Coordinator,
Department of Mental Health, Community, and Administrative Nursing
University of California, San Francisco
San Francisco, California

Catherine A. Chesla, DNSc, RN
Associate Professor, Department of Family Health Care Nursing
University of California, San Francisco
San Francisco, California

Kay K. Chitty, EdD, RN, CS
Adjunct Professor
University of Tennessee at Chattanooga
Clinical Specialist, Private Practice
Chattanooga, Tennessee

Carol Bradley Corpuel, MSN, RN, CS
Assistant Professor, Orvis School of Nursing
University of Nevada, Reno
Psychiatric Clinical Nurse Specialist
St. Mary's Regional Medical Center
Reno, Nevada

Sue DeLaune, MN, RN, C
Instructor, Nursing Department
Loyola University
Instructor, Staff Education Department
Southeast Louisiana Hospital
President, SDeLaune Consulting
New Orleans, Louisiana

Jerry D. Durham, PhD, RN, FAAN
Executive Associate Dean for Educational Services
Professor, Psychiatric-Mental Health Nursing
Indiana University School of Nursing
Indianapolis, Indiana

Anastasia Fisher, DNSc, RN
Assistant Professor, University of San Francisco
San Francisco, California
Adjunct Nurse Researcher, Stanford University Medical Center

Karen Lee Fontaine, MSN, RN, AASECT
Professor of Nursing, Purdue University Calumet
Hammond, Indiana

Susan Hunn Garritson, DNSc, RN
Assistant Clinical Professor, School of Nursing
University of California, San Francisco
San Francisco, California

Sally Hutchinson, PhD, RN, FAAN
Professor, College of Nursing
University of Florida
Jacksonville, Florida

Bethany Phoenix Kasten, MSN, RN
Doctoral Candidate, School of Nursing
University of California, San Francisco
San Francisco, California

Joanne Keglovits, MSN, RN, CS
Clinical Specialist and School Nurse Practitioner
Pleasant Valley School District
Brodheadsville, Pennsylvania

Gloria Kuhlman, DNSc, RN
Professor and Clinical Coordinator, Department of Nursing
Ohlone College, Fremont, California
Geropsychiatric Nursing Consultant

Marilyn Meder, MSN, RN
Adjunct Clinical Instructor
School of Nursing, Widener University
Chester, Pennsylvania

Maryruth Morris, MS, RN, CS
Supervisor, Dually Diagnosed Family Support Program
Monsignor Carr Institute
Buffalo, New York

Beth Moscato, PhD, RN
Research Associate
Department of Social and Preventive Medicine
State University of New York at Buffalo
Buffalo, New York

Noreen King Poole, EdD, ARNP, RN, CS
Professor Emeritus
Palm Beach Community College
Lake Worth, Florida

Marlene Reimer, PhD, RN
Associate Professor, Faculty of Nursing
The University of Calgary
Calgary, Alberta, Canada

Elizabeth A. Riley, MS, RN, CS
Assistant Clinical Director, Adult Inpatient Services
Four Winds Hospital
Private Practice
Saratoga Springs, New York

Susan Simmons-Alling, MSN, RN, CS
Advanced Practice Nurse, Clinical Specialist
Private Practice
Spring Lake Heights, New Jersey

Eileen Trigoboff, MS, RN, CS
Doctoral candidate, State University of New York at Buffalo
Clinical Specialist in Psychiatric Nursing
Buffalo Psychiatric Center
Private Practice
Buffalo, New York

Sandra J. Weiss, PhD, DNSc, RN, FAAN
Professor and Director, Center for Family Health Studies
University of California, San Francisco
San Francisco, California

Lorraine M. Wheeler, MSN, RN, CS
Director of Nursing
El Castillo Residences for Retirement
President, Wheeler/Wheeler Consulting
Albuquerque, New Mexico

Reviewers

Dorothy S. Bonner, MN, RN
LSUMC School of Nursing
New Orleans, Louisiana

Anita Deitrick, MSN(c), RN
Professor, Health and Public Services
Des Moines Area Community College
Ankeny, Iowa

Sharon D. Dettenrieder, MSN, RN
Associate Professor, Department of Nursing
Hartwick College
Oneonta, New York

Karen Espeland, MSN, RN, CCDN
Medcenter One College of Nursing
Bismark, North Dakota

Mary Jo Gorney-Lucero, PhD, RN
Professor, School of Nursing
San Jose State University
San Jose, California

Wendy Hollis, MN, RN
Professor, Nursing Department
Los Angeles Harbor College
Wilmington, California

Alice B. Jehle, MS, RN
Associate Professor, Department of Nursing
Berkshire Community College
Pittsfield, Massachusetts

Carolyn Poole Latham, MS, RN, CARN
Decker School of Nursing
State University of New York at Binghamton
Binghamton, New York

Diana McDonald, MSN, RN, FNP
Nursing Instructor, Health Sciences Department
Los Medanos College
Pittsburg, California

Linda Nance Marks, EdD, RN
School of Nursing
University of Texas, Arlington
Arlington, Texas

Sharon Moore, PhD, RN
Coordinator, Post-Basic Mental Health Nursing
Center for Health Studies
Mount Royal College
Calgary, Alberta, Canada

Evelyn M. O'Reilly, EdD, RN, C
Dorthea Hoffer School of Nursing
Mt. Vernon, New York

Pat Patterson, MAEd, RN
Department of Nursing, Fanshawe College
London, Ontario, Canada

Deborah Ann Rorick, MSN, RNC
Assistant Professor, Department of Nursing
Lakeland Community College
Mentor, Ohio

Marjorie Thiel Ryan, RN, MSN
Associate Professor, Department of Nursing
Miami University
Oxford, Ohio

Leslie West Sands, DSN
Professor, Department of Nursing
Jackson State Community College
Jackson, Tennessee

Sandra Schuler, MSN, RN
Professor, Department of Nursing
Montgomery College
Takoma Park, Maryland

Judith Sutherland, PhD, RN, CS, LCDC
Abilene Intercollegiate School of Nursing
Abilene, Texas

Margaret Trimpey, MSN, RN, C
Associate Professor, School of Nursing
University of Tennessee, Chattanooga
Chattanooga, Tennessee

Betty Whigham, MEd, RN
Professor, Health Sciences Department
Hillsborough Community College
Tampa, Florida

PREFACE

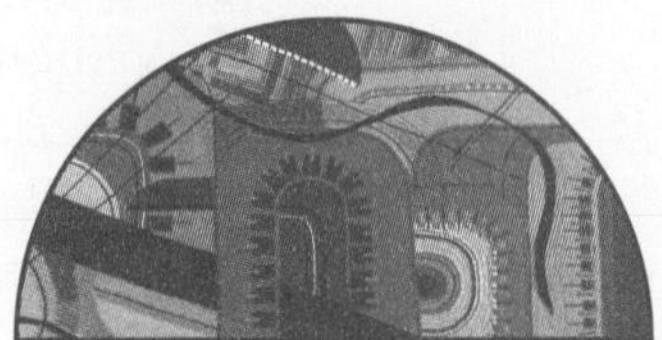

Introduction to Psychiatric Nursing's *Fifth Edition*

This fifth edition of *Psychiatric Nursing* continues to set the standard for psychiatric mental health nursing practice established with the publication of its first edition in 1979. We have written it with three key points in mind: 1) These are complex and changing times in our field of knowledge and practice; 2) psychiatric mental health nurses must be prepared with critical thinking and clinical judgment skills to address clients with dual diagnoses and comorbidities, and to work effectively in community-based as well as hospital settings; and 3) comprehensive and contemporary theory and processes are best learned when presented in a clear, clinically relevant style.

Since publication of the fourth edition, the following advances have influenced our practice. New *Standards for Psychiatric Mental Health Nursing* have been published by the American Nurses Association (1994). The *Diagnostic and Statistical Manual of Mental Disorders (DSM-IV, 1994)* has been fully revised by the American Psychiatric Association. Advances in neurochemistry, neuroendocrinology, and psychoimmunology have occurred at an accelerated pace, adding to our theoretic knowledge of mental disorders. New psychiatric medications have become available, adding to the treatment repertoire for psychiatric clients. The cultural diversity of clients has broadened, presenting new challenges to provide culturally relevant and sensitive care. Psychiatric nursing competence has been acknowledged as central to the care of community-based HIV/AIDS clients, the growing population of older adults, and to other vulnerable populations including the homeless and those addicted to substances. And finally, the available options for care and treatment are being shaped by cost-containment measures such as managed mental health care.

If the 1990s are the decade of the brain for psychiatry, then they must be the decade of the mind for psychiatric nursing. Responding to the complex challenges, content-rich domains, time-constrained decision-making, and high stakes outcomes requires both a comprehensive knowledge base and the habits of mind known as critical thinking. The need for critical thinking holds true whether psychiatric mental health nurses work in an emergency room, an AIDS hospice service, a drug detoxification unit, a nursing home, or a mental health clinic or hospital.

We have designed and written the fifth edition of Psychiatric Nursing to develop and empower the critical-thinking skills of interpreting meaning, examining ideas, assessing truth claims, tolerating divergent views, drawing conclusions based on evidence, explaining rationales, and self assessment. We have also presented the most thorough and up-to-date knowledge relevant to caring practice in our field.

New to Psychiatric Nursing's *Fifth Edition*

New features designed to empower the psychiatric mental health nurse in this edition of *Psychiatric Nursing* include

- Each chapter begins with a Critical Thinking Challenge focused on developing clinical judgment. Analysis and discussion points are presented in an appendix.
- Nursing Self-awareness boxes extend opportunities to use critical thinking in examining possible biases.
- Mind-Body-Spirit Connection boxes acknowledge the growing interest in the relationship of spirituality to mental health and support a fully holistic perspective.
- Globe icons call attention to content that is particularly relevant to cultural diversity. 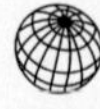

- All the new DSM-IV multi-axial codes, diagnostic categories, and a cultural assessment formulation as well as glossary of culture-bound syndromes appear in the appendices.
- The 1994 ANA Standards and the 1995-96 NANDA-approved diagnoses are used throughout the text.
- An increased emphasis on psychobiologic knowledge is reflected in the fully revised chapter on psychobiology; a separate chapter on psychotropic medications, completely updated, perforated, pocket-sized drug cards; drug appendix; and the use of a drug icon to call attention to medication-relevant information.
- Full-color plates of brain scan images and the most commonly-used psychiatric medications offer additional new resources for client-family teaching.
- Detailed critical pathways appear in the psychiatric disorders chapters and reflect the emphasis on time-linked client outcomes, quality of care, resource utilization, and cost containment in the practice world.
- Four entirely new chapters address contemporary psychiatric nursing concerns, including epidemiology of mental disorders and prevention levels; clients who have a dual diagnosis; clients with sleep disorders; and managed mental health care.

Features Retained from Prior Editions

Psychiatric Nursing retains many strengths that have kept it on the cutting edge of the field for nearly two decades:

- Competencies (behavioral objectives or "ends-in-view") begin each chapter.
- Chapter cross-references.
- New Research boxes in each chapter.
- Rich use of client profiles and clinical examples.
- The nursing process as an organizing format in the disorders chapters.
- Case studies drawn from actual client stories.
- Nursing care plans organized in a standard format that includes expected client outcomes.
- A glossary with terms bold-faced in the text.
- Client/Family Teaching boxes and Nutrition boxes.
- Fully updated references for each chapter.
- An index to locate quickly topics in the text.

The Package

The package includes an instructor's guide with a test bank and resource directory for audio-visual, programmed instruction, and computer-based interactive teaching/learning materials. A computerized test bank is also available.

An Answer to the Complex Realities of the Psychiatric Nursing Field

In this edition of *Psychiatric Nursing*, we hope to continue our tradition of offering a text that is comprehensive and sensitive to cultural concerns, and that promotes critical thinking in a clear, readable style to students preparing for the full range of generalist nursing practice, specialty practice, and to nurse practitioners. We have worked to prepare a textbook that presents the latest in scientific developments while retaining the values of caring. We trust that in reading and studying this book, you will see the relevance of psychiatric nursing knowledge and competencies to holistic caring for all clients.

Acknowledgments

Have you ever looked up to the sky in the autumn when you heard the persistent honking of Canadian geese heading south for the winter? Geese travel thousands of miles with ease and precision by flying in V-formation. As each bird moves its wings, it creates an updraft for the bird following; flying in formation is 70% more efficient than flying alone. Although it appears that the flock is guided by a single leader, the lead bird rotates back into formation when it tires, and another flies at the point position. The drumming sound of the great wings beating together and the encouraging honking energizes the whole formation.

That is the sort of team effort that it took to bring this book into its present form. The journey through the writing of any book is always a collaborative enterprise. It is a pleasure for us to be able to thank all of the team members who provided their lifting power, encouragement, and energy.

Special thanks to Peggy Adams, our sponsoring editor and a warm and caring person, who provided guidance, advocacy, and sensitivity. She facilitated early stages of this revision. Karen Gulliver was responsible for shepherding this book through the production stage. Karen provided a calming presence, a keen eye, and an organized mind. We are thankful for the supportive milieu she created.

The contributors to this book are astute clinicians and academicians whose high standards are evident in their work. We cherish our relationships with them and their commitment to this book.

Despite living on opposite coasts, we have now been friends and colleagues for 30 years and continue to learn from one another.

To all of you, our deepest thanks.

Holly Skodol Wilson
Carol Ren Kneisl

BRIEF CONTENTS

DETAILED CONTENTS

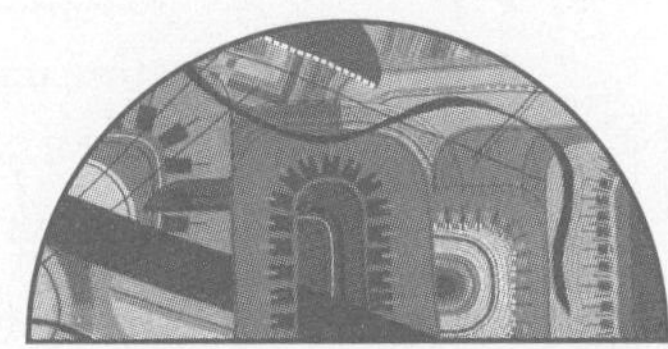

SUMMARY OF SPECIAL FEATURES

Intervention Boxes

Case Studies and Nursing Care Plans

Research Notes

(Each chapter has a Research Note)

PART ONE

THE THEORETIC BASIS FOR PSYCHIATRIC NURSING

CONTENTS

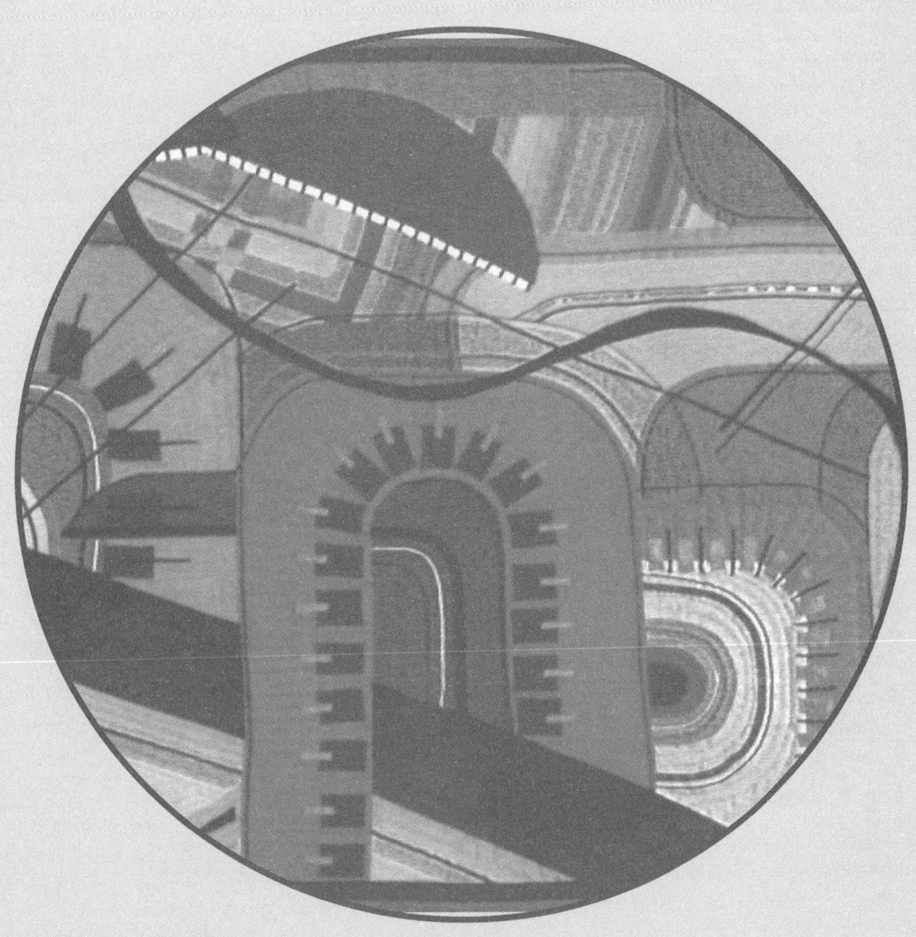

CHAPTER 1

THE PSYCHIATRIC NURSE'S PERSONAL INTEGRATION AND PROFESSIONAL ROLE

Carol Ren Kneisl
Holly Skodol Wilson

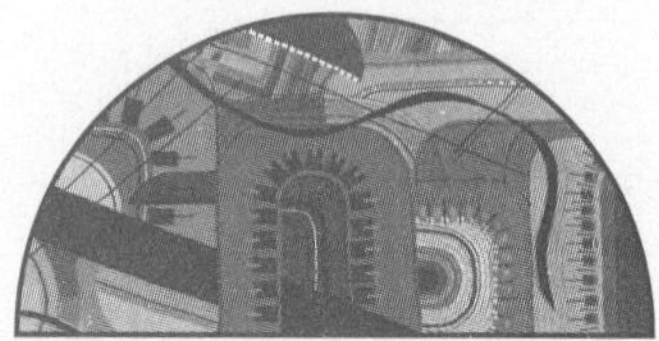

COMPETENCIES

- *Explore the concept of personal integration as it relates to the self and to psychiatric nursing practice.*
- *Discuss the qualities that enable psychiatric nurses to practice the use of self artfully in therapeutic relationships.*
- *Discuss the use of empathy in psychiatric nursing practice.*
- *Describe the roles of the psychiatric nurse and other members of the mental health team.*
- *Identify how the mental health team achieves collaboration.*
- *Explain six qualities associated with power and excellence in real-world situations.*

Cross-References

Other topics relevant to this content are: Ethics, Chapter 10; Nurses' role with the chronically mentally ill, Chapter 21; Nurses' role in family therapy, Chapter 32; Nurses' role in groups, Chapter 31; Nurses' role in milieu therapy, Chapter 9; Nurses' role in one-to-one relationships, Chapter 28; Relaxation and stress management techniques, Chapter 29.

Critical Thinking Challenge

You find your psychiatric nursing clinical experience professionally challenging, intellectually stimulating, and personally rewarding. You are considering becoming a psychiatric nurse upon graduation and have discussed your feelings with a classmate; with your neighbor, a critical care nurse; and with your family physician.

Your classmate says you won't be a real nurse and that you'll forget all the skills you learned in school. Your neighbor, the critical care nurse, thinks you'll be bored as a psychiatric nurse. The high drama, split-second decisions, and high-tech atmosphere of the critical care unit is, she says, the setting where a good student like you would be the happiest and could make the greatest contribution. Your family physician suggests that you should be cautious. With the explosion in psychobiologic research and the discovery of more effective psychopharmacologic agents, she thinks it will be likely that in a few years there will be no need for psychiatric nurses and you'll be out of a job.

What do you think?

The value of self-knowledge is a recurring theme in both the popular and the professional literature. Libraries are stocked with volumes dealing with the undiscovered self, the expansion of human awareness, values clarification, strategies for self-realization, and the like. A common thread in all these is the idea that the quality and nature of a person's relationship with others are strongly influenced by the person's self-view. Consider the following comments made by students in their psychiatric nursing clinical experience:

I just can't take it. . . . I feel myself getting confused about who is the crazy one. There's such a fine line. Sometimes I think I'll be a patient here.

I hated psych—it just didn't seem like nursing to me. I really like to keep busy. When you change someone's dressing, you really feel like you've helped them. Here it's all so uncertain.

All I kept thinking about was that a lot of the patients had done really weird things. This one guy had lived in an apartment with his dead mother's body for three months before they brought him in. Another had tried to shoot the governor. I never felt safe even turning my back on them.

This chapter explores some dimensions of self-knowledge through an examination of the concepts of personal integration and professional role. Specifically, we will examine recurring problems that pertain to the nurse's identity and some strategies for coping with them. Our goal is to enhance the nurse's interactions with psychiatric clients.

The Nurse's Personal Integration

Many students and practitioners faced with relating to people whose behavior they view as offensive, frightening, curious, or socially inappropriate find that their personal attitudes, expectations, myths, and values make it difficult for them to fulfill their professional roles. This was the case in the following example:

Penny, a baccalaureate nursing student, had selected a clinical placement at a methadone clinic in the community. Despite her initial interest, she developed a pattern of absences from the clinic. When her faculty adviser discussed this observation with her, Penny blurted out that, much to her surprise, she was unable to assist with the group meetings for pregnant heroin addicts. The thought of addicting babies before their births—babies who would ultimately suffer because of their mothers' self-indulgence—horrified Penny. She found herself judging their choices constantly and avoiding interaction with them. "I feel like they should be shot instead of given all this free support and sympathy."

For many nurses, confrontation with **deviance** (behavior outside the social norm of a specific group; should not be construed to mean negative behavior) reinforces a personal sense of stability. Others are threatened by such confrontation.

One psychiatric nurse, in recalling her childhood experiences with community deviants, commented on the intense and sometimes morbid excitement that she and her friends found in taunting "Crazy Helen" to run out on her porch and shout incoherently at the neighborhood children or in telling bizarre stories about a grotesque old man called "Charlie-No-Face," who walked along a road late at night chain smoking from the gaping hole that had once been a mouth.

The interest these characters held for the children, along with "Vince-the-Window-Peeper" and "Red-the-Bum," was reawakened in her as she approached her first psychiatric nursing experience. It was all very frightening, yet seductive and stimulating at the same time. The nursing students gossiped about the bizarre histories of their assigned clients as if to reaffirm their separateness from them—their sense of being normal and OK.

Dealing with people whose personal integration is fragmented, dissolving, divided, or alienated puts the nurse's own identity on the line as well. To respond with both compassion and the critical distance necessary to be effective, psychiatric professionals must confront their own identity; separate it from another's identity, which may indeed be dissolving; and finally integrate different values and behaviors comfortably in the therapeutic relationships they develop with clients.

This personal quality is called *detached concern*—the ability to distance oneself in order to help others. It is an essential quality not only in avoiding *burnout,* a problem discussed later in this chapter, but also in *values clarification,* in ethical dilemmas, in using appropriate *assertiveness* when collaborating with colleagues, and in maintaining *empathic abilities* in highly stressful situations.

In the conventional focus on the client, the nurse is regarded as the caregiver, the provider of services, the therapist. Little attention is paid to the stresses psychiatric nurses experience attempting to relate fully to clients while maintaining their own personal integration. This chapter is an attempt to explore that aspect of psychiatric nursing.

Negotiated Reality

Nurses often find that encounters with psychiatric clients are distancing experiences. The nurses become acutely aware of their difference and separateness from clients. They reaffirm their own subjective view of reality and rationalize their actions to keep these actions consistent with their sense of self as healthy, normal people.

Because people are constantly building and protecting their own self-images, they try to get others to see their image of themselves. However, it is impossible to see another's self-image or world view exactly as that person experiences it. Despite this fact, psychiatry has traditionally attempted to get certain people, labeled *crazy,* to assume the perspective of certain other people, called *therapists.*

A more acceptable alternative seems to lie in the creation of some common ground, a mutually understood, **negotiated reality.** Even to this common ground the nurse and the client bring their own conceptions, feelings, and attitudes toward and images of each other and themselves. In many instances, the nurse's image of the client—how the nurse expects the client to act or feel—is not the same as the client's self-image. This is confusing to both client and nurse and hinders the establishment of therapeutic relationships and effective communication.

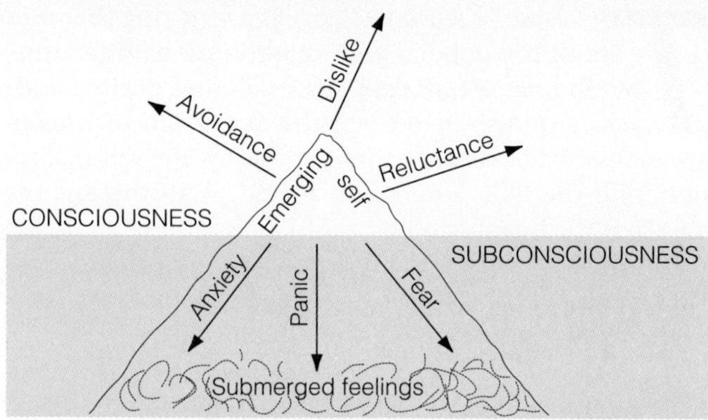

Figure 1–1 Self-awareness of feelings. Superficial feelings are visible; deeper feelings are submerged.

Feelings: The Affective Self

The ultimate effectiveness of efforts to relate to and communicate with others depends on how well people know themselves and develop the capacity for empathy. **Self-awareness** and empathic caring seem to go hand in hand. At the root of social interaction is people's ability to empathize with each other and to understand each other's attitudes and feelings. Because each human being is unique, empathizing is a difficult and challenging task. One way to develop this ability is to practice it. Learning to be aware of one's responses to expression of feelings from another person is a starting point.

Josh is a middle-aged man who sought out nursing as a career. Although he is highly proficient in technical skills and charming and engaging in relationships with most clients, he discovers a surprising intolerance for some of the tears, complaints, and self-preoccupation of depressed clients. He finds himself responding with admonitions to stop it, to bite the bullet, to grow up. He personally has seldom allowed himself to experience his own sadnesses but jokingly characterizes himself as a firm believer in repression and denial. The need to empathize with people unable to control their feelings evoked such discomfort that he found himself unable to work with such clients.

Self-Awareness of Feelings Feelings seem like icebergs: Only the tips stick up into consciousness, and the deeper parts are submerged (Figure 1–1). One such feeling is fear. The conscious part may be experienced as dislike, avoidance, or reluctance. At a deeper level, the feeling is reported as anxiety. Even deeper, the person may acknowledge, "I feel scared." Deeper yet, the person may experience genuine panic. Such an iceberg may well explain Josh's attitude toward tearful, depressed clients. His annoyance, irritation, sarcasm, and disdain may represent the tip of the iceberg of Josh's fear of depression.

The iceberg comparison also applies to other feelings, such as love, hurt, and guilt. A person feeling love may be aware only of a liking or attraction for another. Beneath the tip of that iceberg are feelings of warmth and affection. Deeper are feelings of love, and at the deepest level may be feelings of fusion or ecstasy.

Problems with Submerged Feelings One characteristic of icebergs of feeling is that at the tip the feelings lose their experiential quality and become translated into impulses to act. For example, a person with submerged guilt may express it by frequent worrying and explaining and may be completely unaware of the underlying feelings. The behavior is the only outward manifestation.

People lose touch with their feelings over time as they shape their sense of self. They hear such messages as "boys don't cry" or "girls are too sensitive" and incorporate these injunctions into their emerging self-system, especially into the "me" or "self for others." Not being sufficiently aware of one's feelings has several disadvantages:

- What people don't know *can* hurt them. Repressed feelings may reappear in behaviors that are difficult to alter. For example, hidden anger may emerge in migraine headaches or the use of sarcasm. (See also the Mind-Body-Spirit Connection box in Chapter 4.)
- People who are not aware of their feelings find it difficult to make decisions. It is hard to tell a "should" from a wish. Without some awareness of their real wants, they may have trouble saying no or requesting something they need. They are more likely to rely on others—experts, authorities, rules and regulations, and so forth—for guidance.
- People who, like Josh, are "out of touch with" or unaware of their feelings may find it difficult to be really close to and empathic toward others. Intimacy and empathy demand the expression of here-and-now feelings, whether positive or negative.

Most people realize the value of thinking clearly. They understand that it is a learned ability and takes practice. Feeling clearly (authentically) can also be practiced and learned.

Dominant Emotional Themes Nurses need to explore the dominant emotional themes in their personalities. If they find that they respond to many situations with the same feelings, they are probably narrowing their range of potential feelings.

Whatever the occasion, Marge used it to be tired or bored. Fatigue and chronically depressed states were routine for her. Holidays, vacations, dinner engagements all evoked the same predictable response.

Joan was afraid of everything. When she met her brother at the plane, her first question was, "Aren't you afraid of flying?" She was afraid driving home from the airport. The prospect of starting back to school scared her. She was fearful about wearing a bikini to the swimming club.

People who feel the same way in a variety of situations may be missing a lot of what is happening in those situations. They perceive only what will fit a narrowed range of feelings. Becoming aware of limited emotional themes is a way to begin to widen the range of feelings.

Acceptance of Disapproved Feelings Most people have been taught to block off an awareness and expression of certain feelings. Children are taught that being rude or ungrateful or cranky is rarely acceptable. To retain love and approval, they usually comply, not by stopping the feelings but by acting as if they didn't have them. Nursing students often get similar messages from teachers. It is not acceptable to find a client repulsive, to dislike someone who is sick and dependent, to express anger at or criticism of the teacher. Positive feelings of attraction and love may also seem unacceptable. Failure to recognize these feelings can interfere with interactions.

Recognizing and accepting their own feelings make nurses less vulnerable to other people's ideas about how they should feel. Nurses often feel guilty when they don't feel what others imply they should feel. Instead, nurses need to realize that others merely disapprove of the way they do feel. Nurses who can allow themselves the right to their own feelings can also allow clients the right to have and express theirs.

Beliefs and Values

Beliefs and values take three major forms:

1. Rational beliefs are beliefs that are supported by available evidence.
2. Blind belief is belief in the absence of evidence.
3. Irrational belief is belief held despite available evidence to the contrary.

Dogmatic belief (opinions or beliefs held as if they were based on the highest authority) includes both blind and irrational belief. Dogmatically held beliefs are not based on personal experience. Operating on the basis of dogmatically held beliefs often causes nurses to distort their personal experiences of the world to fit their preconceptions. The following are examples of strongly held beliefs about behaviors that are labeled "mental illness" and about the people who do and don't engage in those behaviors:

- Most clients in mental hospitals are dangerous.
- People who are mentally disordered let their emotions control them.
- Normal people think things out.
- If parents loved their children more, there would be fewer mental disorders.
- When a person has a worry, it is best not to think about it.
- Many people become mentally disordered just to avoid the problems of life.
- Most psychiatric clients are lazy.
- People would not become mentally disordered if they avoided bad thoughts.
- A woman would be foolish to marry a man who has had a mental disorder.
- Anyone who is in a hospital for a mental disorder should not be allowed to vote.
- To become a psychiatric client is to become a failure in life.
- If a man in a mental hospital attacks someone, he should be punished so that he doesn't do it again.
- Most clients in mental hospitals don't care how they look.
- One of the main causes of mental disorders is a lack of moral strength.

Most research on strongly held beliefs indicates that people usually know more about the things they believe than about those they don't believe. The process works like this: If people let themselves find out about those things they don't believe, they might find some validity in the statements. Then they would have to question the beliefs they already hold. By staying ignorant about anything they don't already agree with, they can avoid changing. This posture cuts off personal growth and learning that could be derived from the unknown. Obviously, clients are better served by nurses who are aware of their own dogmatically held beliefs and then challenge those beliefs.

Attitudes and Opinions A feeling is a transitory experience. A feeling held over a period of time is called an attitude. An attitude linked to an idea or belief becomes an opinion. An opinion, then, involves both thinking and feeling. Research in this area has shown that people are more comfortable when their beliefs are consistent with their attitudes. People do several things to keep their attitudes and beliefs consistent:

- They repress any belief or attitude that seems inconsistent.
- They distract their awareness from conflict either physically (such as by leaving the room) or psychologically (such as by daydreaming).
- They distort their perceptions to fit an existing attitude or belief.

Similar maneuvers take place to keep actions consistent with attitudes or beliefs. Nurses often justify treating psychiatric clients inhumanely or unkindly by arguing that the clients deserved it or were asking for it.

Nurses need to be careful that their self-image—as people who act intelligently—does not keep them from seeing the world clearly. Some attitudes are inconsistent with beliefs or actions. It is probably preferable to acknowledge this point than to engage in the elaborate self-deceptions necessary to avoid it.

Arriving at Values Every day, each person meets life situations that call for thought, opinion forming, decision making, and action. At every turn in their personal and professional lives, nurses are faced with choices. Their choices are based on the values they hold, but often those values are not really clear. People actively value something to the degree that they are willing to put energy into doing something about it. Their values are shown in their interests, preferences, decisions, and actions.

In talking with colleagues, Susan, a psychiatric nurse, claims to value interacting with clients more than doing paperwork. Yet a quick assessment of how she spends her time—all excuses taken into account—reveals that she acts on other values.

Mel, a nurse working in a state hospital ward for profoundly retarded children, claims that he believes these clients are human beings, despite their uncommunicative, immobile forms. He demonstrates this value in the hours he spends trying to communicate his presence and concern for them, using acupressure and touch performed slowly and with genuine feeling.

The distinction in the above examples is between *cognitive* and *active values*. Susan verbally subscribes to values but fails to act on them. These are cognitive values. Mel's actions demonstrate that he gives more than lip service to the idea of the dignity of all living beings. He follows active values.

People may learn values in a number of ways:

- Moralizing is a direct, although sometimes subtle, method of inculcating desired values in someone else.
- The laissez-faire approach leaves people alone to forge their own set of values. This may create unnecessary frustration, conflict, and confusion, especially in young people or people being socialized into a profession such as nursing.
- Modeling, in which actions follow professed values, transmits values by setting a living example for a learner to follow.
- Values clarification is a systematic, widely applicable method of teaching the process of valuing rather than the content of any specific values. It uses strategies and exercises to engage learners in becoming aware of their beliefs and values, choosing among alternatives, and matching stated beliefs with actions (see Wilson and Kneisl 1988).

The small amount of research comparing these four methods of learning values highlights the advantages of the fourth method. People who engage in values clarification are more zestful and energetic, more critical in their thinking, and more likely to follow through on their decisions than those who learn values in other ways. However, values clarification must be undertaken in circumstances that allow for sufficient follow-up with students who may uncover uncomfortable or disturbing values.

Taking Care of the Self

Knowing who they are is just a beginning for nurses. Taking care of others requires that nurses respect and care for themselves. Assertiveness, the need for solitude, maintaining physical health, and attending to cues of personal stress are actions crucial to preserving the nurse's personal integration.

Assertiveness

Have you ever had difficulty expressing yourself in a staff meeting? Did you find yourself feeling hopeless, resentful, angry? Were you wishing you had the courage to speak up? Hoping someone else would?

Are you intimidated by the high-pressure tactics of supervisors, physicians, teachers? Do you have trouble standing up to these sacred cows? Do you remain silent but seething? Do you speak up but sound defensive? Do you say yes when you mean no?

Have you ever needed to give someone counseling? Did you avoid the problem, hoping things would change? Did you find yourself beating around the bush? Or did you find yourself being overly harsh when you finally gave the correction?

These questions are from a manual written specifically to help nurses cope with on-the-job stressors by using assertiveness techniques to express themselves more effectively (Muff 1984, pp. 239–240). Often people are either so timid that they do not get what they want or so aggressive and belligerent that they offend and alienate others. **Assertive behavior** is asking for what one wants or acting to get it in a way that respects other people. It is midway between **nonassertive behavior** (timid holding back) and **aggressive behavior** (inconsiderate, offensive aggression). Assertiveness training exercises are designed to teach people to ask for what they want and also to refuse someone without feeling guilty.

Compare the nonassertive, aggressive, and assertive behaviors listed in Table 1–1 to see which descriptions best characterize your behavior with others. Fortunately, old behaviors can be unlearned, and new behaviors can be learned.

Nurses need to recognize their rights as nurses before they can assume responsibility for asserting them. The list below was originally designed to help women health care professionals recognize their rights (Chenevert 1992). They are, however, applicable to health care professionals of both sexes:

- You have the right to be treated with respect.
- You have the right to a reasonable workload.
- You have the right to an equitable wage.
- You have the right to determine your own priorities.
- You have the right to ask for what you want.
- You have the right to refuse without making excuses or feeling guilty.
- You have the right to make mistakes and be responsible for them.
- You have the right to give and receive information as a professional.
- You have the right to act in the best interest of the client.
- You have the right to be human.

Remembering that you have rights is not enough; you must assert them.

Solitude

Most people need time alone to assimilate what has happened in time spent with other people. They also need it for relief from responding to the demands of others. Aloneness need not mean physical distance. People can be alone in a crowded library. The crucial factors are that they are making no demands on others and that no one is making demands on them. After a sanctioned time away, most people return refreshed to their relationships, work, and usual circumstances. Planning for time alone is highly preferable to reaching a breaking point and then aggressively and irresponsibly running away from others.

Personal Physical Health

An important way of taking care of oneself is to provide for the physical health of the body. A proper diet, adequate rest, and exercise rejuvenate and restore the body. All these activities potentially make nurses more alive and better able to share this quality of aliveness with their clients.

Table 1–1 Comparison of Nonassertive, Aggressive, and Assertive Behaviors

Nonassertive	*Aggressive*	*Assertive*
Denies anger/experiences fear	Denies fear/experiences anger	Recognizes both fear and anger
Does not respect self	Does not respect others	Respects both self and others
Destroys relationships as avoidance and resentment build	Destroys relationships through angry outbursts, self-aggrandizement, and need to control	Builds relationships
Wastes energy by repeating situations that were not adequately resolved	Wastes energy in bluster and argument	Uses energy constructively
Fails to achieve goals	Occasionally achieves goals through intimidation	Achieves goals
Is stressful (low self-esteem, helplessness, hopelessness, depression)	Is stressful (power struggles, painful arguments, need to be ever vigilant)	Is stressful (defying traditional stereotypes; pain of being conscious)

Source: Muff 1984, p. 248.

Attending to Internal Stress Signals

Nursing students encountering emotionally disturbed clients commonly begin seeing in themselves all the "symptoms" about which they are learning. This perception is probably due more to heightened awareness of and attention to emotional aspects of their lives than to anything else. However, it is important for nurses to learn to recognize and respond to their own genuine stress signals. All people have times in their lives when they feel a little crazy. They may become very upset at small disturbances or see things out of proportion to their ultimate importance. These feelings are significant warning signals that the person is not coping adequately with stress.

"Crazy" times can be important turning points in people's lives. They are strong messages that change is needed. It is foolish to ignore these messages. In their daily lives, nurses are often tempted to handle their own symptoms of stress by suppressing them with tranquilizers or other drugs. They could serve themselves better by really experiencing their feelings and attending to what the signals are saying. Help in managing stress creatively is the subject of Chapter 29. Using the techniques recommended in Chapter 29 will help nurses to gain control of their lives and ease tension before it becomes unmanageable.

Pain and suffering are sources of some of the most intensely experienced stresses in life. Events such as the death of loved ones, divorce, illness, separation from loved ones, and failure are all part of the cycle of life's experience. Being told that they deserve it, or that they really don't have it so bad and therefore have no right to feel the way they feel, does not help people cope with pain and suffering. They need to find ways of handling their suffering without being destroyed by it. Classmates, friends, and family members can be great sources of support. Being able to both give and receive support strengthens the individual.

According to an old Buddhist teaching, a third of people's suffering is inevitable but they themselves create the rest of it. Realizing that pain and hardship are part of what it is to be a human being makes the pain a bit gentler. Pain is often a response to losing or the fear of losing something or someone valued: a job, a mate, money, self-respect. People want to continue what *was* instead of living with what *is*. It is important to attend to genuine feelings about the loss or prospective loss. These feelings give messages about what the sufferer needs to do. Some people need to replace what they have lost with something similar. Others need to explore a new dimension in their lives.

The alternative to experiencing pain is to live on the surface, out of touch with the joyful experiences in life as well as the painful ones. A more life-enhancing approach is to experience all aspects of life.

Qualities of Effective Psychiatric Nursing

According to the American Nurses Association (ANA), **psychiatric nursing** is "a specialized area of nursing practice that employs theories of human behavior as its science and the purposeful use of 'self' as its art. It is the diagnosis and treatment of human responses to actual or potential mental disorders and their long-term effects. Interventions include the continuous and comprehensive primary mental health care services necessary for the promotion of optimal mental health, the prevention of mental illness, rehabilitation from mental disorders, and health maintenance" (1994, p. 45). Self-awareness, empathy, and moral integrity all enable psychiatric nurses to practice the use of self artfully in therapeutic relationships. Some characteristics of artful therapeutic practice are respect for the client, availability, spontaneity, hope, acceptance, sensitivity, vision, accountability, advocacy, and spirituality (see the Research Note).

Respect for the Client

The behavior of many psychiatric clients indicates their loss of self-respect. Some may appear dirty and disheveled. Others may plead, beg, or cry. Still others may try to do physical harm to themselves. A relationship in which they experience a sense of dignity and receive messages of respect is of inestimable value. The nurse can convey respect in relationships with clients by:

- Taking the time and energy to listen.
- Taking care not to invalidate clients' experience of their world with comments such as, "It's not so bad," "Don't be that way," "Time heals all wounds," or "Keep a stiff upper lip."
- Giving clients as much privacy as possible during examinations and treatments or when they are upset.
- Minimizing experiences that humiliate clients and strip them of identity, thus allowing them to make as many of their own choices and be in control of as much of their own lives as possible.
- Being honest with clients about medicines, privileges, length of stay, and so on, even when the truth may be difficult to handle.

Availability

Of all the members of the mental health team, the nurse has the richest opportunity to be available to clients when needed, at any time of day or night. Because they are with clients on a relatively constant basis, nurses have the responsibility for:

- Creating a nurturing, healing milieu.

RESEARCH NOTE

Citation

Johnson JL: A dialectical examination of nursing art. *Adv Nurs Sci* 1994;17(1):1–14.

Study Problem/Purpose

Recognizing that the literature on *nursing as an art* is extremely diverse and that understanding the art of nursing has the potential to provide direction in achieving excellence in nursing practice, this study was conducted to identify the distinct conceptions of nursing art as represented in the nursing literature. The goal was to formulate patterns of agreement and disagreement and report in an impartial way various ideas contained in a many-sided discussion.

Method

The method used in this study is called a *dialectical approach.* It is used in philosophical research to examine controversies that surround ideas such as the meaning of freedom or the definition of equality. The aim of the method is to systematically examine and identify controversies in discourse (literature or speeches). This investigator analyzed the works of 41 writers, representing a sample of nursing authors who wrote about the subject of *the art of nursing* between 1860 and 1992.

Findings

The examined discourse revealed five distinct conceptualizations that have been identified as nursing art. These are: (1) grasping meaning in client encounters, (2) establishing a meaningful connection with the client, (3) skillfully performing nursing activities, (4) rationally determining an appropriate course of action, and (5) morally conducting one's nursing practice.

Implications

Although the five themes identified in this study represent general areas of agreement among nursing authors, some disagreements exist as well. In general, however, this analysis supports a conception of an artful nurse as one who can grasp what is really significant in a particular patient situation; one who is able to be genuine, recognizing that attempts to mask or hide feelings will distance the nurse from the client and threaten the integrity of their relationship; one whose actions are not automatic or blind but rather are grounded in critical thinking and a knowledge base; and one who is motivated by care and concern for others. In summary, this research supports the qualities emphasized in this chapter.

- Assisting suffering clients to meet their basic human needs.
- Collecting and conveying crucial data about clients that will influence decisions around them.

Spontaneity

Many nurses have come to believe that therapeutic relationships with psychiatric clients require them to be stiff, stilted robots uttering clichés from a list of unnatural-sounding communication "techniques." Nurses who are comfortable with themselves, aware of therapeutic goals, and flexible about using a repertoire of possible interventions for any particular clinical problem find that being natural and spontaneous, while keeping therapeutic goals uppermost in their minds, is their most effective "technique." Clients experience such nurses as authentic. Each nurse is unique and necessarily brings a different personal style to practice. We have different ways of putting the words together to convey to clients that we accept and care about them. Sometimes we say it with nonverbal behavior: keeping promises, being on time, touching, and staying with a client who needs someone. We need to trust our own natural styles, combined with sound communication principles such as those discussed in Chapter 7, in working toward therapeutic goals.

Hope

Effective psychiatric nursing practice is characterized by hope and optimism that all clients, no matter how debilitated, have the capacity for growth and change. Even clients whose most marked attributes are chronicity and deterioration can be helped to some optimal level of well-being by a nurse who believes in their possibilities and is willing to search for some strengths to build on. In one day treatment center, a client joined in a partnership with a creative nurse to assist less able clients toward self-care. It is not unusual in such a situation for the healing to become a source of help to the healer-client.

Acceptance

There is a distinction between acceptance and approval. Acceptance means refraining from judging and rejecting a client who may behave in a way the nurse dislikes. Therapeutic work requires that clients be able to examine, explore, and understand their coping mechanisms without feeling the need to cover up or disguise them to avoid negative judgments or punishments. Nurses who tell clients what they should say or do or feel deny these clients the acceptance they need to explore their problems.

Sensitivity

Genuine interest and concern provide the basis for a therapeutic alliance. Clients recognize the falseness of memorized phrases and assumed postures. The nurse conveys general interest and concern by trying to understand the client's perspective, working with the client on mutually formulated goals, and persisting even when breakthroughs and improvements are subtle and slow instead of dramatic and quick.

Vision

Because psychiatric nurses focus their work on enhancing the quality of life for all human beings, they must come to terms with a personal and professional vision of what quality means. Some conditions of life associated with high quality are influence or power, freedom, accountability, self-determinism, openness to gratifying experience, action, mastery, a sense of purpose or meaning, privacy, hope, stability, nonviolence, and intimacy.

Accountability

According to Peplau (1980), the need for personal accountability—professional integrity—is greater in psychiatric practice than in any other type of health care. Clients in mental health settings are usually more vulnerable and defenseless than clients in other health care settings, particularly because their conditions hinder their thinking processes and their relationships with others. Psychiatric nurses are accountable for the nature of the effort they make on behalf of clients and answerable to clients for the quality of their efforts. As Peplau puts it, "Personal accountability is an attitude—a quality of the heart and mind of those professionals who are competent and determined that every psychiatric patient will have the best problem-resolving assistance possible" (1980, p. 133).

Psychiatric nurses are also accountable to themselves, their peers, their profession, and the public. Accountability to self involves bringing personal behavior under conscious control so that the nurse becomes the person-as-nurse she or he wants to be. Accountability to peers involves engaging in peer review with nurse colleagues to give and receive feedback intended to improve the quality of care. Accountability to the profession involves clarifying the role of the psychiatric nurse, keeping current with changes in the field, and encouraging self-regulation to protect the public and enhance the quality of care. Accountability to the public requires keeping abreast of knowledge in the field, becoming credentialed according to level of competence, applying the ANA Standards of Psychiatric–Mental Health Nursing Clinical Practice, and protecting the rights of clients and their families.

Advocacy

Throughout history, psychiatric–mental health nurses have been ardent supporters of a neglected, ignored, and forgotten population—the mentally ill. In the mid-1990s and into the twenty-first century, there is a need for new energy and political activism (American Nurses Association 1994). In this era of health care reform, there is an especially important concern—ensuring that the needs and the rights of mentally disordered people are not overlooked or ignored while the nation's health care system is being overhauled. (See Chapter 35 on managed mental health care for a discussion of these issues.)

A newly energized political activism calls for nurses to speak out publicly for the health, welfare, and safety of their clients; to take steps to protect their rights; to write articles for the popular press; to lobby their congressional representatives; and to run for political office. The power that such a large group of citizen nurses could wield on behalf of their clients would be awesome.

Spirituality

Spirituality, the search for meaning in life and a belief in a higher power, is at the core of each person's existence. Spirituality varies in strength from person to person. Some people already have a meaningful philosophy of life. Others, on a spiritual journey, search for life's meaning and purpose. Still others experience hopelessness, despair, and spiritual distress.

Some of your clients will have maladaptive behavior that involves religiosity. (To differentiate between religiosity and spirituality, see the Mind-Body-Spirit Connection box.) They may attempt to resolve internal conflicts or conflicts with others through religious rituals or practices. For such clients, their spirituality becomes a central focus in their treatment.

Helping clients in their search for meaning and purpose is possible when nurses have beliefs that sustain them rather than beliefs that are sources of conflict. You must meet your own spiritual needs satisfactorily before you can have a meaningful relationship with your clients.

MIND-BODY-SPIRIT CONNECTION

Spirituality: The Connection Between Mental Health and Mental Illness

Spirituality is the third part of the triad known as mind-body-spirit in the holistic practice of nursing. In ancient times, spirit meant breath—as essential to life as air. Spirituality is that part of every person that yearns to share the beauty, love, and joyfulness of the universe.

We take our spirituality from many sources: Nature, God, Buddha, Higher Power, Goddess, Krishna, B'ahaullah, Mohammed, Yahweh, and others. Although many of these sources are incorporated into organized religions, spirituality is not religion, nor is religion spirituality. Religion is the organization of a set of beliefs, practices, and rituals, whereas spirituality is a reflection of one's "spirit" and its relationship to the rest of the universe.

Some people develop their spirituality throughout life with prayer, meditation, and reflection. Others may leave the spiritual path because of conflicts with religious beliefs, values, and practices, because of toxic family relationships, or because they are too busy trying to survive physically and mentally.

Even though spirituality is one of the three central aspects of the holistic practice of nursing, the physical, emotional, mental, and social aspects get most, if not all, of the mental health specialist's attention.

Spirituality may be an important connection between mental health and mental illness. In mental illness, most clients describe feeling "disconnected" from their families, their friends, the universe itself, and from their "faith." For example, clients describe depression like being in a gray or black tunnel with a profound sense of disconnectedness.

Imagine what it would be like to go for 24 hours or longer without sleep. How would you look? Would you feel disconnected or disoriented? Ask someone with mania what that's like. Have you ever awakened suddenly and not known where you are? How would it be to feel like that for an hour, a whole day, or a month? Ask someone with schizophrenia what that's like. Perhaps you've driven down the road and realized that you're confused about where you are and how you got there. And what if you had voices inside your head at the same time? Would this be frightening? Would you feel disconnected?

It may be that a psychiatric crisis has also brought forth a spiritual crisis. The client may, for the first time, be faced with looking at the three spiritual questions of life.

1. What have I placed on life's altar?
   "Of what value is my life? Why was I born, anyway? I have nothing to give." These are the words of someone who is depressed and someone who is actively suicidal.
2. What do I hold to be sacred?
   What things are important to the client, what things have meaning?
3. How do I know what's true?
   The client with anxiety or psychosis has great difficulty sorting out what's real and what's not real, determining what's true and what's not true. Life as we know it has many dichotomies. The unanswerable becomes even more of a challenge when a psychiatric crisis emerges.

Recall what happened to your relationships with friends and family when you were in a personal crisis. Did the relationships change? Our cognitive sphere, our affective sphere, and our relational sphere are all affected. We lose our centering of purpose, of sacredness, of reality. We lose our spirit and become disconnected. Do you think your clients' relationships change when they are in a crisis?

Helping clients rediscover their spiritual path is a fulfilling role for psychiatric–mental health nurses. You can help clients find out who they *really* are, beyond, for example, simply husband, father, lover, candlestick maker. Help them identify the source of their inner energy and how to get in touch with their "center" or their "soul." Keep in mind that spirituality is a deeply personal inner experience as opposed to a set of behaviors tied to an externally imposed doctrine or ritual. By offering a simple spirituality inventory, such as that in the spiritual health assessment box in Chapter 8, you will encourage clients to look at the strength of their faith, which will help them with their recovery. Faith is a way of being—being open to possibilities, and to healing.

Grace D. Dreyer, MSN, RN, CS

To help you on your journey of spiritual growth, contemplate these questions:

1. What is the meaning, purpose, and direction of my life?
2. To what extent have I evolved on my life's journey?
3. Am I achieving what I want to achieve in my life?
4. What brings me pleasure, and what causes me pain?
5. Am I doing what brings me pleasure and satisfaction in life? If not, why not, and how can I change my situation?
6. How are my values made operational in my daily living?
7. Can I become still enough to listen to the quiet inner voice that directs my being?
8. How can I grow more fully? (Keegan 1994)

Answering these questions, eventually fully, will make you a spiritual activist for yourself and for your clients.

The Use of Empathy in Psychiatric Nursing

Psychiatric nurses are instructed to engage in "therapeutic use of self." They are told that their "relationship" with a client is the primary therapeutic tool, that they should demonstrate qualities of sensitivity and caring. For many beginning students, these instructions are mysterious jargon quite unlike the clear-cut step-by-step procedures they learn for some physical treatments.

I found myself watching the nurses on the unit and my instructors closely when they talked with the clients. Somehow I thought maybe by imitating things that they did or said I'd figure out what "being therapeutic" was supposed to mean. I knew it had something to do with things the nurse said or didn't say when she talked with the clients. But it all got very fuzzy to me beyond that very elementary grasp of it. I used to latch onto ideas like "Agreeing is untherapeutic. So is giving advice or opinions." The only entries I felt safe in putting down in my process-recording were stiff-sounding reflections, like "You sound angry."

Comprehension of and ability to use the process of empathy give the nurse one strategy for responding to the feelings of aloneness often experienced by people who are psychiatric clients. Nurses are taught skills of active listening. But listening without empathy is not enough. Empathic understanding not only increases the nurse's grasp of the client's difficulties but also helps the nurse offer feedback on how the client affects others. Perhaps the most important function of empathic understanding is to help the psychiatric mental health nurse give the client the very precious feeling of being understood and cared about.

Defining Empathy

Empathy is a pervasive phenomenon in the life experience of all people. It allows a person to feel what others feel and respond to and understand the experience of others on their terms. A nurse who empathizes with a client momentarily abandons the personal self and relives the emotions and responses of someone else. People in everyday life tend to empathize most with those to whom they feel closest. In psychiatric practice, nurses often seek to empathize with those from whom they feel most separate or whose closeness threatens the nurses' own sense of integration.

Empathy has been defined as a subtle imitation through which people assume an alien personality. They become aware of how it feels to behave in a certain way and then feed back into the other person's consciousness this awareness and sensitivity to what the behavior feels like. Empathy characteristically develops early in an infant's pattern of relating to the parents. Tension in the parent, for example, induces anxiety in the baby.

Psychiatric Concepts of Empathy

PSYCHOANALYTIC THEORY Intimacy is closely related to empathy. Psychoanalytic theory postulates the development of empathy as a process of "mutual incorporation." The mother compensates for her loss of biologic oneness with her infant at birth by establishing a primitive unity—an emotional bonding—with the child during the first weeks and months of life. Children likewise incorporate the mothering parent into the self. Once children begin to see the mothering parent as a being separate from the self, identification replaces incorporation. At this point, the child experiences the mother as someone to imitate in order to secure love and comfort. From identification comes the capacity for empathy. Identification allows human beings to achieve a clear sense of self, to gain another person's point of view, and to establish an intimate association with others. Adults can empathize through past, present, and future identifications.

SOCIAL INTERACTIONIST THEORY Social interactionists discuss empathy as *role taking,* a process through which people feel with one another. They are able to sense the feelings of another because they have evoked in themselves the attitude of the person to whom they are relating.

People form an image of themselves because they have learned to assume the roles of others and have developed the ability to see themselves as others see them. A faulty ability to take on roles is the result of limited opportunity for role experimentation. Individuals who have not experimented enough do not develop a clear sense of their own integration and thus cannot shift from the role of participant to that of observer.

The capacity for empathy relies on personal integration. Whether problems with empathy are seen as the loss of primitive instincts for imitation in the psychoanalytic framework, or as the result of inadequate opportunities for role experimentation in the social psychologist's view, the conclusion is the same. A firm sense of self is necessary for a person to be a good empathizer. As people continue to interact with others, they learn to be sensitive to others without losing their own integration.

Therapeutic Use of Empathy

From time to time, we hear accounts of dramatic and surprising breakthroughs with psychiatric clients. There are instances in which the usual tools of systematic, logical problem solving and the application of theory seem to be getting nowhere. Instead, therapists fall back for a moment on their empathic sensitivity and get an inside comprehension of some complex emotion. This empathic understanding may be a key to establishing trust with a sullen, withdrawn, suspicious adolescent, or beginning verbal interaction with a chronically mute institutionalized person, or controlling the violent flailing rage of an emotionally disturbed child. In all these instances, empathy is used as a therapeutic tool.

The term *empathy* is often mistakenly used synonymously with *sympathy*. Empathy contains no elements of condolence, agreement, or pity. When nurses sympathize, they assume that there is a parallel between their feelings and those of the client. The perceived similarity makes good judgment and objectivity difficult.

Phases of Therapeutic Empathizing

The process of empathic understanding has four phases:

1. *Identification.* Through the relaxation of conscious controls, we allow ourselves to become absorbed in contemplating the client and the client's experiences.
2. *Incorporation.* We take in the experiences of the client rather than attribute our own experiences and feelings to the client.
3. *Reverberation.* We interplay the internalized feelings of the client and our own experiences or fantasies. While fully absorbed in the identity of the client, we still experience ourselves as separate personalities.
4. *Detachment.* We withdraw from subjective involvement and totally resume our own identity. We use the insight gained from the reverberation phase as well as reason and objectivity to offer responses that are useful to the client.

A nurse's empathic involvement with troubled clients can have a number of stressful consequences. Problems can arise at any phase in the empathy process. The nurse may overidentify and lapse into sympathy for the client. The nurse may fail to incorporate the client's feelings and instead project personal ones. The nurse may bypass the reverberation phase and substitute gut-level intuitions for rational problem solving. At the detachment phase, the nurse may experience overdistancing or burnout. Each of the common obstacles to achieving an empathic concern for clients can be understood as a failure to cope with one of the four phases of achieving empathy. Burning out has been given particular attention here because it is common and is less psychologic than circumstantial. It therefore is not inevitable and can be prevented with thoughtful planning.

Burnout as a Consequence of Empathy

After hours, days, and months of listening to other people's problems, something inside you can go dead and you don't care anymore. That's when you'd rather sit at the desk and do the paperwork than be out talking to clients on the floor.

This nurse verbalizes one of the possible consequences of using empathy when working intensely with troubled people. **Burnout** is the name given this phenomenon, and it happens to poverty lawyers, social workers, clinical psychologists, childcare workers, prison personnel, and others who struggle to retain both their objectivity and their empathic concern for the people with whom they work.

Burnout is a condition in which health care professionals lose their concern and feelings for their clients and come to treat them in detached or even dehumanized ways. It is an attempt to cope, by distancing oneself, with the stresses of intense interpersonal work. It hurts not only clients but also psychiatric professionals, in that they become ineffective and dissatisfied.

One nurse noted that her emotions shifted dramatically, first toward cynical feelings, then negative ones about her clients. "I began to despise every one of them and couldn't conceal my contempt for them." Another reported, "I found myself caring less and less and feeling really negative about the clients here." In many cases, burning out involves not only thinking in derogatory terms about the clients but also believing that somehow they deserve any problem they have. Benner and Wrubel (1989) caution us not to make the mistake of thinking that caring is the cause of burnout and thus try to prevent the "disease" of burnout by protecting oneself from caring. According to them, the sickness is the loss of caring, and the return of caring is the recovery.

There is little doubt that burnout plays a major role in the poor delivery of psychiatric care. It is also a key factor in low staff morale, absenteeism, and high job turnover.

Cues to Burnout Cues to burnout can be found in the language used to describe clients. Burnout victims may refer to their clients as "crocks," "vegetables," "wackos," "brown baggers," and so forth, or they may become highly analytic and abstract: "That's just a manifestation of his primary process thinking."

Another cue is lack of involvement with clients. Some nurses "hide" in the nurses' station or staff conference room to avoid interacting. Some openly reject bids for human contact.

Another withdrawal technique involves "going by the book" rather than considering the unique factors in a situation. It is a way of minimizing personal involvement with the client. By rigidly applying the rules, the nurse can avoid thinking about the client's specific problems. Burnout can transform an original and creative nurse into a mechanical bureaucrat.

Another cue to burnout is joking put-downs among staff members, which makes their work less frightening and overwhelming.

When the nurse is asked where Mr. G is, she laughingly reports that he's taking a shower in preparation for his MMPI test. Everyone in the nurses' station breaks up in gales of laughter.

In a discharge conference, the psychiatrist says he'd like to discharge E, a young male client with a history of violent outbursts. The nurse replies, "With or without baseball bat?" and everyone chuckles.

Reducing Burnout Most research indicates that the causes of professional burnout are rooted not in the permanent psychologic characteristics of individuals but rather in the social context of their work. Most nurses usually expect the presence of negative conditions: large client loads, time pressures, and daily confrontation with suffering, pain, and death. It is the absence of positive factors—a sense of significance, rewarding interpersonal relationships, the appreciation of others, challenge, and variety—that is most distressing. The strategies listed below can be used to reduce and modify the occurrence of burnout:

- Keep staff-client ratios low. Staff members can then give more attention to each client and have time to focus on the positive, nonproblem aspects of the client's life.
- Provide for sanctioned breaks rather than guilt-provoking escapes from the work situation for staff members.
- Provide some relief from prolonged direct client contact, through shorter work shifts or rotating work responsibilities, so that certain staff members are not always working directly with clients.
- Set up formal or informal programs in which staff members can talk over their problems to get advice and support when they need it.
- Encourage staff members to express, analyze, and share their feelings about burning out. This lets them get things off their chest and gives them the chance to get constructive feedback from others and perhaps a new perspective as well.
- Encourage staff members to understand their own motivations in pursuing a psychiatric career and to recognize their expectations for work with clients. Nurses can be on a variety of "ego trips," whose primary purpose is to deal with their own personal problems, not those of the clients.

The Nurse's Professional Role

As society and society's needs change, so do the roles and functions of the psychiatric nurse and the other members of the interdisciplinary mental health team. The role of the psychiatric nurse has changed over the years from that of custodian to a multifaceted one. In 1994, the ANA revised the guidelines for psychiatric–mental health nursing clinical practice. These standards of care and standards of professional performance demonstrate the multifaceted role of the psychiatric–mental health nurse (see the accompanying box; see also Chapter 6). The timeline in this chapter illustrates the history of psychiatric nursing (see page 20).

A central concern of psychiatric–mental health nurses is rehumanizing psychiatric care in a technologic society. It requires a judicious blending of "high touch" with "high tech," a person-to-person, human experience.

Members of the Mental Health Team

Role definitions have become increasingly blurred among mental health care workers as various members of the mental health team have taken on tasks traditionally assigned to other disciplines. This blurring of roles has increased the quantity and raised the quality of care in mental health care settings. Some of the role changes have created anxiety among nurses who have become more interpersonally involved, more autonomous, and more responsible for the quality of mental health services delivered to the consumer. Psychiatrists, the traditional heads of mental health teams, have suffered some anxiety as other mental health care workers and clients have sought to share in decision making and as other capable professionals have assumed administrative functions. Clinical nurse specialists, social workers, and psychologists, among others, have more direct influence than ever before. Roles are less specifically defined, and in many settings, mental health professionals take on whichever functions they do best.

The descriptions below of the education and tasks of mental health team members reflect traditional distinctions. Students should keep in mind that many of the functions are now shared across disciplines when the team member has been educated for the task and when laws permit the sharing of functions.

The Psychiatric–Mental Health Nursing Generalist

The *psychiatric nurse generalist* may have received basic nursing preparation in a diploma, associate degree, or baccalaureate program. Essentially a generalist who works in a specialized setting, this nurse provides the bulk of the nursing care to clients in inpatient settings and many outpatient settings. Registered nurses offer direct and indirect care through the nurse-client relationship. They have major responsibility for the milieu and have contact with clients at all stages of daily life. Nurses at this level may be certified as generalists through the ANA.

According to the American Nurses Association (1994), the basic psychiatric–mental health nursing clinical practice functions include:

- Health promotion and health maintenance (including health assessments; health teaching; stress management; and targeting at-risk situations, potential complications of mental illness, and adverse treatment effects, among others).
- Intake screening and evaluation (including physical and psychosocial assessments, planning for care, recognizing the need for additional clinical data, and referring the client for more specialized testing and evaluation).
- Case management (coordination of health and human services, comprehensive care planning, enhancing self-sufficiency and progress toward optimal health through culturally relevant interventions).
- Provision of a therapeutic environment (assessing and developing the therapeutic potential of institutional and supervised community-based residential or day treatment settings, and practicing the use of self as a therapeutic resource).
- Facilitating self-care activities (tracking clients and assisting them with self-care activities to help clients move toward more independent living).
- Administering and monitoring psychobiologic treatment regimens (including prescribed psychopharmacologic agents and their effects, relaxation techniques, nutrition/diet regulation, exercise and rest, and other somatic treatment regimens).
- Health teaching (including constructive role modeling and providing experiential learning opportunities).
- Crisis intervention (including direct crisis intervention services and serving as a member of a crisis team).
- Counseling (using a problem-solving approach to an immediate difficulty related to health or well-being).
- Home visits (including private residences, prisons, halfway houses, homes for the disabled, nursing homes, foster care residences, and homeless shelters).
- Community action (designing activities to ameliorate the sociocultural factors that adversely affect mental health; working with community planning boards, advisory groups, paraprofessionals, and other key people to mobilize community resources).
- Advocacy (including joining consumer and professional groups to reduce the stigma associated with mental illness; lobbying on behalf of better mental health and psychiatric care; becoming politically active at the local, state, and federal level; running for political office).

Colleagues who are clinical nursing specialists may supervise the registered nurse's therapeutic work and provide consultation.

The Psychiatric–Mental Health Nursing Clinical Specialist

The **clinical specialist in psychiatric–mental health nursing** is a graduate of a master's program providing specialization in the clinical area. A number of universities provide graduate study in adult, child, adolescent, and family psychiatric nursing and in community mental health as well. Nurses may also pursue a doctoral degree in two to four more years of study. Although funds have become more scarce, the National Institute of Mental Health (NIMH) funds some programs, providing stipends and tuition-free study for qualified full-time students.

Clinical specialists may also seek **certification,** the recognition of an advanced level of competence by a professional nursing organization. A means of protecting consumers, certification at the advanced level exists nationally through the ANA.

In addition to the generalist role functions, the certified clinical specialist has expertise in and carries out role functions at the advanced level. According to the American Nurses Association (1994), these functions include:

- Psychotherapy (including individual therapy, couple/marital therapy, group therapy, and family therapy in inpatient, outpatient, community mental health, and private practice milieus).

text continues on page 18

1994 ANA Standards of Psychiatric–Mental Health Clinical Nursing Practice

Standards of Care

Standard I. Assessment

The psychiatric–mental health nurse collects client health data.

Rationale: The assessment interview—which requires linguistically and culturally effective communication skills, interviewing, behavioral observation, database record review, and comprehensive assessment of the client and relevant systems—enables the psychiatric–mental health nurse to make sound clinical judgments and plan appropriate interventions with the client.

Standard II. Diagnosis

The psychiatric–mental health nurse analyzes the assessment data in determining diagnoses.

Rationale: The basis for providing psychiatric–mental health nursing care is the recognition and identification of patterns of response to actual or potential psychiatric illnesses and mental health problems.

Standard III. Outcome Identification

The psychiatric–mental health nurse identifies expected outcomes individualized to the client.

Rationale: Within the context of providing nursing care, the ultimate goal is to influence health outcomes and improve the client's health status.

Standard IV. Planning

The psychiatric–mental health nurse develops a plan of care that prescribes interventions to attain expected outcomes.

Rationale: A plan of care is used to guide therapeutic intervention systematically and achieve the expected client outcomes.

Standard V. Implementation

The psychiatric–mental health nurse implements the interventions identified in the plan of care.

Rationale: In implementing the plan of care, psychiatric–mental health nurses use a wide range of interventions designed to prevent mental and physical illness, and promote, maintain, and restore mental and physical health. Psychiatric–mental health nurses select interventions according to their level of practice.

[Note: Va–Vg are basic level interventions. Vh–Vj are advanced practice interventions.]

Standard Va. Counseling

The psychiatric–mental health nurse uses counseling interventions to assist clients in improving or regaining their previous coping abilities, fostering mental health, and preventing mental illness and disability.

Standard Vb. Milieu Therapy

The psychiatric–mental health nurse provides, structures, and maintains a therapeutic environment in collaboration with the client and other health care providers.

Standard Vc. Self-Care Activities

The psychiatric–mental health nurse structures interventions around the client's activities of daily living to foster self-care and mental and physical well-being.

Standard Vd. Psychobiological Interventions

The psychiatric–mental health nurse uses knowledge of psychobiological interventions and applies clinical skills to restore the client's health and prevent further disability.

Standard Ve. Health Teaching

The psychiatric–mental health nurse, through health teaching, assists clients in achieving satisfying, productive, and healthy patterns of living.

Standard Vf. Case Management

The psychiatric–mental health nurse provides case management to coordinate comprehensive health services and ensure continuity of care.

Standard Vg. Health Promotion and Health Maintenance

The psychiatric–mental health nurse employs strategies and interventions to promote and maintain mental health and prevent mental illness.

Standard Vh. Psychotherapy

The certified specialist in psychiatric–mental health nursing uses individual, group, and family psychotherapy, child psychotherapy, and other therapeutic treatments to assist clients in fostering mental health, preventing mental illness and disability, and improving or regaining previous health status and functional abilities.

Standard Vi. Prescription of Pharmacologic Agents

The certified specialist uses prescription of pharmacologic agents in accordance with the state nursing practice act, to treat symptoms of psychiatric illness and improve functional health status.

Standard Vj. Consultation

The certified specialist provides consultation to health care providers and others to influence the plans of care for clients, and to enhance the abilities of others to provide psychiatric and mental health care and effect change in systems.

Standard VI. Evaluation

The psychiatric–mental health nurse evaluates the client's progress in attaining expected outcomes.

Rationale: Nursing care is a dynamic process involving change in the client's health status over time, giving rise to the need for new data, different diagnoses, and modifications in the plan of care. Therefore, evaluation is a continuous process of appraising the effect of nursing interventions and the treatment regimen on the client's health status and expected health outcomes.

Standards of Professional Performance

Standard I. Quality of Care

The psychiatric–mental health nurse systematically evaluates the quality of care and effectiveness of psychiatric–mental health nursing practice.

Rationale: The dynamic nature of the mental health care environment and the growing body of psychiatric nursing knowledge and research provide both the impetus and the means for the psychiatric–mental health nurse to be competent in clinical practice, to continue to develop professionally, and to improve the quality of client care.

Standard II. Performance Appraisal

The psychiatric–mental health nurse evaluates own psychiatric–mental health nursing practice in relation to professional practice standards and relevant statutes and regulations.

Rationale: The psychiatric–mental health nurse is accountable to the public for providing competent clinical care and has an inherent responsibility as a professional to evaluate the role and performance of psychiatric–mental health nursing practice according to standards established by the profession and regulatory bodies.

Standard III. Education

The psychiatric–mental health nurse acquires and maintains current knowledge in nursing practice.

Rationale: The rapid expansion of knowledge pertaining to basic and behavioral sciences, technology, information systems, and research requires a commitment to learning throughout the psychiatric–mental health nurse's professional career. Formal education, continuing education, certification, and experiential learning are some of the means the psychiatric–mental health nurse uses to enhance nursing expertise and advance the profession.

Standard IV. Collegiality

The psychiatric–mental health nurse contributes to the professional development of peers, colleagues, and others.

Rationale: The psychiatric–mental health nurse is responsible for sharing knowledge, research, and clinical information with colleagues, through formal and informal teaching methods, to enhance professional growth.

Standard V. Ethics

The psychiatric–mental health nurse's decisions and actions on behalf of clients are determined in an ethical manner.

Rationale: The public's trust and its right to humane psychiatric–mental health care are upheld by professional nursing practice. The foundation of psychiatric–mental health nursing practice is the development of a therapeutic relationship with the client. The psychiatric–mental health nurse engages in therapeutic interactions and relationships which promote and support the healing process. Boundaries need to be established to safeguard the client's well-being and to prevent the development of intimate or sexual relationships.

Standard VI. Collaboration

The psychiatric–mental health nurse collaborates with the client, significant others, and health care providers in providing care.

Rationale: Psychiatric–mental health nursing practice requires a coordinated, ongoing interaction between consumers and providers to deliver comprehensive services to the client and the community. Through the collaborative process, different abilities of health care providers are used to solve problems, communicate, and plan, implement, and evaluate mental health services.

→

1994 ANA Standards of Psychiatric–Mental Health Clinical Nursing Practice

(continued)

Standard VII. Research

The psychiatric-mental health nurse contributes to nursing and mental health through the use of research.

Rationale: Nurses in psychiatric–mental health nursing are responsible for contributing to the further development of the field of mental health by participating in research. At the basic level of practice, the psychiatric–mental health nurse uses research findings to improve clinical care and identifies clinical problems for research study. At the advanced level, the psychiatric–mental health nurse engages and/or collaborates with others in the research process to discover, examine, and test knowledge, theories, and creative approaches to practice.

Standard VIII. Resource Utilization

The psychiatric–mental health nurse considers factors related to safety, effectiveness, and cost in planning and delivering client care.

Rationale: The client is entitled to psychiatric–mental health care which is safe, effective, and affordable. As the cost of health care increases, treatment decisions must be made in such a way as to maximize resources and maintain quality of care. The psychiatric–mental health nurse seeks to provide cost-effective quality care by using the most appropriate resources and delegating care to the most appropriate, qualified health care provider.

Source: American Nurses Association, 1994.

- Additional psychobiologic interventions (including prescribing psychoactive medications and ordering appropriate diagnostic and laboratory tests according to the state nurse practice act and state and federal regulations).
- Clinical supervision/consultation (providing education and consultation to other mental health care providers and provider-trainees).
- Consultation-liaison (including making psychiatric and psychosocial diagnoses, implementing interventions with physically ill or disabled clients and their families, and serving as a consultant and educator to nurses and other health care providers in physical care delivery systems).

The Psychiatrist

The *psychiatrist* is a physician whose specialty area is mental disorders. Certification in psychiatry by the American Board of Psychiatry and Neurology requires a three-year approved psychiatric residency, two years of clinical psychiatric practice, and successful completion of an examination. Certification in neurology requires further preparation through a two-year neurology residency and an additional examination.

Psychiatrists are responsible for diagnosis and treatment. Some are oriented primarily toward biologic therapies, others are psychotherapeutically oriented, and a few are chiefly interested in community psychiatry. In traditional medical model settings and in many inpatient settings, the psychiatrist is usually the team leader or administrator. This is not true in milieus where role distinctions are less clearly defined.

The Psychoanalyst

In the United States, a person must be a physician in order to become a psychoanalyst. *Psychoanalysts* are trained at psychoanalytic institutes that provide programs only in psychoanalysis. Most psychoanalysts are in private practice in large urban settings. They may also be certified in the practice of psychiatry, neurology, and/or psychoanalysis. There are nonphysician analysts, called *lay analysts,* who are also trained at psychoanalytic institutes. Some nurses become lay analysts.

The Clinical Psychologist

The *clinical psychologist* is a psychologist specially educated and trained in the area of mental health. To be certified, clinical psychologists must earn a doctoral degree in a program approved by the American Psychological Association and must have completed a one-year psychology internship at an approved clinical facility.

Clinical psychologists perform psychotherapy; plan and implement programs of behavior modification; select, administer, and interpret psychologic tests; and carry out research.

The Psychiatric Social Worker

The *psychiatric social worker* is a graduate of a two-year master's program in social work with an emphasis in the field of psychiatry. Social workers deal with the social problems that confront clients and their families. Their goals are to help clients and their families cope more effectively; identify appropriate community resources for clients; help the hospitalized person maintain relationships with family, friends, and the community; and facilitate the client's return to the community. With the blurring of traditional mental health care roles, social workers have undertaken counseling and psychotherapeutic roles in various settings, including private practice.

The Mental Health/Human Service Worker

The newest addition to the psychiatric team is the *mental health/human service worker.* The growing need for mental health services, the manpower crisis, the widespread popularity and economy of community college programs, and the documented effectiveness of these workers are responsible for the emergence of more than 400 mental health/human service training programs at the certificate, associate, and baccalaureate levels.

Paraprofessionals

Paraprofessionals provide much of the direct service to hospitalized people, particularly in large public facilities. These nonprofessional workers are known by a variety of titles, including *psychiatric aide, psychiatric technician,* and *psychiatric attendant.* Most agencies that employ psychiatric aides provide in-service training programs to help them use their interpersonal potential. Because a large number of the personnel who work in inpatient settings are psychiatric aides, it is extremely important that they maintain a therapeutic milieu under the supervision of professional nurses.

The Occupational Therapist

Occupational therapists in mental health care settings use manual and creative techniques to elicit desired interpersonal and intrapsychic responses. In some settings, they may participate in preparing clients for the return to community living by teaching self-help activities or, in sheltered workshop settings, help clients prepare to seek employment. The occupational therapist, registered (OTR) has a bachelor's degree in occupational therapy or a master's degree in occupational therapy after receiving a bachelor's degree in another field. The OTR also supervises certified occupational therapy assistants (COTA). A COTA is a graduate of an associate degree program and helps clients follow treatment plans.

The Recreational Therapist

The *recreational therapist,* taking into consideration the therapeutic needs of clients, plans and guides recreational activities to provide not only socialization and healthful recreation but also desirable interpersonal and intrapsychic experiences. With increasing frequency, recreational therapists are being prepared in university physical education and health education programs.

The Creative Arts Therapist

Creative arts therapists use art, music, dance, and poetry to facilitate personal experiences and increase social responses and self-esteem. Although creative arts therapists are not found in all settings, they are becoming valued and recognized members of the mental health team. Creative arts therapists have their own programs of study in colleges and universities as well as their own professional organizations, such as the American Art Therapy Association, the American Dance Therapy Association, and the National Association for Music Therapy. Chapter 31 discusses art, music, dance, and poetry therapy groups.

Collaborating on the Mental Health Team

Psychiatric nurses, whether practicing in institutions or in private practice settings, must plan and share with others to deliver maximum mental health services to clients. The purpose of collaboration is to make the best use of the different abilities of mental health team members so that the client receives the most effective service available. Relationship problems among mental health team members must be worked through to avoid distorting the team's efforts on behalf of the client.

Cooperation Versus Competition

The key to working together on a problem with a common purpose is cooperation rather than competition. Working together in cooperation ensures movement toward the common goal, whereas inappropriate competition hinders goal achievement and may be destructive to the competing individuals.

The History of Psychiatric Nursing

1860s

- Florence Nightingale founds school at Saint Thomas Hospital in London. Nightingale among the first to note that the influence of nurses on their clients transcends physical care.
- Linda Richards directs the first American school for psychiatric nurses at the McLean Psychiatric Asylum in Waverly, Massachusetts.

1890s

- Trained nurses attend to the physical needs of clients and do not pursue systematic interpersonal work.
- Psychiatric nursing practice is primarily custodial, mechanistic, and directed by psychiatrists.
- A ratio of 1 trained nurse to 140 clients is not unusual.

1920s

- *Nursing Mental Diseases*, the first psychiatric nursing text, is written by Harriet Bailey and remains the standard textbook in psychiatric nursing for 20 years.
- Most textbooks are written by psychiatrists; only a few pages address psychiatric nurses in such procedures as tube and rectal feeding and preparing treatment trays.

Emergence of the Discipline of Psychiatric Nursing

Most of our present understanding of cooperative and competitive behavior has come from the efforts of game theorists, who have researched player behavior. According to game theorists, players can be identified and placed in categories as follows:

- Maximizers—those interested only in their own gain.
- Rivalists—those interested only in defeating their partners.
- Cooperators—those interested in helping both themselves and their partners.

Maximizers and rivalists jeopardize the client's welfare because they put themselves first and the client last. Rivalists direct their energies toward being "one up" through put-downs of others. They are concerned not with the client but with the process of winning. Cooperators are interested in helping both themselves and their colleagues to aid the client. Participants who actively recognize the importance of each individual member of the mental health team can influence maximizers and rivalists to become cooperators.

Respect for the Positions of Others

Most nursing textbooks and nursing instructors emphasize the need to respect and accept the client and to act in ways that demonstrate personal trustworthiness. They less often consider the need to respect, accept, and trust one's colleagues. Yet effective collaboration is based on re-

1930s

- National League for Nursing Education recommends that psychiatric nursing content and clinical experience be part of the curriculum in all basic nursing programs.
- Psychiatric nursing activities continue to be custodial nursing care, including housekeeping tasks and keeping the keys to locked wards, cabinets, and even toilet tissue containers.

1940s

- New medical surgical procedures (deep sleep therapy, insulin shock therapy, psychosurgery, and electroshock therapy) promote the role of psychiatric nurses as participants in psychiatric treatment.
- Nursing leaders recommend elimination of single-focus schools marking the beginning of the mainstreaming of psychiatric nursing.
- National Institute of Mental Health (NIMH) established; National Mental Health Act helps develop psychotherapeutic roles for nurses.

1950s

- Hildegard Peplau emphasizes psychodynamic concepts and counseling techniques; Gwen Tudor Will demonstrates nursing interventions with a sociopsychiatric base.
- Frances Sleeper advocates psychiatric nurses as psychotherapists.
- First doctoral program in nursing is based on June Mellow's system of psychiatric nursing therapy.
- National League for Nursing introduces the concept of psychiatric nurse specialist; first NIMH grants to integrate mental health concepts into nursing curriculum.

Movement of Psychiatric Nursing into the Mainstream of Nursing

Confirmation of Psychiatric Nursing as a Specialty

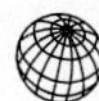

spect for the position from which another participant acts. Our values and our culture direct our beliefs and the climate in which we operate. Knowing this, we can become aware of the values and culture of others, and, in turn, respect them.

Unfortunately, the process of socialization into a profession may make it difficult for a person to respect, accept, and trust the position of another. As students become committed to a profession through the process of socialization, they tend to view members of other disciplines with suspicion. Nursing is particularly susceptible in this regard because nurses have had to struggle to become colleagues with other health care professionals. They may not yet have gained the degree of comfort and professional self-esteem that permits them to be extended the nonthreatening respect, acceptance, and trust of others. As lines become blurred and once-sacred tasks and functions are shared, other colleagues may experience anxiety about respecting, accepting, and trusting the psychiatric nurse.

Supervision, support, and self-exploration are recommended for the expansion of nursing roles within and beyond traditional relationships. The clinical supervision of nurses by nurses can help pinpoint times when traditional caretaking roles are appropriate and when they inhibit growth. Administrative and peer support creates an atmosphere in which nurses are free to share their knowledge, skills, and evolving ideas. Such support increases creativity, depth, and perspective in nursing. Self-exploration and self-assessment, through reading and dialogue with other nurses, can help nurses consider alternatives to traditional stereotyped roles.

The History of Psychiatric Nursing *(continued)*

1960s

- The Community Mental Health Centers Act pushes trend in psychiatric nursing toward expanded and specialized roles.
- First textbook to address group therapy techniques in nursing practice written by Shirley Armstrong and Sheila Rouslin.
- Shirley Burd and Margaret Marshall write and edit the first compilation of psychiatric nursing papers suitable for graduate students in psychiatric nursing.

1970s

- The first master's level certification programs for advanced psychiatric nursing practice are developed by the New Jersey and New York State Nurse's Association.
- The psychiatric nurses who developed and implemented the early certification programs recognized the need to acknowledge expertise, distinguish generalist from specialist roles, and safeguard the public.
- Certification in psychiatric nursing becomes the responsibility of the ANA.

Confirmation of Specialist Roles

Engaging the Client in Collaboration

Include clients in the collaborative process of the mental health team whenever possible. Client participation in their own health care assures nurses that their clients are informed consumers of mental health services.

Clients can also be invited to participate in case conferences. These conferences often have an important place in the functioning of mental health agencies and may have a number of purposes. Encourage clients to participate in case conferences that involve collaboration among several agencies or several mental health care workers moving toward similar goals.

Consult the client about the information to be shared with other members of the mental health team. It is not always easy for the nurse to determine exactly how much to share and with whom. When the boundaries of confidentiality are not clear, confer with the supervisor or a colleague to determine what should be shared. Decisions should take into consideration what agreement exists between nurse and client about sharing information and how the person or agency receiving information will use that information in the client's best interest.

Excellence and Power in Practice

According to Benner (1984), the *competencies* of a psychiatric nurse can be differentiated from *goals* (how the nurse generally uses psychosocial knowledge to achieve an objective or realize an intention in a therapeutic relationship) and from *practice strategies* (how the nurse interacts

1980s

Period of Decline and Retrenchment

- NIMH funding for educational programs cut; federal budget further decreases funding; psychiatric nursing is on the verge of period of retrenchment that remains in evidence today.
- ANA Council of Specialists in Psychiatric and Mental Health Nursing develops a classification system for Psychiatric Nursing Diagnosis.
- Psychobiologic knowledge explodes.
- Psychiatric nursing leaders recommend incorporating new psychobiologic knowledge into clinical practice.

1990s

The Decade of the Brain

- Several psychiatric nurses appointed to President Clinton's task force on health care reform.
- ANA *Psychiatric Mental Health Nursing Psychopharmacology Project* published, intended to increase knowledge of psychobiology and improve client care.
- Psychiatric nursing leaders urge nurses to use the challenging circumstances posed by burgeoning information, reduced funding, and health care reform to clarify nursing's unique contribution to mental health care.

to help clients move in the direction of growth). Both goals and practice strategies are clearly influenced by the psychiatric nurse's personal and professional philosophies. Benner's exemplars (nurses who served as examples in her study) of excellence revealed the following about psychiatric nurses. They consistently

- Acted as psychologic and cultural mediators to help confused people "carve a path into a more shared, less idiosyncratic world" (p. 67).
- Used goals therapeutically in that goals were realistic, workable, and aimed toward improved social and psychologic functioning.
- Worked to build and maintain a therapeutic community for working out the issues of trust, conflict, and cooperation.

Exemplars of excellence in practice challenge nurses to implement their caring power and professional philosophy even under conditions that act as barriers and constraints in the everyday world.

Barriers and Constraints to Excellence

Aspiring toward therapeutic client relationships that are caring, sensitive, holistic, meaningful, and nonjudgmental can be stressful. The nurse must work under conditions that are influenced by economics, legislation, multiple levels of bureaucracy and paperwork, competition among members of the interdisciplinary mental health team, increased reliance on psychotropic medication, hasty discharges, limited follow-up care, a revolving-door pattern of hospital use, and short hospital stays.

Toward a New Entitlement

As Benner (1984) concludes, achieving excellence under the constraints described above requires a philosophy of commitment and involvement, but it also requires power. She advocates six strategies for balancing professional/philosophic mandates with the constraints of the context in which we practice. At the root of these strategies is the nurse's power to implement change through caring and expertise. In Benner's view, the nurse needs the following:

1. *Transformative power,* by which the nurse helps clients transform their views of self or others.
2. *Integrative caring,* through which the nurse helps clients continue with meaningful life activities despite disability and disorders.
3. *Advocacy power* to remove obstacles or stand alongside and enable.
4. *Healing power* to create a climate that mobilizes hope, to find interpretations of situations that are acceptable and clarifying to clients and families, and to help clients use sources of social, emotional, and spiritual support.
5. *Participative/affirmative power,* in which engagement and involvement are sources of energy.
6. *Problem-solving expertise* to grasp the problem rapidly, seeing it in relation to similar or dissimilar situations met in the past, yet not overlooking creative search and cue sensitivity (Benner 1984, pp. 210–215).

The chapters that follow in this text offer sources of excellence and power in the practice of humanistic psychiatric nursing.

Chapter Highlights

- The psychiatric nurse's capacity for empathy and ability to collaborate on the mental health team are related to the nurse's consciousness of meaning, use of language, willingness to negotiate, definitions of reality, awareness of feelings, ability to take care of self, and own self-view.
- Psychiatric nurses experience significant stresses in attempting to relate fully to clients and still maintain their own personal integration.
- Burning out is an attempt to cope with the stresses of intense interpersonal work by a form of distancing.
- The causes of professional burnout are most likely rooted in the social context of the work situation, not in the psychologic characteristics of the individual.
- To preserve personal integration, nurses can develop assertiveness, recognize the need and plan for some time alone, maintain personal physical health, and attend to cues of personal stress.
- Characteristics of artful therapeutic practice include respect for the client, availability, spontaneity, hope, acceptance, sensitivity, vision, accountability, advocacy, spirituality, and empathy.
- Phases in the development of empathic understanding are identification, incorporation, reverberation, and detachment.
- The psychiatric nurse's professional role includes providing direct client and family care, using the environment constructively, teaching self-care, coordinating the diverse aspects of care, providing continuity of care, advocating on behalf of clients and their families, engaging in primary prevention activities, and rehumanizing psychiatric care.
- Members of the mental health team who frequently practice in North America include the psychiatric–mental health nursing generalist, the psychiatric–mental health nursing clinical specialist, the psychiatrist, the psychoanalyst, the clinical psychologist, the psychiatric social worker, the mental health/human service worker, the paraprofessional, the occupational therapist, the recreational therapist, and the creative arts therapist.
- The quality of mental health services depends on cooperation among health care team members and across disciplines, knowledge about each member's contribution, inclusion of the client in decision making, and respect for the position of others.
- Despite barriers and constraints to implementing a professional philosophy in real-world situations, psychiatric nurses can and do find sources of power.

References

American Nurses Association: *A Statement on Psychiatric–Mental Health Clinical Nursing Practice and Standards of Psychiatric–Mental Health Clinical Nursing Practice.* American Nurses Publishing, 1994.

Benner P: *From Novice to Expert: Excellence and Power in Clinical Nursing Practice.* Addison-Wesley, 1984.

Benner P, Wrubel J: Coping with caregiving, in *The Primacy of Caring: Stress and Coping in Health and Illness.* Addison-Wesley, 1989, 365–406.

Bottorff JL, Morse JM: Identifying types of attending: Patterns of nurses' work. *Image: J Nurs Scholarship* 1994;26(1): 53–60.

Carlson-Catalano J: Empowering nurses for professional practice. *Nurs Outlook* 1992;40(3):139–141.

Chenevert M: *STAT: Special Techniques in Assertiveness Training for Women in the Health Professions,* ed 4. Mosby, 1992.
Cosgray RE, et al.: A day in the life of an inpatient: An experiential game to promote empathy for individuals in a psychiatric hospital. *Arch Psychiatr Nurs* 1990; 4(6): 354–359.
Cronin-Stubbs D, Brophy EB: Burnout: Can social support save the psychiatric nurse? *J Psychosoc Nurs* 1985;23(7): 8–13.
Dumas RG: Psychiatric nursing in an era of change. *J Psychosoc Nurs* 1994;32(1):11–14.
Dunn JK: Medical skills and knowledge: How necessary are they for psychiatric nurses? *J Psychosoc Nurs* 1993; 31(12):25–28.
Floyd JA: Nursing students' stress levels, attitudes toward drugs, and drug use. *Arch Psychiatr Nurs* 1991;5(1):46–53.
Foster SW: The pragmatics of culture: The rhetoric of difference in psychiatric nursing. *Arch Psychiatr Nurs* 1990; 4(5):292–297.
Girgenti JR, Mathis AC: Putting psychiatric nursing standards into clinical practice. *J Psychosoc Nurs* 1994;32(6):39–42.
Glotz N, Johnsen G, Johnson R: Advancing clinical excellence: Competency-based patient care. *Nurs Management* 1994;25(1):42–44.
Heinrich K, Killeen K: The gentle art of nurturing yourself. *Am J Nurs* 1993;93(10):41–44.
Hellwig K: Psychiatric home care nursing: Managing patients in the community setting. *J Psychosoc Nurs* 1993;31(12): 21–24.
Hicks LL, Stallmeyer JM, Coleman JR: *Role of the Nurse in Managed Care.* American Nurses Publishing, 1993.
Johnson JL: A dialectical examination of nursing art. *Adv Nurs Sci* 1994;17(2):1–14.
Kahn S, Saulo M: *Healing Yourself: A Nurse's Guide to Self-Care and Renewal.* Delmar, 1994.
Keegan L: *The Nurse as Healer.* Delmar, 1994.
Kilkins SP: Self-assertion and nurses: A different voice. *Nurs Outlook* 1990;38(3):143–145.
Krauss J: *Health Care Reform: Essential Mental Health Services.* American Nurses Publishing, 1993.
Lynch VA: Forensic nursing: Diversity in education and practice. *J Psychosoc Nurs* 1993;31(11):7–14.
McBride AB: Psychiatric nursing in the 1990s. *Arch Psychiatr Nurs* 1990;4(1):21–27.
McConnell EA: *Burnout in the Nursing Profession.* Mosby, 1982.
Miller MP, Duffey J: Planning and program development for psychiatric home care. *JONA* 1993;23(11):35–41.
Muff J: Balancing communication, in Smythe EEM (ed): *Surviving Nursing.* Addison-Wesley, 1984.
Peplau HE: The psychiatric nurse—accountable? To whom? For what? *Perspect Psychiatr Care* 1980;18(3):128–134.
Peter E, Gallop R: The ethic of care: A comparison of nursing and medical students. *Image: J Nurs Scholarship* 1994; 26(1):47–51.
Robinson A: Spirituality and risk: Toward an understanding. *Holistic Nurse Pract* 1994;8(2):1–7.
Talley S, Brooke PS: Prescriptive authority for psychiatric clinical specialists: Framing the issues. *Arch Psychiatr Nurs* 1992; 6(2):71–82.
Thompson J, Strand K: Psychiatric nursing in a psychosocial setting. *J Psychosoc Nurs* 1994;32(2):25–29.
Trygstad LN: The need to know: Biological learning needs identified by practicing psychiatric nurses. *J Psychosoc Nurs* 1994;32(2):13–18.
Warner SL: Humor: A coping response for student nurses. *Arch Psychiatr Nurs* 1991;5(1):10–16.
Wilson HS, Kneisl CR: *Learning Activities in Psychiatric Nursing,* ed 3. Addison-Wesley, 1988.

References for Mind-Body-Spirit Connection Box

Muller W: *Legacy of the Heart.* Simon and Schuster, 1992.

CHAPTER 2

PHILOSOPHY AND THEORIES FOR INTERDISCIPLINARY PSYCHIATRIC CARE

Holly Skodol Wilson

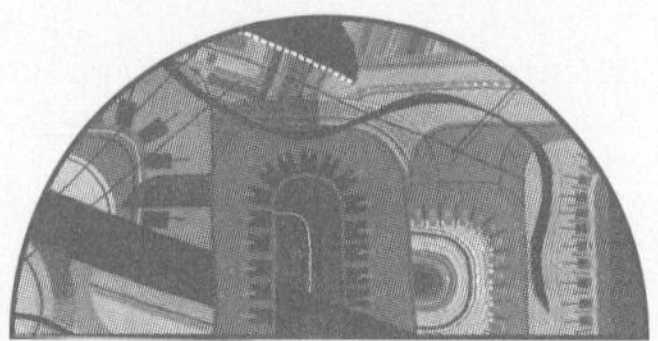

COMPETENCIES

- *Identify the major ideas of interactionism.*
- *Identify the major principles of humanism.*
- *Recognize the influence of the knowledge explosion in psychobiology.*
- *Relate the premises of humanistic interactionism and psychobiology to psychiatric nursing.*
- *Identify the assumptions and key ideas of medical-biologic, psychoanalytic, behaviorist, social-interpersonal, and nursing theories.*
- *Comprehend the implications each theory has for psychiatric nursing practice.*

Cross-References

Other topics relevant to this content are: Contemporary roles of psychiatric nurses, Chapter 1; Cultural considerations in mental health care, Chapter 5; Ethics, Chapter 10; Legal aspects of confinement, Chapter 11; Psychobiology, Chapter 3.

Critical Thinking Challenge

Despite the numerous theories concerning the causes and dynamics of mental disorders (including those you will be reading about in this chapter), psychiatric nurses often lament that practice is rarely based on theory or research in real-world clinical settings. Think of the many possible reasons that contribute to this theory-practice gap in providing mental health services. Then consider what changes in psychiatric nursing research, mental health care economics, and service delivery systems will be necessary in order to begin basing psychiatric nursing interventions on theory and research.

To practice psychiatric nursing humanistically, nurses must devote themselves to understanding what makes people human, how they express their joy of living, their sadness, their desire to love, their hopes for growth. Understanding these phenomena becomes even more crucial when psychiatric nurses must explain how the joy of living suddenly turns to the desire to die, how love of self and others turns to violence and hate, how the hope for growth turns to withdrawal and despair, and how alterations in the brain relate to these human experiences.

This chapter introduces you to a holistic philosophy that includes humanism, interactionism, and the knowledge explosion in psychobiology. In this chapter, we also compare the basic assumptions and implications for practice in the dominant theories for interdisciplinary psychiatric care. These are:

- Medical-biologic theory
- Psychoanalytic theory
- Behaviorist theory
- Social-interpersonal theories
- Nursing theory

Clinicians choose one or a combination of these theories in determining what information to assess about clients, what intervention goals and approaches to recommend, and what ultimate evaluation criteria to set. Your approach to understanding psychiatric clients is influenced by your philosophy. Theories, on the other hand, provide the conceptual tools to formulate that understanding and to interpret clinical data.

Humanistic Interactionism and Psychobiology: The Mind-Body-Spirit Connection

Scope of Practice

All nurses are concerned with the quality of human life and its relationship to health. The psychiatric nurse is especially concerned with the relationship between the individual's optimal psychobiologic health and feelings of self-worth, personal integrity, self-fulfillment, and creative expression. Just as important are the satisfying of basic living needs, comfortable relationships with others, and the recognition of human rights. These elements collectively define **mental health.** The psychiatric nurse's scope of practice is broad enough to include issues such as alienation, identity crises, sudden life changes, and troubled family interactions. It can encompass individual protests or mass confrontations. It may deal with poverty and affluence, the experiences of birth and death, the loss of significant others, or the loss of body parts. It is concerned with sustaining and enhancing the individual and the group. Yet it also must address basic life issues of eating, sleeping, grooming, and hygiene.

This broad-ranging, humanistic, interactional, and psychobiologic view of the scope of psychiatric nursing is dramatically different from the exclusively medical or behavioral science orientation of the last forty years. The classic psychiatric and psychologic approaches have described and classified signs and symptoms of *illness,* then accounted for it by individual psychologic dynamics such as character disorder, weak ego, or failed defense mechanisms. The basis for this text is a new synthesis of psychosocial knowledge and psychobiologic knowledge required for practice in the twenty-first century (See the Research Note on the next page).

Defining the Concept of Mental Disorder

We believe that concepts such as "mental disorder" and "mental health" are interactional and derive their meaning not only from changes in brain biochemistry but also from the definitions given to certain behavior by certain people. We advocate looking at the social conditions under which someone is called "mentally ill." We view mental illness and mental health as outgrowths of intra- and interpersonal processes.

Determining that someone is mentally ill is often a matter of judgment, even when brain chemicals are altered. The appropriateness of behavior depends on whether it is judged plausible or not according to a set of social, ethical, and legal rules that define the limits of appropriate behavior and reality. For example, if a man on a street corner says he is Napoleon, people will not believe him and will consider his statement symptomatic or disturbed. If a man at a masquerade party says he is Napoleon, people reach a different conclusion. Alterations in brain biochemistry may be present in both social contexts.

With the preceding as philosophic background, we support the concept of **mental disorder** as defined by the American Psychiatric Association's *Diagnostic and Statistical Manual of Mental Disorders (DSM-IV):*

> A clinically significant behavioral or psychological syndrome or pattern that occurs in an individual that is typically associated with either a painful symptom (distress) or impairment in one or more important areas of functioning (disability) or with a significantly increased risk of suffering, death, pain, or loss of freedom. In addition, this syndrome or pattern must not be merely an expectable and culturally sanctioned response to a particular event, for example, the death of a loved one. . . . Neither deviant behavior (e.g., political, religious, or sexual) nor conflicts that are primarily between the individual and society are mental disorders unless the deviance or conflict is a symptom of dysfunction in the individual as described above (APA 1994, pp. xxi–xxii).

Psychiatric nurses are concerned with the care of clients who have identified mental disorders. However, our concerns extend to the wide range of human responses to mental distress, disability, and disorder (Loomis et al. 1987). For example, an addicted parent may not only suffer from shame, unemployment, and abusive outbursts of anger but may also lose a sense of purpose and meaning, and experience a disturbed self-concept. These responses have detrimental effects on the health of children, partners, and other significant people in the person's life. Individual, family, and community responses vary with interpretations of meaning and culture.

Like many concepts in the human sciences, the concept of mental disorder lacks a definition that covers all

RESEARCH NOTE

Citation

Trygstad LN: The need to know: Biological learning needs identified by practicing psychiatric nurses. *Psychosoc Nurs* 1994;32(2):13–18.

Study Problem/Purpose

The purpose of this study was to describe the current practice and identify the perceived learning needs of practicing psychiatric nurses regarding the biologic (rather than intra- or interpersonal) aspects of practice.

Methods

This descriptive study design used participant observation and interview methods for data collection and theme analysis on 23 units in 12 inpatient psychiatric facilities chosen specifically for diversity. Public, private, for-profit, and nonprofit settings were included. Two of the settings were long-term and 10 were acute. The client population included both voluntary and involuntary patients who represented a wide variety of DSM diagnoses.

Findings

Evident in all 12 psychiatric settings was the inpatient population trend toward older clients who have concomitant chronic and acute medical problems, physical limitations, and represent cultural diversity. The nurses were consistent in noting a perceived need for practicing psychiatric nurses to steadily increase their knowledge about medications, physical care, and environment. Five specific areas of learning needs included the following: knowledge of medications; recognition of interactions of client physical conditions and medication with other substances such as nicotine, illegal drugs, and over-the-counter medications; skills to manage acute and chronic medical conditions in the psychiatric milieu; the ability to maintain safety and environmental factors such as sensory stimulation; stress management and self-care strategies for psychiatric nurses.

Implications

Biological psychiatry is a reality. Prelicensure nursing education programs and textbooks like this one must incorporate psychobiological knowledge, as do graduate specialist programs and continuing education. Of particular importance are biologic theories of mental disorders, neuroanatomy, circadian rhythms, psychopharmacology, and immunology.

situations. Faced with such a diverse array of human problems, the psychiatric nurse is challenged to synthesize a holistic philosophy for practice that can be the basis for care. See Figure 2–1 on page 30 for approaches to mental disorder throughout history.

Basic Premises of Interactionism

One central idea in the approach we advocate has come to be known as **symbolic interactionism**, a term introduced by Herbert Blumer (1969) to describe an approach to the study of human conduct. It is based on three philosophic premises:

1. Human beings act toward things (other people, events) on the basis of the meaning that the things have for them. Life experiences may have different meanings for different people.
2. The meaning of things in a person's life is derived from the social interactions that person has with others. We learn meanings during our experiences with others.
3. People handle and modify the meanings of the things they encounter through an interpretive process. They come to their own conclusions.

Implications for Psychiatric Nursing Practice

The First Premise: Different Meanings for Different People We believe that all behavior has meaning. The psychiatric nurse must be wary of interventions that ignore, discount, or discredit the meaning an experience has for the client in favor of the nurse's own definition of the situation. Thus, nurses must develop skill in observing, interpreting, and responding to the client's lived experiences in the hope of arriving at a common ground of negotiated meanings and authentic communication.

The Second Premise: Meanings Arise in One's Social World We believe meanings arise in the *process* of interaction with others. It is essential, therefore, that psychiatric nurses take into account the social and cultural environment of each client. A holistic assessment of a client accounts for the interaction patterns in that person's social world.

A shaved head, black leather clothing, and tattoos may appear bizarre in a milieu of upper-middle-class bankers and businesspeople, yet they represent rather strict adherence to dress and demeanor codes of the "heavy metal" subculture. Those who are called "paranoid" or "neurotic" or who are said to be "using alcohol or drugs as emotional crutches" cannot be understood outside their unique social context.

Similarly, it is within interpersonal interaction that clients can learn new definitions for life situations and new repertoires for action. This is the heart of the psychiatric nurse's therapeutic and caring role. The sensitive, intelligent, and humanistic use of self within interpersonal relationships is a key part of the psychiatric nurse's skill. Nurses have a particular potential for helping clients redefine their experiences in more satisfying ways, learn new patterns of coping with stress, and generally enhance the quality of their lives and social worlds.

The Third Premise: Meaning Is a Basis for Behavior We believe that people handle situations in terms of what they consider vitally important about the situation. To understand clients' actions, the psychiatric nurse must identify the meanings those actions have for them.

Nurses need to keep this premise in mind when responding to an expression of human distress. A nurse may say, "I wouldn't worry about it," or "Don't feel that way," "You are reacting inappropriately," or "It's not so bad." Such clichés are not usually helpful, not because they are inherently "untherapeutic" but because in voicing them the nurse neglects the basic premise that people interpret the world in their own way to act in a specific situation.

Interactionism offers psychiatric nursing a perspective of human beings as having purpose and control over their lives, even if they have altered brain chemistry and stressful environments. Interactionism as interpreted here provides the premise for a philosophy of caring with a strong humanistic cast. Interactionism acknowledges the interaction of psychology, biology, and sociocultural context.

Basic Premises of Humanism

One of the purposes of this chapter is to specify a philosophic basis for subsequent chapters. The three premises of interactionism provide us with a partial orientation. A theory of life centered on human beings, termed **humanism**, adds to the philosophic perspective.

The central concept of humanism is that the chief end of human life is to work for well-being within the limitations of life in today's world. Humanism is a philosophy of service to benefit humanity through reason, science, and democracy.

The humanistic perspective has the following eight central propositions:

1. The human being's mind is indivisibly connected with the body.
2. Human beings have the power or potential to solve their own problems.
3. Human beings, while influenced by the past, possess freedom of creative choice and action and are, within certain limits, masters of their own destinies.
4. Human values are grounded in life experiences and relationships, and our highest goal must be the happiness, freedom, and growth of all people.
5. Individuals attain well-being and a high quality of life by harmoniously combining personal satisfactions with activities that contribute to the welfare of the community.
6. We should develop art and awareness of beauty so that the aesthetic experience becomes a pervasive reality in people's lives.
7. We should apply reason, science, and democratic procedures in all areas of life.
8. We must continually examine our basic convictions, including those of humanism.

See Lamont's classic book (1967) for an elaboration of these propositions.

Implications for Psychiatric Nursing Practice As a philosophy underlying psychiatric nursing practice, humanism means devotion to the interests of human beings wherever they live and whatever their status. It reaffirms the spirit of compassion and caring toward others. It is a constructive philosophy that wholeheartedly affirms the joys, beauty, and values of human living.

The subsequent chapters in this text attempt to show how these basic premises can be put to use in psychiatric nursing practice. Some fundamental concepts are described briefly in the following sections.

A Holistic View of the Mind-Body Relationship Our humanistic interactional view is that physical and mental factors are interrelated and that a change in one may result in a change in another. For example, anger may result in increased blood pressure. An invading organism, a decrease in a neurotransmitter, or a structural change in the body can alter thought processes. Low self-esteem can result in hunched shoulders and severe skeletal muscle contractures.

The implications for psychiatric nursing are clear. Healing and caring must be approached **holistically**. The psychiatric nurse deals with the biologic aspects of a primarily psychologic or emotional pattern and the psychologic or emotional aspects of biologic experiences.

The History of Psychiatry

Preliterate Times
Era of Magico-Religious Explanations

- Mental and physical suffering not differentiated.
- "Spirits of torment" acting outside the body are responsible for ills.
- No distinctions made between medicine, magic, and religion.
- Primitive healers address spirits by appeal, prayer, bribery, intimidation, appeasement, punishment.
- Healing methods include exorcism, magical ritual, incantation.

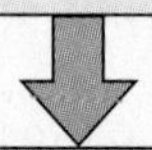

Early Civilization
Era of Organic Explanations

- Hippocrates (460–370 BC) rejects demonology and proposes that psychiatric illnesses caused by imbalances in "body humors:" blood, black bile, yellow bile, and phlegm.
- Psychiatric suffering comes within the realm of medical practice.
- Imbalances in body humors often corrected by bloodletting.

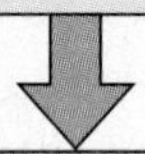

The Medieval Period
Era of Alienation

- Return to the magic, mysticism, and demonology of preliterate times.
- Madness viewed as dramatic encounter with secret powers and influenced by the moon (lunacy).
- *Malleus Maleficarum (The Witches' Hammer)* by Dominican monks Johann Sprenger and Heinrich Kraemer published 1487 rationalized mental illness in terms of magical explanation.
- Violent insane shackled in prisons or sent to sea "in search of reason."

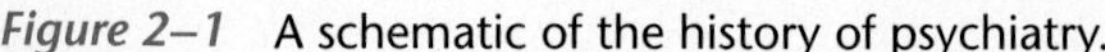

The Renaissance
Era of Confinement

- In 1656 Hôpital Générale in Paris founded to confine the mad, poor, and various deviants.
- The "insane" have no recourse to appeal.
- Madness not linked to medicine; could only be mastered by discipline and brutality.
- Radical physicians like Johann Weyer (1515–1588) believed that "those illnesses whose origins are attributed to witches come from natural causes."

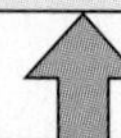

Late Eighteenth and Early Nineteenth Centuries
Era of Moral Treatment

- Physicians classify symptoms of mental disorders without understanding the sources of mental suffering.
- In 1794 Philippe Pinel (1745–1826) treated inmates in the French institutions Bicetre and Salpetriere with humanity and was thus considered mad.
- In England, William Tuke (1732–1822) focused on "moral treatment" in a humane milieu called the York Retreat.
- In America, Benjamin Rush (1746–1813) focused on humanitarianism and moral treatment at the Pennsylvania Hospital.

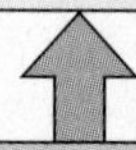

Late Nineteenth and Early Twentieth Centuries
Era of Public Mental Hospitals

- Dorthea L. Dix (1802–1887) founds or enlarges over 30 mental hospitals.
- Moral treatment replaced by custodial care.
- Clifford Beers (1876–1943) published his book describing his own intense suffering and mental anguish, leading to the development of preventative psychiatry and the formation of child guidance clinics.

Figure 2–1 A schematic of the history of psychiatry.

Early Twentieth Century
Era of Psychoanalysis

- Emil Kraepelin (1856–1926) creates system of distinct disease entities and differentiates bipolar disorder from schizophrenia.
- Sigmund Freud (1856–1939) explains human behavior in psychological terms and demonstrates that behavior can be changed through psychoanalysis.

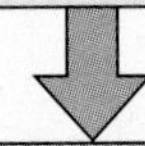

Mid-Twentieth Century
Era of Ideologic Expansion

- From the mid-1940s to the mid-1950s, a strong rift between biologic orientation and dynamic orientation develops.
- By the early 1950s several drugs for the treatment of mental disorder were in common use.
- In 1946 the National Institute of Mental Health (NIMH) opened for research, training, and provision of preventive, therapeutic, and rehabilitative psychiatric services.
- Harry Stack Sullivan (1892–1949) developed the interpersonal theory of psychiatry.
- By 1960 family therapy had become both a diagnostic tool and a mode of treatment.
- Erik Erikson formulated his psychosocial theory of development.
- Psychotropic drugs help staff members manage large numbers of clients in crowded conditions.
- Group therapy and short-term therapy recognized as options to costly long-term therapy or hospitalization.
- Milieu therapy developed by Maxwell Jones in England.

Late-Twentieth Century
Deinstitutionalization and the Community Mental Health Movement

- In 1961 the Joint Commission on Mental Illness and Health presented *Action for Mental Health* to Congress calling for a shift from institutional to community-based care, more equitable distribution of mental health services, preventative services, consumer participation in planning and delivery of mental health workers, education of more mental health professionals, public support for research, shared federal, state, local funding for construction and operation of community mental health centers.
- Congress passed the *Mental Retardation Facilities and Community Mental Health Centers Construction Act.*
- Between 1955 and 1975 the number of resident clients in state mental hospitals decreased nearly 66 percent.
- The *Community Mental Health Systems Act* of 1980 authorized funding of community mental health centers, services to high-risk populations, ambulatory mental health care centers, rape research and services, but was repealed in 1981 and replaced by the *Omnibus Budget Reconciliation Act*, placing mental health programs into an alcohol, drug abuse, and mental health services block grant.

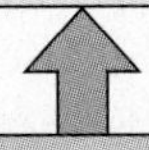

The 1990s: The Decade of the Brain

- The primary innovation of the 1990s is the "biologic revolution:" collaboration of science and technology to expand concepts of mental disorder proposed by psychological, behavioral, and psychoanalytic theories.
- A report by the National Advisory Health Council calls the gains made in research-based knowledge about the epidemiology, diagnosis, treatment, and prevention of major mental illnesses a "quantum leap in understanding the brain."
- Client advocacy groups welcome psychiatry's shift toward psychosocial rehabilitation for client self-care.
- The National Alliance for the Mentally Ill (NAMI), establishes a separate research foundation to study the biologic basis of major mental illness.

Psychiatric nursing care can be given not only in mental health care settings but also in general health care settings and may be directed toward clients whose immediate problems are primarily physical.

An Expanded Role for Nurses The humanistic interactional perspective on mental disorders implies an expanded role for psychiatric nurses. We believe that psychiatric nurses should be prepared to work for change within social and political systems. Psychiatric nursing can no longer be limited to client-oriented activities designed exclusively to control symptoms and increase the capability of individuals to adjust satisfactorily to the existing social condition. Instead, psychiatric nursing must be involved in social goals that advance health holistically. Because psychiatric nursing has political consequences, it is essential that nurses begin to develop a philosophic and ethical framework to guide and evaluate the political outcome of therapeutic intervention.

Negotiation and Advocacy In this book, the model for intervention and change is one of negotiation and advocacy. The responsibility for change remains with the person who seeks psychiatric help or consultation. Clients are held accountable for their own behavior. They are not the passive recipients of care given by psychiatric professionals. Instead, they are empowered in the process of developing new perspectives and encouraged to weigh alternatives and make self-directed choices. They and their families are educated about their disorder and their medications.

Basic Premises of the Psychobiologic Revolution

The last decade has seen major breakthroughs in knowledge about the brain, the mind, the spirit, and behavior. This knowledge explosion has been termed the **psychobiologic revolution** in psychiatry. Research has generated new understanding of how genetics, immunology, biorhythms, brain structure, and brain biochemistry influence mental disorders. New imaging techniques make it possible to view what has never been seen before. New drugs to correct biochemical imbalances in the brain are being studied. Researchers are exploring such psychobiologic interventions as exposure to bright light and white noise, and the restriction of nutrients and non-nutrients believed to affect behavior.

Some authorities argue that psychiatric nurses should continue to focus on the human aspects of care as psychiatry moves toward "remedicalization." They fear that by embracing the biologic sciences we will diminish the art of psychiatric nursing. Others, ourselves included, contend that, to bring a contemporary holistic perspective to psychiatric nursing care, we must integrate the rapidly accumulating knowledge in psychobiology. We do not give up our humanistic, psychosocial, and interactional premises simply because we recognize the value of the breakthroughs being made in psychobiology. Instead, as we redefine the traditional art of psychiatric nursing care and caring in the "Decade of the Brain," our practice and research must integrate "high tech" and "high touch," nature and nurture, the biologic sciences and the behavioral sciences.

Theories for Interdisciplinary Psychiatric Care

Medical-Biologic Theory

The medical-biologic model in psychiatry originated in the era of classification. The classification of mental disturbances brought the emotional and behavioral aspects of people into the domain of the medical doctor. During this period, the systematic observation, naming, and classification of symptoms were emphasized. Emil Kraepelin's monumental descriptive diagnostic classification system is acknowledged as the first comprehensive medical model. It included the notions that the cause of mental illness was organic, that it was located in the central nervous system, that the disease followed a predictable course, and that treatment should be based on accurate diagnosis. Contemporary research findings in the field of psychobiology lend support to some of these early ideas but advance them and make them specific in important ways.

Dominant social attitudes and philosophic viewpoints have influenced the understanding and approaches to mental disorder throughout history, and concepts that may be considered modern may have roots in earlier eras (see Figure 2–1).

Assumptions and Key Ideas Medical-biologic theories, now redefined as psychobiologic, view emotional and behavioral disturbances like any physical disease. Thus, abnormal behavior is directly attributable to a disease process, a lesion, a neuropathologic condition, a toxin introduced from outside the body, or (most recently) a biochemical abnormality of neurotransmitters and enzymes. This position can be summarized as follows:

- The individual suffering from emotional disturbances is sick and has an illness or defect.
- The illness can, at least presumably, be located in some part of the body (usually the brain's limbic system and the central nervous system's synapse receptor sites). Factors related to mental disorders include excesses or deficiencies of certain brain neurotransmitters, alterations in the body's biologic rhythms, including the

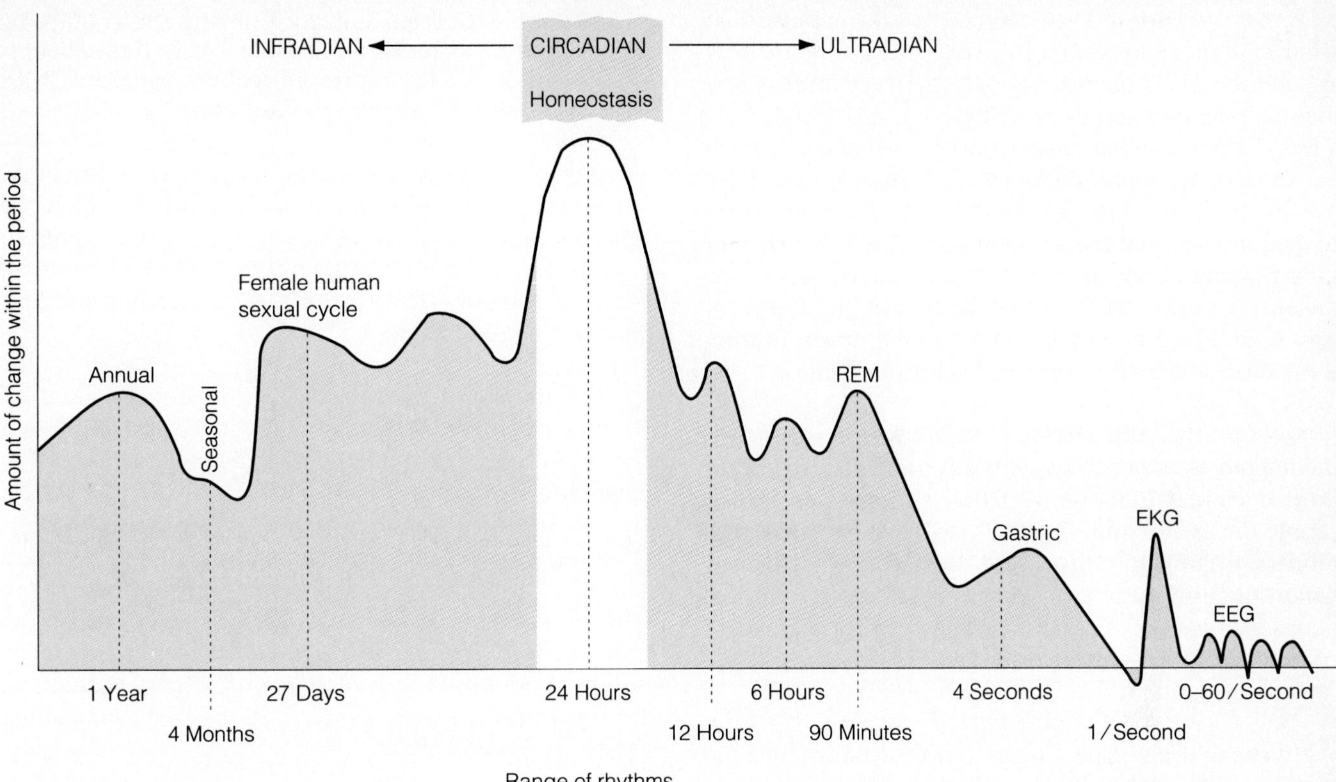

Figure 2–2 The spectrum of human biorhythms.

sleep-wake cycle (Figure 2–2); and genetic predispositions.

- The illness has characteristic structural, biochemical, and mental symptoms that can be diagnosed, classified, and labeled.
- Mental diseases run a characteristic course and have a particular prognosis for recovery.
- Mental disorders respond to physical or somatic treatments, including drugs, chemicals, hormones, diet, or surgery.
- Biologic explanations of mental disorders can reduce the stigma often associated with them, and can discourage claims that mental disorders result from a lack of willpower or moral character.

Implications for Psychiatric Nursing Practice Nurses who were first involved in the care of psychiatric clients were primarily responsible for the client's physical wellbeing. Their responsibilities included administering drugs prescribed by the physician and caring for clients undergoing treatments such as insulin shock, electroshock therapy, or hydrotherapy.

Biologic-medical theories are the conceptual basis for the continued use of biologic therapies in the care of psychiatric clients, the hospital as the setting for care, research into the genetic transmission of mental illness, research on biochemical and metabolic variables among diagnosed psychiatric clients, and dominance of the medical doctor—the psychiatrist—in the mental health team. As long as psychiatric clients are admitted to and reimbursed for care according to medical diagnoses, knowledge of this framework is crucial. Furthermore, as long as biologic knowledge expands, psychiatric–mental health nurses are responsible for translating that knowledge into care practices that recognize the biologic factors related to mental disorders.

Psychoanalytic Theory

Psychoanalytic theory is usually credited to the Viennese physician Sigmund Freud (1962b). Freud believed that all psychologic and emotional events, however obscure, were understandable. For the meanings behind behavior, he looked to childhood experiences that he believed caused adult neuroses. Psychoanalytic therapy consists of clarifying the meaning of events, feelings, and behavior and thereby gaining insight about them. Freud's work shifted the focus of psychiatry from classification to a dynamic view of mental phenomena.

Assumptions and Key Ideas The basic principles of psychoanalytic theory are discussed below.

Psychic determinism states that no human behavior is accidental. Each psychic event is determined by the ones that preceded it. Events in people's mental lives that seem random or unrelated to what went before are only apparently so. Thus, psychoanalysts never dismiss any mental phenomenon as meaningless or accidental. They always search for what caused it, why it happened. For example, people commonly forget or misplace things. They usually view this as just an accident. Psychoanalysts seek to demonstrate that the accident was caused by a wish or intent of the person involved. Psychoanalysts also view dreams as subject to the principle of psychic determinism, each dream and each image in each dream bearing some relationship to the rest of the dreamer's life.

Role of the Unconscious Significant unconscious mental processes occur frequently in normal as well as abnormal mental functioning. These processes are called simply the *unconscious*. Much of what goes on in people's minds is unknown to them, and this accounts for the apparent discontinuities in their mental life. If the unconscious motivation of some behavioral symptoms is discovered, the apparent discontinuities disappear, and the cause becomes clear.

Psychoanalysis The most powerful and reliable method for studying the unconscious is the technique that Freud evolved over several years called **psychoanalysis.** The basic logic behind psychoanalysis is as follows:

1. The client underwent a *traumatic experience* that stirred up intense and painful emotion.
2. The traumatic experience represented to the client some ideas that were incompatible with the dominant ideas constituting the ego. Thus, the client experienced a **neurotic conflict.**
3. The incompatible idea and the neurotic conflict associated with it force the ego to bring into action **defense mechanisms** that manifest themselves as neurotic symptoms (see Chapter 4).
4. Therapy is directed toward resolving the conflict by uncovering its roots in the unconscious. If the client is able to release the **repressed feelings** associated with the conflict, the symptoms disappear.

Strategies used in psychoanalysis are hypnosis, the interpretation of dreams, and free association, in which the client is encouraged to express every idea that comes to mind—no matter how insignificant, irrelevant, shameful, or embarrassing—ignoring all self-censorship and suspending all judgment.

Topography of the Mind Freud classified mental activities according to regions or systems of the mind in a body of thought now referred to as *topographic theory.* Any mental event that occurred outside of conscious awareness represented the **unconscious** region. Mental events that could be brought into conscious awareness through an act of attention were said to be **preconscious.** Those that occurred in conscious awareness were regarded as the **conscious** surface of the mind. This topographic model, although still used to classify mental events in terms of the quality and degree of awareness, has been supplanted by the structural model.

Structure of the Mind With the publication of *The Ego and the Id* in 1923, Freud abandoned the topographic model of the mind for the *structural model* (1962a). The structural model of the mind contends that there are three distinct entities: the id, the ego, and the superego. The **id** is a completely unorganized reservoir of energy derived from drives and instincts. The **ego** controls action and perception, controls contact with reality, and, through the defense mechanisms, inhibits primary instinctual drives. One of its fundamental functions is also the capacity for developing mutually satisfying relationships with others. The **superego** is concerned with moral behavior. Frequently, the superego allies itself with the

Table 2–1 Freud's Psychosexual Stages

Stage	*Age Span*	*Task*	*Key Concept*
Oral	0–18 months	Satisfaction and anxiety management from oral activity	Oral activity gives pleasure and is a source for learning
Anal	18 months–3 years	Learning muscle control for toilet training	Delayed gratification and rule internalization
Phallic	3–6 years	Gender identification and genital awareness	Repression of attraction to the opposite-sex parent, leading to same-sex identification
Latency	6–12 years	Repression of sexuality	Oedipal conflict resolved with a shift to other interests and friends
Genital	12 years–young adult	Channeling sexuality into relationships with members of the opposite sex	Reemerging sexuality to motivate behavior

ego against the id, imposing demands in the form of conscience or guilt feelings. The id in a child operates according to what Freud called the **pleasure principle:** the tendency to seek pleasure and avoid pain. This is not always possible, so the demands of the pleasure principle have to be modified by the **reality principle.** The reality principle is a learned ego function by which people develop the capacity to delay the immediate release of tension or achievement of pleasure.

Drives Freud believed that psychic energy was derived from **drives.** He used the word **cathexis** to refer to the attachment of psychic energy to a person or a thing. The greater the cathexis, the greater the psychologic importance of the person or object. Freud accounted for the instinctual aspects of a person's mental life by assuming the existence of two drives, the *sexual drive* and the *aggressive drive.* The former gives rise to the erotic component of mental activity, and the latter gives rise to the destructive component. The sexual drive came to be known as the **libido.** Table 2–1 presents the stages of psychosexual development according to Freud.

Erikson's Eight Stages of Man Freud's stages of personality development were called stages of psychosexual development because of the shifting emphasis of sources of pleasure or gratification. Erik Erikson, a neo-Freudian, also formulated a developmental theory of personality that attempted to take into account not just biologic instincts but also cultural and interpersonal tasks that have to be accomplished in order to move forward developmentally (Table 2–2). Erikson's developmental theory is also considered more optimistic than Freud's because he believed that clients in therapy could return to a developmental task that had not been accomplished and relearn it.

IMPLICATIONS FOR PSYCHIATRIC NURSING PRACTICE Psychoanalytic theory has historically provided a very limited treatment role for the nurse. Psychoanalytic clients are usually seen in the analyst's office as private clients. With the emergence of psychoanalytically oriented settings such as Chestnut Lodge in Rockville, Maryland, nurses became somewhat more involved, sharing at least in the psychoanalytic language, concepts, and speculations about client dynamics and personality development.

Behaviorist Theory

Behaviorist theory in psychiatry has its roots in psychology and neurophysiology. To the behaviorist, symptoms associated with neuroses and psychoses are clusters of learned behaviors that persist because they are somehow rewarding to the individual. One of the most important

Table 2–2 Erikson's Eight Developmental Stages

Age	*Stage of Development*	*Task/Area of Resolution*	*Concepts/Basic Attitudes*
Birth–18 months	Infancy	Trust versus mistrust	Ability to trust others and a sense of one's own trustworthiness; a sense of hope; withdrawal and estrangement
18 months–3 years	Early childhood	Autonomy versus shame and doubt	Self-control without loss of self-esteem; ability to cooperate and to express oneself; compulsive self-restraint or compliance; defiance, willfulness
3–5 years	Late childhood	Initiative versus guilt	Realistic sense of purpose; some ability to evaluate one's own behavior; self-denial and self-restriction
6–12 years	School age	Industry versus inferiority	Realization of competence, perseverance; feeling that one will never be "any good," withdrawal from school and peers
12–20 years	Adolescence	Identity versus role diffusion	Coherent sense of self; plans to actualize one's abilities; feelings of confusion, indecisiveness, possibly antisocial behavior
18–25 years	Young adulthood	Intimacy versus isolation	Capacity for love as mutual devotion; commitment to work and relationships; impersonal relationships, prejudice
25–65 years	Adulthood	Generativity versus stagnation	Creativity, productivity, concern for others; self-indulgence, impoverishment of self
65 years to death	Old age	Integrity versus despair	Acceptance of the worth and uniqueness of one's life; sense of loss, contempt for others

SOURCE: Childhood and Society, *2nd ed. by Erik H. Erikson, W. W. Norton & Company, Inc. Copyright © 1950, 1963. Renewed 1978 by Erik H. Erikson.*

contributions to this framework was made by Pavlov (1849–1936), who in 1902 discovered a phenomenon he called the **conditioned reflex** in a famous experiment with a dog and a bell. The basic principle of the conditioned reflex is this:

1. A response is a reaction to a stimulus.
2. If a new and different stimulus is presented with or just before the original stimulating event, the same response reaction can be obtained.
3. Eventually the new stimulus can replace the original one, so that the response occurs in reaction to the new stimulus alone.

The conditioned or learned response is viewed as the basic unit of all learning, the unit on which more complex behavioral patterns are constructed. Such construction occurs through a process called **reinforcement**, in which behaviors are rewarded and persist. Pavlov's theories have continued into the present and are valued for their simplicity, concreteness, and objectivity. Some behaviorists see them as the key to understanding and controlling the whole range of undesirable human behavior.

ASSUMPTIONS AND KEY IDEAS The fundamental premises of behaviorist theory are as follows:

- Human beings are merely complex animals. The difference between humans and other animals is one of degree and not kind. Thus the use of animal experience as an analog to human experience is clearly justifiable.
- The self in humans is the sum or repository of past conditionings or simply the behavioral repertoire. Therapists can know clients only by the clients' behavior.
- Behavior is the way in which an animal acts. It can be observed, described, and recorded.
- There is no autonomous person. People are what they do and what they are reinforced for doing by conditions in their environment.
- The self is a structure of stimulus-response chains or hierarchies of habit. It is possible to know and predict conditions under which behavior will occur.
- The symptoms of a mental disorder are, in fact, the substance of that person's troubles. There is no hidden motive, no underlying cause, no internal pathogenic process. There is only the symptom or the behavior, and the aim of behaviorist therapy is to change the behavior.
- The classification of mental illness is meaningful only to provide legal labels. It provides little or no assistance in prescribing a treatment program.
- People can control others whether others want to be controlled or not. Control is neither good nor bad in and of itself.
- The therapist determines what behavior should be changed and what plan should be followed. Change is effected by identifying events in the client's life that have been critical stimuli for the behavior and then arranging interventions for *extinguishing* those behaviors. A changed way of acting precedes a changed way of thinking, according to behaviorist theory.

Both Joseph Wolpe (1956) and B. F. Skinner (1953, 1971) are associated with psychiatric treatment approaches that represent one form of **conditioning** and reflect the above assumptions. Wolpe defined *neurotic behavior* as unadaptive behavior acquired in anxiety-generating situations. He based his therapeutic method on the introduction of a response that inhibits anxiety when situations occur that ordinarily evoke anxiety. Relaxation, for example, was considered incompatible with anxiety and, therefore, effective in inhibiting it. Thus, Wolpe would direct his intervention to a counter-conditioning technique, usually putting the client under hypnosis and using various techniques for gradual **desensitization.** For example, a man afraid of dying might gradually attempt to overcome his anxiety at seeing a coffin, attending a funeral, and so on, by trying to relax in these situations.

Skinner's approach, called **operant conditioning**, emphasizes discovering why the behavioral response was elicited in the first place and what actively reinforces it. The key concept in operant conditioning is reinforcement. Skinner originally used the term **positive reinforcement** to describe an event that increases the probability that the response will recur—a reward for behavior. A **negative reinforcement** was defined as an event likely to decrease the possibility of recurrence because it penalizes the behavior.

Other contemporary behaviorists have redefined Skinner's original terms and introduced some new ones. Positive reinforcement is still an environmental event that rewards and thus increases the probability of a behavioral response. Negative reinforcement can mean removal of an adverse stimulus (such as an electric shock to animals or the restriction of people's privileges) to increase the likelihood of a behavior's recurrence. *Positive punishment,* in contrast, is the introduction of aversive stimuli to decrease the likelihood of the recurrence of a behavior. *Negative punishment* removes something that has been a prior reinforcer, thus again decreasing the likelihood of such behaviors as smoking, drug abuse, truancy, temper outbursts, and abuse. Table 2–3 lists examples of each of these behaviorist concepts.

The term for an intervention designed to change a client's behavior is **shaping.** It is a procedure of manipulating reinforcement to bring the person closer to the desired behavior. There are, according to Skinner, times in a client's life when responses are accidentally reinforced by

Table 2–3 Examples of Behaviorist Concepts

Concept	*Purpose*	*Example*
Positive reinforcer	Increase recurrence of the behavior through reward	Leave of absence from the hospital, per contract with the client
Negative reinforcer	Increase recurrence of the behavior by removing aversive consequences	Removal of restrictions on phone calls or visitors, per contract with client
Positive punishment	Decrease the behavior by adding aversive consequences	Quiet time
Negative punishment	Decrease the behavior by withdrawing a reinforcer or reward	Withdrawal of privileges, such as recreational outings in a residential milieu

a coincidental pairing of response and reinforcement. This accidental pairing may play a role in the development of phobias (irrational fears) and other distressing and/or dysfunctional behaviors.

Implications for Psychiatric Nursing Practice Most psychiatric nurses acknowledge that the application of principles of behavior modification to clients is quite complex. The use of this approach raises issues of control, responsibility for behavior, and the morality of using negative or punitive stimuli in a therapeutic context, to name only a few. Therapists who successfully resolve such basic philosophic issues have designed and implemented successful behavior-modification plans with disturbed, overtly aggressive children, developmentally disabled clients, and violently self-destructive people.

In many institutional environments, clients follow prescribed schedules for daily living that include a **token economy.** Clients are rewarded for desired behavior by token reinforcers, such as food, candy, and verbal approval. The movement toward community-based psychiatric treatment has made plain some of the shortcomings and economic realities of therapies aimed toward resolving everyone's intrapsychic conflicts. The movement has instead attempted to replace maladaptive behavior with behavior that allows people to function effectively within their natural environment. When parents or others in the client's environment are taught to implement the behavior change procedures, therapy moves away from the artificial situation of the therapist's office into the client's total environment. It no longer requires the presence of highly trained, often expensive experts and thus makes treatment more affordable.

Psychiatric nurses have had a special role in teaching behaviorist principles to people with little training so that they can act as change agents. Nonprofessional staff on psychiatric wards can be taught the effective use of behaviorist principles to eliminate chronic, maladaptive behavior. Hyperactive children or children with borderline intelligence can be treated in the home by their parents when nurses teach the parents to use approaches such as frequency counts on specific behaviors to be modified, time-outs (short periods of isolation) for undesired behavior, and the bestowal of attention, praise, and affectionate physical contact as rewards.

Social-Interpersonal Theories

Social-interpersonal theories of psychiatry grew out of a general dissatisfaction with approaches that account for mental illness in terms of either intrapersonal mechanisms (the symptoms of a disease) or individual personality dynamics such as anxiety, ego strength, and libido. Advocates of this perspective assert that other theories neglect the crucial social processes and cultural variation involved in the development, identification, and resolution of disturbed human responses.

Assumptions and Key Ideas Three separate but philosophically congruent schools of thought contribute to social-interpersonal theories. These are the labeling theory, the interpersonal-psychiatric, and the general systems approaches. The assumptions and key ideas of each are discussed below.

The Labeling Theory School The labeling theory approach is summarized partially by sociologist Kai Erikson (1962): "Deviance is not a property inherent in certain forms of behavior; it is a property conferred upon these forms by audiences which directly or indirectly witness them." Thus, mental illness is a *label* applied to certain behaviors that violate the rules of conduct imposed by others.

The Interpersonal-Psychiatric School Psychiatrists Adolf Meyer (1948–1952) and Harry Stack Sullivan (1953) made significant contributions to social-interpersonal theory in the first half of the twentieth century. Sullivan trained with William Alanson White and Adolf Meyer rather than Freud. He is viewed as the least reductionist of psychiatric theorists and emphasizes modes of interaction as the real focus of psychiatric inquiry. Sullivan became the theoretic and ideologic leader of the interpersonal school of psychiatry often associated with the William Alanson White Foundation.

One concept that plays a crucial role in the organization of behavior, according to Sullivan, is the **self-system** or *self-dynamism*. The self-system provides tools that enable people to deal with the tasks of avoiding anxiety and establishing security. The self is a construct built from the child's experience. It is made up of **reflected appraisals** the person learns in contact with significant others. The self develops in the process of seeking physical satisfaction of bodily needs and security. To feel secure, the self essentially requires feelings of approval and prestige as protection against anxiety. Rewarding appraisals from others yield what Sullivan calls the *good-me* aspect of the self. Anxiety-producing appraisals result in the *bad-me*. The *not-me* exists normally in dreams and in aspects of experience that are poorly understood and later experienced as dread, horror, and loathing among mentally disordered people. In summary, Sullivan emphasizes the pervasive interaction between the organism and the environment.

Sullivan emphasizes effects of culture on the development and functioning of the personality (Table 2–4). Nonetheless, Sullivan has little to say about the impact on behavior of specific variations in the social or cultural scene. Like Sullivan, other advocates of the interpersonal school of psychiatry, such as Karen Horney (1950) and Erich Fromm (1941), stress the general climate in the immediate family. Alfred Adler (1971), however, attempts to understand more of the social and cultural conditions influencing behavior. The interpersonal school of psychiatry in general focuses less on social context than the labeling theory perspective and takes a developmental-interpersonal view of the self. The **self-actualization** and hierarchy of needs theories of Abraham Maslow (1962) belong squarely in this school (Figure 2–3).

The General Systems School **General systems theory**, when applied to living systems (people), provides a conceptual framework for integrating the biologic and social sciences with the physical sciences. In psychiatry, it offers a resolution of the mind-body dichotomy, an integration of biologic and social approaches to the nature of human beings, and an approach to psychopathology, diagnosis, and therapy. Karl Menninger (1963) views normal personality functioning and psychopathology in terms of general systems theory. His work addresses four major issues:

1. Adjustment or individual-environment interaction.
2. The organization of living systems.
3. Psychologic regulation and control, known as *ego theory* in psychoanalysis.
4. Motivation, which is often called *instinct* or *drive* in the psychoanalytic framework.

A salient point of Menninger's theory is the idea of **homeostasis** (equilibrium). He asserts that the greater the threat or stress on a system, the greater the number of system components involved in coping with or adapting to it. Therefore, pathology can exist at various levels, from the cell and organ level to the group and community level. An example of the former might be the behavioral changes that follow cellular alterations due to addictive drugs, to a blood clot, or to a tumor. Examples of pathology at the group level include family violence. At the community level, overpopulation, pollution, homelessness, and poverty are instances of pathology. In general

Table 2–4 Sullivan's Stages of Interpersonal Development

Age	*Stage*	*Task/Key Concept*
Birth–18 months (to appearance of speech)	Infancy	Experiences anxiety in interaction with mother figure; learns to use maternal tenderness to gain security and avoid anxiety
18 months–6 years (from first speech to need for playmates)	Childhood	Learns to delay gratification in response to interpersonal demands; uses language and action to avoid anxiety
6–9 years	Juvenile	Develops peer relationships and uses environment outside the family to shape self
9–12 years	Preadolescence	Develops a caring relationship with same-sex peer, chum relationship
12–14 years	Early adolescence	Develops interest in opposite-sex relationships
14–21 years	Late adolescence	Has satisfying relationships; directs sexual impulses
21 years +	Adulthood	Establishes a love relationship

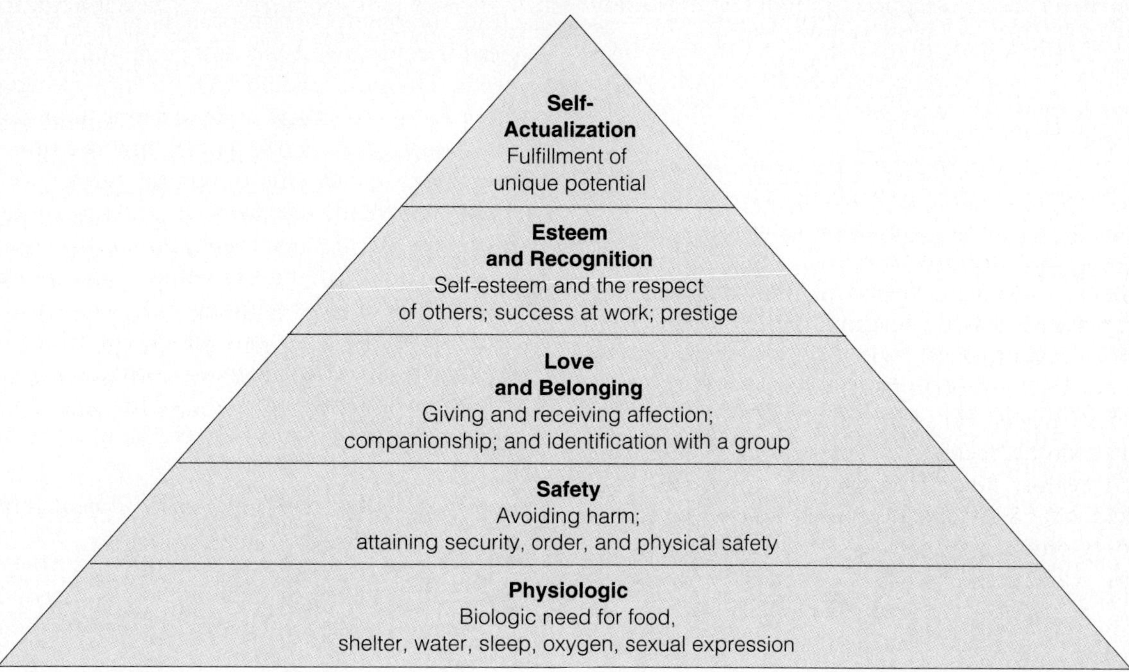

Figure 2–3 Maslow's hierarchy of needs.

systems theory, all represent abnormalities or stresses on matter-energy processes and would be included within the domain of psychiatric professionals.

In Menninger's view, a system's well-being depends on the amount of stress on it and the effectiveness of its coping mechanisms. He asserts that "mental illness" is an impairment of self-regulation in which comfort, growth, and production are surrendered for the sake of survival at the best level possible but at the sacrifice of emergency coping devices. Therapists using the general systems approach emphasize current conflicts, restoration of impaired systems of functioning, and subsequent reintegration of the restored function into future coping strategies.

Implications for Psychiatric Nursing Practice Social-interpersonal theories give independent and collaborative psychiatric nursing clear theoretic direction and support. Nursing roles are associated with shifts in the delivery of psychiatric services variously termed *case management, social psychiatry, community psychiatry, psychoeducation,* and *milieu therapy.* All are associated with efforts to provide psychiatric services more efficiently to large groups of people, particularly those previously neglected, and attempts to counteract the debilitating effects of long-term institutionalization. All are also associated with a movement to address the client's social context in providing psychiatric care. According to these orientations, all social, psychologic, and biologic activity, including research developments in psychobiology, affecting the mental health of the population is important to professionals in community psychiatry. Therapeutic interventions may include programs for social change, political involvement, community organization, social planning, family support groups, and education about medications, symptom management, and family environment. Many implications for practice can be derived from this theoretic model:

- Clients are approached in a holistic way, reflecting the interrelationship and interaction between the biophysical, psychologic, and socioeconomic-cultural dimensions of human life. This increases the number of factors the nurse must assess when caring for a client.
- Because of the increased number and diversity of variables to be considered, graduate and undergraduate content in psychiatric nursing education must be revised. Curricula must include concepts, theories, and research findings to support extended thinking about mental health, culture, social systems, ethnicity, deviant behavior, social support, psychobiology, and the human condition. These new content areas drawn from the social and natural sciences must then be integrated with conventional psychiatric nursing content to form an internal coherent knowledge base.
- Definitions of the client must include the concept of the client system. A family, a couple, an aggregate, or even a community may collectively constitute the client.
- Intervention strategies include **primary prevention** achieved through psychoeducation, social change, and research.

- Therapy focuses on helping troubled people gain a useful perspective on their lifestyle and social environment and develop coping skills and resources, rather than on exclusively repressing and controlling their symptoms.
- The psychiatric nurse must be prepared to function as an autonomous member of the mental health team and to assume more responsibilities. There is a shift away from the dominance of the physician in decision making and toward diffusion of roles. Practitioners' roles are based less on background discipline than on availability and interest in helping the client. For example, a cadre of mental health professionals who could become chronic care experts is sorely needed, particularly those who can synthesize psychobiologic knowledge with psychosocial rehabilitation skills and psychoeducation.

Once clients are viewed as becoming dysfunctional in the context of unhealthy or problem-filled interpersonal relationships, establishing healthy, constructive interpersonal relationships becomes important in their care. Psychiatric nurses can apply concepts of milieu therapy, primary prevention, social psychiatry, community psychiatry, and psychobiologic interventions to implement this fundamental idea. The following case example is an illustration:

Mrs. S is a 67-year-old, upper-middle-class woman in good physical health. She has become increasingly untidy, forgetful, reclusive, sad, and suspicious since the death of her aggressive, bank president husband from a heart attack six months ago. She recently sold the large house where she had lived for the past 45 years and moved into a two-bedroom apartment in a nearby town. Because of apartment rules, she was unable to take her 12-year-old cat. She sold the house because her husband had told his lawyers that she should do so. (He had made all the family decisions while he lived.) Mrs. S has taken to skipping meals except for candy bars because she must rely on a friend to drive her to the grocery store. (Her husband never felt she needed to learn to drive.) Her younger sister (age 59), seeking advice about Mrs. S's behavior, phoned the community mental health center on the suggestion of the family physician.

The social-interpersonal psychiatric nurse assessing this situation would tend not to view Mrs. S's symptoms as psychologic conflicts reflecting her ambivalence toward her dead husband or as manifestations of a mental disorder, such as major, single-episode depression. Instead, the nurse would focus on the way Mrs. S is functioning in her current interpersonal situation and her holistic human responses to it. In this analysis, the nurse does not view Mrs. S as "diseased" and therefore in exclusive need of a somatic treatment such as medication. Instead, treatment consists of helping Mrs. S develop strategies for coping with her new situation and satisfying her needs. The nurse would seek out the younger sister and other family members in an attempt to enhance Mrs. S's social support network. Efforts may be directed toward mobilizing other environmental forces (including the nurse) to provide company, stimulation, and proper nutrition for Mrs. S, since the absence of all three contributes to her symptoms and discomfort. The clinical situation would undoubtedly reinforce the psychiatric nurse's political efforts to point out the potential consequences of lifelong passive dependence of some adult women. The nurse may also become involved in community organizations working for better services for older clients.

An Overview of Psychiatric Nursing Theories

The concept of nursing as primarily technologic has been replaced by the idea that nursing is theory-based. Still, nursing remains more divergent than convergent when it comes to identifying the theories to be applied. Most authorities concur that *theoretic pluralism*—the simultaneous refinement and testing of numerous contenders for nursing's dominant theory—is highly appropriate for the present phase in nursing's scientific and intellectual history. Let's briefly examine a few of the best-known theorists and identify the concepts and principles most relevant to psychiatric nursing. Most of these theorists accept the focal concepts for nursing as *people, nursing, health,* and *society.*

In the early 1950s, Lydia Hall, Virginia Henderson, and Hildegard Peplau had already published precursors to contemporary nursing theories, and Faye Abdellah had begun observations that led to the formulation of her theory by 1955.

Table 2–5 presents a comparison of the traditional theories upon which psychiatric nurses base their plans of care.

HALL Lydia Hall's (1959) theory is best represented by three interlocking circles depicting what she called the "aspects of nursing." Hall's three aspects of nursing were the person (the core), the disease (the cure), and the body (the care). She developed her theory at the Loeb Center for Rehabilitation primarily for the adult client recuperating from a physical illness in a residential treatment center. She showed relationships among the three concepts by varying the size of the three circles to represent the amount or proportion of nursing time focused on each. Most psychiatric nursing practice would focus on the core component of her theory.

HENDERSON Virginia Henderson (1966) contributed the now-famous definition of nursing:

Table 2–5 Major Features of Traditional Psychiatric Theories Compared

Theory	*Assessment Base*	*Problem Statement*	*Goal*	*Dominant Interventions*
Medical-biologic	Individual client symptoms	Disease	Symptom management; cure	Psychopharmacology and other biologic therapies
Psychoanalytic	Intrapsychic; unconscious	Conflict	Insight	Psychoanalysis
Behaviorist	Behavior	Learning deficit	Behavior change	Behavior modification or conditioning
Social-interpersonal	Interactions between individual and social contexts	Interpersonal dysfunction	Enhanced awareness and quality of interpersonal interactions	Group, family, and milieu therapies

> Nursing is primarily assisting the individual (sick or well) in the performance of those activities contributing to health or its recovery (or a peaceful death) that he would perform unaided if he had the necessary strength, will, or knowledge.

Henderson identified fourteen activities to be addressed in basic nursing care. Nurses, she proposed, either help the client with the activities or provide conditions under which the client can perform them unaided. The first nine activities encompass a version of basic physiologic human needs. The remaining five include needs for communication, spirituality, work, play, and learning—the categories that are emphasized by psychiatric nurses.

PEPLAU Hildegard Peplau published her nursing theory in the classic book *Interpersonal Relations in Nursing* (1952). She defined nursing as a significant therapeutic interpersonal process, and the core concepts of her theory were the four phases of the nurse-client relationship:

1. Orientation
2. Identification
3. Exploitation (or working)
4. Resolution

Some say that these phases are ancestors of the phases of the nursing process. Psychiatric nurses continue to use Peplau's theory to understand and guide decisions in the one-to-one therapeutic relationship.

ABDELLAH Faye Abdellah (1960) presented a list of twenty-one nursing problems that she developed over a five-year period during the late 1950s. The list includes physiologic as well as psychosocial needs and resembles both Henderson's fourteen nursing care components and Maslow's hierarchy of needs.

OREM Dorothea Orem's (1971) theory of self-care was originally introduced around 1959 and identified ten universal self-care requisites, divided into six categories that encompass both physical and psychosocial human needs. Orem also introduced a second order of concepts originally called health deviation self-care demands to refer to care required in the event of illness, injury, or disease. Nursing, a second key component of her scheme, was divided into compensatory, partially compensatory, and supportive-educational systems of care that could be matched to the client's assessed level of self-care functioning in each area. This theory firmly established the notion of a goal of self-care as integral to the discipline of nursing's perspective on the meaning of health. Orem's theory is particularly well adapted to meeting nursing care needs of the severely and chronically mentally ill.

ROGERS Martha Rogers (1970) drew on knowledge from anthropology, sociology, religion, philosophy, mythology, and general systems theory to define nursing as a holistic science of human nature and development. Rogers's key nursing principles, called the principles of homeodynamics, view human beings holistically. Changes in life processes are irreversible, nonrepeatable, and rhythmic and indicate patterns of increasing complexity and organization. Most of her concepts have counterparts in general systems theory, but she has added the notions of life processes, change, and human-environmental interaction to the concepts central to nursing. Rogers's work gives psychiatric nurses a mandate to use holistic principles as a guide to practice and to consider physical as well as psychosocial problems and needs.

ROY Sister Callista Roy's (1976) adaptation theory views people as constantly faced with the need to adapt to focal, contextual, and residual stimuli. She identifies four modes of human adapting: *physiologic needs, self-concept, role function,* and *interdependence*. Obviously, these adaptive modes again include physiologic, psychologic, and social aspects of people. The notion of coping or adapting to stimuli again relates nursing to people in interaction with their environment. Self-concept, role function, and interdependent areas of coping all lend themselves to the conceptualization of the practice of psychiatric nursing.

OTHERS The theories presented here in no way represent all the theories about nursing practice. Ida Jean Orlando (1961) stresses the interaction of meanings between nurse and client. Ernestine Wiedenbach's (1964) work presents an example of a "situation-producing" theory that conceptualizes a goal and a nursing prescription for fulfilling the goal. Myra Levine (1967) uses four conservation principles to conceptualize nursing interventions: *conservation of energy, conservation of structural integrity, conservation of personal integrity,* and *conservation of social integrity.* Imogene King (1971) discusses concepts of social systems, perceptions, interpersonal relations, and health and their impact on people.

A review of these theories indicates some clear differences in emphasis and perspective and some intriguing similarities. From these theories the parameters of our discipline emerge. Such parameters provide the beginnings for directing practice, focusing nursing research, and providing a framework of concepts integral to the teaching of professional students. For additional information on nursing theories, see A. I. Meleis's authoritative book, *Theoretical Nursing* (1991).

Choosing a Theory for Practice

Psychiatric nurses use one or a combination of theoretic frameworks to guide the application of the nursing process to their practice. In this text, we use the humanistic interactional approach in combination with new knowledge in psychobiology. As mentioned earlier, this approach synthesizes strengths derived primarily from social-interpersonal and biologic theories and allows for the evolution of nursing theories as our body of knowledge grows. In clinical work, however, the selection of a theoretic framework may be influenced by various factors. Among them are the nurse's education, the philosophy of the setting in which clients are treated, the nature of the client's present problem, the available treatment, the need to be efficient and practical, and even client attributes such as social class and gender.

The failure to effect a "cure" according to the principles of any one theory may induce clinicians to recast the problem in different theoretic terms, adopting different treatment options. For example, a psychotic client who does not respond to medication may respond to a well-planned behavior-modification program. Approaches associated with two or more different theories are often used in combination. For example, bizarre, self-destructive behavior may be controlled with medications so that the client is more available for group or individual therapy. Such a combined or eclectic approach demands that a clinician be capable of functioning according to all theories of care, depending on which is best for the client and best fits the resources and limitations of the situation. If nurses give adequate consideration to the theoretic framework of their psychiatric nursing, they will foster practice-oriented research and clinical judgments that can be articulated and taught to others. Research is a tool for developing psychiatric nursing theory that synthesizes the most useful elements of these theories.

Chapter Highlights

- A philosophy that integrates humanism, interactionism, and the knowledge explosion in psychobiology provides a holistic perspective for psychiatric nursing.
- The choice of a theory for psychiatric nursing care determines information assessed, goals and interventions recommended, and evaluation criteria set.
- Theories traditionally include the medical-biologic, the psychoanalytic, the behaviorist, the social-interpersonal, and various nursing theories.
- In medical-biologic theory, emotional and behavioral disturbances are viewed as diseases.
- Psychoanalytic theory developed by Freud holds that all psychologic events have meaning and are understandable.
- Psychoanalytic theory states that much of what goes on in people's minds is unknown to them, or unconscious, and accounts for apparent discontinuities in their lives that are due to unresolved conflicts in stages of psychosexual development.
- In behaviorist theory, the self and mental symptoms are viewed as learned behaviors that persist because they are rewarding to the individual.
- In behaviorist theory, the nurse's role is expanded to planner, counselor, and educator, but therapeutic goals are limited to symptom control through behavior-modification techniques that raise ethical issues.
- In social-interpersonal theories, treatment occurs within an interpersonal context; mental illness is a label applied to certain behaviors by others; the clinician views deviant behavior in its broader context and uses a general systems approach to integrate biologic and sociocultural data.

- In the social-interpersonal framework, treatment is likely to include helping clients develop strategies for coping, mobilizing social support networks, and involving the therapist in community organization and planning.
- The psychiatric nurse's role in the social-interpersonal framework is expanded to include social and political action and community intervention as well as direct intervention with individuals, families, and groups.
- Concepts serving as the focus for contemporary nursing theories are people, nursing, health, and society.
- Research that develops nursing theory by focusing on the effectiveness of therapeutic approaches on client outcomes can synthesize the most useful ideas from all the dominant theoretic frameworks for psychiatric care.

References

Abdellah FG, et al.: *Patient-Centered Approaches to Nursing.* Macmillan, 1960.

Adler A: *The Practice and Theory of Individual Psychology.* Translated by P. Radin, 1929; reprinted, Humanities Press, 1971.

American Psychiatric Association: *Diagnostic and Statistical Manual of Mental Disorders,* ed 4. APA, 1994.

Blumer H: *Symbolic Interaction: Perspective and Method.* Prentice-Hall, 1969.

Erikson E: *Childhood and Society,* ed 2. Norton, 1963.

Erikson K: Notes on the sociology of deviance. *Soc Prob* 1962;9:308.

Freud S: *The Ego and the Id.* Norton, 1962a.

Freud S: *The Standard Edition of the Complete Psychological Works of Sigmund Freud.* Hogarth Press, 1962b, 24 vols.

Fromm E: *Escape from Freedom.* Irvington Publishers, 1941.

Hall L: *Nursing—What Is It?* Publication of the Virginia State Nurses' Association, Winter 1959.

Henderson V: *The Nature of Nursing.* Macmillan, 1966.

Horney K: *Neurosis and Human Growth.* Norton, 1950.

King IM: *Toward a Theory of Nursing: General Concepts of Human Behavior.* Wiley, 1971.

Lamont C: *The Philosophy of Humanism.* New York: Frederick Ungar Publishing, 1967.

Levine ME: The four conservation principles of nursing. *Nurs Forum* 1967;6:45–59.

Loomis M., et al.: PND-I: A classification of phenomena of concern for psychiatric-mental health nursing. *Arch Psychiatr Nurs* 1987;1(1):16–24.

Maslow A: *Toward a Psychology of Being.* Van Nostrand, 1962.

Meleis AI: *Theoretical Nursing.* Lippincott, 1991.

Menninger K: *The Vital Balance.* Viking Press, 1963.

Orem DE: *Nursing: Concepts of Practice.* McGraw-Hill, 1971.

Orlando IJ: *The Dynamic Nurse-Patient Relationship: Function, Process and Principles.* Putnam, 1961.

Peplau HE: *Interpersonal Relations in Nursing.* Putnam, 1952.

Rogers ME: *The Theoretical Basis of Nursing.* FA Davis, 1970.

Roy C: *Introduction to Nursing: An Adaptation Model.* Prentice-Hall, 1976.

Scheff T: *Being Mentally Ill: A Sociological Theory.* Aldine, 1966.

Skinner BF: *Beyond Freedom and Dignity.* Knopf, 1971.

Skinner BF: *Science and Human Behavior.* Macmillan, 1953.

Stevens BJ: *Nursing Theory,* ed 2. Little, Brown, 1984.

Sullivan HS: *The Interpersonal Theory of Psychiatry,* Perry HS, Gawel ML (eds). Norton, 1953.

Wiedenbach E: *Clinical Nursing, A Helping Art.* Springer, 1964.

Wolpe J: Learning versus lesions as the basis of neurotic behavior. *Am J Psychiatry* 1956;112:923–931.

CHAPTER 3

PSYCHOBIOLOGY

Susan Simmons-Alling

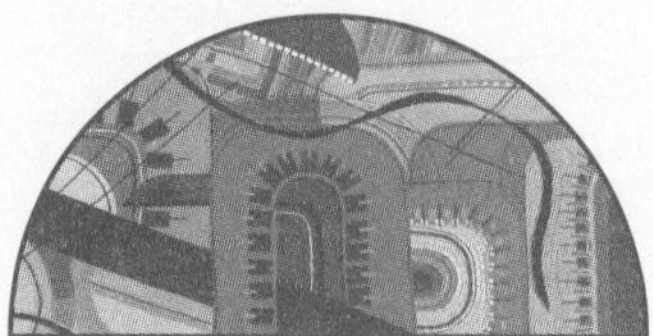

COMPETENCIES

- *Identify the functions of the neuroanatomical structures involved in psychiatric illnesses.*
- *Correlate the alterations of neuromessengers with the development of psychiatric disorders.*
- *Relate how genetic variables influence the development and progression of psychiatric disorders.*
- *Discuss the communication between the endocrine and immune systems.*
- *Critique how psychobiology promotes advocacy and critical thinking.*
- *Describe how communication in your practice is a psychobiologic process.*

Cross-References

Other topics relevant to this content are: Stress, anxiety, and coping, Chapter 4; Advocacy, Chapter 11; Delirium/Dementia, Chapter 12; Schizophrenia, Chapter 14; Mood disorders, Chapter 15; Anxiety disorders, Chapter 16; Sleep, Chapter 19; Psychophysiologic conditions, Chapter 22; Stress management, Chapter 29; Psychopharmacology, Chapter 33.

Critical Thinking Challenge

Psychiatric clinicians are expected to provide rapid assessment and interventions that move the client quickly through the system due to constraints on resources and costs. Standardized care plans based on a template of outcome criteria tend to focus interventions under these conditions. Individualized assessments of clients' needs are pared to the minimum, and interventions are becoming increasingly biologic (medication). However, if major psychiatric illnesses are brain diseases that affect behavior, cognition, learning, and emotion, can you expect to improve function without considering each client's unique biologic, environmental, and psychosocial strengths and weaknesses? Does the psychobiologic necessarily exclude the humanistic, individualized approach in psychiatric nursing? Can you integrate the psychologic, interpersonal, cultural, and spiritual considerations when you address the psychobiology of mental disorders?

Psychobiology is neither a new concept nor a recent discovery. It has existed since the birth of humankind and has been a subject of discussion for at least the last 2000 years. What *is* new in psychobiology is a broader understanding of the biologic basis of the mind and behavior. Current knowledge about the biologic components of behavior is revolutionizing not only psychiatry but also our view of behavior, temperament, and psychiatric disorders and their treatment.

A comprehensive definition of psychobiology is diffi-

The author wishes to acknowledge Geoffry McEnany for his scholarship and vision in the previous editions of this chapter.

cult at best. Psychobiology encompasses an enormous body of information that is growing almost exponentially. For this reason, the conceptual "face" of psychobiology is changing. With these thoughts in mind, we can offer the following definition: **Psychobiology** is the study of the biochemical foundations, molecular and genetic, of cognition, mood, emotion, affect, and behavior and the interactions among them. It takes into consideration both internal and external influences across a person's life span, including genetics, the effects of other body systems such as the endocrine and immune systems, temperament, and the environment.

In this chapter, we strive to give you an overview of psychobiology and make the psychobiologic principles fit with those of nursing. It is impossible in one chapter to even touch upon all of the facets of psychobiology in any detail; this chapter is an attempt to motivate you to apply psychobiologic principles in your professional work.

Nursing's standards (ANA 1994) urge the inclusion of biologic therapies along with the use of the more traditional psychotherapy, psychosocial therapies, and combination therapies (Krauss 1993). The shift to a system of community-based mental health care is being emphasized in health care reform. However, the setting will not be the essential consideration; it will be the needs of the client at any given time in the health care continuum.

A major barrier that inhibits clients and families from seeking care is stigma. Stigma results from the lack of knowledge and misunderstanding of the etiology of severe mental illness. Bad parenting and lack of character can no longer be blamed as contributors to mental illness. Understanding the working hypotheses of psychobiology is a social imperative for removing the guilt and stigma associated with psychiatric disorders. "Quick fixes" are not applicable to chronic illnesses or unbalanced states of emotion.

Your attitude about the underlying neurobiology of behavior can influence therapeutic outcomes. It follows that if you view biologic or somatic therapies ambivalently, you will communicate your attitude to the client and family. If your approach is dualistic—mind versus brain, or nature versus nurture—then your ability to deliver individualized psychoeducation positively and be an advocate will be limited.

Contemporary psychiatric nursing uses both the neurobiologic and the psychosocial and behavioral therapies. Because the 1990s have been recognized by Congress and the National Institute of Mental Health as the "Decade of the Brain," outcomes of studies conducted in this era will provide new strategies for assessments and interventions with clients who experience emotional and behavioral problems. Psychiatry has shifted to include the neurobiologic domains; nursing must also shift and integrate psychobiologic concepts with our traditional practice to provide holistic caring for both clients and their families.

A New Era of Communication

Communication has been a basis for psychiatric nursing ever since the role began. All behavior is communication, and all communication affects behavior (Watzlavick, Beavin, Jackson, 1967). Through neurobiologic discoveries, communication now has a molecular, anatomical, and chemical basis. Who we are originates from order or disorder at the molecular level. The common unit at all levels is communication (Restak 1994).

The brain encodes or decodes information through complex interactions of neuromessengers, chemical processes, and anatomic systems. When clients say that health care providers told them their symptoms were "a nervous breakdown" or "all in their head," you can reframe those communications and put the message in context with current neurobiologic knowledge. For example, panic attacks are real; they result from the triggering of an overreactive alarm center in the brain, which sends a message of fear via the release of a neurotransmitter, causing a racing heart and shortness of breath.

To help integrate psychobiologic principles into your clinical practice, we will focus on the brain (structure) and the substances and processes (function) that play key roles in behavior and emotional communication.

Brain, Mind, and Behavior

Neuroanatomy: An Overview

Volumes have been written about the anatomy of the brain and the other components of the nervous system. This overview will focus on the structures relevant to communication processes in contemporary psychiatric nursing practice. For clarification, you may assume the brain and mind are not separate, and that the "mind is what the brain does" (Restak 1994). We will focus on the structures of the brain believed to be involved in the formation of cognition, behavior, and emotion. We'll begin with neuroanatomy, move on to genetics, and then explore physiology.

The brain is defined in various ways. The definition that best suits the perspective of this chapter is that the brain is that part of the central nervous system (brain and spinal cord) encapsulated by the skull. The brain is the core of our humanity. Intercommunications among different parts of the brain yield the experiences of love, hate, joy, and sadness. The brain provides the underlying biology for will, determination, hopes, and dreams.

THE CEREBRUM The **cerebrum** comprises the largest part of the human brain. It is divided into two seemingly equal components, the *cerebral hemispheres*. The deep furrow that divides the hemispheres is known as the *longitudinal* *sulcus*. A small but important piece of tissue, the *corpus callosum,* connects the two hemispheres medially and allows communication between them. In the past, scientists believed that each hemisphere had separate functions, such as logic or creativity and spatial accommodation. With the advent of new technologies such as positron emission tomography (PET), it is now possible to assess metabolic activity in the brain as it occurs (see the accompanying box). Scientists are able to observe brain activity and have come to realize that creative as well as logical activities require input from both cerebral hemispheres.

The brain in general, and the cerebral hemispheres in particular, are well protected not only by the skull but also by a protective fluid, called cerebrospinal fluid (CSF),

Tools of Psychobiology

Brain Imaging

- *Computed tomography (CT).* An X-ray beam (radiation exposure) is passed through serial sections of the brain to look at structural images.
- *Magnetic resonance imaging (MRI).* Reconstructs detailed images of cerebral anatomy from multiple perspectives, including subcortical structures, using radiofrequency signals emitted by relaxing hydrogen atoms. It delineates gray and white matter. New instruments image elements other than hydrogen, allowing MRI to be used for structural, functional, and metabolic imaging. Contraindication for clients with any metal objects in their bodies such as pacemakers, due to the presence of a magnetic field.
- *Positron emission tomography (PET).* Imaging of active neurochemical substrates and physiologic processes; regional localization of metabolic functions through the measurement of radioactive labels or tags attached to molecules as glucose; density of neuroreceptors; regional cerebral blood flow (rCBF) of the brain. Operates on the principle that blood rushes to the busiest area of the brain to deliver oxygen and nutrients to the active neurons.
- *Single photon emission computed tomography (SPECT).* Measures rCBF; visualizes and measures the density of neuroreceptors, using tracer isotopes such as xenon, a gas; iodine 123; or technetium.

Neurophysiologic Techniques

- *Electroencephalogram (EEG).* Measures electrical activity patterns of the brain from leads connected to surface electrodes placed on the scalp and nasopharyngeal area.
- *Polysomnography (sleep EEG).* Measures electrical brain activity data during all-night sleep.
- *Brain electroactivity mapping (BEAM).* Extends the EEG by generating computerized maps of brain electrical activity to produce images; permits visualization of the brain performing tasks or specific functions. Useful with children.
- *Event related potential (EPs).* Repeated auditory or visual stimuli associated with tiny electrical events in the cerebral cortex or subcortical structures, measured by surface electrodes.

Pharmacologic Challenge

The use of a drug (challenge) to provoke a neuronal system for better understanding of its physiologic effects and changes. Examples are the Dexamethasone suppression test (DST), thyrotropin-releasing hormone (TRH) challenge, or giving a drug known to have specific receptor affinity such as clonidine to examine the alpha2 adrenergic system in panic disorder.

Molecular Genetics

- *Linkage map.* A genetic map that represents the relationship between two genes, often revealed by the inheritance of traits in families, to determine the relative position of genes on a given chromosome.
- *Restriction fragment length polymorphisms (RFLPs).* Method of molecular genetics using restriction enzymes, which cuts a DNA strand at sites where the enzyme recognizes a sequence between coding information. Differences in the lengths of these restriction fragments are believed to be inherited. The transmission can be mapped within families and a genetic pattern of transmission identified.
- *Candidate genes.* Identification of a specific gene thought to have pathophysiologic relevance to the illness being studied.

that circulates around and within the brain. Deep within the brain are three spaces, or *ventricles,* that aid in the circulation of CSF. CSF volume is about 125 mL in the normal adult and is replaced approximately four times in 24 hours. The CSF reflects neurochemical activity of the brain and is one method for studying in vivo (within the living organism) communications. The purpose of a spinal tap is to measure the volume and pressure of the CSF; to look for trauma, blood, or infection; and to measure **metabolites**, the products or substances produced from the breakdown of metabolic processes of the brain's neuromessengers.

The cerebral hemispheres are divided into four lobes, named after the parts of the skull under which they lie: frontal, parietal, temporal, and occipital (see the accompanying box and Figure 3–1). All of the lobes contain many *gyri* (ridges), *fissures,* and *sulci* (grooves) that maximize the surface area of the brain.

The cerebral hemispheres consist of both white and gray matter. Gray matter consists of fibers that are referred to as *nerves;* bundles of nerves are called *tracts*. The cerebral cortex consists solely of gray matter with underlying white matter. The cerebral cortex works much like the processing unit of a computer. The cortex is the part of the brain that makes sense out of the volumes of input. It processes and synthesizes information, thought, reasoning, will, and choice and is the seat of dreams.

As essential as the cerebral hemispheres are to emotional, intellectual, and biologic functioning, they must interact with other components of the brain. For example, people need input from and clear communication between different brain structures to produce efficient and purposeful behavior. The **limbic system**, often referred to as "the emotional brain," is believed to be responsible for the experience and expression of emotion, as well as memory and some aspects of attention. The limbic system consists of structures from the cerebral hemispheres and the *diencephalon,* a part of the brain located between the cerebrum and midbrain (Figure 3–2).

Two limbic structures play an especially important role in the enactment of emotion: the amygdala and the hippocampus. The **amygdala** gauges certain emotional reactions and plays a role in social behavior. It serves as the behavioral awareness center and helps pattern appropriate behavioral responses. With the hippocampus, the amygdala generates emotions from perceptions and thoughts, and plays a role in the sense of smell. Does the smell of baking cookies trigger a pleasant childhood memory of being in your grandmother's kitchen when she baked cookies for you? This is the combined effect of amygdala and hippocampal functions. The **hippocampus** is also involved in emotional reactions and in learning, by helping to process, store, and retrieve information in memory. It provides new information for permanent storage. Weak stimuli in this area can cause epileptic seizures. Hallucinations may in part originate from hyperexcitability of psychomotor effects of olfactory, visual, auditory, and tactile stimulation in this region.

The functions of the limbic system are not discrete, and the neuronal connections are so widespread and intricate within the brain that their complex interactions involve many different areas. Other neuronal groups that participate with the limbic system are the thalamus, hypothalamus, and the pituitary gland.

Gross Functions of the Cerebral Lobes

Frontal Lobes

- Responsible for movement; the right frontal lobe controls the left side of the body's movements, and vice versa.
- Contain the premotor cortex, which organizes complicated movement.
- Contain prefrontal fibers with capacities for the ability to plan and problem-solve; also responsible for social judgment, volition, attention, learning, spontaneity, thinking, and affect.

Parietal Lobes

- Contain the sensory cortex, which interprets contact sensations such as touch and pressure.
- Facilitates spatial orientation.

Temporal Lobes

- Involved in hearing, memory, language comprehension, and emotions.
- Connect with the limbic system (the "emotional brain") to allow for the expression of such emotions as rage, fear, sexual and aggressive behavior, and possibly love.

Occipital Lobes

- Facilitate the interpretation of visual images and visual memory.
- Involved in language formation.
- Collaborate with many other brain structures in the formation of memory.

THE THALAMUS AND HYPOTHALAMUS Other limbic structures are located in the diencephalon and include the thalamus and the hypothalamus. The **thalamus** functions as a relay station, receiving many impulses from the

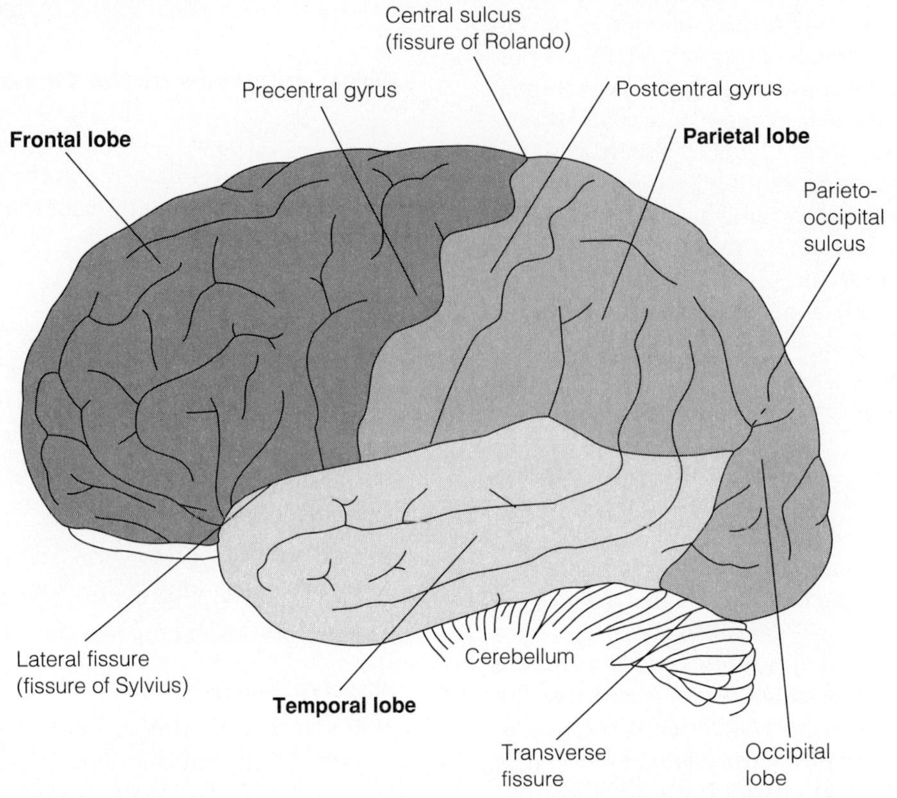

Figure 3–1 Delineation of the cerebral lobes.

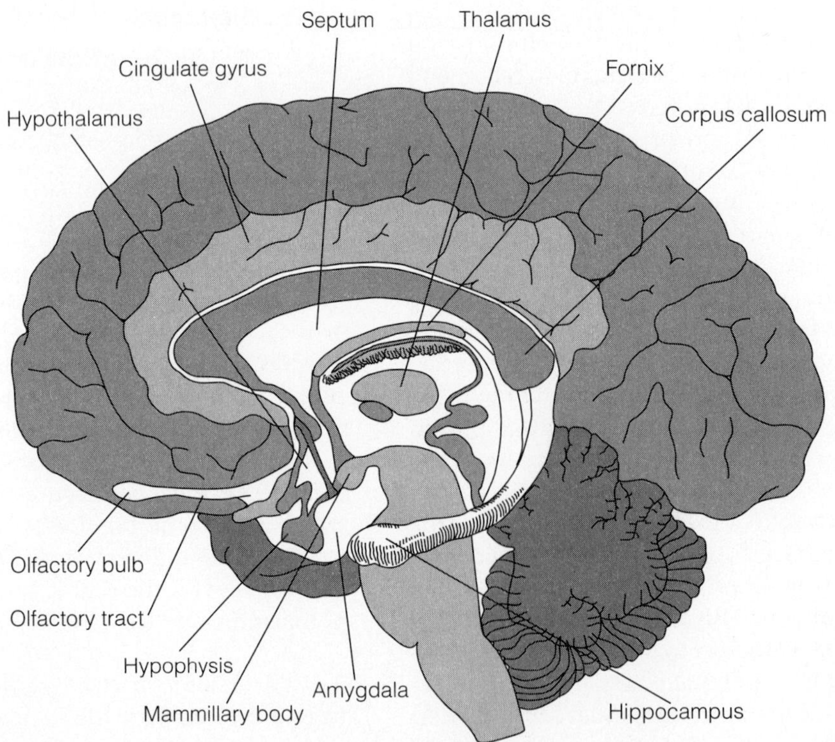

Figure 3–2 Structures of the limbic system.

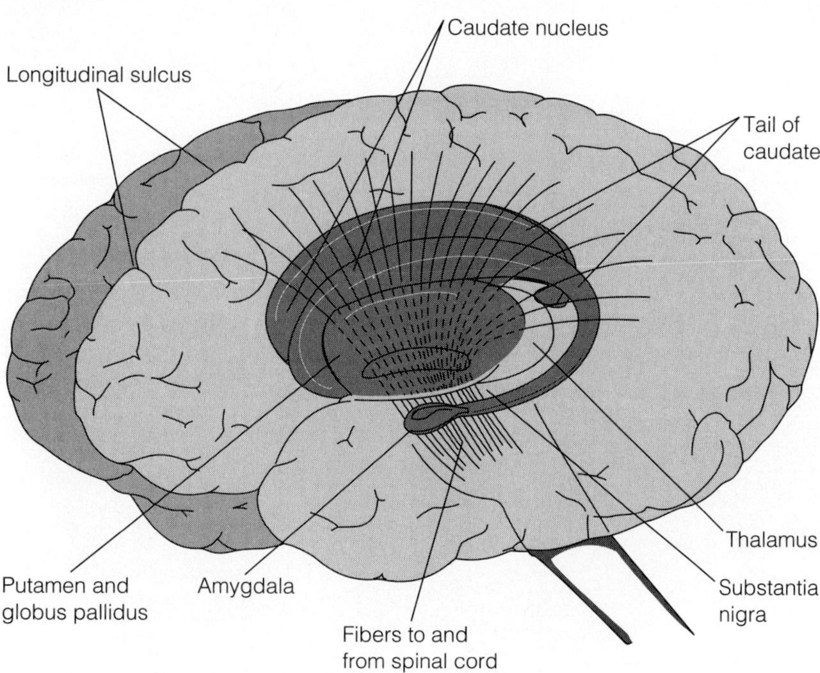

Figure 3–3 Anatomical relationships of the basal ganglia to the cerebral cortex and thalamus.

spinal cord, brain stem, and cerebellum. With the aid of many connections in the cerebral hemispheres and cortex, the thalamus regulates activity and movement, sensory experience (except smell), and emotional expression.

The **hypothalamus** is a "hub" between the mind and body, giving physical form to thoughts and emotions. It weighs approximately 4 g and accounts for less than 1% of the total volume of the brain. However, its size is not a good indication of importance. The hypothalamus regulates many of the body's critical activities, including hormone levels, appetite (hunger), body temperature (thermoreceptors), sex drive (libido), water balance (thirst), circadian rhythms, pleasure, and pain.

The hypothalamus is the critical link between the cerebral cortex, the limbic system, and the endocrine system. It serves as a pipeline to the brain stem and acts as a conduit for control of the autonomic nervous system.

The **pituitary gland**, under the direction of the hypothalamus, secretes hormones, which, carried through the bloodstream, trigger the activities of other glands. The mamillary bodies, located at the back of the hypothalamus, help transfer information about the activities of the hypothalamus to other parts of the brain. The pituitary also receives input from the fornix and includes connections to the thalamus, which in turn communicates to and from the frontal cortex (see Figure 3–2).

THE BASAL GANGLIA The **basal ganglia** are collectively a complex of structures that include the caudate nucleus, putamen, globus pallidus, and substantia nigra (Figure 3–3). Their functions include initiating and terminating movement, planning motor activities, mediating hallucinations and delusions, and processing emotions and memories. The basal ganglia have a high concentration of dopamine receptors, acetylcholine, gamma-aminobutyric acid, and peptides. A deficit of dopamine from this area is associated with Parkinson's disease. Parkinson's disease is characterized by rhythmic tremors of the extremities, slurred speech, and an unchanging facial expression much like that of former boxer Muhammad Ali, who sustained numerous blows to his head, resulting in damage to the basal ganglia.

THE CEREBELLUM The **cerebellum** lies below the posterior section of the cerebrum. It is the second-largest structure within the brain (Figure 3–4). Like the cerebral hemispheres, the cerebellum has an outer layer of gray matter and is mainly composed of underlying white matter. The main function of this highly specialized part of the brain is movement, posture, balance, and sensory-motor coordination. The hand-eye coordination of a diamond cutter, the fluid movements of a ballerina, and the success of a quarterback's moves all depend on cerebellar functions.

THE BRAIN STEM Beneath the limbic, hypothalamic, and thalamic areas is the brain stem. The brain stem consists of three smaller structures: the medulla oblongata, the pons, and the midbrain (see Figure 3–4). The **medulla oblongata** (Latin for "oblong marrow") is the connecting piece of tissue between the brain stem and the spinal

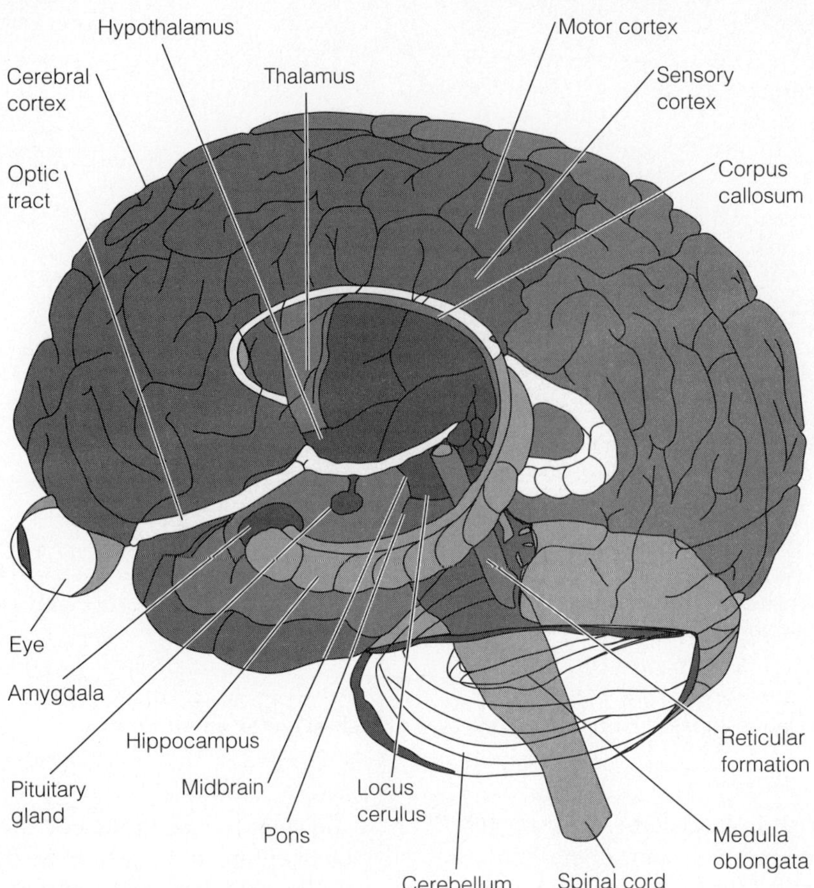

Figure 3–4 The cerebellum, brain stem, and associated structures.

cord. It is less than 5 cm long but is responsible for the control of many vital functions, including respiration, regulation of blood pressure, and partial regulation of heart rate. It also controls the perception of pain, vomiting, swallowing, and some aspects of talking. Incoming fibers from the spinal cord cross over in the medulla, yielding left cerebral hemispheric control of the right side of the body, and vice versa.

Within the brain stem are areas called the **autonomic nervous system (ANS).** There are two divisions: the sympathetic division and the parasympathetic division. In stressful emotional circumstances, the sympathetic division of the ANS (also called the sympathetic nervous system) prepares for fight or flight; the parasympathetic initiates the relaxation response with the aid of the endocrine system. Researchers have established that prolonged stress can weaken the immune system and may trigger mood disorders (Chrousos and Gold 1992; Post 1992). The goal of meditation and other forms of stress management is to inhibit the sympathetic response and strengthen the parasympathetic response.

Pons means "bridge," and bridging is its function. The pons contains conduction paths between the spinal cord and the brain. It also contains reflex centers that mediate sensations of the face, chewing, abduction of the eyes, facial expressions, balance, and the regulation of respiration. Located within the pons is the **locus ceruleus,** a tiny oval structure that contains 70% of the neurons (nerve cells) that release norepinephrine, the influence of which extends throughout the brain. One projection is to the amygdala, resulting in emotional and cardiovascular control. Activation of the locus ceruleus is associated with fear, pain, and alarm.

The **midbrain** is above the pons and below the cerebral hemispheres. The midbrain is a reflex center for the regulation of eye movement, visual accommodation, and regulation of pupil size. The midbrain is also essential for relaying impulses to the cerebral cortex and sending behavior-producing messages back to the rest of the body.

Certain portions of the brain function in concert with other parts to create a system with a given function; the limbic system is a good example. Other systems that are of special interest to psychiatric nurses include the reticular activating system and the extrapyramidal system.

The **reticular activating system (RAS)** consists of nerve pathways that originate in the spinal cord and connect in the reticular formation, a system of neurons that modulates awareness and states of consciousness. By screening stimulation from the environment, the RAS enables us to concentrate. The RAS also permits routine inattention, allowing for sleep. During sleep, excitatory neurons of the RAS gradually become more and more excitable because of prolonged rest, while inhibitory neurons of sleep centers become less excitable because of their overactivity, leading to a new cycle of wakefulness. This helps explain the rapid transitions between sleep and wakefulness. Arousal, as experienced by people with psychiatric conditions, can be the insomnia that occurs when a person's mind becomes preoccupied with a thought. In states of mental illness, there is obviously some biologic disequilibrium of the RAS because it involves motivation and levels of arousal. However, the details of this imbalance are complex and not well understood at this time.

The **extrapyramidal system** consists of tracts of motor neurons from the brain to parts of the spinal cord. This system has complex relays and connections to areas of the cortex, cerebellum, brain stem, and thalamus. These tracts play an important role in gross movements and responses of emotional tone, such as smiling and frowning.

Antipsychotic drugs create side effects that affect the extrapyramidal system; hence the term *extrapyramidal side effects,* or *EPS.* The four general classes of EPS are parkinsonism, dyskinesias and dystonias, akathisias, and tardive dyskinesia.

A Review of Genetics

Often clients may tell you that others in their family experience "moodiness," "crazy thoughts," or that they "can't work." These disclosures are important clues about how major psychiatric disorders tend to run in families. A new area of research is exploring the genetic material to find clues to a possible heritable basis of behavior. What are the molecular consequences of abnormal genes? To begin to answer this question, a review of the chemical composition of genes and certain aspects of cell structure and function is necessary.

Gene Structure The **nucleus,** the cell's information center, holds the genes that make up chromosomes. The **gene** is the functional unit of information of the **chromosome.** The human genome consists of 23 pairs of chromosomes, one from each parent; 22 pairs are the somatic chromosomes, and one pair is the sex chromosomes (XX female, XY male). Genes are segments of **DNA** (deoxyribonucleic acid), the complex molecule that makes up chromosomes. **RNA** (ribonucleic acid) is another complex molecule that plays a role in translating DNA's coding instructions for making protein. Each strand of the complex molecule of DNA is compactly formed into a double helix. The strand of DNA is composed of chemical nucleotides consisting of one sugar molecule (DNA or RNA), one phosphate group, and one of four nitrogen bases. The **nucleotides** are adenine (A), thymine (T), guanine (G), and cytosine (C). The nucleotides line up next to each other like two sides of a zipper, with the phosphate and sugar forming the outer strand; the bases (A, T, G, and C) act like interlocking teeth. The sequence of amino acids, which are proteins, is coded by genes. The sequence or code is like a language and is not arbitrary. The nucleotides, or two sides of the zipper, can only fit together in one way: A pairs with T, and G pairs with C. This base pairing allows for the known sequence of one strand to predict the partner strand. Each strand of the double helix thus specifies its complement and allows for the duplication of genetic information in dividing cells.

Gene Function Structure determines function, and function determines behavior. Variations in the chemical composition of the genes can produce abnormal structural proteins or enzymes, altering the sending or receiving of signals and resulting in dysfunction or disease. The main component of all living matter is proteins, which are large molecules or long chains of amino acids linked together. The sequence of amino acids along the chain determines each protein's physical and biologic properties, acting as information molecules.

The transfer of DNA from the nucleus requires messenger RNA (mRNA), which serves as the instructor for the making of proteins outside the nucleus (Figure 3–5). Ribosomes, which float in the cytoplasm or sit on the rough endoplasmic reticulum, translate the mRNA into proteins. Also in the cytoplasm are the mitochondria, which generate energy, via ions and adenosine triphosphate (ATP), from the oxidation of fats and sugars, and also contain RNA and DNA. The process of protein synthesis is diagrammatically illustrated in Figure 3–6.

Instructions for the synthesizing and metabolizing of the molecular messengers of the brain are coded in the DNA. One of the premises of neurobiology is that major mental illnesses are brain diseases. Without DNA, there would be no organism; and without protein, the organism would not be alive or able to respond to its internal world or the outer world of experience (the environment) (Restak 1994). A typical protein has a useful life of about two days; thus, new protein molecules are constantly being synthesized. This concept may help explain how a client's symptoms or behavioral expression can change over time. New messages among the complex combinations of proteins change the code in the physical environment, resulting in different expressions of temperament, behavior, and individuality.

New technologies enable researchers to modify DNA and RNA so that both the messages and the expression of the messages can be manipulated experimentally. DNA markers, from fragments of DNA (restriction fragment

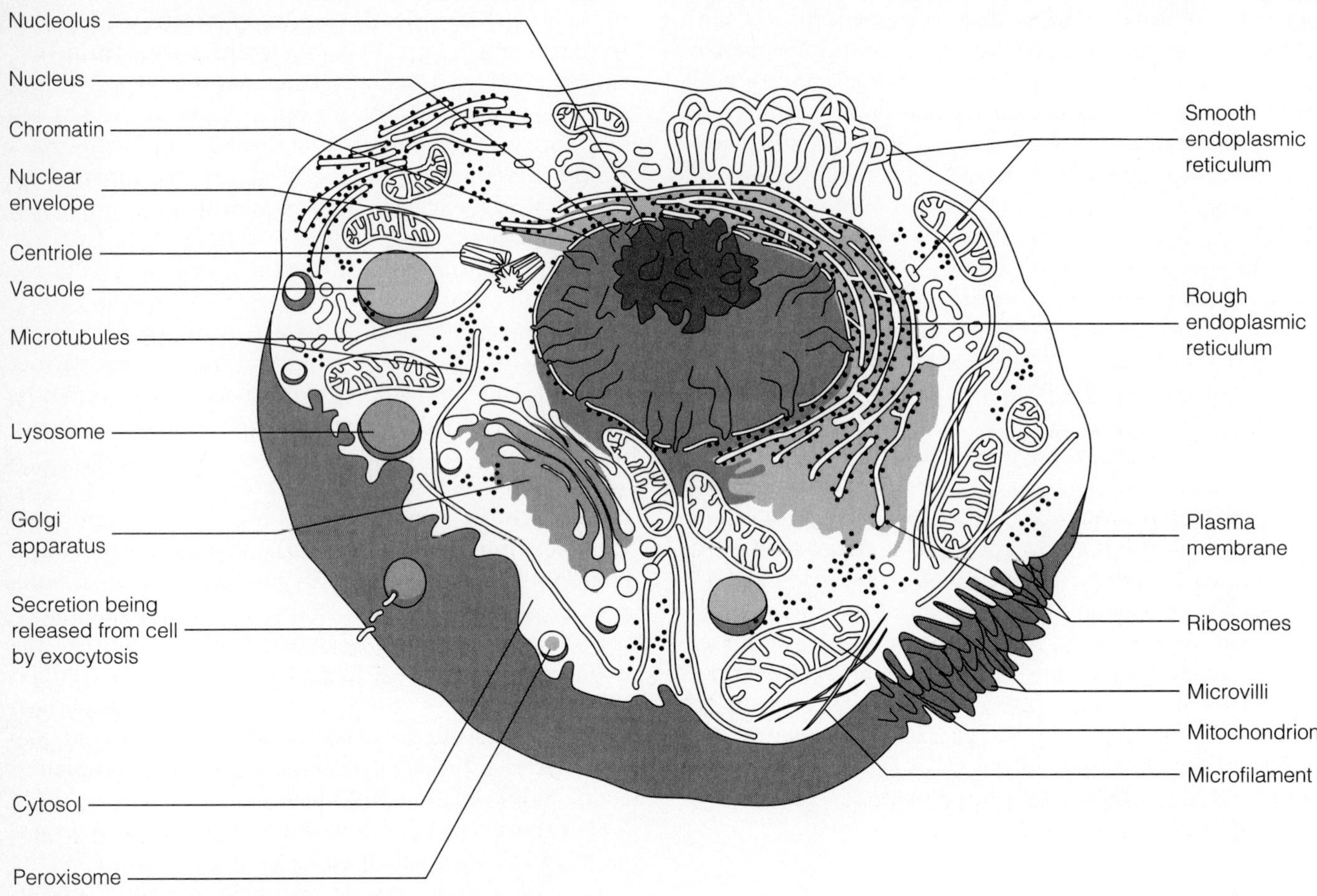

Figure 3–5 Basic cell structures.

length polymorphisms, or RFLPs), are making it possible to identify and localize the genes involved in a disease process. This helps us understand the molecular and cellular pathophysiology of the disease and its treatment, and possibly, in the future its prevention (Malcespina, Quitkin, Kaufmann 1992).

Linkage studies will make it possible for nurses to be involved in genetic counseling. The ethical implications of this process are controversial, and nurses need to be familiar with the concepts to help clients avoid the potential stigma associated with genetic diseases (see Chapter 10, Ethical Reasoning).

THE GENETIC BASIS OF PSYCHIATRIC ILLNESS Research on the genetic basis of inherited psychiatric illnesses remains elusive. In all the genetic models, the role of environmental influences, perinatal events, trauma, infections, or stress have to be considered. This concept suggests that even though some mental illnesses are familial, the single-gene location may apply only to a few families, while several chromosomal locations (polymorphisms) may account for heritability in other families. Following is a summary of the genetic findings for some of the major heritable disorders.

Mood Disorders Family studies show that affective illness runs in families with a risk of 3–7% for bipolar disorder and 11–16% for unipolar disorder, compared with the general population risk of 0.8% for bipolar and 3.7% for unipolar (Bowman and Nurnberger 1993). Although chromosome 11 was first suggested as being involved in mood disorders, it did not replicate in other studies. Currently two candidate genes, the corticotropin receptor and the alpha subunit of a G protein, located on chromosome 18, suggest susceptibility for bipolar disorder (Berrettini et al. 1994). In addition, the absence of male-to-male transmission of bipolar disorder in some families may account for an X-linked subtype of transmission. The relatives of people with early-onset illness generally are at higher risk than late-onset relatives. No definitive biologic marker currently exists, but sensitivity to rapid eye movement (REM) sleep induction is found in twins and families with mood disorders, supporting that sleep disturbance is common in depression.

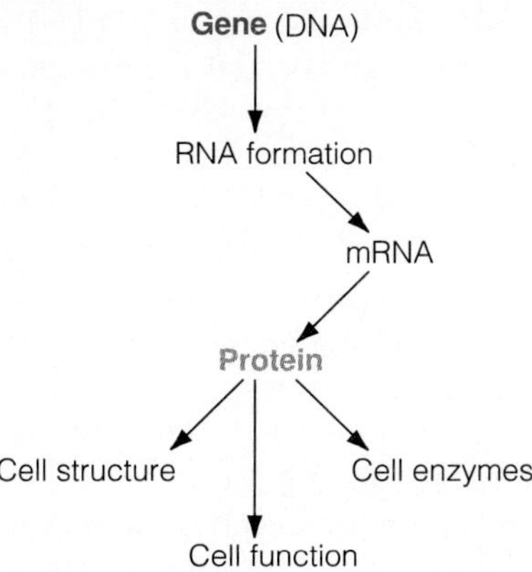

Figure 3–6 Protein synthesis.

Schizophrenia Pooled twin studies show that monozygotic (MZ) or identical twin concordance is 33%, compared with 8% dizygotic (DZ) twins. The risk for siblings of people with schizophrenia is 8–10%, 12% for children of a parent with schizophrenia, and 46% for children of two ill parents (Bowman and Nurnberger 1993). To date, no chromosomal linkage has been identified in replicated findings. A promising biologic marker found in ill and healthy relatives is smooth pursuit eye movement deficits. It may link with attentional deficits and a dominant inheritance pattern.

Panic Disorder Panic disorder family studies show a 22–55% risk of panic in first-degree relatives compared with 2% controls. MZ twin concordance for panic disorder is about 31%. These findings are not found in generalized anxiety disorder, showing that panic attacks are a separate disorder. Few large family studies have been conducted, and what is inherited might be a predisposition to a biologic deficiency, rather than a single-gene abnormality.

Obsessive-Compulsive Disorder (OCD) Few systematic family studies have been conducted for OCD, but clinical and familial studies suggest heritability. There is increasing incidence of OCD in families of young children; one in four have a first-degree relative with OCD. The rate of OCD is significant in families of people with Tourette's disorder, regardless of whether the person has concomitant diagnosis of OCD. OCD itself occurs more frequently in female relatives of people with Tourette's disorder, suggesting some sex-related expression of the syndrome. Males are more likely to express Tourette's and tics, and females express OCD in the absence of tics.

Alcoholism The risk of alcohol dependence is 3 to 4 times greater in first-degree relatives of people with alcohol dependence. The risk is 25–35% for male relatives and 5–10% for female relatives. MZ twins show a higher concordance rate for alcoholism than DZ twins. Linkage studies have yet to find a chromosome for alcoholism. Biologic markers reported to be associated with alcoholism include male alcoholics and their sons showing a decreased slow-wave activity on EEGs. Sons have also been found to have reduced behavioral and endocrine responses to alcohol, as compared to controls (Bowman and Nurnberger 1993).

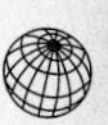

A cultural biological marker regarding the activity of the alcohol-metabolizing enzyme aldehyde dehydrogenase (ALDH) is under genetic control. An inherited ALDH I deficiency in 25–50% of Japanese, Korean, and Chinese individuals is associated with a flushing response when they consume alcohol. This leads to a lower rate of alcoholism as compared with other Asian persons (Bowman and Nurnberger 1993).

Alzheimer's Disease (AD) For early-onset families a genetic basis has been established, the risk for men and women being equal. Although rare, in some families of early onset a dominant trait is linked with chromosome 21, which is near the beta-amyloid precursor protein, which is found in high amounts in the brains of persons with AD. In addition, chromosome 14 has been linked with an early onset familial pattern for a small number of families. For late-onset AD (60 years or older) chromosome 19, the loci for apolipoprotein E, form 4, relates with excess risk (Bowman and Nurnberger 1993).

The application of these genetic strategies to clinical practice will bring many new challenges and ethical dilemmas. Alterations in genetic coding, or designer genes, are currently being used with diseases such as cancer and cystic fibrosis to supply healthy genes or block a defective gene. In mental illness perhaps the following questions will be answered in the next decade:

Do the same genes but a different environment result in depression or an anxiety disorder?

Which neurochemical system, when recoded, will provide a better drug treatment for schizophrenia?

Does a stressful life event trigger genetically vulnerable neurons to promote rapid cycling mood disorder or panic disorder?

How do shy children with blue eyes and hay fever receive the inhibition trait?

Pathophysiological traits and genetic linkage markers will assist families in getting answers as to who is at risk; are there cultural differences, and can the illness be prevented?

Neurons, Synapses, and Neurotransmission

The brain's structural complexity increases as one considers the biochemical processes that occur with every thought, emotion, memory, dream, or hope. Thought and feeling are made possible by complex interplays and communications between cells in the central nervous system in response to stimuli in the environment. The specialized cells of the nervous system are called **neurons.** Like other cells in the body, each neuron has a cell body that contains the cytoplasm and the nucleus. Unlike other cells, a neuron has at least two other extensions: an axon and one or more dendrites. An **axon** is the portion of a neuron that conveys electric impulses *from* the cell body to other neurons. Axons are covered with a white myelin sheath and compose the white matter in the brain and spinal cord. **Dendrites** are unmyelinated and conduct electrical messages *to* the cell body. There are approximately 100 billion neurons in the brain and nearly an equal number of supporting (glia) cells.

Neurons are classified according to the direction in which they conduct impulses. *Sensory neurons,* also known as afferent neurons, send messages from the periphery to the brain. For example, if you place your foot into a tub of scalding water, the message that the water is too hot is sent to your brain via sensory neuron pathways. *Motor neurons,* or efferent neurons, carry messages that originate in the brain and yield a behavioral change in the periphery. In the example of your foot in the hot water, the message from the brain is to remove the foot (quickly!) from the hot water; this message travels via motor neuron pathways. Interneurons, specialized neurons that communicate between sensory and motor neurons, help produce a given, desirable behavior.

Communication among and between neurons is complex and specific. This communication is believed to be the basis of behavior. Each neuron forms anywhere from 1000 to 10,000 synaptic connections. The **synapse** is a gap in the synaptic cleft between neurons (Figure 3–7). These reciprocal synapses form positive and negative feedback loops. Neurons are arranged in networks or pathways whereby neuronal communication is facilitated by repetition. Interneuron communication is electrical and chemical and occurs at synapses, or points of contact between neurons, as well as along the neuron itself.

SYNAPTIC TRANSMISSION *Neuromessenger* is a collective, generic term for neurotransmitters, neuromodulators, and neurohormones. **Neurotransmitters (NT)** are neuromessengers that are rapidly released at the presynaptic neuron upon stimulation, diffuse across the synapse between two neurons, and have either an excitatory or inhibitory effect on the postsynaptic neuron (see Figure 3–7). The membrane of the axon terminal of a neuron contains many saclike projections called **synaptic vesicles,** which contain the NT molecules that transmit the message across the synapse.

Neurons are encased in cell membranes that function as a complex regulation site. The membranes contain proteins, some of which are phospholipides, enzymes and ion channels. **Ion channels** are water-filled molecular tunnels that pass through the cell membrane and allow electrically charged atoms (ions) or small molecules to enter or leave the cell. The neuron exists in a state of tension because of the various ions in its membrane. Changes in ion concentrations cause the nerve impulse, or **action potential,** which transmits information between neurons. The four major ions are sodium, potassium, calcium, and chloride. Each ion passes in or out of the neuron via its own channel. Nerve impulses involve the opening or closing of the ion channels by gates.

Once the action potential reaches the end of the axon, the electrical transfer of the information ends, and messages are then conveyed by the chemicals, the NT molecules. The signal is mediated by binding to specific receptors on the cell surface (Guyton 1991). Depending on the type of channel, the action potential is excitatory, influencing the neuron to fire, or inhibitory, preventing it from firing. Presynaptic axon terminals contain large numbers of calcium channels, which determine the quantity of NT that is released into the synaptic cleft.

At the synapse, the membrane of the postsynaptic neuron contains receptor proteins. **Receptors** are highly specialized proteins embedded in the membrane of the neuron that are in part exposed to the extracellular fluid and recognize the neuromessenger. Receptors are presynaptic (axon) or postsynaptic (dendrite), depending on their location. Neurotransmitters and receptors vary in their affinity for each other, depending on the NT involved. They may bind like a lock and key, or the outcome may depend on what is available. Every neuron is more or less sensitive to a constant amount of neuromessenger, and this is an important principle in pharmacology. The NT that remains in the synapse after the postsynaptic response is either dissolved by synaptic enzymes or reabsorbed for recycling by the presynaptic neuron, a process known as reuptake.

NEUROTRANSMITTERS There are three classes of NT: biogenic amines (monoamines), amino acids, and peptides (Table 3–1). The biogenic amines include dopamine (DA), norepinephrine (NE), epinephrine, serotonin (5-hydroxytryptamine, or 5-HT), acetylcholine (Ach), and histamine (H). They are synthesized in the axon terminals and released into the synapse. Identification of these neurotransmitters began the era of neuropsychopharmacology. Functional imaging techniques now enable researchers to visualize the pathways of neuron clusters at work, to better understand their functional association with behavior. The original belief that a neuron contained only one NT is no longer valid. Figure 3–8 illustrates the basic pathways of three of the major biogenic amines.

Dopamine **Dopamine (DA)** is found in the basal ganglia area, where it is associated with the control of

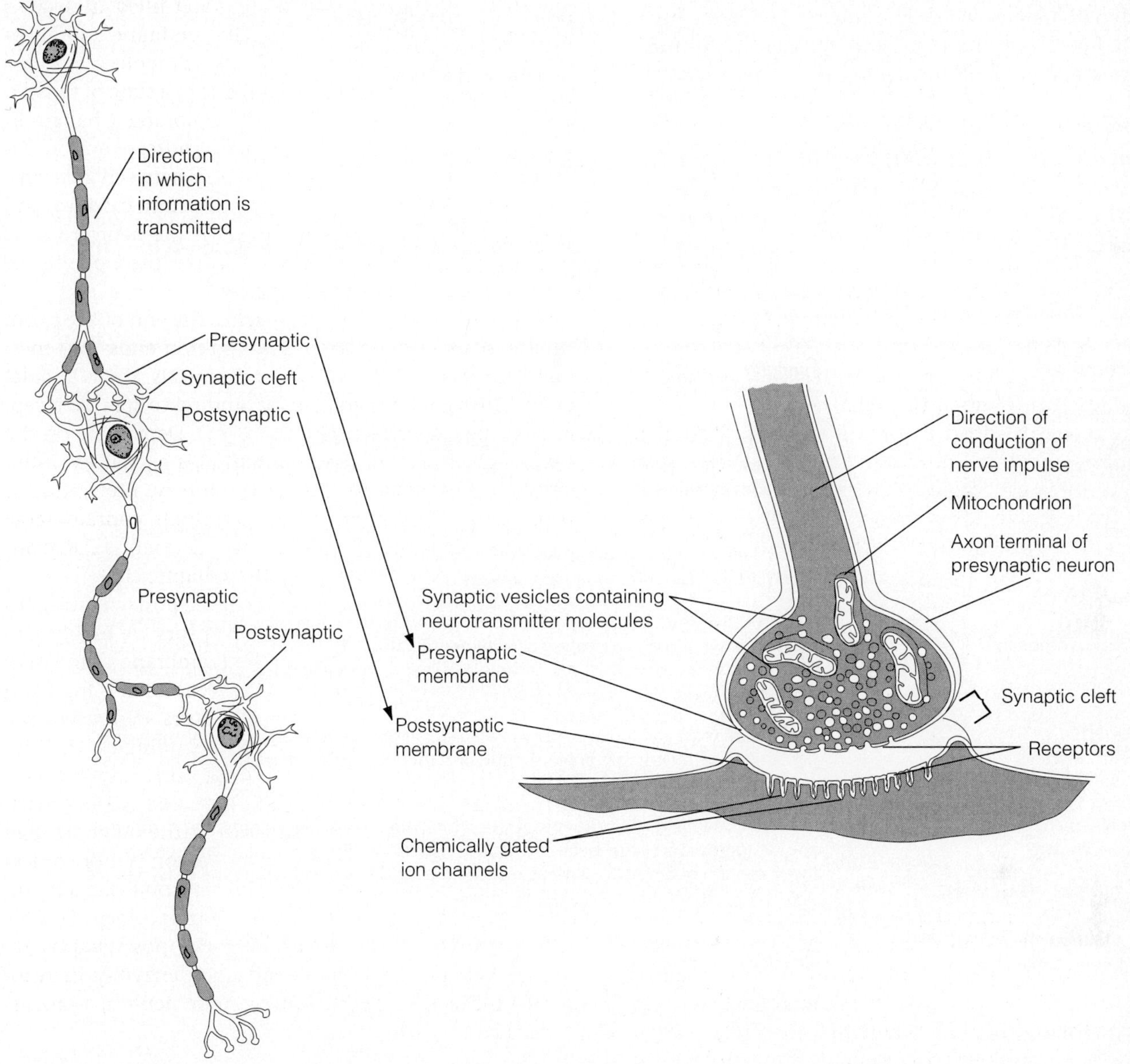

Figure 3–7 Neurons and synaptic transmission. A single neuron can be a presynaptic neuron at one synapse and a postsynaptic neuron at another. When a nerve impulse arrives at an axon terminal, neurotransmitter molecules are released. The molecules diffuse across the synaptic cleft and bind to receptor proteins on the membrane of the postsynaptic neuron. This binding alters the three-dimensional shapes of the receptors, initiating a series of events that influence the response of the postsynaptic neuron.

complex movement; in the limbic system, where it is associated with memory, mood, reward, pleasure, and motivation; in the hypothalamic tract, where it is associated with endocrine functions, circadian rhythms, food and water intake, and temperature; and in the frontal cortex pathway, where it is associated with insight, judgment, problem solving, inhibition, and social awareness. Because of the projections of the pathways to these areas, DA disturbance is involved in psychosis. The efficacy of neuroleptic or antipsychotic drugs used to treat psychoses is correlated with their ability to block DA receptors.

Norepinephrine Receptors for **norepinephrine (NE)** are located in the pons, specifically the locus ceruleus, where NE is associated with the stress response, arousal, and alertness; in the cerebral cortex, where it affects cognitive functioning; the limbic system, where it is associated with emotional responses, the ability to focus or learn, pleasure, reward, and the regulation of mood; and in the hypothalamus, where it influences endocrine functions, temperature, appetite, and biological rhythms. NE plays a major role in mediating mood disorders and anxiety.

Serotonin **Serotonin (5-HT)** has the opposite effect of NE, which is a stimulator; 5-HT has a calming effect. The 5-HT neurons arise in the raphe nuclei and project to the same areas as the NE pathways. Serotonin appears to be a modulator. Its effects include and influence the temperature, sensory, sleep, and assertiveness areas of the brain; it serves as a chemical mediator in pain perception, normal and abnormal behaviors, moods, drives, the regulation of food intake, and in neuroendocrine functions. Receptor subtypes decrease cerebral blood flow during a migraine episode and increase the response to pain.

Acetylcholine The first chemical to be identified as a true neurotransmitter, **acetylcholine (Ach)** is the "grand

Table 3–1 The Major Known Neurotransmitters

Neurotransmitter	*Function*
Biogenic Amines (Monoamines)	
Dopamine (DA) Precursor: tyrosine	Integrates thoughts and emotions; regulates pleasure and reward-seeking stimuli; control of complex movement; motivation; cognition; stimulates hypothalamus to release hormones affecting adrenal, thyroid, and sex hormones.
Norepinephrine (NE) Precursor: tyrosine	Stimulates sympathetic division of the ANS; role in stress response; fluctuates with sleep and wakefulness; role in attention and vigilance, arousal, ability to focus or learn, feeling of reward, regulation of mood and anxiety.
Serotonin (5-HT) Precursor: tryptophan	Inhibits activity and behavior; role in level of arousal; increases sleep time; reduces aggression, play, sexual, and eating activity; temperature regulation; pain control; mood states; role in circadian rhythms; sensory regulation; helps focus the brain; regulates pituitary.
Histamine (H) Precursor: histidine	Mediates allergic and inflammatory responses; smooth muscle constriction; stimulates gastric acid secretion; role in biorhythms and thermoregulation; role in second messenger transmission.
Acetylcholine (Ach) Precursor: choline	Attention; memory; promotes preparation for action; conserves energy; thirst; defense and/or aggression; sexual behavior; mood regulation; REM sleep; stimulates parasympathetic division of the ANS; controls muscle tone in balance with DA in the basal ganglia.
Amino Acids	
Gamma-aminobutyric acid (GABA) Precursor: glutamic acid	Reduces aroused aggression, anxiety, and excitation; sedation; anticonvulsant and muscle-relaxant properties.
Glycine Precursor: serine	Inhibitory.
Glutamate	Excitatory; role in learning and memory; neural degeneration.
Aspartate	Excitatory.
Peptides (Neuromodulators)	
Somatostatin	Mood disorders; Alzheimer's disease; negative feedback control of thyrotropin secretion; role in positive symptoms of schizophrenia. Excites limbic neurons.
Neurotensin	Role in schizophrenia.
Substance P	Excitatory; role in pain syndromes, mood, and movement disorders.
Cholecystokinin (CCK)	Role in schizophrenia; eating and movement disorders; panic disorder.
Vasopressin	Role in mood disorders.
Corticotropin-releasing hormone (CRH)	Stress, mood, memory, and anxiety.
Opioids: endorphins and enkephalins	Alters emotional behavior; pain control; hallucinations; pleasure; motor coordination; water balance.

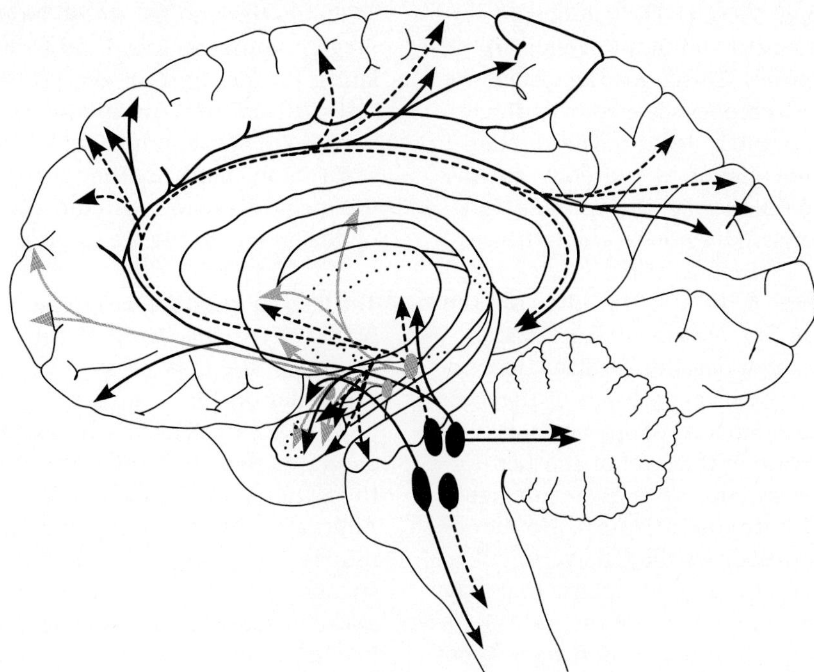

Figure 3–8 Common neurotransmitter pathways. Blue = DA, black = NE, dashed line = 5-HT. Dotted line indicates pons.

parent" of neurotransmitters. DA and Ach share a concentration of activity within the basal ganglia, and drugs that are used to block EPS are cholinergic stimulants, suggesting a reciprocal relationship between these two neurotransmitters in the modulation of movement and possibly psychosis. Ach plays a major role in the encoding of memory and in cognition. It also plays a mediation role in mood disorders, stress, and sleep regulation. It is considered to be highly significant in neuromuscular transmission.

Histamine The role of histamine (H) in psychiatric illness is less understood. It is a chemical messenger that mediates a wide range of cellular responses, including allergic and inflammatory reactions, gastric acid secretions, and neurotransmission. Some psychiatric medicines, the neuroleptics, block H receptors, resulting in the side effects of sedation, weight gain, and drowsiness.

Amino Acids These neurotransmitters are natural substances found throughout the brain and body and in the proteins of the food we eat. **Gamma-aminobutyric acid (GABA)** is the most prevalent inhibitory NT. GABA neurons are widely distributed in the central nervous system. Glycine, also an inhibitory NT, is primarily in the brain stem, spinal cord, and cerebellum. GABA has a prominent role in arousal; when the neuron is stimulated, GABA acts as a brake, decreasing neuronal excitability. Benzodiazepines act by binding with GABA and benzodiazepine receptors to produce antianxiety, sedative, anticonvulsant, and muscle-relaxant properties.

Glutamate and aspartate are the two primary excitatory amino acid neurotransmitters. Glutamate is primarily located in the cerebral cortex and hippocampus and has a role in long-term memory and learning. Too much glutamate can be a neurotoxin, as seen in Huntington's chorea and phencyclidine (PCP) psychosis.

SECOND MESSENGERS Psychopharmacologic strategies are becoming more specific with increased understanding of signal transduction. When the NT receptor complex results in a direct change in the membrane potential, it is called first messenger transmission. A rapid, direct membrane change can also initiate a series of intracellular reactions triggering a **second messenger transmission. G proteins** (G for guanine) are large families of receptors that are the links in second messenger cascades. Second messengers are membrane proteins that relay nerve signals from the NT complex through a chain of chemical reactions to the nucleus. Drugs acting at this level allow for greater selectivity in targeting specific enzymes associated with behavior. This cascade of signals is a major mechanism for switching proteins on or off.

Psychoendocrinology and Psychoneuroimmunology

This section will challenge the concept of mind-body dualism by examining the interaction of the brain with two subsystems: the body's endocrine system and the immune system.

The Role of the Endocrine System The **endocrine system** functions through neurochemical messengers in the bloodstream called **hormones.** The endocrine system is a communication system. Hormones secreted from the hypothalamus instruct the pituitary to stimulate the target tissues, glands. The major glands of the body are the adrenals, the gonads, and the thyroid; their primary function is releasing hormones. Hormones act as triggers. Each component of the **neuroendocrine axis** can feed back into any component of the system, including the cortex and limbic system. The amount of hormone produced is partly regulated by a negative feedback mechanism. Feedback regulation exists at all levels of the axis. Thus the rise or fall in the blood level of one hormone can cause an increase or decrease in the level of another hormone. The immune and endocrine systems are integrated through a shared set of hormone receptors. Hormones have a broader range of responses than nerve impulses and require seconds to days to cause a response that may last from weeks to months.

Irregularities of neuroendocrine function have been linked to depression, postpartum psychosis, schizophrenia, polydipsia in clients with psychosis, panic disorder, OCD, anorexia nervosa, Alzheimer's disease, and circadian rhythms. Psychopharmacologic challenge tests, as described in the Tools of Psychobiology box, to help our understanding of the pathophysiology of these conditions are becoming more common in psychiatric assessment. One of the most common is the **Dexamethasone Suppression Test (DST),** which attempts to assess the hypothalamic-pituitary-adrenal (HPA) axis (Figure 3–9). Dexamethasone, a synthetic glucocorticoid, is given by mouth at 11:00 PM to "challenge" the axis. By measuring blood samples of the hormone cortisol drawn at 4:00 PM the day before the pill is taken, and at 8:00 AM (highest level of normal rhythm), 4:00 PM (lowest level of rhythm), and 11:00 PM the day after the pill is taken, one can assess a relationship between the pituitary and the hypothalamus. Dexamethasone "turns off" ACTH secretion at the pituitary, which in turn suppresses cortisol secretion from the adrenals. In a normally functioning axis, cortisol is reduced for the next 24 hours. However, nonsuppression, or "escape," is observed by a rise in the 4:00 PM level, when it should be low, in many psychiatric conditions. There are no side effects or long-lasting changes as a result of taking the pill. The results are *not* diagnostic of the illness but suggest some pathology in the HPA axis function. A new perspective of DST results is to inform the clinician that the pathophysiology is likely to be responsive to certain heterocyclic or monoamine oxidase (MAO) inhibitors (drugs used in treating depression), and warrants further study (Greden 1993).

Hormones secreted by the hypothalamus and pituitary are **peptides,** large, complex chains of amino acids linked together and synthesized by ribosomes in the neuronal cell body through the transcription of DNA. Their physiology is complex; they bind to specific receptors, modulating the response of the postsynaptic cell to the NT. These effects are slow, involving such prolonged actions as changes in the number of receptors, synapses, and closures of ion channels. They also have an important role in the memory process (Guyton 1991). The most commonly understood peptides are summarized in Table 3–1.

The Role of the Immune System **Psychoneuroumminology (PNI)** is the study of the links between thoughts, emotions, the nervous system, and the immune system. The relationships between these systems have been known by clinicians for a long time. New research is being dedicated to further the *why* of the interactions. In 1992, the National Institutes of Health (NIH) set up an Office of Alternative Medicine to investigate methods and techniques previously untested and misunderstood by mainstream medicine. This field holds much potential for you and clinicians in all specialties to determine how ethnic healing practices, therapeutic touch, massage, guided imagery, relaxation, and nutritional counseling influence the healing process. This area of practice extends to psychiatry, as we strive to understand the influence stress has on mental illness. The most common psychologic problems medical clients suffer are reactive depression and anxiety, and they account for heavier usage of medical services. Stress-related symptoms account for 60% of all primary care visits.

Our understanding of chemical communication between the brain and immune system comes from the study of receptors. Cells in the limbic system have many receptors for neuropeptides such as endorphins, and immune system cells contain receptors for endorphins and other peptides such as corticotropin-releasing hormone (CRH) (Hellhammer and Wade 1993). Macrophages, white blood cells that ingest and destroy invading cells, produce interleukin-1 (IL-1), a molecule called a cytokine, which stimulates the HPA axis, where sleep is promoted and body temperature is raised. The brain can directly influence the immune system by sending messages along nerve cells. The series of communications affects the cell nucleus, producing changes in the DNA and RNA that alter the shape of the neuron or even cause cell death (Chrousos and Gold 1992). In the fight-or-flight response, immune system function is slowed, and energy is directed toward helping the body meet the immediate challenge.

Kindling and Behavioral Sensitization

Kindling is the repeated administration of a subconvulsant stimulus to the neuron (Post 1992). The stimulus may be a chemical cascade from stress, which results in sensitizing the neuron rather than tolerance of the stimulus. *Behavioral sensitization* is a chemical phenomenon

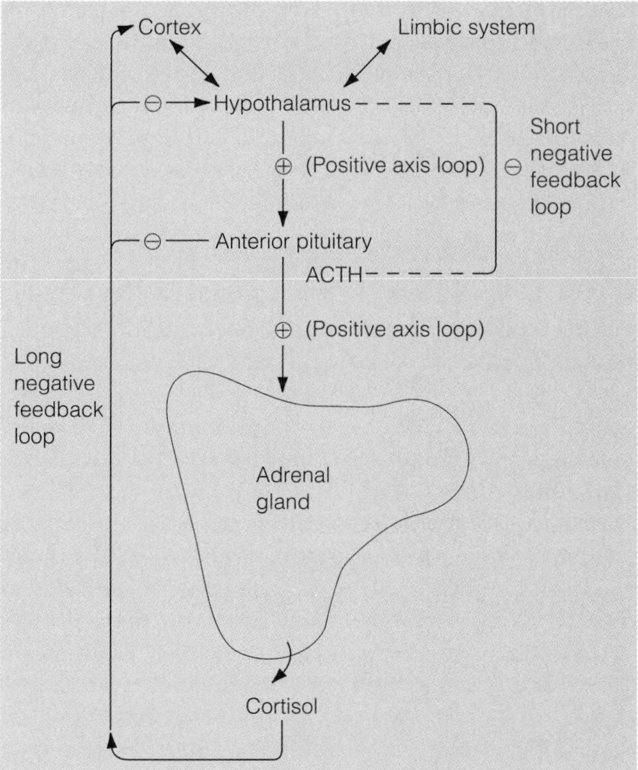

Figure 3–9 Example of neuroendocrine feedback. The positive loop in the axis is depicted by the hypothalamus. Upon stimulation from the cortex or limbic system, the release of trophic peptide CRH (corticotropin-releasing hormone) tells the pituitary gland to signal the adrenal cortex, via ACTH (adrenocorticotropic hormone), to release the glucocorticoid cortisol. Cortisol released into the bloodstream provides negative feedback to the hypothalamus or anterior pituitary. Additionally ACTH can provide negative feedback to the hypothalamus.

whereby changes occur in behavior as part of short-term and long-term memory. Following a series of these "seizures," the neuron requires less stimulus to produce the seizurelike response. Kindling appears to be a kind of learning, independent of cognition, and it can set off an autonomous process.

Although kindling has not been demonstrated definitively in humans, there is indirect support for these biological interactions. Alcohol withdrawal, posttraumatic stress disorder (PTSD), panic disorder, and rapid-cycling mood disorders are similar in that stress or a chemical substrate produces kindled seizures in the amygdala region, which over time produce behavior changes (Post 1992). Carbamazepine, an anticonvulsant, and the benzodiazepines act on kindled episodes. Future clinical implications of this research require more formal conceptualization. But it applies as a working hypothesis because bipolar disorder correlates with a stressful life event around the first episode about 60% of the time. Thus, repetitions of illness (episode sensitization) may trigger further psychopathology and also provide some explanation for why people with rapid-cycling mood disorders become refractory to medications over time. The neuron changes, so different drugs or combinations are required to stabilize the progressive course.

Circadian Rhythms

Biological rhythms, or biorhythms, program our 24-hour day-night cycles. **Chronobiology** is the relationship between time and biological rhythms and their effect on living systems. There are rhythms in endocrine secretion, NT synthesis, receptor number, enzyme levels and affinities, brain electrical activity, duration of cell cycle times, and the transcription regulation of DNA (Kaplan and Sadock 1991). Rhythms can have different cycle lengths: less than 24 hours, **ultradian**; 24 hours, **circadian**; more than 24 hours, **infradian**. Zeitgebers, time cues or synchronizers, set the biological rhythms.

One of the major functions of circadian timing is the sequencing and coordination of metabolic/physiologic events. The **suprachiasmatic nucleus (SCN)**, a cluster of neurons in the hypothalamus, is the body's own internal synchronizer for temperature and sleep. External influences include the light-dark cycle, mealtime patterns, and work schedules.

One theory of depression is that it represents a phase advance disorder, as evidenced by early morning awakening, decreased onset of REM sleep, and neuroendocrine changes. Research into the question of whether estrogen shortens the circadian period, lengthening the sleep phase, advancing sleep onset, and consolidating sleep would help our understanding of the phenomenology of depression and menopause related to changes in the sleep-activity cycle for women (Leibenluft 1993). Symptoms of people with seasonal affective disorder (SAD) vary, but the common ones are increased sleep and appetite, decreased energy, weight gain, low self-esteem, and negativism. A common treatment for this desynchronization is exposure to broad-spectrum light. Melatonin, a hormone of the pineal gland, is a marker of circadian phase position. Light suppresses nighttime melatonin production. Recent findings support a flexible schedule for time of light exposure (Wirtz-Justice et al. 1993). You can teach clients who have a recurrent pattern of winter depression to begin preparing for their symptoms by seeking treatment in the early fall.

Additional preventive strategies include cautioning students who have bipolar disorder to not stay up all night studying or partying as that disrupts the sleep-wake cycle; helping postpartum mothers with a history of mood disorders to have alternatives for night feedings to avoid becoming sleep-deprived; and advocating that people with mood disorders not work irregular shift patterns.

The Americans with Disabilities Act supports the idea that people with psychiatric disabilities should have a "reasonable" work schedule.

As our understanding of biorhythms grows, we can expect that certain clinical decisions such as when it is best to perform surgery and the optimal time to administer medications will change. Knowing a client's circadian patterns will help you administer appropriate medication dosages, resulting in greater efficacy and minimal side effects (Nagayama 1993).

Psychobiology and Mental Disorders

This section examines current hypotheses about the psychobiologic basis of schizophrenia, mood disorders (major depression and bipolar disorder), anxiety disorders (panic disorder and OCD), and Alzheimer's disease.

Schizophrenia

The evolution of the diagnosis of schizophrenia has been dramatic: a shift from a narrowly focused definition of the illness to the requirement of specific criteria of quantifiable symptoms over time. No single neurobiologic hypothesis as the etiologic variable exists. Different domains of psychopathology are directing clinical decisions using multifocal treatments.

LOSS OF NEURONS Researchers are trying to determine why there is a loss of neurons in the brain tissue of people with schizophrenia. There are fewer nerve cells overall but more pyramidal cells (containing DA, Ach, and glutamate) that are excitatory in nature, bringing sensory inputs (sights, sounds, thoughts) to the cerebral cortex. This suggests that the illness may result from an increased flow of activity up to the cortex, explaining why people with schizophrenia become overwhelmed by stimuli such as hallucinations and misperceptions. Studies of DA receptors, especially DA type II (D_2) receptors, provide clues to the neuropathology of schizophrenia. Most D_2 receptors are in the basal ganglia, as observed in in vivo neuroimaging studies. The presence of D_2 receptors in structures with receptors having connections to the limbic and cortical pathways helps link the functions or behaviors of the cognitive and emotional aspects of schizophrenia. Postmortem studies and PET scans are trying to unravel the issue of whether the postmortem findings are a result of antipsychotic drug treatment or primary to the pathophysiology of the disease syndrome.

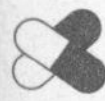

The standard antipsychotic drugs haloperidol and fluphenazine bind to block D_2 receptors in the basal ganglia and target the symptoms of hallucinations, delusions, and loose associations (also referred to as positive symptoms). From the application of molecular genetics techniques, the cloning of other DA receptors (D_3, D_4, and D_5) has led to more specific psychotropic medications. New atypical antipsychotics clozapine and risperidone are targeting such behaviors as restricted emotional expression, attention deficits, poor grooming, lack of motivation, social withdrawal, and poverty of speech (collectively called negative symptoms). They are referred to as atypical because they are selective for receptor subtypes other than D_2 and have less risk in causing EPS. The Research Note reviews the relationship between DA and 5-HT receptors and the new antipsychotic medications and their clinical implications.

STRUCTURAL ABNORMALITIES A second major hypothesis about schizophrenia is that there are structural brain abnormalities associated with the syndrome. Brain CT scans show enlarged ventricles and widened sulci and fissures that appear to have been present from the *onset* of symptoms and are thus not a result of treatment. In twins in which the ventricles appear normal in size, the ventricles of the twin with schizophrenia are larger. Postmortem and MRI studies support a left-sided brain abnormality, as seen in a bilateral reduction in the temporal cortex, reduced hippocampal and amygdala regions (Kleinman and Hyde 1993). A prenatal injury, postnatal maturational change in brain cells, or delayed myelination of nerve cells may explain the delay of the syndrome until adolescence. Myelin forms the insulating lining of axons and is associated with the maturation of behavior during normal development.

Neurochemical findings implicated in schizophrenia show increases in glutamate receptors and decreased 5-HT subtype receptors in the cortical and mesolimbic neurons. This may explain the increase in suicide rates among members of this population; further research is currently trying to validate this connection.

Contemporary treatment of schizophrenia is primarily influenced by a stress-diathesis model (a biologic predisposition to a disease). What might be the interactions between the psychobiologic vulnerability and environmental events that stress the person's adaptive abilities and precipitate the onset of the syndrome or the recurrence of symptoms? Nurses should target interventions that alter the neurochemical systems with pharmacotherapy and psychosocial treatments (as social skills, case management, and family education) for the external stressors or negative symptoms. O'Connor (1994) proposes a comprehensive intervention model for use with clients with schizophrenia.

Mood Disorders

Because of the variability in genetics and symptoms of major depression and bipolar disorder, the psychobiologic basis of mood disorders is difficult to determine. Research has focused on 5-HT and NE receptors. Brain stem nuclei that project to the amygdala, hippocampus, mamillary bodies, and cerebral cortex help account for the symptoms of appetite change, insomnia, depressed affect, loss of interest (anhedonia) and pleasure, decreased problem-solving skills, and suicide attempts. Postmortem findings show reduced 5-HT reuptake sites in the hypothalamus and hippocampus. Because decreased 5-HT is associated with aggression, it may account for the suicide potential of this population.

NEUROCHEMISTRY Neuroendocrine challenge tests report increased cortisol, blunted ACTH response, hypothalamic-pituitary-thyroid axis alterations, and a higher-than-expected rate of autoimmune thyroiditis. When clients ask you what these results indicate you can emphasize they are state-dependent findings, markers which occur while the person is in a depressed mood (state), not diagnostic or a genetic characteristic of the illness.

Recent neurotransmitter studies suggest that complex interactions among NE, 5-HT, DA, Ach, GABA, peptides,

RESEARCH NOTE

Citation

Marder, SR, Meibach RC: Risperidone in the treatment of schizophrenia. *Amer J Psych* 1994;151(6): 825–836.

Study Problem/Purpose

Finding drugs that are more effective in treating all the symptoms associated with schizophrenia and that have less subjective distress and fewer EPS has been a challenge. Risperidone blocks both DA and 5-HT receptors. The goal of this study was to investigate the safety and efficacy of risperidone in the treatment of schizophrenia and to determine the optimal dose.

Methods

In this double-blind trial, 388 hospitalized men and women with schizophrenia (verified by *DSM-III-R* criteria) were given fixed doses of risperidone (2, 6, 10, and 16 mg/day), placebo, or haloperidol (20 mg/day). After informed consent was obtained and enrollment into the study was completed, all meds were stopped and a one-week placebo period to eliminate any drugs from their systems began. Medication to control EPS and sleep were permitted if needed. The main measure of efficacy was the Positive and Negative Symptom Scale, but the Clinical Global Impression Scale and EPS Rating Scale were also used. Following the medication-free week, clients were randomly assigned to one of the medication treatment groups for 8 weeks. During the first week, clients on risperidone were gradually raised to their assigned dose and then remained on that dose. Improvement (efficacy) was defined as a 20% reduction from baseline total Positive and Negative Symptom Scale score to the score at the end of the study.

Findings

This multicenter study demonstrated that risperidone is a safe and effective antipsychotic medication, effective for both positive and negative symptoms of schizophrenia. The optimal daily dose of risperidone, 6 mg, offered few EPS and was effective for the positive and negative symptoms, for some people, by the end of one week. The 16 mg dose of risperidone was as effective for symptoms but was associated with EPS.

Implications

The possible role of 5-HT in contributing to the efficacy of DA in psychosis is encouraging. Since 5-HT is implicated in aggressive and suicidal behavior, perhaps risperidone will have an impact over time on these aspects of schizophrenia. The drug was well tolerated; it contributed to less subjective distress, fewer side effects, and better adherence to the treatment plan. The fact that the negative symptoms were improved provides more hope in psychosocial and vocational adjustment for people with schizophrenia. As with any study, the results have elements of caution in generalizing them for all clients.

The trial had a small sample size and was conducted for only 8 weeks on inpatients. Further study could address whether it is possible that refractory clients, one subgroup, may do better at low doses (6 mg), while recently relapsed clients require higher doses (16 mg). The results of this study are exciting and offer the potential for new antipsychotic medications that can be taken at lower doses, that are more specific in their target symptoms, and that have fewer side effects.

and second messengers contribute to bipolar disorder. There may be as many as six different types of bipolar disorder; further research to distinguish between them will refine our assessments and clinical treatments. Bipolar disorder tends to accelerate over time if left untreated. Early episodes tend to be precipitated by stress, but once recurrent episodes have occurred, the illness accelerates independently of external causes. Even with a genetic predisposition, there can also be changes in gene expression based on life experiences. The genetics, pathophysiology, and neurochemistry studies will yield more effective outcomes.

Somatic therapies other than medications are used in the treatment of mood disorders. **Electroconvulsive therapy (ECT)** is used for psychotic depression and mania. Exactly how ECT works is not well understood. Evidence suggests that it may resynchronize circadian rhythms, like a "brain defibrillator"; it may act as an anticonvulsant like carbamazepine; or it may restore the equilibrium between cerebral hemispheres. Contrary to popular belief, ECT causes no tissue damage or neuronal cell loss (structural brain damage). Most clients report general improvement in cognition in addition to relief from depression, several weeks following ECT. Another somatic therapy that relates to circadian rhythms is *sleep deprivation.* Total or partial sleep deprivation for one night has antidepressant effects but should be used only with careful supervision and assessment.

Because of the various clinical symptoms associated with mood disorders, you have an excellent opportunity to assess clients for their unique psychobiological profile. The outcome of this specific assessment with each client over time will promote improved efficacy of treatment for the target symptoms and potentially prevent disruptive episodes.

Anxiety Disorders

Anxiety disorders have many subtypes, and a complete review is not feasible in this chapter. As discussed earlier, the question of whether anxiety disorders are a separate type of disorder or a variant of a depressive spectrum is still unanswered. MRI and PET scans reveal right hippocampal changes, high brain metabolism, and an abnormal sensitivity to hyperventilation in people with panic disorder.

NEUROCHEMISTRY Neurochemical changes are associated with NE, 5-HT, GABA, and peptides in panic disorder. The discharge of NE in the brain stem, chemoreceptors in the medulla, and 5-HT set off a series of communications that extend through the limbic system, rich in benzodiazepine receptors, to the prefrontal cortex. This pathway may explain the rapid pulse from the NE discharge being interpreted by the cortex as a life-threatening heart attack. These neural connections allow for a hypervigilant cognitive appraisal or inability to integrate the sensory information with any biologic sensation. The behavioral outcome is anticipatory anxiety and avoidance of stimuli that might be the associated precipitant of the arousal (an inappropriate behavioral response).

PET scans show higher metabolic rates in the left prefrontal cortex and caudate nuclei in people with OCD. The caudate or "gating station" dysfunction may lead to overactive circuits that fail to properly integrate cognitive, emotional, and motor responses to sensory inputs. The prefrontal hyperactivity may be related to the tendency to ruminate and plan excessively, as well as to think in an abstract way. Increased frontal lobe activity manifests as a heightened sense of judgment (guilt and worry), intense affect (depression), and hyperjudgmental rigidity (Insel and Winslow 1990).

Abnormal regulation of the 5-HT subsystem has a role in the pathophysiology of OCD. This hypothesis is supported by the improved treatment response to selective serotonin inhibitors. In addition, increased levels of arginine vasopressin, somatostatin, and CRH are found in the CSF of people with OCD. These neuropeptides promote grooming activity and perseverative motor behaviors and increase arousal (anxiety), which are part of the OCD symptomatology.

How do nurses differ in their approaches to mildly anxious clients versus clients with moderate, high, or crisis levels of anxiety? Provided that nurses assess the client's anxiety accurately, how *prescriptive* are the interventions, and what *objective* evaluative measures of anxiety control do nurses use? Anxiety is a psychobiologic condition that responds to both behavioral and pharmacologic interventions; it is recognized as amenable to nursing care. Although many nurses have written about or researched anxiety and its related behaviors in clients, we need to use this knowledge in clinical settings more fully, allowing for more consistent assessment and more prescriptive interventions.

Alzheimer's Disease

People with Alzheimer's disease show a decrease in cerebral blood flow or metabolic function in the posterior temporoparietal regions. It is the only major mental illness to show this characteristic pattern of hypometabolic function. Thus, PET and SPECT studies may be useful in differentiating Alzheimer's from other disorders that include confusion and intellectual deterioration as symptoms. Structural neuronal degeneration occurs, producing **neurofibrillary tangles** and amyloid deposits, or **plaques.** The nerve receptor density and the distribution studies offer promise for improved diagnostic accuracy.

Decreases in cholinergic neurons in a region of the basal ganglia that connect to the amygdala, hippocampus, and cortex are seen. Functionally, this results in the

NURSING SELF-AWARENESS

Promoting Psychobiologic Nursing

To assist you in examining your views and feelings about psychiatric clients, answer the following:

- What terminology do you use to refer to people with psychiatric behaviors: "crazy"; schizophrenic/manic-depressive, that is, the diagnosis; mentally ill; disabled; victim?
- Would you mind living next door to a transitional living facility for people with psychiatric problems?
- How do you feel about someone in your family who has a psychiatric illness?
- Are the "manipulations" of manic behaviors biologic or psychologic?
- Are people with psychiatric problems more violent than the general population?
- Do you blame the client in noncompliance?
- Is "manipulation" wanting too much or a lack of social skill in dealing with people?
- Can people with psychiatric problems contribute positively in their family?
- Is the client the expert, or is it the care provider?
- Should you avoid touching people with psychiatric problems?
- Can a person with a mood disorder control his or her illness or behavior?
- Do you feel hopeless about people with persistent mental illness?
- Can people cure their cancer by thinking positive thoughts?
- Is psychopharmacology the only answer for chronic psychiatric conditions?
- Can diet, exercise, and a regular daily pattern of living enhance mental health?
- Couldn't depressed people try harder to get going?
- Can people intent on suicide be helped?
- Do you want to work with people who have psychiatric problems?

short-term memory loss characteristic of the disease. While the deficits are considered central, there are other NT systems involved in the pathology. These include NE, 5-HT, DA, peptides, and nerve growth factor. If receptors in the limbic structures are affected, depression or labile mood results; a decrease in social skills, inhibition, and impaired judgment can also be a part of the behavioral pattern.

In assessing and intervening with these people, be aware that disorientation results in fear and agitation. Thus, any *change,* such as bed reassignment or facility transfer, is a major stressor. For those with parietal involvement, walking down a hall with a patterned carpet, stepping up on a weight scale, or managing steps is difficult because they cannot orient themselves in relation to the space around them.

Working with clients suffering from AD and their family caregivers calls for your creativity and knowledge of the structure and function of the brain in order to assist with their needs.

Psychobiology and Nursing

Integrating psychobiologic principles into your psychiatric nursing practice will link the body, mind, brain, and behavior. Because you practice holistically, you will recognize that your practice begins and ends with your clients, with their dysfunctions and disorders, their temperaments and aspirations. What are the facts that count, and why are behaviors the way they are? You must not cease to question. To understand client needs necessitates the full synthesis of communication, from molecular to verbal. An understanding of clients' physical and social environment rounds out the mind-body connection. Be aware of your dualistic issues, as presented in the Nursing Self-Awareness box, and how your attitudes may diminish your ability to be an advocate and support person to clients and their families.

The trend of integrating psychobiology does not equate with only administering medications, nursing neglect, or abdicating the valued roles of psychiatric nurses. Incorporating psychobiology will enable you to fine-tune your assessments, diagnoses, interventions, and evaluations of human response patterns. The synthesis of this critical thinking will provide clients and families with *quality* care cost-effectively.

Nursing science is still evolving, and you are positioned to move the knowledge base from intuition to science. We profess that psychoeducation assists in client compliance—how? How do people with positive symptoms learn? What clinical decision-tree do you use to assess whether a client needs a PRN medication for agitation, is having EPS, is anxious, wants "attention," or is trying to communicate? Which client populations can benefit from humor? Which stress-management interventions are best for someone with panic disorder versus someone in crisis? What early interventions in circadian dysregulation can promote healing for abused individuals (Glod 1992)? Does a caffeine challenge trigger physiologic arousal in PTSD as in people with panic disorder (Wolfe 1994)?

Change is an opportunity for you to be flexible, creative, and visionary. Keep a diary of how you made a difference for a client. Was a biologic variable involved? Communicate how you made a difference, and link it with cost-effectiveness. The care of people with psychiatric illness rarely uses technology, but often incorporates the technology to find the neuropathology. Your practice is the nurse-patient relationship and *all* the communication involved.

The exact biologic determinants for psychiatric disorders and behaviors remain elusive. To date there is no definitive biologic test to identify a psychiatric disorder. However, multifocal and multidisciplinary care incorporating psychobiologic dimensions will advance our ability to offer new, more effective assessments and less stigmatized interventions for our clients.

Chapter Highlights

- Anatomic systems within the brain such as the cortex and limbic system are associated with functions including memory, affect, and problem-solving. These may be dysfunctional in major psychiatric illnesses.
- From a psychobiologic perspective, the brain is the source of behavior, emotion, cognition, and "humanness." Molecules make each of us unique.
- One aspect of mood or behavior may be linked to more than one neuromessenger, and a single neuromessenger may be associated with more than one brain activity or behavior.
- Proteins, which are under the control of the genetic code, serve as information molecules to specify form and function of cells which determine behavior.
- Individuality and life experiences that modify basic personality result from various combinations of amino acids and the four nucleotides that make up proteins.
- The intercommunication between the endocrine and immune systems can promote coping during stress or facilitate psychiatric conditions.
- Understanding how the mesocortical neuromessengers interact provides you with the ability to predict negative symptom behaviors in clients with schizophrenia so that you can provide social skills training to supplement pharmacotherapy.
- Using the emerging data from psychobiology, such as the effect of biological rhythms on behavior, or negative symptom association with dopamine and serotonin, enables the psychiatric nurse to understand and advocate for the unique needs of the client.
- The communication pattern between DNA transcription from heritability, second-messenger reactivity, stress, and receptor signaling over time provides a model that changes pharmacologic responsivity for persons with bipolar mood disorder.

References

American Nurses Association: *A Statement on Psychiatric–Mental Health Clinical Nursing Practice and Standards of Psychiatric–Mental Health Clinical Nursing Practice.* American Nurses Association, 1994.

Berrettini WH, Ferro TN, Goldin LR, Weeks DE, Detera-Wadleigh S, Nurnberger Jr JI, Gershon ES: Chromosome 18 DNA markers for manic-depressive illness: Evidence for a susceptibility gene. *Proc Natl Acad Sci* 1994;91:5918–5921.

Bowman ES, Nurnberger Jr JI: Genetics of psychiatric diagnosis and treatment, in Dunner DL (ed): *Current Psychiatric Therapy*. Saunders, 1993.

Chrousos GP, Gold PW: The concepts of stress and stress syndrome disorders. *JAMA* 1992;267(9) :1244–1252.

Glod C: Circadian dysregulation in abused individuals: A proposed theoretical model for practice and research. *Arch Psychiatr Nurs* 1992;VI(6):347–355.

Goleman D, Gurin J (ed): *Mind/Body Medicine*. Consumer Reports Books, 1993.

Greden JF: The laboratory in psychiatry, in Dunner DL (ed): *Current Psychiatric Therapy*. Saunders, 1993.

Guyton A: *Textbook of Medical Physiology*, ed 8. Saunders, 1991.

Hellhammer DH, Wade S: Endocrine correlates of stress vulnerability. *Psychother Psychosom* 1993;60(1):8–17.

Insel TR, Winslow JT: Neurobiology of obsessive-compulsive disorders, in Jenike MA, Baer L (eds): *Obsessive-Compulsive Disorders: Theory and Management.* Year Book Publishers, 1990.

Kaplan HI, Sadock BJ: *Synopsis of Psychiatry: Behavioral Sciences, Clinical Psychiatry*, ed 6. Williams & Wilkins, 1991.

Kleinman JE, Hyde TM: Structural foundations of mental illness and treatment: Neuroanatomy, in Dunner DL (ed): *Current Psychiatric Therapy*. Saunders, 1993.

Krauss JB: *Health Care Reform: Essential Mental Health Services*. American Nurses Association, 1993.

must produce enzymes and absorb nutrients; and breathing stresses the respiratory system, which must exchange carbon dioxide and oxygen. More broadly and holistically, **stress** designates a broad class of experiences in which a demanding situation taxes a person's resources or coping capabilities, causing a negative effect. This broader definition approximates the humanistic perspective of this textbook. In this view, stress is a person-environment interaction. The source of the stress, the demanding situation, is known as a **stressor**. The internal state the stress produces is one of tension, anxiety, or strain.

There is no universally accepted definition of stress among stress theorists and researchers. An interactional view of stress, such as the one given above, is consistent with how nurses view human experiences. The theories of stress that follow are the perspectives in common use. Although they do tell us a great deal about responses to stressful situations, it is crucial for nurses to recognize that these explanations are not necessarily consistent with nursing's orientation. Such factors as causes, the situational context in which the stressful event occurs, and the psychologic interpretation of the demanding situation must be considered in a holistic, humanistic approach to the client. Axis IV of *DSM-IV* offers some general parameters for assessing the severity of stress.

Conflict as a Stressor

The concept of conflict is useful in identifying the stresses that help cause disturbed coping patterns. Conflict often explains such observable behaviors as hesitation, vacillation, blocking, and fatigue. **Conflict**—the coexistence of opposing desires, feelings, or goals—is frequently seen in the behavior of psychotic clients, who may have difficulty making even the simplest decisions.

These conflicts are the most likely to cause stress:

- Conflicts that involve social relations with significant people.
- Conflicts that involve ethical standards.
- Conflicts that involve meeting unconscious needs.
- Conflicts that involve the problems of everyday family living.

A conflict proceeds according to these four steps:

1. The person holds two goals simultaneously.
2. The person moves in relation to both of the goals, using (a) approach-avoidance movements or (b) avoidance-avoidance movements.
3. The person shows hesitation, vacillation, blocking, or fatigue.
4. Resolution occurs either temporarily or permanently.

Conflict with Approach-Avoidance Movements When a person holds two incompatible goals at the same time, the goals usually constitute an either-or situation. If the person chooses one goal, the other goal is rejected or abolished automatically. This situation is called a double approach-avoidance conflict. Here is an example:

Mrs R holds two goals. She wants to talk with the nurse about her fears of going back to work. At the same time, she wants not to be perceived as weak or "a bother." Mrs R makes a movement in relation to her first goal—talking to the nurse—by walking up to her. When the nurse stops and turns toward her, Mrs R asks some superficial question about her supper. In this way she avoids discussing her real concerns. When the nurse offers an opening to talk further, Mrs R avoids the conversation she needs by saying she wants to rest. An hour later, she rings the bell with an apologetic but vague question about her medication.

Vacillation describes Mrs R's behavior.

Principles That Explain Vacillation To understand how vacillation comes to be the manifest behavior and what is going on during a conflict situation like the one that was described above, we need to understand the following four key principles:

1. As you near a desirable goal, the approach tendency is strengthened.
2. As you near an undesirable goal, the avoidance tendency is strengthened.
3. The strength of the avoidance tendency always increases more rapidly with nearness to the goal than does the strength of the approach tendency.
4. The strength of both tendencies varies with the strength of the need basic to the tendencies. That is, an increased need can strengthen both tendencies and intensify the conflict, whereas a decreased need can weaken both tendencies and lessen the conflict.

Avoidance-Avoidance Conflict In avoidance-avoidance conflict, a person is faced with two undesirable goals at the same time. The person attempts to avoid the nearer of these two goals, but with the retreat from the nearer goal, the tendency to avoid the second goal increases. Unless the tendency to avoid one of the goals overpowers the tendency to avoid the other goal, or unless there is a third way out of the conflict, the person feels trapped by the conflict.

Robert P, the 35-year-old son of well-to-do parents, was strongly attracted to "the good life." He wanted to live in a creative, esthetic environment, read good books, attend the opera, drink quality wine. Simultaneously he wanted both to avoid working to earn the money for the lifestyle he desired

and to not depend on his parents for support. His lifestyle became one of waiting to find a resolution to his conflict. He neither worked nor accepted "handouts" from his family, but his preferred lifestyle became one that he talked about rather than lived.

The Fight-or-Flight Response to Stress

Beyond the routine and essential stress of everyday life, humans risk encountering undesirable or excess stress that threatens well-being and may even be life threatening. They cope with such threats through either a **fight** (aggression) or **flight** (withdrawal) response. The fight-or-flight response was first discussed by the physician Walter Cannon in 1932, when he identified stress as an actual cause of disease. Consider the following situation of extreme stress: A woman is walking down a dark, deserted street when a man with a knife emerges from the shadows just in front of her. Does she try to defend herself? Does she run away? Whichever action she takes is a result of a variety of physiologic responses to extreme danger. According to Mason (1980), when a person faces such a situation

- The heartbeat increases to pump blood throughout the necessary tissues with greater speed, carrying oxygen and nutrients to cells and clearing away waste products more quickly.
- Blood pressure rises as the heart rate increases.
- Breathing become rapid and shallow.
- Epinephrine and other hormones are released into the blood.
- The liver releases stored sugar into the blood to meet the increased energy needs of survival.
- The pupils dilate to let in more light; all the senses are heightened.
- Muscles tense for movement, for either flight or protective actions, particularly the skeletal muscles of the thighs, hips, back, shoulders, arms, jaw, and face.
- Blood flow to the digestive organs is greatly constricted.
- Blood flow to the brain and major muscles is increased.
- Blood flow to the extremities is constricted, and the hands and feet become cold. This response is protection against bleeding to death quickly if the hands or feet are injured in fight or flight and allows blood to be diverted to more important areas of the body.
- The body perspires to cool itself, because increased metabolism generates more heat.

Although these physiologic responses seem appropriate for the situation described, imagine the wear and tear on the body if humans responded to all stress in all of these ways.

Selye's Stress-Adaptation Theory

Hans Selye, a Canadian endocrinologist and the most well-known and widely recognized stress researcher, developed another framework for understanding how people respond to stress. According to Selye, each person has a limited amount of energy to use in dealing with stress. How quickly it is used and, therefore, how quickly one adapts to stress depend on several factors such as heredity, mental attitude, and lifestyle, among others.

Selye defines stress as the rate of wear and tear on the body (1956). He disputes the idea that only serious disease or injury causes stress. Selye thinks that any emotion or activity requires a response or change in the individual. Stressors can be physical, chemical, physiologic, developmental, or emotional. Playing a game of tennis, going out in the rain without an umbrella, having an argument, and getting a promotion are all examples of stressful events. Life itself is basically stressful because it involves a process of adaptation to continual change. Though the experience of adaptation is stressful, it is not necessarily harmful. Indeed, it can be exciting and rewarding under certain circumstances; and although we cannot avoid the stress of living, we can learn to minimize its damaging effects.

While a medical student, Selye made an interesting and important observation that became the cornerstone of his stress-adaptation theory. He observed that, regardless of the diagnosis, most clients had certain symptoms in common; they lost their appetite, they lost weight, they felt and looked ill, they were anxious and fatigued, and they had aches and pains in their joints and muscles. A long series of experiments (1956) led to more objective evidence of actual body damage: enlargement of the adrenal glands; shrinkage of the thymus, spleen, and lymph nodes; and the appearance of bleeding gastric ulcers.

Feelings of anxiety, fatigue, or illness are subjective aspects of stress. Though stress itself cannot be perceived, Selye found that it can be objectively measured by the structural and chemical changes that it produces in the body. These changes are called the **general adaptation syndrome (GAS)** because when stress affects the whole person, the whole person must adjust to the changes. The GAS occurs in three stages: alarm, resistance, and exhaustion. An example of the GAS can be found in combat soldiers. These men are exposed to ever-present threats of death and mutilation. They also experience the severe psychologic shock of witnessing the destructiveness of war. Other psychologic and interpersonal factors, such as the loss of personal freedom and separation from loved ones, contribute to their overall stress load. The experiences of combat soldiers can be used to illustrate the three stages of the GAS, which are summarized in Table 4–1.

Table 4–1 The General Adaptation Syndrome

Stage	*Physical Change*	*Psychosocial Changes*
Stage I: Alarm reaction Mobilization of the body's defensive forces and activation of the fight-or-flight mechanism	Release of norepinephrine and epinephrine causing vasoconstriction, increased blood pressure, and increased rate and force of cardiac contraction; increased hormone levels; enlargement of adrenal cortex; marked loss of body weight; shrinkage of the thymus, spleen, and lymph nodes; irritation of the gastric mucosa	Increased level of alertness; increased level of anxiety; task-oriented, defense-oriented, inefficient, or maladaptive behavior may occur.
Stage II: Stage of resistance Optimal adaptation to stress within the person's capabilities	Readjustment of hormone levels; reduction in activity and size of adrenal cortex; lymph nodes return to normal size; weight returns to normal	Increased and intensified use of coping mechanisms; tendency to rely on defense-oriented behavior
Stage III: Stage of exhaustion Loss of ability to resist stress because of depletion of body resources	Decreased immune response with suppression of T cells and atrophy of thymus; depletion of adrenal glands and hormone production; weight loss; enlargement of lymph nodes and dysfunction of lymphatic system; with continued exposure to the stressor, cardiac failure, renal failure, or death may occur.	Exaggerated defense-oriented behaviors; disorganized thinking; disorganization of personality; misperception of sensory stimuli with appearance of illusions; reduced reality contact with appearance of delusions or hallucinations; with continued exposure to the stressor, stupor or violence may occur.

ALARM REACTION When soldiers first encounter the stress of war, they experience the *alarm reaction.* During the alarm reaction, the body undergoes biochemical reactions, such as the production of the adaptive hormones adrenocorticotropic hormone (ACTH), cortisone, and aldosterone. Biochemical reactions also enlarge the adrenal cortex and lymph nodes. These changes lower the person's overall resistance. For example, soldiers may show such behavioral changes as increased irritability, sleep disturbances, and recurrent nightmares. Soldiers are described as being hypersensitive to minor stimuli. For instance, they will leap up in fright at the sound of a branch cracking. This behavior generally indicates a failure to maintain psychologic integration.

STAGE OF RESISTANCE Many soldiers are able to adjust to combat. As they do so, the next stage, *resistance,* occurs. During this stage, biologic changes in hormone levels, the adrenal cortex, and lymph nodes are reversed. These soldiers can maintain their psychologic integrity. They may become used to killing and may even take pride in it. They may be able to maintain a fatalistic attitude about their own and their comrades' survival. Soldiers who have made this adjustment may be able to resign themselves to fate and believe that they are serving in the military for an important purpose, even though they cannot fully understand it. They may take comfort in the thought that combat will not last long, or that they will soon be rotated out of the combat area to take on a less stressful role.

The nature of this adaptation seems to depend on many psychologic and social factors. These include the stability of the soldier's personality, the morale of the combat unit, the sense of security and control provided by the leadership, and the friendships the soldier forms with other soldiers, which provide emotional support.

STAGE OF EXHAUSTION The third stage, *exhaustion,* occurs if stress continues over a prolonged period. It also occurs when multiple stressors are active simultaneously, or when the person undergoes repeated or overwhelming stress. When too many life changes occur within a short time, there is not enough time for the body to accommodate and adjust. Adaptive energy is exhausted, and the body surrenders to stress. The adrenal glands again enlarge and then are depleted. The lymph nodes enlarge, producing a subsequent dysfunction of the lymphatic system. There is an increase and then a decrease in hormone levels.

The longer soldiers are in combat, the more vulnerable and anxious they are likely to feel. Prolonged combat lowers tolerance to stress. It may produce increased anxiety, depression, tremulousness, and impairment of judgment and self-confidence. This decompensation results in disturbances in interpersonal relationships. The soldier may lose all sense of loyalty to comrades. In some cases, the residual effects of combat exhaustion persist for a long time. Combat experience may continue to disturb former soldiers after they return to civilian life. They may experience guilt about killing and have nightmares about war experiences.

Exhaustion may be reversible if the total body is not affected and if the person can eventually eliminate the source of stress. However, if stress is unrelieved, or if the body's defenses are totally involved, the person may not regain psychologic stability and may become physically ill.

Selye's theory has stimulated extensive research on the neuroendocrine mechanisms underlying stress. The consequent research into psychoendocrinology has brought Selye's model into question (McCain and Smith 1994). Some research has demonstrated that neuroendocrine response differs for different stressors, and that there is individual variance in the sensitivity to psychosocial stimuli (Lazarus and Folkman 1984; Smith 1993).

Life Changes as Stressful Events

Most people are accustomed to thinking of untoward events as stressful, but they do not realize that desirable events such as job promotions, vacations, or outstanding personal achievements may also prove stressful. Holmes and Rahe (1967) studied life changes as stressful events to learn the amount of social readjustment required to cope with them. These authors believe that life events that require coping behavior tend to decrease a person's ability to handle illness or subsequent stress. Since Holmes and Rahe began their research, other investigators have raised cautions about applying this model indiscriminately. These cautions are discussed later in this section.

Their research assigned ratings to forty-three different life changes, called *life change units* (*LCUs*). They asked subjects to indicate what life changes had occurred in the past year and then to add up the points assigned to each one. According to these researchers, a low score indicated that the subject was not likely to have an adverse reaction. A "mild" score meant that there was a 30% chance that the person would manifest the impact of stress through physical symptoms. People in the "moderate" category had a 50% chance of a change in health status, and a "high" score meant an 80% chance of major illness in the next two years. High LCU scores also correlated with an increased probability of accidental injury. This example demonstrates the LCU model:

Marcia M, a 22-year-old woman in group therapy, had recently been divorced from her husband (LCU 73) after attempting to achieve a marital reconciliation (LCU 45). Marcia's pregnancy (LCU 40) earlier in the year was uneventful, and the couple's healthy son was born on June 2 (LCU 39). At 6 weeks of age, the child suddenly and unexpectedly died in his crib (LCU 63). The Ms began to argue frequently (LCU 35) before they made the decision to divorce. After the divorce, Marcia found herself short of funds (LCU 38) and went to work as a waitress in a pizza restaurant (LCU 36). She found it necessary to move to a less expensive apartment (LCU 20). In the period of one year, Marcia accumulated an LCU score of 390 and was in the high-risk group.

In the early 1970s, other researchers correlated life stress events and mental health. In a study of 720 households in a metropolitan area, Meyers and his associates (1972) found a relationship between a high number of life changes and changes in the mental status of individuals. For example, an increase in the number of life changes preceded worsening of psychiatric symptoms, whereas a decrease in life changes brought improvement. The more stressful the life changes, the greater the likelihood of mental illness. Meyers and his associates also found that entrance-related life events (those involving the addition of a new person into one's social sphere, perhaps through marriage or the birth of a child) produced less symptomatology than did exit-related events (those associated with the loss of a valued individual or status).

APPLICATION TO CLINICAL PRACTICE Nurses applying the Holmes and Rahe model should be aware of the following cautions. This model is based on several assumptions that depict a person as a passive recipient of stress.

- It assumes that events affect all people in the same way, regardless of how the individuals perceive the event.
- It assumes that there is a common threshold beyond which disruption occurs.
- It assumes that the same amount of adaptation is required for each event among all people.
- It equates "change" with "stress" (Lyon and Werner 1987).

To understand the effects of life changes on health, the nurse needs to identify what each individual perceives as stressful. Only then can the nurse use the Holmes and Rahe model to help people become aware of the stress they face in their lives. It is also useful in planning for the future. To return to the example of Marcia M who had accumulated an LCU score of 390:

During the course of group therapy, Marcia shared her desire to return to college and complete the junior and senior years of a medical technology program in which she had been enrolled before her marriage. To do so, she would have to make a number of changes: move to an apartment close to the college because she could not afford to own a car, change her working hours or job so that she could attend day classes, change her sleeping habits, change her recreational and social activities, and reduce her other expenses to pay school costs. The changes required would add almost 200 LCUs to her score.

In group, Marcia was able to consider this information and reevaluate her goals. She decided to delay her return to school until she could get on her feet financially. She chose not to make any other changes in her life for the present time.

Clients can use this information, much as Marcia did, to help decide when it is advantageous or disadvantageous to engage in a life change. This knowledge helps them make responsible decisions about the directions their lives will take. You can assist clients by incorporating the guidelines below in your practice:

- Help clients recognize when a life change occurs.
- Encourage clients to think about the meaning of the change and identify some of the feelings associated with the change.
- Discuss with clients the different ways they might best adjust to the event.
- Encourage clients to take time in arriving at decisions.
- If possible, encourage clients to anticipate life changes and plan for them well in advance.
- Encourage clients to pace themselves. It can be done, even if they are in a hurry.
- Encourage clients to consider the accomplishment of a task as a part of daily living and to avoid looking at such an achievement as a stopping point or a time for letting down.

Stress as an Interaction

Richard Lazarus, a pioneering theorist and researcher in stress, coping, and health, is known for his interactional approach to understanding stress. His view is reflected in the definition of stress given at the beginning of this chapter. Lazarus (1966, 1976) sees perceived threat—what the person appraises as taxing or exceeding his or her resources and endangering his or her well-being—as the central characteristic of stressful situations, and in particular, a threat to a person's most important goals and values. Once a person has perceived a threat, the person evaluates it by thinking about it. This process is termed *cognitive appraisal*. According to Lazarus, the process works like this:

1. The person assesses the potential for benefit, harm, loss, threat, or challenge in a situation. This is termed *primary appraisal*.
2. The person then evaluates his or her coping resources and options in the situation. This is termed *secondary appraisal*.
3. The person applies the coping resources and options at his or her disposal. This is termed *coping*.
4. The person engages in ongoing reinterpretation of the situation based on new information. This is termed *reappraisal*.

Cognitive appraisal and coping style are influenced by the person's culture. Providing culturally sensitive care requires understanding the client's perspective and recognizing that a client's cognitive appraisal of a situation may, and probably will, differ from your own.

Lazarus believes that stress depends not only on external conditions but also on the person's physical vulnerability and the adequacy of that person's coping styles.

Psychoneuroimmunology Framework

Psychoneuroimmunology (PNI) offers a comprehensive framework for understanding the relationship between stress and disease and the biopsychosocial nature and complexity of the stress process. As discussed in Chapter 3, PNI is concerned with interaction among the neurologic, endocrine, and immune systems and takes into account the nature of the influence of psychosocial factors on immune function and health outcomes. Cells in the brain and the endocrine and immune systems produce neuropeptides, the chemical messengers that are links between the mind and the body.

Neuropeptide manufacture is activated by positive mental states and suppressed by negative mental states. Several stress and coping-related studies have suggested that some people have *self-healing personalities,* while others have *disease-prone personalities*. Self-healers are emotionally stable people who bounce back from stressful situations (Friedman and VandenBos 1992). These are people whom others describe as enthusiastic, joyful, secure, energetic, alert, and content. They are likable and have close, warm relationships with others. Borysenko (1993) reports a doubling of N-K cell activity (natural killer lymphocytes that attack virally infected cells and tumor cells in the body) in people with a sense of connectedness as opposed to people who are lonely and isolated.

A now classic study on hardiness and health found that individuals who have strong feelings of confidence in their ability to control circumstances, a willingness to see life events as challenges rather than as obstacles, and a strong commitment to the experiences and demands of daily living have fewer illnesses than those who lack these qualities (Kobasa 1979).

Disease-prone personalities, on the other hand, tend to display negative emotions. They are suspicious of others and tend to be chronically anxious, angry, or depressed. These chronic negative emotional patterns are linked with various physiologic changes such as activation of the sympathetic nervous system, increase in the level of cortisol, and suppression of the immune system, leading to increased vulnerability to illness (Rogers et al. 1994).

As you can see, each of the theories discussed previously contributes to our understanding of stress and coping. However, none is complete in and of itself. PNI offers a comprehensive framework for understanding stress-disease relationships by taking the best of what these theories offer and integrating them with the increasing body of evidence on how stress can alter immunologic functioning and, consequently, disease susceptibility and pathology. The Mind-Body-Spirit Connection box in

Chapter 27 is an example of the multifaceted nature of this framework.

Anxiety

Anxiety is a state of varying degrees of uneasiness or discomfort. It is frequently coupled with guilt, doubts, fears, and obsessions. Beyond the mild level, anxiety is often described as a feeling of terror or dread; anxiety is believed to be the most uncomfortable feeling a person can experience. In fact, anxiety is so uncomfortable that most people try to get rid of it as soon as possible.

Anxiety is a potent force because the energy it provides can be converted into destructive or constructive action. When used constructively, anxiety can stimulate the action necessary to alter a stressful situation, fill a painful need, or arrange a compromise. A client who understands the source of anxiety is best able to use it constructively.

The Neurobiologic Basis of Anxiety

Contemporary thinking about anxiety includes a neurobiologic component. Anxiety is now thought to result, at least in part, from dysregulation of one or more neurotransmitters and their receptors. Most research has focused on the BZ-GABA-chloride complex, although several other neurotransmitters and their receptors such as serotonin, norepinephrine, and the neuropeptide cholecystokinin may play a role in the development of anxiety (Salzman et al. 1993). The neurobiologic component of anxiety is more fully discussed in Chapter 16.

Sources of Anxiety

Anxiety is an inevitable result of the attempt to maintain equilibrium in a changing world. People experience anxiety in many different situations and interpersonal relationships. However, the general causes of anxiety have been classified into two major kinds of threats:

1. Threats to biologic integrity: actual or impending interference with basic human needs such as the needs for food, drink, or warmth.
2. Threats to the security of the self:
   a. Unmet expectations important to self-integrity.
   b. Unmet needs for status and prestige.
   c. Anticipated disapproval by significant others.
   d. Inability to gain or reinforce self-respect or to gain recognition from others.
   e. Guilt, or discrepancies between self-view and actual behavior.

It is crucial to understand that either actual *or* impending interference may cause anxiety; actual interference with a biologic or psychosocial need is not a necessary condition. All that is necessary is the *anticipation* of one of these major threats.

Threats to biologic integrity or to the fulfillment of such basic human needs as food, drink, warmth, and shelter are a general cause of anxiety. Threats to the security of self are not as easily categorized. In some instances, they are obvious; in others, they are more obscure because each person's sense of self is unique. To one person, power and prestige may be essential; to another, independence; to a third, being of service to others.

Consider the last category—being of service to others. Suppose that Mrs C, a nurse, is convinced that a client would feel much better if he expressed his fears to her. But no matter how often she provides the opportunity, he insists, "This is not the time to talk about it," and thwarts her attempt. She is not able to help him in a way that is important to her sense of self. In addition, she believes that the unit's head nurse (whose communication skills she admires) expects her to have been successful in this endeavor. When unmet needs or expectations related to essential values (such as being of service to the client) are coupled with the actual or anticipated disapproval of others who are important (the head nurse), anxiety is generated.

Anxiety as a Continuum

Many theorists conceptualize anxiety as a continuum (Figure 4–1). Mild to moderate anxiety can be functionally effective in that it helps us focus our attention and generates energy and motivation. Thus, anxiety is an aspect of problem solving in that it alerts us to the need to concentrate our resources. However, severe anxiety and panic narrow our attention to a crippling degree. Under these conditions alertness is greatly reduced, and learning does not usually take place.

Mild Anxiety Mild anxiety (+) helps one deal constructively with stress. A mildly anxious person has a broad perceptual field because mild anxiety heightens the ability to take in sensory stimuli. Such a person is more alert to what is going on and can make better sense of what is happening with others and the environment. The senses take in more; the person hears better, sees better, and makes logical connections between events. The person feels relatively safe and comfortable. Because learning is easier when one is mildly anxious, mild anxiety helps clients learn, for instance, how best to administer their own insulin. Mild anxiety can also help a nursing student review psychiatric–mental health nursing before a final examination.

Moderate Anxiety In moderate anxiety (++), a person remains alert, but the perceptual field narrows. The

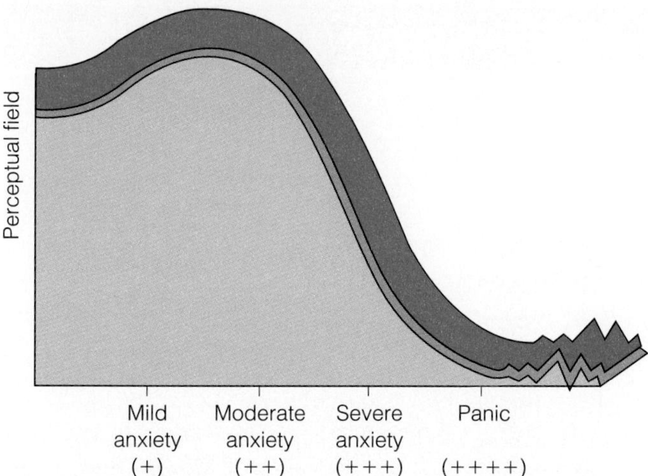

Figure 4-1 The effect of anxiety on the perceptual field. Notice that the perceptual field is increased in mild anxiety, becomes increasingly constricted as anxiety increases, and is completely disrupted at the panic level.

moderately anxious person shuts out the events on the periphery while focusing on central concerns. For example, a nursing student who is moderately anxious about the final examination may be able to focus so intently on studying that she or he is not distracted by an argument between roommates, loud music on the stereo, and a rousing chase scene on television. The student shuts out the chaos in the environment and focuses on what is of central personal importance—preparing for the exam. This process of taking in some sensory stimuli while excluding others is called **selective inattention.**

People also use selective inattention to cope with anxiety-provoking stimuli. This phenomenon may account for the anxious preoperative client who fails to remember what the nurse said about postoperative pain or the need to cough and deep-breathe after surgery.

Although the perceptual field is narrowed and the person sees, hears, and grasps less, there is an element of voluntary control. Moderately anxious individuals can, with direction, focus on what they have previously shut out.

SEVERE ANXIETY In severe anxiety (+++), sensory reception is greatly reduced. Severely anxious people focus on small or scattered details of an experience. They have difficulty in problem solving, and their ability to organize is also reduced. They seldom have the complete picture. Selective inattention may be increased and may be less amenable to voluntary control. The person may be unable to focus on events in the environment. New stimuli may be experienced as overwhelming and may cause the anxiety level to rise even higher.

The sympathetic nervous system is activated in severe anxiety, causing an increase in pulse, blood pressure, and respiration and an increase in epinephrine secretion, vasoconstriction, and even body temperature. A multitude of physiologic changes may be observed, which are described in the section that follows.

PANIC The panic level of anxiety (++++) is characterized by a completely disrupted perceptual field. Panic has been described as a disintegration of the personality experienced as intense terror. Details may be enlarged, scattered, or distorted. Logical thinking and effective decision making may be impossible. The person in panic is unable to initiate or maintain goal-directed action. Behavior may appear purposeless, and communication may be unintelligible.

Assessing Anxiety

Anxiety can be assessed in the physiologic, cognitive, and emotional/behavioral dimensions. This observation illustrates the relationship between the mind and the body. Anxiety is a multidimensional phenomenon in that the total person is involved in every aspect of it. Objective data, particularly nursing observations, may be critical because of the nature of anxiety. Selective inattention and dissociation interfere with the client's awareness of anxiety and ability to give accurate reports. Families and friends also can contribute data useful to the assessment of anxiety.

PHYSIOLOGIC DIMENSION Observations of the client's physiologic state are likely to indicate autonomic nervous system responses, particularly sympathetic effects. Various organs may be affected, such as the adrenal medulla, heart, blood vessels, lungs, stomach, colon, rectum, salivary glands, liver, pupils of the eyes, and sweat glands (See Figure 16–1 in Chapter 16). Anxious clients may have an increased heart rate, increased blood pressure, difficulty breathing, sweaty palms, trembling, dry mouth, "butterflies in the stomach" or a "lump in the throat," as well as other symptoms.

Laboratory tests are not routinely done to evaluate anxiety because observation is faster and more accurate. However, anxiety affects the results of laboratory tests done for other purposes. Blood studies may show increased adrenal function, elevated levels of glucose and lactic acid, and decreased parathyroid function and oxygen and calcium levels. Urinary studies may indicate increased levels of epinephrine and norepinephrine.

COGNITIVE DIMENSION Assessment of cognitive function may indicate difficulty in logical thinking, narrowed or distorted perceptual field, selective inattention or dissociation, lack of attention to details, difficulty concentrating, or difficulty focusing. The level of anxiety determines the extent to which cognitive function is affected. Mild, moderate, severe, or panic level of anxiety is assessed according to the descriptions earlier in this chapter.

EMOTIONAL/BEHAVIORAL DIMENSION In the emotional/behavioral dimension, clients may be irritable, angry, withdrawn, and restless, or they may cry. The affective response can often be assessed through the client's subjective description. Clients may describe themselves as "on edge," "uptight," "jittery," "nervous," "worried," or "tense." They may feel dizzy or faint and may experience a feeling of impending doom as if something terrible were about to happen.

Coping with Stress and Anxiety

Nurses can be helpful if they understand the changes their clients are undergoing. Reactions to threatening situations, such as illness and hospitalization, can be divided into two general categories: task-oriented responses and defense-oriented responses. When we feel competent to deal with stress and the situation is not too threatening to our sense of self, our behavior tends to be task-oriented. Task-oriented behavior is geared toward problem solving. Consider the situation of a student who is majoring in mathematics and fails his courses. If he is not too frightened by the possibility that he may not be suited for a career in this field, he can assess the situation and change his major. This is a task-oriented reaction. It is based on a realistic appraisal of the situation and involves a series of carefully thought-out judgments about what course of behavior would be most effective.

When we feel inadequate to cope with stress and the situation is extremely threatening to our sense of self, we tend to engage in defense-oriented behavior. The diagnosis of a terminal illness, for instance, may be so overwhelming that a person must temporarily defend against acknowledging this reality. Everyone uses defense-oriented behavior from time to time as a protective measure. Such behavior becomes harmful only when it is the predominant means of coping with stress. In such cases, problem-solving and reality-based behavior are continually avoided.

Coping strategies are a set of behaviors people under stress use in struggling to improve their situations. Coping strategies can be thought of simply as ways of getting along in the world.

Everyday Ways of Coping with Stress

Everyday coping strategies offer an immense repertoire of defenses to maintain control and balance in the face of stress. A person can cope on different levels, including

RESEARCH NOTE

Citation

Cooper CL, Faragher EB: Psychosocial stress and breast cancer: The inter-relationship between stress events, coping strategies and personality. *Psychol Med* 1993;23:653–662.

Study Problem/Purpose

These investigators had previously studied the relationships between disease severity in women with breast cancer and the occurrence of stressful life events. The purpose of this study was to gather all potential psychosocial factors explored in previous studies in order to examine the relationships between disease severity in women with breast cancer and stressful life events, personality predisposition, and coping strategies.

Methods

A four-part questionnaire was completed by 2163 women. The questionnaire included a demographic section, a 42-item life events inventory, an adapted Type A behavior inventory, and a list of 36 coping strategies. The subjects were assigned to one of four categories according to their breast condition diagnosis: cancer, cyst, benign, and normal.

Findings

The cancer group tended to be older, widowed smokers who were retired or employed only part-time, and had experienced losses. The most surprising finding was that women who are regularly exposed to high amounts of stress are not at highest risk for breast cancer. The mediating factor was the women's ability to express emotions such as anger. The ability to express emotions appears to reduce the risk of developing serious breast disease.

Implications

This study validates the importance of the counselor and educator roles for nurses in helping clients modify illness-generating behaviors. Helping clients learn to express feelings, to reframe life events so that the possible positive benefits of change can be appreciated, and to lead an engaged, socially interactive life are important nursing intervention strategies.

physical, social, cognitive, and emotional levels. However, the devices people choose to cope with stress depend on many factors. Among them are the external circumstances, the suddenness and intensity of the stress, the resources available to the person, and the person's predisposition to certain coping patterns, established over the course of one's development. One man who is late for an appointment because he gets caught in a traffic jam may react with a furious outburst of anger. Another may begin to daydream and forget where he is going. A third may use the time to solve some problem.

Most often, individuals use behaviors that have worked well for them in the past. Sometimes they behave in a certain way because it is the only method they have of coping with stress or because other coping strategies failed to work. Some people learn to turn to others for protection and nurturance; some learn to turn to chemicals or food; some rely on self-discipline and keeping a stiff upper lip; others feel better after the intense expression of feelings; some withdraw physically and/or emotionally; still others exercise or talk the problem out. Common coping methods are discussed below.

TURNING TO A COMFORTING PERSON The earliest coping strategy is probably the familiar method of turning to a nurturing person for soothing and protecting. Receiving love is being reassured that one is lovable. Love from supportive others may take the form of physical touching, rocking, patting, or verbal reassurances of various kinds ("Don't be afraid, I'll stay with you"). Bible study or listening to religious tapes is comforting to many people. This category also includes eating in times of stress and for general support. Alcohol, nicotine, and other chemicals are often used to enhance well-being in the face of stress. Many theorists view these alternatives as substitutes for the dependent comfort of being a baby in the care of a nurturing parent.

RELYING ON SELF-DISCIPLINE Whereas some people under stress tend to turn to the comfort of friendly company, food, or alcohol, all of which are reminiscent of childhood dependence, others rely on self-discipline. Self-control ranks high in the value system of many cultures and subcultures. This coping style involves pride in the ability to laugh off problems, endure frustrations, and discount anxiety. Keep a stiff upper lip, bite the bullet, and get over it are all admonitions that people address to themselves when self-discipline is their patterned response to stress. These people are unlikely to want the company of supportive others and may even push them away. They are often unresponsive when others seek comfort from them, for they see such dependent behavior as weak.

INTENSE EXPRESSION OF FEELING Crying, swearing, and laughing all tend to relieve tension. Swearing loses its usefulness as an escape valve if it becomes a habit. This is less true of both crying and laughing. Crying and laughing tend to release energy and exert a soothing effect on a person who is experiencing tension.

AVOIDANCE AND WITHDRAWAL While some people find it hard to sleep when they are under tension, others react to worries, bad news, or an argument with somnolence. Still others respond with a form of waking sleep like apathy or emotional withdrawal, which accomplishes the same thing.

TALKING IT OUT Many people relieve tension by talking it out. Talking implies establishing and maintaining a contact of sorts with another human being. In addition, it enables new ideas to emerge and new perspectives to be entertained. Obviously, this device is the medium of most therapeutic intervention. One research study found that over 50% of the study population reported that their preferred method of coping was to talk to someone (Ziemer 1982). This finding has profound implications for nursing because nurses are the health care providers who spend the most time with clients. It also has profound implications for clients whose communication is dysfunctional or whose ability to communicate freely is restricted. Psychiatric clients generally fall into these categories.

PRIVATELY THINKING IT THROUGH Some people believe that the unexamined life is not worth living. When faced with a problem that causes them anxiety, these individuals become introspective about it. The rationalizations that emerge serve as effective tension relievers.

WORKING IT OFF Physical activity to relieve tension may range from simple gestures like finger tapping, floor pacing, and door slamming to activities purposely designed to alter the tension-producing circumstances, such as aerobic exercise. In addition, some tense individuals feel a lot of aggressive energy. Physical exertion in the form of demanding sports, like jogging or racquetball, or manual labor, like scrubbing the floor, is a way to use this energy constructively.

USING SYMBOLIC SUBSTITUTES Stress may be relieved by ascribing symbolic values to acts or objects. These acts or objects may or may not have other meanings. There are symbolic devices for the management of tensions in religious practices such as confession, prayer, or sacrifice. For some people, the automobile has a symbolic significance; others ascribe symbolic significance to their annual income or their physical appearance.

The list is almost endless, but the principle is always the same. Some people attach a meaning beyond the obvious one to objects, experiences, and people, through which they find a means to reduce their tensions.

SOMATIZING Many organs of the body have an expression and communication function. This is sometimes known as *somatizing* or *organ language*. Some organs communicate their messages only to their owner. For example, the heart may communicate by means of palpitation. Other demonstrations are public, such as blushing or stuttering. Urination and defecation, increased sweating, and altered sexual activity are other familiar examples of organ language.

Coping Resources

Early research on coping was concerned with how people respond to specific stresses in a laboratory setting. More recent studies that consider the whole being in interaction with the environment have led to viewing coping as a dynamic process that involves the demands and restrictions on a person as well as the resources available.

GENERALIZED RESISTANCE According to Antonovsky (1980), people stay healthy or cope adequately with stress because they possess what he calls *generalized resistance resources (GRRs),* factors in the person, group, or organization that help in managing tension.

Physical and biochemical GRRs are physiologic characteristics, such as genetic features and levels of immunity. These GRRs also include interaction of the nervous and endocrine systems that help in adaptation; for example, interactions involving ACTH, thyroid-stimulating hormone or TSH, vasopressin, norepinephrine, and insulin and their influence on human behavior. Not only are individuals different in their genetic and biochemical makeup, but the physiologic effects of illness and stress may also alter a person's ability to use physical and biochemical GRRs positively.

Material goods and relative wealth constitute the *artifactual and material GRRs;* having these attributes makes it easier to cope with illness. Money helps to ensure the best health care available. Effective coping is often interrelated with one's socioeconomic status simply because the higher the status, the greater the resources to help the person cope. For example, household help not only relieves an ill person's worries but also reduces the practical burden.

Cognitive GRRs have to do with intelligence and knowledge. When people know about stressors, they can avoid them. They can also predict when periods of stress are imminent and thus reduce their impact. Knowing what community services are available is also a cognitive GRR.

People who are self-aware—who know their own capacities and potentials and have a well-developed sense of themselves—possess *emotional GRRs*. Emotional GRRs determine the extent of psychologic hardiness. In general, they have to do with how competent and self-assured one feels.

Valuative and attitudinal GRRs are the products of a person's culture and environment. People are apt to respond in learned ways. The attitudinal aspect also is related to how flexible, rational, and farsighted the person is. The more rational or accurate one's appraisal of a threatening situation and the more flexible one is in approaching the situation and envisioning the consequences, the greater one's resources for coping.

Interpersonal-relational GRRs are available social support systems. The greater a person's social contacts, the greater the social resources available to augment the ability to deal with stress. Love, affection, and nurturance are hallmarks of interpersonal-relational GRRs.

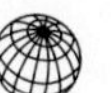

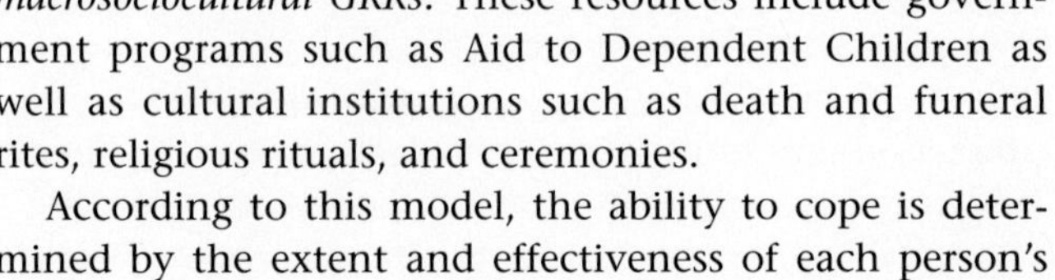

Institutional structures that facilitate coping are called *macrosociocultural GRRs*. These resources include government programs such as Aid to Dependent Children as well as cultural institutions such as death and funeral rites, religious rituals, and ceremonies.

According to this model, the ability to cope is determined by the extent and effectiveness of each person's generalized resistance resources. Yet the actual process of coping remains unclear. Theorists and researchers still do not fully understand exactly which personal resources should be mobilized and under which conditions.

Defense-Oriented Ways of Coping: Defense Mechanisms

The coping strategies described above are considered normal. They are simply ways of getting along. In some people, however, what passes for a normal adjustment is actually a very tenuous one with few outlets for controlled aggression, few love objects, few opportunities for satisfaction and growth. These people find it more and more difficult to cope with additional stress. Ultimately, the external stress the person is trying unsuccessfully to ward off is matched by a mounting internal stress. The person suffers both from increased anxiety and from the strain on overworked stabilizers. And what happens to the person who has no one to talk with, who can't jog five miles, or who can't laugh off the problem?

When a person is unable to ward off stress or reduce tension in the usual way, anxiety mounts as the person feels increasingly inadequate to cope with the situation. Under these circumstances, the person is more likely to engage in *defense-oriented behavior.* Defense-oriented behavior is not a specific attempt to solve a problem; it consists of using mental mechanisms to lessen uncomfortable feelings of anxiety and to prevent pain regardless of cost. These characteristic mental mechanisms are commonly called **defense mechanisms.** They are automatic psychological processes that protect the self by allowing the person to deny or distort a stressful event or to restrict awareness and reduce the sense of emotional involvement. But they can also interfere with rational decision making. People who use defense mechanisms are excluding some information about the situation they are in.

They are also denying their own feelings about it.

Defense mechanisms are primarily unconscious and often inflexible coping patterns that protect a person through intrapsychic (coming from within) distortions that are really self-deceptions. The person usually has little awareness of what is happening or even less control over events. Although these reactions may help keep the lid on anxiety, they also limit the ability to grow from and savor the experience, they interfere with rational decision making and the ability to work productively, and they impair and erode interpersonal relationships. Even adaptive devices can go wrong.

Because human behavior is so complex and varied, defense mechanisms can be classified in many ways. Often, they are classified according to whether they are simple or complex, whether they are most likely to arise in a specific phase of development, or whether they are commonly associated with a particular form of psychopathology. Definitions of various defense mechanisms overlap, and the same observed behavior may often be explained by more than one type of defense. And people do not use one method of defense at a time; they usually rely on a combination of defenses. For study purposes, the common defense mechanisms discussed here are repression, suppression, dissociation, identification, introjection, projection, denial, fantasy, rationalization, reaction formation, displacement, and intellectualization. They are summarized in Table 4–2.

REPRESSION **Repression**, the basis of all defense mechanisms, is the dynamic behind much of "forgetting." When people repress, they unconsciously exclude distressing emotions, thoughts, or experiences from awareness. Repression bars access to conscious awareness of feelings and thoughts that would cause anxiety and disrupt the self-concept. It also affords protection from a

Table 4–2 Defense Mechanisms

Name	*Definition*	*Example*
Repression	Unconsciously keeping unacceptable feelings out of awareness.	A man is jealous of a good friend's success but is unaware of his feelings.
Suppression	Consciously keeping unacceptable feelings and thoughts out of awareness.	A student taking an examination is upset about an argument with her boyfriend but puts it out of her mind so she can finish the test.
Dissociation	Handling emotional conflicts, or internal or external stressors, by a temporary alteration of consciousness or identity.	A woman has amnesia for the events surrounding a fatal automobile accident in which she was the speeding driver.
Identification	Unconscious assumption of similarity between oneself and another.	After hospitalization for minor surgery, a girl decides to be a nurse.
Introjection	Acceptance of another's values and opinions as one's own.	A woman who prefers a simple lifestyle assumes the materialistic, prestige-oriented values of her husband.
Projection	Attributing one's own unacceptable feelings and thoughts to others.	A man who is quite critical of others thinks that people are joking about his appearance.
Denial	Blocking out painful or anxiety-inducing events or feelings.	A manager tells an employee he may have to fire him. On the way home, the employee shops for a new car.
Fantasy	Symbolic satisfaction of wishes through nonrational thought.	A student struggling through graduate school thinks about a prestigious, high-paying job she wants.
Rationalization	Falsification of experience through the construction of logical or socially approved explanations of behavior.	A man cheats on his income tax return and tells himself it's all right because everyone does it.
Reaction formation	Unacceptable feelings disguised by repression of the real feeling and by reinforcement of the opposite feeling.	A woman who dislikes her mother-in-law is always very nice to her.
Displacement	Discharging pent-up feelings on people less dangerous than those who initially aroused the emotion.	A student who has received a low grade on a term paper blows up at his girlfriend when she asks about his grade.
Intellectualization	Separating an emotion from an idea or thought because the emotional reaction is too painful to be acknowledged.	A man learns from his doctor that he has cancer. He studies the physiology and treatment of cancer without experiencing any emotion.

MIND-BODY-SPIRIT CONNECTION

Repressed Memories: Controversial, Unusual, and Sometimes Bizarre Occurrences

At the turn of the century, Sigmund Freud proposed that we actively and deliberately bury painful or dangerous memories beyond the reach of consciousness. He called this process repression.

According to Freud, repressed memories influence behavior, thinking, and emotions, and produce mental symptoms. Early in his career Freud wrote that sexual abuse in childhood was common and was the cause of repression. This abuse, and the resulting repression, caused the "hysteria" he diagnosed in his patients. After 1897, Freud abruptly abandoned his theory on repression. Instead, he said, children have fantasies of being seduced. These imagined seductions, according to Freud, cause internal conflict, and repression is a way of coping with this internal conflict.

It is unclear why Freud abandoned his theory. Some of his critics believe that Freud bowed to social pressure and the threat of professional ostracism because the notion of rampant childhood sexual abuse was outrageous. Others of his critics believed that Freud himself distorted his patients' stories because of his own psychological problems.

To understand the concept of repression, we need to understand how memory works. Memories are stored in a portion of each of the thousands of neurons in the brain. Each neuron represents a little bit of memory. Because the brain is such a complex organ, it parcels out bits and pieces of an experience to different parts of the brain. For example, memories of sound are parceled out to the auditory cortex, memories of appearance to the visual cortex, memories of sensation to the sensory cortex, memories of smell to the olfactory cortex, and source memory to the frontal cortex. All scattered memory fragments remain physically linked. It is the limbic system that takes on the job of assembling these bits and pieces. The limbic system actually acts as a neural file clerk by pulling memory fragments from various file drawers. Intensely traumatic events produce unusually strong nerve connections.

Memory can go awry if the terror of an experience is so great that the biological processes underlying information storage are disrupted. However, the right biological stimulus can set the nerve circuits firing and trigger fear. The source of the fear is *not* remembered. Memory blocks come at great cost. They leave a person without an explanation for bewildering emotional distress that causes turmoil.

Memory can also be confounded; that is, snippets

sudden trauma until the person can deal with the shock. From the individual's point of view, a repressed memory is "forgotten" and cannot be deliberately brought to awareness (see the Mind-Body-Spirit Connection box). Although the repressed feelings remain unconscious, they continue to exert pressure for expression. The self tries to maintain the repression, but in people experiencing extreme stress or anxiety, or in febrile (feverish) or toxic states, repression may begin to fail. Clients who are intoxicated by alcohol or drugs or who are emerging from anesthesia may verbalize feelings that they usually repress.

Susan was raped. She was brought to an outpatient clinic by her roommate. Susan said she felt very anxious and could not recall the circumstances surrounding her rape or what the rapist looked like. Her use of repression protected her from facing her fears and humiliation.

Nursing Intervention Strategies Nursing intervention in such cases should be supportive and protective of the client's defenses. After the initial shock has lessened and the client's anxiety level has been reduced, you can help the client examine the traumatic event.

SUPPRESSION **Suppression** is an intentional act that helps keep thoughts, feelings, wishes, or actions that cause anxiety out of conscious awareness. Suppression is the conscious form of repression.

A woman, who is an only child, learns that her elderly widowed mother has been diagnosed with cancer. The woman recognizes that she will be the sole support of her mother during this trying time. She also has some professional responsibilities that cannot be put off. The woman decides to put off worrying about what the future may bring or anticipating her mother's death until her mother's diagnostic studies are completed, an accurate staging of the cancer can be performed, the first chemotherapy sequence has been completed, and a realistic prognosis is made of her mother's chances for a remission. As she puts it: "I've got too much to do and can't afford to fall apart right now."

MIND-BODY-SPIRIT CONNECTION *(continued)*

of memory from a real event can be interwoven with snippets of an imagined event. Recent research by Elizabeth Loftus has demonstrated that the mere suggestion that you could have once been lost in a shopping mall can leave a memory trace in the brain. This memory trace can then become linked to the memory of a friend's or sibling's story of being lost, a fairy tale such as Hansel and Gretel, as well as actual memories of shopping malls. Under stress and over time, the knowledge that being lost in a mall was only a suggestion deteriorates. If you're asked at a later time if you were ever lost in a mall, your brain will activate these assorted images, and eventually you "remember" being lost in a mall as a child.

These findings—that memories are open to faulty recollection or that they can be created through a suggestion from another—have caused great distress for survivors of childhood sexual abuse who experience the phenomenon called **recovered memory.** Recovered memories of childhood sexual abuse are those that emerge into consciousness after being repressed for a period of time, sometimes for years. Imagine what it must be like having recalled long-forgotten memories of painful and humiliating sexual abuse by a trusted or loved adult. Imagine further what it must be like to have your unsettling memories viewed with suspicion. You might feel helpless, hopeless, and lost. Your sense of self would be fragmented, and your self-esteem diminished; your spiritual distress would be heightened.

The recent rise in reported cases of recovered memory has led to a large number of lawsuits against perpetrators accused of having committed acts of abuse years ago. An organization, the False Memory Foundation, assists those claiming to be wrongly charged with abuse. (The False Memory Foundation is more completely discussed in Chapter 23.) Essentially, people who have recovered repressed memories are pitted against alleged perpetrators who claim these memories are actually manufactured **false memories.** Therapists who work to help people recover repressed memories are pitted against memory researchers who claim that false recovered memories are fabricated in the highly charged atmosphere of mental health therapy.

Psychiatric nurses need to be aware of both sides of the issue. Remember that many persons who have experienced sexual abuse have a history of not being believed by parents or others they love or trust. Expressing disbelief will only cause the client further pain. Being compassionate will help clients in the struggle to examine their own lives.

Carol Ren Kneisl, MS, RN, CS

Clients may refuse to consider their difficulties by saying that they "don't want to talk about it" or that they will "think about it some other time." This, too, is suppression.

Nursing Intervention Strategies Suppression can be dealt with in the same way as repression. Suppression is generally easier to deal with because the material remains conscious. You can be somewhat more directive in assessing why the client avoids talking about a situation. Suggest that the client try to look at the situation because it affects future plans. Offering information about the situation may help clients look at their situations objectively. As they learn more, they may feel less threatened.

DISSOCIATION In **dissociation,** the individual handles emotional conflicts, or internal or external stressors, by a temporary alteration of consciousness or identity (see Chapter 16 for specific mental dysfunctions in which dissociation is the major mental mechanism). Dissociation resembles repression, but it has a different origin. The self is formed through the process of disapproval and approval from significant other people. Therefore, the self *dissociates,* or refuses awareness of, the expression of personal qualities and experiences of which significant others disapprove. These feelings come to exist separately from the person's self-concept. A little girl with artistic abilities that are not validated by her parents will not think of herself as artistic. She may deny her abilities even when other people point them out.

People who dissociate do not "notice" what they are doing. This limitation of awareness is maintained because the person experiences anxiety whenever permissible levels for the self are trespassed.

Ms T consciously believes that sexual overtures are wrong, yet she behaves seductively toward men. She cannot understand why men see her behavior as a sexual invitation. The use of dissociation complicates Ms T's problems. She needs to ignore or deny aspects of her situation to feel comfortable in it. Other people notice and point out Ms T's seductive behavior, but she cannot recognize it because it is not a part of

her self-concept. If Ms T admitted her sexual feelings, she would experience severe anxiety and personality disorganization.

For a discussion of nursing intervention strategies for dissociation, see Chapter 16.

IDENTIFICATION **Identification** is the wish to be like another person and to assume the characteristics of that person's personality. It represents a turning away from our own personality. Identification is unconscious. In this it differs from *imitation,* which is the conscious copying of another person's qualities. Identification with people we admire can serve an important function in maturation by evoking latent qualities. For instance, a little girl who identifies with her mother and sisters thus learns the behavioral characteristics of womanhood.

The most primitive type of identification is seen in the infant's relationship with the mother. Infants seem to perceive no difference between their mothers and themselves and only gradually become aware that their mothers exist apart from them. Small children deal with people in terms of how these people meet their needs. They do not see them as separate individuals with needs of their own. Such identifications may persist into adult life in people who have not differentiated themselves psychologically from seemingly powerful parents.

One specific manifestation of identification is passiveness in relationships. People who feel they have no resources of their own will overvalue the resources of others and expect to be taken care of. People who are most identified with their parents tend to be people who were not allowed to develop their own individuality. Part of the process of self-realization occurs in adolescence, when we discard, with much anxiety and insecurity, our identification with the parents on whom we have been so dependent. Some clients may not have achieved a degree of self-identity sufficient to do this. Identification can inhibit our usefulness, because it prevents us from focusing on our own capacities.

Identification can be seen in clients who rely heavily on the nurse's advice and support. They expect that all their needs will be met and that nothing will be expected of them.

Mr L is diabetic. He is not interested in learning about the diet he must follow and the medication he must take. He expects the nurse to take responsibility for seeing that he gets the right food and medicine. Identification prevents him from being self-reliant.

Nursing Intervention Strategies Nurses who work with clients like Mr L should clarify what the client's expectations of the nurse are and then correct any misperceptions about the nurse's role. It is important to help Mr L increase his own skills and take responsibility for his own care. Initially, you can offer the client collaboration and interdependence. The long-term goal in dealing with identification is for the client to formulate a self-care plan independently.

INTROJECTION **Introjection** is closely related to identification. It is the process of accepting another's values and opinions as one's own if they contradict the values one had previously held. A man whose employer engages in shoddy workmanship may introject his employer's values even though they are contrary to his own moral beliefs because he is afraid of losing his job. Introjection also occurs in severe depression following the death of a loved one. The depressed person may assume many of the deceased person's characteristics, and in so doing lose some self-awareness. As a nurse, you can treat introjection like identification, remembering that introjection is more primitive and more intractable. It originates in our experience of being fed as infants. We incorporate people and objects into ourselves in the same way that we swallowed food. We felt a sense of oneness with everything in the external world and could not differentiate ourselves from others. Because thinking processes are not involved in the first experience of introjection, this defense mechanism tends to be difficult to explore on the verbal level.

PROJECTION **Projection** is an unconscious means of dealing with personal difficulties or unacceptable wishes by attributing them to others. We blame other people for our shortcomings or see them as harboring our own unacceptable feelings or thoughts. In the course of development, the child, needing parental approval, will identify with the parents and will also deny what they seem to condemn or fail to acknowledge. For instance, if her parents do not openly express and recognize angry feelings, a little girl will tend to regard anger as dangerous. She will then deny awareness of her own anger. Anger in others will disturb her, and she will tend to condemn in others the anger she cannot accept in herself. It is common knowledge that people often tend to criticize others for their own unacknowledged inferiorities. The person who fears being taken advantage of is often an opportunist.

In adult life, projection can be destructive if it interferes with our ability to acknowledge our own feelings. The tendency to attribute our own undesired feelings to others also blurs the boundaries between ourselves and others. This, in turn, makes it difficult to understand other people's feelings. People who make excessive use of projection tend to attribute to others hostile or seductive motives that do not actually exist. This prevents them from forming trusting and reciprocal relationships.

Linda G is wary and suspicious of every man she meets. Regardless of how they behave toward her, Linda says: "They

only want one thing." She interprets their behavior as sexually suggestive but has no awareness of her own sexual interest in them.

A tendency to projection may also interfere with problem solving. A young woman who believes she is failing a course because of her teacher will not focus her energies on her studies.

Nursing Intervention Strategies Clients who must deal with the stress of serious illness may shift the blame for their condition onto you, the nurse. They may complain of poor nursing care to a nurse who is actually very skillful. These clients may actually fear that they have caused their own problems by neglecting their health. They may believe that they are being "paid back" for wrongdoing in the past. If you feel that such a client is accusing you falsely, do not show anger or retaliate but show, through consistency and attention, that you respect the client and are concerned about his or her welfare.

As clients feel more secure in the nurse-client relationship, encourage them to explore the realistic aspects of their situation. For example, you can help a man who blames his family for his alcoholism objectively explore what is known about the etiology of alcoholism. This may help him come to terms with his feelings of guilt and anger. This type of intervention helps the client separate his own feelings from the objective facts of the situation.

DENIAL **Denial** of reality is one of the simplest of the defense mechanisms. In denial, painful or anxiety-producing aspects of awareness are blocked out of consciousness. The reality of a situation is either completely disregarded or transformed so that it is no longer threatening. Denial is one of the most common defenses against the stress of diagnosis and illness and is typically present in the first few minutes of adjustment to the death of a loved one. It may be helpful as a temporary protection against the full impact of a traumatic event.

A father reacts with denial when he shouts, "No, it can't be true; there must be a mistake," when told his 8-year-old son has just died in the trauma unit of injuries incurred when his bicycle collided with an automobile.

A young woman admitted to a psychiatric hospital because of acute anxiety and frightening hallucinations says she just "needs a rest."

Nursing Intervention Strategies Sometimes denial is the best solution for the client. In such situations, support the denial. A terminally ill client who believes she will soon recover and who cannot think about her illness should be allowed the protection of denial. Not all clients need to face up to reality. You should recognize that the use of denial may be preventing serious personality disorganization.

Sometimes, however, denial is directly harmful to the client, as when a man refuses to take medication that is crucial to his survival. In such cases, the motivation for the client's behavior should be assessed. After discovering the protective function the denial is serving, focus on helping the client meet these needs in a way that is not self-destructive. You can also help by not reinforcing patterns of denial but rather focusing on instances when the client seems to be dealing with reality.

FANTASY **Fantasy** is a form of nonrational mental activity that enables the individual to temporarily escape the demands of the everyday world. Fantasies are not confined by the reality considerations of cause and effect and time and space. Fantasy normally characterizes the thinking of children before they are able to engage in consensually validated communication. Adults revert to fantasy during times of stress to obtain a symbolic satisfaction of wishes.

A businesswoman facing financial difficulties temporarily escapes by daydreaming that she is enjoying a luxurious vacation on a Caribbean island.

Another woman with advanced multiple sclerosis imagines herself a famous ballerina with complete control of her body.

A man whose wife has told him she wants a divorce imagines how much his wife will appreciate him now that he has been diagnosed with cancer.

Fantasy may offer temporary relief from pressures, but people who spend too much time in fantasy may be unable to meet the requirements of reality.

Clients who are very ill may fantasize that when they recover, many good things will happen to them. They may imagine that they will receive special recognition in their work or that they will get along better with their families. These fantasies may help such clients deal with the deprivations caused by illness. However, they may also create unrealistic expectations. The fantasies may make one feel good temporarily but interfere with problem solving.

Nursing Intervention Strategies Clients who engage in fantasy related to their illness need gradual help in assessing the responses others are likely to make and the achievements they themselves may realistically expect. Clients who fail to adjust to reality will be disappointed when their expectations are not met.

A helpful approach that will not devastate clients who need to hold on to some fantasy is to ask them to discuss their specific future plans. Examining the details of work and interpersonal adjustment may help a person relinquish unrealistic expectations and make more realistic plans. For example, the man who believes that a diagnosis of cancer will improve his marriage because his wife will appreciate him more fully must recognize that this is improbable. He needs to examine the real effects his illness will have on her. He must plan how to make specific improvements in their communication by anticipating problem areas.

Imagination does have a creative aspect, however. Fantasies have a richness and variety that is lacking in the everyday world. Certain artists, such as Dalí and Picasso, enriched their works of art through fantasy. Evidence also exists that insights leading to scientific discovery do not come about as the result of step-by-step logical thinking. Rather, they are created through fantasy.

RATIONALIZATION **Rationalization** is the attribution of "good" or plausible reasons for questionable behavior to justify it or to deal with disappointment. Rationalizing helps us avoid social disapproval and bolster flagging self-esteem.

A nurse fails to return to the bedside of the elderly nursing home client despite a promise to do so before leaving work. She feels her behavior is justified because the client has problems with recent memory and probably wouldn't remember anyway.

Many people use rationalization because they wish to prove to themselves or others that their actions are governed by reason and common sense, even though they may not fully understand the reasons for their own behavior. Such explanations may be essential to maintaining personal integrity. They are not destructive as long as they do not prevent one from solving everyday problems.

Rationalization becomes more of a hindrance when it prevents us from making necessary changes in our behavior by interfering with our ability to examine that behavior. One sign of rationalization is an active search for reasons to justify our behavior or beliefs. Another is an inability to recognize inconsistencies in our beliefs. A third is being upset when our reasons are questioned, since each questioning threatens our defenses.

Clients may use rationalization to soften the blow of losses caused by illness. For instance, a man who is ill may give up work prematurely after rationalizing that he wouldn't have been successful in that field anyway. Such unnecessary restrictions deprive us of possible achievements.

Nursing Intervention Strategies Nurses must respect the client's need to rationalize fears and insecurities they cannot face. However, hold out to clients the possibility for change. You can help clients face the reality of their situation by encouraging them to explore ways they can change to deal with it more effectively. One way is to help them explore in detail past instances in which they did change to cope with a stressful situation. Believing and recognizing that we have real strengths helps us face our areas of insecurity.

REACTION FORMATION **Reaction formation** is a defense whereby we keep an undesirable impulse out of awareness by emphasizing its opposite. To protect ourselves from recognizing dangerous feelings, we develop conscious attitudes and behavior patterns that are just the opposite of those feelings. Hostility may be concealed behind a facade of love and kindness. The desire to be sexually promiscuous may be concealed behind a moralistic demeanor. People who use this defense are not conscious of their true feelings.

Some people who crusade passionately against alcohol or pornography may have an underlying wish to enjoy these things. Clues that reaction formation is occurring are an inappropriate intensity of feeling and the inability to consider alternative points of view. A person who is always unnaturally sweet and loving and cannot consider the possibility of being angry is probably using this excess of feeling to counteract an unacceptable degree of anger.

Reaction formation can be useful. It can help us maintain socially approved behavior and avoid the awareness of desires that are not socially acceptable. But this defense, too, results in self-deception, because it is not under conscious control. Therefore, it may result in exaggerated or rigid behaviors that leave us ill-equipped to deal with crisis. People who feel they can never express annoyance and discomfort may need to be "good" clients, who never question their care or make demands. Such clients may not be able to allow themselves to depend on others. They may not be able to acknowledge their needs and seek fulfillment. This rigid stance is a reaction formation against the unconscious wish to be completely dependent. It also prevents the person from meeting a crisis with flexibility, because many possible actions are blocked from awareness. People who use this defense may also be excessively harsh in dealing with other people's weaknesses. They may be unable or unwilling to help others because they think people should be able to solve their own problems.

Nursing Intervention Strategies A client manifesting reaction formation requires essentially the same approach as one manifesting repression. Respect and support the client's defenses while providing a secure relationship in which to explore feelings and new behavioral alternatives. Also be aware that it is easy to be annoyed at clients who cannot face their true feelings. The rigid and excessive display of what seems to be an insincere emotion can be frustrating. Remember that these clients are not "lying" or pretending. They are unconsciously protecting themselves against recognizing threatening feelings.

DISPLACEMENT **Displacement** is the discharging of pent-up feelings, generally hostility, on an object less dangerous than the object that aroused the feelings. This defense is used when emotions are aroused in a situation where it would be dangerous to express them.

John has just failed an important examination. He believes his failure was the instructor's fault. He cannot express the full extent of his anger, because that would get him into worse trouble with the instructor. John goes quietly back to the dormitory. But when his roommate turns the stereo on too loud, John explodes. He doesn't fear retaliation from his roommate—they are peers and friends.

In some cases, we turn our anger toward another person inward on the self. When this happens, we experience exaggerated self-accusations and guilt.

Nursing Intervention Strategies Clients may express inappropriate anger to the nurse when they are actually angry at someone or something else. The client may feel more secure with the nurse, who offers a safe target for displaced feelings. Displacement differs from projection in that people who use displacement are not distorting their feelings and attributing them to someone else. The feelings are clear, and the person acknowledges them. They are simply being directed at the wrong person. Therefore, it may be easier to help these clients acknowledge the real situation by remaining calm and accepting during an angry outburst. For example, after the outburst is over, say, "You seem so angry; I wonder if you really are angry because your breakfast is cold or if there might be some other reason." Opening up the possibility for a discussion of anger may help these clients to sort out just why and at whom they are angry.

INTELLECTUALIZATION **Intellectualization** is the process of separating the emotion aroused by an event from ideas or opinions about the event because the emotion itself is too painful to acknowledge. The painful emotion is avoided by means of a rational explanation that divests the event of any personal significance. Failures are less significant if one believes that the situation could have been worse.

A woman whose husband recently died deals with her grief by telling her friends in a rational manner that it was better that he died suddenly by heart attack rather than to have died at the end of a long, chronic illness.

A boy who breaks his pelvis while skiing consoles himself after the accident by saying, "I would rather have a broken hip than a broken neck."

Clients may use intellectualization to blunt the emotional impact of their problems. This may be difficult for the nurse to perceive, because such clients often seem to know a great deal about their condition. They may be able to discuss in great detail the metabolic processes in diabetes or the psychodynamics of anxiety. At the same time, they cannot apply these concepts to their own situation in an emotional sense.

Nursing Intervention Strategies Intellectualization resembles rationalization in that it provides a verbal means of dealing with anxiety. Its use closes off the possibility of accepting and working out problems. Clients often use intellectualization at the onset of a crisis, and the need for this defense may decrease in a supportive nurse-client relationship. You can help the client relate emotionally to a problem by not forcing the expression of feeling. This will only frighten the client further. Asking these clients to explain how their knowledge relates to them personally may encourage them to accept and explore their emotional reactions.

Chapter Highlights

- Stressful situations tax a person's resources or coping capabilities, causing a negative effect. The source of the stress is known as a stressor.
- Selye's stress-adaptation theory can be used to explain the physiologic effects of stress.
- In the psychobiologic view, stress is a function not only of external conditions but also of the physical vulnerability of the person and the adequacy of that person's coping styles.
- Anxiety is an uncomfortable feeling that stems from threats to biologic integrity and the security of the self.
- Nurses can expect clients and their families to become anxious in the face of unknown or potentially painful, dangerous, or disfiguring events.
- Stress, life changes, and threats to one's self-concept cause anxiety and place additional coping demands on the individual.
- The choice of coping strategy often depends on external circumstances, the suddenness and intensity of the stress, the resources available to the person, and a predisposition to a certain coping pattern.
- People cope with stress in a variety of ways that seem to have worked in the past. Some talk it over with others; some jog; others pray or laugh off the problem.

- When someone is unable to ward off stress or reduce anxiety in the usual way, tension mounts. People may have to rely on largely unconscious and inflexible coping patterns that are self-deceptive.
- Anyone may use defense mechanisms to cope with anxiety or stress, but a healthy person tends to use problem-solving methods more often.
- Defense mechanisms include repression, suppression, dissociation, identification, introjection, projection, denial, fantasy, rationalization, reaction formation, displacement, and intellectualization.

References

Ader R, Felton DL, Cohen N (eds): *Psychoneuroimmunology,* 2nd ed. Academic Press, 1991.

Aldwin C, Revenson TA: Does coping help? A reexamination of the relation between coping and mental health. *J Pers Soc Psychol* 1990; 41:131–134.

Antonovsky A: *Health, Stress, and Coping.* Jossey-Bass, 1980.

Barnfather JS, Lyon BL (eds): Stress and coping: State of the science and implications for nursing theory, research and practice. Sigma Theta Tau International, Center Nursing Press, 1993.

Benner P, Wrubel J: *The Primacy of Caring: Stress and Coping in Health and Illness.* Addison-Wesley, 1989.

Borysenko J: *Fire in the Soul: A New Psychology of Spiritual Optimism.* Warner Books, 1993.

Botsis AJ, Soldatos CR, Liossi A, Kokkevi A, Stefanis CN: Suicide and violence risk: I. Relationship to coping styles. *Acta Psychiatr Scand* 1994;89:92–96.

Cohen LJ: Psychiatric hospitalization as an experience of trauma. *Arch Psychiatr Nurs* 1994;8(2):78–81.

Cooper CL, Faragher EB: Psychosocial stress and breast cancer: The inter-relationship between stress events, coping strategies and personality. *Psychol Med* 1993;23:643–662.

Cousins N: *Head First: The Biology of Hope.* Dutton, 1989.

Dahl J, O'Neal J: Stress and coping behavior of nurses in Desert Storm. *J Psychosoc Nurs* 1993;31(10):17–21.

Eysenck H: Personality, stress, and disease. *Psychological Inquiry* 1991; 2:221–232.

Floyd JA: Nursing students' stress levels, attitude toward drugs, and drug use. *Arch Psychiatr Nurs* 1991;5(1):46–53.

Friedman H, VandenBos G: Disease-prone and self-healing personalities. *Hosp Comm Psychiatr* 1992;43(12):1177–1179.

Godbey KL, Courage MM: Stress-management program: Intervention in nursing student performance anxiety. *Arch Psychiatr Nurs* 1994;8(3):190–199.

Holmes TH, Rahe RH: The social readjustment rating scale. *J Psychosom Res* 1967;11:213–218.

Kiecolt-Glaser JK, Glaser R: Psychoneuroimmunology: Can psychological interventions modulate immunity? *J Cons Clin Psychol* 1992;50:569–575.

Kobasa SC: Stressful life events, personality, and health; An inquiry into hardiness. *J Pers Soc Psychol* 1979;37:1–11.

Kobasa SC, Maddi SR, Kan S: Hardiness and health: A prospective study. *J Pers Soc Psychol* 1982;42:168–177.

Lazarus RS: *Patterns of Adjustment.* McGraw-Hill, 1976.

Lazarus RS: *Psychological Stress and the Coping Process.* McGraw-Hill, 1966.

Lazarus RS, Folkman S: *Stress, Appraisal, and Coping.* Springer, 1984.

Lyon BL, Werner J: Stress: Ten years of practice-relevant research, in Werley H, Fitzpatrick J (eds): *Annual Review of Nursing Research.* Springer, 1987.

Mason LJ: *Guide to Stress Reduction.* Peace Press, 1980.

McBride AB: Mental health effects of women's multiple roles. *Am Psychol* 1990;35:381–384.

McCain NL, Smith JC: Stress and coping in the context of psychoneuroimmunology: A holistic framework for nursing practice and research. *Arch Psychiatr Nurs* 1994;8(4): 221–227.

Meyers J, et al: Life events and mental status. *J Health Human Behav* 1972;1:398–406.

Outlaw FH: Stress and coping: The influence of racism on the cognitive appraisal processing of African Americans. *Issues Ment Health Nurs* 1993;14:399–409.

Peebles-Kleiger MJ, Kleiger JH: Re-integration stress for Desert Storm families: Wartime deployments and family trauma. *J Traumatic Stress* 1994;7:173–193.

Pennebaker JW: *Opening Up: The Healing Power of Confiding in Others.* Morrow, 1990.

Rahe RH: Life change events and mental illness: An overview. *J Human Stress* 1979;5:2–10.

Rogers M, et al.: Prevalence of medical disorders in patients with anxiety disorders. *Int J Psychiatry in Medicine* 1994;24(1):83–96.

Salzman C, Miyawaki EK, Le Bars P, Kerrihard TN: Neurobiologic basis of anxiety and its treatment. *Harvard Rev Psychiatr* 1993;1(4):197–206.

Selye H: *Stress Without Distress.* American Library, 1974.

Selye H: *The Stress of Life.* McGraw-Hill, 1956.

Smith JC: *Understanding Stress and Coping.* Macmillan, 1993.

Tache J, Selye J: On stress and coping mechanisms. *Issues Ment Health Nurs* 1985;7:3–24.

Tartasky DS: Hardiness: Conceptual and methodological issues. *Image* 1993;25(3):225–229.

Vollhardt LT: Psychoimmunology: A literature review. *Am J Orthopsychiatr* 1991;61(1):35–47.

Wade SL, Monroe SM, Michelson LK: Chronic life stress and treatment outcome in agoraphobia with panic attacks. *Am J Psychiatr* 1993;150:1491–1495.

Warner SL: Humor: A coping response for student nurses. *Arch Psychiatr Nurs* 1991;5(1):10–16.

Williams JM, Hogan TD, Andersen MB: Positive states of mind and athletic injury risk. *Psychosom Med* 1993;55: 468–472.

Williams R, Williams V: *Anger Kills.* Harper, 1994.

Wolinski K: Self-awareness, self-renewal, self-management. *AORN* 1993;58(4):721–730.

Ziemer MM: Coping behavior: A response to stress. *Top Clin Nurs* 1982;2(4):8.

References for Mind-Body-Spirit Connection Box

Kneisl CR: Authentic recovered memory or reconstructed false memory? Today's biggest story in psychiatry. *Capsules and Comments in Psychiatric Nursing* 1994;1(2):1–3.

LeDoux JE: Emotion, memory and the brain. *Sci Am* 1994;270:50–57.

Loftus EF: The reality of repressed memories. *Am Psychol* 1993;48:518–536.

Ofshe R, Watters E. *Making Monsters: False Memories, Psychotherapy, and Sexual Hysteria.* Charles Scribner's Sons, 1994.

Terr L: *Unchained Memories: True Stories of Traumatic Memories, Lost and Found.* Basic Books, 1994.

CHAPTER 5

PSYCHIATRIC EPIDEMIOLOGY IN A CULTURALLY DIVERSE SOCIETY

Beth Moscato

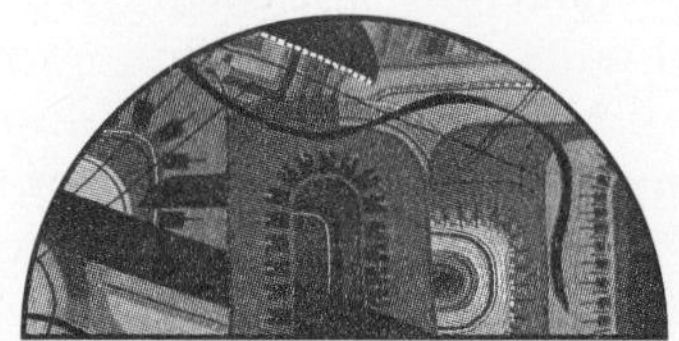

COMPETENCIES

- *Define and identify three uses of psychiatric epidemiology.*
- *Explain the natural history of disorder, including its four stages.*
- *Describe the three levels of prevention, and give one example of how each level may be used by psychiatric nurses.*
- *List four risk factors associated with mental disorders, demonstrating sensitivity to cultural diversity.*
- *Define prevalence rate, and name the two most prevalent mental disorders as reported by the National Comorbidity Survey.*
- *Define comorbidity, and discuss research findings concerning a highly comorbid group in the general population.*
- *Specify three care-seeking patterns related to the use of mental health services.*
- *Evaluate when and how you might apply epidemiologic principles in your psychiatric nursing practice.*

Cross-References

Other topics relevant to this content are: Psychobiology, Chapter 3; Assessment, Chapter 8; Communication skills, Chapter 7; Ethics, Chapter 10; Nurse's values, Chapter 1; Psychiatric theories, Chapter 2; Culture-bound syndromes, Appendix C; Clients with a dual diagnosis, Chapter 25.

Critical Thinking Challenge

Psychiatric nurses often focus on a particular client in a clinical setting. Does such a client represent "what kind" and "how much" mental disorder is "out there" in the community? Are you willing to expand your nursing skills by considering the community itself as a potential "client" for mental health assessment and services? How can you apply principles of psychiatric epidemiology to your psychiatric nursing experiences for population groups as well as individual clients? How might a client's cultural and ethnic background influence this process?

The practice of psychiatric nursing traditionally focuses on the individual, group, family, and therapeutic use of the surrounding environment (milieu). Various disciplines, such as psychiatric nursing, can be grouped according to their underlying principles and methods. Epidemiology represents an emerging specialty that focuses on human populations rather than on individual clients per se. "Epidemiology" consists of these three Greek word roots: *epi,* meaning "among"; *demos,* meaning "people"; and *logos,* meaning "doctrine"—the doctrine of what is among or happening to people.

Epidemiologists often study the psychobiosocial factors that influence health status in populations. Epidemiologic principles and methods may be applied to determine the cause of a disorder (such as HIV), to assess risks associated with a harmful exposure (such as rape), to determine whether a particular treatment (such as behavior therapy) is effective, and to identify health service utilization needs and trends. Psychiatric epidemiology is particularly useful to the psychiatric nurse as the basic discipline for preventive and community psychiatry.

Hundreds of millions of people worldwide in both developing and developed countries suffer from psychiatric disorders causing personal suffering, social disruption, and economic losses. The worldwide occurrence of psychiatric disorders prompts nurses to address multicultural diversity as principles of psychiatric epidemiology are applied to various human populations. The United States represents a multiethnic country consisting of numerous subgroups who have brought unique cultural traits with them from waves of immigration over years. Minority subcultures include, but are not limited to, African Americans, Hispanics (Mexican Americans, Puerto Ricans, Cuban Americans), Asian Americans (Chinese, Japanese, Koreans, Pacific Islanders), and native Americans (American Indians, Eskimos). General considerations of cultural diversity that may influence the experience, expression, reporting, and evaluation of psychiatric disorders will be discussed within this chapter.

Psychiatric Epidemiology: An Overview

An important premise of psychiatric epidemiology is that mental illness is not randomly distributed across populations. Not all people are at equal risk for developing mental disorders. One client may be depressed, another may be psychotic, while a third may suffer from debilitating physical illness. Such differences in the occurrence of mental disorders are of prime interest in epidemiology. A brief overview of psychiatric epidemiology will serve as a foundation for the subsequent application of epidemiologic principles to your work in psychiatric nursing.

This chapter focuses on an overview of mental disorders in general. Examples of important concepts frequently emphasize depression because it is among the most common disorders in the United States today.

Psychiatric epidemiology is the study of the distribution and determinants of mental disorders (or other health-related conditions or events) in human populations. Purposes include prevention, surveillance (monitoring), and the control of mental disorders. Epidemiology traditionally investigated the cause of disease. More recently, "disease" has been generalized to include a wide variety of mental disorders and health-related problems. Health-related conditions or events may include injuries; exposure to environmental pollutants, natural and man-made disasters, and traumatic or violent events; behavioral problems; and the nonuse or misuse of mental health services. This chapter uses the word "disorder" rather than "disease" to reflect current perspectives in the field of psychiatric epidemiology.

A psychiatric epidemiologist is an investigator who studies mental disorders or other health-related conditions or events in defined populations to develop a comprehensive picture of mental health problems and to evaluate interventions. An advanced professional degree (masters or Ph.D.) from a school of public health or similar institution is required. Epidemiologists ask, "Which characteristics among individuals (such as genetic) or their environment (such as exposure to stressful life events) explain differences in morbidity from specific mental disorders?" Nursing provides an excellent background for investigating disease occurrence and its relation to various characteristics of individuals or their environment.

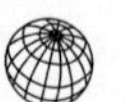

Within the context of psychiatric epidemiology, **cultural diversity** refers to a sensitivity to cultural and ethnic background that may influence the expression, reporting, and evaluation of mental disorders. Considerations of cultural diversity related to mental disorders will be interwoven throughout this chapter.

Uses of Psychiatric Epidemiology

Psychiatric epidemiology is used to do the following:

- Determine causative factors for specific disorders.
- Identify groups of people (populations) at high risk of developing specific disorders.
- Recognize changes in health problems, especially the emergence of new problems.
- Plan for current health needs and predict future needs.
- Evaluate preventive and therapeutic measures.

It is important to note that both the patterns of occurrence of mental disorders in a community and the patterns of delivery of psychiatric care are studied. The services offered influence and are influenced by the amount and nature of the disorders and by changes in modes of therapy.

Historical Perspectives

Historically, epidemiology as a science evolved from the study of epidemics such as cholera. Past interest focused mainly on acute infectious diseases with short duration. In the past few decades, increasing attention has been focused on the epidemiology of chronic diseases, such as cancer, coronary heart disease, and mental disorders.

Initial Studies Prior to World War II A primary objective of a community-based study is to provide information about the proportion and range of mental disorders as they appear in the general population. The first investigation regarding the frequency of mental disorders in the United States was conducted by Dr. Edward Jarvis in Massachusetts (Jarvis 1972). Community leaders and hospital records were surveyed to estimate the frequency of "insanity" and "idiocy," the two major psychiatric classifications at that time. Approximately sixteen community studies were carried out prior to World War II using agency records and key informants to identify cases of mental disorder. When information was collected in this manner, the median for all types of disorders among studies was only 3.6% (Dohrenwend and Dohrenwend 1982).

Epidemiologic Studies Following World War II World War II stimulated interest in mental health issues because psychiatric problems were cited as the largest factor in nonacceptance by the armed forces. Rates of psychiatric reactions (combat fatigue, "shell shock," and situational stresses such as extreme deprivation in concentration camps) varied in relation to combat stress. This growing public awareness of mental disorders prompted epidemiologic studies in the general population. Most of the sixty studies conducted during this time relied on direct interviews using symptom scales to measure overall mental impairment. Such measures were economical, easy to administer, and avoided traditional diagnostic categories. When information was collected in this manner, the median for all types of mental disorders among studies was 20% (Dohrenwend and Dohrenwend 1982).

The studies described thus far were not uniform and could not easily be compared. There was no consensus among researchers regarding the definition of mental disorders, mental disorder assessment tools, or specific research methods. These studies did not produce estimates of specific psychiatric disorders to address public health concerns in the United States.

Epidemiologic Catchment Area (ECA) Studies The landmark ECA studies, funded by the National Institute of Mental Health, were carried out at five different geographic sites to comprehensively study mental disorders in both community and institutionalized populations. These extensive studies had the following noteworthy characteristics: improved case definition, improved research design, improved diagnostic criteria *(DSM-III)*, standardized diagnostic interviews, and computerized data processing (Eaton et al. 1984; Regier et al. 1984).

The primary objective of the ECA studies was to estimate prevalence rates for specific mental disorders, that is, to indicate "how much" and "what kind" of mental disorders were of public health concern. A **prevalence rate** measures the number of people in a population who have a disease or disorder at a given time (Rothman 1986). Prevalence estimates may be established for varying time periods, such as one year or a lifetime. A lifetime prevalence estimate measures the number of people who have *ever* experienced a particular disorder. Emphasis was placed on specific mental disorders to obtain information regarding etiology (cause), clinical course, and treatment responses of each major disorder.

The following summarizing statements highlight major findings from the ECA studies (Robins, Locke, and Regier 1991):

- 32.2% of the population (18 years and older) met criteria for at least one mental disorder in their lifetime.
- Alcohol abuse/dependence, phobia, drug abuse/dependence, and major depression were the most common disorders.
- There is an increase in affective and anxiety disorders in women.
- Antisocial personality and alcohol abuse/dependence predominated in men.
- Young adults (age 25–44) had the highest prevalence estimates for most disorders.

One of the important results of the ECA studies has been to question the excess of mental disorders among women compared to men in earlier studies. In those earlier studies, less attention was given to substance abuse and antisocial personality, which are more prevalent in men.

Key Epidemiologic Concepts

Several key concepts commonly used in epidemiology may serve as a foundation for applying epidemiologic principles to your work in psychiatric nursing. Knowledge of these terms is also useful when reviewing current medical literature. Nursing students are referred to *Epidemiology in Nursing and Health Care* (Valanis 1992) for additional information regarding general epidemiologic concepts and their applications. Also note that *Episource* (Bernier and Mason 1991) serves as a general practical guide to resources in epidemiology.

Prevalence

Here is the formula for determining prevalence rate (Mauser and Kramer 1985):

$$\text{Prevalence rate} = \frac{\text{Number of existing cases of disorder at a point in time}}{\text{Total population}}$$

Prevalence rates may be used for the following purposes:

- To express the burden of a disorder in the population.
- To identify population subgroups (by age, sex, etc.) for prevention strategies.
- For the planning and evaluation of mental health services.
- To track changes in patterns of a disorder over time.

Incidence

An **incidence rate** measures the number of *new* cases of a disease or disorder in a population over a period of time. Here is the formula for determining incidence rate (Mauser and Kramer 1985):

$$\text{Incidence rate} = \frac{\text{Number of new cases of disorder over a period of time}}{\text{Population at risk}}$$

Incidence is a direct measure of the rate at which individuals in a given population develop a disease or disorder. Thus, incidence is a direct measure of risk. Clues to the causes of a disorder may be obtained as new "incident" cases are studied.

Studies of chronic diseases, such as schizophrenia, generally use prevalence measures; studies of acute disorders or events, such as rape, generally use incidence measures. One can examine prevalence or incidence rates by age, sex, race/ethnicity, and other psychobiosocial factors to determine which subgroups are at greatest risk for specific diseases. The identification of vulnerable subgroups may be the first step in the development of intervention strategies that target resources for people at greatest risk.

Risk Factors

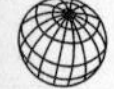

A critical issue related to cultural diversity in psychiatric epidemiology is that important factors reflecting varying cultures need to be assessed in clinical practice and research. Ethnicity, race, dietary patterns, the use of alcohol and drugs, health and healing practices, other lifestyle habits, religious or spiritual beliefs, the use of time, and migration patterns may differentially affect the experience, expression, reporting, and evaluation of mental disorders among culturally diverse groups. The field of research has been criticized in retrospect for studying white males and, to a lesser extent, white females, and then generalizing the results to all other groups.

The notion of biopsychosocial risk factors is common in psychiatric literature. A **risk factor** is a factor whose presence is associated with an increased chance or probability of mental disorder. Some risk factors cannot be modified, such as age. Other risk factors are susceptible to change, such as personal lifestyle habits regarding the use of alcohol and tobacco. A limited review of numerous risk factors associated with the occurrence of many psychiatric disorders is outlined by Bromet and Parkinson (1992).

Risk Factors That Cannot Be Modified The following risk factors for mental disorders cannot be modified: gender, age, and a positive family history. The impact of each factor is briefly highlighted.

Gender Differences in rates between males and females are found for substance abuse, anxiety disorders, and depression. The male-to-female ratios are estimated at 6:1 for alcoholism, 1:2 for depression, and 1:2 for phobias.

Age Age is associated with the occurrence of mental disorders. An important finding from the ECA studies was that young adults (age 25–44) had the highest prevalence estimates for most disorders. Alcoholism is known to peak in the early forties. Heavy drinking associated with driving or fighting while intoxicated appears to peak in the early twenties.

Positive Family History Depression and schizophrenia appear related to a history of such disorders in the family. Evidence points to a genetic vulnerability for developing alcoholism. There is some evidence that alzheimer's disease may show a familial pattern. Findings regarding bipolar disorder (manic depression) and anxiety disorders are currently controversial with regard to family history. Recent developments in genetics may contribute to further understanding regarding the contribution of family history to the development of mental disorders.

Risk Factors That Can Be Modified Risk factors for mental disorders that are susceptible to change are divided into the following four groups: demographic status, physical health status, social environment, and agents in the physical environment.

Demographic Factors Lower *social class* status is associated with increased rates of depression, alcohol and other substance abuse, and antisocial personality disorder. Although risk factors vary among mental disorders, a recent study examined the effect of poverty on psychiatric health (Bruce, Takeuchi, and Leaf 1991). A key finding was that adults in poverty, as defined by federal poverty guidelines, had twice the risk for an episode of at least one mental disorder compared with those not in poverty.

Ethnicity appears to be indirectly associated with mental disorders because different ethnic groups share different social and physical environments. The ECA studies found similar prevalence rates for most mental disorders between blacks and whites. For major depression, white men tended to have higher rates than black men, while black women had higher prevalence rates than white women. Whites of all ages have higher suicide rates than blacks, with Native American youth at increased risk for suicide.

Marital status, especially being single, may be associated with psychiatric disorders such as schizophrenia. The highest rates of depression occur among those recently divorced or separated. Married women are more depressed than nonmarried women. In contrast, married men are less depressed than unmarried men.

Physical Health Status The link between physical and mental health is noteworthy. Studies provide evidence that psychiatric patients may have an increased mortality rate. Medically hospitalized patients have increased rates of mental disorder as well. Major depression is associated with many chronic medical conditions and is predictive of shortened life expectancy.

Social Environment Higher levels of stress associated with particular events in one's social environment may be associated with increased rates of mental disorder. Loss of life or property is a risk factor related to *natural disasters,* such as earthquakes, floods, and tornadoes. *Single traumatic events,* such as bereavement or unemployment, may produce adverse mental health consequences. The diagnosis of posttraumatic stress disorder (PTSD) represents a response to an unusual, intense stressor. *Adverse life events* are known to contribute to some forms of depression. A stressful family environment is an established risk factor for behavioral problems in children.

Physical Environment High-level *chemical exposures* to mercury, carbon monoxide, carbon disulfide, and lead are related to serious central nervous system disturbances. Environmental exposure to lead is related to deleterious effects on children. When considering *homelessness,* rates of mental disorder among homeless adults and children are remarkably high.

It is important to note that the presence of one particular risk factor does not inevitably lead to the development of a mental disorder. Rather, a number of factors occurring in a defined time period may cause a disorder. **Multifactorial causation** is the term used to describe the requirement that a combination of causes or factors may be needed to produce the disorder.

Table 5–1 Risk Factors Associated with the Occurrence of Psychiatric Disorders

Risk Factors That Cannot Be Modified	***Risk Factors That Can Be Modified***
Gender Age Positive Family History	Demographic Factors • Low social class status • Ethnicity • Marital status Physical Health Status Social Environment • Disasters • Single traumatic events • Adverse life events Physical Environment • High-level chemical exposures • Homelessness

CULTURALLY DIVERSE LIFESTYLE HABITS
These may influence the experience, expression, reporting, and evaluation of mental disorders. Lifestyle habits may include dietary patterns, use of alcohol and drugs, health and healing practices, religious and spiritual beliefs, use of time, and migration patterns.

Keep these nonmodifiable and modifiable risk factors in mind as you apply the nursing process in your clinical work. (See Table 5–1.) Targeting specific risk factors for intervention is one goal of primary prevention.

The Natural History of Disorder

Many disorders, especially chronic disorders, have a natural life history. The **natural history of disorder** refers to the course of disorder over time in the absence of intervention. Chronic disorder may be viewed in a sequence of stages. Risk factors favoring the development of a disorder may be present early in life, preceding the appearance of symptoms by many years. It is important to note that we do not have a complete understanding of the natural history of many psychiatric disorders. (As mentioned earlier, the word "disorder" rather than "disease" is used here, although general epidemiologic texts commonly refer to the natural history of disease.) Every disorder has its own life history, but in general, disorders have these four basic stages: stage of susceptibility, stage of presymptomatic disorder, stage of clinical disorder, and stage of disability (Figure 5–1).

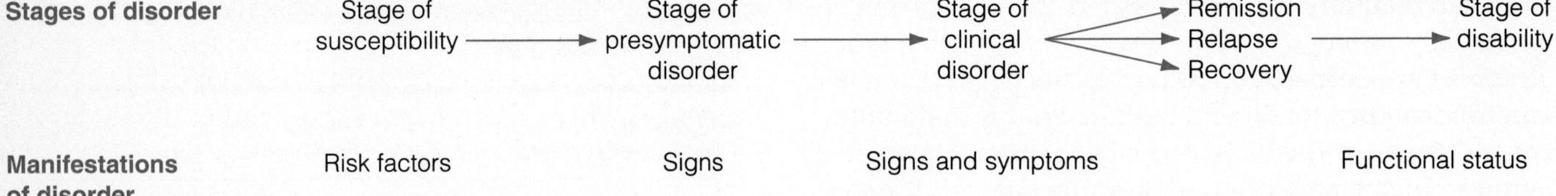

Figure 5–1 Stages in the natural history of disorder.

Stage of Susceptibility During this stage, the groundwork has been laid by the presence of risk factors that favor the occurrence of disorder. The individual is susceptible to the disorder, but the disorder has not yet developed. Identification of those at high risk for developing a disorder is a major mental health care challenge. For example, the following risk factors may "set the stage," placing a woman at increased risk for depression: lack of a primary relationship, not employed outside the home, have three or more children under the age of 6, and have endured the loss of a parent in childhood.

Stage of Presymptomatic Disorder During this stage, there is no apparent disorder, but pathological changes have started to occur. The disorder has begun but remains unrecognized because it may be asymptomatic. If signs of the disorder are present, they may be considered to be the ordinary discomforts of daily living. Mild depression serves as an example of this presymptomatic stage.

Stage of Clinical Disorder This stage is characterized by recognizable signs and symptoms of disorder. For some disorders, people regularly come under nursing or medical care at some point over the course of an illness. These disorders are "high-profile" because they cause such symptoms as peculiar behavior, failure to thrive, severe or chronic distress, or pain. Classification may be based on laboratory findings or on functional or therapeutic considerations. Cancer is usually classified by the location, extent, and type of tumor. The most current source of classification of psychiatric disorders is the fourth edition of the American Psychiatric Association's *Diagnostic and Statistical Manual of Mental Disorders,* or *DSM-IV* (American Psychiatric Association 1994). *DSM-IV* criteria for psychiatric disorders rely on a descriptive diagnostic classification scheme. It is important to note that "clinical disorder" describes a disorder that has come under nursing or medical care and is then treated in a variety of ways that may alter the subsequent course of events.

Stage of Disability Some disorders run their course and resolve completely, either spontaneously or in response to therapy. However, some disorders leave residual impairment or disability of short or long duration. While there is a substantial amount of disability associated with acute disorders, the extended disability resulting from chronic disorders is of greater significance to society.

Levels of Prevention

Understanding the stages of the natural history of disorder can serve as a basis for applying prevention strategies. Emphasis here is on preventive, rather than curative, nursing interventions. Prevention simply means keeping the disorder from occurring. The meaning of the word has been extended to include measures that interrupt or slow the progression of disorder. Three levels of prevention are usually possible, depending on when clinical efforts are made. Although these concepts apply to mental disorders in this chapter, they may be effectively applied to any medical disease or condition.

Primary Prevention **Primary prevention** involves avoiding the occurrence of disorder by removing the risk factors. The goals of primary prevention are mental health promotion and the prevention of disorder. Mental health promotion addresses conditions at home, work, and school that favor healthy living. Emotional support, adequate shelter, a safe environment, and good nutrition are examples. Mental health education programs, including counseling in preparation for major life events (such as independent living programs and parent training in child development) are an integral aspect of mental health promotion. The prevention of disorder is usually carried out through specific protective measures. These may involve training in specific skills and competence building for high-risk individuals (stress-management seminars, Big Brother/Big Sister programs) or may emphasize healthy behaviors (lifestyle counseling, Students Against Drunken Driving programs, and "Say No to Drugs" programs).

It is important to note that primary prevention is often accomplished outside the mental health care system. Nurses may be directly involved in many primary prevention activities, including client referral to specific appropriate community resources to reduce the risk of mental disorder.

Secondary Prevention **Secondary prevention** involves the early detection and prompt treatment of disorder. An important caution is that *prognosis is affected by the duration of any mental disorder.* Thus, secondary prevention strategies are crucial in mental health care. Because of a current inability to prevent certain disorders, efforts to control many of these disorders focus on secondary prevention. In the presymptomatic stage, screening surveys by health departments and other community agencies may target individuals to order to alter the natural history of the condition detected. At the stage of clinical disorder, prompt, thorough diagnosis and treatment are essential. A large number of secondary prevention services include inpatient units, emergency services, outpatient clinics, and day treatment programs. Psychiatric case-finding efforts in walk-in clinics, primary practice, and hospital settings are further examples of secondary prevention strategies that can be employed.

In general, there are three clinical outcomes regarding mental disorders: remission, relapse, or permanent recovery. Much of your effort as a psychiatric nurse will focus on achieving the overall goal of secondary prevention, that is, termination or limitation of the course of a mental disorder.

TERTIARY PREVENTION **Tertiary prevention** involves the limiting of disability and rehabilitation when a disorder has occurred. Ideally, this level of prevention is restorative in nature; in reality, the emphasis may be on sustaining basic functions. Goals of tertiary prevention include restoring functional status, limiting progression, and preventing complications. An interdisciplinary team addressing nursing care, medical care, rehabilitation (physical, vocational), occupational therapy, and other support services may be involved. Two specific examples of tertiary prevention are suicide prevention associated with an inpatient's severe major depressive episode, and independent living programs for the frequently admitted chronic psychiatric patient.

The interrelationships between the stages of the natural history of disorder and the levels of prevention are illustrated in Figure 5–2. Mauser and Kramer (1985) is a reference for the natural history of disorder, and Kaplan, Sadock, and Grebb (1994) is a good resource for information on specific levels of prevention. *Treatment of Mental Disorders* (Sartorius et al. 1993) provides a comprehensive section emphasizing World Health Organization perspectives on prevention. Orlandi (1992) serves as an excellent resource for evaluating community-based alcohol and other drug abuse prevention programs specific to several cross-cultural community groups (African American, Hispanic, American Indian and Alaska natives, and Asian/Pacific Island-American). Likewise, Owan (1985) evaluates mental health treatment, prevention, services, training, and research specific to Southeast Asian refugees.

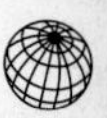

Types of Studies

A brief summary of two types of epidemiologic studies may serve as a resource to nurses who consult the current literature but do not have a background in research (see Research Note). Two common types of studies that examine the distribution and determinants of mental disorders are descriptive studies and cross-sectional studies.

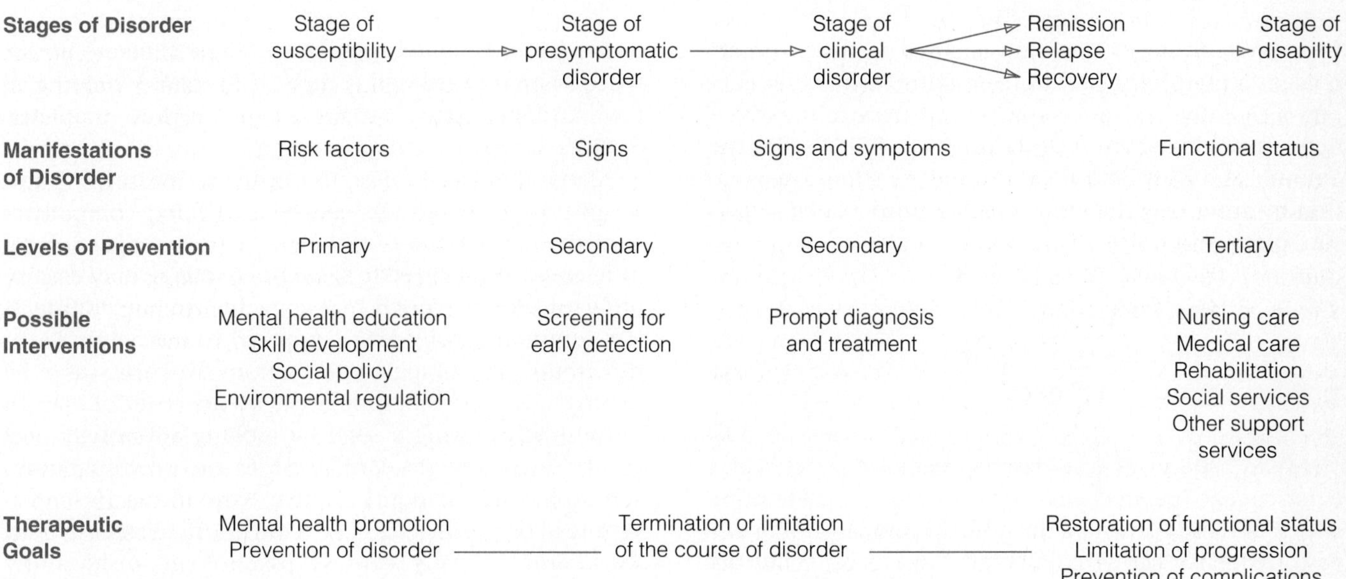

Figure 5-2 Stages in the natural history of disorder, with corresponding levels of prevention, possible interventions, and therapeutic goals.

RESEARCH NOTE

Citation

Kessler R, McGonagle K, Zhao S, et al. Lifetime and 12-month prevalence of DSM-III-R psychiatric disorders in the United States: Results from the National Comorbidity Survey. *Arch Gen Psychiatr* 1994;51:8–18.

Study Problem/Purpose

The National Comorbidity Survey (NCS) is a congressionally mandated survey designed to estimate the prevalence of psychiatric disorders in a representative national sample of the U.S. population. This landmark study focuses on the comorbidity of substance use disorders and non-substance psychiatric disorders in order to investigate risk factors, course of illness, and the utilization of services that are associated with comorbidity.

Methods

This cross-sectional (prevalence) study involved approximately 10,000 subjects representing the noninstitutional U.S. household population (age 15–54 years). A complex sampling design was used to provide information on demographic correlates of disorder (gender, age, race, socioeconomic status, urbanicity, and region). Data were collected by lay interviewers administering structured psychiatric interviews. DSM-III-R psychiatric disorders were generated using a revised version of the Composite International Diagnostic Interview.

Findings

The NCS represents the largest and most extensive research on psychiatric disorders in the United States to date. There is more psychiatric disorder than previously thought. Nearly half of subjects report at least one disorder in their lifetime. The most common psychiatric disorders are major depression and alcohol dependence, followed by social and simple phobias. Mental disorder is highly concentrated in approximately one-sixth (14%) of the population who had a history of three or more comorbid disorders. The majority of individuals with psychiatric disorder fail to seek treatment. Additional findings are forthcoming in the literature.

Implications

Prevalence rates allow estimates of the national public health burden of psychiatric morbidity and comorbidity. Findings point to the need for community-based preventive programs aimed at more outreach. There is also a need for more research on barriers to mental health services.

Descriptive Studies Knowing about patterns of occurrence is a useful first step in identifying factors that may play a causative role or otherwise contribute to the development of a disorder. A **descriptive study** identifies the amount and distribution of a disorder within a population by answering the following questions related to person, place, and time:

- *Who* is affected? (person)
- *Where* do the cases occur? (place)
- *When* do cases occur? (time)

"Who" addresses important personal characteristics (such as age, gender, and ethnicity/race) to determine which of these characteristics differ in comparisons of disease frequency across populations. Age is generally the most important personal characteristic associated with disorders. Gender is also a factor among disorders; depression, for example, shows male-female differences in patterns of disorder and death. Rates of depression are almost twice as high in women compared to men. Women also have a higher rate of attempted suicide, but completed suicides are more common in men.

Many disorders differ markedly in frequency and severity by racial group. Like race, ethnicity may influence the development of disorder. For example, cultural differences are believed to influence use of alcohol among different groups, which may explain why alcoholism is less common among Jews compared to many other ethnic groups. Psychologic stress among Hispanics may be related to Mal de Ojo, thought to be the result of a witch purposefully casting a spell by looking admiringly at a child. Native Americans may suffer such culture-bound syndromes as Pibloqtok (active, convulsive hysterical seizures) or Ghost sickness (confusion, dizziness, and fear). Some Asians express psychologic disharmony through somatic complaints (headaches, stomach aches, and palpitations).

"Where" addresses the geographic location where dis-

orders are clustered. Variations in location can provide clues to factors associated with the occurrence of disorders. International comparisons are widely used to assess relative progress in the control of disorders. "Where" also may address political subdivisions, such as entire nations, states, counties, and towns. Location, such as a remote rural setting, may influence access to mental health services.

"When" addresses the occurrence of disorders by time, which is usually expressed on an annual or lifetime basis. Prevalence rates are commonly presented in terms of lifetime and one-year periods for various disorders. Incidence rates may be reported in terms of a one-year time span. Seasonal fluctuations in the frequency of disorders may also be noted, such as the seasonal patterns associated with some mood disorders.

CROSS-SECTIONAL STUDIES A **cross-sectional study** is conducted at one point in time. The prevalence of disorder is measured by surveying a group that consists of some people with and some without a disorder. These studies, often called prevalence studies, are relatively inexpensive, simple to carry out, and may provide clues to factors associated with disorder. Cross-sectional studies are among the most common types of research designs reported in the psychiatric literature.

Often the ideal population to be studied is either too large or too spread out over time, and there is a need to select a smaller group of individuals for study. A sample or representative portion of the population may actually participate in the study. A *representative sample* resembles the population in relation to important characteristics such as age and gender. If the study sample is truly representative of the larger population, then the results of the study can be safely extended to that population. (This chapter's Research Note is an example of a national cross-sectional study based on a large representative sample.)

Recent Developments

Several recent developments in psychiatric epidemiology are diagnostic and treatment advances in relation to cultural diversity, key findings from major recent studies, and patterns in the use of mental health services.

Cultural Diversity in DSM-IV Classifications

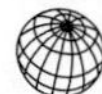

In psychiatric epidemiology, a case is a person in the population or study group identified as having a particular mental disorder. The definition of a case in epidemiology is not necessarily the same as the ordinary clinical definition. Cases may be identified by clinical nursing diagnoses, by psychiatrists' clinical diagnoses, by clinical records, by surveys of the general population, and by population screening (Last 1988).

As previously noted, the most current classification of psychiatric disorders is found in the *DSM-IV.* Although discussions regarding the *DSM-IV* are incorporated throughout this textbook, *DSM-IV* features relating to cultural diversity deserve emphasis.

Twelve *DSM-IV* field trials were carried out in more than 70 diverse sites. Representative groups of subjects were selected from a range of sociocultural and ethnic backgrounds to test diagnostic categories as a whole, as well as specific items within each category. A *DSM-IV* section entitled "Specific Culture, Age, and Gender Features" systematically offers guidance concerning variations in the presentation of each disorder that may be attributable to one's cultural setting. The section also provides information on differential prevalence rates related to culture.

Cultural Diversity in Assessment and Treatment

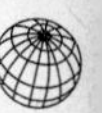

"Culture not only builds its own vulnerabilities (and strengths), but also plays a part in how these vulnerabilities find expression (Tseng and McDermott, p. 22)." Thus culture can influence the experience, expression, reporting, and evaluation of mental disorders. Symptoms related to major depression, as highlighted by the *DSM-IV*, may illustrate this point. Depression may be experienced in somatic terms, rather than with sadness or guilt, in some cultures. People of Latino and Mediterranean cultures may complain of headaches and "nerves." People of Chinese and Asian cultures may emphasize weakness and tiredness. Middle Easterners may refer to problems of the "heart." The Hopi may express the depressive experience by being "heartbroken." Cultures may differ regarding the seriousness placed on symptoms and share distinctive culture-specific experiences (such as the feeling of being hexed).

Guidelines for a detailed cultural assessment are offered in the *DSM-IV* to provide a systematic review of the client's cultural and ethnic background and to identify ways in which the cultural context influences nursing care. A glossary of culture-bound syndromes is provided to help identify any local patterns of experience that may or may not be linked to a specific *DSM-IV* category (see Appendix C). Campinha-Bacote (1992) provides a review of one specific culture-bound syndrome in African-American culture (voodoo illness) and subsequent nursing interventions. DeLeon Siantz (1994) highlights cultural influences in relation to mental health issues for a particular subgroupof Mexican-American migrant farmworker families. The accompanying Nursing Self-Awareness inventory on page 94 applies principles of psychiatric epidemiology

NURSING SELF-AWARENESS

Applying Principles of Psychiatric Epidemiology

Attempt to identify the following concerns regarding a particular population that is served:

- Which groups of people (such as children, elderly, or homeless) are at high risk for the development of specific psychiatric disorders?
- Are there any changes in health problems at this setting, especially the emergence of new problems?
- In what ways might I be involved in the identification of current health needs of this population, and the prediction of future needs of this population?
- Are there particular care-seeking patterns related to the utilization of mental health services (including nonuse or misuse of services) that I need to be aware of?
- How might I be involved in the evaluation of preventive and therapeutic measures aimed at this population?

Attempt to answer the following questions regarding a particular client that is served:

- Have I assessed which risk factors associated with psychiatric disorders may relate to this client? Have I identified which risk factors can and cannot be modified?
- Have I obtained information of this client's cultural and ethnic identity as part of my psychiatric nursing assessment?
- Do I have an understanding of this client's lifestyle habits which may impact on mental health care (such as health and healing practices, religious and spiritual beliefs, and use of alcohol and drugs)?
- Can I identify cultural resources that might be useful in the planning and provision of mental health services for this client?
- Am I able to formulate goals targeting one or more of the three levels of prevention (primary, secondary, tertiary)?

to a particular clinical setting and client with emphasis on cultural and ethnic assessment.

Refer to the World Health Organization book that examines diverse cultural influences entitled *Treatment of Mental Disorders* (Sartorius et al. 1993). This text includes Jilek's cross-cultural evaluation of traditional medicine, folk therapy practices that operate outside official health care systems. Finally, *Ethnicity and Disease* is an international journal on population differences in disease patterns.

Cultural Diversity and Instrument Development

Several instruments are used to define a case in psychiatric epidemiology. Two current instruments of merit are the Composite International Diagnostic Interview (CIDI) and Center for Epidemiologic Studies Depression Scale (CES-D). The CIDI is a structured interview developed by the World Health Organization (WHO) and the Alcohol, Drug Abuse, and Mental Health Administration (ADAMHA) in an effort to standardize definitions of mental disorders for epidemiologic research throughout the world (World Health Organization 1993). The performance of the CIDI was evaluated in international field trials and holds promise for use in culturally diverse groups.

The CES-D is a 20-item, self-report scale useful in detecting depressive symptoms in the general population (Radloff 1977). It may be self-administered and takes less than five minutes to complete. The CES-D scale is suitable for use with people across a wide range of ages, education levels, geographic areas, and social classes (Radloff and Locke 1986). The CES-D is emphasized because it is found to be suitable for black, white, Hispanic, and Asian English-speaking American populations.

Instruments for measuring mental disorders are sometimes translated into another language for international use. It is important to note that words in one language do not always translate into words in another language, subtle meanings of words may be different, and people in other cultures may be unfamiliar with American psychiatric procedures.

Key Findings from Recent Major Studies

Key findings from recent major studies on mental disorders are relevant to psychiatric nurses in these areas: mortality, morbidity and comorbidity, and the use of mental health services.

MORTALITY Information on mortality associated with psychiatric diagnoses is important for two reasons. First, an increased risk of mortality represents a serious negative outcome that may contribute information about the natural history of disorder. Second, information on mortality may be used to identify high-risk groups in community settings. Researchers recently followed a community sample of adults who were first interviewed in 1980 as part of the ECA study in New Haven, Connecticut (Bruce et al. 1994). Nine years later, the researchers determined who was living or deceased. A key finding was the greater risk of mortality among adults with the following disorders: major depression, alcohol abuse or dependence, and schizophrenia. The high prevalence of depression and of alcohol-related disorders emphasize the great impact these problems have on community health in general.

Morbidity and Comorbidity There is increasing awareness of the issue of comorbidity among people with mental disorders, particularly depression, anxiety, and alcohol and other substance abuse. **Comorbidity** is defined as the occurrence of two or more psychiatric disorders over an individual's life span.

The National Comorbidity Survey (NCS) The landmark National Comorbidity Survey, a congressionally mandated survey conducted with a representative national sample, is the most extensive and current research regarding psychiatric disorders to date (Kessler et al. 1994). The goals of the NCS included:

- Carrying out a national survey to estimate the prevalence of psychiatric morbidity and comorbidity in the United States.
- Investigating the implications of comorbidity for mental health service utilization and course of illness.
- Investigating the risk factors for comorbidity.

More specifically, this survey of the noninstitutionalized U.S. household population (age 15–54) reported on about 10,000 subjects using a study design that enabled investigation of seasonal variation in the prevalence of mental disorders. A structured psychiatric interview was used to generate DSM-III-R psychiatric diagnoses.

The prevalence of psychiatric disorders was greater than previously thought. Nearly half the subjects reported at least one mental disorder in their lifetime. The most common disorders were major depression and alcohol dependence. The following findings were consistent with previous research:

- Women had higher rates of affective and anxiety disorders.
- Men had higher rates of substance abuse disorders and antisocial personality disorder.
- Most disorders declined with age and with higher socioeconomic status.
- Fewer than 40% of those with a lifetime disorder had ever received professional treatment.

A most striking finding is that mental disorders are more highly concentrated than previously recognized in approximately one-sixth (14%) of the population who have had a history of three or more comorbid disorders. When severity is considered, this group also includes the great majority of those with severe disorders. Less than 50% of this highly comorbid group ever obtained specialty mental health treatment, despite the number and severity of their disorders.

The Epidemiologic Catchment Area (ECA) Studies Additional findings from the ECA studies provide information from community and institutional samples regarding the comorbidity of mental disorders related to alcohol and other drug abuse. Regier et al. (1990) reported that, in general, 37% of those with a mental disorder also had an alcohol abuse disorder. Among mental disorders associated with alcoholism, anxiety disorders were most prevalent (19%), followed by antisocial personality disorder (14%) and depressive disorder (13%). The relationship between mental disorder and drug abuse (other than alcohol) is also noteworthy: A comorbid mental disorder was found among more than half of those with drug (other than alcohol) abuse disorders.

Expressed in terms of risk, those having a mental disorder in their lifetime had more than twice the risk of having an alcohol abuse disorder and over four times the risk of having another drug abuse disorder. Individuals treated in specialty mental health and addictive disorder clinics were at significantly higher risk for having comorbid disorders. Helzer and Pryzbeck (1988) found that comorbidity of alcoholism with other disorders was more common for women compared to men. Issues related to comorbidity will receive significant attention in future psychiatric research.

The Use of Mental Health Services Care-seeking patterns need to be especially addressed in the conduct of epidemiologic studies. Patterns may be summarized as follows:

- Most people with mental disorders do not seek professional treatment.
- Comorbidity increases the likelihood that a person will seek treatment. Still less than half of the highly comorbid group identified in the National Comorbidity Study ever obtained specialty mental health treatment, despite the number and severity of their disorders.
- When seeking treatment, most people with mental disorders seek treatment from primary care physicians, who prescribe the majority of psychotropic

medications. Yet there is a current decrease in primary care physicians, especially in impoverished and rural areas.

- Individuals with chronic mental disorders comprise the majority of those who seek treatment.
- Psychiatrists tend to treat individuals with severe disorders, yet there is a current undersupply of psychiatrists in the United States.

Awareness of these care-seeking patterns is essential in order to address the nonuse or misuse of mental health services. Knowledge of such patterns is also useful for selection of the most appropriate subjects for a given epidemiologic study. Pivotal issues are the availability, accessibility, cost, and quality of mental health services, especially since prognosis is affected by the duration of any mental disorder.

Cost is the most frequently addressed mental health topic in current literature on medical care organization. A recent national estimate of expenditures for the treatment of mental health problems was $18 billion based on a 1987 national survey (Freiman, Cunningham, and Cornelius 1994). Financial incentives appear to drive the services provided to those with mental disorders, and funding sources appear to drive the entire health care industry. Insurance coverage for mental health care appears to lag behind that for other medical care. Following are severely underserved groups in relation to mental health services:

- The substance abuser.
- Older adults (especially if minority).
- The uninsured.
- The homeless.

Current mental health policy appears reactive rather than proactive, situational rather than long-term and strategic, and rehabilitative rather than preventive.

Implications for Psychiatric Nursing Practice

In general, epidemiologic principles extend nursing skills by considering the community itself as a potential "client" for mental health assessment and services. More specifically, epidemiologic principles may be applied to each step of the nursing process. Assessment may include collecting information on the natural history of disorder, potential risk factors, and the client's cultural and ethnic background. Nursing diagnoses may involve the use of one or more psychiatric instruments as part of diagnostic procedures. The levels of prevention may serve as a comprehensive framework for planning and implementing nursing interventions, as well as for evaluation and outcome criteria.

Because most people with mental disorders never seek professional treatment, there is a need for more outreach to ensure availability, accessibility, reasonable cost, and quality of mental health services for all subgroups of the population. Psychiatric nurses may advocate for more outreach aimed at high-risk groups, such as the impoverished, the homeless, and those with comorbid conditions.

Nurses are critically evaluating nursing practice to provide quality care to culturally diverse clients seeking health care services. Johnston and Baumann (1992) assert that nurses must systematically evaluate currently existing conceptual models for cultural relevance and sensitivity. Wright (1994) viewed counseling in its cultural context and suggests that nursing theories, techniques, and the profession itself are cultural phenomena reflecting American society's culture, history, beliefs, and values.

Implications for Psychiatric Nursing Research

The results from studies suggest that the causes and consequences of high comorbidity should be the focus of continued research. More research on potential barriers to professional care seeking is needed, including care-seeking patterns that consider ethnic and cultural differences.

The research contains gaps. There appears to be a lack of systematic, evaluative study aimed at determining which treatments are most effective for which disorders in which groups at any given time. Research into productivity and efficiency is important: Most clients, especially those with severe or persistent mental disorders, have found a fragmented, underfinanced, uncoordinated, and frequently inaccessible system of care.

Following are potential areas for future nursing research: expanded cross-national comparisons; genetics and neurobiology; environmental factors (such as physical illness, traumatic life events, lack of support, and lack of physical exercise); the development of preventive programs; advances in psychopharmacology; children and adolescent studies; the use of various study designs; and the development of brief interview instruments for use in screening programs.

Chapter Highlights

- Psychiatric epidemiology is the study of the distribution and determinants of mental disorders (or other health-related conditions or events) in human populations. Uses include identifying causative factors for specific disorders, identifying groups at high risk, recognizing changes in health problems, identifying preventive strategies, planning for services related to mental disorders, and predicting future needs.

- Mental illness is not randomly distributed across populations. Prevalence rate measures the number of people in a population who have a disease or disorder at a given time. The most prevalent mental disorders in the United States associated with increased morbidity and mortality are depression and alcohol dependence.
- Risk factors related to mental disorders include those that cannot be modified (gender, age, and positive family history) and those that can be modified (demographic factors, physical health, social environment, and physical environment).
- The natural history of disease is the course of disease or disorder over time in the absence of intervention. The stages of the natural history of disorder are a basis for understanding the three levels of prevention.
- Primary prevention involves avoiding the occurrence of disorder by removing the risk factors. The goals of primary prevention are general health promotion and specific protective measures.
- Secondary prevention involves the early detection and prompt treatment of disorder. The goal of secondary prevention is termination or limitation of the process of a mental disorder.
- In general, there are three clinical outcomes regarding mental disorders: remission, relapse, or permanent recovery. Prognosis is affected by the duration of any mental disorder.
- Tertiary prevention involves the limiting of disability and rehabilitation when a disorder has occurred. Goals of tertiary prevention include restoring functional status, limiting progression, and preventing complications.
- Culture can influence the experience, expression, reporting, and evaluation of mental disorders. A sensitive and systematic review of the client's cultural and ethnic background is an important part of the psychiatric nursing process.
- Comorbidity is the occurrence of two or more mental disorders over an individual's life span. Mental disorders are frequently associated with alcohol abuse and other drug use.
- Women have higher rates of affective and anxiety disorders. Men have higher rates of substance abuse disorders and antisocial personality disorder.
- Mental disorders are highly concentrated in approximately one-sixth of the population who have a history of three or more comorbid disorders.
- Most people with mental disorders never seek treatment. Comorbidity increases the likelihood that an individual will seek treatment.

References

American Psychiatric Association: *Diagnostic and Statistical Manual of Mental Disorders,* ed 4. American Psychiatric Association, 1994.

Bernier RH, Mason VM (eds): *Episource: A Guide to Resources in Epidemiology.* The Epidemiology Monitor, 1991.

Bromet E, Parkinson D: Psychiatric disorders, in Last J,Wallace R (eds): *Maxcy-Rosenau-Last Public Health & Preventive Medicine.* Prentice Hall, 1992.

Bruce M, Leaf P, Rozal G, Florio L, Hoff R: Psychiatric status and 9-year mortality data in the New Haven Epidemiologic Catchment Area Study. *Am J Psychiatr* 1994;151(5):716–721.

Bruce M, Takeuchi D, Leaf P: Poverty and psychiatric status. *Arch Gen Psychiatr* 1991;48:470–474.

Campinha-Bacote J: Voodoo illness. *Perspect Psychiatr Care* 1992;28(1):11–17.

deLeon Siantz M: The Mexican-American migrant farmworker family. *Nurs Clin North Am* 1994;29(1):65–72.

Dohrenwend B, Dohrenwend B: Perspectives on the past and future of psychiatric epidemiology: The 1981 Rema Lapouse Lecture. *Am J Public Health* 1982;72:1271–1279.

Eaton W, et al.: The design of the Epidemiologic Catchment Area surveys: The control and measurement of error. *Arch Gen Psychiatr* 1984;41:942–948.

Freiman M, Cunningham P, Cornelius L: Use and expenditures for the treatment of mental health problems (AHCPR Pub. No. 94-0085). National Medical Expenditure Survey Research Findings 22, Agency for Health Care Policy and Research. Public Health Service, July 1994.

Helzer JE, Pryzbeck TR: The co-occurrence of alcoholism with other psychiatric disorders in the general population and its impact on treatment. *J Stud Alcohol* 1988;49(1):219–224.

Jarvis, E: *Insanity and Idiocy in Massachusetts: Report of the Commission on Lunacy, 1855.* Harvard University Press, 1972.

Johnston N, Baumann A: Selecting a nursing model for psychiatric nursing. *J Psychosoc Nurs* 1992;30(4):7–11.

Kaplan H, Sadock B, Grebb J: *Kaplan and Sadock's Synopsis of Psychiatry,* ed 7. Williams & Wilkins, 1994.

Kessler R, McGonagle K, Zhao S: Lifetime and 12-month prevalence of DSM-III-R psychiatric disorders in the United States: Results from the National Comorbidity Survey. *Arch Gen Psychiatr* 1994;51:8–18.

Last J: *A Dictionary of Epidemiology,* ed 2. Oxford University Press, 1988.

Mauser J, Kramer S: *Epidemiology—An Introductory Text,* ed 2. Saunders, 1985.

Orlandi, MA (ed): (1992). *Cultural Competence for Evaluators: A Guide for Alcohol and Other Drug Abuse Prevention Practitioners Working With Ethnic/Racial Communities.* U.S. Department of Health and Human Services. Public Health Service. Alcohol, Drug Abuse, and Mental Health Administration and the Office for Substance Abuse Prevention. DHHS Publication No. (ADM) 92-1884.

Owan, TC (ed): (1985). *Southeast Asian Mental Health: Treatment, Prevention, Services, Training, and Research.* U.S. Department of Health and Human Services. National Institute of Mental Health. Public Health Service. Alcohol, Drug Abuse, and Mental Health Administration in collaboration with Office of Refugee Resettlement. DHHS Publication No. (ADM) 85-1399.

Radloff L: The CES-D Scale: A self-report depression scale for research in the general population. *Appl Psychol Meas* 1977;1(3):385–401.

Radloff L, Locke B: The Community Mental Health Assessment Survey and the CES-D Scale, in Weissman M, Myers J, Ross C (eds): *Community Surveys of Psychiatric Disorders.* Rutgers University Press, 1986.

Regier D, et al.: Comorbidity of mental health disorders with alcohol and other drug abuse. *JAMA* 1990;264:2511–2518.

Regier D, et al.: The NIMH Epidemiologic Catchment Area Program: Historical context, major objectives, and study population characteristics. *Arch Gen Psychiatr* 1984;41:934–941.

Robins LN, Locke BZ, Regier DA: An overview of psychiatric disorders in America, in Robins LN, Regier DA (eds): *Psychiatric Disorders in America.* Free Press, 1991.

Rothman K: *Modern Epidemiology.* Little, Brown, 1986.

Sartorius N, DeGirolamo G, Andrews G, German G, Eisenberg L (eds): *Treatment of Mental Disorders: A Review of Effectiveness.* American Psychiatric Press, 1993.

Streiner D, Norman G, Blum H: *Epidemiology.* B.C. Decker, 1989.

Tseng, W-S, McDermott, Jr, JF: *Culture, Mind and Therapy: An Introduction to Cultural Psychiatry.* Brunner/Mazel, 1981.

Valanis B: *Epidemiology in Nursing and Health Care.* Appleton and Lange, 1992.

World Health Organization. Composite International Diagnostic Interview (CIDI): Core Version 1.1. World Health Organization, 1993.

Wright J: Counselling at the cultural interface: Is getting back to roots enough? *J Adv Nurs* 1991;16:92–100.

PART TWO

PROCESSES FOR CLINICAL PRACTICE IN PSYCHIATRIC NURSING

CONTENTS

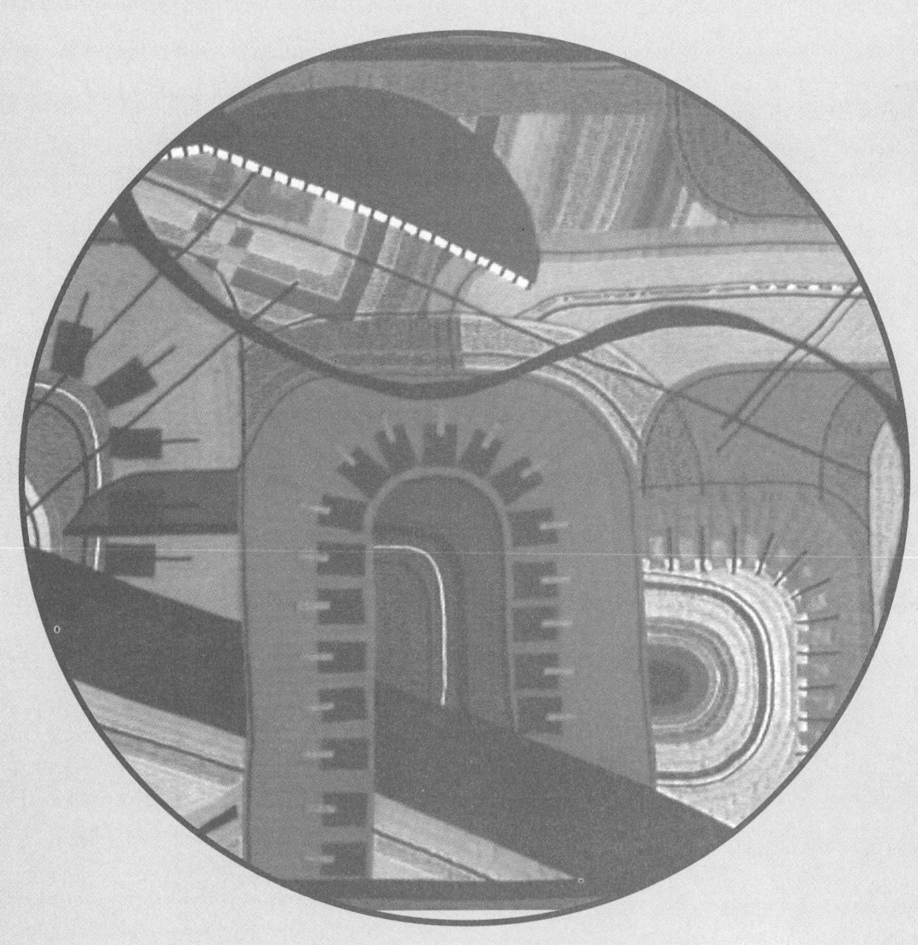

CHAPTER 6

APPLYING THE NURSING PROCESS

Holly Skodol Wilson

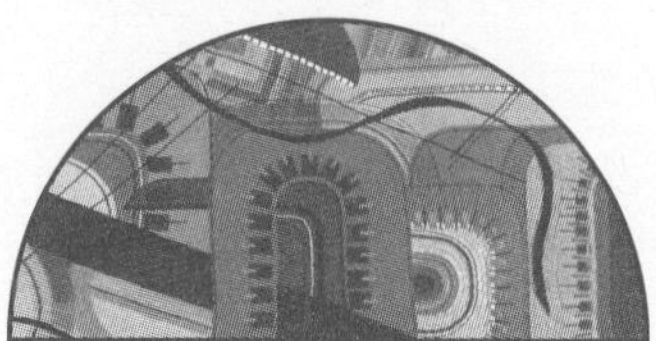

COMPETENCIES

- *Discuss the steps of the nursing process in relation to the 1994 Standards of Psychiatric–Mental Health Clinical Nursing Practice.*
- *Apply the nursing process to situations involving clients with psychiatric–mental health diagnoses.*

Cross-References

Other topics relevant to this content are: Psychiatric nursing standards, Chapter 1; Assessment, Chapter 8; Theories, Chapter 2.

Critical Thinking Challenge

Imagine yourself as charge nurse on an unlocked psychiatric inpatient unit committed to maintaining high standards of care. A 55-year-old man with a 30-year history of alcohol abuse and cigarette smoking is admitted for alcohol detoxification. Because he had pulled out his IV fluids on the preceding shift, managed to get hold of a cigarette lighter in order to smoke, and fallen out of bed, he is now in a posey vest (soft restraints). Your assessment of his current mental status, and his background history and mental status examination results, convince you that he is at risk for harming himself. Your hospital policies justify one-to-one supervision because he meets the criteria. Yet the staff situation is such that you are unable to assign a member of your nursing team to be with him constantly. What are your options? What would you do to provide an acceptable standard of care for this client?

How does a nurse approach the following clinical problems? Obviously, there are no quick and easy formulas for responding to situations that involve genuine human complexities. The 1994 ANA Standards of Psychiatric–Mental Health Clinical Nursing Practice reflect the current state of knowledge in the field and offer some guidance in providing nursing care to clients like those described below.

Diane S, a 23-year-old woman, is admitted to a medical unit with severe anorexia nervosa and thoughts of suicide. She is agitated and tearful and says life looks so bad that she just wants to get out of it.

B. J. is a 27-year-old man who walked into the hospital emergency room because he sees the walls sparkling and weaving around, he feels like people are laughing at him, and he tastes petroleum in his mouth, which he describes as the "taste of afterbirth." He was on his way to jump off the George Washington Bridge when he saw the hospital and decided to come in for help.

The client is a 52-year-old, disheveled woman dressed in ragged street clothes and wearing a turban on her head. She believes that there are radio waves in her teeth reporting of a plot to have her committed to mental hospitals. She has lived on the streets for the past two years with all her possessions and clothing in four large brown paper bags. She speaks in an uninterrupted monotone and is hostile toward the nurse.

The six standards of psychiatric and mental health care presented in Chapter 1 are the focus of this chapter. Together they guide the nurse in the use of the nursing process to make clinical decisions in the practice of psychiatric–mental health nursing. The word *process* suggests movement toward a goal in phases or stages. The **nursing process** is the conscious, systematic set of cognitive and behavioral steps that make up the clinical act of nursing practice. It is adapted from the scientific approach to problem solving. The steps are:

1. Assessing the client's health status from objective and subjective data (collecting and reviewing data).
2. Formulating a psychiatric nursing diagnosis (identifying problems).
3. Identifying outcomes individualized for the client.
4. Developing a plan for interventions (prescriptions to attain outcomes).
5. Implementing the planned interventions (putting the plan in action).
6. Evaluating the nursing care (judging the effectiveness of the plan in achieving outcomes and changing it when needed).

This chapter describes the ways that the nursing process approach is applied to psychiatric nursing practice. We urge that the nursing process become the way in which you think about clients, with the human responses discussed in other chapters of this text. Nursing process is currently used in most nursing curricula and included in most nurse practice acts. The nursing process is flexible and adaptable. It can be applied in a variety of settings with individual clients, families, groups, and aggregates. It requires you to use judgment and creativity in caring for clients in an organized and systematic way. (See the Research Note on this page.)

RESEARCH NOTE

Citation

Becker HA, MacCabe N: Indicators of critical thinking, communication and therapeutic intervention among first-line nursing supervisors. *Nurse Educator* 1994;19(2):15–19.

Study Problem/Purpose

The purpose of this investigation was to identify indicators of communication, critical thinking, and therapeutic intervention skills from first-line nursing supervisors' descriptions of exemplary and substandard nursing practice in an attempt to determine what behaviors make up these critical outcome skills identified by the National League for Nursing.

Methods

Six critical incidents with both positive and negative outcomes in each of the skills areas were contributed by a total of 19 nursing supervisors from four different hospitals and a private mental health agency. Each critical incident was reviewed in order to specify the nursing behaviors involved.

Findings

A total of 442 specific behaviors were generated from the 109 critical incidents described. From these, 40 behavioral indicators were identified as falling within the three NLN-defined skill areas. Among the indicators were "accurately assesses client's current condition,""communicates effectively," and "independently manages a plan of care."

Implications

The behaviors identified, derived from critical incidents, are useful in establishing a dialogue between nursing education and nursing service; they serve as a basis for future research on nurses' competence in critical thinking, communication, and therapeutic intervention.

Standard I: Assessing

Standard I of the 1994 Standards of Psychiatric–Mental Health Clinical Nursing Practice states that the psychiatric–mental health nurse collects client health data.

Rationale

The assessment interview—which requires linguistically and culturally effective communication skills, interviewing, behavioral observation, database record review, and comprehensive assessment of the client and relevant systems—enables the psychiatric–mental health nurse to make sound clinical judgments and plan appropriate interventions with the client.

Measurement Criteria

1. The priority of data collection is determined by the client's immediate condition or need.
2. The data may include but are not limited to:
   a. Ability to remain safe and not be a danger to oneself and others.
   b. Client's central complaint, symptoms, or focus of concern.
   c. Physical, developmental, cognitive, mental, and emotional health status.
   d. History of health patterns and illness.
   e. Family, social, cultural, and community systems.
   f. Daily activities, functional health status, substance use, health habits, and social roles, including work and sexual functioning.
   g. Interpersonal relationships, communication skills, and coping patterns.
   h. Spiritual or philosophical beliefs and values.
   i. Economic, political, legal, and environmental factors affecting health.
   j. Significant support systems, both available and underutilized.
   k. Health beliefs and practices.
   l. Knowledge, satisfaction, and motivation to change, related to health.
   m. Strengths and competencies that can be used to promote health.
   n. Other contributing factors that influence health.
3. Pertinent data are collected from multiple sources using various assessment techniques and standardized instruments as appropriate. Multiple sources of assessment data can include not only the client, but also family, social network, other health care providers, past and current medical records, and community agencies and systems (with consideration of the client's confidentiality).
4. The client, significant others, and interdisciplinary team members are involved in the assessment process to the extent possible.
5. The client and significant others are informed of their respective roles and responsibilities in the assessment process and data analysis.
6. The assessment process is systematic and ongoing.
7. Date collection is based on clinical judgment to ensure that relevant and necessary data are collected.
8. The database is synthesized, prioritized, and documented in a retrievable form.

Data collection requires astute observation, purposeful listening, a broad knowledge of human behavior, and an understanding of what needs to be known and where to obtain the information. The tools used in psychiatric assessment of individual clients include the following:

- Psychiatric history
- Mental status examination
- Psychosocial assessment, including culture
- Neurologic assessment
- Psychologic testing

These assessment tools, among others, are discussed in Chapter 8.

Subjective Data **Subjective data** are reported by the client and significant others in their own words. An example is the **chief complaint** expressed by clients in the course of an intake interview or psychiatric history. Here are some examples of chief complaints:

I was in "warp 5" and pretending to be an undercover cop.

My brother doesn't think I take good enough care of myself.

My husband has been beating me and I think I am losing my mind.

Objective Data **Objective data** are collected and verified by people other than the client and family. Here are some examples:

- Physical examination findings, such as hearing loss.
- Neurologic examination findings, such as those observed when testing for reflexes or observing for tremors.
- Results of psychometric tests, such as the Temporal and Personal Orientation Test or the Global Cognitive Function and Language Comprehension Tests used to assess functional status among the elderly.
- Scores on rating scales developed to quantify the severity of disabilities among the chronically mentally ill.
- Laboratory test results, including complete blood count, sedimentation rate, blood chemistry, thyroid function studies, serum vitamin B_{12}, folate levels, computed tomography brain scan, chest X-ray films, and electrocardiograms.

The Nursing History The nursing history is the foremost method of collecting data from the primary source (the client). Nursing histories summarize client information that the nurse can use to individualize care. They differ from medical or psychiatric histories, which are records of pervious illness and hospitalizations, in that they focus on *client perceptions and expectations* related to their illness, hospitalization, and care.

The **primary data source** is the client. **Secondary data sources** include laboratory and psychologic test results, family members, and other members of the mental health team. Together, these data sources provide a rationale for determining the client's nursing diagnosis and a basis for planning, implementing, and evaluating nursing care. The assessment phase of the nursing process culminates in the formulation of a nursing diagnosis.

Standard II: Diagnosing

Standard II states that the psychiatric–mental health nurse analyzes the assessment data in determining diagnoses.

Rationale

The basis for providing psychiatric–mental health nursing care is the recognition and identification of patterns of response to actual or potential psychiatric illnesses and mental health problems.

Measurement Criteria

1. Diagnoses and potential problem statements are derived from assessment data.
2. Interpersonal, systemic, or environmental circumstances that affect the mental well-being of the individual, family, or community are identified.
3. The diagnosis is based on an accepted framework that supports the psychiatric–mental health nursing knowledge and judgment used in analyzing the data.
4. Diagnoses conform to accepted classifications systems, such as North American Nursing Diagnosis Association (NANDA) Nursing Diagnosis Classification, *International Classification of Diseases* (WHO 1993), and the *Diagnostic and Statistical Manual of Mental Disorders,* 4th ed. (APA 1994), used in the practice setting.
5. Diagnoses and risk factors are validated with the client, significant others, and other health care providers when appropriate and possible.
6. Diagnoses identify actual or potential psychiatric illness and mental health problems of clients pertaining to:
   a. The maintenance of optimal health and well-being and the prevention of psychobiologic illness.
   b. Self-care limitations or impaired functioning related to mental and emotional distress.
   c. Deficits in the functioning of significant biologic, emotional, and cognitive systems.
   d. Emotional stress or crisis components of illness, pain, and disability.
   e. Self-concept changes, developmental issues, and life process changes.
   f. Problems related to emotions such as anxiety, aggression, sadness, loneliness, and grief.
   g. Physical symptoms that occur along with altered psychologic functioning.
   h. Alterations in thinking, perceiving, symbolizing, communicating, and decision making.
   i. Difficulties in relating to others.
   j. Behaviors and mental states that indicate the client is a danger to self or others or has a severe disability.
   k. Interpersonal, systemic, sociocultural, spiritual, or environmental circumstances or events that have an effect on the mental and emotional well-being of the individual, family, or community.
   l. Symptom management, side effects/toxicities associated with psychopharmacologic intervention and other aspects of the treatment regimen.
7. Diagnoses and clinical impressions are documented in a manner that facilitates the identification of client outcomes and their use in the plan of care and research.

The Two-Component Statement of a Nursing Diagnosis

Most authorities propose that the nursing diagnosis statement have two components:

1. The client's potential or actual unhealthful response.
2. The reasons for or possible etiology of the client's unhealthful response.

These authorities believe that incorporating both components gives clearer direction to the planning, implementation, and evaluation steps of the nursing process. Others maintain that cause-and-effect relationships are premature given the current state of nursing research, and that the etiology component of the diagnosis statement is therefore purely speculative. This text acknowledges the lack of consensus on the issue of etiology and presents nursing diagnosis as a name for a perceived difficulty organized by a classification system. A compromise position is to give the name of a difficulty and add a "related factor" phrase.

Toward a Classification System for Psychiatric Nursing Diagnoses

NANDA The **North American Nursing Diagnosis Association (NANDA)** solicits proposed new nursing diagnoses for review by the association. Such proposed diagnoses undergo a systematic staged review that concludes with a mail vote by the entire membership. If the proposed diagnosis is accepted, it is included in NANDA's official list of diagnoses. Such acceptance indicates NANDA's view that the diagnosis is ready for use and continuing development.

To assist interested parties in submitting proposed diagnoses, the NANDA Diagnoses Review Committee has prepared a set of guidelines for submission. These guidelines ensure consistency, clarity, and completeness of submissions. Submitted diagnoses that do not meet the guidelines are returned to the person submitting them for revision so that the review process can begin. Proposed diagnoses are reviewed by the Diagnoses Review Committee, the Clinical Technical Review Task Forces, and the NANDA board prior to review and comment by the General Assembly and membership vote. An example of a proposed nursing diagnosis in the required NANDA format appears in the accompanying box.

The most current (1994) list of NANDA nursing diagnoses, which appears in Appendix D, is organized into nine "human response patterns." These are:

Pattern 1: Exchanging—mutual giving and receiving
Pattern 2: Communicating—sending messages
Pattern 3: Relating—establishing bonds
Pattern 4: Valuing—assigning relative worth
Pattern 5: Choosing—selecting alternatives
Pattern 6: Moving—activity
Pattern 7: Perceiving—receiving information
Pattern 8: Knowing—meaning associated with information
Pattern 9: Feeling—subjective awareness of information

NANDA nursing diagnoses have the following three components:

- Definition
- Defining characteristics
- Related factors

The Eleventh Conference on Classification of Nursing Diagnoses was held in 1994 in Nashville. The review process was changed in two important ways: (1) New diagnoses are now reviewed in different stages when they meet different criteria to encourage their continued development. (2) Diagnoses included in the classification

NANDA Nursing Diagnosis: Hopelessness

Definition

A subjective state in which an individual sees limited or no alternatives or personal choices available and cannot mobilize energy on own behalf.

Defining Characteristics

Major: Passivity
Minor: Lack of initiative; decreased verbalization; decreased affect; verbal cues (despondent content, "I can't," sighing); turning away from speaker; closing eyes; shrugging in response to speaker; decreased appetite, increased sleep; lack of involvement in care/passively allowing care.

Substantiating/Supportive Materials

Eisman, R. (1971). Why did Joe die? *American Journal of Nursing,* March.

Farberow, N.L. (1981). Suicide prevention in the hospital. *Hospital and Community Psychiatry,* 32(2), 99–104.

Jalowiec, A., Powers, M.J. (1981). Stress and coping in hypertensive and ER patients. *Nursing Research,* January–February.

Jourard, S. (1970). Suicide, an invitation to die. *American Journal of Nursing,* February, 70(2).

Kritek, P. (1981). Patient power and powerlessness. *Supervisor Nurse,* 12(6), 26–29, 32–34.

Lambert, Lambert. (1981). Role theory and the concept of powerlessness. *Journal of Psychosocial Nursing,* September.

Miller, C., Denner, P., Richardson, V. (1976). Assisting the psychosocial problems of cancer patients: A review of current research. *International Journal of Nursing Studies.*

Related Factors

Prolonged activity restriction creating isolation; failing or deteriorating physiologic condition; long-term stress; abandonment; lost belief in transcendent values/God.

Source: NANDA Diagnosis Review Committee Correspondence.

will be reviewed again in light of relevant research literature and changes in the field.

DSM-IV The standard interdisciplinary psychiatric diagnosis manual, or *DSM-IV*, is used by the whole mental health team. *DSM-IV* provides a label for a client's psychiatric disorder and thus facilitates communication among team members. The NANDA diagnosis for a psychiatric client is the conceptualization of a client's human response from the unique nursing perspective. Psychiatric nurses must be knowledgeable about both psychiatric diagnostic nomenclature and the expanding efforts of nurses to develop our own diagnostic nomenclature. Both are essential for communication with colleagues and for developing an individualized nursing care plan. Table 6-1 compares a sample DSM-IV diagnosis and related psychiatric nursing diagnoses according to NANDA.

Standard III: Identifying Outcomes

Standard III states that the psychiatric–mental health nurse identifies expected outcomes individualized to the client.

Rationale

Within the context of providing nursing care, the ultimate goal is to influence health outcomes and improve the client's health status.

Measurement Criteria

1. Expected outcomes are derived from the diagnoses.
2. Expected outcomes are client-oriented, therapeutically sound, realistic, attainable, and cost-effective.
3. Expected outcomes are documented as measurable goals.
4. Expected outcomes are formulated by the nurse and the client, significant others, and interdisciplinary team members, when possible.
5. Expected outcomes are realistic in relation to the client's present and potential capabilities.
6. Expected outcomes are identified with consideration of the associated benefits and costs.
7. Expected outcomes estimate a time for attainment.
8. Expected outcomes provide direction for continuity of care.
9. Expected outcomes reflect current scientific knowledge in mental health care.
10. Expected outcomes serve as a record of change in the client's health status.

Table 6–1 A Comparison of DSM-IV and NANDA Nursing Diagnoses

DSM-IV Diagnosis	*NANDA Nursing Diagnoses*
209.1x Primary degenerative dementia Alzheimer's type, presenile onset	6.5.2 Bathing/Hygiene Self-Care Deficit
	8.3 Altered Thought Processes
	5.1.1.1 Ineffective Individual Coping
	3.2.1 Altered Role Performance
	3.1.1 Impaired Social Interaction

Standard IV: Planning

Standard IV states that the psychiatric–mental health nurse develops a plan of care that prescribes interventions to attain expected outcomes.

Rationale

A plan of care is used to guide therapeutic intervention systematically and achieve the expected client outcomes.

Measurement Criteria

1. The plan is individualized, tailored to the client's mental health problems, condition, or needs, and it:
   a. Identifies priorities of care in relation to expected outcomes.
   b. Identifies effective interventions to achieve the outcomes.
   c. Specifies interventions that reflect current psychiatric–mental health nursing practice and research.
   d. Includes an education program related to the client's health problems, treatment, and self-care activities.
   e. Indicates responsibilities of the psychiatric–mental health nurse and the client, and may include responsibilities for interdisciplinary team members to carry out the plan of care.
   f. Gives direction for client-care activities delegated by the psychiatric–mental health nurse to other care providers.
   g. Provides for appropriate referral and case management to ensure continuity of care.
2. The plan is developed in collaboration with the client, significant others, and interdisciplinary team members, when appropriate.
3. The plan is documented in a manner that allows access to it by team members and modification of the plan as necessary.

Properties of an effective nursing plan of care are listed in the accompanying box. A sample plan is shown in the Nursing Care Plan box, below.

Hints for Negotiating Goals

The first step is to determine whether to try to convince the client that your goals are the right goals or to alter your goals. One way to do so is to ask clients what their goals are and how you can help them achieve their goals. Some clients respond that they just came along to appease a significant other who is the one with the real problem. Others believe they are there for a "rest" or a "checkup." Some want to be taken care of and protected, and some believe they have been tricked or betrayed and locked up against their will. Having asked, you must *listen*. Sometimes the simple experience of being heard and understood without being invalidated and dismissed out of hand becomes the basis for subsequent negotiations and eventual agreement about mutually determined goals.

Properties of an Effective Nursing Care Plan

- Identifies priorities of care.
- States realistic outcomes in measurable terms with an expected date of accomplishment.
- Is based on identifiable principles.
- Indicates which client needs are the primary responsibility of the psychiatric nurse and which will be referred to others with appropriate expertise.
- Reflects mutual goal setting and shared responsibility for goal attainment at the level of the client's abilities.
- Forms the basis for client care activities performed by others under the nurse's supervision.

NURSING CARE PLAN

Sample Format

Nursing Diagnosis (NANDA)

Impaired Social Interaction related to Altered Thought Processes

Expected Outcome

By Day 2 client will be able to tolerate limited interaction with staff (at least 5 minutes 3 times/shift.)

Nursing Interventions

- Introduce self each shift.
- Attempt to meet needs despite client's inability to verbalize them.
- Set up 3 times/shift to be with client.
- Spend the time in structured ways, e.g., do grooming tasks, go for a walk. Client does not tolerate intense verbal interaction and becomes more inappropriate with direct questions.
- If client starts to giggle, allow client time to be alone.
- Help client join activities.
- Redirect client from situations with too many stimuli.
- Give encouragement and positive feedback when appropriate.
- Role model social interaction and use group activities to increase social skills.
- Use nurse-client relationship to help client learn new social skills.

Outcome Met If

On discharge, client tolerates limited interaction with others in a structured environment as evidenced by ability to follow schedule.

Nursing Diagnosis

Bathing/Hygiene Self-Care Deficit related to cognitive impairment

Expected Outcome

Client will:

- Be up, dressed, and shaved by 9:00 AM
- Make bed and clean area by 9:30 AM
- Do laundry Monday and Thursday PM
- Shower Monday, Wednesday, and Friday PM

Nursing Interventions

- Arrange hygiene schedule with client
- Review schedule early in the shift and give reminders as necessary of tasks to be done.
- Monitor and give further assistance if needed.
- Give positive feedback for all tasks accomplished.
- Allow client to do as much as possible for self.
- Be alert for progress and allow as much independence as the client tolerates.

Outcome Met If

At discharge, client performs self-care tasks independently.

Once a nursing diagnosis has been identified and clear, unambiguous goals have been set and listed in order of priority, you can consider possible solutions by using what are known as "predictive principles." Bower (1985) calls predictive principles "guides for developing realistic alternatives of action or action hypotheses that tell the nurse what will promote or inhibit progress toward a desired goal." You select one intervention from many choices based on a prediction of the likely or probable consequences of each option. The use of predictive principles cuts down on trial-and-error and the rigid use of standard operating procedures.

Standard V: Implementing

Standard V states that the psychiatric–mental health nurse implements the interventions identified in the plan of care.

Rationale

In implementing the plan of care, psychiatric–mental health nurses use a wide range of interventions designed to prevent mental and physical illness, and promote, maintain, and restore mental and physical health. Psychiatric–mental health nurses select interventions according to their level of practice. At the basic level, the nurse may select counseling, milieu therapy, self-care activities, psychobiologic interventions, health teaching, case management, health promotion and health maintenance, and a variety of other approaches to meet the mental health needs of clients. In addition to the intervention options available to the basic-level psychiatric–mental health nurse, at the advanced level the certified specialist may provide consultation, engage in psychotherapy, and prescribe pharmacologic agents where permitted by state statutes or regulations.

Measurement Criteria

1. Interventions are selected based on the needs of the client and accepted nursing practice.
2. Interventions are selected according to the psychiatric–mental health nurse's level of practice, education, and certification.
3. Interventions are implemented within the established plan of care.
4. Interventions are performed in a safe, ethical, and appropriate manner.
5. Interventions are documented.

Work is ongoing by a large research team at the University of Iowa to develop **The Nursing Interventions Classification (NIC)**, the first comprehensive classification of all treatments and interventions that nurses perform (McCloskey and Bulecheck 1994). SNOMED, a structured nomenclature and classification used in human and veterinary medicine, will include NIC as well as NANDA nursing diagnoses in its next edition. SNOMED contains elements needed for a computerized client record.

Standard VI: Evaluating

Standard VI states that the psychiatric–mental health nurse evaluates the client's progress in attaining expected outcomes.

Rationale

Nursing care is a dynamic process involving change in the client's health status over time, giving rise to the need for new data, different diagnoses, and modifications in the plan of care. Therefore, evaluation is a continuous process of appraising the effect of nursing interventions and the treatment regimen on the client's health status and expected health outcomes.

Measurement Criteria

1. Evaluation is systematic and ongoing.
2. The client, significant others, and team members are involved in the evaluation process, as possible, to ascertain the client's level of satisfaction with care and evaluate the cost and benefits associated with the treatment process.
3. The client's responses to interventions are documented.
4. The effectiveness of interventions in relation to outcomes is evaluated.
5. Ongoing assessment data are used to revise diagnoses, outcomes, and the plan of care as needed.
6. Revisions in the diagnoses, outcomes, and the plan of care are documented.
7. The revised plan provides for continuity of care.

If interventions are discontinued because of a nursing judgment, documentation is needed. Included in this documentation are changes in client behavior as an outcome of the interventions and as evidence that the goal was attained. Such documentation is essential not only to ensure good quality client care but also to minimize legal liability. Nursing care plans that are updated on working tools such as the Kardex should also be updated in the client's permanent record. New developments in the field of *nursing informatics* that address the use of infomation and technology by nurses are resulting in computerized systems for care planning and systems of cost accounting.

Putting Psychiatric Nursing Standards into Practice

The contemporary climate for psychiatric–mental health care is one that demands accountability in terms of client outcomes and cost containment. While the therapeutic use of self and the art of caring remain the cornerstones of practice, Billings (1993) correctly points out that caring goes beyond an innocent feeling and a sensitive act. It is based on an informed decision-making process that has a theoretical and research base. In her words, "We have moved from innocence and instinct to autonomy and accountability" (p. 174). Applying the nursing process, as described in this chapter, is a critical competency basic to excellence in state-of-the-art professional practice in psychiatric–mental health nursing.

Chapter Highlights

- The nursing process provides a scientific way of planning care for psychiatric clients.
- Phases of the nursing process include assessing, diagnosing, identifying outcomes, planning, implementing, and evaluating.
- The 1994 ANA Standards for Psychiatric–Mental Health Clinical Nursing Practice reflect the current state of knowledge and base practice on theory.
- The nursing process is a conscious, deliberate, yet flexible and adaptable systematic set of cognitive and behavioral steps that describe the clinical act in nursing practice with individuals, families, groups, and aggregates.
- Effective nursing depends on accurate, systematic, and continuous data collection.
- Nursing diagnoses express conclusions about clients' human responses supported by recorded assessment data, current scientific premises, and humanistic principles.
- The nursing care plan is used to guide therapeutic intervention and achieve desired outcomes; it should reflect agreement between client and professional on short- and long-term goals.
- The implementation phase of the nursing process is characterized by continued data collection and observation, as well as modification in intervention strategy and timing, if necessary.
- Evaluation completes the nursing process and occurs so that the database, expected client outcomes, nursing diagnosis, and nursing care plan can be revised.

References

American Nurses Association: *A Social Policy Statement.* ANA, 1980.

American Nurses Association: *Standards of Psychiatric–Mental Health Clinical Nursing Practice.* ANA, 1994.

American Psychiatric Association: *Diagnostic and Statistical Manual of Mental Disorders,* ed 4. APA, 1994.

Baradell JG: Cost-effectiveness and quality of care provided by clinical nurse specialists. *Psychosoc Nurs* 1994; 32(3): 21–24.

Billings CV: Psychiatric mental health nursing progress notes. *Arch Psychiatr Nurs* (June) 1993;7(3):174–181.

Bower F: *The Process of Planning Nursing Care,* ed 4. Mosby, 1985.

Girgenti JR, Mathis AC: Putting psychiatric nursing standards into clinical practice. *Psychosoc Nurs* 1994;32(6):39–42.

Lederer JR, et al.: *Care Planning Pocket Guide,* ed 5. Addison-Wesley, 1993.

McCloskey JC, Bulecheck GM: Standardizing the language for nursing treatments: An overview of the issues. *Nurs Outlook* 1994;42(2):56–63.

Neal MC, et al.: *Nursing Care Planning Guides for Psychiatric and Mental Health Care.* Wadsworth, 1980.

Romano CA: Diffusion of technology innovation. *Adv Nurs Sci Nursing Informatics.* 1990; 113(2):11–21.

Townsend MC: *Nursing Diagnoses in Psychiatric Nursing,* ed 2. F. A. Davis, 1991.

World Health Organization: *International Classification of Diseases,* ed. 10. WHO, 1993.

CHAPTER 7

THERAPEUTIC COMMUNICATION

Carol Ren Kneisl

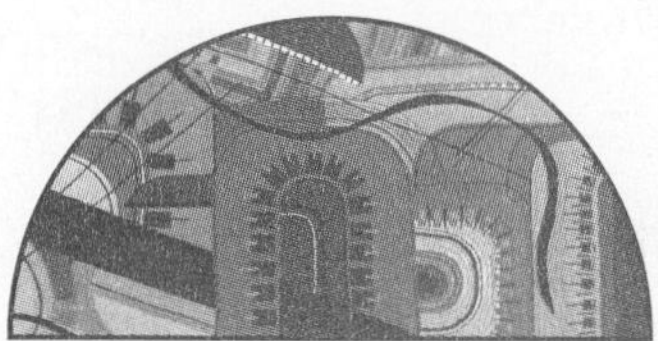

COMPETENCIES

- *Describe the process of human communication.*
- *Compare linear, interactional, and transactional models of communication.*
- *Discuss verbal and nonverbal modes of communication.*
- *Relate three major theories of communication to humanistic psychiatric nursing practice.*
- *Identify the concepts of facilitative communication that are essential ingredients of interpersonal relationships.*
- *Apply skills that foster effective communication throughout the nursing process.*

Cross-References

Other topics related to this content are: Empathy, Chapter 1; Influence of territoriality and personal space on communication, Chapter 31; Role of human values in the communication of the nurse, Chapter 1.

Critical Thinking Challenge

You are about to embark upon your first inpatient psychiatric nursing experience. You feel anxious because although you've read the facilitative communication techniques described in this chapter, you feel uncomfortable about using them. They seem artificial, stilted, and "not you." What can you do to help make your psychiatric nursing experience a positive learning experience for you as well as for your clients?

When John Bowlby (1951) discovered that infants in foundling homes were literally dying for lack of contact and affection, the scientific community began to attach new importance to the old saying that *people need people*. We recognize today that the mechanism for establishing, maintaining, and improving human contacts is interpersonal communication. Communication is a very special process and the most significant of human behaviors. Moreover, it is the main method for implementing the nursing process.

The therapeutic interpersonal relationship in psychiatric–mental health nursing practice often develops through a storytelling experience. Telling stories is as natural and human as breathing. When they tell "their story," clients explain themselves, the events of their lives, and the circumstances they face. Psychiatric nurses help clients tell their stories, help them explore the circumstances of their lives, and help them resolve the things that have gone wrong. However, the process of communication is so complex and has so many dimensions that it cannot be reduced to a few simple steps that nurses can memorize and perform.

The Process of Human Communication

Communication is an ongoing, dynamic, and ever-changing series of events, each of which affects and is affected by all the others. Unfortunately, some people define communication simply as the transfer of information or meaning from one human being to another. However, meaning cannot be transferred; it must be mutually negotiated, because meaning is influenced by a number of significant factors.

Variables That Influence Communication

Perception A person's image or perception of the world is an essential element in communicating. The term **perception** refers to the experience of sensing, interpreting, and comprehending the world in which one lives. This makes perception a highly personal and internal act.

People process through their senses all the information they have about the world around them. However, seeing is not always believing. Contemporary communication specialists have discovered that because of human physiologic limitations, the eye and brain are constantly being tricked into seeing things that are not really what they seem; these are called **illusions**. Figure 7–1 shows an illusion that reflects physiologic constraints. Before continuing to read, stare at Figure 7–1 for 20 seconds. The illustration will appear to swing back and forth. You can verify that the movement is an illusion by checking your visual perception against your tactile sensations.

What people "see" or sense is strongly influenced by many factors. Stop reading here, and look at Figure 7–2.

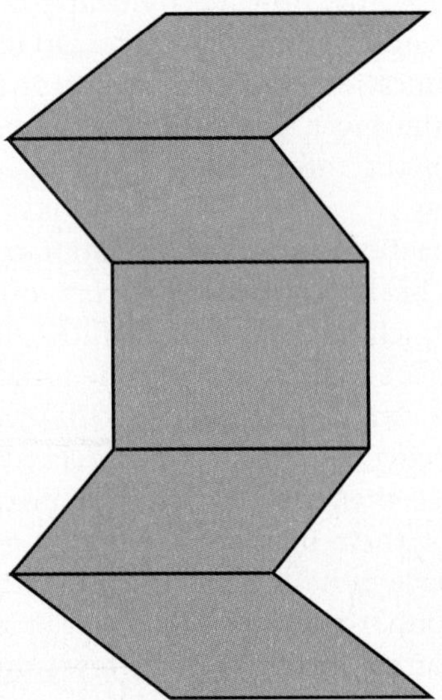

Figure 7–1 A perceptual illusion.

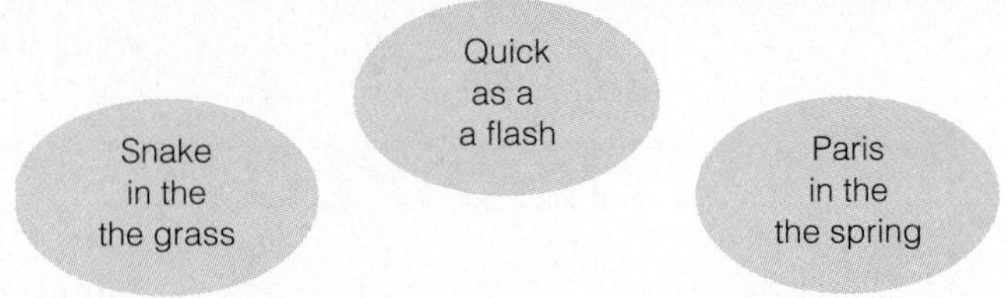

Figure 7–2 The influence of past experience on perception.

Past experiences have prepared us to see things, people, and events in particular ways. When we read the sayings in Figure 7–2, past experience encourages us to see them inaccurately as the familiar sayings "Snake in the grass," "Quick as a flash," and "Paris in the spring." The words actually are "Snake in *the the* grass," "Quick as *a a* flash," and "Paris in *the the* spring."

People tend to observe more carefully when a purpose guides the observation. The purposes or reasons for engaging in an observation also determine what we observe. The nurse in an intensive care unit observes a cardiac surgery client differently than a family member does.

Finally, when understandings differ, you and I can look at the same object and see different things. Mental set helps determine how and what a person perceives. Before you read any further, look at the picture of the young woman in Figure 7–3. Do you see the silhouette of a young woman? Do you also see the face of an elderly woman? Using the phrase "the picture of the young woman in Figure 7–3" encouraged you to perceive the illustration in a particular way. Now you should also be able to see the elderly woman in the illustration.

As the illustrations demonstrate, the old axiom might be better stated: "Believing is seeing." Because we tend to perceive in terms of past experiences, expectations, and goals, perceptions may be a prime obstacle to communication. No two individuals perceive the world in exactly the same way, and the meanings of events differ because people's perceptions of them differ. Perceptions of other human beings are of particular importance because human communication is inevitably affected by participants' perceptions of one another. To see others at all as they are, people need to know themselves and to know how the self affects the perceptions of others.

Values Values are concepts of the desirable. People value what is of worth to them. Values influence the process of communication because people's values, like their perceptions, differ.

Value systems differ for a number of reasons. Age is one. Children's values shift when they become teenagers. The college or work experience generally influences values in yet other directions. Marrying or being a parent or grandparent may cause other value changes or shifts.

Psychiatric nurses must ultimately come to terms with

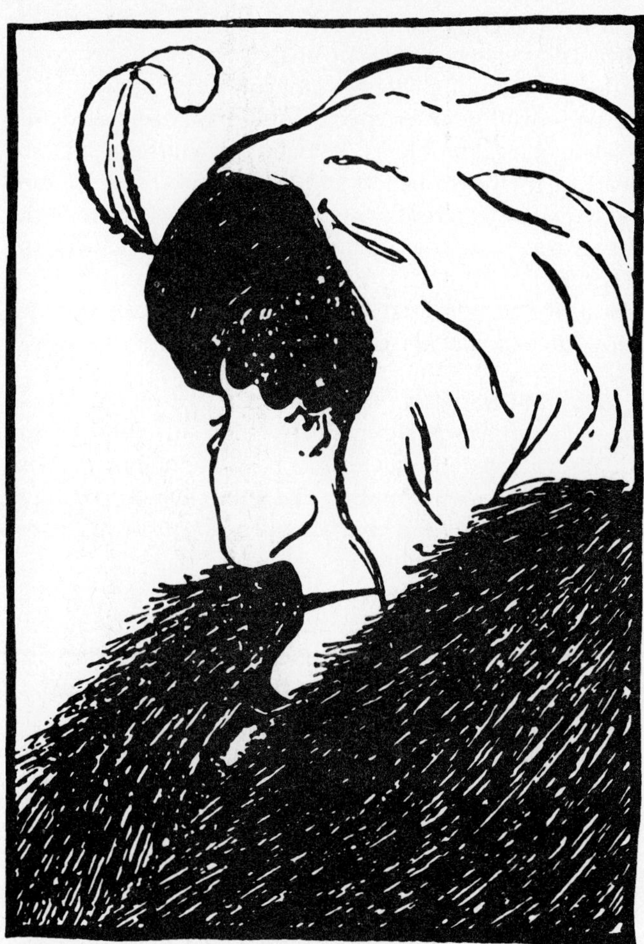

Figure 7–3 The influence of mental set on perception.

the problem of values, because conflicting value systems among mental health professionals expose clients to uncertainty and confusion. Consider the following examples:

The parents of a 15-year-old girl were upset to find a small plastic bag of marijuana in her dresser drawer. She had been playing hooky from school and wore jeans that her parents considered sloppy. After a series of lengthy, angry discussions with her parents, she was confined to her room. During this period she refused to eat or drink.

When the teenager was seen by a mental health treatment team, the members' opinions were divided. Some said that her behavior signaled an emotional disturbance. They labeled her antisocial, depressed, and anxious. Others believed the parents were too rigid in attempting to force her to accept their values.

In another instance, a 35-year-old man was firmly committed to prayer. Most of his spare time involved church-related activities. Staff members at a mental health clinic where he sought counseling told him that he was resorting to an early infantile attitude about God as the magic worker.

Clearly, these staff members were influenced by their own values.

The daily roles people take also influence their values. In any one day a man may be a student, husband, father, nurse, citizen, speaker, artist, son, and teacher.

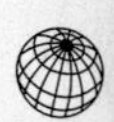

CULTURE Each culture provides its members with notions about how the world is structured and what it means. These preconceptions, learned at an early age, are so subtle that they often go unrecognized. They nonetheless set limits on communication and interaction with others. Relying on culturally determined generalizations or stereotypes can have profound effects on one's relationships with others.

Subculture Communication is culture-bound in a wide variety of ways. The culture and the **subculture** (the culture within the culture) teach people how to communicate through language, hand gestures, clothing, and even in the ways they use the space around them.

There is some controversy about what constitutes a culture and a subculture, or culture within a culture. Recently researchers have referred to the "culture" of the hospital, the operating room, or the nursing school and the "subculture" of the mentally ill, the physically handicapped, or the elderly. Anthropologists point out that simply sharing some common characteristics does not make people members of a culture or subculture. There must be considerably more homogeneity in the group for it to be considered a culture or a subculture. For example, the Choctaw Indians living on a reservation in Philadelphia, Mississippi, are a subculture because they share a language, values and beliefs, and behavioral patterns. They are part of the larger American Indian culture. In contrast, the physically handicapped are not a subculture because they have various disabilities, come from different socioeconomic levels, and may only rarely come into contact with other physically handicapped people.

A case can be made for viewing a hospital or part of it as a culture or subculture. The transient inhabitants of the hospital share a language, standards of acceptable behavior, and a similar world view. This can be seen even more clearly in specialty units, such as intensive care or psychiatric units. People can be viewed as working within a hospital culture while living within the American culture. Applying the term *culture* or *subculture* to these environments may help us understand a hospital, an emergency room, a school, or a church. Some nurse anthropologists view nursing as a subculture (the health care providers subculture) and document its definite set of beliefs, practices, habits, rituals, and values, often stemming from dominant American cultural values.

The nurse who does not know that "run it by me" means to explain something, that a "close-knuckle drill" is a fistfight, or that "hit on a broad" means to sweet-talk a female may be confused by conversations with members of certain subcultures—adolescents and street people, for example. The nurse who overhears two clients talking about "angel dust" is likely to come to erroneous conclusions if unaware that the term refers not to a Christmas decoration but to PCP—an animal tranquilizer. In some cultures, belching after dinner is a compliment to the host and is considered proper etiquette. In other cultures, belching may be thought uncouth or an insult. When Americans make a circle with thumb and forefinger and extend the other fingers, they mean "OK." To Brazilians, the same gesture is an obscene sign of contempt.

These examples make it obvious that communicating with meaning requires that the participants take culture well into account. How people communicate with others who do not share similar histories, heritages, or cultures is of critical importance in humanistic psychiatric nursing practice.

World View A **world view** is the way a group of people (culture or subculture) see their social world, symbolic system, and physical environment and their own place in each. World view is revealed in people's religion, art, language, values, and health care beliefs and practices. A people's world view provides a sense of identity as an American Indian, a Puerto Rican, or a Masai tribesman. It promotes a group's survival and gives members a generally useful picture of the universe.

Ethnocentrism **Ethnocentrism** is the belief that one's own culture is more important and better than any other culture. It frequently takes the form of negative value judgments or selective reporting that criticizes or emphasizes negative aspects of other cultures.

Health care providers need to confront their own ethnocentric, medicocentric, psychocentric views. The following are examples of medicocentric beliefs:

- The doctor or nurse knows best.
- Clients must be compliant if they want to get better.
- If clients aren't compliant they don't want to get better and therefore are not worthy of our time.
- Psychiatric clients can be classified according to the DSM-IV.
- Because of the nature of their illness, psychiatric clients are often noncompliant.
- The description of feelings and thoughts is very important in mental health.

These views are responsible for such professional beliefs as, "Why bother explaining her medication to her; she is ignorant," or "Hispanics have those crazy beliefs in their own witchdoctors. They never do what we say." Such ethnocentric beliefs, spoken or unspoken, inevitably create antagonism among clients and health care personnel. In the present litigious environment, antagonism can easily escalate to legal problems. To avoid this, nurses need to be aware of their own beliefs and values and recognize how these may be different from, not better than, those of the clients they care for. Taking a holistic view reduces the likelihood of ethnocentrism. In addition, a nurse who is aware of the potential for ethnocentrism can use this knowledge to educate and be a role model for others.

Cultural Relativism **Cultural relativism** is the fundamental anthropologic concept that all cultures are equally valued. It argues against passing judgments about practices that are unfamiliar, strange, or even shocking to us, suggesting instead that all cultures can be evaluated only on their own values in context.

Combating ethnocentrism is not easy. It takes energy and work and constant assessment of oneself and society. Client problems need to be seen from a cultural relativist's perspective; that is, what does the problem seem like to the client? Only by understanding the client's view can nurses provide effective care.

Levels of Communication

Communication takes place on at least three different levels: intrapersonal, interpersonal, and public. Psychiatric nurses are more concerned with intrapersonal and interpersonal communication. **Intrapersonal communication** occurs when people communicate within themselves. A nurse who walks into a client's room and thinks, "The first pint of blood is almost finished. I'd better get the next one ready for infusion," is communicating intrapersonally.

Interpersonal communication, which this chapter discusses in depth, takes place in dyads (groups of two people) and small groups. This level of person-to-person communication is at the heart of psychiatric nursing.

Public communication is communication between a person and several other people. Its most common form is the presentation of a public speech. Communications through the mass media are other forms of public communication.

Theories and Models of Human Communication

One of the easiest ways to illustrate the nature of human communication and the elements of the process is through a model, or visual representation.

People use models frequently for many purposes. They might use a map, which is a visual representation of a geographic location, to find their way to the community mental health center they plan to visit. Health professionals use EEGs to see a visual representation of the electrical activity in the brain. However, models provide incomplete views—a map does not show all the trees, buildings, or park statues in the territory; and an EEG tracing does not show the color, size, or blood supply of the brain. It is important to keep this in mind when looking at models. They sometimes make a process look simpler than it is.

Communication as an Act

Viewing human communication as an act is to see it as a one-way phenomenon: Person A talks to person B. Communicators who follow this concept attempt to transfer the thoughts or ideas in their heads into someone else's head. Communication then becomes something that is done *to* another person.

Two major assumptions behind this view are that skill is all-important, and that meaning is transferable. Such a model fails to take into account the variables discussed earlier: perception, values, and culture. It suggests that the receiver plays a passive role and does not affect the communicator. It places primary emphasis on the selection of "correct" messages. When misunderstandings occur, either the communicator is faulted for failing to send the correct message, or the receiver is faulted for having allowed something to interfere with the transmission of a correct message. Both people become preoccupied with laying blame and achieving the impossible—constructing "perfect messages." These implications and assumptions are evidence that the model of communication as an act is inadequate.

Communication as an Interaction

Communication as an interaction takes into account the process of mutual influence in communication. In this view, when two people interact, they put themselves into each other's shoes. Each tries to perceive the world as the other perceives it, in order to predict how the other will respond. In other words, communication is not a one-way process. It is a circular process in which the participants take turns at being communicator and receiver: Person A (communicator) talks to person B (receiver), and person B (communicator) talks to person A (receiver).

Clearly, this model accounts for more factors than the previous one. However, it still oversimplifies human communication because it treats it as a series of causes and effects, stimuli and responses.

Communication as a Transaction

MUTUAL INFLUENCE BETWEEN COMMUNICATORS In communication as a transaction, the participants are both communicators. No one is labeled as either communicator or receiver. Communication is viewed as a process of simultaneous mutual influence rather than as a turn-taking event.

In a transactional perspective, participants are who they are in relationship to the other person with whom they are communicating. For example, in each dyadic (two-person) communication event there are at least *six* people involved: A's A, A's B, A's impression of the way B sees A, B's B, B's A, and B's impression of the way A sees B. Therefore, in addition to the content message, a relationship message also exists. Suppose A passes B in the corridor and A says, "Hi, how are you." B answers, "Just fine, thanks," moving down the corridor and away from A as quickly as possible. B's behavior is a comment on the relationship between A and B. Their subsequent communication will be affected by how A perceives B's response. If A thinks B walked away because B wanted to get home before a rainstorm hits, A is likely to respond one way to B the next time they meet. If A believes B is angry with A, A is likely to respond quite differently at the next encounter. The symbolic interactionist model described next helps explain what takes place between A and B.

A SYMBOLIC INTERACTIONIST MODEL OF COMMUNICATION A symbolic interactionist model is based on a transactional perspective. It views human communication on the social-interpersonal level and accounts for the whole persons involved in the process. The participants are products of their social system and integral parts of it. In the communication, some events take place *within* the participants (they are intrapersonal), and some take place *between* the participants (they are interpersonal).

A model constructed by Hulett (1966) according to symbolic interactionist principles, and adapted for this text, is shown in Figure 7–4. It shows five phases in each person's communication sequence: input, covert rehearsal, message generation, environmental event, and goal response.

During the phase of *input*, the person is motivated through some stimulus, either external or internal, toward some goal that requires engaging in a social interaction with another. Let's say that Jeff is attracted to Sarah and would like to get to know her better.

In the *covert rehearsal* phase, the person moves to make sense of the input received and develops and organizes a message *before* generating it. Figure 7–5 on page 115 represents the covert rehearsal phase of the symbolic interactionist model. The individual first scans the information about self and others (Jeff enjoys theater and remembers hearing Sarah tell a friend that she'd really like to see the new musical comedy in town) and then mentally rehearses possible actions to take (role playing) and possible reactions of the other (role taking). This gives Jeff the chance to think of four or five different ways to approach Sarah. This process is represented by the intrapersonal feedback loop.

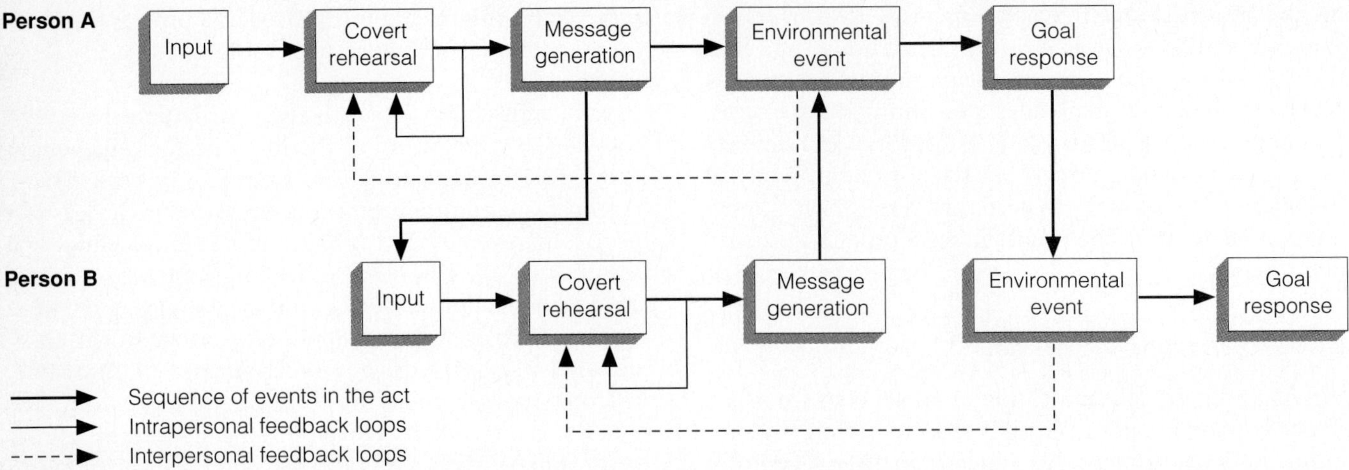

Figure 7–4 A symbolic interactionist model of communication. *SOURCE: Adapted from Hulett 1966, p. 14.*

The covert rehearsal phase is really the core of the communication process. In it, Jeff decides what to say, how to say it, and even whether to send the message to Sarah at all.

During *message generation*, the third phase, the instrumental act of giving a message is performed. (Jeff asks Sarah to the theater.) A message generated by one person serves as the input or the stimulus for another person. (Sarah thinks about Jeff's invitation, decides whether she wants to go to the theater with him, and considers what response to make to Jeff.) Once the second person completes the covert rehearsal and generates a message, this message becomes an *environmental event* for the first person. In our example, the environmental event is the fourth stage in the sequence for Jeff, whose *goal response* serves as an environmental event for Sarah, and so on.

A second, or interpersonal, feedback loop connects the person's environmental event phase to the covert rehearsal stage. It allows the person an opportunity to determine whether he or she has made an error in the approach to the other and to make appropriate corrections by repeating the covert rehearsal and devising an altered message. (Jeff carefully considers Sarah's response. He listens to what she says and watches her behavior toward him. If her response is less than enthusiastic, he will try to determine what went wrong and how to correct it.)

In summary, the symbolic interactionist view of communication includes the following concepts:

- People run through a series of internal trials in the process of organizing a message.
- People select and transmit the message that will, in their view, have the highest probability of success.
- Success depends on the accuracy and completeness of the cognitive map and the accuracy and efficiency of the intrapersonal and interpersonal feedback loops.
- Communication is a dynamic (ever-changing) process that is unrepeatable and irreversible.
- Communication is complex.
- The meaning of messages is not transferred; it is mutually negotiated.

Communication is, at the very least, a very complicated process.

Biologic Factors

Looking at communication in its broadest sense requires us to go beyond the spoken word, the written word, and motor activity to the molecular level. In this broad view, communication can also be thought of as "the swirl of neurotransmitters within a synapse between neurons" (Restak 1994, p. 7). Neurobiology researchers believe that communication at the molecular level may be the root of all brain functioning, including communication.

The neuron, the functional unit of the brain, differs from other cells in the body in that it is specialized for the function of information processing. The flow of information from one nerve cell to another involves the passage of electrically charged chemical particles—sodium, potassium, calcium, and chloride—across the cell membrane of the neuron. Neurotransmitters released by the presynaptic membrane of the axon cross the synaptic cleft and bind to their receptors on the postsynaptic membrane of the dendrite of the target cell.

Therefore, brain activity can also be thought of in terms of messages and receptors or communicators and receivers. It makes sense to acknowledge that when communication is disrupted at one level—for example, when a crucial chemical in the brain undergoes an alteration—the end result can be felt at other more obvious communication levels of the individual (such as verbal and

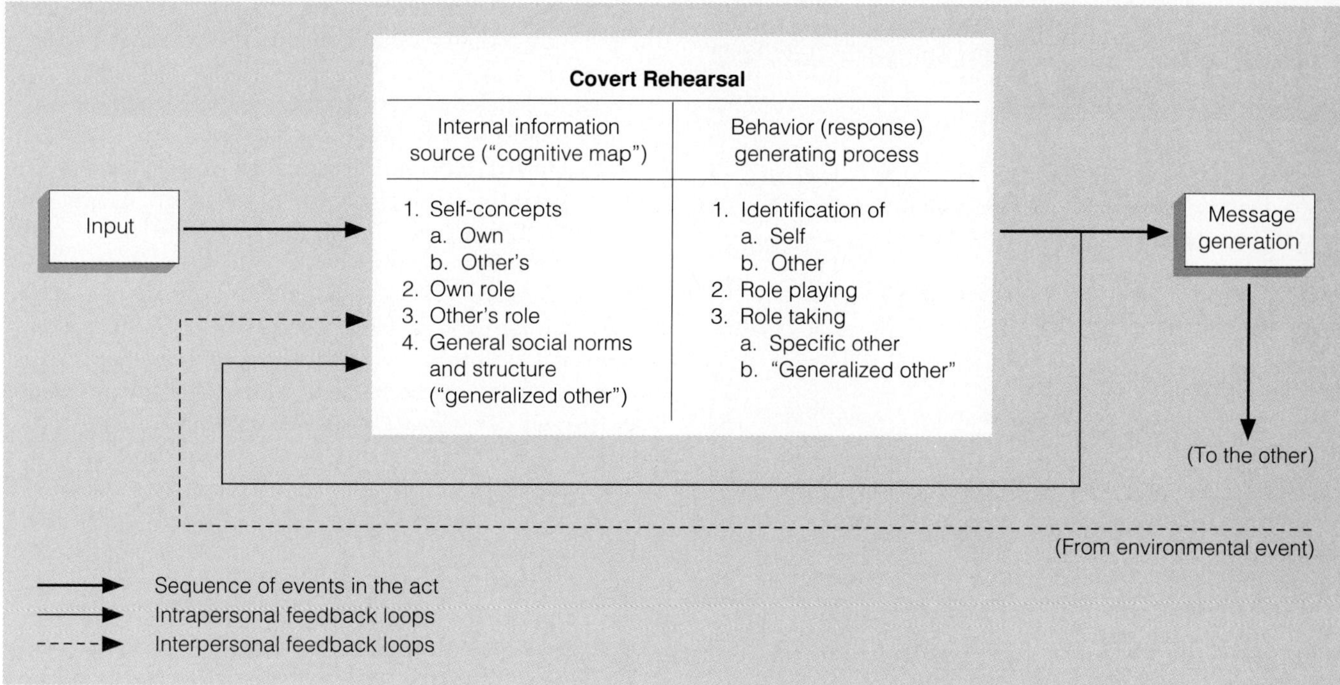

Figure 7–5 The covert rehearsal phase of the symbolic interactionist model.
Source: Hulett 1966, p. 18.

nonverbal communication and intrapersonal and interpersonal communication). The Research Note on the next page is an example. To put this into perspective, your understanding of the words on this page is related not only to your understanding of written English, but also to the chloride ion channel activity on the membranes of millions of your brain cells.

Modes of Communication

The Spoken Word

Verbal language, the ability to utter the spoken word, makes people human and distinguishes them from other animals. Yet problems arise when we discover that words mean different things to different people. That is, *words* do not "mean" something; *people* do.

If communication between nurse and client is to be mutually negotiated, the nurse at least must understand the four concepts discussed next.

Denotation and Connotation A *denotative meaning* is one that is in general use by most people who share a common language. A *connotative meaning* usually arises from a person's personal experience. While all Americans are likely to share the same general denotative meaning of the word *pig*, the word may have completely different connotations for a farmer, a butcher, a consumer of meat, a person of the Moslem faith, an orthodox Jew, a college student, a prisoner, and a police officer. These positive and negative connotative meanings can evoke powerful emotions.

Private and Shared Meanings For communication to take place, meaning must be shared. This bewildering conversation between Alice and Humpty Dumpty shows what happens when meaning is not shared:

> "There's glory for you!"
>
> "I don't know what you mean by 'glory.'" Alice said.
>
> Humpty Dumpty smiled contemptuously. "Of course you don't—till I tell you. I meant 'there's a nice knock-down argument for you!'"
>
> "But 'glory' doesn't mean 'a nice knock-down argument,'" Alice objected.
>
> "When I use a word," Humpty Dumpty said, in rather a scornful tone, "it means just what I choose it to mean—neither more nor less." (Carroll 1965, p. 93)

By assigning meanings to a word without agreement, Humpty Dumpty essentially created a private language.

People can use private meanings to communicate with others only when the parties agree about what the word means. The private meaning then becomes a shared meaning. It is common for families, two friends, or members of larger social groups (military personnel, drug users, adolescents) to use language in highly personal and

RESEARCH NOTE

Citation

Liehr P: Uncovering a hidden language: The effects of listening and talking on blood pressure and heart rate. *Arch Psychiatr Nurs* 1992;6(5): 306–311.

Study Problem/Purpose

Three specific research questions were addressed:

1. What is the cardiovascular effect of listening as compared with talking?
2. What is the effect of gender on cardiovascular changes during listening and talking?
3. What is the effect of story content on cardiovascular changes during listening?

Methods

One hundred nine government employee subjects from a large eastern U.S. city were monitored by an automatic blood pressure cuff while they remained quiet, listened to either an allegory or a personal story, and spoke about their usual daily activities.

Findings

Cardiovascular arousal was higher during talking than it was during listening. It made no difference whether subjects heard an allegory or a personal story. Subjects who talked first had higher blood pressure during talking than those who listened before they talked.

Implications

The strongest implication for practice emerges from observed cardiovascular changes during talking; that is, blood pressure and heart rate changes were statistically significant during talking about a nonstressful topic. This suggests that nurses should use caution when urging clients to "ventilate," especially when the topic is stressful and the client has a history of cardiovascular disease. The results also suggest that it may be physiologically useful to ease into requests for client narrative by allowing the client time before talking. Although listening to standardized stories does not result in clinically significant cardiovascular change, the effects of listening to and talking about meaningful information shared in an interpersonal relationship requires further study.

private ways. Problems arise when the assumption is made that people who are outside the group share these meanings.

People labeled schizophrenic may use language in an idiosyncratic way or may use a private, unshared language referred to as **neologisms**. Such people are unaware that others don't share this use of language. People who use neologisms expect to be understood and may become upset when they are not.

A young man who was hospitalized on a psychiatric unit complained to other clients and staff members that he had been *odenated,* and he became increasingly frustrated and anxious when it became apparent that he wasn't being understood. With some help he was able to explain that he was upset about having been moved to a private room. The room was, he said, so dark and dingy that it looked like a cave. Animals live in caves that are called *dens.* In his view he had been *o-den-ated*—put in a cave.

In trying to make private meanings shared, the nurse should make an effort to reach mutual understanding of the client's message. It is insufficient, and quite possibly inaccurate, to attach meaning based solely on the nurse's (or the client's) interpretation of an event, a word or phrase, or a nonverbal gesture.

Nonverbal Messages

Most researchers agree that **nonverbal communication** channels carry more social meaning than verbal channels. Nonverbal cues help us judge the reliability of verbal messages more readily, especially in the presence of a **mixed message** (inconsistency between the verbal and nonverbal components).

There is a wide variety in nonverbal channels: body movements, including facial expressions and hand gestures; pitch, rate, and volume of the voice; the use of personal and social space; touch; and the use of cultural artifacts (such as clothing and cosmetics).

Body Movement The study of body movement as a form of nonverbal communication is called *kinesics*. Facial expressions, gestures, and eye movements are the most commonly used categories.

Facial expressions are the single most important source of nonverbal communication. They generally communicate emotions. The silent film comedians—blank-faced Buster Keaton and comic, endearing Charlie Chaplin—and the great mime Marcel Marceau communicate not only isolated acts but complete sequences of behavior with kinesics alone.

Body movements and gestures provide clues about people and about how they feel toward others. Hand gestures can communicate anxiety, indifference, and impatience, among other things. Foot shuffling and fidgeting may express the desire to escape. Body position gives cues about how open a person is to another person, or how interesting and attractive one person is to another. People tend to position their bodies according to their feelings about the person with whom they are communicating.

Eye contact is another very important cue in communicating. For example, proper sidewalk behavior among Americans is for passers-by to look at each other until they are about eight feet apart. At this distance, both parties look downward or away so they will not appear to be staring. Several common but unstated rules about eye contact are:

- Interaction is invited by staring at another person on the other side of the room. If the other person returns the gaze, the invitation to interact has been accepted. Averting the eyes signals a rejection of the looker's request.
- A looker's frank gaze is widely interpreted as positive regard.
- Greater mutual eye contact occurs among friends.
- People who seek eye contact while speaking are usually perceived as believable and earnest.
- If the usual short, intermittent gazes during a conversation are replaced by gazes of longer duration, the person looked at is likely to believe that the person gazing considers the relationship between the two people to be more important than the content of the conversation.

Voice Quality and Nonlanguage Sounds *Paralinguistics* or *paralanguage* refers to something beyond or in addition to language itself. The two principal components are *voice quality*, such as pitch and range, and *nonlanguage vocalizations*, such as sobbing, laughing, or grunting—noises without linguistic structure.

Vocal cues can differentiate emotions. Who hasn't heard the injunction, "Don't speak to me in that tone of voice!" Sometimes people use vocal cues to make inferences about personality traits. For example, people who increase the loudness, pitch, timbre (overtones), and rate of their speech are often thought to be active and dynamic. Those who use greater intonation and volume and are fluent are thought to be persuasive. Status cues in speech are based on a combination of word choice, pronunciation, grammar, speech fluency, and articulation, among other factors.

Use of Personal and Social Space *Proxemics* is the study of space relationships maintained by people in social interaction. It includes the dimensions of *territoriality* (fixed and permanent territory that is somehow marked off and defended from intrusion) and *personal space* (a portable territory surrounding the self that others are expected not to invade).

Knowing something about proxemics is useful, for example, in planning the physical space in which communication is to occur. Nurses can arrange furniture to increase or decrease interpersonal distance. Nurses should be especially sensitive to the constraints imposed on communication by physical objects. Nurses can use proxemics to decipher verbal communication by paying attention to how others use interpersonal space.

Touch Touching behaviors, because they tend to personalize communication, are extremely important in emotional situations. In American society, the use of touch is governed by strong social norms. Unwritten guidelines control who, when, why, and where people touch.

Most of the taboos against touching seem to stem from the sexual implications of touching behavior. However, although touching is a physical act, it may or may not be sexual in nature. A realization of the importance of touch and an understanding that touching is not necessarily a sexual behavior may make this channel of communication available to more people. It is equally important to be sensitive to the other person's disposition toward touching, so as not to alienate another by infringing on the person's right not to be touched.

Cultural Artifacts Artifacts are items in contact with interacting people that may function as nonverbal stimuli: clothes, cosmetics, perfume, deodorants, jewelry, eyeglasses, wigs and hairpieces, beards and mustaches, and so on.

Think about what information is communicated through artifacts such as a full-length mink coat, hair that is dyed purple, a gold band on the third finger of the left hand, a military uniform, or a Phi Beta Kappa key.

Relationships Between Verbal and Nonverbal Systems

The verbal and nonverbal elements of human communication are inextricably linked. Six different ways in which verbal and nonverbal systems interrelate are discussed below.

1. A nonverbal cue may *repeat* a verbal cue but in a different way. The deep-sea fisherman who verbally describes the size of the sailfish he caught may also extend both hands to indicate its length. The gesture repeats the idea.
2. Nonverbal behavior may also *contradict* verbal behavior. Consider the woman who meets a college roommate she hasn't seen for quite some time. She says, "You haven't changed a bit," but her tone of voice and facial expression convey sarcasm. When verbal and

nonverbal cues contradict one another, it is usually safer to put more faith in the nonverbal cues.

3. Nonverbal messages that *add to or modify* verbal messages are said to be complementary. When a man says he is a "little" irritated about being kept waiting, his tone of voice and body actions may indicate a more profound anger.
4. Certain nonverbal cues *accent or emphasize* verbal cues. A woman shrugs her shoulders when she says she doesn't really care which movie she and her companion see. A master of ceremonies holds up his hand when he asks for quiet. These gestures and body movements emphasize the words.
5. Cues that *regulate,* such as those that tell people when to start talking or when to stop talking, are usually nonverbal. A woman who keeps opening and closing her mouth briefly while others are talking is indicating that she wants a turn too.
6. Sometimes nonverbal cues are used to *substitute* for words. A wave from a friend at a distance replaces "hello." Applause at the end of a play tells the actors that they have pleased the audience.

Biopsychosocial Communication Theories

Ruesch's Theory of Therapeutic Communication

The psychiatrist Jurgen Ruesch (1961) developed a theory of therapeutic communication. In his view, communication includes all the processes by which one human being influences another. Ruesch's theory takes into account the perceptions and interpretations that influence one person's view of the other. Further, Ruesch assumes that, to survive, the individual must communicate successfully.

According to Ruesch, communication is one of the hardest human skills to master. It takes a long time to learn because it occurs in a series of steps, each building on the previous one. To communicate effectively requires decades of continuous practice. It is believed that interference hampers development and leaves an indelible mark.

BASIC CONCEPTS The basic concepts of Ruesch's theory are as follows:

- Communication occurs in four different settings: intrapersonal, interpersonal, group, and societal.
- The ability to receive, evaluate, and transmit messages is influenced by perception, evaluation (which involves memory, past experiences, and value systems), and the transmission quality of messages (amount, speed, efficacy, and distinctiveness).
- Messages achieve meaning when they are mutually validated or verified between the two parties. (In Ruesch's view, however, it is the psychiatric therapist's reality that verifies a message. The definition is not mutually agreed upon by client and therapist.)
- Correction through feedback is basic to adaptive, healthy behavior and successful communication.

CHARACTERISTICS OF SUCCESSFUL AND DISTURBED COMMUNICATION The four formal criteria for successful communication are efficiency, appropriateness, flexibility, and feedback. When these criteria are not met, communication is disturbed.

Efficiency Simplicity, clarity, and correct timing are all components of efficient messages. Psychiatric nurses and other mental health professionals may find themselves using complex and scientific words or professional mental health jargon to convey messages. Obscure or clumsy language and irrelevant or useless information may also prevent others from understanding a message.

Clear messages give a sense of order or structure and reduce ambiguity by narrowing the number of possible interpretations of meanings. Emphasizing the important ideas helps.

Proper timing is also important. It is best to give messages when the other person is able to "hear" them, when there are no intervening noises or inputs, and when the other person can interpret them without undue haste. Problems occur if the interval between the messages is either too short or too long.

Appropriateness Messages are appropriate when they are relevant to the situation at hand and when there is mutual fit of overall patterns and constituent parts. Communication is inappropriate when it does not fit the circumstance, is irrelevant, or is misconstrued.

Communication can also be inappropriate in amount. Since every individual has both high and low tolerance levels for stimulation, a person's ability to cope with ideas, make decisions, and act is affected by the amount and rate of sensory input received. Exceeding a tolerance level is called **overload**. A person who is overloaded by too many messages or by messages too closely spaced cannot handle incoming messages. **Underload** occurs when delay or lack of information interferes with a person's ability to comprehend the message of another.

The **tangential reply** is another example of inappropriateness. A tangential reply to a statement disregards the content of the message and is directed toward either an incidental aspect of the initial statement, the type of language used, the emotions of the sender, or another facet of the same topic.

Flexibility People cannot always be sure how a message will be received, because each person with whom they communicate is unique and changing. Since they cannot expect constancy from others, people need to be flexible. In communication, lack of flexibility manifests itself as either exaggerated control or exaggerated permissiveness. Both extremes increase the likelihood of frustrating, ungratifying, or disturbed communication.

Maintaining flexibility can be difficult if doing so requires a person to abandon or temporarily lay aside a carefully planned goal. To be flexible, a person must have the ability to set new priorities and to move to meet immediate goals. People who practice humanistic psychiatric nursing work to achieve flexibility in their relationships with clients and colleagues.

Feedback **Feedback** is the process by which performance is checked and malfunctions corrected. It performs a regulatory function in the communication process. Feedback allows people to decide which messages have been understood as intended. It requires the cooperation of two people—one to give it, and one to receive it.

Under certain circumstances of disturbed communication, feedback either fails or functions poorly. When messages do not get through or are distorted, appropriate replies cannot be obtained, and corrective feedback does not occur. Content that elicits anxiety, fear, shame, or any of several other strong emotions is likely to hamper feedback. Feedback is discussed in greater depth later in this chapter.

The Theory of Pragmatics of Human Communication

Watzlawick, Beavin, and Jackson (1967) base their theory of human communication on the assumption that communication is synonymous with interaction. These authors maintain that, in the presence of another, all behavior is communicative. This theory is concerned with the pragmatics, or the behavioral effects, of human interaction. What makes this theory particularly useful for this book is its conception of human communication as a reciprocal process.

Some Axioms of the Theory According to this theory, one cannot *not* communicate. Both activity and inactivity, verbalizations and silences, convey messages. This communication occurs on two levels. The *content level* of a communication is the report aspect, in which information is conveyed. The *relationship level* is communication about a communication.

All interchanges can be viewed as either **symmetric** (based on equality) or **complementary** (based on difference). In symmetric relationships, the partners usually mirror each other's behavior, thus minimizing difference. Complementary relationships, in contrast, maximize difference.

Disturbances in Human Communication Communication can be disturbed when a person attempts *not* to communicate. In this framework, the basic dilemma in schizophrenia is the schizophrenic person's attempt not to communicate. However, because it is impossible not to communicate, schizophrenics are faced with the need to deny that they are communicating while denying that this denial is a communication.

Another disturbance occurs when a person communicates in a way that invalidates the messages sent to or received from the other person. Such communications, called *disqualifications*, include a wide range of behavior such as self-contradictions, inconsistencies, subject switches, incomplete sentences, and misunderstandings.

A person may communicate in a way that confirms, rejects, or disconfirms the other person's view of self. Confirmation of one person's self-view by another is thought to be the greatest single factor in ensuring mental development and stability. Rejection of the other's definition of self essentially conveys this message: "You're wrong." Disconfirmation, by contrast, conveys this message: "You don't exist." Disconfirmation questions the other's authenticity. Disconfirmation leads to alienation and has been found to occur with some regularity in interactions between people labeled schizophrenic and the members of their families.

Although all relationships are necessarily either symmetric or complementary, *runaways* (exaggerations to the point of disturbance) may occur in either of the patterns. For example, the danger of competitiveness is ever-present in symmetric relationships. Symmetric interactions that lose their stability may enter a spiral in which each individual attempts to run just a little bit "more equal" than the other. Runaways are seen in quarrels between people or wars between nations, behaviors that are relatively open. Rejection of the other's self generally occurs when a symmetric relationship breaks down.

Breakdowns in complementary relationships, however, are generally characterized by disconfirmation of the other. For this reason, they are usually viewed as more serious.

Neurolinguistic Programming Theory

Neurolinguistic programming (NLP) is a communication model developed in the early 1970s by Richard Bandler and John Grinder (1975, 1976). The model is derived from theory in linguistics, neurophysiology, psychology, cybernetics, and psychiatry. Relatively new to nursing, NLP first appeared in the nursing literature in 1983 (Brockopp 1983; Knowles 1983).

Bandler and Grinder first observed psychotherapists who were known as expert communicators to discover what made them so effective as therapists. They concluded that people take in, or *access,* information in three sensory modalities: auditory, visual, and kinesthetic. Further, each person prefers one mode over the others. Sounds may facilitate communication with one person, while touch or sight may be more effective with another person. In addition, people *process* information, or make sense out of it, according to the representational system (the NLP phrase for sensory modality) through which they receive it.

They also found that the expert communicators they observed were able to adapt themselves to match the client's representational system and to imitate the client in a natural and respectful way. Bandler and Grinder theorized that by tuning in to and then using the other person's preferred sensory mode, one could greatly enhance the ability to establish rapport. The most effective communicators, according to NLP theory, are those who can use all three modalities and easily move from one representational system to another.

ASSESSMENT

Preferred Predicates

Auditory	*Visual*	*Kinesthetic*
Argue	Appear	Attach
Chant	Bright	Breathless
Debate	Colorful	Calm
Eavesdrop	Glimpse	Excite
Hassle	Image	Fondle
Hear	Observe	Hurt
Listen	Pretty	Rough
Overhear	Scan	Sharp
Praise	Sight	Soft
Quiet	Spy	Sore
Scream	Stare	Support
Silent	Ugly	Tension
Tell	View	Throw
Whine	Watch	Touch
Whisper	Wink	Warm

Determining the Representational System To determine whether a client's representational system is auditory, visual, or kinesthetic, one identifies the client's:

- Preferred predicates (verbs, adjectives, adverbs that tell something about the subject)
- Eye-accessing cues
- Gross hand movements
- Breathing pattern
- Speech pattern and voice tones

Preferred Predicates The accompanying Assessment box categorizes predicates according to the auditory, visual, and kinesthetic modes. A necessary first step before attempting to link words with nonverbal behavior is observing the client to see which set of predicates is preferred.

Eye-Accessing Cues Eye-accessing cues correlate with an individual's thinking process. People who are visualizing generally turn their eyes upward or look straight ahead, focusing on nothing. Someone processing auditory information usually moves the eyes from side to side. A person engaging in intrapersonal communication usually focuses the eyes down in the direction of the nondominant hand. A person in the kinesthetic mode looks down toward the dominant hand when experiencing sensations or emotions.

Gross Hand Movements Gross hand movements also give clues to the client's sensory mode. People have a tendency to point toward or touch the sense organ that matches their current sensory mode. The person in a visual mode often points toward the eye, and the person in an auditory mode often points toward or touches the ear.

Breathing Pattern Assessing the breathing patterns helps the observer understand the client's representational model. Shallow, thoracic breathing is often associated with visual accessing. Even breathing or prolonged expiration is associated with auditory accessing, and deep abdominal breathing is associated with kinesthetic accessing.

Speech Pattern and Voice Tones Visual accessing often correlates with quick bursts of words that are high pitched, strained, or nasal. Auditory accessing is often associated with a clear, midrange voice tone or with a rhythmic tempo and clearly enunciated words. Kinesthetic accessing is associated with a slow voice and a low volume or deep tone, or with a breathy tone and long pauses.

Therapeutic Use of NLP Using NLP theory in psychiatric nursing practice gives us yet another way to empathize with clients by "trying on" their style. People tend to be less anxious with the familiar. Nurses who mirror the client's sensory mode are likely to be experienced as more comfortable and safer to be with, conditions that facilitate rapport.

Knowles (1983) suggests that nurses can use mirroring to help the client follow the nurse's lead. For example, with an anxious client, the nurse might begin by mirroring the behaviors that indicate the client's anxiety and then shift into a more relaxed posture and less anxious behaviors. According to Knowles, the nurse can lead the client from a more anxious state to a less anxious state by employing the NLP principles discussed here.

An important benefit of the NLP approach is that it allows nurses to assess the client's style and preferred sensory mode and to communicate more effectively with clients by using both verbal and nonverbal communication in the client's preferred mode. Brockopp (1983) gives these examples of how to express the same nursing intervention with different predicates, depending on the client's preferred mode:

> Visual—"Yes, I can *see* that you are much better. You *look* good, your eyes are *clear,* your *appearance* has certainly changed."
>
> Auditory—"Yes, I can *hear* from the *sound* of your voice that you are better. *Talking* with you today is quite different from yesterday."
>
> Kinesthetic—"Yes, you do seem to be *feeling* much better today, you're *holding* your head up, and your *grasp* is certainly *firmer* than yesterday." (p. 1014)

By expanding their abilities to communicate with clients in all three modes, nurses can become more effective communicators.

Facilitative Communication

Facilitative communication aims at initiating, building, and maintaining fulfilling and trusting relationships with other people. Communicating ideas and feelings with clarity, efficiency, and appropriateness helps a person be interpersonally effective. In reading the rest of this chapter, try to relate the therapeutic communication principles and practices discussed earlier to these ideas about facilitative communication.

Social Superficiality Versus Facilitative Intimacy

Most relationships between people begin at the level of social superficiality. In a nurse-client relationship, we try to develop facilitative intimacy, which differs from social intimacy. For example, the interdependence that characterizes the social relationship is greatly reduced. In social relationships, participants may "tell their stories" to one another. In facilitative relationships that have therapeutic goals, only the client is engaged in storytelling with the nurse. The progress is specifically focused. Clients not only explain themselves, the events of their lives, and the circumstances they face, they do so with a purpose in mind—understanding the circumstances through exploring them and moving to improve the circumstances of their lives.

Movement toward therapeutic intimacy may be difficult at first. For one thing, such intimacy violates certain social taboos. For example, at a party it may be socially incorrect to comment on a person's anxiety, stuttering, or facial tic. During facilitative and therapeutic communication, all messages, including these nonverbal ones, are heeded and may be discussed.

Therapeutic intimacy also requires that the participants move beyond social chitchat into meaningful areas of concern for the client. Therapeutic intimacy requires high involvement and commitment.

Essential Ingredients

Several interpersonal principles and practices are essential to the achievement of facilitative intimacy.

Responding with Empathy Most theorists believe that empathy is the most important dimension in the helping process. Without a high level of empathic understanding, nurses have no real basis for helping. Empathy facilitates interpersonal exploration.

Responding with Respect Responding with respect demonstrates that the nurse values the integrity of the client and has faith in the client's ability to solve problems, given appropriate help. By encouraging clients to put forward possible plans of action, the nurse conveys respect for their ability to take charge of their own destiny. Giving advice, by contrast, conveys a directly opposite message.

Responding with Genuineness Genuineness refers to the ability to be real or honest with another. To be effective, genuineness must be timed properly and based on a solid relationship. Honesty is not always the best policy, especially if it is brutal or if the client is not capable of dealing with it.

Clients who can experience the authenticity of the nurse can risk greater genuineness and authenticity themselves. The nurse who is genuine is more likely to deal with and eventually help the client resolve real problems, rather than just those that are safe or socially acceptable.

Responding with Immediacy Responding with immediacy means responding to what is happening between the client and the nurse in the here-and-now. Because this dimension may involve the feelings of the client toward the nurse, it can be one of the most difficult to achieve. For example, the client may confront the nurse with overt or implied criticism of the nurse's role or competence. If the nurse responds in a defensive or evasive way, the relationship may be threatened. If the nurse is open, reasonable, and concerned, the relationship may be strengthened. However, by focusing attention on the relationship too early, the nurse can hinder the formation of an adequate base.

Responding with Warmth Warmth is so closely linked with empathy and respect that it is seldom communicated as an independent dimension. It is important, however, to note some additional points about the expression of warmth. Effusive, chatty, "buddy-buddy" behavior should not be confused with warmth. Warmth is most often conveyed in communications of respect and empathy.

The nurse should be aware of and accept the client's right to maintain distance. Warmth and intimacy cannot be forced. Initially high levels of warmth can be counterproductive for clients who have received little warmth from others in their lives or have been taken advantage of by others. Warmth alone is insufficient for building a relationship and solving problems.

Facilitative Communication Skills

Presenting a how-to manual or a "cookbook" of communication skills goes against the thrust of this book. Using a set of communication skills as a sort of relationship "magic" will probably doom you to failure. Relationships, and the people in them, are unique and much too complex to rely on a formula for facilitative communication. The following skills are therefore presented with many misgivings. It is important to remember that a holistic approach essentially precludes the rigid, inflexible application of communication techniques. Those presented here should be viewed as having the potential to foster effective communication. They must be adapted individually for each human encounter.

Actively Listening **Actively listening** is paying undivided attention to what the client says and does. Paying undivided attention is the major goal of active listening. A common error made by inexperienced psychiatric nurses is being too busy planning what they are going to say next. Focusing on yourself prevents you from hearing what the other person is saying and gives the client the nonverbal message that what he or she is saying is not very important. In fact, what the client is saying is very important. If you don't listen, you won't be able to comprehend the message. If you don't comprehend the message, you will not be able to effectively use the facilitative communication techniques that follow.

Active listening is best accomplished when environmental distractions are minimized. Consider finding a quiet place, turning off the television, or closing the door. Avoid taking extensive notes; they take your attention away from the client, and you will miss some of what is being said on the verbal level and done on the nonverbal level. Face the client, use eye contact, show interest, and listen objectively while minimizing your own personal responses.

Using Silence Do not feel obligated to respond after every statement a client makes. **Using silence** goes beyond active listening and can be a very effective facilitative technique when it encourages the client to communicate, when it allows the client time to ponder what has been said or a connection the client has made, when it allows the client time to collect his or her thoughts, or when it allows the client time to consider alternatives. Looking interested while maintaining an open posture or a questioning look will encourage the client to use the time effectively.

Uncomfortable silences should be broken and analyzed. You would not want a client to become increasingly anxious or resistive. (See Chapters 4 and 16 for suggestions on handling anxiety and Chapter 28 for suggestions on handling resistance.)

Remember, silence is an effective communication technique only when it is used as an appropriate and purposeful therapeutic intervention. Nurses who are silent because they are uncomfortable or because they lack the knowledge or the skill to communicate effectively must seek an experienced clinical supervisor to help them analyze their own personal and professional growth needs.

Reflecting **Reflecting** is repeating the client's verbal or nonverbal message for the client's benefit.

Reflecting Content Reflecting the *content* of the message basically repeats the client's statement. This gives clients the opportunity to hear and mull over what they have told you.

- "You believe things will be better soon."
- "You think it would be better to take a part-time job."

Content reflection is perhaps one of the most misused and overused methods in mental health counseling. It loses its effectiveness when used for lack of other choices.

Reflecting Feelings Reflecting *feelings* is verbalizing the implied feelings in the client's comment.

- "Sounds like you're really angry at your brother."
- "You're feeling uncomfortable about being discharged from the hospital."

In reflecting feelings, you attempt to identify latent and connotative meanings that may either clarify or distort the content. Reflection is useful because it encourages the client to make additional clarifying comments.

Imparting Information **Imparting information** is helping the client by supplying additional data. This therefore encourages further clarification based on new or additional input.

- "Group therapy will be held on Tuesday evening from 6:30 until 8:00."
- "I am a psychiatric nurse."

It is not constructive to withhold useful information from the client or to reply "What do you think?" to a straightforward, information-seeking question. However, be careful not to cross the line between giving information and giving advice, or give information as a way of avoiding an area of interpersonal difficulty. Also, the nurse who gives personal, social information may move out of the realm of therapeutic intervention.

Remember that clients' participation in decision making begins when they take in and understand information about their own condition. The goal of imparting information should be to provide effective education that empowers clients and their families. Studies have shown that an educated, empowered client is more likely to achieve positive mental health outcomes and less likely to need admission or readmission to an acute care facility (Weaver and Wilson 1994). You can help clients by utilizing each teachable moment.

Clarifying **Clarifying** is an attempt to understand the basic nature of a client's statement.

- "I'm confused about. . . . Could you go over that again, please?"
- "You say you're feeling anxious now. What's that like for you?"

Asking the client to give an example to clarify a meaning helps you understand the client's intended message better. A person who describes a concrete incident is more likely to see the connections between it and similar occurrences. Illustrations are very useful qualifiers.

Paraphrasing In **paraphrasing**, the nurse assimilates and restates what the client has said.

- "In other words, you're fed up with being treated like a child."
- "I hear you saying that when people compliment you, you feel embarrassed. If they knew the real you, they'd stay away."

Paraphrasing gives you the opportunity to test your understanding of what a client is attempting to communicate. It is reflective in nature, in that it lets the client know how another person is understanding the message.

Checking Perceptions **Checking perceptions** means sharing how one person perceives and hears another. After sharing perceptions of the client's behaviors, thoughts, and feelings, ask the client to verify the perception.

- "Let me know if this is how you see it too."
- "I get the feeling that you're uncomfortable when we're silent. Does that seem to fit?"

Nurses use perception checks to make sure that they understand a client. An effective perception check conveys the message, "I want to understand. . . ." It gives the other person the opportunity to correct inaccurate perceptions. It also allows you to avoid actions based on false assumptions about the client.

Questioning **Questioning** is a very direct way of speaking with clients. But when used to excess, questioning controls the nature and range of the client's responses. Questions can be useful when you are seeking specific information. When your intent is to engage the client in meaningful dialogue, however, questions should be limited.

When using questions, it is best to make them open-ended rather than closed. An *open-ended question* focuses the topic but allows freedom of response.

- "How were you feeling when your mother said that to you?"
- "What's your opinion about . . . ?"

The *closed question* limits the client's choice of responses, generally to "yes" or "no" ("Were you feeling angry when your mother said that?"). Closed questions limit therapeutic exploration.

"Why" questions usually have the same effect. They are often impossible to answer and rarely lead to a clearer understanding of the situation. However, "who," "what," "when," and "how" questions may be helpful when used judiciously.

Structuring **Structuring** is an attempt to create order or evolve guidelines. It helps the client become aware of problems and the order in which the client might deal with them.

- "You've mentioned that you want to improve your relationships with your wife, your sister, and your boss. Let's put them in order of priority."
- "No, I won't be giving you advice, but we can discuss the possible solutions together."

Structuring is particularly useful when clients introduce a number of concerns in a brief period and have little idea of which to begin work on. Nurses use structuring not

INTERVENTION

Characteristics of Helpful, Nonthreatening Feedback

Strategy	Rationale
Focus feedback on behavior rather than on client.	Refer to what client actually does rather than how nurse imagines client to be.
Focus feedback on observations rather than inferences.	Refer to what nurse actually sees or hears client do; inferences refer to conclusions or assumptions nurse makes about client.
Focus feedback on description rather than judgment.	Report what occurred rather than evaluating it in terms of good or bad, right or wrong.
Focus feedback on "more or less" rather than "either/or" descriptions of behavior.	"More or less" descriptions stress quantity rather than quality (which may be value-laden).
Focus feedback on here-and-now behavior rather than there-and-then behavior.	The most meaningful feedback is given as soon as it is appropriate to do so.
Focus feedback on sharing of information and ideas rather than advice.	Sharing ideas and information helps client make decisions about own well-being; giving advice takes away client's freedom to be self-determining.
Focus feedback on exploration of alternatives rather than answers or solutions.	Focusing on a variety of alternatives for accomplishing a particular goal prevents premature acceptance of answers or solutions that may not be appropriate.
Focus feedback on its value to the client rather than on catharsis it provides nurse.	Feedback should serve needs of client, not needs of nurse.
Limit feedback to amount of information client is able to use rather than amount nurse has available to give.	Overloading will decrease effectiveness of feedback.
Limit feedback to appropriate time and place.	Excellent feedback presented at an inappropriate time may be ineffective or harmful.
Focus feedback on what is said rather than why it is said.	Focusing on why things are said or done moves away from observations and toward motive or intent (which can only be assumed, unless verified).

only to explore content but also to delimit the parameters of the nurse-client relationship and to identify how the nurse will participate with the client in the problem-solving process.

PINPOINTING **Pinpointing** calls attention to certain kinds of statements and relationships. For example, you may point to inconsistencies among statements, to similarities and differences in the points of view, feelings, or actions of two or more people, or to differences between what one says and what one does.

- "So, you and your wife don't agree about how many children you want."
- "You say you're sad, but you're smiling."

LINKING In **linking**, the nurse responds to the client in a way that ties together two events, experiences, feelings, or people. You can use linking to connect past experiences with current behaviors. Another example is linking the tension between two people with current life stress.

- "You felt depressed after the birth of both your children."
- "So, the arguments didn't really begin until after you got your promotion."

GIVING FEEDBACK **Feedback** helps others become aware of how their behavior affects us and how we perceive their actions. Responding with feedback can be therapeutic self-disclosure. It allows the nurse to offer clients constructive information that makes them aware of their effect on others. Total self-disclosure by the nurse is inappropriate in the nurse-client relationship. It places a burden of interdependence on the client and limits the time and energy available to work on the client's concerns. Reciprocal self-disclosure is more appropriate in friend and colleague relationships.

- "When you wring your hands, I feel anxious."
- "Sometimes when you turn your head away from me, I think you're angry."

It is important to give feedback in a way that does not threaten the client, resulting in increased defensiveness. The more defensive the client, the less likely the client will hear and understand the feedback. The accompanying Intervention box lists some characteristics of helpful, nonthreatening feedback.

CONFRONTING Constructive confrontations often lead to productive change. **Confronting** is a deliberate invitation to examine some aspect of personal behavior that indicates a discrepancy between what the person says and what the person does. Confrontation requires careful attention to nonverbal communication and the discrepancies between nonverbal and verbal messages.

Confrontations may be informational or interpretive, and they may be directed toward both the resources and the limitations of the client. An **informational confrontation** describes the visible behavior of another person. An **interpretive confrontation** expresses thoughts and feelings about the other's behavior and draws inferences about the meaning of the behavior.

- "You say you're 'the dummy in the family,' yet none of your brothers or sisters made the honor roll like you did."
- "Ever since Sally and Joe criticized the way you conducted the meeting, you haven't spoken to them. It looks like you're feeling angry."

Six skills to be incorporated in constructive confrontations are:

1. Use of personal statements with the words *I, my,* and *me.*
2. Use of relationship statements expressing what the nurse thinks or feels about the client in the here and now.
3. Use of behavior descriptions (statements describing the visible behavior of the client).
4. Use of description of personal feelings, specifying the feeling by name.
5. Use of responses aimed at understanding, such as paraphrasing and perception checking.
6. Use of constructive feedback skills (see the Intervention box).

SUMMARIZING **Summarizing** is the highlighting of the main ideas expressed in an interaction. Both the client and the nurse benefit from this review of the main themes of the conversation. Summarizing is also useful in focusing the client's thinking and aiding conscious learning.

- "The last time we were together you were concerned about. . . ."
- "You had three main concerns today."

You can use this technique appropriately at different times during an interaction. For example, it is useful to summarize the previous interaction in the first few minutes you and the client spend together. Early summarizing helps the client recall the areas discussed and gives the client the opportunity to see how you have synthesized the content of a previous session. Summarizing is useful because it keeps the participants directed toward a goal.

Injudicious use of summarizing is a common pitfall. You may rush to summarize despite other, more pressing and immediate client concerns. In this instance, summarizing is likely to meet your needs for structure but does nothing to address the client's here-and-now concerns.

PROCESSING **Processing** is a complex and sophisticated technique. Process comments direct attention to the interpersonal dynamics of the nurse-client experience. These dynamics are illustrated in the content, feelings, and behavior expressed.

- "It seems that important things that need to be taken care of come up in the last five minutes we have together in our session."
- "Today is the first day our session has started out with silence. Last week it seemed there wouldn't be enough time."

Processing is most useful when therapeutic intimacy has been achieved.

Ineffective Communication Styles

The three clinical situations presented below are meant to show some unhelpful or even harmful ways of responding to clients (adapted from Gazda 1973, pp. 62–65). They illustrate a few of the common response styles that do not facilitate constructive communication. An example of a helpful response is given at the end of each of the situations.

Situation 1

Client: "They wouldn't let me join their pinochle game!"

Responses that are not helpful:

Detective: "Who wouldn't?"

Detectives are eager to track down the facts of the case. They grill the client about the details of what happened and respond to this factual content instead of paying attention to feelings. Detectives control the flow of the conversation, often putting the client on the defensive.

Magician: "It's time to eat dinner, so it doesn't matter now, does it?"

Magicians try to make the problem disappear by telling the client it isn't there. This illusion is not lasting. Denying the existence of a problem denies the validity of the client's own experience and perception.

Manager: "Would you help me get everyone together for the picnic?"

Managers believe that they can make the client forget the problem by keeping the client too busy to think about it. This conveys the message that the task the manager has assigned is more important than the client's problem. Effective nurses let clients know that they are aware of the magnitude of any particular problem to the client.

Judge: "Remember yesterday when you didn't play fair? Of course they wouldn't want to play with you today!"

Judges give rational explanations to show that the client's past actions have caused the present situation—that the client is the guilty party. Although such responses may be accurate, they are rarely helpful because they are premature; they are being given before the client is ready to accept and use them.

Responses that are helpful:

"It hurts to be turned down!" and "That hurt!"

Situation 2

Client: "You asked me to chair the community meeting next week, but I can't do that. Please get somebody else. Anybody would be better than me."

Responses that are not helpful:

Drill sergeant: "Later tonight, figure out what each person should do. Give them assignments and make sure they work on it some each day. Get organized now and it will come out fine."

Drill sergeants give orders and expect them to be obeyed. Because they know just what the client should do, they see no need to give explanations, listen to the client's feelings, or explain their commands to the client.

Guru: "You won't find out what you can do if you don't try new things. It's better to try and fail than not to try at all."

Gurus dispense proverbs and clichés on every occasion, as though they were the sole possessors of the accumulated wisdom of the ages. Unfortunately, their words are too impersonal and general to apply to any individual's situation with force or accuracy, and often the sayings are too trite to be noticed at all.

Magician: "You don't *really* mean that do you?"

Response that is helpful:

"You're sort of afraid to accept this responsibility. It looks like more than you can handle."

Situation 3

Client: "I don't know what to do with my kids! They won't listen!"

Responses that are not helpful:

Detective: "What's causing the problem?"

Florist: "With all your ability? I can't believe that! Why, you're such a good parent."

Florists are uncomfortable talking about anything unpleasant, so they gush flowery phrases to keep the client's problem at a safe distance. Florists mistakenly think that the way to be helpful is to hide the problem under bouquets of optimism.

Judge: "You know, you got off to a bad start with your kids. You are going to have a hard time changing them."

Sign painter: "You're a born pessimist!"

Sign painters think that naming a problem solves it. They have an unlimited inventory of labels to affix to people and their problems.

Drill sergeant: "First get them all tested psychologically. Then write up some behavior contracts. Keep your kids busy with simple projects. Then. . . ."

Guru: "Things always look the worst before they get better."

Prophet: "If you don't get some results with them pretty soon, there will be trouble!"

Prophets know and predict exactly what is going to happen. By declaring the forecast, prophets relieve themselves of responsibility. They sit back to let the prophecy come true.

Magician: "You're imagining things. They're good kids, and you know it. They're a lot better than you give them credit for!"

Response that is helpful:

"I guess it gets you down when you do all you know how and then don't get results."

Culturally Aware Communication Strategies

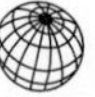

Cultural and social class differences between client and nurse may impede a nurse's best intentions. Quality nursing care is culturally sensitive; that is, the nurse is aware of cultural issues that are important to the client and may affect the client's response to treatment. In planning nursing interventions the nurse does not follow a predetermined plan but plans care that is culturally congruent for each person. For example, if a Hispanic teenage girl is obese and wants to lose weight, the nurse would not hand her a printed 500-calorie diet plan but would work with her and a nutritionist to plan a diet based on the foods she prefers. The nurse would also discuss the care plan with the girl's father and would expect many family members at visiting time. If an Asian client who is a Buddhist wants time each day to meditate, the nurse would allow for that time in the care plan rather than imposing our frenetic Western pace in which every hour is filled with "constructive," "growth-producing" activity.

Taking a client's culture into consideration when planning care is not an easy task. It is time-consuming and requires patience, insight, and creativity on the part of the nurse.

Understanding One's Own Sociocultural Heritage Gaining awareness of sociocultural differences requires that nurses first come to understand their own backgrounds and the influence of that background on their practice. Nurses are better able to meet the sociocultural needs of a client when they acknowledge that a culture and a society influence their beliefs, values, attitudes, and behavior. The questions in the Nursing Self-Awareness box are designed to facilitate acknowledgment of the nurse's own sociocultural heritage. Answering these questions honestly and completely is the important first step in self-awareness. The second step involves exploring beliefs and attitudes that may be different from or the same as those held by the client.

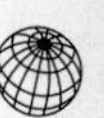

Avoiding Misdiagnosis Clients from different cultures may be misdiagnosed by Western health care providers. Culturally sensitive nurses can play a role in assessing clients' social, psychologic, and behavioral symptoms in the light of clients' own cultural norms. For example, a psychiatrist may diagnose a man who talks to the dead as schizophrenic, but for a Puerto Rican who believes in espiritismo, talking to the dead is a common practice. A client who is a charismatic Christian may lapse into an altered state of consciousness and speak in tongues. To interpret these behaviors as evidence of schizophrenia is inappropriate. Likewise, categorizing a refugee child who has experienced trauma and violence as mentally ill is revictimization. Obtaining a cultural profile helps to prevent misdiagnosis.

Assessing Communication Style An excellent model for obtaining a client's comprehensive cultural profile is Fong's (1985) CONFHER model. The selected questions below from Fong's model are designed to elicit relevant information specifically in relation to communication style.

- Does the client speak English fluently? If not, how limited is the client's ability to communicate in English?
- Does the client understand common health terms such as *pain, fever,* and *nausea*?
- Would the client like an interpreter or to have the question rephrased in simple English?
- Can the client read and write in English?

NURSING SELF-AWARENESS

Questions That Acknowledge Sociocultural Heritage

- What ethnic group, socioeconomic class, religions, age groups, and community do you belong to?
- What experiences have you had with people from ethnic groups, socioeconomic classes, religions, age groups, or communities different from your own?
- What were those experiences like? How did you feel about them?
- When you were growing up, what did your parents and significant others say about people who were different from your family?
- What about your ethnic group, socioeconomic class, religion, age, or community do you find embarrassing or wish you could change? Why?
- What sociocultural factors in your background might contribute to being rejected by members of other cultures?
- What personal qualities do you have that will help you establish interpersonal relationships with persons from other cultural groups?
- What personal qualities may be detrimental?
- What assumptions do you hold about the people who populate our world?

- Are there ethnic behaviors or styles of nonverbal communication to which the client adheres (e.g., the bowing of the head to show respect in the traditional Japanese culture, or frequent smiling and speaking softly in the Southeast Asian culture)?
- Does the client mean what he or she says, or does the client give a pleasant, agreeable answer when a literal, factual answer might be unpleasant and embarrassing?
- How much physical touching is appropriate in the client's culture?

The nurse can emphasize similarities to form a close therapeutic relationship. Differences may serve as topics for discussion. An open, ongoing dialogue is beneficial for both parties because it promotes understanding of the other culture.

Circumventing the Language Barrier When English is not the client's primary language and you are a monolingual provider, it will help if you select the words you use carefully, avoiding buzz words and jargon. Speak clearly, pacing yourself to be neither too fast nor too slow. Words that are slurred, have many syllables in them, or are too technical make communication more difficult. Speaking too fast may overload the client and make it difficult for the client to follow. Speaking too slowly may lose the client's attention.

Select the gestures you use with care, using your nonverbal behavior to underscore your words and your actions. The proper use of gestures can clarify a message, and drawings can sometimes be helpful. Be careful however; as discussed earlier in this chapter, not all gestures mean the same thing in all cultures.

Listen to your client's words and watch your client's gestures carefully. Do your best to understand and validate the meaning they have for you. Listening carefully to the client helps you avoid focusing on what you will say or do next and demonstrates your genuine concern for the client's distress.

If the client attempts to speak English, his or her thoughts may appear distorted when language is the real problem. There have been a number of documented instances in which people have been diagnosed as mentally disordered and confined to a mental hospital because mental health professionals erroneously diagnosed a language problem or value difference as disordered thinking or psychosis.

An interpreter may be necessary if language is a barrier. If the client does not have his or her own interpreter, you may be able to enlist the aid of a bilingual staff member. Health and social services departments, international institutes, college language departments, neighborhood houses, or cultural centers will often know of people who are willing to volunteer as interpreters.

INTERVENTION

Guidelines for Monolingual Providers in a Cross-Cultural Environment

- Unless you are thoroughly effective and fluent in the target language, always use an interpreter.
- Avoid using family members as interpreters.
- Learn basic words and sentences in the target language. Asking interpreters about words or comments that have not been translated prompts attention to detail.
- Use dictionaries of languages used by your client population. Beware of brief "definitions" that serve only as labels.
- Become familiar with special terminology. Specific beliefs, practices, and traditions are often referenced by indirect language or special terms. Local beliefs and moral tenets may lead to overemphasis on or underreporting of certain symptoms, issues, and events.
- Check the quality of translated health-related materials by having them back-translated.
- Meet with your interpreters on a regular basis. They will provide both a window and a mirror when you deal with another language and another culture.
- Personal information is often closely guarded and difficult to obtain. Clients often request a specific interpreter or even bring their own.
- Evaluate the interpreter's style and approach to clients. For special situations and problem cases, try to match the interpreter to the task.
- Be patient. Careful interpretation often requires the interpreter to use long explanatory phrases.

Source: Adapted from R. Putsch 1985.

The three Intervention boxes provide specific guidelines for circumventing the language barrier and working with interpreters.

An interpreter may be necessary if language is a barrier.

INTERVENTION

Guidelines for Nurse-Interpreter-Client Interactions

- Address clients directly. Avoid directing all of your commentary to and through the interpreter.
- Be certain the interpreter is thoroughly involved with the client during an interview.
- Develop alternatives to gathering information by direct questions. People who are strangers to direct, Western-style inquiry may respond better to conversational modes.
- Invite correction and induce the discussion of alternatives: "Correct me if I'm wrong, I understand it this way . . . Do you see it some other way?"
- Pursue seemingly unconnected issues raised by the client. These issues may lead to crucial information or uncover difficulties with the interpretation.
- Come back to an issue if you suspect a problem and get a negative response. Be certain the interpreter knows what you want. Use related questions, change the wording, and come at the issue indirectly.
- Provide instructions in list format. Ask clients to outline their understanding of the plans.
- If alternatives exist, spell each one out.
- Emphasize by repetition.
- Clarify your limitations. The willingness to talk about an issue may be viewed as evidence of "understanding" it or the ability to "fix" it.
- Rumors, jealousy, privacy, and reputation are crucial issues in closely knit communities. Acknowledge the problem and assure the client of confidentiality.
- Unless the correct circumstances are devised, it may be impossible to address certain male/female problems by way of discussion or physical examination.

Source: Adapted from R. Putsch 1985.

INTERVENTION

Guidelines for Language Use in Interpreter-Dependent Interviews

- Use short questions and comments. Technical terminology and professional jargon, such as "psychotropic medication" should be reduced to plain English.
- When lengthy explanations are necessary, break them up and have them interpreted piece by piece in straightforward, concrete terms.
- Use language and explanations the interpreter can handle.
- Make allowances for terms that do not exist in the target language.
- Try to avoid ambiguous statements and questions.
- Avoid abstraction, idiomatic expressions, similes, and metaphors. It is useful to learn about these usages in the target language.
- Plan what you want to say ahead of time. Avoid confusing the interpreter by backing up, inserting a proviso, rephrasing, or hesitating.
- Avoid indefinite phrases using *would, could, if,* and *maybe*. These can be mistaken for actual agreements or firm approval of a course of action.
- Ask the interpreter to comment on the client's word content and emotions.

Source: Adapted from R. Putsch 1985.

Chapter Highlights

- Communication is an ongoing, dynamic, and ever-changing series of events, each of which affects all others; it is the mechanism by which people establish, maintain, and improve their human contacts.
- Meaning cannot be transferred form one human being to another but must be mutually negotiated between people. Words and gestures do not "mean" something; people do.
- Communication takes place on intrapersonal, inter-

personal, and public levels and includes nonverbal messages that are interrelated with the spoken word.

- Relationships with clients are initiated, built, and maintained through the vehicle of interpersonal communication.
- To help clients deal with problems, nurses need to be aware of how their own perceptions, values, and culture influence the way they process information about the world.
- In developing the nurse-client relationship, a major focus is the development of facilitative intimacy.
- Facilitative intimacy is enhanced when nurses respond with empathy, respect, genuineness, immediacy, and warmth.
- Relationships are unique and too complex for a set of rigid, inflexible communication techniques to be consistent with humanistic psychiatric nursing practice.
- Communication skills that may foster facilitative communication include actively listening, using silence, reflecting content, reflecting feelings, imparting information, clarifying, paraphrasing, checking perceptions, questioning, structuring, pinpointing, linking, giving feedback, confronting, summarizing, and processing.

References

American Society for Training and Development: *Neurolinguistic Programming Resource Manual*. The Society, 1986.

Bandler R, Grinder J: *The Structure of Magic*, vol. 1. Science and Behavior Books, 1975.

Bandler R, Grinder J: *The Structure of Magic*, vol. 2. Science and Behavior Books, 1976.

Becker HA, MacCabe N: Indicators of critical thinking, communication, and therapeutic intervention among first-line nursing supervisors. *Nurse Educ* 1994;19(2):15–19.

Bloch D: *Words That Heal*. Bantam Books, 1990.

Bowlby J: *Maternal Care and Mental Health*, ed 2. World Health Organization, 1951.

Bradley JC, Edinberg MA: *Communication in the Nursing Context*, ed 3. Appleton & Lange, 1990.

Brockopp D: What is NLP? *Am J Nurs* 1983;83:1012–1014.

Carroll L: *Through the Looking Glass and What Alice Found There*. Random House, 1965.

Cunningham A: The good, the bad and the phony: Why women smile. *Lear's* 1993 (March);6:112–115.

Elder J: *Transactional Analysis in Health Care*. Addison-Wesley, 1978.

Fong C: Ethnicity and nursing practice. *Topics Clin Nurs* 1985;7:1–10.

Gazda GM: *Human Relations Development*. Allyn and Bacon, 1973.

Gazda G, Childers W, Walters R: *Interpersonal Communication: A Handbook for Health Professionals*. Aspen, 1982.

Grainger RD: Eye movements: A new psychotherapeutic tool. *Am J Nurs* 1992;92:18.

Hulett JE Jr: A symbolic interactionist model of human communication. *A V Communication Review* 1966;14:5–33.

Knowles RD: Building rapport: Through neurolinguistic programming. *Am J Nurs* 1983;83:1011–1014.

Liehr P: Uncovering a hidden language: The effects of listening and talking on blood pressure and heart rate. *Arch Psychiatr Nurs* 1992;6(5):306–311.

Miller LE: Modeling awareness and feeling: A needed tool in the therapeutic workbox. *Perspect Psychiatr Care* 1989; 25(2):27–29.

Nigro A, Maggio J: A neglected need: Health education for the mentally ill. *J Psychosoc Nurs* 1990;28(7):15–19.

Northouse PG, Northouse LL: *Health Communication: Strategies for Health Professionals*, ed 2. Appleton & Lange, 1992.

Putsch R: Cross-cultural communications. *JAMA* 1985;254: 3344–3348.

Restak RM: *Receptors*. Bantam Books, 1994.

Rosenberg L: The use of therapeutic correspondence: Creative approaches in psychotherapy. *J Psychosoc Nurs* 1990; 28(11):29–33.

Ruesch J: *Therapeutic Communication*. Norton, 1961.

Ruesch J, Bateson G: *Communication: The Social Matrix of Psychiatry*. Norton, 1968.

Sharf BF: Teaching patients to speak up: Past and future trends. *Patient Ed Couns* 1988;11:95–108.

Sherman KM: *Communication and Image in Nursing*. Delmar, 1994.

Sluder H: The write way: Using poetry for self-disclosure. *J Psychosoc Nurs* 1990;28(7):26–28.

Tommasini NR: The use of touch with the hospitalized psychiatric patient. *Arch Psychiatr Nurs* 1990;4(4):213–220.

Watzlawick P, Beavin J, Jackson D: *The Pragmatics of Human Communication*. New York: Norton, 1967.

Weaver SK, Wilson JF: Moving toward patient empowerment. *Nurs Health Care* 1994;15(9):480–483.

CHAPTER 8

ASSESSMENT

Holly Skodol Wilson
Carol Ren Kneisl

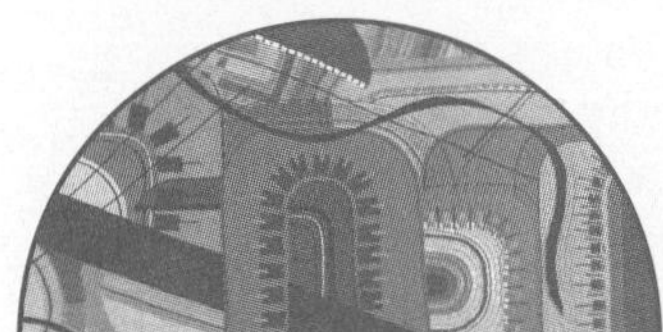

COMPETENCIES

- *Describe the processes of psychiatric history-taking, mental status examination, biologic and neurologic assessment, brain imaging, and psychologic testing.*
- *Discuss the DSM-IV multiaxial system for making a psychiatric diagnosis.*
- *Describe the process of individual psychosocial and cultural assessment.*
- *Discuss the differences between source-oriented and problem-oriented systems of recording.*
- *Identify methods of recording nurse-client interactions.*
- *Comprehend the organization and function of the process recording.*

Cross-References

Other topics relevant to this content are: Brain imaging, Chapter 3; Assessing clients with mood disorders, Chapter 15; Assessing clients with delirium or dementia, Chapter 12; Assessing clients with substance-related disorders, Chapter 13; Assessing clients with schizophrenic disorders, Chapter 14; Family characteristics and dynamics, Chapter 32; Group process, Chapter 31; Nursing process, Chapter 6; Suicide assessment, Chapter 24; DSM-IV Cultural assessment formulation, Appendix C.

Critical Thinking Challenge

Most guidelines for conducting a mental status intake examination emphasize the importance of conducting a suicide assessment. This assessment, however, is customarily limited to asking questions like, "Have you ever thought of ending it all?" or "Have you ever considered suicide?" "Do you plan to hurt yourself?" Consider a situation where you are responsible for an intake assessment for a 35-year-old male client being admitted to inpatient care because he has been transferred from an emergency room after driving his car off a freeway ramp into a building. His psychiatric diagnosis is major depression with psychotic features and he has had prior hospitalizations for what in his chart are termed "suicidal gestures." He is single, unemployed, and has a problem with alcohol abuse. In your interview you ask if he is considering hurting himself again, and he says "no." He seems anxious and does express feelings of hopelessness. He also wishes he will find a new life because of his hospitalization. What recommendations do you make for his first few days on the psychiatric inpatient unit, and why?

The systematic scientific approach known among nurses as the *nursing process* has evolved as the cornerstone of clinical practice. The nursing process begins with assessment for the purpose of collecting and analyzing objective and subjective data about the clients with whom nurses work. The primary sources of client data in most instances are the clients themselves. Psychologic tests, nurses' notes, physicians' orders, and other secondary data sources can enlarge, clarify, and substantiate data obtained directly from the client.

Collecting and Assessing Client Data

The Psychiatric Examination

Systems of collection and assessment vary among mental health agencies. The psychiatric examination consists of two parts: the psychiatric history and the mental status exam. It is most often done during initial or early interactions with a client. The traditional psychiatric examination is discussed in this chapter because it is still used in settings in which psychiatric nurses work and is considered the counterpart of the physical examination and history.

INITIAL CONTACT FORM The initial contact form (Figure 8–1 on page 133) is filled in before the history and mental status exam are done. It provides basic demographic and problem information at the time the client requests service or is referred by another person or agency. This information should provide the clinician with enough data to make some early key decisions.

- How urgent is the situation? (See the accompanying Assessment box.)
- Who is to be assigned responsibility for proceeding with the next step?
- What type of response is indicated as "the next step"?

This form is used chiefly by the intake worker who is the member of the mental health team designated to handle all incoming calls and requests for service during a specified period of time.

ASSESSMENT

Crisis Rating: How Urgent Is Your Need for Help?

- *Very urgent:* Service request requires an immediate response within minutes. Examples: crisis outreach; medical emergency, requiring an ambulance to be called (overdoses); severe drug reaction; police contacted if situation involves extreme suicidal danger or weapons.
- *Urgent:* Response requires rapid but not necessarily immediate response, within a few hours. Examples: low risk of suicide; mild drug reaction.
- *Somewhat urgent:* Response should be made within a day (approximately 24 hours). Example: a planning conference in which key people are not available until the following evening.
- *Slightly urgent:* A response is required within a few days. Example: the client's funding runs out within a week, and the client needs public assistance.
- *Not urgent:* A situation has existed for a long time and does not warrant immediate intervention; a week or two is unlikely to cause any significant difference. Examples: a child with a learning disability; certain types of marital counseling.

The Psychiatric History

DATA SOURCES Not all data gathered during psychiatric history-taking are obtained from the client. There are several other sources. Family, friends, police, mental health personnel, and others may contribute data to the **psychiatric history.** When the sources are varied, the psychiatric history focuses on the perceptions of others: how they see the client, and the circumstances of the client's life. The sources of the psychiatric history and their relationship to the client should always be clearly indicated. Information given by these sources should be reviewed and understood in terms of that relationship.

CATEGORIES OF DATA The psychiatric history generally includes the following information:

- *Complaint*—the main reason the client is having a psychiatric examination. The client may have personally initiated the psychiatric examination, or others (courts, hospital staff, family, referral from school or industry) may have initiated it. The "chief complaint" should be recorded verbatim and indicated as such with quotation marks in the write-up ("I just don't want to live any longer" or "My drug use has become unmanageable").
- *Present symptoms*—the nature of the onset and the development of symptoms. These data are usually traced from the present to the last period of adaptive functioning.
- *Previous hospitalizations and mental health treatment.*
- *Family history*—generally, whether any family members have ever sought or received mental health treatment.
- *Personal history*—the person's birth and development; past and recent illnesses; schooling and educational problems; occupation; sexual development, interests, and practices; marital history; the use of

INITIAL CONTACT SHEET

Today's Date 12-4-96
Time 9 AM
PM

Walk-in
Phone ✓
Outreach
Written

ID #
SS # 123-45-6789
Welfare/
Medicaid #

SERVICE REQUESTED FOR
Client's NAME Maria (First) Jane (Middle) Bianco (Last)

Address 5601 Valleyview Dr. (Street) Rockford, NY 10101 (City/Town) Zip County
Permanent ✓
Temporary
Catchment Area

Phone # 666-1234 Means of Transportation Auto
Directions to home
(if outreach)
Sex Male
Female ✓
Date of Birth 1-14-43 Age 53

SERVICE REQUESTED BY
☐ AGENCY Name Phone #
☐ OTHER Address Time(s) seen by
☑ SELF If Agency-Contact Person the agency

PRESENTING SITUATION/PROBLEM - What made you decide to seek help today?
(use other side if needed)

Feeling depressed about relationship with husband and life in general. Difficulty sleeping, low energy level, "I need to get help."

Have you talked with anyone about this? Yes Who?
Address No ✓ Phone #
Date of last contact

Are you taking ANY medication now? Yes ✓ What? 1. Valium
(if more than 3 begin list on MH-2) No
2. Dalmane
3. Aspirin

CRISIS RATING How urgent is your need for help?
☐ Immediate (within minutes)
☐ Within a few hours
☐ Within 24 hours
☐ Within a few days
☑ Within a week or two

Comments

Articulate woman with marital problems—would probably benefit from counseling and perhaps couples group later

DISPOSITION (Check all that apply)
☐ Crisis
☐ Medical Emergency
☐ Assessment (specify)
☐ Discharge Planning
☐ Expediting/Advocacy
☐ Other (explain)
☑ Referral made to Individual counseling Confirmed Yes ✓ No Date 12-14-96
Date of Next Contact 12-15-96 Assigned to
Date of Assignment Request taken by

Figure 8–1 Initial contact sheet. *Source: Reproduced by permission of the Erie County Department of Mental Health; Mental Health Services, Erie County, Corporation IV, South East Corporation V, and Lakeshore Corporation VI.*

alcohol, drugs, and tobacco; and religious or spiritual practices.

- *Personality*—the client's relationships with others, moods, feelings, interests, and leisure activities.

The main purpose of history-taking is to gather information, although it is often effective in establishing rapport with a client. The interviewer can promote rapport by avoiding an interrogative approach and allowing the client's story to unfold naturally.

The Mental Status Examination*

The **mental status examination** (MSE) is usually a standardized procedure in agencies that use it. Its primary purpose is to help the examiner gather more objective data to be used in determining etiology, diagnosis, prognosis, and treatment, and to deal immediately with any risk of violence or harm. The sections of the mental status examination that deal with *sensorium* and *intellect* are particularly important in determining the existence of delirium, dementia, amnestic, and other cognitive disorders. The purpose of this examination differs from that of the psychiatric history in that it identifies the person's *present* mental status.

The mental status examiner generally seeks the following categories of information, not necessarily in the sequence presented here.

1. *General behavior, appearance, and attitude*—a complete and accurate description of the client's physical characteristics, apparent age, manner of dress, use of cosmetics, personal hygiene, and responses to the examiner. Postures, gait, gestures, facial expression, and mannerisms are included in the description. The examiner also notes the client's general activity level.

A 35-year-old white male, dressed in torn, disheveled jeans. Presented a blank facial expression, slouched posture, shuffling gait, generally low activity level, and sullen behavior.

Other descriptors that may be used include "frank," "friendly," "irritable," "dramatic," "evasive," "indifferent," and so forth. Details should be sufficient to identify and characterize the client.

2. *Characteristics of talk*—the form, rather than the content, of the client's speech. The speech is described in terms of loudness, flow, speed, quantity, level of coherence, and logic. A sample of the client's conversation with the examiner may be included in quotation marks. The goal is to describe the quantity and quality of speech to discern difficulties in thought processes. The following patterns, if present, should be particularly noted.

a. **Mutism**—no verbal response despite indications that the client is aware of the examiner's questions.

b. **Circumstantiality**—cumbersome, convoluted, and unnecessary detail in response to the interviewer's questions.

c. **Perseveration**—a pattern of repeating the same words or movements despite apparent efforts to make a new response.

d. **Flight of ideas**—rapid, overly productive responses to questions that seem related only by chance associations between one sentence fragment and another. Associated with flight of ideas might be *rhyming, clang associations, punning,* and *evidence of distractibility.*

e. **Blocking**—a pattern of sudden silence in the stream of conversation for no obvious reason but often thought to be associated with intrusion of delusional thoughts or hallucinations.

3. *Emotional state*—the person's pervasive or dominant mood or affective reaction. Both subjective and objective data are included. Subjective data are obtained through the use of nonleading questions, for instance, "How are you feeling?" If the client replies with general terms, such as "nervous," the interviewer should ask the client to describe how the nervousness shows itself and its effect, since such words may mean different things to different individuals. The examiner should observe objective signs, such as facial expression, motor behavior, the presence of tears, flushing, sweating, tachycardia, tremors, respiratory irregularities, states of excitement, fear, and depression. The attitude of the client toward the examiner sometimes offers valuable clues. Attitudes of hostility, suspiciousness, or flirtatiousness, a desire for bodily contact, or outspoken criticisms should be noted.

The psychiatric client is apt to have a persistent emotional trend reflective of a particular emotional disorder, such as depression. If this is true, the examiner should probe further to discover the intensity and persistence of this reaction, in keeping with *DSM-IV* criteria.

It is desirable to record verbatim the replies to questions concerning the client's mood. The relationship between mood and the content of thought is particularly significant. There may be a wide divergence between what clients say or do and their emotional state as expressed by attitudes or facial expressions.

Note whether intense emotional responses accompany discussion of specific topics. **Shallowness** or **flattening of the affect** is indicated by an insufficiently intense emotional display in association with ideas or situations that ordinarily would call for a stronger response.

Dissociation or *disharmony* is often indicated by an inappropriate emotional response, such as smiling or silly

**Reprinted with permission of Sandoz Pharmaceuticals, Division of Sandoz, Inc. From Small 1980.*

behavior, when the attitude should be one of concern, anxiety, or sadness.

It is difficult to evaluate emotional reactions in clients who use *simulation* or play-acting. Clients who are trying to cover up a deep depression may feign cheerfulness and good spirits. The reverse may also be true.

The client's emotional reactions may be constant or may fluctuate during the examination. Try to specify the ease or readiness with which such changes occur in response to pleasant or unpleasant stimuli. Use such terms as the following to indicate intensity of response:

- Composed, complacent, frank, friendly, playful, teasing, silly, cheerful, boastful, elated, grandiose, ecstatic.
- Tense, worried, anxious, pessimistic, sad, perplexed, bewildered, gloomy, depressed, frightened.
- Aloof, superior, disdainful, distant, defensive, suspicious.
- Irritable, resentful, hostile, sarcastic, angry, furious.
- Indifferent, resigned, apathetic, dull, affectless.

Pay attention to the influence of content on affect, and note especially disharmony between affect and content or thought. Also important is constancy or change in the emotional state.

4. *Content of thought: special preoccupations and experiences*—delusions, illusions, or hallucinations, depersonalizations, obsessions or compulsions, phobias, fantasies, and daydreams. You can elicit these data by asking such questions as, "Do you have any difficulties?" or "Have you been troubled or ill in any way?"

Delusions are false beliefs. If the client has delusions of being the object of environmental attention, some of the following questions might reveal them: "Do people like you?" "Have you ever been watched or spied upon or singled out for special attention?" "Do others have it in for you?"

Delusions of *alien control* (passivity) are feelings of being controlled or guided by external forces. If you suspect these delusions, ask the client such questions as, "Do you ever feel your thoughts or actions are under any outside influences or control?" "Are you able to influence others, to read their minds, or to put thoughts in their minds?"

A client with *nihilistic delusions* more or less completely denies reality and existence. The client states that nothing exists, or that everything is lost. Statements such as "I have no head, no stomach," "I cannot die," or "I will live to eternity" suggest nihilistic delusions.

Delusions of *self-deprecation* are often seen in connection with severe depressions. The client describes feeling unworthy, sinful, ugly, or foul-smelling.

Delusions of grandeur are associated with elated states such as great wealth, strength, power, sexual potency, or identification with a famous person or even God.

Somatic delusions are focused on having cancer, obstructed bowels, leprosy, or some horrible disease. These are to be distinguished from a preoccupation with normal, visceral, or peripheral sensations.

Hallucinations are false sensory impressions with no external basis in fact. Try to elicit the clearness of the projection to the outside world—for example, the source of the voices (from outside or inside the head), the clarity and distinctness of the perception, and the intensity. Be subtle in approaching the client for evidence of hallucinatory phenomena, unless the client is obviously hallucinating. In the case of obvious hallucinations, it's appropriate to ask about them directly.

Obsessions are insistent thoughts recognized as arising from the self. The client usually regards them as absurd and relatively meaningless, yet they persist despite endeavors to get rid of them.

Compulsions are repetitive acts performed through some inner need or drive and supposedly against the client's wishes, yet not performing them results in tension and anxiety.

Fantasies and **daydreams** are preoccupations that are often difficult to elicit from the client. The difficulty may be that the client misunderstands what the examiner wants, but often people are ashamed to talk about them because of their content.

5. *Orientation*—**orientation** in terms of time, place, person, and self to determine the presence of confusion or clouding of consciousness. You may introduce such questions by asking, "Have you kept track of the time?" If so, "What is today's date?" Clients who say they don't know should be asked to estimate approximately or to guess at an answer. Many clinicians begin the mental status exam with these questions because disorientation should cause the examiner to question the validity and reliability of data obtained subsequently.

6. *Memory*—the person's attention span and ability to retain or recall past experiences in both the recent and the remote past. If memory loss exists, determine whether it is constant or variable and whether the loss is limited to a certain time period. The examiner should be alert to **confabulations**—invented memories to take the place of those the client cannot recall. It is useful to introduce questions relating to memory by some general statement such as "Has your memory been good?" or "Have you had difficulty remembering telephone numbers or appointments?"

a. *Recall of remote past experiences.* Ask for a review of the important events in the client's life. Then compare the response with information obtained from other sources during the history-taking.

b. *Recall of recent past experiences,* such as the events leading to the present seeking of treatment.

c. *Retention and recall of immediate impressions.* The examiner might ask the client to repeat a name, an address, or a set of objects—for example, car, coin, and telephone—immediately and again after 3–5 minutes. Another test is to have the client repeat three-digit numbers at a rate of one per second, or to repeat a complicated sentence.

d. *General grasp and recall.* You might ask the client to read a story and then repeat the gist with as many details as possible. In a classic, concise guide for conducting a psychiatric examination, S. M. Small (1980) includes the following story as an example:

> A cowboy from Arizona went to San Francisco with his dog, which he left at a friend's while he purchased a new suit of clothes. Dressed in the new suit, he went back to the dog, whistled to him, called him by name, and patted him. The dog would have nothing to do with him in his new hat and coat, but gave a mournful howl. Coaxing had no effect, so the cowboy went away and donned his old garments. Then the dog immediately showed his wild joy on seeing his master as he thought he ought to be.

7. *General intellectual level*—a nonstandardized evaluation of intelligence. The examiner looks for the person's ability to use factual knowledge in a comprehensive way.

a. *General grasp of information.* You may ask the client to name the five largest cities of the United States, the last four presidents, or the governor of the state.

b. *Ability to calculate.* Tests of simple multiplication and addition are useful for this purpose. Another test consists of subtracting from one hundred by sevens until the person can go no further (serial sevens test).

c. *Reasoning and judgment.* A common test of reasoning is to ask clients what they might do with a gift of $10,000. Examiners must be particularly careful to correct for their own biases and values in assessing each client's answer.

8. *Abstract thinking*—the distinctions between such abstractions as poverty and misery or idleness and laziness. It is common to ask the client to interpret simple fables or proverbs, like "Don't cry over spilled milk."

9. *Insight evaluation*—whether clients recognize the significance of the present situation, whether they feel the need for treatment, and how they explain the symptoms. Often it is helpful to ask clients for suggestions for their own treatment.

10. *Summary*—the important psychopathologic findings and a tentative diagnosis. Any pertinent facts from the medical history and/or physical examination should be added to the summary.

Table 8–1 lists some of the mental status examination findings differentiating dementia or delirium, psychosis, and mood disorders.

Biologic Assessment

As the summary of the mental status examination and Table 8–1 suggest, nurses must carefully consider the possibility that a client's symptoms may have a biologic, particularly neurologic, basis. In some reported instances, clients with brain tumors or bromide intoxication have been hospitalized on psychiatric units and treated exclusively for their seemingly psychiatric symptoms. Such a critical oversight obviously delays and seriously hampers appropriate treatment of a biologic or neurologic problem. The value of careful screening for biologic disorders cannot be overemphasized. In many community settings, psychiatric nurses are the only mental health care providers prepared to undertake a biologic and neurologic assessment and interpret the results.

The objectives of a biologic and neurologic assessment are:

1. Detection of underlying and perhaps unsuspected organic disease that may be responsible for psychiatric symptoms.
2. Understanding of disease as a factor in the overall psychiatric disability.
3. Appreciation of somatic symptoms that reflect primarily psychologic rather than physiologic problems.

Biologic History-Taking Of several procedures that enlighten the nurse who is attempting to account for biologic aspects of psychiatric symptoms, the client's history is certainly a major one. The nurse should inquire into two primary areas of biologic history:

1. Facts about known physical diseases and dysfunction.
2. Information about specific physical complaints.

Information about previous illnesses may provide essential clues. Clients with comorbidities of substance abuse and mental disorder are particularly challenging. For example, suppose the presenting symptoms include paranoid delusions and the client has a history of similar episodes. During each previous episode, the client responded to diverse forms of treatment and demonstrated no residual symptoms. This history suggests a strong possibility of amphetamine- or other drug-related psychosis, and a drug screen laboratory test may be indicated. An occupational history may provide information about exposure to inorganic mercury, leading to symptoms of psychosis; or exposure to lead, resulting in mental disorder.

The second area of emphasis in biologic history-taking is eliciting information from the client about specific

Table 8–1 Differentiation of Mental Status Examination Findings

	Delirium	*Dementia*	*Manic Episode*	*Schizophrenic Disorder*	*Depressive Disorder*
Appearance and Behavior	Fluctuating impairment of consciousness, restlessness	May show deterioration of personal habits but state of consciousness not clouded	Hyperactive, elated, assertive, boisterous, with rapid emphatic speech; may be suddenly angry or argumentative	Variable	Dejected, slowed, slumped, troubled
Mood	Anxiety, fear, lability	Irritability, lability	Elation, sometimes anger and irritability	Blandness, impoverishment or inappropriateness of affect	Depression, hopelessness
Thought Processes and Perceptions					
Coherence and relevance	May be confused, incoherent	May become confused	Rapid association of ideas that may seem illogical	Often incoherent, disorganized	
Thought content	May have delusions		May have delusions and feelings of persecution	May have feelings of unreality, depersonalization, persecution, influence and reference; delusions that are bizarre and symbolic	May have delusions, often involving guilt, self-deprecation, somatic complaints
Perceptions	May have illusions, hallucinations		May have illusions, rarely hallucinations	May have hallucinations and illusions, often bizarre and symbolic	May have illusions, rarely hallucinations
Cognitive Functions					
Orientation	May be disoriented	May be disoriented	Well-oriented	Usually but not always well-oriented	Well-oriented
Attention and concentration	Poor	Poor	Distractable		
Recent memory	Poor	Poor		Usually well-preserved; difficult to test because of inattentiveness and indifference	
Remote memory	May become poor	May become poor		Usually well-preserved; difficult to test be-cause of inattentiveness and indifference	
Information	Preserved until late	Preserved until late			
Vocabulary	Preserved until late	Preserved until late		Concrete, may be bizarre	
Abstract reasoning	Concrete	Concrete			
Judgment	Poor	Poor			
Perception and coordination	May be poor	May be poor			

Source: Adapted from Bates 1983, pp. 312–313. Reprinted by permission of Lippincott/Harper & Row.

TIME & DATE	PUPILS			L.O.C.	S-R	T.R.	MOTOR				TOTAL
	R	< = >	L				RUE	RLE	LUE	LLE	MAX. 25

Explanation of Codes

Pupils

Reaction time, right (R) and left (L)

(2) Reacts briskly

(1) Reacts slowly

(0) No reaction

Size

(=) Equal

(<) Right lesser than left

(>) Right greater than left

Level of Consciousness (L.O.C.)

(5) Alert and oriented x 3 = awakens easily; oriented to person, place, time

(4) Alert and partially oriented = awakens easily but oriented in only one or two of the three spheres

(3) Lethargic but oriented = slow to arouse, possibly slurred speech, but oriented x 3

(2) Lethargic and disoriented = slow to arouse, oriented in only one or two spheres or completely disoriented

Figure 8–2 Neurologic assessment guide. *Source: Copyright © 1977. American Journal of Nursing Company. From American Journal of Nursing, September, Vol 77, No. 9.*

physical complaints. Again, it is crucial for the nurse to consider symptoms in terms of both psychiatric conditions and physical diseases. Symptoms that are atypical of psychiatric disorders are particularly revealing clues. For example, suppose a client with hallucinations and delusions also complains of a severe headache at the onset of the symptoms. The symptoms together suggest possible brain disease and call for careful and repeated neurologic assessment and use of brain imaging techniques. History-taking should also include information about medications the client currently takes. Digitalis intoxication may result in impairment. Reserpine may produce symptoms generally considered psychiatric in nature.

Observation Observation also yields important data bearing on the possible presence of organic disorders.

- An unsteady gait may suggest diffuse brain disease or alcohol or drug intoxication.
- Asymmetry—dragging a leg or not swinging one arm—might be a sign of a focal brain lesion.

OR

(2) Restless/combative (confused) = spontaneously thrashing about in bed; striking out at others; inattentive to commands

(1) Responds to stimulation only = exhibits only some type of withdrawal or posturing in response to stimulation

(0) Unresponsive = gives no response of any kind

Stimulus-Response (S-R)

(5) Responds to commands = gives appropriate responses to orientation questions, complies with instructions on hand grasp, toe wiggling, etc.

(4) Responds to name = opens eyes to name or gives some indication that he or she hears (nods, moves, etc.), but does not follow all commands

(3) Responds to shaking = responds only to vigorous physical stimulation

(2) Responds to pinprick = responds to light pain applied with pin to trunk or extremities to elicit either withdrawal or posturing

(1) Responds to deep pain = responds only to mandibular pressure, periorbital rub, sternal rub, or pinch

(0) Unresponsive = gives no response to any stimulus

Type of Response (T.R.)

(3) Complex withdrawal = withdrawal and attempt to remove stimulus

(2) Simple withdrawal = withdrawal from stimulus alone

(1) Posturing = decorticate—head, arms, and hands flexed; decerebrate—head extended, arms extended and pronated, back arched

(0) Flaccid = no response

Motor

Right Upper Extremity (RUE)
Right Lower Extremity (RLE)
Left Upper Extremity (LUE)
Left Lower Extremity (LLE)

(2) Full spontaneous use = moves designated extremity or extremities with or *without* any stimulus

(1) Moves to stimulus only = responds only to touch, pin, or deep pain

(0) No movement = does not respond to any stimulus

Weakness of an extremity is indicated by writing "weaker" under the appropriate column.

Figure 8–2 *(continued)*

- Although inattention to proper hygiene and dress, particularly mismatched socks or shoes, is common in people with emotional disorders, it is also a hallmark of dementias.
- Frequent, quick, purposeless movements are characteristic of anxiety, but they are equally characteristic of chorea and hyperthyroidism.
- Tremors accompanied by anxiety may point to Parkinson's disease.
- Recent weight loss, although often encountered in depression and schizophrenia, may be due to gastrointestinal disease, carcinoma, Addison's disease, and many other physical disorders.

The psychiatric nurse should observe skin color, pupillary changes, alertness and responsiveness, and quality of speech and word production, keeping in mind the possibility of delirium, dementia, substance intoxication, or other medical conditions.

Neurologic Assessment A careful neurologic assessment is mandatory for each client suspected of having brain

Table 8–2 Common Psychologic Tests in Clinical Use

Name of Test	*Description*	*Method*
Stanford-Binet Intelligence Test	A general intelligence test based on an age-level concept from 2 years to about 15 years. It is particularly useful to test children and to evaluate mental retardation.	The client is asked to do a graded series of tasks designed to correlate with the abilities of children of a particular age group. Each set is more difficult than the one before it.
Wechsler Adult Intelligence Scale (WAIS)	A general intelligence test for people 16 and older. It is the most widely used and best standardized intelligence test.	The client completes 11 subtests, which yield both verbal and performance scores as well as full-scale IQs. Subtest raw scores may also be compared to reveal variability in functioning. The subtests are: information, comprehension, arithmetic, similarities, memory for digits, vocabulary, digit symbol, picture completion, block design, picture arrangement, and object assembly.
Wechsler Intelligence Scale for Children (WISC)	A general intelligence test for children ages 5–15.	Similar to the Wechsler Test for adults, this test asks the client to complete 10 subtests, which yield separate verbal, performance, and full-scale scores.
Rorschach Test	A projective test that is the most highly developed of the personality tests. It reveals personality features and symptoms and is commonly used as a diagnostic tool.	The client responds to 10 cards, one at a time, consisting of black-and-white or colored standardized inkblots. Responses include the impressions, thoughts, and associations that come to mind while the client looks at the inkblot.
Thematic Apperception Test (TAT)	A projective test offering a standardized set of stimuli for exploring the client's emotional life. Themes and interpersonal problems emerge in the client's responses.	The client is shown a series of ambiguous pictures of people in various emotionally significant situations and is asked to respond by describing what is happening in the picture and telling a story about it. Adaptations have been designed for use with children. In these, the central figure is a child or the pictures are cartoons of animals.
Minnesota Multiphasic Personality Inventory (MMPI)	A self-administered objective (as opposed to projective) personality test designed to yield a broad examination of personality functioning that is amenable to statistical interpretation, such as self-attitudes, certain aspects of ego functioning, and profiles of symptoms or psychopathology.	The client responds to 550 statements by indicating either "true," "false," or "cannot say." The client's personality profile is sketched in terms of: • Preoccupation with body diseases • Depression • Hysteria • Antisocial personality • Masculine or feminine features • Paranoid qualities

dysfunction. Its goal is to discover signs pointing to circumscribed, focal cerebral dysfunction or diffuse, bilateral cerebral disease. A guide for evaluating the presence of signs of central nervous system disorders or "neurologic soft signs" is presented in Figure 8–2 on page 138.

Brain Imaging Techniques As previously introduced in Chapter 3, a range of brain imaging techniques are now available for viewing the living brain to detect seizure activity; evaluate Sleep Disorders; detect disorders such as multiple sclerosis; detect tumors, trauma, and strokes; examine the blood flowing to the brain; and identify cerebral atrophy, cerebral hemorrhage, cerebral infarct, hematomas, and abscesses. All of these conditions may present as psychiatric or behavioral symptoms. The most frequently used brain imaging techniques are described in the Tools of Psychobiology box in Chapter 3.

Authorities in mental health practice consistently remind clinicians of the need for thorough biologic and

Table 8–2 (continued)

Name of Test	Description	Method
Minnesota Multiphasic Personality Inventory (MMPI) *(continued)*		• Anxiety, phobias, and psychogenic fatigue • Schizophrenic features • Manic features
Draw-a-Person Test	A projective test used with both adults and children to elicit information on the client's body image or perception of self and the client's relationship to the environment. It is also used as a screening device to detect the presence of brain impairment. With children it may be used to compare the age level of expression with the child's chronologic age for a rough approximation of intelligence.	The client is asked first to draw a human figure and later to draw a person of the opposite sex. The test may be expanded by asking the client to draw a picture of a house and a tree as well (called the House-Tree-Person Test), an animal, or a family.
Sentence Completion Test	A projective test designed to elicit conscious associations to specific areas of functioning, thus illustrating the fears, preoccupations, ambitions, and idiosyncrasies of the client.	The client is asked to spontaneously complete sentences such as "I feel guilty about . . . ," "Sex is . . . ," "My mother . . . ," "Sometimes I wish . . . ," Both mood and content are noted.
Bender-Gestalt Test	A test of visual-motor coordination most useful with adults as a screening device to detect the presence of brain impairment. It may also be used to evaluate the level of maturation in the coordination of intellectual, muscular, and visual functions in children.	The client is asked to copy 9 separate geometric designs onto plain white paper, one at a time. Sometimes the client is asked to draw the design from memory after an interval of 45–60 seconds.
Blacky Test	A projective test used most frequently with children (although also designed for adults) to determine the level of psychosexual development.	The client is shown various cartoons about a dog (who may be identified as male or female) and the dog's family and is asked to make up a story about each cartoon.
Wechsler Memory Scale	A psychologic test for immediate, short-term, and long-term memory.	The client is asked to do 7 memory tests, including current information, orientation, mental control, logical memory, digits forward and backward, visual reproduction, and associate learning. A memory quotient (MQ) score is useful in the determination of brain mental syndrome.
Word Association Test	A projective test similar in form and organization to the Sentence Completion Test, designed to elicit associations to areas of conflict.	The client is asked to respond spontaneously to a series of 50 or more words, presented one at a time. Words presumed to be related to the conflicts of the specific client are mixed with words that generally produce an emotional reaction.

neurologic assessment of clients seen in psychiatric settings. The psychiatric literature abounds with stories of clients whose symptoms were initially considered exclusively psychiatric but ultimately proved medical, especially neurologic. Assessment errors occurred not because the features did not suggest medical disease but because such features were given too little weight or were misinterpreted. Changes in the APA's *DSM-IV* (1994) require that both medical condition and substance abuse be ruled out as conditions resulting in psychiatric symptoms.

Psychologic Testing

Clinical psychologists administer and interpret a wide variety of psychologic tests. There are two types of psychologic tests: those concerned with intelligence and those concerned with personality. Both intelligence and personality tests are typically included in a comprehensive psychologic evaluation. Both types of tests are summarized in Table 8–2 above.

INTELLIGENCE TESTS **Intelligence tests** may be useful particularly in evaluating the presence and degree of mental retardation. Commonly used intelligence tests are the **Stanford-Binet Test**, the **Wechsler Adult Intelligence Scale**, the **Wechsler Intelligence Scale for Children**, the Gesell Developmental Schedules, and the Vineland Social Maturity Scale.

PERSONALITY TESTS Personality tests are also called **projective tests** because they evoke projection in the responses of the person being tested.

The Rorschach Test Hermann Rorschach, a Swiss psychiatrist, developed the **Rorschach Test** in 1921. It consists of ten standardized inkblots in black and white or color on separate cards, displayed one by one. Clients are asked to respond in terms of their associations, thoughts, and impressions. Because each card contains only inkblots, clients' responses are *projected,* that is, they come from within the clients themselves. People may see people, animals, insects, objects, anatomic parts, or other things. The examiner scores the response using a system of symbols in relation to the following:

- *Location.* Where on the blot area was the response seen?
- *Content.* What did the client see?
- *Determinant.* What characteristic of the blot prompted the response?
- *Form-level.* How closely did the response correspond to the contour of the blot area used?
- *Originality.* How common a response is it?

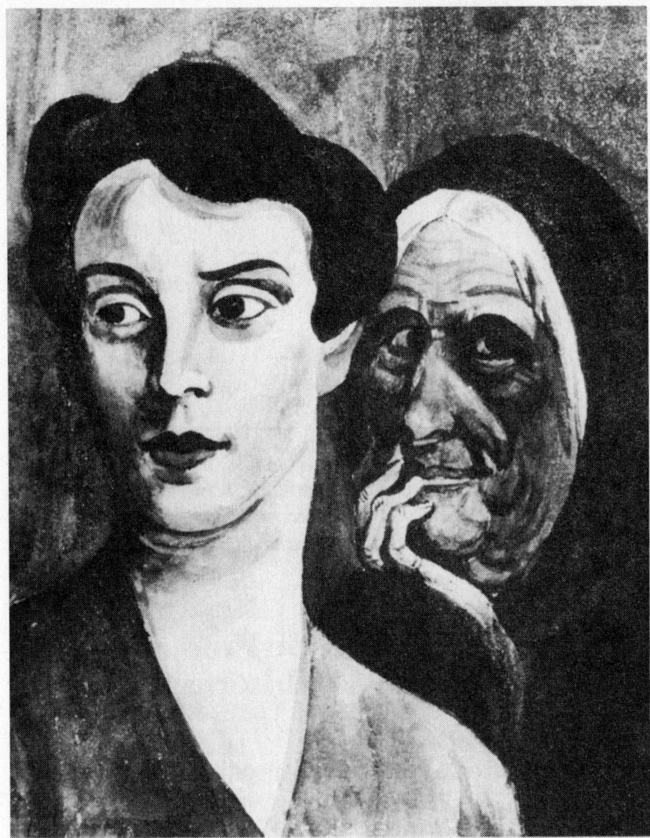

Figure 8–3 Card 12 GF of the Thematic Apperception Test. *SOURCE: Reprinted from Murray 1943. Copyright © 1943 by the President and Fellows of Harvard College; 1971 by Henry A. Murray. Reprinted by permission.*

Interpretation is based on a complicated system of scoring symbols and analyzing content. The Rorschach is the most highly developed of all the projective tests used to evaluate the personality.

The Thematic Apperception Test (TAT) The TAT also consists of a series of cards shown one by one. However, TAT cards are pictures of people in various emotional situations (Figure 8–3). Clients are asked to describe what seems to be happening in the picture or to tell a story about it. Because the pictures are ambiguous, the responses reveal aspects of the clients' own emotional lives. The psychologist who interprets and scores the TAT looks for themes, threads, and patterns in the response. Some adaptations of the TAT for use with children are available.

The Minnesota Multiphasic Personality Inventory (MMPI) The **MMPI** is a complex and lengthy test consisting of 550 questions. Scoring is done in relation to nine areas: preoccupation about body diseases; depression; hysteria; antisocial personality; masculine or feminine features; paranoid qualities; anxiety, phobias, and psychogenic fatigue states; schizophrenic features; and manic features. A clinical profile of personality structure is drawn from the client's responses in these areas.

Since the MMPI is largely self-administered and can be scored quickly on computers, it has been advocated as a screening measure for colleges and universities, industry and business, and government agencies, among others. The large-scale collection and use of such information are alarming because of the negative labeling that such psychologic testing may lead to.

The Draw-a-Person Test In the **Draw-a-Person Test,** clients are asked first to draw a human figure and then, usually, to draw a figure of a member of the opposite sex (Figure 8–4). The drawings may be interpreted to give information about clients' concepts of their own bodies and personality structures; their relationships with members of the opposite sex, the same sex, and parents; and their views of the roles of men and women.

PET Scan Brain Images

PET scans are a tool for assessment of cortical and subcortical brain functions. The scans reveal "cool" versus "hot" metabolic areas in the brain based on individualized spectrums of color (blue = low end of the metabolic range; yellow = intermediate metabolic range; red = high end of the metabolic range).

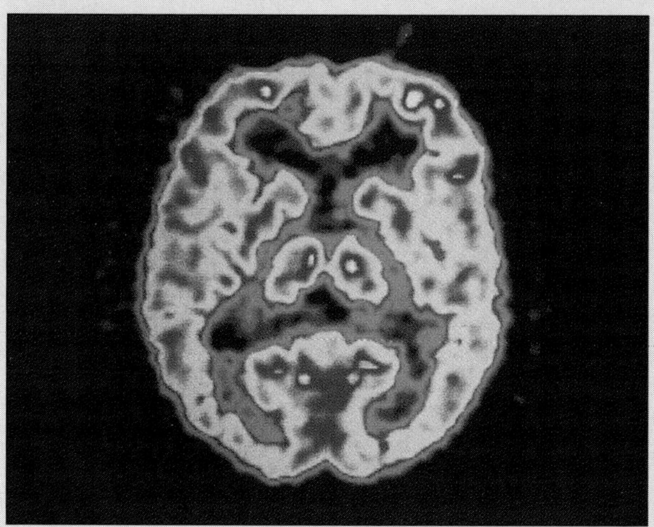

(A)

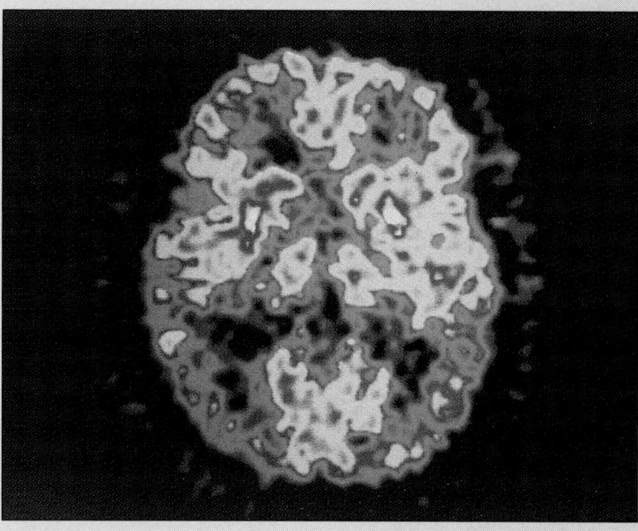

(B)

Dementia Compare a normal brain scan (**A**), with (B), the brain of a person with Alzheimer's disease. (**A**) The red and yellow areas indicate normal metabolic rates. (**B**) Note the blue areas indicating abnormally low metabolism in the parietal and temporal lobes of the person with Alzheimer's disease. *Courtesy of Laboratory of Neuroscience, National Institute on Aging.*

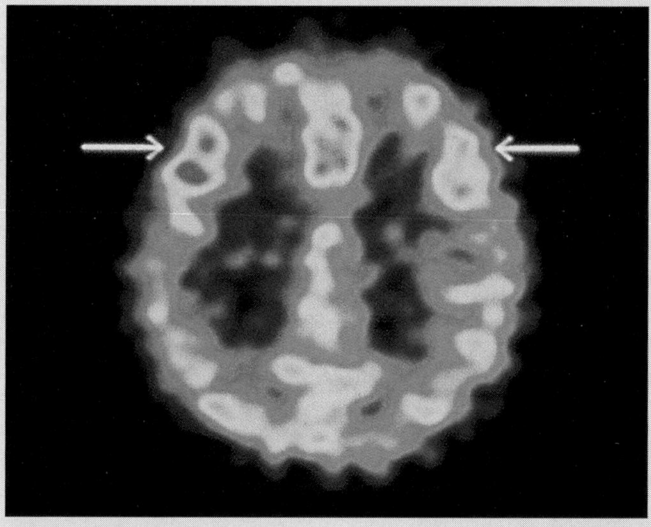

(A)

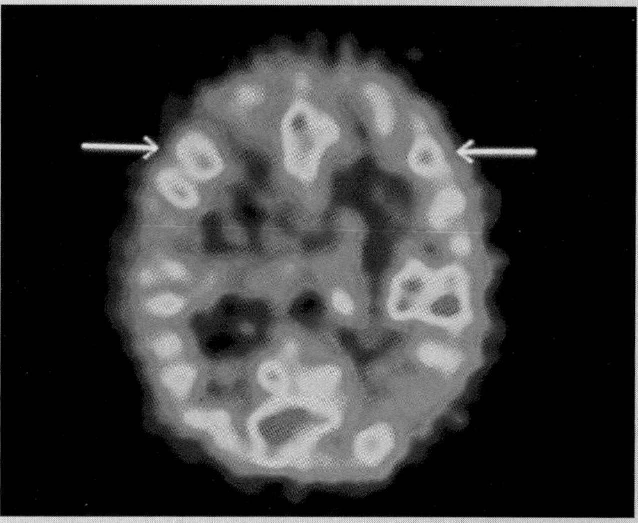

(B)

Schizophrenia PET scans of discordant monozygotic twins taken during a test to provoke activity and measure regional cerebral blood flow. (**A**) Arrows indicate areas of normal blood flow and brain activity in unaffected twin. (**B**) Arrows indicate areas of lower blood flow and brain activity in schizophrenic twin. *Courtesy of Dr. Karen F. Berman, Clinical Brain Disorders Branch, National Institute of Mental Health.*

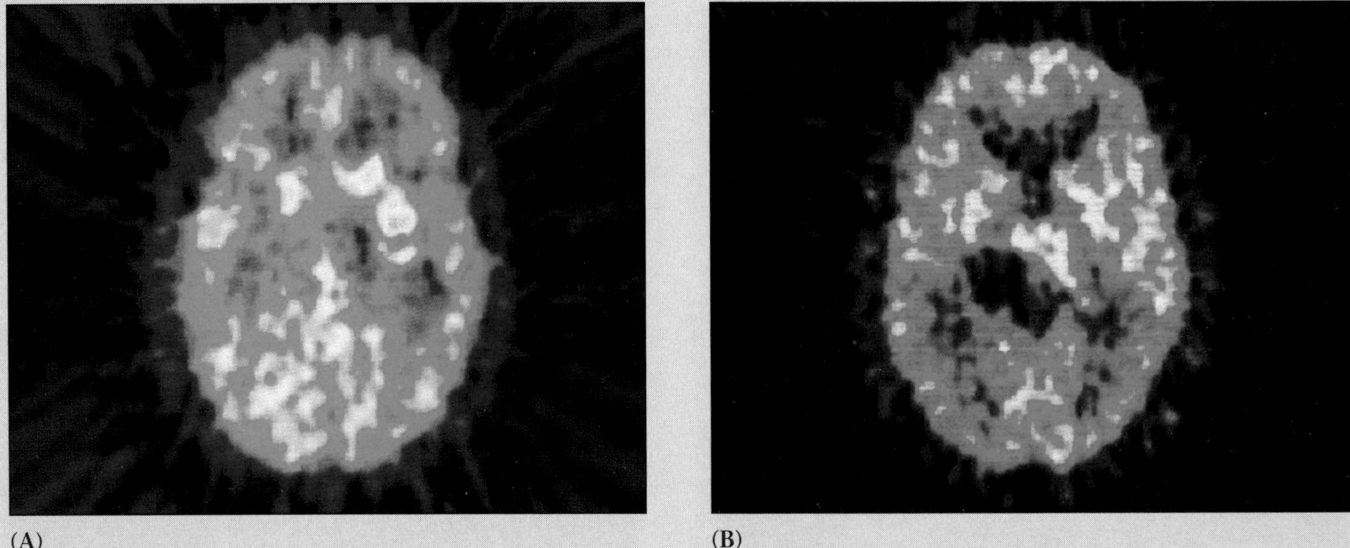

(A) (B)

HIV Disease PET scans facilitate a diagnosis by distinguishing between metabolically hot lymphomas and metabolically cold toxoplasmosis. (**A**) PET scan of an HIV-related lymphoma, the metabolically hot tumor on the right side of the scan. (**B**) In contrast, this scan shows HIV-related toxoplasmosis, indicated by the dramatic "hole" of a metabolically cold area. *Courtesy of Dr. Giovanni DiChiro and Dr. Ramesh Raman of the Neuroimaging Branch, National Institute of Neurological Disorders and Stroke, National Institute of Health.*

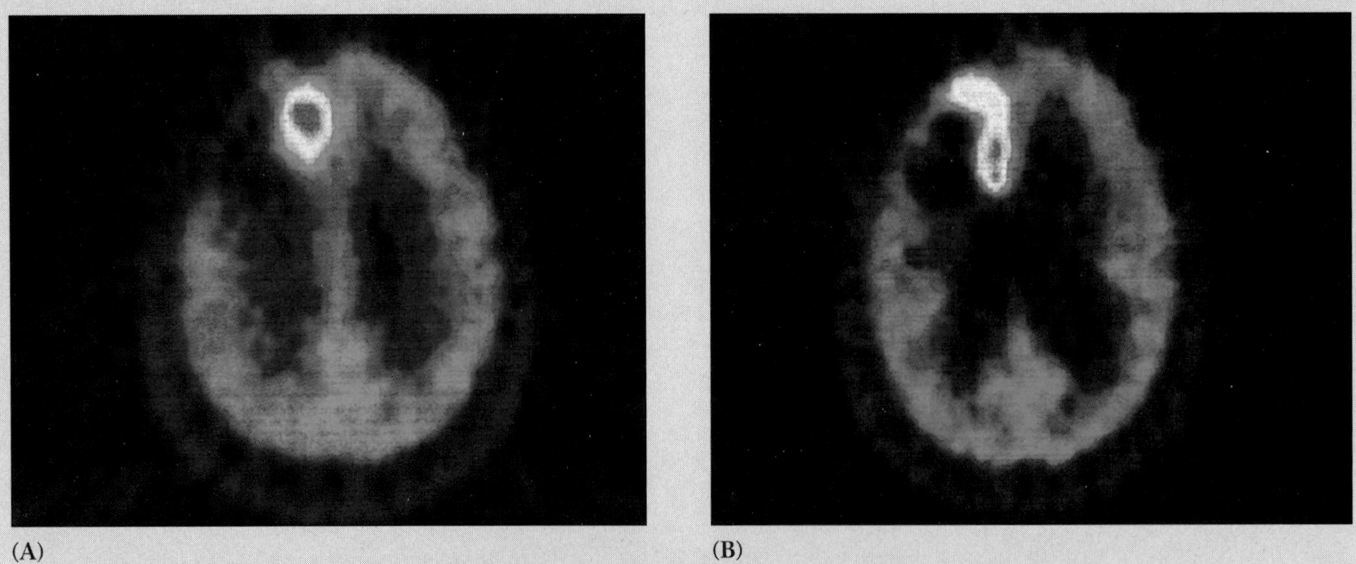

(A) (B)

Glioma This frontal lobe glioblastoma multiforme, a primary brain tumor, is metabolically very hot. (**A**) Note the large red area of the tumor. (**B**) The same tumor at a different level in the brain. *Courtesy of Dr. Giovanni DiChiro and Dr. Ramesh Raman of the Neuroimaging Branch, National Institute of Neurological Disorders and Stroke, National Institute of Health.*

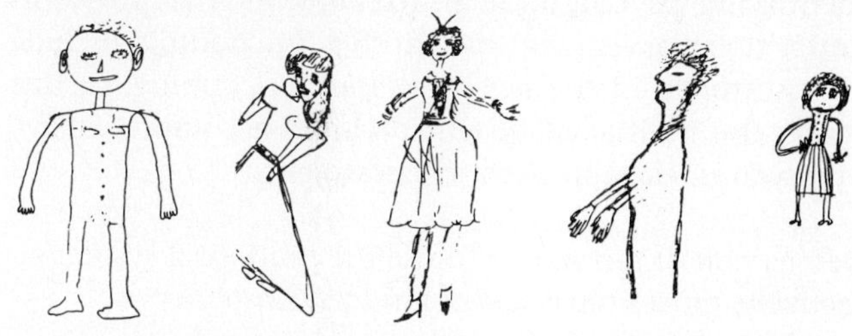

Figure 8–4 Examples of the Draw-a-Person Test done by five women who had been hospitalized for two years. *Source: Spire 1967 pp. 243, 248, 249, 251, 256.*

The Sentence Completion Test The **Sentence Completion Test** asks clients to complete an extensive series of incomplete sentences with the first thoughts that come to mind. The sentences are designed to elicit responses concerning fantasies, fears, daydreams, and aspirations, among other things.

The Bender-Gestalt Test The **Bender-Gestalt Test** asks clients to reproduce, as best they can, nine geometric designs that are printed on separate cards. Because this test can be used to evaluate memory, it may be particularly helpful in identifying brain damage. It is also used to evaluate the maturation level of children in the coordination of visual, motor, and cognitive functions. For an example of a Bender-Gestalt design series, see Figure 8–5.

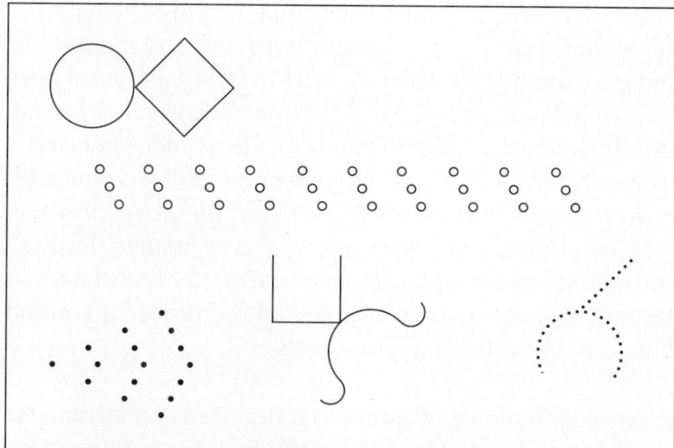

Figure 8–5 Examples of figures to be copied on a Bender-Gestalt Test. Clients are asked to copy the figures on a single sheet of paper and then to draw them from memory. The clinician looks for distortion of the figures in terms of incompleteness, rotation, oversimplification, perseveration (giving more than is present in the stimulus). The interpreter looks at the use of space on the page. Recall drawings also test for memory deficits. *Source: Bender 1938.*

Psychiatric Diagnostic Practice According to the DSM-IV

The first edition of the *Diagnostic and Statistical Manual* was published by the American Psychiatric Association (APA) in 1952. The second edition, published in 1968, attempted compatibility with the International Classification of Diseases, Injuries, and Causes of Death (ICD-9) published by the World Health Organization. *DSM-II* was widely criticized for its low reliability and tendency to reflect an individual psychiatrist's philosophy or such client characteristics as social class rather than actual clinical data.

The APA published a third edition entitled the *Diagnostic and Statistical Manual of Mental Disorders* in 1980 and a revised edition in 1987. Important features distinguished the *DSM-III-R* from its predecessors. It used specified diagnostic criteria to improve the reliability of diagnostic judgments and offered a multiaxial or multidimensional approach to clinical assessment of psychiatric clients in which five different classes of data are collected and assessed.

The *DSM-IV* represents the current state of knowledge about diagnosing mental disorders. It is composed of a list of all the official numeric codes and terms for all recognized mental disorders, along with a comprehensive description of each and specified diagnostic criteria that must be present in order to make each diagnosis. (For a complete list of codes and diagnoses according to the *DSM-IV,* see Appendix A.)

Basic Principles of the Multiaxial System The multiaxial framework for client assessment provided by *DSM-III* and *DSM-III-R* and retained and strengthened in *DSM-IV* is congruent with holistic views of people, recognizes the role of environmental stress in influencing behavior, and requires that the clinician collect data about client adaptive strengths as well as about symptoms or problems. One of the most important features of the *DSM-IV* is increased interclinician reliability resulting from the use of specified observable criteria that have been field-tested for interrater reliability. Its multiaxial approach is undoubtedly of significance to psychiatric nursing.

The following example illustrates the principle behind a multiaxial system:

A 35-year-old man came to an outpatient mental health clinic for evaluation. He came in for treatment of a severe fear and avoidance of flying that amounted to a phobia. However, he also had a long-term personality disturbance and suffered from eczema. Suppose three different clinicians were asked to evaluate this man. A biologically oriented clinician would certainly diagnose the eczema but might fail to notice the personality disturbance and make little of the phobia. A psychodynamically oriented clinician would be sure to diagnose the personality disorder but might overlook the eczema and the phobia, considering them to be merely manifestations of the underlying personality disturbance. Finally, a clinician who was behaviorally oriented would notice the phobia but might fail to diagnose the personality disturbance and the eczema. It is clear, then, that because of their differing theoretic orientations, these clinicians have a rather high likelihood of diagnostic disagreement.

Now suppose this same man were presented to the same three colleagues, but this time the clinicians were required to evaluate him in each of three different areas of functioning: behavioral or psychologic, personality, and physical functioning. In this case, all three clinicians would be much more likely to diagnose all three conditions and thus agree on the total evaluation of the individual.

In the *DSM-IV* multiaxial system, every person is evaluated on five axes, each dealing with a different class of information about the client. A multiaxial evaluation system provides a much more comprehensive evaluation of an individual and increases the likelihood that clinicians will agree among themselves about the condition of the person being evaluated.

The *DSM-IV* multiaxial system includes the five axes listed in the accompanying box. Axes I and II include all the mental disorders in the *DSM-IV* and therefore might be said to represent the intrapersonal or *psychologic* area of functioning. Axis III is for recording general medical conditions related to understanding the cause of psychiatric symptoms or managing the individual and thus represents the area of *physical* functioning. Axes IV and V, for identifying psychosocial and environmental problems and a global assessment of adaptive functioning, include an assessment of the person's *social* functioning. In this sense, the multiaxial system provides a comprehensive biopsychosocial approach to assessment.

DSM-IV Axes

Axis I:	Adult and Child Clinical Disorders
	Conditions not attributable to a mental disorder that are a focus of clinical attention (V-codes)
	Additional codes
Axis II:	Personality Disorders
	Mental Retardation
Axis III:	General Medical Conditions
Axis IV:	Psychosocial and Environmental Problems
Axis V:	Global Assessment of Functioning (GAF)

DESCRIPTION OF THE AXES To use the multiaxial system effectively, nurses must understand its components.

Axes I and II: Adult and Child Clinical Disorders, V-Codes, Personality Disorders, and Mental Retardation Axes I and II comprise all the mental disorders and other conditions that are a focus of clinical attention (called V-codes). The easiest way to differentiate between these first two axes is to focus first on Axis II. On Axis II are personality disorders, usually diagnosed in adults, and developmental disorders including mental retardation, diagnosed in children and adolescents. Axis II is also used to report maladaptive personality traits. All the remaining mental disorders of adults and children and associated conditions are recorded on Axis I. The classes of disorders on Axis II were given their own axis because their usually mild and chronic symptomatology is often overshadowed by a more florid Axis I condition. *DSM-IV* clarifies the conceptual distinction between Axis I and Axis II by noting that Axis II conditions

- Have an early onset.
- Have a stable, not episodic, course.

In addition to the other mental disorders, Axis I includes the **V-codes.** V-codes include such conditions as marital problems, occupational problems, and parent-child problems, in which the problem being evaluated or for which clinical care is sought is not due to a mental disorder. *A* ***mental disorder*** *is differentiated from other problems in living as a clinically significant behavioral or psychological syndrome or pattern that occurs in an individual and is associated with either a painful symptom (distress) or impairment in functioning (disability), or with an increased risk of suffering, death, pain, disability, or loss of freedom.* Further, the distress or disability does not primarily reflect a sanctioned response to an event, deviant behavior, or conflict between an individual and society.

If a man with bipolar disorder that has been in remission for many years develops marital difficulties for reasons unrelated to his psychiatric history or condition (perhaps, for example, because his wife wants to resume a career), both "Marital problem" and "Bipolar disorder in remission" could be recorded on Axis I. If, however, the bipolar disorder is not in complete remission, and marital conflict develops as a result of his changeable moods and other symptoms associated with the mental disorder, the marital problem would

not be recorded in addition to the bipolar disorder, since the marital problem in this case is due to the person's mental disorder.

Examples of evaluations using only Axes I and II are presented in the box below.

Examples of DSM-IV Multiaxial Evaluation on Axes I and II

Example 1

Axis I:	303.90	Alcohol dependence, in remission
Axis II:	301.70	Antisocial personality disorder

Example 2

Axis I:	V71.09	No diagnosis
Axis II:	301.22	Schizotypal personality disorder

Axis III: General Medical Conditions (from ICD-9CM) Clinicians use Axis III to record physical disorders and medical conditions that must be taken into account in planning treatment, or that are relevant to understanding the etiology or worsening of the mental disorder. A clinician might also want to record other significant physical findings, such as "soft" neurologic signs or even a single symptom (such as vomiting). An example of an evaluation done through Axis III is presented in the box below.

Example of DSM-IV Multiaxial Evaluation on Axes I, II, and III

Axis I:	312.8	Conduct disorder, socialized, aggressive
Axis II:	V71.09	No diagnosis
Axis III:		Diabetes

In this example, the client, a child in this case, will probably not be very compliant with the diabetes treatment regimen because of psychologic problems (conduct disorder, noted on Axis I).

If there is a lack of information on Axis III, that fact should be stated: "No information" or "Diagnosis deferred—not evaluated" or "Referred to Dr. Smith for evaluation." In any event, *something* should be noted on this axis; omitting it for lack of information undermines the purpose of a holistic multiaxial system. Of course, recent advances in psychobiologic knowledge make Axis III findings particularly important for psychiatric mental health nursing.

Axis IV: Psychosocial and Environmental Problems Axis IV provides the categories of psychosocial problems that may affect the diagnosis and treatment of mental disorders, shown in the box below.

Axis IV: Psychosocial and Environmental Problems

Problems with primary support group
Problems related to the social environment
Educational problems
Occupational problems
Housing problems
Economic problems
Problems with access to health care services
Problems related to interaction with the legal system/crime
Other psychosocial and environmental problems

In addition to identifying the type of problem(s), evaluators should also note in their own words the specific problems that they consider pertinent. Thus, a multiaxial evaluation, up through Axis IV, might look like the example in the box below.

Example of a DSM-IV Multiaxial Evaluation on Axes I, II, III, and IV

Axis I:	300.01	Panic disorder
Axis II:	301.83	Borderline personality disorder
Axis III:		No diagnosis
Axis IV:		Unemployment

Global Assessment of Functioning (GAF) Scale

Consider psychological, social, and occupational functioning on a hypothetical continuum of mental health–illness. Do not include impairment in functioning due to physical (or environmental) limitations.

Code	(Note: Use intermediate codes when appropriate, e.g., 45, 68, 72.)
100–91	Superior functioning in a wide range of activities, life's problems never seem to get out of hand, is sought out by others because of his or her many positive qualities. No symptoms.
90–81	Absent or minimal symptoms (e.g., mild anxiety before an exam), good functioning in all areas, interested and involved in a wide range of activities, socially effective, generally satisfied with life, no more than everyday problems or concerns (e.g., an occasional argument with family members).
80–71	If symptoms are present, they are transient and expectable reactions to psychosocial stressors (e.g., difficulty concentrating after family argument); no more than slight impairment in social, occupational, or school functioning (e.g., temporarily falling behind in schoolwork).
70–61	Some mild symptoms (e.g., depressed mood and mild insomnia) OR some difficulty in social, occupational, or school functioning (e.g., occasional truancy, or theft within the household), but generally functioning pretty well, has some meaningful interpersonal relationships.
60–51	Moderate symptoms (e.g., flat affect and circumstantial speech, occasional panic attacks) OR moderate difficulty in social, occupational, or school functioning (e.g., few friends, conflicts with peers or coworkers).
50–41	Serious symptoms (e.g., suicidal ideation, severe obsessional rituals, frequent shoplifting) OR any serious impairment in social, occupational, or school functioning (e.g., no friends, unable to keep a job).
40–31	Some impairment in reality testing or communication (e.g., speech is at times illogical, obscure, or irrelevant) OR major impairment in several areas, such as work or school, family relations, judgment, thinking, or mood (e.g., depressed man avoids friends, neglects family, and is unable to work; child frequently beats up younger children, is defiant at home, and is failing at school).
30–21	Behavior is considerably influenced by delusions or hallucinations OR serious impairment in communication or judgment (e.g., sometimes incoherent, acts grossly inappropriately, suicidal preoccupation) OR inability to function in almost all areas (e.g., stays in bed all day; no job, home, or friends).
20–11	Some danger of hurting self or others (e.g., suicide attempts without clear expectation of death; frequently violent; manic excitement) OR occasionally fails to maintain minimal personal hygiene (e.g., smears feces) OR gross impairment in communication (e.g., largely incoherent or mute).
10–1	Persistent danger of severely hurting self or others (e.g., recurrent violence) OR persistent inability to maintain minimal personal hygiene OR serious suicidal act with clear expectation of death.
0	Inadequate information

The rating of overall psychological functioning on a scale of 0–100 was operationalized by Luborsky in the Health-Sickness Rating Scale (Luborsky L: Clinicians' judgments of mental health. Archives of General Psychiatry *7:407–417, 1962). Spitzer and colleagues developed a revision of the Health-Sickness Rating Scale called the Global Assessment Scale (GAS) (Endicott J, Spitzer RL, Fleiss IL, Cohen J: The Global Assessment Scale: A procedure for measuring overall severity of psychiatric disturbance.* Archives of General Psychiatry *33:766–771, 1976). A modified version of the GAS was included in* DSM-III-R *as the Global Assessment of Functioning (GAF) Scale.*

Axis V: Global Assessment of Functioning (GAF) This axis provides the rating scale shown in the box above. One of the most accurate indicators of clinical outcome is the level of premorbid functioning that an individual sustained. For this reason, Axis V provides a **Global Assessment of Functioning (GAF) Scale** to rate the highest level of psychologic, social, and occupational functioning that an individual was able to sustain for at least a few months during the past year as well as at the time of evaluation. Examples of full multiaxial DSM-IV diagnoses appear on page 147.

THE DSM'S USEFULNESS TO PSYCHIATRIC–MENTAL HEALTH NURSING From the perspective of psychiatric nursing, the *DSM-IV* represents some progress toward values that mental health nurses have espoused for decades. They

Examples of How to Record Results of a DSM-IV Multiaxial Evaluation

Example 1

Axis I	296.23	Major depressive disorder, single episode, severe without psychotic features
	305.00	Alcohol abuse
Axis II	301.6	Dependent personality disorder
		Frequent use of denial
Axis III		None
Axis IV		Threat of job loss
Axis V	GAF = 35	(current)

Example 2

Axis I	300.4	Dysthymic disorder
	315.00	Reading disorder
Axis II	V71.09	No diagnosis
Axis III	382.9	Otitis media, recurrent
Axis IV		Victim of child neglect
Axis V	GAF = 53	(current)

Example 3

Axis I	293.83	Mood disorder due to hypothyroidism, with depressive features
Axis II	V71.09	No diagnosis, histrionic personality features
Axis III	244.9	Hypothyroidism
	365.23	Chronic angle-closure glaucoma
Axis IV		None
Axis V	GAF = 45	(on admission)
	GAF = 65	(on discharge)

Example 4

Axis I	V61.1	Partner relational problem
Axis II	V71.09	No diagnosis
Axis III		None
Axis IV		Unemployment
Axis V	GAF = 83	(highest level past year)

- Provide a framework for interdisciplinary communication.
- Base revisions on a series of formative evaluations.
- Represent a collaborative achievement.
- Represent progress toward a more holistic view of mind-body relations.
- Provide for diagnostic uncertainty.
- Incorporate biologic, psychologic, and social variables.
- Have achieved positive results in extensive field testing for validity and reliability.
- Consider adaptive strength as well as problems.
- Reflect a descriptive, phenomenologic perspective rather than any psychiatric theory.

The Research Note on the next page gives an example of the rigorous scientific work on which *DSM-IV* decisions were made.

Psychosocial Assessment

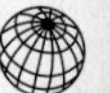

Psychosocial assessment is a dynamic process. It begins during the initial contact with the client, and it continues throughout the nurse-client experience. Psychosocial assessments may be made of an individual, a family, or a group. In any case, they begin with the identifying characteristics, such as name, sex, age, marital status, and ethnic and cultural origins. Problem identification and definition are also necessary phases in the assessment process. The method for assessment described below has

RESEARCH NOTE

Citation

Skodol AE, Oldham JM, Gallaher PE, Bezirganian S: Validity of self-defeating personality disorder. *Am J Psychiatr* 1994;151:560–567.

Study Problem/Purpose

This study set out to investigate the validity of a separate personality disorder currently termed self-defeating personality and historically known as masochistic personality. This condition is associated with a pattern of self-punishment and self-sabotage: choosing people and situations that lead to mistreatment, inciting angry, rejecting responses, and avoiding people who treat one well. The diagnosis of masochistic personality, according to vocal feminist critics, has been disproportionately applied to women, fails to consider interactional power relations, and obscures problems of domestic violence and date rape by blaming the victim.

Methods

This rigorous clinical study enrolled 100 applicants for inpatient treatment of personality disorders and 100 for psychoanalysis and used the Structured Clinical Interview for *DSM-III-R* and the Personality Disorder Examination instrument to conduct independent assessments.

Findings

Self-defeating personality disorder did not appear to be a valid separate personality disorder. This particular diagnostic label had only fair internal consistency, a degree of measurement difficulty, overlap with other Axis I and Axis II disorders, and no relationship to validators.

Implications

This study is a noteworthy example of the new scientific standard required if mental disorders are to be included in the *DSM*. The Axis II personality disorders are among the most muddled of the categories. It seems important to make decisions about what to include and what to exclude based on science, such as that represented in this research, rather than on politics and rhetoric.

been adapted from the classic problem-solving model of Compton and Galaway (1979, pp. 250–251).

INDIVIDUAL ASSESSMENT During the individual assessment, the nurse considers the following factors:

1. *Physical and intellectual.*
   a. Presence of physical illness and/or disability.
   b. Appearance and energy level.
   c. Current and potential levels of intellectual functioning.
   d. How the client sees personal world and translates events around self; client's perceptual abilities.
   e. Cause-and-effect reasoning, ability to focus.
2. *Socioeconomic factors.*
   a. Economic factors—level of income, adequacy of subsistence: their effect on lifestyle, sense of adequacy, and self-worth.
   b. Employment and attitudes about it.
   c. Racial, cultural, and ethnic identification; sense of identity and belonging (see Appendix C). 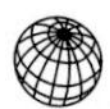
   d. Religious identification and link to significant value systems, norms, and spiritual practices. See the Spiritual Health Assessment box, opposite, for sample questions.
3. *Personal values and goals.*
   a. Presence or absence of congruence between values and their expression in action; meaning of values to individual.
   b. Congruence between the individual's values and goals and the immediate systems with which the client interacts.
   c. Congruence between the individual's values and the assessor's values; the meaning of this for the intervention process.
4. *Adaptive functioning and response to present involvement.*
   a. Manner in which the individual presents self to others—grooming, appearance, posture.
   b. Emotional tone and change or constancy of levels.
   c. Style of communication—verbal and nonverbal; ability to express appropriate emotion, follow train of thought; factors of dissonance, confusion, uncertainty.
   d. Symptoms or symptomatic behavior.
   e. Quality of relationships the individual seeks to establish—direction, purposes, and uses of such relationships for the individual.
   f. Perception of self.
   g. Social roles that are assumed or ascribed; competence in fulfilling these roles.
   h. Relational behavior.
      (1) Capacity for intimacy.
      (2) Dependence/independence balance.
      (3) Power and control conflicts.
      (4) Exploitiveness.
      (5) Openness.

Spiritual Health Assessment

For these 5 statements, indicate whether you *never, sometimes, often,* or *nearly always* agree.

1. I trust myself.
2. I feel my life has meaning and purpose.
3. Other people give meaning to my life.
4. I trust other people.
5. I have close friends.
6. I have experienced the following in my life:

   Loss ____ Separation ____ Divorce ____ Geographic moves ____ Rejection ____ Death ____
7. Do *religion* and *spirituality* mean the same thing to you? If not, what are the differences to you?
8. With 1 being the lowest and 10 the highest, place an X on the scale below to indicate your relationship with your higher power, and circle the place on the scale that you feel would be ideal for your relationship with your higher power. Explain why you chose each of these points.

   1 2 3 4 5 6 7 8 9 10

   (no relationship) (turn only problems over) (turn total self over)
9. My religious upbringing and background can be described as (check as many as apply):

   Nurturing ____ Helpful ____ Strict ____ Conservative ____ Liberal ____

   Punishing ____ Negative ____ Had very little ____ Had none ____

Grace D. Dreyer, MSN, RN, CS

5. *Developmental factors.*
   a. How role performance is equated with life stage.
   b. How developmental experiences have been interpreted and used.
   c. How the individual has dealt with past conflicts, tasks, and problems.
   d. Whether the present problem is unique in the person's life experience.

THE PLACE OF ASSESSMENT IN PRACTICE Assessment is essential in clinical practice and serves several purposes:

- Identifying problems.
- Identifying client motivations, strengths, and resources.
- Identifying forces (both internal and external to the client) that may hinder the therapeutic plan.
- Setting reasonable goals.
- Determining appropriate intervention strategies.
- Providing continuous evaluation of the process and indicating when the therapeutic plan should be changed.

Assessment is an ongoing, dynamic process that Compton and Galaway once described as a "squirming, wriggling, alive business" (1979, p. 287). It provides an opportunity for nurse and client to engage in a partnership based on mutual definition of problems and goals.

Systems of Recording

Nurses must communicate adequately in writing to inform members of the mental health team of the client's problems and patterns of interaction. Recording is an important process; it should provide the basis for:

- Altering a treatment plan.
- Determining appropriate intervention strategies.
- Allowing communication among members of the mental health team or mental health agencies.
- Providing around-the-clock data on hospitalized clients.

- Evidence in court.
- Research.

An often unrecognized or disregarded purpose of recording is to provide quality accountability of psychiatric nursing practice. Recorded data can be used to give nurses feedback about their practice, through processes such as the psychiatric audit (discussed later in this chapter). Careful recording is also critical to avoiding legal exposure in a lawsuit. Exactly what system of recording is used depends on the agency.

Essential Recording Principles

The most significant events the nurse records are the behavior patterns and interpersonal interactions of the client. It may also be important to record other significant information: the client's sleeping, eating, and elimination patterns; physical appearance; somatic treatments and medications; and so on. *Any changes in a client's suicide potential should be carefully and regularly assessed and documented according to agency policies and the standard of care.*

The following types of notes should be made:

- *Intake interview and mental status exam results.* Be sure to include a suicide and violence assessment, a drug abuse assessment, and a medical condition history.
- *Progress over time.* Mental health agencies may require that notes be entered at specific times, such as at the end of each 8-hour shift or at the end of each 24-hour period. When events of special significance occur, they should be recorded as soon after the event as possible, not held until the 8 or 24 hours have elapsed. In the case of special observation precautions, some form of recording may be necessary every 15 minutes. Such recording is crucial in the case of a suicidal client so that increased observation levels can be ordered when necessary.
- *Nurse-client relationship.* Notes are often made after each session with the client in individual, group, or family therapy. These notes summarize what occurred during the experience.
- *Summary report.* Summary reports are usually made at the termination of contact with the client, that is, when individual, group, or family therapy has ended. The summary report presents a clear and concise picture of the highlights of the experience.

Behavior and interaction notes should include examples rather than interpretations. Instead of writing "Ms W is hallucinating," it is preferable to write "Ms W states she hears Moses telling her not to get dressed today or leave her room."

The mental health field is rich in terms that nurses must learn if they are to speak the language in which mental health professionals converse. However, too much jargon may cloud meaning. The language of mental health, which relies heavily on words and phrases from psychology, has also borrowed from public health, sociology, anthropology, philosophy, and the federal government. Nurses should use jargon sparingly. The glossary at the end of this book may be particularly useful.

Source-Oriented Recording

Source-oriented records are becoming less common as more agencies institute problem-oriented methods of recording. Source-oriented recording usually consists of a clinical record or chart that includes unassembled chronologic notations made by individual mental health team members. Physicians write orders and progress notes in one place, and nurses chart their notes in another. Other members of the team may not contribute in writing at all. Laboratory findings are kept in a third isolated section of the chart. Source-oriented recording hinders close communication among members of the mental health team. Such systems often duplicate efforts and fail to pull information about the client into a logical whole.

Problem-Oriented Recording

The problem-oriented system of recording is a major improvement over the source-oriented system. It is a way of organizing the same raw data into a comprehensive whole that can be used for assessment, planning, evaluation, research, and health care audits. The process stimulates mental health team members to gather, document, and describe data.

There are four necessary elements in problem-oriented recording systems:

1. *Database.* The database consists of all the information gathered at the initial contact with the client. It includes psychiatric history, psychosocial assessment, laboratory and physical findings, and the results of mental status examinations and psychologic tests. Figure 8–6 shows the mental health supplement to the standard defined database used in one mental health facility.

2. *Problem list.* The problem list emerges from the database and summarizes the problems of the client. It should also include the client's assets. It is continually updated to present an accurate picture of the client's current situation. In the case of many psychiatric clients, safety risk must be considered as an essential problem.

3. *Initial plans.* A section of the record delineates the therapeutic plans for the client. Plans are formulated in terms of the problems to which they relate. Plans often include outcome behaviors and target dates. See, for example, the critical pathways in this book.

text continues on page 153

MEDICAL RECORD	SUPPLEMENT DEFINED DATA BASE

SUPPLEMENT TO (*Check only one*) PART ☐ I ☐ II ☐ III ☐ IV ☐ V ☐ VI

PREPARED BY (*Signature & Title*)	SERVICE	DATE
T. Kim, R.N., Clinical Specialist	Emergency	12-23-96

CHIEF COMPLAINT: In patient's own words and your impressions.

Gaunt, disheveled man in mid-thirties complains, "I have no purpose in life."

HISTORY AND DEVELOPMENT OF COMPLAINT

A. Date of onset and circumstances under which complaint developed.

Since resigning responsible position as electronics engineer 10 years ago, client has been drifting aimlessly, living at minimal level of subsistence. Brought in by police who found him living in his car in a school parking lot.

B. Previous hospitalizations and treatment-response to psychotropic drugs.

Unknown

C. Previous history of violent behavior, suicidal behavior, alcohol and drug abuse, previous arrests, and treatment by alcohol, drug and forensic program.

Experimentation with LSD and marijuana for 10 years at least 3x per week . . . often once per day, with related impairment of social & occupational function. (No job, no dating relationships or social life)

MENTAL STATUS EXAMINATION

A. Overall general appearance. Thin, unshaven dirty man in mid-thirties with poor nutrition, hygiene and tearful expression.

B. Attitude and degree of cooperativeness.

Generally despondent but passively cooperative

C. Thought content and process—what patient thinks about—how patient thinks over and underproductive, spontaneous, circumstantial.

Thought content focuses on discovering solution to life's mysteries....finding the key or answer.

Thought processes are vague and disconnected. Long periods of silence between verbalizations.

SUPPLEMENT
DEFINED
DATA BASE

VA FORM 10-7978g

Figure 8–6 A mental health supplement to the standard database. *Source: Veterans Administration Hospital, Buffalo, NY.*

D. Motoric behavior—overactive, underactive, inappropriate.

Slow, underactive bordering on catatonic low energy level

AFFECT

A. How the patient feels—shallow, anxious, depressed appropriate, inappropriate.

Depressed and discouraged—feelings of inadequacy

SENSORIUM MENTAL GRASP AND CAPACITY

A. Orientation / memory

Oriented to time, place & person

B. Abstract thinking

Can interpret proverbs but ponderously

C. Judgment / insight, adequate, complete, incomplete, distorted

Questionable

D. Cognitive disorder—hallucinations and delusions

No data available at this time

E. Estimate of intelligence

Average or above

DIAGNOSTIC IMPRESSION

Substance use disorder, dysthymic disorder, possible borderline personality

TREATMENT PLAN PROBLEMS	GOALS	TREATMENT
Poor nutritional status	Improve status	Offer balanced, high cal diet suited to his vegetarian preference.
Poor hygiene status	Improve status	Encourage daily bathing. Refer to Dentist
Dependence on Cannabis	Decrease usage	Refer to group therapy
Depression	Control Sx	Prescribe anti-depress. medication. Refer to psych. therapist for individual counseling

Figure 8–6 (continued)

4. *Progress note.* Progress notes parallel items in the problem list. They are used to monitor the plans, identify the need for modification, and provide a follow-up. The progress notes include narrative notes, flow sheets, and a discharge summary.
   a. Narrative notes are written in SOAP style, an acronym for *subjective* (the problem as perceived by the client), *objective* (clinical findings or observations), *assessment* (what is suggested by an analysis and synthesis of the subjective and objective data), and *plan* (proposed solutions for the identified problems).
   b. Flow sheets are used to tabulate information in graphic form. They are useful when some factor must be monitored frequently.
   c. The discharge summary is a summary of each problem area and the level of resolution reached. It provides the essential data for community follow-up services.

Figure 8–7 demonstrates how one mental health facility uses problem-oriented progress notes.

Nursing Care Plans

Nursing care plans are a means of providing nursing personnel with information about the needs and therapeutic plans for each client. They are of major importance when an agency uses source-oriented recording methods, because they provide an ongoing, up-to-date record of goal-directed, individualized nursing care. When problem-oriented recording methods are used, nursing care plans may be an outgrowth of the record.

Critical Pathways

Critical pathways are an innovation on the more familiar and traditional nursing care plan. They are usually concisely formatted in columns and emphasize patient outcomes (short-term goals) tied to target dates. The critical pathways included in this text specify the following categories of information:

1. Daily patient outcomes (short-term goals).
2. Assessments, tests, and treatments.
3. Knowledge deficit (daily prescriptions for nursing interventions focused on client teaching).
4. Diet (daily prescriptions).
5. Activity (daily prescriptions for nursing interventions).
6. Psychosocial considerations (daily prescriptions for nursing interventions).

The precise format for critical pathways may vary from setting to setting or be based on the client's condition. As is the case with nursing care plans, critical pathways are not set in stone and must be modified based on changes in client assessment data. Furthermore, standardized critical pathways should always be individualized for individual clients.

Algorithms

Algorithms are behavioral steps, or step-by-step procedures, for the management of common problems. Algorithms have proved to be useful protocols, particularly in settings that employ large numbers of paraprofessionals. At intake points in community mental health settings, such as walk-in neighborhood clinics, mental health workers often make the initial psychosocial assessment and may plan and implement treatment strategies. Clinical algorithms for common mental health problems provide the nonprofessional with structured, standardized guidelines for decision making.

Professional nurses in nonpsychiatric settings find clinical algorithms particularly useful. Algorithms for depression and suicidal lethality have been found to be reliable and valid in these circumstances.

Psychiatric Audits

The **psychiatric audit** is one way to evaluate the quality of mental health services consumers receive. The client's chart is reviewed to compare criteria for quality care with actual practice. Problem-oriented recording systems provide the descriptive documentation necessary for such a program. Although documentation may not always accurately indicate the quality of the care given, it is an important part of the process because it keeps the mental health care workers accountable to consumers of their services.

Process Recordings

A **process recording** is a verbatim and progressive recording of the verbal and nonverbal interactions between client and nurse within a given period of time. It is a means of communication between nurses or nursing students and their clinical supervisors, consultants, or instructors about their client relationships. To learn the function of therapeutic intervention, nurses must study and objectively review verbal and nonverbal communications to learn their potential significance. These interactions may reveal the existence of problems or attempts at resolution of these problems.

PURPOSES The process recording serves these purposes:

- It helps nurses sharpen their skills of observation and listening by providing an opportunity to find clues that were not recognized during the face-to-face encounter.

MEDICAL RECORD | PROBLEM-ORIENTED PROGRESS NOTES

PROBLEM		Format—Problem title (Do not abbreviate) S-Subjective O-Objective A-Assessment P-Plans. (All notes must have signature and title of person making entry.) Continue on reverse.
DATE	NO.	
12-4-96	3	Problem Title: Angry and agitated.
		Subjective: "I can't take anymore of this — I have to get out!"
		Objective : Client is pacing, crying, waving his hands, yelling at nursing
		staff and other patients. Looks very upset.
		Assessment: Client has just completed interview with his private
		therapist, who told him his wife has filed for
		divorce, and won't talk to him about it.
		Plan: 1. Give client time and space to decrease agitation
		2. Offer him use of quiet room
		3. Keep him in eye contact, but do not engage him at this time
		4. If he is not quieter in 1 hr offer PRN medication
		T. Kim, RN
		Clinical Specialist

PROBLEM-ORIENTED

PROGRESS NOTES

VA FORM 10-7978i

Figure 8–7 A sample form for problem-oriented progress notes. *Source: Veterans Administration Hospital, Buffalo, NY.*

- It promotes the communication skills of nurses. By examining their words, gestures, and nonverbal communication, nurses can reduce their use of clichés, double messages, and stereotyped automatic comments.
- It gives the nurse a tool for assessing nurse-client interactions and gives the instructor, clinical supervisor, or consultant a tool for assessing and guiding the nurse in clinical work. It supplements memory, facilitates evaluation, and acquaints the student with rudimentary applied research skills.
- It provides data from which nurses can assess their own behavior in interactions with clients. By encouraging nurses to examine their personal reactions to client behavior, the process recording enriches their self-understanding and experience. An added advantage is that it allows nurses to look at the dynamics of nurse-client behavior when they are away from the interpersonal situation.
- It helps nurses plan nursing interventions. By evaluating the effectiveness of therapeutic strategies in actual clinical situations and linking their observations to theory, nurses can identify additional or alternative nursing interventions.

Data Collection An excerpt from a sample process recording appears in Figure 8–8. The raw data or verbatim recording can be obtained in a number of ways.

On-the-Spot Recording The nurse may make brief notes on the spot, perhaps using some shorthand code of symbols and abbreviations, in a stenographer's notebook. There are several advantages to this form of recording. Notes on verbal communication can be made easily, it is a more accurate technique than attempting to recall after the experience, and it prevents the nurse from unwittingly omitting important material. It also demonstrates that the nurse is paying close attention to what the client says and does. However, the nurse usually interacts less freely and becomes less spontaneous when recording on the spot, because of the need to attend to the note-taking task. It may also limit observation of the nonverbal components of the client's communication.

After-the-Fact Recording When the nurse gathers data by recall, it is important to record them as soon as possible after the interaction with the client. The most successful method is for nurses to structure their time so that they can begin writing in a quiet area immediately. The longer the time between interaction and recording, the less able nurses are to remember words and actions and their sequence. If it is difficult to set aside enough time, the nurse should record only raw data at once and delay analysis. A delay may actually improve analysis. It may allow a more objective interpretation, because time and distance make nurses less protective of their original behavior.

The advantage of this method is that it does not require the nurse to take notes while paying close attention to the client. It thus does not curtail the nurse's spontaneity. The major disadvantage is that the nurse may not remember completely and thus distort the interaction. Nurses using this method of recording tend to omit or shorten important details.

Tape Recording The most common form of mechanical recording is by audiotape. Tape recorders are now smaller, less expensive, and less obtrusive than earlier models were. Videotape recordings may also be used. Although now available in portable form, they are costly and are less commonly used.

Tape-recorded data can be transcribed, and they provide a more accurate record of verbal interactions than notes do. The recording avoids unintentional editing or condensation of important content. Nurses who use a tape recorder can reexperience tones of voice, pauses, silences, speaking rates, actual words, and sequences of responses. Because tapes force nurses to listen to themselves as they actually are rather than as they would like to be, using a tape recorder may cause anxiety. Clients may fear being "on tape" and refuse to give the nurse permission to tape the session. Other disadvantages are that tape recording does not pick up visual cues, and transcribing the tape can be costly and/or time-consuming.

Confidentiality and Comprehensiveness When recording client data, the nurse has the responsibility to protect the client from unwarranted exposure. The client's name should not appear on the process recording, and the record should not be treated carelessly or left lying about. The nurse's respect for the client's self-disclosures is one way for the client to gauge the nurse's trustworthiness.

The client, Jennie, is a 26-year-old woman who lives with her 5-year-old daughter. Scott, her husband, moved out of the house last month. Jennie was briefly hospitalized in a psychiatric unit three years ago with a diagnosis of "obsessive-compulsive reaction."

INTERACTION (VERBAL AND NONVERBAL)	*NURSE-CENTERED ANALYSIS*	*CLIENT-CENTERED ANALYSIS*
(Jennie arrives fifteen minutes late.)		
Nurse: Hi, Jennie.	Non judgmental beginning	
Jennie: Hi. The cab was a little late.		
Nurse: You took a cab?	Reflecting to encourage client to elaborate	
Jennie: Yeah. It's freezing out and I knew that. . . I. . .didn't feel like walking up (laugh), plus I. . . I was. . . um. . . (quietly) getting ready at the last minute, anyway.		Evades responsibility
Nurse: Ah hum. Sometimes you have trouble getting going?	Paraphrases to encourage elaborations by client	Assumes responsibility
Jennie: Yes!		
(Silence.)		
Nurse: So how are things going?	Open-ended question that leaves topic up to client	
Jennie: Um. . . last night. . . not so well.		
Nurse: Not so well?	Reflecting back to client	
Jennie: Oh. . .(low voice) I don't know, I guess. It happened after I ate dinner. I just, I don't know if it's the low blood sugar or nerves or what. I mean it *acts* like low blood sugar.		Focusing on physical problems perhaps to avoid emotional issues
Nurse: How's that? You mentioned this before—with low blood sugar you have certain symptoms, and you feel like you know when it's happening. How does it feel?	Open-ended question	
Jennie: Well . . . like, first, I guess, first I notice that my thinking was getting worse. And, like, it was harder to *think* and harder to concentrate. And, like, I never realized . . . I thought some of that business was just emotions and being upset, and then, after reading this book I have on low blood sugar, it explains that . . . like, if your blood sugar is low, well it's low for your whole body, so your brain is only half nourished.		Describing experience attributed initially to physical cause

Figure 8–8 Excerpt from a sample process recording.

Chapter Highlights

- The nursing process begins with assessment, and the primary source of client data in most instances is the client.
- Correct problem identification and intervention strategies often depend on the quality of information sharing.
- Psychiatric client information is gathered, assessed, and communicated through psychiatric history-taking, mental status examination, biologic and neurologic assessment, psychologic testing, psychosocial assessment, and process recordings.
- Traditionally, history-taking has followed a medical model and is most concerned with gathering information about a client's psychiatric problem.
- The mental status examination is used to identify a person's general behavior and appearance, characteristics of talk, emotional state, special preoccupations and experiences (particularly suicidal ideation and intent), sensorium or orientation, memory, general intelligence, abstract thinking, and insight. Its primary purpose is to gather data to formulate a psychiatric diagnosis, prognosis, and treatment plan.
- Psychologic tests are tests concerned with intelligence and personality.
- It is particularly important for the nurse to rule out a biologic or neurologic basis for psychiatric symptoms by conducting a thorough history, directly observing the client, completing a neurologic assessment, and comprehending brain imaging techniques.
- The *DSM-IV* is the APA's most recent system for diagnosing and classifying mental disorders and is more congruent with holistic views of people than were prior editions of the *DSM*.
- In conducting a psychosocial assessment to determine a client's problems, the nurse should include physical, intellectual, socioeconomic, and developmental factors; personal values and goals; adaptive functioning; and response to present involvements.
- Recording provides the basis for altering the treatment plan, determining intervention, linking mental health team members, gaining around-the-clock data on hospitalized clients, evidence in court, and research.
- The nurse uses psychiatric jargon sparingly, recognizing its inadequacies for understanding the depth and variety of human problems.
- Problem-oriented systems of recording are comprehensive and logically structured; they can be used in performing the psychiatric audit, developing nursing care plans, formulating critical pathways, and devising algorithms.

References

American Psychiatric Association: *Diagnostic and Statistical Manual of Mental Disorders*, ed 4. American Pscyhiatric Press, 1994.

Bates B: *A Guide to Physical Examination*, ed 3. Lippincott, 1983.

Bender L: *A Visual-Motor Gestalt Test and Its Clinical Use*. Research monograph 3. American Orthopsychiatric Association, 1938.

Compton BR, Galaway B: *Social Work Processes*, ed 2. Dorsey Press, 1979.

McFarland GK, Wasli EL: *Nursing Diagnosis and Process in Psychiatric Mental Health Nursing*. Lippincott, 1986.

Murray HA: *Thematic Apperception Test*. Harvard University Press, 1943.

Patient assessment: Neurological examination. (Programmed instruction.) *Am J Nurs* 1975;75 (Part I, September): PI, pp. 1–24. 1975;75 (Part II, November): PI, pp. 1–24. 1976;76 (Part III, April): PI, pp. 1–25.

Raichle ME: Visualizing the mind. *Sci Am* 1994 (April): 58–64.

Small SM: *Outline for Psychiatric Examination*. Sandoz, 1980.

Spire RH: An experimental study of the use of photographic self-image confrontation as a nursing procedure in the care of chronically ill schizophrenic female patients. Project in partial fulfillment of MS degree, State University at Buffalo, 1967.

Wilson HS: Is *DSM-IV* the gold standard for psychiatric diagnosis? *Capsules & Comments Psychiatr Nurs* 1994; (1)3:1–3.

Wilson HS, Skodol AE: Overview and examination of DSM-IV. *Arch Psychiatr Nurs* 1994; (8)6:340–347.

CHAPTER 9

ESTABLISHING AND MAINTAINING A THERAPEUTIC ENVIRONMENT

Susan Hunn Garritson

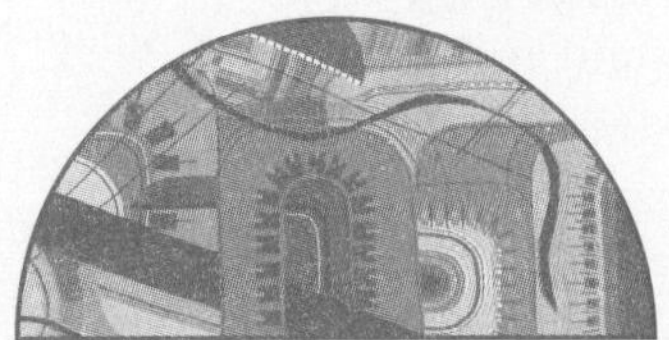

COMPETENCIES

- *Define therapeutic environment.*
- *Describe five characteristics of the therapeutic environment that are managed by nurses and that provide opportunities for nursing interventions.*
- *Discuss the impact of such events as short length of inpatient treatment and high acuity on current views of the therapeutic environment.*
- *Identify three social interaction therapy principles.*
- *Identify three behavior modification principles.*
- *Explain how you feel when implementing interventions intended to maximize safety but that require you to control another's freedom of movement and self-determination.*

Cross-References

Other topics related to this chapter are: Behaviorism, Chapter 2; Era of moral treatment, Chapter 2; Ethics, Chapter 10; Group therapy, Chapter 31; Legal issues, Chapter 11; Violence and victimatology, Chapter 34; Managed care, Chapter 35.

Critical Thinking Challenge

The therapeutic environment is derived from moral therapy values of kind, nonpunitive intervention and milieu therapy principles of utilizing all aspects of the social and physical environment for therapeutic purposes. Currently, managed mental health care and utilization review standards limit acute care access to the most seriously disturbed clients and reward brief stays and behavior control through psychopharmacology. How can these treatment approaches be integrated to maximize the therapeutic potential of the inpatient setting? In what ways do these approaches conflict? How can you, as the nurse, balance and blend these treatment philosophies within your practice?

In this chapter, **therapeutic environment** is broadly interpreted to reflect the therapeutic potential of people, resources, and events in the client's immediate environment to promote optimal functioning in the activities of daily living, the development or improvement of interpersonal skills, and the ability to manage outside the institutional setting. Various terms such as *therapeutic milieu, therapeutic community,* and *milieu therapy* have been applied to discussions of the treatment environment. While some argue that different strategies and theoretical perspectives are associated with these labels, the terms are often used interchangeably and refer to the impact of the authority structure and the roles and relationships on decision making and client interactions.

Typically, interpersonal conflicts are discussed as they occur in order for clients to develop social skills and to promote personal growth. The traditional biomedical model, in which the physician is responsible for diagnosis and prescribing treatment while the client assumes a "sick role," contrasts with milieu therapy models in which organizational hierarchy is flattened, therapeutic potential is seen in multiple relationships, and the client assumes personal responsibility for behavior. Originally, therapeutic milieu programs were at least several months long and had homogenous client populations.

A nurse's 24-hour daily contact with clients provides a unique opportunity for creating and managing the therapeutic environment as a special domain. No other discipline literally shares with clients the living space of the treatment unit. Nurses individually influence the environment through their presence. Nurses provide human contact, support, and direction; they share philosophy and values; and they establish collaborative work relationships. Nurses can indirectly influence client behavior by the assessment and manipulation of both the physical and social environment.

While many milieu principles remain relevant in current treatment environments, trends such as short lengths of stay, high patient acuity, and resurgence of the biomedical model require reexamination of the relevance of the assumptions of the therapeutic community in acute inpatient care. The emergence of subacute treatment settings and community-based rehabilitation programs also offers new arenas to implement therapeutic environment principles. Psychiatric nursing's current challenge is to synthesize a new model that includes the best aspects of both the biologic and the therapeutic milieu models.

Current Ideas About the Therapeutic Environment

Current ideas about the therapeutic potential of the treatment environment include attention to the general organizational culture, restrictiveness, extent of the client's utilization of treatment resources, and application of therapeutic environment principles across treatment settings.

A variety of external factors have affected the therapeutic environment since the days of its precursor, milieu therapy (see the accompanying box). These issues have an impact on the treatment environment in several ways. It is more difficult to develop group cohesiveness and involvement with other clients' progress when group membership changes frequently. Symptom acuity may also limit a client's ability to be actively involved with the treatment issues of others. Staff roles may be more traditional and typical of medical care settings, and this may create more hierarchical relationships.

Despite these significant changes in inpatient services, are there characteristics in common to historic and current therapeutic treatment environments?

External Factors That Affect the Therapeutic Environment

- Client groups are not homogenous.
- Clients frequently have dual diagnoses, such as psychiatric and substance abuse problems or psychiatric and medical problems.
- Managed mental health care organizations increasingly limit access to inpatient care to those who are a danger to themselves or others.
- Lengths of inpatient stay have decreased to an average of about seven days.
- Treatment is closely monitored to determine the need for medication, seclusion, restraint, or other intensive supervision.
- Case managers quickly assess discharge planning needs and obstacles and coordinate access to other levels of services.
- There has been a resurgence of the medical model of care as psychopharmacology and electroconvulsive therapy offer specialized treatment approaches to symptom reduction.
- Clients with multiple medical problems and dementias may also require more traditional medical interventions.
- Staff members now have diverse and specialized training and are expected to work as multidisciplinary teams to address individualized treatment goals.
- Regulatory agencies, client rights groups, and professional practice standards establish criteria for the therapeutic environment.

Organizational Culture

Watson (1992) describes four traditional qualities of a therapeutic community:

1. *Democratization*—the ability of clients and staff members to have input into their treatment and their work.
2. *Permissiveness*—tolerance of deviant behavior while upholding the need for control.

3. *Reality confrontation*—giving information and sharing feelings in a nonhostile way with the intent of helping others learn to modify their behavior.
4. *Communalism*—an emphasis on the sharing nature of the community through the sharing of tasks, living areas, and opinions.

These are not discrete variables, and they may be apparent in varying degrees in given treatment environments depending on staff, client, and setting characteristics. In actual practice, these qualities will also be influenced by the program's attitude toward privacy, autonomy, safety, and group well-being.

PRIVACY Individuals routinely vary their patterns of contact with and withdrawal from others, as well as the information they share about themselves. The very nature of psychiatric hospitalization conflicts with the need for privacy. Intimate personal details are examined and discussed, and there may be no opportunity to escape staff surveillance or social contact. Nurses must respect a client's privacy by keeping surveillance and monitoring to the minimum necessary for client safety, honoring the confidentiality of personal information, and maintaining routine social practices such as knocking on the door and waiting for an answer before entering a bedroom or bathroom.

AUTONOMY The rules and schedules that characterize psychiatric treatment settings usually promote the management of groups of people and may interfere with the personal decision making and autonomy of the individual client. Although the ability of mentally ill clients to carry out age-appropriate roles may be significantly impaired, the therapeutic environment provides opportunities for normal functioning according to each client's abilities.

SAFETY Mentally ill clients may pose significant safety hazards to themselves or others because of suicidal or assaultive behaviors, poor judgment, or confusion. A nurse's efforts to maintain client safety may deprive clients of privacy and autonomy. For example, clients requiring close surveillance have little or no privacy; nurses may intervene to override decisions made by clients whose judgment is impaired.

GROUP WELL-BEING A client's behavior may be disruptive or detrimental to the overall well-being of other clients. Nurses may need to monitor or manage certain clients to maximize the common good. As with the concept of safety, the individual's privacy and autonomy may be violated when group well-being is considered primary. (Some philosophers, however, consider that the group's well-being enhances the individual's autonomy.) Individual autonomy, individual well-being, and group well-being are often conflicting issues. Nurses must be sensitive to situations in which clashes occur.

The **Moos Ward Atmosphere Scale** is a tool that measures dimensions of the therapeutic environment. These dimensions include: involvement, support, spontaneity, autonomy, practical focus, personal focus, order, clarity, control, and the expression of anger. Moos has demonstrated that these factors vary with treatment setting, client needs, unit philosophy, and life cycle of the unit, and he supports research to link the treatment environment to client outcomes (Kahn and Frederick 1988). The Research Note for this chapter indicates that clients and staff members may have different perceptions of the ward atmosphere's dimensions.

Restrictiveness

The **restrictiveness** of the treatment environment is characterized according to physical, psychologic, and social dimensions. The physical environment includes the nature of the setting, such as location in the community, security, and options for behavior control (e.g., seclusion). The psychologic environment is composed of staff and client backgrounds, behavior, attitudes, and values. The social environment consists of the rules and regulations that govern the operation of the setting as well as the treatment standards for managing client behavior.

The importance of evaluating a program's restrictiveness stems from mental health legislation mandating care according to the least restrictive alternative. This concept is heavily influenced by ethical and legal theories that hold individual autonomy paramount. Thus, program rules or staff attitudes that interfere with a client's autonomy would be considered more restrictive than a program that supported autonomy and self-determination.

A facility's physical structure is a major focus of attention in pursuing the least restrictive alternatives for treatment. Physical restrictiveness is ranked according to the degree of interference with client independence. Based on their research, Krauss and Slavinksy (1982) propose the following order:

1. *Most restrictive:* Total institutions (state hospitals).
2. Nearly total institutions (nursing homes).
3. Institutions with partially independent residents (halfway homes).
4. Institutions with independent but isolated residents (single-room-occupancy hotels).
5. Family of origin, friends, other relatives.
6. *Least restrictive:* Family of orientation (family resulting from marriage or other relationship).

The physical structure of many institutions—such as locked doors, communal living arrangements, and limited access to community resources—interferes with client freedom of movement and individuality. Thus, fa-

RESEARCH NOTE

Citation

Caplan C: Nursing staff and patient perceptions of the ward atmosphere in a maximum security forensic hospital. *Arch Psychiatr Nurs* 1993;7: 23–29.

Study Problem/Purpose

Are there differences between nursing staff members and clients' perceptions of the ward atmosphere in a forensic hospital?

Methods

The Moos Ward Atmosphere Scale was used to measure nursing staff and client perceptions of ward environment in four treatment units of a forensic hospital that detained offenders who had mental disorders. A convenience sample of direct nursing care staff members from all three shifts were asked to participate; 69% (n = 70) completed the questionnaire. All clients who were in the hospital more than three days were asked to participate; 62% (n = 39) consented and completed the questionnaire.

Findings

Staff members had significantly higher scores than clients on the subscales of involvement, order and organization, and program clarity. Clients had significantly higher scores than staff on support and staff control. Staff and clients had equal mean scores on the subscales for spontaneity and anger/aggression.

Implications

Nursing staff members perceived an emphasis on the importance of planning activities and following schedules and routines. Clients perceived an emphasis on compliance with ward routine and staff control. Nurses perceived that they communicated their expectations clearly, but clients felt they did not always understand the rules or expectations. Clients perceived staff members as strict enforcers of hospital regulations, although staff members believed they exerted only minimal control over client behavior. Both groups perceived that there was minimal tolerance for the open expression of feelings, particularly anger or disagreement. In a forensic hospital, nursing staff are authorized to maintain a therapeutic environment while guaranteeing safety and security with a population of clients who have a high potential for violence. They may place particular emphasis on orderliness and compliance with strict behavioral standards as a means to balance their therapeutic and security roles.

cilities located in huge hospital complexes, which do not interface with the community's shopping, religious, or entertainment activities or provide for client privacy, have a more restrictive environment than community-based settings.

The physical structure of mental institutions has been linked to the problem of **institutionalization**, in which the client's ability to function declines. "Institutionalized" clients become apathetic about discharge, resigned toward institutional life, and dependent on the setting for their total care. Goffman (1961) theorized that clients grew unable to negotiate and manage daily living activities outside institutions that provided for all aspects of their lives and prevented access to the community by high walls, barred windows, or geographic isolation.

Client Utilization of Treatment Resources

Allen et al. (1988) extend the concept of the **therapeutic alliance** from the psychotherapy relationship to hospital treatment. Alliance in hospital treatment is primarily characterized by the client's collaboration in the treatment process. Collaboration is the extent to which the client actively utilizes treatment opportunities as resources for constructive change. The collaboration concept has three dimensions:

1. Goal orientation—thoughtful, reflective, and purposeful participation in hospital treatment.
2. Involvement—communication with staff members.
3. Use of structure—utilization of the prescribed treatment program.

Collaboration is highly correlated with severity of psychopathology as well as treatment outcome. In inpatient treatment, collaboration is multidimensional and influenced by the variety of treatment relationships characteristic of the therapeutic environment.

The Therapeutic Environment Framework

Kahn and White (1989) propose a framework for acute, short-term treatment programs that incorporates biologic

INTERVENTION

Guidelines for Working with Clients in the Therapeutic Environment

Strategy	*Rationale*
Safety	
• Appropriate structural security, including locked doors, nonbreakable glass, seclusion room, silent alarms, devices such as concave nonbreakable mirrors to view blind spots.	• Security must be appropriate to client acuity and type of treatment program.
• Unit rules and staff policy related to acceptable conduct.	• Rules should be clearly stated.
• Procedures and training for use of time-outs, seclusion, restraint, special precautions, search and management of client personal belongings such as razors.	• Staff training promotes consistency and safe implementation of security and client management techniques.
Structure	
• Client orientation to behavior expectations through multiple sources, including handbook, bulletin boards, community meeting, identification of a primary nurse.	• Clients are unfamiliar with expectations; new information may need to be repeated.
• Delineation of program schedule and expectations for client participation.	• Clear expectations and written schedule promote client independence.
Support	
• Staff visibility and availability to guide and monitor client activities.	• Demonstrates role-modeling skills and provides an opportunity for informal assessment and interaction.
• Implementation of least restrictive interventions such as confirming messages, calming, personal control, setting limits, and medication to minimize the need for more restrictive behavior management.	• Least restrictive interventions promote client autonomy and demonstrate respect.
• Enhance normality of the environment through use of clocks, calendars, furniture.	• Reduces the institutional qualities of environment.

and psychosocial perspectives to achieve an intensely supportive treatment environment. This environment maximizes the use of multidisciplinary therapeutic opportunities. Following are the principles of this acute care framework:

- Establish a consistent, caring environment characterized by:
  - safety
  - structure
  - support
  - socialization
  - self-understanding
- These elements are fostered through the philosophy, policies, and procedures that define the treatment program. Staff members promote safety by clearly stating expectations for conduct and maintain it through such interventions as suicide precautions, time-outs, seclusion, and restraint. Structure is established through client orientation, activity schedules, and methods to address noncompliance. Staff members create a positive social climate by observing the ward atmosphere, assessing staff attitudes and parallel issues, establishing clear goals and accountability, promoting communication, and intervening in disruptive events.
- Provide graduated therapy with levels individualized to the client's phase of illness, resources, and support systems. A graduated therapy program involves: orientation to the program and development of goals; education about the illness, treatment, and coping skills; and integration of the illness and hospital experience into the client's self-concept and postdischarge plans.

INTERVENTION *(continued)*

Strategy	*Rationale*
• Promote opportunities for self-care decision making, and activities that prepare for return to community.	• Reduces dependence on hospital; promotes positive transition to community.
• Integrate client's existing social supports, including family and spiritual support system to reinforce goals and interventions.	• Promotes family involvement and empowerment; extends opportunities for positive outcome by involving social supports.
• Monitor and discuss staff concerns to promote communication, identify parallel issues, ensure a positive social climate.	• Staff interactions affect the general atmosphere and capacity for therapeutic interventions.
• Support cultural diversity and staff self-awareness related to issues of client rights and social control.	• Demonstrates respect and supports client autonomy and independence.
Socialization	
• Orient client and family to the steps and process of inpatient psychiatric treatment.	• Clients and family may be unfamiliar with psychiatric treatment; may have misinformation.
• Identify fears and stereotypes client/family may have about "brain surgery, shock treatment, or padded cells," as well as concerns about how psychotherapy works.	• Reduces fear and engages in treatment.
• Educate client/family about legal rights of psychiatric clients and confidentiality of information.	• Engages client and family in treatment process.
• Encourage client participation in determining and evaluating treatment goals.	• Promotes involvement and empowerment.
Self-Understanding	
• Encourage formal and informal group participation.	• Provides opportunities to gain social skills.
• Emphasize commonalities of experience.	• Reduces sense of isolation and hopelessness.
• Identify skills gained through hospital experience.	• Offers hope and focuses on the future.
• Instill hope and social connectedness.	• Reduces isolation.
• Encourage client feedback about satisfaction with treatment and hospital experience.	• Promotes empowerment.

- Emphasize commonalities between clients' experiences to instill hope, promote interpersonal feedback, achieve mastery over a crisis, and regain social connectedness.

Kahn and White's dimensions provide a framework for establishing a therapeutic environment in an acute psychiatric hospital setting. The factors of the Moos Ward Atmosphere Scale and the dimensions of restrictiveness are ways to describe the environment and influence it by altering aspects of the physical, psychologic, or social structure. Assessment of collaboration is a way of evaluating the efficacy of the therapeutic alliance and progress of the overall hospital treatment. Together, these allow the nurse to establish and maintain a therapeutic environment and evaluate the client's progress to promote a positive outcome.

Assessment and Management

Some of the current ideas about the therapeutic environment, particularly the philosophic values, do not easily lend themselves to quick evaluation or manipulation. Assessment is complicated by the need to consider the clients' levels of functioning as well as the discrete features of the structural environment. What is suitable for one group of clients may be too strict or too lenient for another (see the Intervention box above).

Safety

When evaluating the environment, first consider the physical plant. Restrictive aspects such as the type of building or its location have already been discussed. While building features are theoretically significant, they are also beyond the nurse's ability to influence. However, other aspects of the physical structure are open to the nurse's intervention. Safety is a primary characteristic of the therapeutic environment. The physical plant contributes to safety through levels of security and space allocated for privacy. Locked doors and the availability of seclusion rooms are typical security features of many inpatient settings. Other aspects of security are more subtle. For example, are the doors to bedrooms, bathrooms, kitchen, laundry, or lounges locked to control client access? Have doors or curtains to bedrooms or bathrooms been removed? As the nurse, you should

1. Evaluate whether security is sufficient.
2. Assess the advantages and necessity of the security.
3. Assess whether the security has any detrimental impact.
4. Consider whether the security advantages could be accomplished through some other intervention that would not have the associated disadvantages.

SECURITY BASED ON AN UNCLEAR RATIONALE In this example, a structural control implemented for a specific reason was no longer relevant yet had not been discontinued.

A 15-bed unlocked ward had laundry facilities so that clients could care for their own clothes. A psychotic and confused client put a potted plant through a wash cycle, causing major damage to the washing machine. Staff members locked the laundry facilities to prevent future damage to the machines. The doors remained locked even after this client was discharged, preventing any independent client access to the facilities. Preventing possible future damage to machines became a predominant staff concern.

While locking laundry room doors was intended to be a short-term structural solution to avoid further environmental damage, the solution became permanent and created a new problem of interference with self-care performance by more independent clients.

A voluntary, unlocked unit has a progressive nursing philosophy emphasizing client self-care, autonomy, and independence. The client dining room has a small kitchenette, and clients frequently prepare their own snacks. The clients' refrigerator had always been located in the locked medication room. Thus, any independent meal preparation or simple decision to have a glass of juice required the client to request access to the refrigerator. Despite the inconvenience of having to unlock the door, staff members were initially reluctant to move the refrigerator. They rationalized that they could better monitor clients' intake by controlling access to the refrigerator. Once the refrigerator was moved to the kitchenette, however, staff were more likely to discuss food and fluid intake with their clients. This elimination of a structural control provided an opportunity for client-staff communication and improved staff's counseling and education related to clients' diets.

In this example, the unit security was not based on any rationale. This control actually interfered with client autonomy and self-care.

THE IMPACT OF CHANGES IN SECURITY Changes in the security of the environment, such as unlocking the door of a normally locked unit or locking the door of a normally unlocked unit, have been noted to increase client agitation.

Mrs A is a 72-year-old woman hospitalized for evaluation of a sudden onset of confusion and forgetfulness. Nurses locked the unit's main door to keep Mrs A from inadvertently wandering off the ward. Other clients were free to come and go but were inconvenienced by relying on staff members to unlock the door.

Staff members noticed an increase in irritability and demanding behavior of several clients soon after the door was locked. Small cliques of clients collected near the door, while others paced nearby.

The staff decided that the impact of the locked door on the overall milieu was detrimental. A nurse was assigned to keep Mrs A within eye contact at all times to ensure her safety, and the unit door was unlocked. The ward atmosphere soon returned to normal.

In this example, the nurse assessed Mrs A as being confused and forgetful. The nurse made the nursing diagnosis of Altered Thought Processes. The staff initially intervened by locking the unit's main door to maintain Mrs A's safety. This action, however, was evaluated as being detrimental to other clients. Therefore, the door was unlocked and an alternative intervention, one-to-one supervision, was successfully implemented.

SECLUSION AND RESTRAINT Seclusion and restraint represent interventions that use structure to control client behavior. Studies indicate that seclusion and restraint are frequently used within a few hours of admission, possibly to control behavior until medications take effect or to intervene in agitated behavior before it escalates (Kirkpatrick 1989). Other factors linked to the use of seclusion are unit philosophy, staff attitudes and education, client-staff ratios, and level of unit disturbance. Because seclusion and restraint are highly restrictive interventions that interfere with client autonomy and freedom of movement, it is important to implement alternative steps whenever possible.

Klinge (1994) studied staff opinions about seclusion and restraint at a state forensic hospital. In this study, staff members preferred to treat clients in ways that they themselves would want to be treated. More educated staff considered seclusion, restraint, and medications to be overused. About two-thirds of the respondents preferred to treat with medications primarily because these were interpreted as the "least restrictive" intervention. Male and female staff viewed the reinforcement value of seclusion and restraint significantly differently. Female staff felt that clients received more attention from other clients while in seclusion and that this was positive. Male staff felt that clients received more attention from other clients when in restraints and that this was negative. Consistency and rationale for implementation of seclusion and restraint and identification of alternative ways to manage unacceptable behavior were recommended.

Nurses at one psychiatric hospital were able to drastically reduce seclusion and restraint hours (Craig et al. 1989). A multivariate program was undertaken with hospital administration and interdisciplinary staff involvement. The program included:

- Structural renovation of the seclusion-restraint rooms to maximize staff access, reduce external stimulation, and ensure client privacy.
- Development of a conceptual nursing model that defined seclusion and restraint as intensive care, and identification of interactions to reduce fear and helplessness.
- Improvement of registered nurse staffing, and the use of alternative interventions such as flexible barriers (opened and closed doors), personal distance, and selected interactions to provide intensive care.
- Training in assaultiveness management, crisis theory, and alternative interventions.
- Involvement of staff members from other disciplines in recommending behavior interventions for management problems and in reviewing restrictive treatment lasting longer than 12 hours.

During the first 12 months of this program, restraint decreased more than 600 hours per month. There was a combined seclusion-restraint decrease of over 950 hours per month.

ALTERNATIVE STRATEGIES Wilson (1982) studied "infracontrol" phenomena at Soteria House, an experimental personal growth community for people with schizophrenia. Conventional control mechanisms such as locked doors, medications, and strict regulation of activity or property were avoided in this setting. Soteria's ideology emphasized self-regulation, tolerance for deviance, and group cohesiveness. However, an ideology of eliminating structural control did not eliminate the need to maintain safety or the problem of social control of psychotic clients' behavior.

Wilson studied how problems of social control are solved in the absence of conventional psychiatric control structures. The process of *presencing* was identified as a key mechanism to manage resident behavior. Staff and residents spent a great deal of daily living time together, and the basic *presence* of people with individual patterns of tolerance and interaction guided and limited behavior. Such a milieu might well be characterized as "low EE," or low *expressed emotion*. Nurses frequently use the presencing technique by sitting with or listening to clients, although they are apt to describe it as "providing support" or "the therapeutic use of self." The example of Mrs A illustrated how the use of presencing not only kept her safe but also improved the environment by allowing the unit door to remain unlocked.

The structural environment should not *dehumanize* its inhabitants; moreover, is should actively contribute to their improved functioning and comfort. **Reality-orientation resources** such as the following contribute to a sense of normality:

- Clocks and calendars to promote time orientation.
- Newspapers to encourage an awareness of social events.
- Ramps and rails to promote movement.
- Furniture arranged to promote interaction.

Healthy people may take these for granted, but they are critical resources to the impaired client.

Mrs T is a 47-year-old woman with severe depression. She is very agitated and is having trouble sleeping. Although sleep medication has been ordered, Mrs T has been in and out of bed and is pacing. As a result of her restlessness, the sheets and blankets are strewn about and the plastic mattress cover is exposed. The rumpled bedding and cold mattress further contribute to Mrs T's discomfort. Nurses order a mattress pad and contoured sheets to promote Mrs T's comfort until her symptoms respond to medication.

Deinstitutionalization has changed the location of psychiatric treatment, and walled institutions with barred windows are less common today than they were forty years ago. However, structural controls remain in community psychiatric settings. Lack of access to rooms and equipment and the absence of the free activity of normal life perpetuate the restricted atmosphere of institutions.

NURSING SELF-AWARENESS

Your Attitudes About Organizational Rules

To increase self-awareness about your own attitudes about organizational rules in a treatment setting:

- What kinds of client behaviors make me uncomfortable or angry?
- What unit rules are most important?
- How do I feel when a client breaks a unit rule?
- What do I do in response to a client who breaks a unit rule?

To increase self-awareness about your own attitudes about client autonomy and self-determination:

- Am I comfortable with clients deciding what the program's schedule, activities, or rules will be?
- Am I comfortable with clients deciding their own treatment goals?
- How do I feel when a client chooses a treatment goal that is not the same as the one I would have selected or that I do not think is in the client's "best interest"?
- Should clients be allowed to comment on each other's behavior or treatment goals?

To increase self-awareness about your own opinions about least restrictive interventions for mental illness:

- How do I feel when a client's legal right to leave a treatment setting is deemed more important than the client's need for treatment?
- Should clients be allowed to refuse treatment even when interventions like medication would definitely reduce their symptoms?
- Does society have an obligation to care for the seriously mentally ill even if this requires limiting a client's freedom to refuse treatment?
- How do I feel when I see a person on the street who is gesturing and talking to himself or herself and who is carrying a few belongings in a plastic bag?

Failure to Recognize the Need for Security Just as the staff may fail to notice over time structural controls that are no longer necessary, they may also grow used to potential safety problems. As nurses identify opportunities to make the environment less restrictive, they must also be alert to situations that could present serious hazards to the acute client population.

The side doors to the dining room of a locked unit opened onto a hallway and were used by dietary staff members to make food deliveries and by housekeeping staff to provide access for cleaning. There was no way for these staff members to determine from the hallway whether a client was in the dining room. While the dining room space had been used for alternative activities for years, access by the support staff had never posed a problem. During one recreational games session, staff members entered though the hallway doors to deliver some supplies. A client bolted toward the open door, ran down several flights of stairs, out of the building, and into a busy street.

Program Structure

Program structure, another aspect of the therapeutic environment, is composed of the schedule and expectations for client treatment and participation. Nurses have a number of opportunities to communicate expectations and to address noncompliance, including individual orientation, community meetings, and behavior modification. See the Nursing Self-Awareness box about attitudes toward organizational rules in a treatment setting.

Interaction Methods Some techniques, such as community meetings, client government, and specialty theme groups promote normal functioning through the use of social interaction, group activities, group pressure, and peer expectations. Clients are considered responsible people able to take action and adjust their behavior in a purposeful manner. **Social interaction interventions** are based on the following principles:

- *Expectations* for behavior are clearly communicated in order to maintain or change behavior.
- The acquisition and maintenance of new behaviors depend on the degree of *personal participation and involvement* in learning the necessary new skills.
- The occurrence of a behavior depends on the *sense of being a member* of the group. Group expectations and sanctions have a significant influence on behavior. (Paul and Lentz 1977 pp. 49–51)

Table 9–1 Comparison of Interaction Methods

Social Interaction	*Behavior Modification*
Principles	
Expectations are clearly communicated.	Behavior depends on positive or negative consequences.
Learning new behaviors depends on personal participation and involvement.	Events that occur together will become associated.
Group membership influences behavior.	New behavior may be taught or role modeled.
Techniques	
Community meeting: welcome new members, explain unit rules, plan activities.	Positive reinforcement: praise, tokens/tangible rewards.
Client government.	Negative reinforcement: no response, loss of tokens, removal from group activity.
Individualized contracting for basic expectations.	

SOURCE: *Paul and Lentz 1977.*

Social interaction methods and behavior modification, discussed later, are compared in Table 9–1.

Community Meetings Groups provide an opportunity for clients to solve problems of conflicting interests, experience cooperation with others, share responsibility, and experience leadership in the group. The most common milieu-oriented group is the community meeting. Its functions include:

- Welcoming new members.
- Identifying and discussing unit rules (expectations).
- Discussing aspects of the unit environment such as cleanliness, privacy, radio and television use, or other interpersonal problems that may interfere with the quality of life for the group.
- Planning activities.

Clients usually chair the community meeting and report on assignments, such as checking for cleanliness of areas of responsibility (like the kitchen or bedrooms).

Unit Rules All clients should be given the regulations of the setting either before or as soon after admission as possible. Although written expectations do not automatically ensure acceptable behavior or prevent harmful behavior, they provide a clear baseline, serve as reminders, and provide structure for clients.

Two written documents—the specific no-harm contract (Figure 9–1) and basic expectations (Figure 9–2)—establish behavioral requirements for all clients. These rules reinforce the staff's commitment to basic safety and specify obligations for all members of the setting. Written expectations may be presented to clients at the time of admission, discussed in community meetings, and used as a reference if a client violates a rule.

A 45-year-old depressed and suicidal man is admitted to a voluntary unit. This conversation takes place after the nurse greets the client at the time of admission:

Nurse: **Dr K informed me that you have been very depressed. Have you thought about harming yourself?**

Mr L: **Sometimes I wake up in the middle of the night and I think I can't go on. I just want to sleep, but I am tormented by my thoughts.**

No Harm Contract

I agree that I am in control of my behavior. I understand that intended injury to myself, others, or property is grounds for discharge from this unit or commitment to another psychiatric setting as an involuntary patient.

If I have impulses to harm myself or others, I agree to talk with a staff member, whom I can expect to assist me in controlling my own behavior.

__________ Date   ____________________ Client

____________________ Witness

Figure 9–1 An example of a no-harm contract. SOURCE: *Langley Porter Psychiatric Hospital and Clinics, Nursing Staff, Behavioral Neurosciences Service.*

Basic Expectations Contract

1. Food and Fluid
I agree to:
   A. Eat all meals in the dining room with the client group.
   Exception:———
   B. Report problems with food/fluid intake to primary care nurse.

2. Elimination
I agree to:
   A. Maintain positive elimination habits.
   B. Report problems with elimination promptly to assigned nurse.

3. Personal Hygiene and Body Temperature
I agree to:
   A. Keep myself and my room area (including laundry and linen) clean.
   B. Complete my assigned ward job.
   C. Report problems with body temperature or hygiene to assigned nurse.

4. Rest/Activity
   A. Rest
   I agree to:
      1. Get up by 8:00 A.M. and remain up during the daytime.
      Exception: Scheduled nap time after lunch from______P.M. to______P.M.
      2. Retire to bed no sooner than 9:00 P.M. or later than 12:00 (midnight).
      Exception:______
      3. Remain in bed until 7:00 A.M. "wakeup" except to get water or use the bathroom.
      4. Notify staff if I cannot sleep and work with them, according to the care plan, to try to sleep.
   B. Activity
   I agree to:
      1. Attend all scheduled R.T. activities, group therapy meetings, Thursday R.T. outings, community meetings, and weekend outings.
      2. Accept nursing staff referral to my personal schedule if I have a question about my participation in activities.
      3. Use no alcohol or nonprescribed drugs while on the unit or on passes.

5. Solitude and Socialization
If I have suicidal or self destructive ideas or feelings, I agree to:

   A. Discuss my ideas or feelings only in therapy sessions (individual, group, or family) or with the nurse assigned to my care and not with other clients.
   B. Accept reminders from nursing staff that I have signed the no-harm contract.
   C. Accept assistance from the nurse assigned to my care to learn new ways to manage my feelings and behavior to remain safe.

I can expect the nurse assigned to my care to assist me by:

A. Discussing my immediate feelings and behavior and identifying alternative activities to maintain my safety.
or B. Going to my room with me and sitting with me quietly for five to ten minutes, and then assisting me to get involved in a game (cards, pool) or with other clients in a group situation (television, living room).
or C. Teaching me new coping behaviors such as relaxation techniques, deep-breathing exercises, or writing my thoughts.
or D. Referring me to my primary therapist.

I also agree to discuss other problems—including concerns about medication—in therapy sessions (individual, group, or family).

____
Signature Date

Adapted from Langley Porter Psychiatric Hospital and Clinics, 1985. Nursing Staff, Behavioral Neurosciences Service.

Figure 9–2 A written contract establishes behavior requirements for clients, reinforces the staff's commitment to basic safety, and specifies obligations for all members. *Source: Adapted from Langley Porter Psychiatric Hospital and Clinics, 1985. Nursing Staff, Behavioral Neurosciences Service.*

Nurse: Do you want to kill yourself now?

Mr L: Not this minute. The middle of the night is the hardest time for me.

Nurse: Nursing staff can sit with you or talk to you when you want to hurt yourself, even during the night. It is important that you tell your nurse when you feel suicidal. You are in control of your behavior even though life seems bleak right now.

Mr L: All right.

Nurse: Nursing staff have a written agreement to be available to keep you, and all other clients here, safe. (Hands Mr L the no-harm contract.) Do you feel able to make this commitment to control your behavior?

Mr L: Yes. (Signs contract.)

(Later, in a community meeting:)

Nurse: I would like to introduce and welcome Mr L. (Group members introduce themselves.)

Nurse: Since several new members have come to the unit this week, this might be a good time to discuss the unit's rules.

Mrs A: We all came here for help, but sometimes that means we have to take charge of ourselves.

Nurse: What does "take charge" mean?

Mrs A: I am ultimately responsible for what I do to myself. I know I can't stay here if I cut myself like I did at home. I asked my nurse to sit with me when I first came in.

Group Living The community meeting is also used to solve problems related to living with a large group of people or living in the hospital unit.

Clients on a 25-bed unlocked unit had access to two pay telephones. Both telephones, however, were near the nurses' station, and conversations could be overheard easily. Clients complained in community meeting of the lack of privacy, and a nurse intervened to help them write a letter to the hospital administration. The administration purchased a new cordless telephone, which allowed clients to make and receive calls in any area of the unit.

Client Government Some client community groups also grant clients privileges for completing ward jobs or for demonstrating certain behaviors in the community living groups. Clients are expected to take responsibility for themselves and each other and to learn the consequences of their actions. Involving clients in the management of the unit and receiving therapy with other clients provide opportunities for participation, corrective learning experiences, and the development of new behavior patterns. Feedback is an essential technique for increasing insight and promoting learning. This type of community group, known as **client government**, may be most suitable to intermediate and long-term care settings, where the client group is stable and a group culture evolves over time.

The community meeting group of a 20-bed adolescent program bases recommendations for weekend passes on members' requests and the individual's functioning in the client community. Lisa, 14 years old, has a history of running away from home, lying, drug and alcohol abuse, prostitution, and suicide threats. She requested a Saturday day pass, although she did not have specific plans for how she would spend the time. Other clients commented that Lisa had not completed her ward job of checking the cleanliness of the kitchen, and the staff noted that she continued to withdraw from social contacts. The group agreed that Lisa should not receive a pass until she could demonstrate some improved ability to structure her time and interact with others.

Basic Expectations Nurses develop written basic expectations to help clients take care of themselves (see Figure 9–2). When Lisa complained about not receiving a pass, the following conversation ensued:

Nurse: Perhaps we should review the expectations for how you should act so that you can earn a pass. Do you have your copy? (Lisa finds her copy of the written basic expectations in the back of her nightstand drawer.) The expectations are like directions. They explain what you should do to earn pass privileges.

Lisa: I act OK. I should have gotten a pass. I didn't know I was supposed to check the kitchen to get a pass.

Nurse: The directions say you are expected to complete your ward job. The directions also tell you to participate in the activity program.

Lisa: I lost my schedule for the activities.

Nurse: Let's write a new schedule out together so we can talk about what activities you enjoy doing.

Individualized Written Expectations: Contracts The use of individualized written expectations for clients is described by McEnany and Tescher (1985). They recommend that this technique be used only with carefully selected clients. Clients must have the intellectual capacity to follow through with the contract negotiation process and the motivation to stick with a plan that works toward specific goals. The nurse should be knowledgeable about the client's disorder and its behavioral manifestations, change theory, and teaching-learning principles.

The goals of individualized contracting are to:

- Provide a consistent behavioral approach to the client by all staff members.
- Give the client an opportunity to use personality strengths by making decisions related to hospital care and discharge.
- Give the client an opportunity to learn behaviors that enhance coping skills and ability to function.

The following case example illustrates an intervention using an individualized behavioral contract to comply with the unit's Basic Expectations Agreement:

Beverly is a 30-year-old white female admitted to an inpatient psychiatric unit following an overdose of trifluoperazine. This twice-married, twice-divorced woman has two

children in foster homes. She has a long history of alcohol, marijuana, and cocaine use; multiple psychiatric hospitalizations; and treatment with antipsychotic drugs. On admission, Beverly was poorly groomed, pale, and thin. She denied hallucinations, delusions, or dramatic mood shifts, and her reality testing was intact. She said that after her boyfriend left her alone recently, she experienced her body as disjointed and "falling apart," and she feared leaving her hotel room. She described feeling "suffocated" by her relationships, yet she also described her sense of emptiness. She had no long-term relationships. During hospitalization Beverly was emotionally labile, had difficulty following her schedule, and was easily frustrated by the limits and compromises of living in the hospital. She demanded medication, threatened suicide, and complained of paranoia and various somatic symptoms. Beverly's primary nurse proposed that they work together to identify goals and behaviors for improved personal and interpersonal functioning. Beverly identified problems of emptiness, poor relationships, and anger and chose to focus on the goal of improved social skills. Beverly agreed to the following expectations:

- **I will participate in group therapy and psychodrama to express my feelings verbally.**
- **I will participate in movement therapy to express my feelings physically and learn to control my body.**
- **I will identify uncomfortable situations with other people and discuss the interactions with my nurse at appointed times.**
- **I will continue my routine activities until the appropriate time to meet with my nurse.**

Beverly's social skills improved as she followed through with these expectations.

Sautter et al. (1991) recommend that group and individual interventions be mutually reinforcing. For example, behavioral expectations and goal setting can be addressed in both individual meetings and client groups. New behaviors and other strategies are discussed and practiced in a variety of large and small psychotherapy and expressive arts groups. Feedback on progress toward meeting goals can be provided in community meetings as well as specific goal review meetings. The short length of inpatient hospitalization requires establishing clear priorities for addressing client problems and integrating resources to support problem resolution.

BEHAVIOR MODIFICATION The goal of **behavior modification** is to bring about change in behavior through the use of the environment; however, emphasis is on consequences for actions rather than group pressure and encouragement (see Table 9–1). According to Paul and Lentz (1977), the key principles of behavior modification are as follows:

- The frequency of a behavior depends on positive or negative *consequences.*
- Events that occur together will come to be *associated.*
- New behaviors are developed through others' *teaching and role modeling.*

Positive Reinforcement Positive reinforcement is an environmental consequence that encourages a behavior. For example, praising a client who expresses knowledge about medication encourages the client to demonstrate this knowledge. Praise is positive reinforcement. Sometimes staff actions may also inadvertently encourage a client's symptomatic behavior.

Gustavo becomes increasingly anxious about discharge. As the date approaches, his ability to follow the ward routine and take care of himself declines. Staff members decide he is not ready for discharge. Gustavo's ability to care for himself then improves. A new discharge date is set, and again, Gustavo's behavior deteriorates as the date approaches. The staff again delays the discharge date. The staff's decision to delay discharge positively reinforces the client's anxious behavior as discharge approaches.

Tokens have also been used in behavior modification programs as positive reinforcement. Through acceptable behavior, clients earn tokens that they can exchange for desirable items.

In a treatment center for adolescents with conduct disorder, Alford and Jarenko (1990) studied positive statements that supported the center's rules as a type of positive reinforcement for behavioral self-control. The center used posted behavioral objectives and positive consequences for appropriate behavior and individual progress. The positive rule-supporting statements served as an adjunct to the existing positive behavior-modification program. Clients who participated in both the standard treatment program and the additional positive statements intervention reported less-severe psychiatric symptoms on follow-up than clients who participated only in the standard program. The researchers concluded that the success of the dual-level behavior-modification program was related to the significant influence of verbal support from other residents.

Negative Reinforcement Negative reinforcement is used to decrease or eliminate behavior. Examples of negative consequences include:

- Showing no response to undesirable behavior.
- Removing something of value because of undesirable behavior.
- Removing the client from the situation in which undesirable behavior takes place (called a time-out).

A young woman with no organic illness repeatedly collapses in front of the nurses' station. Staff members initially rush to help her. Over time, this reaction positively reinforces an undesirable behavior. Nursing staff agree to implement a behavior-modification plan based on "no response to undesirable behavior." Subsequently, when the client falls to the floor at the nurses' station, all staff continue with their work.

In some token-based behavior-modification programs, the client may not only earn tokens for desirable behavior but also lose tokens for unacceptable behavior. "Loss of tokens" illustrates a negative reinforcement technique based on the removal of a valued item.

Negative reinforcement can also inadvertently discourage acceptable behavior. For example, a nurse who makes no response to a client exhibiting medication knowledge discourages the client from continuing to verbalize this understanding.

Corrigan and Storzbach (1993) summarize studies of the use of behavior modification to reduce psychiatric symptoms that were unresponsive to medications. Behavioral strategies were successful in reducing both the frequency of delusional speech and reports of hallucinations. Behavior modification for managing psychotic symptoms is limited, however, by the fact that the clinician cannot monitor client symptoms without jeopardizing the behavior-modification strategy. For example, if the strategy is that the client will lose tokens when delusions and hallucinations are discussed, the impact of the strategy is weakened if it is acceptable to discuss these symptoms with the clinician with no loss of tokens. Behavior-modification strategies for symptom management are best used to help clients identify appropriate settings and situations for verbalizing psychotic symptoms.

Behavior-modification plans may combine positive and negative consequences. For example, a 28-year-old male patient had a 12-year history of psychotic symptoms that were only partially controlled with antipsychotic medications. The client's talk about demons reduced his ability to live as independently as he was otherwise capable of doing. The nurse designed a behavior-modification intervention that rewarded the client with five tokens for every 15-minute period that he did not speak about demons (positive reinforcement). In addition, he was fined ten tokens for each comment made about demons during vocational and recreational events. The client's comments about demons substantially decreased.

A Supportive Social Climate

The multiple influences on individual and group behavior may come from external sources such as professional practice standards, regulatory agencies, and laws. The client's attitudes, beliefs, and behaviors, as well as styles of interaction between people, also have an impact on the therapeutic environment.

GENERAL ATMOSPHERE The previous discussion of the Moos Ward Atmosphere Scale and the psychosocial dimensions of restrictiveness provide basic information for understanding the social climate. General comments, concerns, styles of interaction, staff visibility, and client involvement in therapeutic activities provide occasions for observations that reflect the general atmosphere.

Overinvolvement and Loss of Client Autonomy Nursing routines that limit client self-care can be detrimental to the unit atmosphere.

Acutely psychotic and chronically mentally ill men and women are admitted to a 20-bed locked unit in a large county hospital. Nurses on this unit seem rushed and complain of having no time to discuss nursing care issues or write nursing care plans. A nurse consultant observed work patterns for several days and noted that the staff were involved (frequently unnecessarily) in intimate details of the clients' daily activities. This involvement extended to lighting matches for cigarettes and squeezing toothpaste onto toothbrushes. Simple routines that interfered with client autonomy also controlled the staff by preventing professional performance and relationships.

The nurse consultant assessed that the staff's complaint of excessive workload while they helped with daily details of client activities actually created self-care deficits for clients. The consultant recommended that the staff promote client self-care skills to be in accordance with their actual ability. This resulted in improvement of client independence and staff performance.

Parallel Process Once a relationship has begun, each person begins to influence the other in subtle ways. This mutual influencing, called **parallel process**, occurs unconsciously; it is usually active long before it becomes visible. Parallel process only becomes visible (and therefore available for intervention) when it is identified and discussed. Nurses should not assess client behavior as if it occurs in a vacuum. Routinely ask the question: What else is there? When assessing social interactions in the therapeutic environment, consider the following points:

- Conflict often surfaces in a location quite remote from its source.
- Few or no identifiable signs of conflict may exist where it began.
- The relationship between the source of the conflict and the place it surfaces may not be apparent.
- The form of the conflict may change as it changes location. (Lego and Pawlicki 1993)

Parallel process may occur between staff members and clients.

A consulting clinical nurse specialist met with a group of staff nurses from an adolescent treatment unit to discuss an increase in staff absences due to illness. Several staff members complained that administrators' rules limited their ability to make independent decisions. The next day in a group meeting, clients discussed their anger about not receiving weekend passes. That evening, two clients left the unit without passes.

The consultant identified that both staff and clients are angry about restrictions and limited independence. Both groups respond by being absent from the program. Their actions are parallel; that is, each group is responding to anger in the same manner. The consultant's plan is to reduce the avoidance behavior of both staff and clients by discussing their perceptions of decreased autonomy and increasing opportunities for independent decision making for both groups.

Parallel process may also occur between members of the multidisciplinary staff. Intershift conflict within the nursing staff or conflict between disciplines (such as nursing and rehabilitation therapies, or nursing and social work) is not uncommon, yet the source of the conflict is not always clear. By asking "What else is there?" nurses can identify the origin of the disagreement and thereby defuse the parallel interaction process.

Spirituality

Nurses can use the spiritual beliefs of clients to enhance the therapeutic environment. Waldfogel and Wolpe (1993) note that 94% of Americans report believing in God, which makes the United States one of the most religious countries in the industrialized world. They describe six dimensions of religious influence:

1. Ideological: religious beliefs.
2. Intellectual: knowledge (information, stories).
3. Ritual: participation in prayer, ceremony, church attendance, listening to music.
4. Experience: self-report of an encounter with or connection to a Supreme Being.
5. Consequence: health-enhancing behaviors (avoidance of cigarettes or alcohol) as prescribed by formal religion.
6. Support: social support provided through religious affiliation.

Specific assessment of a client's spiritual beliefs and practices provides the nurse an opportunity to understand their clinical impact and to use spiritual resources available to the client to enhance wellness and coping (see the accompanying box). Discussion of beliefs enables the nurse to reassure clients who fear that their beliefs will be challenged or minimized in a psychiatric environment. Finally, acknowledgment of the significant influence of spirituality in American life encourages nurses to recognize and explore their own beliefs in order to minimize the impact of bias in their client interactions.

Incorporating Spirituality into the Therapeutic Environment

Incorporate spirituality into the therapeutic environment by:

- Providing opportunities for ceremonies, such as weekly services or holiday celebrations.
- Facilitating group discussions based on sharing religious or spiritual beliefs.
- Demonstrating tolerance and acceptance of differing beliefs and rituals.
- Encouraging the social support that can be provided by acceptance in a community that shares similar beliefs.
- Being aware of how one's own beliefs may influence client interactions.

Source: Adapted from Waldfogel and Wolpe 1993.

Individualized interventions based on a client's spiritual beliefs and practices can include:

1. Defining a negative life event in terms of an opportunity for spiritual growth or a divine plan.
2. Using spiritual music or ceremonies to promote relaxation and reduce anxiety.
3. Collaborating with clergy or a representative of the client's faith who is accepted by the client to (a) correct misinterpretations of spiritual information that the client may be using maladaptively; (b) translate to clinicians spiritual aspects of a client's decision making; or (c) identify options and alternatives consistent with the faith that support adaptive resolution.

Here is an example:

A 19-year-old gay male was hospitalized for symptoms of major depression with severe guilt and suicidal ideation. He and his family were members of a fundamentalist religious group. They spoke to each other with frequent references to "God's Will" and commented on each other's behavior,

whether it would please or displease God. The family responded to the client's homosexuality by repeatedly telling him that he deserved God's wrath. A minister was able to provide scriptural education to this client to reconsider his family's interpretations and relieve his tremendous guilt.

Socialization

The therapeutic environment is individualized according to the client's phase of illness, resources, and support systems through setting and reviewing treatment goals, education, and integrating the illness and hospital experience into the client's perspective. The accompanying box lists questions the client may ask the nurse about what to expect during an inpatient hospital experience; such questions deserve responses.

Client Orientation

1. What psychiatric treatment can I expect to receive?
2. Will I receive medications? Do I have to take the medications?
3. Do I have to share a room with someone else?
4. Will I have to tell other clients about my problems?
5. Will you write down information that I tell you about myself or my family?
6. Is this unit a safe place for me?
7. Can I leave the unit on passes?
8. What happens if I no longer want to be a client in this hospital?
9. What happens if I have a disagreement with someone?
10. Who are the staff here? Who can I talk to if I have questions?
11. Can I smoke?
12. When is bedtime?
13. What time are the meals? Can I keep my own snacks?
14. Is there a way for me to wash my own clothes?
15. Is there a telephone I can use?
16. When are the visiting hours?
17. Can I write letters and get mail?
18. Can I keep my money with me? Is my personal property safe?
19. Are religious services available?

Answers to these questions can be individualized to reflect each unit's treatment philosophy and the specific legal rights of the client according to the state.

Explanation of Psychiatric Treatment Clients may have a limited understanding of psychiatric treatment, particularly in inpatient settings. Socialization to the treatment program includes explanation of the assessment, treatment, and discharge planning process; use of medications and other types of treatment, such as electroshock therapy (as appropriate); participation in group and family therapy; legal rights; and confidentiality.

Goals and Outcome Measures External regulatory standards require inpatient clinicians to identify behaviors that indicate when a problem area has been effectively treated. Clinical outcome evaluation is also an increasingly common approach to quality assurance monitoring. Nurses can take advantage of goal setting and outcome monitoring to carry out therapeutic environmental principles in the following ways:

- Orient and educate clients about hospitalization and treatment by reviewing the clinical problems, treatments, and behavioral outcomes that are the focus of hospitalization.
- Engage clients in the treatment process by encouraging them to identify personal goals and by participating in the evaluation of the course of their treatment.

Inpatient clinicians generally focus on reducing symptoms that prompted a client's admission; appropriate prescription and administration of medications and treatments; the use of seclusion/restraint; and the absence of events such as suicides or client absences from the unit "against medical advice" as outcomes of psychiatric care. Others view the outcome of mental health care as the client's ability to function in the community. Primary emphasis is placed on data that reflect the client's living arrangements; participation in school, work, or daytime activity; the absence of alcohol or drug use; involvement with the legal system; impairment in the areas of self-care, school, or work performance; family or community relationships; and use of appropriate mental health, physical health, and social services.

Sample Client Satisfaction Questionnaire

	Yes	Some	No
1. Has our program helped you?	1	2	3
2. Would you tell a friend who needed similar help to come to our program?	1	2	3
3. Was the facility clean and well maintained?	1	2	3
4. Did you like the meals and snacks?	1	2	3
5. Were you involved in your treatment planning?	1	2	3
6. Were your ideas written into the treatment plan?	1	2	3
7. Did the staff explain the treatment plan to you to your satisfaction?	1	2	3
8. Did the staff spend time with you and talk to you?	1	2	3
9. Did the staff listen to your ideas and concerns?	1	2	3
10. Were the staff members polite and respectful to you?	1	2	3
11. Were staff members sensitive to your cultural background?	1	2	3
12. Would you come here again if you needed help?	1	2	3
13. Overall, how satisfied were you with our program?	1	2	3

Please comment on any "no" answers:

What I liked most about the program was:

What I liked least about the program was:

Dickey and Wagenaar (1994) comment that the perspectives of the clinician, client, and family should all be considered when evaluating the outcome of mental health care. The clinician evaluates the client's symptoms and illness, the client evaluates his or her own sense of wellness and general functioning, and the family evaluates both the client's general functioning and symptoms and the impact of caring for their family member.

CLIENT SATISFACTION **Client satisfaction** is an important outcome that is independent from other clinical outcomes and goals. Client satisfaction is also an appropriate indication of the success of the therapeutic environment. Considering client satisfaction empowers clients by objectively gathering feedback about their experience with clinicians (professional knowledge, attitude and courtesy, cultural competence), perspectives about the program's usefulness in addressing their individual needs, and suitability of the physical setting and environmental amenities. The Client Satisfaction Questionnaire box presents one way to collect such information.

CLIENT AND FAMILY EDUCATION In addition to educating the client and family about the client's illness and treatment, the nurse also educates them about the principles of the therapeutic environment and its implementation outside the hospital (see the accompanying box).

Chapter Highlights

- The therapeutic environment is the purposeful use of people, resources, and events in the immediate environment to ensure safety, promote optimal functioning in daily activities, develop or improve interpersonal skills, and enhance the capacity to live independently.
- Inpatient psychiatric settings have been dramatically affected by changes in the types of diagnostic prob-

CLIENT/FAMILY TEACHING

Establishing a Therapeutic Environment Outside the Hospital

Goal: To help both client and family reach a mutually agreeable plan for a safe, secure, and supportive living arrangement that meets both the client's and the family's needs.

- Establish a healthy lifestyle and habits.
  Eat a balanced diet.
  Avoid caffeine, alcohol, cigarettes, and illegal drugs.
  Get adequate rest and sleep.
  Exercise at least three times a week: walking, jogging, swimming, aerobics.
- Establish a daily schedule.
  Have a routine to wake up, eat, accomplish daily activities, and rest.
  Identify tasks to be accomplished or skills to be performed; complete these in small, manageable increments.
  Take medications as prescribed.
- Use positive communication skills.
  Give directions appropriate to the client's ability to manage independently, such as verbal prompting and physical assistance, verbal prompting alone, praise for independent performance.
  Avoid criticism, argument, and negative reinforcement.
  Express empathy.
  Help client identify feelings by reflecting and making observations.
- Identify and participate in support groups.
  Recognize signs of family stress and stages of coping.
  Plan for respite; trade off responsibilities with other family members.
  Gather information about resources for the client and the family, including long-term financial, social, and health care resources.
  Select professionals you are comfortable working with.
  Evaluate resource options for client's living arrangements and rehabilitation.
- Recognize symptoms of exacerbation of the client's illness.
  Have a plan for symptom management, such as increasing medication, reducing schedule demands, contacting physician or case manager.
  Have a plan for emergency behavior management such as violence or suicide potential.

SOURCE: *Adapted from Bisbee 1991.*

lems clients have, shortened lengths of stay, and mandates by external regulatory agencies.

- These external factors, as well as increased emphasis on psychopharmacologic treatment, have reduced the role of traditional milieu therapy and challenged nurses to redefine the therapeutic nature of the environment.
- Five aspects of a therapeutic environment are safety, structure, support, socialization, and self-understanding.
- Nursing interventions that take advantage of therapeutic opportunities in the environment are based on principles of least restrictiveness, human dignity, client empowerment, and culture sensitivity.
- While improvement in clinical symptoms remains an important outcome, other indications of outcome include functioning in the community and satisfaction with treatment.

References

Alford B, Jarenko M: Behavioral design of a positive verbal community: A preliminary experimental analysis. *J Behav Therapy Exper Psychiatr* 1990;21:173–184.

Allen JG, Deering D, Buskirk JR, Coyne L: Assessment of therapeutic alliances in the psychiatric hospital milieu. *Psychiatry* 1988;51:291–299.

American Nurses Association: *Standards of Psychiatric and Mental Health Nursing Practice.* ANA, 1992.

Bisbee CC: *Educating Patients and Families About Mental Illness.* Aspen Publishers, 1991.

Caplan C: Nursing staff and patient perceptions of the ward atmosphere in a maximum security forensic hospital. *Arch Psychiatr Nurs* 1993;7:23–29.

Corrigan P, Storzbach, D: Behavioral interventions for alleviating psychotic symptoms. *Hosp Commun Psychiatr* 1993;44:341–347.

Craig C, Ray F, Hix C: Seclusion and restraint: Decreasing the discomfort. *J Psychosoc Nurs Ment Health Serv* 1989;27(7): 16–19.

Dickey B, Wagenaar H: Evaluating mental health care reform: including the clinician, client, and family perspective. *J Mental Health Admin* 1994;21:313–319.

Emrich K: Helping or hurting? Interacting in the psychiatric milieu. *J Psychosoc Nurs Ment Health Serv* 1989;27(12): 26–29.

Garritson SH: Characteristics of restrictiveness. *J Psychosoc Nurs Ment Health Serv* 1987;25(1):10–19.

Gerlock A, Solomons HC: Factors associated with the seclusion of psychiatric patients. *Perspect Psychiatr Care* 1984;21(April–June):46–53.

Goffman E: *Asylums.* Aldine Publishing, 1961.

Joint Commission on Accreditation of Hospitals: Therapeutic environment, in *Consolidated Standards Manual for Child, Adolescent, and Adult Psychiatric, Alcoholism, and Drug Abuse Facilities and Facilities Serving the Mentally Retarded/Developmentally Disabled.* Joint Commission on Accreditation of Hospitals, 1987, pp. 177–182.

Kahn EM, Frederick N: Milieu-oriented management strategies on acute care units for the chronically mentally ill. *Arch Psychiatr Nurs* 1988;2(3):134–140.

Kahn EM, White EM: Adapting milieu approaches to acute inpatient care for schizophrenic patients. *Hosp Community Psychiatry* 1989;40(6):609–614.

Kirkpatrick H: A descriptive study of seclusion: The unit environment, patient behavior, and nursing interventions. *Arch Psychiatr Nurs* 1989;3(1):3–9.

Klinge V: Staff opinions about seclusion and restraint at a state forensic hospital. *Hosp Commun Psychiatr* 1994; 45:138–141.

Krauss, J, Slavinsky A: *The Chronically Ill Psychiatric Patient and the Community.* Blackwell Scientific Publications, 1982.

Lego S, Pawlicki, C: How does parallel process manifest itself in psychiatric nursing practice? *J Psychosoc Nurs* 1993; 31:41–44.

Lowe T: Characteristics of effective nursing interventions in the management of challenging behavior. *J Adv Nurs* 1992;17:1126–1232.

McEnany G, Tescher B: Contracting for care. *J Psychosoc Nurs Ment Health Serv* 1985;23:11–18.

Munetz MR, Geller JL: The least restrictive alternative in the postinstitutional era. *Hosp Commun Psychiatr* 1993; 44:967–973.

Paul GL, Lentz RJ: *Psychosocial Treatment of Chronic Mental Patients: Milieu Versus Social Learning Programs.* Harvard University Press, 1977.

Richardson B: Psychiatric inpatients' perceptions of the seclusion room experience. *Nurs Res* 1987;36(4):234–238.

Rosenblatt A: Concepts of the asylum in the care of the mentally ill. *Hosp Commun Psychiatr* 1984;35:244–250.

Sautter F, Heaney C, O'Neill P: A problem-solving approach to psychotherapy in the inpatient milieu. *Hosp Commun Psychiatr* 1991:814–817.

Schatzman L, Strauss A: A sociology of psychiatry: A perspective and some organizing foci. *Social Problems* 1966; 14:3–16.

Strauss A, Schatzman L, Bucher R, Ehrlich D, Sabshin M: *Psychiatric Ideologies and Institutions,* rev ed. Free Press of Glencoe, 1981.

Waldfogel S, Wolpe PR: Using awareness of religious factors to enhance interventions in consultation-liaison psychiatry. *Hosp Commun Psychiatr* 1993;44:473–477.

Watson J: Maintenance of therapeutic community principles in an age of biopharmacology and economic restraints. *Archiv Psychiatr Nurs* 1992;6:183–188.

Whitehead CC, Polsky RH, Crookshank C, Fik E: Objective and subjective evaluation of psychiatric ward redesign. *Am J Psychiatry* 1984;141(May):639–644.

Wilson HS: *Deinstitutionalized Residential Care for the Mentally Disabled—The Soteria House Approach.* Grune & Stratton, 1982.

CHAPTER 10

ETHICAL REASONING

Holly Skodol Wilson

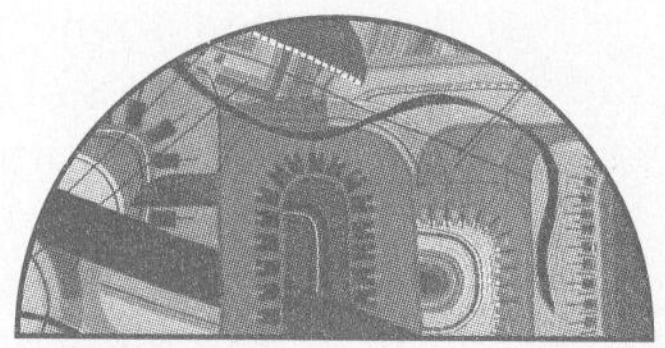

COMPETENCIES

- *Discuss the process of analyzing an ethical issue.*
- *Compare and contrast dominant ethical perspectives.*
- *Define the six major principles of bioethics.*
- *Identify and discuss ethical dilemmas particular to psychiatric nursing.*
- *Apply to practice dilemmas the framework of integrated clinical judgment and the competencies for ethical reasoning presented in this chapter.*

Cross-References

Other topics relevant to this content are: Cultural considerations, Chapter 5; Elder abuse, Chapter 38; Ethics in milieu therapy, Chapter 9; Legal issues, Chapter 11.

Critical Thinking Challenge

Managed care is a cost-cutting approach in which the psychiatric clinician (therapist or case manager) does not control decisions about the type and location of treatment provided to clients. Instead, such decisions are made by managed care monitors employed by insurance companies. Treatment options are typically limited when clients are defined as noncompliant: a person who is severely and persistently mentally ill and refuses to take his or her medication, or a person with the comorbidites of depression and substance abuse who refuses medical detoxification. Critically analyze the ethical dilemmas raised by managed care. What bioethical guidelines might balance the need for the equitable distribution of mental health services with clients' rights?

A young teacher of nursing ethics and philosophy once said, "Reasoning in ethics means bringing all one's faculties in a balanced way to bear on the sincere concern for human well-being in general and the meaning of human experience. Being reasonable in ethics is more like having integrity than like being smart." This chapter describes a framework for analyzing ethical issues and resolving ethical dilemmas in psychiatric nursing. Reason and reflection have always held an important place in the study of ethics, for ethics is more than a personal or inspirational enterprise for answering moral questions. Moral judgments are most highly developed when the *process of arriving at them* and the *reasons for believing in them* are clear and convincing. At the heart of ethical judgments are the reasons for them.

Framework of Questions for Analyzing an Ethical Issue

1. Who are the relevant actors in the situation?
2. What is the required action?
3. What are the probable and possible consequences of the action?
4. What is the range of alternative actions or choices?
5. What is the intent or purpose of the action?
6. What is the context of the action?

Throughout the history of nursing education, teachers and students alike have been concerned with ethical matters. A closer look, however, reveals that the concern has been less with moral principles and ethical dilemmas and more with the legal aspects of practice and what psychiatric nurse–bioethicist Anne Davis refers to as "the etiquette of the profession" (Davis and Aroskar 1978). Nursing has made notable advances toward professional autonomy in recent years. Greater autonomy, however, has increased the need to account for and accept the consequences of professional decisions and actions. Autonomy, according to Aroskar (1980), has to do with the right of self-determination, governance without outside control, and the capacity to exist independently. Professionals do this by:

- Developing codes of ethics that serve as guidelines for defining professional responsibility.
- Setting rigorous qualifications for entry into the profession.
- Establishing peer review procedures.
- Setting standards for practice, such as those described in the ANA's *Standards of Psychiatric–Mental Health Clinical Nursing Practice*.

Professionals must balance the goal of more autonomy in nursing with efforts to achieve what providers and consumers determine is the common and the individual "good" in health care. The goal of this chapter is not to preach right and wrong but to help you develop a way of thinking about complex ethical issues and dilemmas in psychiatric nursing.

Analyzing Ethical Issues

One of the major difficulties in ethical analysis is that there are no definite, clear-cut solutions to ethical dilemmas. For centuries moral philosophers—beginning with Socrates, Plato, and Aristotle—have struggled with two main ethical questions: What is the meaning of right or good? and What should I do? To identify, clarify, define, and defend a stand on an ethical issue, we must engage in a process of ethical reasoning about data that can be gathered by using the framework of six critical questions set out in the accompanying box.

Psychiatric nurses must often identify alternative courses of action and decide what to do when there is a conflict of rights and obligations between clients and families, between themselves and other mental health care workers, or between the client's good and the community or social good.

Dominant Ethical Perspectives

Various ethical perspectives provide different ways of structuring the answers to the questions in the accompanying box, thus leading to different decisions about what is the right action. The dominant ethical perspectives include the following traditions:*

- *Egoism.* The egoist answers questions about the morally right thing to do by saying that something is good because "I desire it." The right act, then, is the one that maximizes the pleasure of the person asking the question.
- *Deontology.* The deontologic or formalist approach suggests that rightness or wrongness depends on the nature or form of the action for moral significance. In this tradition, there are both *act deontologists* and *rule deontologists*—that is, rightness may be based on performing certain morally significant acts properly or adhering to certain preestablished rules or principles. This position requires a commitment to the principle of **universality**—that is, one will make the same moral judgment in any similar situation regardless of time, place, or persons involved. Many rule deontologists believe in the divine command theory—an act is wrong because it is forbidden by God. The difficulty for both believers and nonbelievers in this theory is that sometimes the rules conflict. In an attempt to get out of the problem of conflicting rules, Immanuel Kant, writing in the late eighteenth century, stated that you should act only on a maxim that you can simultaneously will to be a universal law. Unfortunately, Kant's position doesn't help with moral *conflict.* For example, if returning the institutionalized mentally dis-

**Adapted from Davis and Aroskar 1978.*

turbed to the community was identified as a morally good action, Kant would have us ignore any specifics of a particular situation, even though an individual might end up living in a dingy stairwell and stealing food.

• *Utilitarianism.* In the theory of utility, good is "happiness or pleasure," and right is "the greatest good for the greatest number of people." Implicit in this position is the assumption that one can weigh and measure harm and benefit and come out with the best possible balance of good over evil. Among the questions raised by this position is what happens to individual justice when the general welfare is emphasized.

• *Theory of obligation.* The basic principles of the theory of obligation are: (1) the principle of beneficence, which requires that we not just *want* good but *do* good rather than evil; and (2) the principle of justice, which requires that we distribute benefits and burdens equally through society. A problem with this position is what to do when the two principles conflict at the public and individual levels.

• *Ideal observer theory.* This perspective outlines the characteristics of ethical reason as consistency, disinterest, dispassion, omnipresence, and omniscience. These are the qualities of an *ideal observer* or *moral judge.* The ideal observer has only general interests, such as the welfare of all, and does not make decisions on practical or emotional grounds. The questions of who should be the moral judge and where the development of this moral consciousness will occur are left unanswered.

• *Justice as fairness.* The principles of justice as fairness are: (1) each person is to have an equal right to the most extensive liberty for all, and (2) social and economic injustices are to be addressed so that the least advantaged receive the greatest benefit. In this system, the first principle of maximizing liberty for all has absolute priority. Five criteria emerge from this tradition for judging the rightness of any ethical principles:

1. Universality. The same principles hold for everyone.
2. Generality. They must not be geared to specific people or situations.
3. Publicity. They must be known and recognized by all.
4. Ordering. They must order conflicting claims.
5. Finality. They may override the demands of law or custom.

Principles of Bioethics

The preceding ethical traditions or a combination of them operate when nurses reflect on ethical dilemmas. Bioethics is a field that applies ethical reasoning to issues and dilemmas in the area of health care.

Taking a stand on an ethical issue involves much more than merely accepting the moral position or personal values of another. As listed in the accompanying box, bioethicists offer six principles as important guidelines (Davis 1981).

Principles of Bioethics

- *Autonomy*—the right to make one's own decisions.
- *Nonmaleficence*—the intention to do no wrong.
- *Beneficence*—the principle of attempting to do things that benefit others.
- *Justice*—the distribution, as fairly as possible, of benefits and burdens.
- *Veracity*—the intention to tell the truth.
- *Confidentiality*—the social contract guaranteeing another's privacy.

Source: Davis 1981.

Ethical Dilemmas in Psychiatric Nursing

The nurse must protect the rights of the individual client yet mediate between these rights and the interests of the social group. Sometimes the two are in conflict. Ultimately, nurses must reconcile a number of crucial ethical dilemmas with their personal and professional values. Among these issues are:

- The potential stigma of psychiatric diagnostic labels.
- Psychiatry's right to control individual freedom.
- The justification for involuntary treatment.
- The use of restrictive treatment interventions.
- The client's right to suicide.
- The client's right to privacy.

Practicing psychiatric nursing requires ethical responsibility. The quality of a nurse's moral commitment is a measure of professional excellence. However, problems arise when there is conflict about the ground rules for behavior, whether the conflict is between client and social group, nurse and profession, or nurse and agency. These problems are phrased in the ethical language of right and wrong. Circumstances likely to give rise to such problems include the following:

RESEARCH NOTE

Citation

Sullivan MD, Youngner SJ: Depression, competence and the right to refuse lifesaving medical treatment. *Am J Psychiatr* 1994;151(7):971–978.

Study Problem/Purpose

This study explored legal and bioethical literature to examine the clash between ethical and moral perspectives on situations in which depressed clients who have serious medical illnesses refuse life-sustaining treatment.

Methods

This study used methods of document analysis to trace case law, court rulings, and other literature relevant to the issue of competence to refuse life-saving treatment and the possible impact of depression on this refusal.

Findings

In psychiatry, a client's desire to die is considered to be evidence of impaired capacity to make decisions about life-saving treatment. The clinical evaluation of depression's effect on a client's ability to make medical decisions is complex for the following reasons: (1) depression is viewed as a reasonable response to a serious medical illness, (2) depression produces distortions of decision making that are more subtle than those caused by delirium or psychosis, and (3) a diagnosis of major depression is neither necessary nor sufficient to determine that a client has impaired decision-making competence.

Implications

Court rulings have legitimized the right of seriously ill medical patients to refuse treatment and have not treated their decision as suicide. This ethical and legal opinion supporting the right to refuse life-saving treatment in the medical setting has generally not extended to medically ill psychiatric clients. A depressed client's wish to die is assumed to be rooted in psychopathology and characterized as suicide. The clinical and moral pitfalls that accompany the view that a psychiatric client's choice of death is pathological, unreasonable, and ripe for preventive intervention are particularly complex when medically ill patients are also suffering from depression. The authors conclude that mental health professionals need to recognize that some treatment refusals that result in death are legitimate, even if they are accompanied by suicidal intent. It is important to treat depression in the seriously ill client, but these investigators conclude that it is sometimes appropriate to accept the client's decision to refuse life-sustaining treatment.

- The professional and the client are from different social classes and may have different statuses or cultural values.
- The voluntary nature of the client's participation is compromised.
- The client's competence to enter into an agreement about intervention is questionable, or the client does not realize that certain interventions are being implemented. (For a study on competence, see the Research Note.)

Every nursing relationship begins with an unusual burden of ethical responsibility. The following pages explore some of these moral issues.

The Stigma of Psychiatric Diagnoses

The list of stereotypes associated with diagnostic categories is well known to most nurses. Equally familiar are the consequences to people with these diagnoses. People labeled as drug addicts, alcoholics, convicts, paranoids, and so on acquire a discredited social identity because of the character flaws often associated with the labels. To much of society, the labels used in psychiatry suggest decadence, immorality, and wanton disregard for society's values. Sociologist Erving Goffman subtitles his classic monograph on stigma *Notes on the Management of Spoiled Identity* (1963). It is important to consider how and when psychiatric nurses, while advocating humane treatment for clients, indirectly contribute to their spoiled identities by participating in the arbitrary use of oppressive labels.

The Need for Diagnostic Labels Diagnosis has considerable value in psychiatric practice. Putting clients into diagnostic categories makes it easy for health care professionals to communicate with each other about the client. The diagnosis often dictates a particular course of treatment and enables the mental health team to prognosticate about a client's recovery. Diagnostic categories enable nurses to plan comprehensively for client care and to conduct research.

Before the publication of the third edition of the APA's *Diagnostic and Statistical Manual of Mental Disorders* and its revised edition, diagnostic categories such as schizophrenia, paranoia, and sociopathy were not sufficiently precise to give a clear idea of desirable treatment. A person labeled schizophrenic can be treated with drugs, milieu therapy, or behavior-modification techniques. All of these could be justified by one theoretic orientation or another. Nonetheless, the diagnostic label was felt to be the key to subsequent decisions about a client, especially the choice of medication. In some cases when clients failed to respond favorably to the medication indicated by their diagnosis, the diagnosis was changed. Advocates for the criteria-based DSMs believe that their use will greatly improve diagnostic practices.

THE NURSE'S MORAL STANCE ON DIAGNOSES Does labeling with psychiatric diagnoses merely provide psychiatric professionals with some additional sense of control in their dealings with clients? Is it true that a diagnosis gives staff members an increased sense of being able to predict client behavior and a way of calmly viewing what might otherwise be upsetting behavior: "That's just her hysterical personality coming out," or "Those complaints are just paranoid delusions." The consequences of psychiatric labels for clients and their families, however, raise moral questions about their legitimacy when they are used arbitrarily or without current knowledge of diagnostic criteria. Consider the following, adapted from a letter to a newspaper advice columnist:

I am a 12-year-old girl who is left out of all social activities because my father is an alcoholic. I try to be nice and friendly to everyone, but it's no use. The girls at school have told me that their mothers don't want them to associate with me because my father might be dangerous. Is there anything I can do? I am very lonesome because it's no fun to be alone all the time. My mother tries to take me places with her, but I want to be with people my own age. Please give me some advice.

Sincerely,
An Outcast

Nurses have a moral responsibility to question practices that exact a price from clients far in excess of the benefits. Every moment of moral injustice takes its toll on nurses as well as clients. Every moment of moral responsibility strengthens their sense of personal integrity.

Controlling Individual Freedom

Involuntary hospitalization and treatment of psychiatric clients are usually considered humanitarian efforts to help "the mentally ill." Yet any practice that directly and coercively deprives a person of freedom has political implications. In most states, a client who is involuntarily committed to a mental hospital has few of the legal protections that even a criminal offender has. In addition, in some states clients have no guarantee that they will ever be released from the hospital unless they alter their behavior sufficiently to please their "keepers." This ethical issue is further complicated by the fact that psychiatric professionals can no longer argue that involuntary hospitalization is necessary to restore mental health. Instead, the confinement must be justified as necessary to protect the client or others from harm.

VIOLENCE AND SOCIAL CONTROL Violence encountered in psychiatric nursing practice usually involves violence directed toward others or violence directed inward in the form of suicide.

Violence Against Others Psychiatric nurses are faced with the dilemma of trying to be both healer-helpers and agents of social control. In dealing with violently destructive clients, they must balance the value of life against the value of liberty.

Suicide Traditionally, nurses have felt that they should do everything possible to preserve life. They have relied on this imperative to justify intervention in suicide attempts as well as heroic technical measures to avert impending deaths. Recent reconsideration of euthanasia, however, seems to raise questions about a client's right to suicide. *Euthanasia* has been defined as the intentional termination of a life of such poor quality that it is not worth living. The concept of allowing a person to die without the use of life-prolonging treatment is called **passive euthanasia. Active euthanasia,** by contrast, is defined as an act that results in a person's death. The treatment given to dying clients is often in conflict with the treatment they desire. For example, a physician may disregard a client's protests against treatment. The doctor may assert that the client's medical condition is causing the client to behave irrationally. There is not necessarily an ethical difference between clients dying of physical deterioration and clients dying of emotional or mental deterioration. Many of the same ethical questions emerge about the suicidal client:

- How is *quality of life* defined?
- Is the definition limited to physical factors?
- Who should have the right to make the definition?
- How is rationality to be measured?
- Are people always in conscious control of their choices?

An individual's right to choose when and how to die is a complex biomedical issue currently receiving more attention than ever before. The thoughtful professional nurse needs to clarify the issues, give them careful consideration, and search for a personal position. There are many ways in which people can deliberately shorten or end their own lives. They can destroy themselves quickly with a gun, or slowly through the chronic use of drugs such as tobacco or alcohol. When is coercive intervention by psychiatric practitioners justified?

THE USE OF RESTRICTIVE TREATMENTS At some time in their lives, all people experience the kind of excessive stress that makes them feel miserable or even desperate. But some people communicate these feelings in ways that are inappropriate, troublesome, unreasonable, or frightening to others. A young woman who in times of stress mutilates her body by burning it repeatedly with cigarettes; a teenager who breaks everything in sight during violent, destructive outbursts; and a belligerent male who initiates physical fights with anyone and everyone without provocation—all usually become candidates for *symptomatic treatments,* behavioral control measures often used against a person's will.

Psychosurgery The most dramatic of restrictive measures is **psychosurgery**, the surgical removal or destruction of brain tissue with the intent of altering behavior even though there may be no direct evidence of structural disease or damage in the brain. Psychosurgery has become the subject of marked controversy on ethical grounds. Advocates claim that it is done to restore rather than destroy individual freedom. They argue that before psychosurgery, the client is crippled by mental illness. Individual autonomy is compromised by the client's bizarre behavior or internal psychologic state. After the surgery, clients supposedly are more autonomous than before, by their own and others' criteria. Advocates of the selective use of psychosurgery, even against the client's will, outline three conditions that must be met to justify it:

1. The illness being treated is seriously disabling and untreatable by nonsurgical means such as medication or therapy.
2. The treatment is undertaken with some sort of systematic investigative protocol; it is accompanied by evaluation research.
3. The treatment occurs in settings with as many safeguards as possible to arrive at informed consent, if possible, perhaps using a client advocate during the procedure.

Psychotropic Drugs The discovery that certain drugs can radically alter the expression of human emotions has had an enormous impact on psychiatry. The mental hospital is no longer seen as a "warehouse" for storing society's deviants; it is now a "clearinghouse" where clients are sorted, renovated, and dispatched back into their communities with symptomatic behavior under control through one or another of the current psychiatric medications.

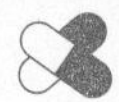

Psychiatric professionals have associated the advent of psychotropic medications with a new optimism and less fear about working with people labeled mentally ill. Conceivably, the impact of the drugs on the attitudes of nurses may increase the amount of humane contact clients are given while in the hospital. Furthermore, it might be argued that the drugs have helped keep people out of the hospital and have decreased the need for other more dramatic measures, such as electroshock treatment.

Drugs that make people feel better, however, can lessen their motivation to confront an oppressive situation. This can have serious implications for the political and moral climate of society. Consider, for example, this common clinical problem:

A woman is married to a domineering and insensitive man. She becomes increasingly unhappy, then intensely anxious. When she is on the verge of fighting back to try to alter her oppressed situation, she becomes more agitated and visits a psychiatric clinic. Her therapist prescribes a medicine that alleviates her tension. As a consequence, the woman has less awareness of her plight and is less inclined to confront her problems. She ultimately continues to submit to her husband's oppressiveness.

It is conceivable that pills could be developed to keep such a woman quietly enslaved throughout her married life. Suppose drugs were coercively given to anyone whose unhappiness was rooted in social oppression?

The cautious and judicious use of drugs with the client's consent can be helpful. Used irresponsibly, they can close off moral and political confrontations. Decisions about the use of drugs must be made in the context of the social situation and environment.

In hospital settings, medications are regularly used to reduce symptoms and make client behavior more manageable. Most staff members justify their use of chemical controls by defining violent or bizarre behavior as an indirect request for limits. By assigning this meaning to the use of drugs, practitioners can feel that their actions to suppress symptoms are based on the needs of the client rather than on the staff's management motives.

After pacing angrily up and down the hall in front of the nurses' station for 20 minutes or so, Carlotta kicks over some mops in a bucket. A male staff member shouts to the nurse to get her PRN medication ready and strides into the hall telling the client to stop it. She cries and shouts, and they begin struggling. Several other staff members rush over to assist. They drag and carry her into her room, where she gets Haldol (10 mg). She continues fighting and screaming. Staff members decide to put her in soft restraints and continue to wrestle with her in her room. Finally they decide to transfer her to the ward downstairs, where she can be put into a seclusion room. In a report, a staff member describes the incident as: "Carlotta blew up and needed controls." In further discussion of the case, it became apparent that the decision to put her into seclusion was made because restrained clients have to be checked and released every 15 minutes, which is a lot of work for the staff.

It is possible that all these controls would not have been necessary had a nurse behind the glass windows of the nurses' station responded to the nonverbal cues of mounting tension that the client communicated before kicking over the mops.

Restraints Even the physical characteristics of psychiatric inpatient settings convey the notion that clients are not expected to be capable of self-control and that staff members have the responsibility for providing it. Many clients view these interventions as forms of abuse, while the staff sees them as "helping people who can't take care of themselves." Consider the following directions on the use of restraints:

> The acutely psychotic client who is delusional, the angry individual who is testing limits, and the intoxicated client are the types of individuals to whom restraints may be applied for their own protection and that of others. These individuals are nonverbally asking for help to control their potentially inappropriate behavior. When all other techniques have failed and it is quite obvious that the client is out of control, the staff must take action and forcibly apply restraints.

All the judgments that must be made about restraints involve moral decisions. What other techniques have been tried? Is the client obviously out of control? How does the nurse decide? Is the client cognitively compromised? What will be the effects on the client of such a dramatic intervention? What are the effects on others in the milieu?

Clients themselves have begun to guard against repressiveness by issuing their own bill of rights, as shown in the box on the next page. This issue captured public attention in the notorious case of Joyce Brown, a homeless New York woman forcibly removed from the streets because of her self-neglect and provocative behavior. She was judged competent, however, to refuse medication despite her status as an involuntary patient. Deciding that impairment is sufficient to deprive a client of the right to *informed consent* is yet another controversy in nursing ethics. The model bill of rights included in the 1980 Mental Health Systems Act passed by Congress appears in Chapter 11.

Client Privacy and Confidentiality

When people seek psychiatric help, they must usually reveal highly personal, possibly embarrassing, and potentially damaging information about themselves. Almost all modes of therapeutic intervention rely on the client's willingness to talk openly and honestly about personal concerns, feelings, or problems. The solo therapist in private practice with voluntary clients is usually able to avoid compromising the client's right to confidentiality. In fact, many private therapists view themselves as vigilant protectors of their clients' privacy. Nurses, however, may encounter a serious ethical conflict in being both the confidant of the client and the employee of the organization. Nurses have dual allegiances—to the client and to the agency.

Clients usually assume that health care professionals have no other purpose than to help them. They lose sight of the fact that nurses are often asked to collect data about them that might be highly influential in determining their medications, their disposition, and even their civil rights. While it is often the psychiatrist who makes final pronouncements about a client's mental health status, diagnosis, prognosis, and the like, such pronouncements rest on information collected and communicated to the doctor by nurses. This information-gathering process merits serious scrutiny.

Information gathering and sharing are part of the psychiatric nurse's role. Thoughtful handling of patient confidentiality is facilitated by three safeguards:

1. Nurses must convey to clients the limit of confidentiality in their exchanges—that is, what the nurses do with the information a client shares.
2. Nurses must attempt to portray accurately to others the reliability, validity, and representativeness of the data they communicate about a client.
3. Strict confidentiality may have to be violated when an innocent third party is endangered.

Managed Mental Health Care in Psychiatric Practice

Managed care refers to cost-containment systems in which a population at risk receives care that is constrained by a specified budget and is held accountable for defined client outcomes or results. In effect, managed

Mental Patient's Bill of Rights

We are ex-mental patients. We have been subjected to brutalization in mental hospitals and by the psychiatric profession. In almost every state of the union, a mental patient has fewer de facto rights than a murderer condemned to die or to life imprisonment. As a human being, you are entitled to basic human rights that are taken for granted by the general population. You are entitled to protection by and recourse to the law. The purpose of the Mental Patients' Liberation Project is to help those who are still institutionalized. This Bill of Rights was prepared by those at the first meeting of MPLP held on June 13, 1971, at the Washington Square Methodist Church. If you know someone in a mental hospital, give him/her a copy of these rights. If you are in a hospital and need legal help, try to find someone to call the number listed below.

1. You are a human being and are entitled to be treated as such with as much decency and respect as is accorded to any other human being.
2. You are an American citizen and are entitled to every right established by the Declaration of Independence and guaranteed by the Constitution of the United States of America.
3. You have the right to the integrity of your own mind and the integrity of your own body.
4. Treatment and medication can be administered only with your consent and, in the event you give your consent, you have the right to demand to know all relevant information regarding said treatment and/or medication.
5. You have the right to have access to your own legal and medical counsel.
6. You have the right to refuse to work in a mental hospital and/or to choose what work you shall do and you have the right to receive the minimum wage for such work as is set by the state labor laws.
7. You have the right to decent medical attention when you feel you need it just as any other human being has that right.
8. You have the right to uncensored communication by phone, letter, and in person with whomever you wish and at any time you wish.
9. You have the right not to be treated like a criminal; not to be locked up against your will; not to be committed involuntarily; not to be fingerprinted or "mugged" (photographed).
10. You have the right to decent living conditions. You're paying for it and the taxpayers are paying for it.
11. You have the right to retain your own personal property. No one has the right to confiscate what is legally yours, no matter what reason is given. That is commonly known as theft.
12. You have the right to bring grievance against those who have mistreated you and the right to counsel and a court hearing. You are entitled to protection by the law against retaliation.
13. You have the right to refuse to be a guinea pig for experimental drugs and treatments and to refuse to be used as learning material for students. You have the right to demand reimbursement if you are so used.
14. You have the right not to have your character questioned or defamed.
15. You have the right to request an alternative to legal commitment or incarceration in a mental hospital.

The Mental Patients' Liberation Project plans to set up neighborhood crisis centers as alternatives to incarceration and voluntary and involuntary commitment to hospitals. We plan to set up a legal aid society for those whose rights are taken away and/or abused. Although our immediate aim is to help those currently in hospitals, we are also interested in helping those who are suffering from job discrimination, discriminatory school admissions policies and discrimination and abuse at the hands of the psychiatric professions. Call the number listed below if you are interested in our group or if you need assistance.

Mental Patients Alliance of Central New York
P.O. Box 158
Syracuse, N.Y. 13201
(315) 947-5822

Source: Mental Patients Alliance of Central New York Inc.

mental health care creates a situation in which the psychiatric professional no longer controls decisions about the type of treatment or the setting (inpatient versus outpatient). Instead decisions, such as two-therapy sessions each week or outpatient drug rehabilitation, are monitored by an agent employed by insurers. Clearly, managed psychiatric care raises serious ethical issues related to client autonomy of choice regarding therapist and site, the integrity of the psychiatric nurse-client relationship, and the risk that noncompliant psychiatric clients may be denied access to additional treatment (Olsen 1994).

Moral Principles for Managed Mental Health Care Harvard psychiatrist James Sabin (1994), director of the Teaching Center at the Harvard Community Health Plan, offers four principles to guide you through the ethical dilemmas posted by managed mental health care systems:

1. Recognize that as a clinician, you are dedicated to caring for clients in a relationship of fidelity and, at the same time, must act as a steward of society's scarce mental health care resources.
2. Recognize that it is ethically correct to recommend the least costly treatment unless you have evidence that a more costly intervention will yield a superior outcome. (Needless to say, this decision is a problematic call in circumstances when hospitals or agencies adopt for-profit stances that risk client health and safety) (McDonald 1994).
3. You need to advocate for the ethical principle of justice in managed mental health care situations so that cost savings with one client are used to meet the mental health care needs of another, not pay off an insurance company's debts.
4. It is your responsibility to discuss the situation openly with your clients so that they understand the reimbursable parameters of their care and can act in their own interests.

A moral debate about the ethics of applying managed care to psychiatric clients is currently emerging. Be prepared to sharpen your ethical reasoning skills and tools.

Clinical Judgment and Ethical Reasoning

The judgments that lead people to label someone's experience as paranoid rather than simply unpopular are based on shifting criteria. Behavior that is considered bizarre or unreasonable in one cultural context may be considered desirable in another. The definitions of those who need psychiatric help are constantly changing. Nurses are necessarily guided in therapeutic work by a belief system—some vision of what kinds of changes would improve a client's life. Nurses are further guided by some moral principles that limit the extent to which they will help a client obtain happiness at the expense of others, and the extent to which they will participate in the oppression of an individual in the interests of societal control. Laws represent yet another source of limits.

Nursing is frequently faced with two goals:

1. Responding to the therapeutic needs of individuals.
2. Serving society by preserving social order.

Often these two goals are in conflict, and nurses must face the dilemma of placing one above the other. The only way to resolve the conflict is for us to clarify our own values through a process of ethical reasoning.

Situations that involve ethical dilemmas require you to understand the concept of **moral claims.** Ethical reasoning is the process you can use when there is a conflict of claims and you have to make a choice favoring one claim over another. Anyone who is responsible for moral choices is obliged to recognize the reason, virtue, ideal, rule, or principle on which he or she makes a decision. Gordon and her colleagues (1994) have developed a useful framework for integrating the process of clinical judgment used in therapeutic and ethical reasoning. Their flow diagram, shown in Figure 10–1, guides the nurse in recognizing cues that suggest the presence of a dilemma, gathering information concerning the relevant parties' ethical claims, and arriving at an ethical choice and plan of action in a manner that is reasoned, disciplined, and systematic.

Competencies Required for Ethical Reasoning

The well-known moral developmentalists Kohlberg (1978) and Rest (1986) suggest that ethical reasoning requires the following competencies:

1. You must be able to interpret a moral situation in terms of possible choice of action and its consequences for the welfare of those involved.
2. You must be able to make a judgment about a morally desirable or required course of action.
3. You must be able to give priority to morally obligatory values above other personal values.
4. You must have the strength, commitment, and skills required to carry out morally correct decisions.

These competencies and preceding framework for clinical judgment provide tools that can be used to address moral dilemmas in both psychiatric nursing practice and research.

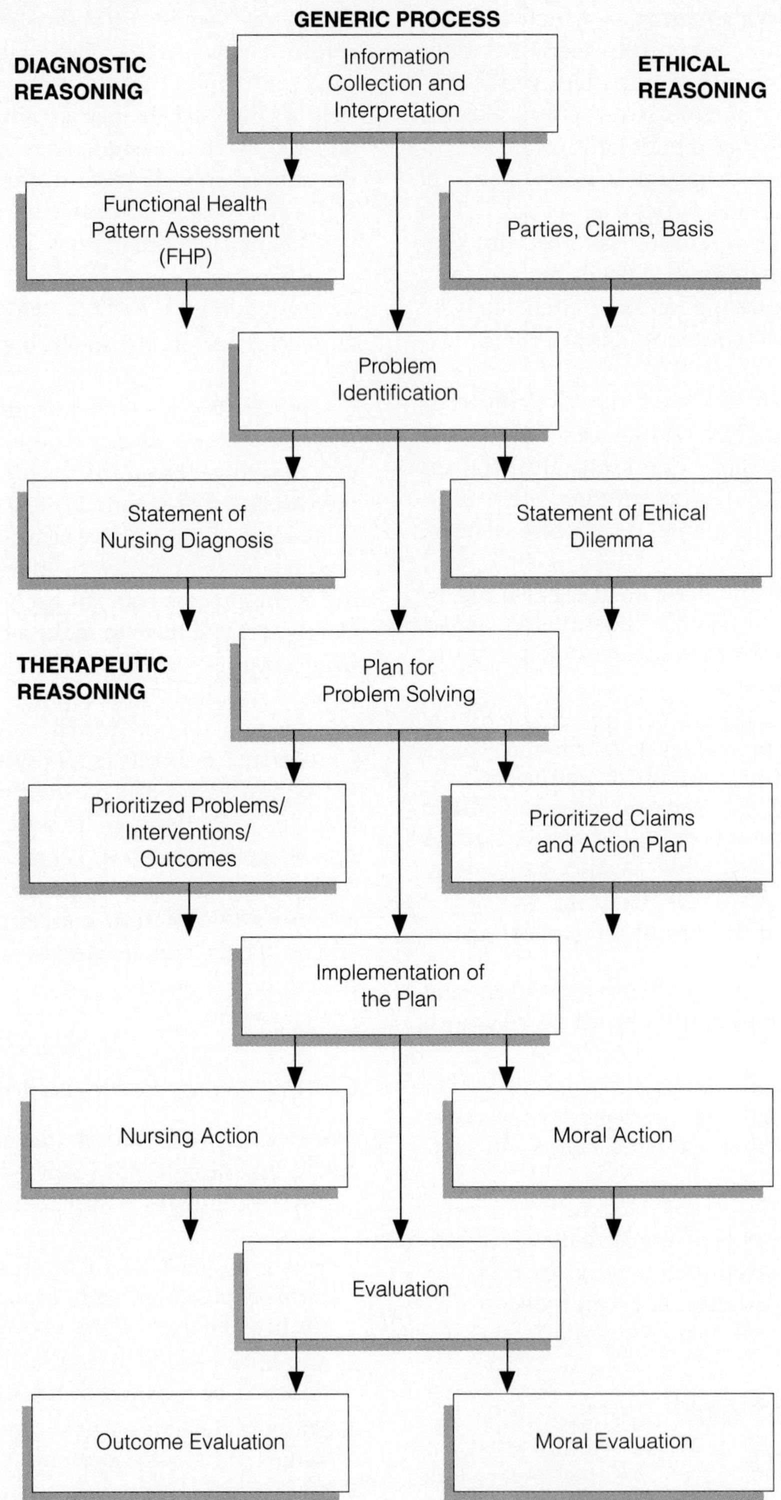

Figure 10–1 An integrated model of diagnostic, therapeutic, and ethical reasoning.
Source: Gordon et al. 1994.

Chapter Highlights

- Ethical reasoning is a process for achieving clear and convincing reasons for making moral decisions rather than discovering a singular right or wrong solution for ethical dilemmas.
- An ethical dilemma is a conflict between two obligations or moral claims.
- Nurses move toward professional autonomy by developing codes of ethics, setting qualifications for practitioners, participating in peer review, setting standards, and accepting consequences for professional decisions.
- Known dominant ethical perspectives include egoism, deontology, utilitarianism, theory of obligation, ideal observer theory, and justice as fairness.
- Principles of bioethics include autonomy, nonmaleficence, beneficence, justice, veracity, and confidentiality.
- Contemporary mental health ethical dilemmas include the effects of psychiatric labeling, the control of personal freedom, the use of restrictive treatments, the rights of the client to privacy and confidentiality, and issues related to managed care in mental health services.
- The nurse must protect the rights of the individual yet mediate between these rights and the interests of the social group, using clinical judgment and ethical reasoning.

References

Aroskar MA: Establishing limits to professional autonomy: Whose responsibility? *Nurs Law Ethics* 1980;1.

Colorado Society of Clinical Specialists in Psychiatric Nursing. Ethical guidelines for competence. *J Psychosoc Nurs* 28(5);1990:38–39.

Davis AJ: Ethical dilemmas in nursing. Recorded at JONA and Nurse Educator's 1981 Joint Leadership Conference, available from Teach'em, Inc., 160 East Illinois Street, Chicago, Illinois.

Davis AJ: Professional obligations, personal values in conflict. *Am Nurs* 1990:7.

Davis AJ, Aroskar MA: *Ethical Dilemmas and Nursing Practice.* Appleton-Century-Crofts, 1978.

Goffman E: *Stigma: Notes on the Management of Spoiled Identity.* Prentice-Hall, 1963.

Gordon M, Murphy CP, Candee D, Hiltunen E: Clinical judgment: An integrated model. *Adv Nurs Sci* 1994;16(4): 55–70.

Kohlberg L: The cognitive-developmental approach to moral education, in Scharf D (ed): *Readings in Moral Education.* Winston Press, 1978.

McDonald S: An ethical dilemma: Risk versus responsibility. *J Psychosoc Nurs* 1994;32(1):19–25.

Mohr WK: The private psychiatric hospital scandal: A critical social approach. *Arch Psychiatr Nurs* 1994;8(1):3–8.

Olsen D: Considerations of managed care in mental health treatment. *J Psychosoc Nurs* 1994;32(3):25–28.

Rest JR: *Moral Development: Advances in Research and Theory.* Praeger, 1986.

Sabin JE: A credo for ethical managed care in mental health practice. *Hosp Comm Psychiatr* 1994;45(9):859–869.

Spencer E: Psychiatric ethics: Entering the 1990s. *Hosp Comm Psychiatr* 1990;41(4):384–386.

Sullivan MD, Youngner SJ: Competence and the right to refuse lifesaving treatment. *Am J Psychiatr* 1994;151(7): 971–978.

CHAPTER 11

ADVOCACY, CLIENT RIGHTS, AND LEGAL ISSUES

Joanne Keglovits
Marilyn Meder

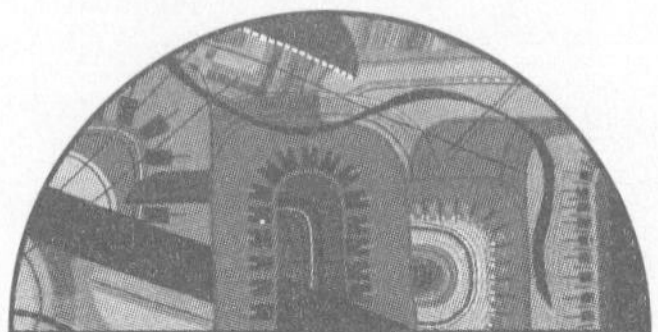

COMPETENCIES

- *Recognize the major components of mental health statutes.*
- *Realize the need for a working knowledge of the mental health law in the state in which you practice.*
- *Identify liability issues and safeguards.*
- *State two factors necessary for client consent.*
- *Describe two models of decision making.*
- *Discuss your duty to intervene in situations where clients are at risk.*
- *Explore the frustrations and challenges you may experience in your work as client advocate.*

Cross-References

Other topics relevant to this content are: Managed care, Chapter 35; Ethical dilemmas, Chapter 10; History of moral treatment, Chapter 2; Milieu aspects, Chapter 9; Monitoring treatment compliance among the chronically mentally ill, Chapter 21.

Critical Thinking Challenge

Most states require that nurses intervene to help clients. Most nurses want to help clients. At times, though, some mental health clients simply refuse to cooperate with treatment. This can be frustrating for nurses and clients. How can you reconcile the desire and duty to help with a client's refusal for treatment? When do you think it is acceptable for a client to refuse to be treated? How do you think refusal to cooperate with treatment should be handled?

Judicial, legislative, political, and economic decisions profoundly influence mental health practice. Many factors bring about changes in the understanding and practice of mental health intervention. These changes challenge the psychiatric nurse to examine central issues, such as the definition of *mental health,* decision making, clients' and society's rights, liability, and accountability. This examination requires a surrender of past ideas and generally improves care, but it often confuses the boundaries of mental health practice and the law. This confusion entraps mental health care professionals, lawyers, families, clients, and the public in a muddle of conflicting policies and procedures.

The individual rights of minority groups, including the mentally disabled, have taken on new meaning over the past twenty years. Many of the values implied by a humanistic perspective are now mandated by law. These values, however, blur the boundaries between public and individual good, voluntary and involuntary treatment, and informed and uninformed consent, and this blurring of boundaries makes the development and implementation of policies difficult. In addition, a client's right to privacy, to receive and refuse treatment, and to define happiness and growth pivot on society's values.

This chapter will bring some clarity to the ever-changing relationship between the law and mental health services so that nurses can not only practice with confidence but also exercise their power as citizens and professionals to influence the direction of mental health care.

An Overview of Mental Health Laws and Judicial Decisions

In the last twenty years, the courts have had an impact on the direction of mental health legislation and state statutes. As a review of history tells us, the courts have traditionally been concerned with the possibility of wrongful commitment. Little attention was paid to the restrictions placed on the legal and civil rights of an individual once hospitalized. In recent years, however, the courts have become more concerned with the substantive rights of a hospitalized individual, including the right to treatment, the right not to perform institutional labor, and retention of civil rights such as the rights to communication, visitation, religious activities, and medical self-determination. This is reflected in many state statutes, along with an emphasis on procedural safeguards focused on involuntary commitment.

A review of mental health laws and judicial decisions underscores the fact that there is great variability from state to state. Because of this variability, it is critical to safe practice that nurses be knowledgeable about the mental health statutes and regulations in the state in which they practice. Most inpatient units maintain copies of these statutes, as do local law libraries. Nurses may also refer to the agency in their state that oversees mental health care.

Admission Categories

The two major categories of hospitalization are **voluntary admission** and **involuntary commitment.** Admission and release procedures differ accordingly. They are described below and compared in Table 11–1.

Voluntary Admission All states except Alabama now have some provision for voluntary admission. Voluntary admission comes about by written application for admission by prospective clients, or someone acting in their behalf, such as a parent or guardian. As the word *voluntary* implies, the client has a right to demand and obtain release. However, all states except California have what is called a "grace period" in which the client agrees to give notice, usually in writing, of the intention to leave. Depending on the statute, this grace period can last from 24 hours (in Arizona) to 15 days (in Oklahoma). It is justified on the grounds that the hospital staff needs time to examine the client to determine whether a change to involuntary status is indicated. The extra time also gives family and staff the opportunity to persuade the client to remain voluntarily. This "conditional provision" is seen by some as a covert form of involuntary hospitalization.

There are now statutory assurances in over half the states, compared with just nine a decade ago, that voluntary clients must be adequately informed of their rights and status.

Informal voluntary admission, an alternative to the structure and personal concessions required in voluntary admission, is an option in several states. This procedure is similar to that required in a medical admission. The prospective inpatient verbally requests admission and is free to leave the institution at any time. Informal voluntary admission procedures are more likely to be an option in general and private facilities than in state institutions, and they account for a small percentage (less than 1–9%) of all admissions in states that have this provision.

Involuntary Commitment The state's ability to hospitalize or *commit* an individual involuntarily is sanctioned by one of two state powers:

1. Police power enables the state to hospitalize people who are considered dangerous to others because of their illness.
2. **Parens patriae** power enables the state to take on the role of protector and assume reponsibility for people considered dangerous to themselves or unable to care for themselves in a potentially dangerous situation because of a mental disability.

Most states provide for more than one involuntary hospitalization procedure. Involuntary hospitalization can come about if the designated body, such as a court, an administrative tribunal, or the required number of physicians find that the prospective client's mental state meets the statutory criteria for involuntary commitment. The criteria vary from state to state according to the type of involuntary hospitalization. However, all state involuntary commitment statutes can be expected to include one or more of the following criteria:

- Dangerous to self or others.
- Unable to provide for basic needs.
- Mentally ill.

In an increasing number of states, involuntary commitment is justified only if the individual is dangerous to self or others because of a mental disorder. The remaining states augment this by stating that the client's need for

Table 11–1 Voluntary and Involuntary Hospitalization Compared

	VOLUNTARY ADMISSION		INVOLUNTARY COMMITMENT		
	Informal	*Voluntary*	*Emergency*	*Temporary*	*Extended*
Released	Anytime	Usually conditional	Average after 3–5 days	48 hours to 6 months	After 60–180 days or an indeterminate time
Use	Limited	Increasing	Increasing	Increasing	Decreasing
Criteria for admission	Client request	Client request	Usually client dangerousness	Client dangerousness or need of care and treatment	Client dangerousness or need of care and treatment

care and treatment may also justify commitment. For specific state laws governing civil commitment, see Parry (1994).

Involuntary hospitalization can be divided into three categories: (1) emergency, (2) temporary or observational, and (3) extended or indeterminate. Civil commitment to outpatient psychiatric treatment is also possible in a number of states. See the Research Note on clients' perception of involuntary hospitalization.

Emergency Emergency involuntary hospitalization is available in all states except Alabama, Arkansas, and Mississippi. It is a temporary measure with limited, short-range goals, and it deals largely with the prevention of behavior likely to create a "clear and present" danger to the client or others. Under common law, any official or private person has the right to detain a dangerous mentally disordered person.

Some formal application is required to initiate emergency detention. In some states, any citizen may make the application. In others, it is limited to police officers, health officers, and physicians. Because this type of involuntary admission is an emergency measure and is warranted only until the appropriate legal steps can be taken, the statutes limit the amount of time an individual can be detained. The limits range from 24 hours in states such as Arizona, Georgia, and Michigan to 20 days in New Jersey. The usual practice is to allow detention for 3–5 days.

Temporary or Observational Temporary or observational involuntary hospitalization is the involuntary commitment of an allegedly mentally deranged individual for a specified period of time to allow for adequate observation so that a diagnosis can be made and treatment instituted. The actual time period can vary from 48 hours (in Alaska) to as long as 6 months (in West Virginia).

In some states, any citizen can make an application for the temporary hospitalization of a person in need of aid. Others require a family member or guardian, a health or welfare officer, or a physician to apply. Temporary hospitalization may be brought about by the medical certification of one or two physicians, or it may require further approval by a judge, justice, or district attorney in some jurisdictions.

At the end of the observation period, several options are available. The treating physician may (1) discharge the client, (2) have the client stay voluntarily, or (3) file an application for extended hospitalization. In at least nine states, observational hospitalization is mandatory before a court ruling may be made in favor of extended hospitalization.

Extended or Indeterminate Indeterminate or extended involuntary hospitalization can come about through either judicial or nonjudicial procedures. *Judicial hospitalization procedures* require that a judge or jury determine whether the person is mentally ill to a degree that requires extended hospitalization. If so, the court orders the client hospitalized for an extended period (60–180 days) or an indeterminate time.

Proceedings are usually initiated by an application for hospitalization of an allegedly mentally ill person. About half the states permit any responsible person or citizen to make or swear to the application. Others allow only one or more of the following groups: relatives, public officers, physicians, and hospital superintendents. Supporting medical evidence may or may not be required at the time of application.

Most states having judicial hospitalization procedures make some provision for a prehearing medical examination in addition to the medical certification required to support the application. In all forty-eight jurisdictions having judicial hospitalization procedures, it is mandatory to notify the person proposed to be hospitalized of the hearing. Most states also require notice to the client's attorney, family, or guardian.

RESEARCH NOTE

Citation

Kinzelman AJ, Taynor J, et al.: Clients' perceptions of involuntary hospitalization. *J Psychosoc Nurs* 1994;32(6):28–32.

Study Problem/Purpose

The purpose of this study was to explore clients' perceptions of involuntary hospitalization.

Methods

A confidential open-ended interview schedule was administered after hospital discharge to 15 self-selected participants from a rural three-county mental health catchment area in the Midwest. The interview schedule was developed with input from the researchers, agency staff, family members, consumers. During the interview, the client's perceptions of the following events were explored: being taken to the hospital, the admission process, role in court proceedings, hospital experience, leaving the hospital, return to the community, then living in the community.

Findings

All participants identified the involuntary hospital experience as an emotionally painful and demanding one and welcomed the opportunity to share their perceptions. Panic levels of anxiety, fear, and confusion were the predominant feelings identified by clients on their way to the hospital. Clients with children remembered being worried about who would care for them in their absence. Shame and a sense of failure were identified by clients who were being readmitted. Helpful responses from nursing staff included a calm, patient manner, and a willingness to give clear explanations. During the admission process, clients continued to feel extreme anxiety. However, the demands of the admission process did little to take this into account. Helpful responses included flexibility on the part of the nursing staff in the admission procedures and attention to the physical needs and habits of the client.

Almost all participants voiced dissatisfaction with the court proceedings. Clients identified a need for more information about the hearing process prior to the proceedings. Also, clients wanted a chance to speak for themselves during the hearing. The predominant feelings during hospitalization were ones of anger, fear, sadness, and being trapped. More than half the clients voiced dissatisfaction with the medication prescribed and as outpatients discontinued the medication. Helpful responses included involvement of the client in treatment planning, including the medication regime. Leaving the hospital and returning to the community were action-oriented times for clients. Helpful responses from case managers focused on coping with the demands of daily living, finances, relationships, and community stigma.

Implications

This study demonstrates that once provided with the opportunity, clients can offer specific ideas about their health care, expectations, and needs. Nurses need to listen to communication such as this and incorporate the information into the planning of activities for clients. At minimum, this study sensitizes the nurse to the need to develop a structured, ongoing plan to elicit feelings from the client about the impact of involuntary hospitalization. In addition, in-hospital groups need to specifically address the issues inherent in the loss of freedom and forced disconnection from significant others. Outpatient groups for clients and families might be formed in order to discuss and facilitate reintegration into community life.

A hearing is mandatory in most states, although a few states leave it to the client to request it. While the client's presence is required at the hearing in a few states, most states merely permit attendance if it is not thought to be harmful to the client's condition or if the client in fact demands it. Few states require the hearing to be held in a courtroom. Most say the place is entirely discretionary.

Jury trials are no longer mandatory in any state, but fifteen states still have provisions for the use of a jury to decide the question of hospitalization.

Nonjudicial hospitalization procedures for extended or indeterminate involuntary hospitalization include both administrative and medical certification, but such procedures are much less prominent on the statute books than they were a decade ago. Three states (Nebraska, South Dakota, and West Virginia) have provisions for administrative hospitalization procedures. Extended hospitalization is brought about by an administrative board, which basically follows the same procedure used in judicial hospitalization.

Involuntary hospitalization by *medical certification,* an alternative to the more traditional judicial commitment, is possible in eight states and the District of Columbia. It is usually advocated for clients who are incapable of consenting to voluntary treatment, although they do not protest hospitalization. The need for hospitalization is usually determined by an examination by one or more physicians and documented by a medical certificate. All states having medical certification provide either for judicial proceedings, if the client contests the hospitalization at any time after certification, or for expanded habeas corpus proceedings.

Involuntary Outpatient Commitment A growing number of states have modified their statutes and regulations to allow for court-ordered outpatient treatment. Although this option is not widely used at present, Perlin (1989) predicts it will be one of the growth areas in involuntary law in the near future. In most states allowing for involuntary outpatient commitment, the criteria are similar to that necessary for inpatient commitment: proof of mental illness and dangerousness. A few states have passed statutes permitting preventive commitment, considered by legal scholars to be a variation of involuntary outpatient commitment. In these instances, outpatient commitment is used to avert a further deterioration of the person's mental health that would require inpatient hospitalization. Geller (1992) found that involuntary outpatient treatment increased client compliance with neuroleptic medications and decreased the need for crisis services and inpatient hospitalization. Involuntary outpatient commitment has been used to ensure that mentally ill offenders follow through with outpatient treatment once they are released from prison. Conditional release, a concept related to outpatient commitment, is discussed later in this chapter.

Dilemmas Associated with Involuntary Commitment Involuntary hospitalization is an exercise of power, and like all forms of power, it can be abused. Because of this potential for abuse, commitment criteria are important. In this country, a person's loss of liberty can be justified only under certain circumstances. Loss of individual freedom through incarceration is generally accepted as justified if one is charged with a crime. In the past, people were quarantined if they had a contagious disease such as tuberculosis. Today debates continue regarding the restriction of activities of HIV-infected individuals and the public's right to safety.

As the review of mental health statutes shows, a degree of "dangerousness" is the favored justification for loss of liberty by involuntary hospitalization. The "dangerousness" criterion is not without its inherent problems. Some of these are considered to be the following:

- Definitions of "dangerousness" vary from state to state.
- It is impossible to predict dangerous behavior reliably.
- In the absence of other criteria, "dangerousness" will be overused to justify admission.
- The stigma of *dangerous* will be added to that of *mentally ill.*
- The stereotype of *mentally disabled* will be reinforced and thus will work against the development of community programs.
- The media will be encouraged to continue selective reporting of instances in which mental illness and criminal behavior appear to be linked.
- Clinical practice shows that "dangerous" individuals are often not treatable, while the most treatable individuals are not dangerous.

Discharge or Separation from a Mental Institution

A client can separate from a mental institution in one of three ways: discharge, transfer, and escape.

DISCHARGE Like admission, discharge from a mental hospital can have various layers of complexity. Discharges occur in one of two ways—conditionally or absolutely.

Conditional As implied by the word *conditional,* complete discharge in this situation depends on whether the person fulfills certain conditions over a specified period of time, usually 6 months to 1 year. Compliance with outpatient care, demonstrated ability and willingness to take medications, and the ability to meet the needs of daily living are a few of the many possible prerequisites.

A person who is unable to meet the specified conditions can be reinstitutionalized without going through any legal admission procedure. An individual committed for an extended or indeterminate time is more likely to be a candidate for conditional than absolute discharge.

Absolute The legal relationship between the institution and the client is terminated by an absolute discharge. If the client should require readmission to the hospital at any time, even a few hours after discharge, a new hospitalization proceeding would be required.

An absolute discharge can be achieved in three ways:

1. An administrative discharge is issued by the hospital officials.
2. A judicial discharge is ordered by the courts.
3. A writ of habeas corpus is ordered by the courts on the client's application.

As a rule, the authority for discharging involuntary clients rests in the hands of the hospital superintendent, and these clients are given administrative discharges. However, a few statutes extend this power to the central agency responsible for supervising mental institutions in the state, such as the Department of Mental Hygiene. The client has no formal method of initiating an administrative discharge.

Twenty-seven states have provisions for judicial discharge, which is initiated by an application to the court by the client, the client's family, or any citizen who is in disagreement with hospital authorities over the client's need to be hospitalized. A few states require the application to be accompanied by a medical certificate supporting the idea that the client is ready for discharge. In many states, judicial discharge does not depend on complete recovery. A degree of improvement may be sufficient. Twenty-one states guard against frequent applications for discharge by the same clients by imposing a 3-month to 1-year waiting period between requests.

All but a few states recognize the right of clients, or persons acting in their behalf, to question, by means of a **writ of habeas corpus**, the legality of their detention in a mental hospital. Dating back to English common law, this document is available not only to mental health clients but also to any person deprived of liberty through illegal detention. The question of the need for continued confinement of the client is not addressed by habeas corpus in most states. Some courts have expanded the writ to include an examination of the client's mental status at the time of the proceedings. In these cases, the basic criterion for further detention or release is the client's present mental status. This expanded use of the writ is reflected in the statutes of at least sixteen states.

TRANSFER Transfers account for approximately 3% of the separations from a mental health care facility. Most are transfers within the state and county mental health system. A smaller number are transfers from state to federal facilities or from one state to another.

ESCAPE A client may take the initiative and decide to terminate the relationship with the institution by informally leaving the hospital grounds. This is commonly referred to as escape, **elopement**, or being AWOL (absent without leave). Voluntary clients cannot generally be returned to the hospital against their will. However, involuntarily committed clients may be brought back to the hospital against their will with the assistance of the police, if necessary.

Rights of Clients

The current concern for client rights has not developed overnight. It actually has been evolving since the 1960s, when there was an increased interest in underrepresented minority groups including blacks, the poor, women, and the mentally disabled.

In 1980 the United States Congress passed the Mental Health Systems Act, which included a model mental health client's bill of rights. This model bill of rights is summarized in the box on the next page. The Omnibus Budget Reconciliation Act of 1981 brought about the repeal of parts of the Mental Health Systems Act but did retain the bill of rights. Mental patients have published their own version of a bill of rights featured on page 184 in Chapter 10.

INFORMED CONSENT A client has the right to understand and participate in the treatment process prior to consenting to treatment. **Informed consent** is required by all states by either case law or statute. The main purpose of the doctrine of informed consent is to encourage individual autonomy and sound decision making. Client self-determination is the basic principle of informed consent.

Key elements of informed consent are **competency**, information, and voluntariness. A client must be cognitively able to understand the situation and the implications of treatment. If a client's competency is in question, a mental status examination may be necessary. The medication record may need to be reviewed to determine if the client received medication that might interfere with cognitive ability. Any deficits in the client's reception and processing of information need to be taken into account. The client must be competent to understand the problem, along with the negative and positive effects from the proposed treatment, and the likely outcome with and without treatment.

Many illnesses impair the ability to acquire new information. At times, this is a response to the biologic components of the illness or the effects of medication. Other times, there may be an educational deficit. For some long-term clients, the presence of a mental illness may have affected the educational experience. This does not mean that intelligence is affected, but that reading and writing skills may not be consistent with chronological age. It is essential for the nurse to develop plans for offering information that would be needed in the decision-making process. It may be necessary to present information in small pieces using simple language and pictures. Several short presentations may be required with some mechanism to assess learning to determine whether the client understands the proposed treatment.

All clients must be offered choices and given the advantages and disadvantages of each. While members of the mental health team can offer suggestions, it must be clear to the client that there is no self-serving bias on the part of the treatment team for one choice or another. The client must have the opportunity to ask questions or gain a second opinion. The client should not be rushed or coerced into giving consent.

Mental Health Systems Act Bill of Rights

1. Right to appropriate treatment in the least restrictive setting.
2. Right to individualized treatment plan, subject to review and reassessment. To include assessment of mental health services needed after discharge.
3. Right to active participation in treatment, with the risk, side effects, and benefits of all medication and treatment to be discussed, as well as treatment alternatives.
4. Right to give or withhold consent. May be treated without personal consent only in emergencies or with the consent of a guardian after incompetency has been determined by a court.
5. Right to be free of experimentation unless it follows the recommendations of the National Commission on Protection of Human Subjects.
6. Right to be free of restraints except in an emergency and unless restraints are specifically part of the treatment plan, always subject to the participation and consent requirements. Applies also to behavior-modification techniques involving restraints and seclusion.
7. Right to a humane environment.
8. Right to confidentiality of mental health information.
9. Right of access to personal treatment records unless two mental health professionals believe it to be detrimental.
10. Right to as much freedom as possible to exercise constitutional rights of association and expression. Restriction of specific visitors is allowed only if fully documented and part of the treatment plan.
11. Right to information about these rights in both written and oral form, presented in an understandable manner at the outset of treatment and periodically thereafter.
12. Right to assert grievances through a mechanism that includes the power to go to court.
13. Right to obtain advocacy assistance.
14. Right to criticize or complain about conditions or services without fear of retaliatory punishment or other reprisals.
15. Right to referral to complement the discharge plan.

Informed consent must be documented in writing through the use of a specific form signed by the client, or by an entry into the client's medical record. While written documentation of informed consent will likely fulfill the legal obligation, it is helpful to think of informed consent as more of a reoccurring process. While hospitalized, clients should be offered many chances to participate in their own care.

At times, it may become clear that the client lacks the ability to offer consent. In this case, it is important to interact with legal counsel to determine what should be done. Some states will allow legal relatives to participate for a client who cannot consent. Other states demand that the client have an advocate appointed to serve as decision maker. For a summary of informed consent requirements, see the accompanying box.

RIGHT TO TREATMENT The first argument for a right to treatment for involuntarily committed individuals came from Morton Birnbaum, a lawyer and a physician, in an article published in 1960. However, the ground-breaking cases did not come from the familiar circles of civil commitment but from people who had been sidetracked from the prison system into hospitals.

Rouse v Cameron The first case to address the right to treatment issue directly and gain national attention was *Rouse v Cameron,* 373 F2d 451 (DC Cir 1966). In 1962, Charles Rouse had been brought to trial for carrying a dangerous weapon, which is a misdemeanor in the District of Columbia and carries a maximum sentence of one year. Instead of being convicted and sent to trial, Rouse pleaded "not guilty by reason of insanity" and was sent to the maximum security pavilion at Saint Elizabeth's Hospital for treatment. Under District of Columbia law, the plea of insanity takes away criminal responsibility and subjects the defendant to an automatic involuntary commitment.

Informed Consent Requirements

Informed consent requires that the client:

- Is of the age of consent.
- Is deemed mentally competent.
- Can state that he or she is acting voluntarily.
- Can repeat the elements of the condition.
- Can repeat the treatment options.
- Can repeat the benefits and consequences of each treatment.
- Can repeat the consequences of inaction.
- Is not impaired by alcohol or other drugs.
- Can complete the specific written forms such as consent forms, treatment plans, and discharge plans.

Four years later, Rouse questioned his detention by means of a writ of habeas corpus on the grounds that he had not received any psychiatric treatment. His lawyer argued that he was entitled to treatment in exchange for loss of liberty. State laws vary tremendously on how the person committed by reason of insanity obtains release. Some state statutes require the person to remain committed until pardoned by the governor. Others require the person to meet the same criteria for discharge as any other civilly committed individual.

Judge David Bazelon, speaking for the United States Court of Appeals for the District of Columbia, stated that involuntary commitment is imposed because it is assumed that the criminal offender needs treatment for a mental condition. If treatment is not given, as in Rouse's case, the court held, the offender is deprived of basic rights. Although Judge Bazelon said Rouse was entitled to treatment on the basis of the present District of Columbia statute, he indicated that there might be a constitutional basis for the right as well. Whenever possible, however, courts will base their decisions in statutory rather than constitutional grounds.

Nason v Bridgewater Another important decision was the Supreme Judicial Court of Massachusetts ruling in *Nason v Bridgewater,* 233 NE2d 908 (Mass 1968). John Nason, a man indicted for murder, had been sent to Bridgewater State Hospital because he was found incompetent to stand trial. After spending five years at Bridgewater, the Massachusetts facility for the dangerously insane, he filed a writ of habeas corpus for his release on the grounds that he was not receiving adequate treatment, and he requested transfer to another facility. Through expert testimony, Nason's attorneys were able to show that staffing at Bridgewater was so grossly inadequate that Nason was simply receiving custodial care. The court acknowledged the existence of a constitutional right to treatment, at least for incompetent people awaiting trial, and even went on to suggest what a proper treatment plan for Nason would be.

While *Rouse* and *Nason* may have had little impact on the actual delivery of care in most institutions around the country, they did articulate the right to treatment and provided a statutory and tentative constitutional rationale for that right.

Wyatt v Stickney The next step in the move to establish a right to treatment through the court system was taken in Alabama in 1970, with the filing of *Wyatt v Stickney,* 344 F Supp 373 (MD Ala 1972). It was the first class-action suit successfully brought against a state's entire mental health care system. The issue was detention without treatment of individuals committed civilly and involuntarily. The court established that involuntary clients have a constitutional right to individualized treatment that will give each of them a realistic chance to be cured or at least improve. The court found that the treatment program in Alabama state institutions was deficient in three fundamental areas. It did not provide (1) a humane psychologic and physical environment, (2) qualified staff to administer adequate treatment, and (3) individualized treatment plans. To remedy these defects, the court promulgated a lengthy and detailed set of standards, including the following:

- Provisions against institutional peonage (the institutional use of clients for work).
- A number of protections to ensure a humane psychologic and safe physical environment.
- Minimum staffing requirements.
- Establishment of a human rights committee at each institution.
- A requirement that every client has a right to the least restrictive setting necessary for treatment.

If the standards could not be met and clients were denied adequate treatment, the court stated, they had to be released from custody. In the words of Judge Johnson, "to deprive any citizen of his or her liberty upon the altruistic theory that confinement is for human therapeutic reasons and then fail to provide adequate treatment violates the very fundamentals of due process" (*Wyatt v Stickney,* 325 F Supp 781, 785 [MD Ala 1971]).

Donaldson v O'Connor Another important development in the constitutional right to treatment controversy was *Donaldson v O'Connor,* 493 F2d 507 (5th Cir 1974). Kenneth Donaldson, an involuntary patient in a Florida mental hospital for over 14 years, brought suit against the hospital superintendent, alleging that the superintendent had maliciously deprived him of his constitutional right to liberty. At trial, the jury found that (1) Donaldson had received not merely inadequate treatment but no treatment at all, (2) he was not dangerous, (3) acceptable community alternatives were in fact available for Donaldson, and (4) the doctor, knowing all this, had "maliciously" refused to release him.

On appeal, the federal court of appeals held that there is a constitutional right to treatment, and it awarded $38,000 in compensatory and punitive damages to Donaldson. However, the United States Supreme Court declined to affirm the court of appeals finding of constitutional right to treatment. The court said that the case raised a single question concerning every person's constitutional right to liberty—that is: Does one have the right to be discharged from custodial care if not dangerous to self or others, the right not to receive treatment if one can survive safely in freedom? The unanimous answer was yes (*O'Connor v Donaldson,* 43 USLW 4929 [1975]).

In February 1977, at the age of 67, Kenneth Donaldson was awarded $20,000 from two defendant psychiatrists. Donaldson's lawsuit had been undertaken in the public interest by the American Civil Liberties Union and the Mental Health Law Project, and a ruling in early May 1977 entitled Donaldson to recover reasonable attorneys' fees. Donaldson has written a book about his confinement, *Insanity Inside Out* (1976).

The concept of right to treatment is an outgrowth of the philosophic point of view that the deprivation of liberty, whether voluntarily or involuntarily, must have an overriding purpose. A review of court cases indicates that the right to treatment came about because there was no overriding purpose: Because of overcrowded conditions, inadequate staffing, financial and programmatic deficiencies, there were not enough resources to deliver the bare minimum of treatment. "Right to treatment" ensures that clients are not in a treatment setting for custodial purposes only. The necessary elements in a treatment-oriented program are:

- Physical examination and psychosocial assessment on admission and then as indicated.
- Treatment plans with clear objectives and interventions.
- Evidence of client participation in treatment planning and consent for all treatment methods.
- Up-to-date medical records.
- Treatment in as normal an environment as possible.
- Staff in adequate numbers and with sufficient training to provide quality care.
- Availability of treatment that meets client needs as identified in the treatment plan.
- Necessary support services such as dental, speech, physical, and rehabilitation therapy.
- Ongoing treatment plan evaluations.
- Programs to help clients develop skills needed for independent versus institutional living.
- Adequate planning for discharge to a less restrictive setting, according to client needs.

Some of the unresolved problems or questions regarding the issue of right to treatment are the cost in tax dollars and the difficulty in providing effective treatment for all conditions. If effective treatment does not exist, is custodial care enough?

Right to Refuse Treatment The courts articulated a committed client's right to treatment over a decade ago. More recently, the courts have been asked to rule on whether the client in a mental institution has the right to refuse treatment.

One of the first cases was *Price v Sheppard,* 239 NW 2d 905 (Minn 1976), in which electroconvulsive therapy was felt to be an "intrusive" treatment and not allowed to be given against a competent client's wishes. The two best known cases are *Rennie v Klein* and *Rogers v Okin.*

Rennie v Klein *Rennie v Klein* was initiated in December 1977 by John Rennie, an involuntarily committed client at a New Jersey state hospital who claimed that the hospital and the New Jersey Department of Human Services were violating his constitutional rights by forcibly administering medication. Rennie had objected to the side effects produced by chlorpromazine (Thorazine) and lithium carbonate.

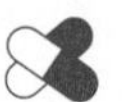

Judge Stanley Brotman ruled that involuntarily committed clients have a qualified right to refuse psychotropic medication (New Jersey statutes already stated that voluntary clients have an absolute right to reject medication). His decision was based on the constitutional right to protect their mental processes from government interference. Judge Brotman, impressed by the side effects of psychotropic medication, stated, "Individual autonomy demands that the person subjected to the harsh side-effects of psychotropic drugs have control over their administration" (*Rennie v Klein* 462 F Supp at 1145).

Judge Brotman did qualify the right to refuse, listing four factors to be considered in overriding a client's objection:

1. *Safety.* Is the client a physical threat to other clients or staff members?
2. *Competency.* Is the client competent to make treatment decisions?

3. *Less restrictive means.* Do less restrictive means of treatment exist, and are they available?
4. *Risk versus benefit.* What are the risks of permanent side effects from the proposed treatment?

In 1979, Rennie's complaint was amended to include class-action allegations, and the court went on to add more specific steps to be followed in implementing an involuntarily committed client's qualified right to refuse treatment. These included:

1. Notify clients that they have a right to refuse medication.
2. Provide clients with information regarding potential side effects of the medication.
3. Obtain written consent prior to initiation of the medication.

If written consent is withheld by a client already declared "legally incompetent" by the court or certified "functionally incompetent" by a treating psychiatrist, the decision to medicate forcibly would be referred to a client advocate. It would be up to the client advocate's discretion to request a hearing before an independent psychiatrist, who would base a decision on the four factors mentioned above. In the case of a competent though involuntarily hospitalized person, a hearing before an independent psychiatrist would be required at which the client would have the right to legal counsel.

Rogers v Okin Another important case in the establishment of a client's right to refuse medication is *Rogers v Okin,* 478 F Supp (D Mass 1979). In 1975 a class-action suit was initiated by clients at Boston State Hospital, who contended that their constitutional rights were being violated by the hospital's practice of using forced seclusion and medication in nonemergency situations. Judge Joseph Tauro issued a temporary restraining order against the use of seclusion and medication without the client's informed consent. In the case of a person declared incompetent by the court, informed consent would need to be elicited from the client's guardian. This restraining order applied to both voluntary and involuntary clients. In 1979, after a lengthy trial, the court made the temporary restraining order permanent.

Judge Tauro based his decision on the constitutional right to privacy (right to be left alone) and the first amendment right to freedom of thought. While Judge Tauro recognized that safety considerations might necessitate forcible administration of medication, he allowed much less discretion on the part of the hospital staff than did Judge Brotman in *Rennie.* Only in emergencies that create a substantial likelihood of physical harm to the client or others could medication be forcibly administered. Judge Tauro did not include a set of procedures to be followed in the case of client refusal, as had been done in *Rennie.* Instead, hospital staff members were directed to apply to the court for a competency hearing and the subsequent appointment of a guardian for clients they believed to be incompetent to make treatment decisions. The decision in *Rogers* is considered to be more far-reaching than that in *Rennie* because it grants competent clients and guardians of incompetent clients an absolute right to refuse medication in nonemergency situations.

Other recent court decisions support a qualified right to refuse psychotropic medication, unless a legitimate emergency exists. It is vital to remember that overriding a client's right to refuse treatment is legally complicated and related to safeguards that are in place to manage such situations. These legal safeguards serve to protect the rights of all people.

Dilemmas Associated with the Right to Refuse Treatment There are a number of areas of judicial disagreement in the right to refuse treatment that will create dilemmas for the mental health care professional. For example, there is no common definition of the term *psychiatric emergency.* The traditional definition of *emergency* refers to an overt and immediate threat to a person's life. The contemporary definition focuses on the immediate, impending, and significant deterioration of the client's condition.

Another area of controversy is: At what point can the state override an involuntarily committed client's right to refuse psychotropic medication in a nonemergency? Is it only when a person has been judged incompetent, or does danger to self or others provide a legitimate reason under the state's police power to administer treatment?

In the case of an incompetent individual, there is disagreement over who should decide for the person and what standard should be used. Is it to be a guardian, the hospital staff, or the judiciary? Is the standard to be what the best interests of the client seem to be as judged by an informed outsider, or is it what the client would want if competent to make the choice?

Here are some criteria a court is likely to use in ruling on a case involving the right to refuse treatment:

- *Client competency.* If the client is competent, informed consent is possible.
- *Intrusiveness of treatment.* As the intrusiveness increases, so does the court's scrutiny.
- *Permanence of treatment effect.* If side effects are adverse and permanent, the court is less likely to override refusal.
- *Experimental nature of treatment.* The treatment must have scientific merit, and the client must give informed consent.
- *Risk-benefit ratio.* The benefits of treatment must outweigh the risk.

- *Motivation for treatment.* The treatment cannot be used to punish or "quiet" the client for the staff's benefit.
- *Motivation for refusal.* Religious objections are usually upheld.

Despite the difficulties and issues raised by the client's right to refuse treatment, some very real positive outcomes are these:

- Clients must be involved in treatment choices, process, and outcome.
- Clients must be informed of choices and offered alternatives.
- Staff members must acquire a second opinion on potentially harmful procedures.

LEAST RESTRICTIVE ALTERNATIVE The idea of least restrictive alternative has become an important component of both the deinstitutionalization and client rights movements. The term **least restrictive alternative (LRA)** generally refers to the placement of clients in the therapeutic setting that will provide care while allowing maximum freedom. Several important cases bear on this topic.

The first of these was *Lake v Cameron,* 364 F2d 657 (DC Cir 1966). Mrs. Lake, a 61-year-old woman, had difficulty caring for herself because of confusion secondary to arteriosclerotic brain disease. While not considered a danger to others, she did wander when confused and was subsequently admitted to St. Elizabeth's Hospital. The court ruled that Lake did not need 24-hour psychiatric supervision and a less restrictive form of treatment should be found. Ironically, even though Lake won her case, she ended up dying at St. Elizabeth's because no other facility was available.

While in principle the right to LRA is relatively straightforward, its implementation is often not clear-cut. Munetz and Geller (1993) propose that LRA can be useful, in this current postinstitutionalization era, only if its complexity is recognized. This means that the LRA for a client cannot be predetermined but must be individually assessed, according to the needs and desires of the client.

The American Nurses Association's Standards of Psychiatric–Mental Health Clinical Nursing Practice expect that the nurse will choose the least restrictive limit and use it only for as long as it is necessary for the safety of the client and others. To help nurses begin to judge the restrictiveness of an intervention, Garritson (1983) suggests consideration of the following dimensions:

- Treatment setting
- Institutional policy
- Enforcement
- Treatment
- Client characteristics

Treatment Setting Treatment setting is evaluated on such criteria as the limitations it places on physical freedom (locked or unlocked), choice of activities, and the presence of "adult status" as shown by locked bedrooms and the unsupervised use of private bathroom facilities. In this scheme, total institutions would be considered the most restrictive, halfway houses less so, and family or independent living the least.

Institutional Policy Institutional policy is the degree of restriction imposed by the rules and regulations necessary to run the institution. Criteria to evaluate a setting would include such items as the amount of supervision in daily living tasks, the amount of client involvement in treatment planning, and the priority of activities that increase the client's autonomy.

Enforcement The enforcement dimension includes the methods sanctioned to enforce the institution's rules. Is coercion or threat of punishment used? Is the standard for socially acceptable behavior higher in the institution than it would be in the client's own environment? For example, a nurse says to a client, "We don't use that foul language here . . . I don't think you're ready for that pass." How readily and to what extent is the client's autonomy compromised to meet organizational needs?

Treatment The treatment dimension has to do with the intrusiveness of the treatment used. Psychosurgery and electroconvulsive therapy would be considered more intrusive than medication. Long-acting medication such as fluphenazine decanoate would be considered more intrusive than oral medication. The clarity of treatment goals is also a consideration. Nebulous or nonexistent goals increase restrictiveness.

Client Characteristics The client's illness characteristics are seen by some as restricting behavior to a much greater degree than any locked door. Some believe it is simplistic to think that moving a client from an institutional setting to the community will automatically result in less restriction. Without effective community-based treatment, including safe housing, many chronically ill clients frequently end up in "psychiatric ghettos" (see Chapter 21).

COMMUNICATION AND VISITATION All but three states (Alabama, Mississippi, and West Virginia) have some statutory provisions on client correspondence. The basis for laws granting communication rights is that such communication can expose cases of wrongful hospitalization. Generally, communication is unrestricted or guaranteed to named public officials or the central hospital agency for the state. Twenty-seven states extend this guarantee to include correspondence with attorneys. Most states require that any correspondence limitation be part of the client's clinical record. Approximately half the states require the client to have reasonable access to writing materials and postage.

All but five states (Alabama, Mississippi, Pennsylvania, Virginia, and West Virginia) have some statutory provisions concerning visitation. However, hospital authorities are generally given broad discretionary powers to curtail this right. Before implementing any restriction in communication or visitation, the nurse should ask: Is it fair and reasonable? Could I defend it to a noninvolved professional?

RESTRAINTS AND SECLUSION Though improvements in treatment have decreased the use of mechanical or physical restraints, such restraints still play a role in some treatment programs. Most states have attempted to regulate their use by statute. Twenty-six states specify that restraints can be used when the client presents a risk of harm to self or others. Eight states also permit the use of restraints for therapeutic purposes. Some states specifically say restraints are not to be used for punishment or staff convenience. In those states not having statutory provisions regarding restraints, the procedures to be followed are usually found in the administrative regulations.

Half the states have laws relating to seclusion. Prevention of harm to self or others is the most common criterion, followed by treatment or therapeutic reasons. Colorado specifically prohibits the use of seclusion but does allow a time-out period. The use of either restraints or seclusion must be documented in the client's medical record in most states.

ELECTROCONVULSIVE THERAPY AND PSYCHOSURGERY In almost all states, electroconvulsive therapy (ECT) is closely regulated by statute. Most state statutes specify that ECT can be administered only if informed consent is obtained from the client. In the case of an incompetent client, consent must be obtained from the guardian or next of kin. The client's right to refuse ECT is specifically mentioned in many state statutes.

Psychosurgery, referred to in various state statutes as "brain surgery," "lobotomy," or "experimental" or "hazardous" procedures, is also closely regulated by state statute. Most state statutes specify that psychosurgery can be performed only if informed consent is obtained from the client. In several states, psychosurgery can be performed only upon a court order if the client is incompetent. The client's right to refuse psychosurgery is also specifically mentioned in many state statutes.

PERIODIC REVIEW Thirty-one states and the District of Columbia have some provision for periodic review of involuntary clients. Periodic review provides some protection for the individual against spending more time than necessary in the hospital. Review is required every 30 days in some states, every year in others. A few states require review "as frequently as necessary," or "from time to time." The actual scope of the review is usually not governed by statute. The trend in recent years has been away from hospitalization for indeterminate periods of time. In New York and California, short-term commitment is the rule, and court review is necessary to extend commitment for another short period.

PARTICIPATION IN LEGAL MATTERS Psychiatric clients have rights to participate as citizens in legal matters.

Contracts Clients committed to a mental hospital generally maintain their right to make a valid contract, unless they have also been judged incompetent. In most states, commitment proceedings are separate from those for competence. Therefore, an individual who is "legally incompetent" is not necessarily subject to commitment, and an individual committed to an institution is not automatically legally incompetent. Even though the issue of contracts may seem clear-cut, in reality a client's right to contract may be restricted by the administrative regulations of hospitals and state mental health agencies. A contested contract would most likely be a matter for the court to decide.

Wills To make a valid will, a person must:

- Be aware of making a will.
- Be familiar with the property being disposed of.
- Know the names, identities, and relationships of the people named in the will.

A person with a psychiatric diagnosis, whether in or out of the hospital, can make a valid will as long as these requirements are met. Psychosis with accompanying delusions does not by itself negate a valid will. The delusions have to produce a significant distortion of the person's perception of the property, family, or personal relationships to invalidate the will.

Marriage and Divorce According to statute and common law, a valid marriage contract hinges on the individual's possession of sufficient mental capacity to give consent. Sufficient mental capacity implies that the person:

- Understands the nature of the marriage relationship.
- Knows the duties and obligations involved.

The statutes of a small number of states prohibit marriage by mentally disordered people because they are believed to be incapable of making a contract. More states, however, prohibit marriage by the mentally disordered on the grounds that they are "insane" or "of unsound mind," without specifically defining these terms. Despite these prohibiting statutes, few states even try to enforce the prohibition outside mental institutions.

Most states have provisions for annulment or divorce on the grounds of prenuptial mental disability. Within the last 25 years, divorce on the grounds of postnuptial mental disability has been incorporated in the statutes of most states.

Voting Most states do not actually prohibit hospitalized people from voting. In fact, some specifically preserve this right by legislation. The institutionalized are eligible to register to vote in twelve states. In eighteen others, the ability to vote depends on a hospitalized client's legal competency. Only in Maryland and Missouri are individuals confined to an institution ineligible to vote. All states except Louisiana allow absentee voting by disabled persons. The hospitalized client's right to vote is probably more restricted by caretaker and community apathy than it is by statute.

Right to Drive Statutes on driving privileges are difficult to interpret. Most states will not issue a driver's license to mentally disturbed people. In some states this restriction also applies to epileptics, drug addicts, and alcoholics. Several states suspend a driver's license as soon as the individual enters a mental institution. Other jurisdictions limit the restriction to those admitted involuntarily, while still others base suspension on legal competency.

Right to Practice a Profession The ability of a hospitalized client to practice a profession is usually impaired simply by the physical confinement. However, most states have some statutes prohibiting the practice of a profession by a mentally disturbed person. The vagueness of the statutes often makes it difficult to know when they are applicable. As a rule, it is up to the professional licensing board to suspend or revoke the license of a member who is believed to be too mentally incapacitated to practice a profession safely, even though not hospitalized.

Rights of Children or Minors

The rights of children, along with those of other groups frequently considered politically powerless, have been the subject of judicial and legislative action over the last twenty years. Up until this time children or minors had few rights of their own. Under early common law, children were the parents' "property" and owed them strict obedience.

In most states, an individual is considered a minor or juvenile if younger than 18 years of age. As a minor the person is considered legally incompetent. Legal consent for medical treatment must come from parents or guardian. There are, however, a number of exceptions to this general rule of presumed legal incompetency in some state statutes. These include the rights to:

- Seek treatment for drug abuse.
- Consent to contraception.
- Seek psychiatric treatment.

Other factors, such as military service, marriage, emancipation, pregnancy, and parenthood, may also affect the age at which a minor may be considered competent.

The most controversial issue of a minor's role in the mental health system involves involuntary commitment. Like adults, minors can be committed to a mental hospital against their will. But, unlike adult admissions, the admission of a minor who objects is considered "voluntary" if the parents have authorized it. Because of the realization that parents may not always be acting in the best interests of the child, a number of lawsuits challenging this practice were filed in the 1970s. It was argued that the "voluntary" admission of minors without procedural safeguards was unconstitutional, and that a court hearing should always be held to determine if commitment is warranted. The Supreme Court had already ruled in 1967 *In re Gault* (387 US 1) that juveniles in the criminal justice system were entitled to some of the same procedural safeguards accorded adult defendants. Many states did not change their commitment statutes to include procedural safeguards. However, in the 1979 case *Parham v J.R.* (442 US 584), the United States Supreme Court upheld the rights of parents to admit their children to psychiatric facilities as long as a "neutral factfinder" (physician) believes medical standards for admission have been met.

The trend for inclusion of procedural safeguards, though slowed by the ruling in *Parham v J.R.*, continues as an increasing number of states have modified their "voluntary" parental commitment statute by one or more of the following factors:

- Lowering the age of required consent. In four states (Alaska, Idaho, Vermont, and Pennsylvania), the age is 15 or older. The majority of states specify age 16–18. In New Jersey, 21 is the age of consent.
- Requiring the consent of the child.
- Providing for a court hearing if the child protests.
- Providing for self-initiated institutionalization for minors. In New Mexico, a child 12 years or older qualifies for self-initiated hospitalization; six other states cite age 14; and the rest are divided between ages 16 and 18 years.

Therapist-Client-Public Relations

Legal conventions provide direction about appropriate action in therapist-client-public relationships.

Confidentiality Almost all states have a specific statute regarding confidentiality of client information, and the specific steps to be taken for release of that information. The confidential nature of the client information is also cited in the American Nurses Association Code of Ethics, as it is in most professional codes.

The goal of confidentiality is to ensure the client's privacy. There is a significant amount of stigma attached to being the recipient of psychiatric treatment. Though professionals may argue that this is unfair, it is a fact. Because of this, it is important that clients be the ones to give out this information about themselves. Instructors, students, supervisors, or team members who receive information about a client in the course of supervision or in providing treatment for the client are also obligated to treat this material as confidential.

In order for the disclosure of information to occur, a client must sign a release form. To be a valid release, the client must be told as specifically as possible what information is to be released. The client should know the following prior to signing.

- What information is going to be released?
- Who needs it?
- Why do they need it?
- When will they need it?
- How will it be used?

Emergency situations may arise. For example, a client may be in a car accident or take an overdose while out on pass and end up being treated in another hospital's emergency room. In these situations, the release of information can occur without the client's approval. It is important to document such a breach of confidentiality.

Confidentiality of information is not easy to maintain. Medical records are generally kept, not in locked files, but at an easy access point in the nurses' station. Medical files usually travel all over the hospital with the client and are often available for the perusal of others not directly involved in the client's treatment. The increased use of computers for communication and data storage, along with the information requested by the government, third-party payers, and employers, often poses a threat to a client's privacy. More mundane incidences of breaches of confidentiality occur when staff members talk about clients in the halls, elevator, and cafeteria.

Privileged Communication **Privileged communication** is a narrower concept than confidentiality. It is established by state statute to protect possibly incriminating disclosures made by the client to specified professionals. Privileged communication has traditionally existed between husband and wife, attorney and client, clergy and church member, and physician and client. In some states, communication between psychologist and client is also accorded privileged status. Arkansas, New York, Oregon, Vermont, and Wisconsin recognize privileged communication between nurse and client. The privilege is the client's and can be claimed only if a therapeutic relationship exists. The professional can reveal the information at the client's request.

Each state that grants a privilege also specifies exceptions to that privilege. The most common exceptions include:

- When the therapist suspects child abuse, elder abuse, or spousal abuse.
- When the therapist is seeking civil commitment.
- When the court orders the exam.
- When the client introduces a defense of mental illness into litigation proceedings (likely to happen in child custody disputes, malpractice suits against therapists, personal injury suits, workers' compensation cases, and will contests).
- When the client poses a danger to others (establishes the therapist's duty to warn).

Disclosure to Safeguard Others An exception to confidentiality and privilege that has developed from a California Supreme Court decision illustrates the competition between two responsibilities of the mental health care professional: (1) confidentiality to the client, and (2) protection of the public from the "violent" client. The court's ruling underlines the mental health care professional's responsibility to balance the two.

In *Tarasoff v Regents of the University of California,* 13 CAL3d 177, 529 P2d 553, 118 Cal Rptr 129 (1974), the parents of Tatiana Tarasoff successfully sued the University of California, claiming that a psychotherapist on the staff of the university's student counseling center had a responsibility to warn their daughter that his client, Prosenjit Poddar, had threatened to kill her when she returned from a trip abroad. At the time, the psychologist did notify campus security officers that he believed his client was dangerous and should be involuntarily committed for observation and treatment. However, Poddar appeared rational to the police and promised them he would stay away from Tarasoff. Poddar terminated treatment, and two months later killed Tatiana Tarasoff.

The suit was brought on two accounts: (1) failure to warn Tarasoff, and (2) failure to detain Poddar for treatment. Although the suit was dismissed by the lower courts, on appeal the California Supreme Court reversed the dismissal, saying that, despite the unsuccessful attempt to confine Poddar, the therapist knew that Poddar was at large and dangerous and had a duty to warn Tarasoff of the danger. The court recognized the client's right to confidentiality but said this must be weighed against the public's need for safety against violent assault, especially when an individual in danger can be identified. The *Tarasoff* concept or at least some version of it has continued to be reaffirmed in several state and federal jurisdictions. In a number of cases, therapists were held liable for not taking some action to protect potential unidentified victims. Douard and Winslade (1994) believe it would be in the best interest of the public and mental health care professionals if the *Tarasoff* principle were expressed and clarified by state statute.

Appelbaum (1985) suggests a change from the idea of a "duty to warn" to that of a "duty to protect." The accompanying Intervention box shows a model to help mental health caregivers decide on a course of action in implementing the duty to warn or protect.

Situations in which reporting by physicians to authorities is required by law include child and elder abuse, knife or gunshot wounds, certain contagious diseases, and the driving of a car by a person with unstable epilepsy. In court cases so far, a client's voicing of suicidal ideation does *not* create a duty to warn. The duty to warn or protect applies only when there is danger to others.

The duty to warn has stirred up controversy in the mental health community. There is a concern about the fact that clients with aggression problems will drop out of therapy, not use it effectively, or be less likely to seek treatment for fear of being betrayed. Remember also that no mental health care professional can reliably predict the future violence of a mentally disordered person.

The Intersection of Psychiatry and Criminal Law

Psychiatry also affects the resolution of such legal questions as the credibility of witnesses, competency to make a will or contract or to stand trial, compensation of injured persons, custody of children, and, most controversial, criminal responsibility. Forensic nursing is a new clinical subspecialty that focuses on evaluating and treating perpetrators and victims of criminal and interpersonal violence and the families of both.

INTERVENTION

A Model for Implementing the Duty to Warn or Protect

Action	*Implementation*
Assess dangerousness	Compare data to factors believed to correlate with dangerous behavior, such as increasing use of drugs and/or alcohol, current and past threats of violence and/or assaultive behavior, presence of command hallucinations.
	Be sure to review past and current treatment records. Interview client, family, and significant others.
	Ask: Is the threat serious? Are the threats repeated? Are the means to carry out the threat available? Can the victim be identified? Is the victim accessible?
Select a course of action to protect the victim	Consider either voluntary hospitalization, or, if necessary, initiate involuntary commitment.
	If the client is already hospitalized, is a more secure unit needed to prevent escape?
	If the client is an outpatient, is medication needed? Are more frequent visits needed? Is a more intensive outpatient care needed, such as a day program?
	Because threats often involve family members, is intensive, systems-oriented therapy indicated to include the intended victim?
	If containment or control is not possible, contact the identified victim. Consider also alerting the police.
Implement decision	Continue to monitor: If initial course of action fails, take other measures. Be sure to document this decision-making process in the client's record.

Competency to Stand Trial

Competency to stand trial is based on our common law tradition that defendants must have the mental capacity to defend themselves in a court of law. The process of determining competency to stand trial is the issue most frequently leading to the hospitalization of individuals in the criminal justice system. Until 1972, pretrial commitment was widely used as the final disposition. The defendant failed to become "competent" and remained in the institution indefinitely.

Such was the case in *Jackson v Indiana*. The defendant was a 27-year-old retarded, hearing-impaired, mute individual accused of stealing property valued at $9 and confined to a maximum security unit awaiting trial. Because of his disabilities, it was doubted that he would ever become competent to stand trial. In its ruling, the United States Supreme Court set out some general limitations on the length of pretrial commitments, saying a person cannot be held more than a "reasonable period of time." If the person is unlikely to become competent to stand trial, the civil commitment standards must be met, or the person must be released.

A psychiatric nurse clinician is qualified in some states to perform competency evaluations by interviewing the defendant to determine his or her understanding of the nature of the legal process, recognition of the consequences of the accusation, and ability to assist counsel in the defense.

A competency evaluation no longer requires an inpatient stay and may be done in a prison outpatient setting. While not many nurses may actually perform competency evaluations, nurses employed in public mental hospitals may work with clients transferred from the prison system for treatment to regain their competency.

The Insanity Defense

All civilized cultures have had some form of insanity defense. It has been recognized in English courts for over 700 years. Insanity tests or rules that are influential or currently in use include wild beast, M'Naghten, irresistible impulse, Durham or "product," and model penal code.

Wild Beast Test The wild beast test, articulated in 1723, essentially said a man must be so totally deprived of his understanding and memory that he knows no more of what he is doing than an infant or wild beast. The wild beast test remained the standard for judging responsibility until a case involving the assassination attempt of a head of state in 1800. The defense successfully argued that if the person's mental condition either produced or caused the criminal act, the person should not be held legally responsible for it. This was considered a landmark decision because it broke with the idea that a person must be totally deprived of reason, and did not link insanity with the inability to tell right from wrong. Subsequent cases did not follow this precedent but reverted to the wild beast test. However, this reasoning is found in the Durham test or "product rule" of 1954.

M'Naghten Rule From the trial of *The Queen v Daniel M'Naghten* in 1843 came rules that have provided the basis for most American federal and state court decisions on the insanity plea. Daniel M'Naghten was a Scottish woodcutter who felt persecuted by the Tories, who were in power. He believed they were following him, preventing him from sleeping, accusing him of crimes, and planning to murder him. He decided to take action and shoot the prime minister, but he mistakenly shot the prime minister's secretary.

The jury found M'Naghten not guilty by reason of insanity. Even though M'Naghten was committed to an asylum and spent the rest of his life there, his acquittal was met with anger and outrage, much like the recent outcry in the Hinckley acquittal (discussed later in this chapter). M'Naghten's attack had been the fifth attempt on a political figure in forty years, and the government and press believed the court's action would not help stem this tide. The fifteen judges of the common law court were called to task for their ruling and asked to clarify and tighten the concept of criminal responsibility. Their clarification has come to be known as the M'Naghten rule, which states that for an insanity plea to be valid, the defendant at the time of committing the offense must have been functioning under such a defect of the mind, or reasoning power, as not to know the nature and quality of the act or that it was wrong.

The M'Naghten rule was adopted in the federal court and most state courts in the United States by 1851. Until recently, only New Hampshire had judged insanity pleas by a rule not in line with the M'Naghten formula.

Irresistible Impulse Test The claim that the M'Naghten rule focused exclusively on cognition led to the development of the irresistible impulse doctrine as a supplement to the M'Naghten rules in some states. The irresistible impulse test refers to a person's inability, because of a mental disorder, to control behavior even though that person may know it is wrong. A popular question asked in making the determination is: Would the person have yielded to that impulse had a policeman been at his (her) elbow?

Durham Test or "Product Rule" In 1954, the Supreme Court of Appeals for the District of Columbia handed down its decision in *Durham v U.S.*, discarding the M'-Naghten rule and introducing another basis for determining criminal responsibility. Known as the "product rule," this had actually been articulated by the New Hampshire Supreme Court in 1870. The rule stated that a person is not criminally responsible if the behavior at the time of the crime was a "product" of mental illness. The Durham rule did not gain wide acceptance and was generally discarded in 1972.

American Law Institute's Model Penal Code In 1955, the American Law Institute (ALI) drafted the Model Penal Code test, which states that a person is not responsible if because of a mental disorder he or she lacks the capacity either to appreciate the criminality (wrongfulness) of an act or to conform his or her conduct to the requirements of the law. The ALI formulation includes both cognitive (knowledge) and volitional (control) criteria. It is used in all federal circuit courts and was used in the Hinckley case. More than half the states also use these criteria. Approximately one-third of the states use some variation of the M'Naghten rule and irresistible impulse test. New Hampshire is the only state still using the product rule.

Despite its infrequent use, the insanity defense has been the subject of much debate ever since the 1982 "not guilty by reason of insanity" verdict in the trial of John Hinckley, Jr., would-be assassin of President Ronald Reagan. The verdict drew a mixed reaction from the American public. Some believed Hinckley to be insane. Others felt frustrated that punishment had not been administered. To some people the success of the insanity plea seemed linked to the ability to afford an expensive legal defense.

Prior to the Hinckley verdict, the insanity defense had been raised in a number of other sensational cases. The media focus on the "Twinkie defense," so named because of the argument that junk food affected Dan White's mental functioning and diminished his responsibility in the murder of a San Francisco mayor and councilman, did not exactly portray psychiatry in a positive light. David Berkowitz, a bizarre multiple murderer known as Son of Sam, was initially found incompetent to stand trial. Once competent, he surprisingly pleaded guilty to second-degree murder, and the insanity issue was never presented at trial.

Prior to more effective treatment of mental disorders, a verdict of not guilty by reason of insanity (NGRI) saved a person from the death penalty but not from lifelong incarceration. With modern treatment, however, individuals who are found NGRI are often released or discharged quite early. Movie and television portrayals of former psychiatric clients as "mad killers" and "homicidal maniacs" have primed the public to fear the worst.

Since the Hinckley verdict there have been various proposals to drastically limit or abolish the insanity defense. Montana and Idaho have already done so. The National Commission on the Insanity Defense was an independent commission established by the National Mental Health Association to broaden the public debate on the insanity defense and make recommendations of its own. From its investigations, public hearings, and analysis, the commission concluded that much of the outcry for change in the insanity defense is based more on myths and displaced frustration over the multiple problems of the criminal justice system than on facts. The myths and realities of the insanity defense are summarized in the accompanying box.

In 1994, the U.S. Supreme Court let stand Montana's law by refusing to review it. At present, states are free to abolish the insanity defense.

Liability and the Psychiatric Nurse

Criminal and civil are the two main classes of law. *Criminal law* pertains to behavior considered to be a threat to the order of society as a whole, such as murder, assault, and robbery. *Civil law* is concerned with the legal rights and duties of private parties.

An important division of civil law is known as *tort law*. The term **tort** comes from the Latin word for "twisted." A tort is a wrongful act resulting in injury for which the injured party files a civil suit requesting legal redress, usually in the form of monetary damages. Torts may be intentional, as in assault, battery, defamation of character, invasion of privacy, false imprisonment, fraud, and misrepresentation; or unintentional, as in negligence.

Negligence

The concepts of duty and responsibility permeate human relationships. In healthy relationships, expectations are negotiated between individuals that delineate the responsibilities of each person. People who experience times of stress and illness may have difficulty forming realistic expectations, accepting responsibility for actions, and understanding the roles and limits of those who would like to help.

There are times when two people may experience problems understanding and meeting the duties and responsibilities of the relationship. The resolution of such problems is often a therapeutic issue. At times, however, the legal system may become involved. This is particularly true if the client, or the client's family, perceives that the nurse failed to provide the quality of care expected.

All nurses are responsible for determining the quality of care as experienced by their clients. If lapses in the quality of care occur, they should be addressed. The term **negligence** is used whenever a nurse fails to act in a manner in which most reasonable and prudent nurses would act. How does one determine what is reasonable and prudent? First, the nurse is accountable to external legal authorities such as the nurse practice acts of the state in which she or he practices, and civil and criminal codes. The nurse is also accountable to the Standards of Psychiatric–Mental Health Clinical Nursing Practice (1994) published by the American Nurses Association, to the em-

The Insanity Defense: Myths and Realities

Myth: Many criminal defendants plead insanity and most are acquitted.
Reality: The insanity plea is rarely used; acquittals are extremely rare.

Myth: The insanity defense causes major problems for the criminal justice system.
Reality: The insanity defense has a minor practical role in the criminal justice system but a very important moral role.

Myth: Mentally ill people are dangerous and are capable of violent behavior at any time.
Reality: The overwhelming majority of the 35 million mentally ill people in this country are neither dangerous nor unpredictable; they are victims of stigma.

Myth: Most insanity defendants are murderers who commit random acts of violence.
Reality: Most of the crimes committed by insanity defendants are nonviolent crimes. Only 14% of insanity defendants are charged with homicide or other violent crimes, most of which are directed not at strangers but at family members and authority figures.

Myth: The insanity defense allows defendants to fool juries and escape punishment.
Reality: The overwhelming majority of acquittees suffer from the most serious forms of mental illness.

Myth: The insanity defense is a rich man's defense.
Reality: Most insanity defendants are likely to be as poor as most other criminal defendants.

Myth: Insanity trials are a "circus" of conflicting expert testimony that confuses the jury.
Reality: Most insanity cases reflect agreement among the experts, the defense, and the prosecution; few go to trial, and even fewer go to a jury. The celebrated cases are the exception, not the rule.

Myth: Most insanity acquittees go free immediately or within a short time after trial.
Reality: The majority of acquittees are confined for significant periods of time.

Myth: Insanity acquittees repeat the same crime when they are released.
Reality: Crimes committed by insanity acquittees upon release tend to be less violent in nature. Recidivism rates are no higher than for convicted felons.

Myth: The "guilty but mentally ill" verdict means that the defendant will receive mental health treatment.
Reality: A "guilty but mentally ill" verdict does not guarantee treatment beyond what a convicted felon would receive.

ploying agency or hospital, and to current journal and textbook information related to the care of mental health clients.

CONDITIONS FOR ESTABLISHING NEGLIGENCE A simple breach in the quality of care does not necessarily mean that a nurse was negligent. Certain conditions must be met to determine negligence and hold the nurse accountable.

1. A contract for care must have been established between the nurse and the client. A nurse may also begin this contract by accepting a client assignment, discussion with the client, offering information, education, providing treatment, serving as a group leader, accepting a client into an activity, or supervising the activities of a mental health worker. It is important to note that entering into a therapeutic relationship creates a legally binding contract between the nurse and the client.
2. There must be identifiable, explicit, and manifest duty of care in which the intentions of the nurse are to help the client. This intention to help is termed *good faith.* One example is the "good faith" use of the nursing process, including pertinent and timely assessment, planning, intervention, and evaluation of the client. Another example is a nursing care policy that indicates a course of action. A policy of a given hospital might state that each nurse must perform an assessment that includes information related to the emotional, physical, and social health of each client. Failure to use the nursing process and to follow the procedure to provide such an assessment (and take actions based upon this assessment) might be grounds for a charge of negligence. Ignorance of a policy or procedure is not an acceptable rationale for not following a policy or procedure. For example, all nurses are expected to assess clients for the potential to commit suicide. All reasonable, prudent nurses perform an assessment for suicide potential. The nurse must act to safeguard the life of the client within the limits of the law. Failure to perform such an assessment or take actions to protect the client might be deemed negligent, if harm is present.
3. The client must suffer harm that can be directly linked to the failure of the nurse to act in a reasonable and

Determination of Negligence

- Did a contract for care exist?
- Was the care reasonable and prudent?
- Did the care follow that which is suggested by external sources such as nurse practice acts, the ANA Code of Ethics, the ANA Standards for Psychiatric–Mental Health Clinical Nursing Practice, the state Mental Health Act?
- Did the care offered follow the care suggested by internal sources such as policies and procedures of the agency or physician orders?
- Was there evidence of thorough assessment of the client, including old records and interviews with family members?
- Did the action taken reveal appropriate ongoing monitoring of the client's condition?
- Did harm result to the client?

prudent manner. A nurse who fails to assess for suicide potential, thus failing to protect the client, can be held negligent only if the client suffers harm in a suicide attempt or dies as a result of self-inflicted action.

4. There may be no written policy or procedure, nor a law to guide a practitioner in acting, but there is strong indication for action based on what is generally considered *common practice*. Consider a client who lacks any contact with reality. The client cannot perform activities of daily living such as eating, bathing, toileting, or making decisions about safety. It is common practice to provide care in which the nurse will perform the activities of daily living for the client. Conversely, it is common practice to encourage clients to do as much for themselves as possible. Mental health care nurses generally do not bathe clients who can bathe alone. Another example concerns the boundaries of personal relationships between clients and mental health care professionals. Some states fail to define the boundaries of personal relationships between clients and mental health care professionals. In these cases, each nurse must define the nature of the nurse-client relationship. Nurses do not form social relationships with mental health clients with whom there is or has been a professional relationship. This implies that nurses do not date nor engage in sexual activity with a client. Any suggestion or promise that the relationship might be personal can be considered negligence—the failure to explain the limits of the relationship to the client and to act within the boundaries of that relationship.
5. There are times when clients contribute to the harm they suffer. A client may be informed of the dangers of certain actions and yet may decide to act against the advice of the nurse. Each client maintains the civil rights of freedom of speech, movement, and action unless there are grounds to curtail these rights, as in the case of harm to self and others. Consider, for example, a client who had been beaten by her boyfriend and was informed about the pattern of escalating abuse, given the phone numbers of agencies that were available on a 24-hour basis, encouraged to form a safe plan, and offered alternative living arrangements. She decided to return to her boyfriend and suffered paralysis from another beating. She claimed the staff did not act to protect her. Use the accompanying box to help you determine if the staff was negligent.

Medical Malpractice

Medical **malpractice** refers to the negligent acts of health care professionals when they fail to act in a responsible and prudent manner in carrying out their professional duties.

As the practice of nursing moves toward greater independence and accountability, nurses are more likely to be named as defendants in lawsuits. Some reasons for increases in claims against mental health care professionals are:

- The emphasis on client rights in recent court decisions.
- The public's more open attitude and greater expectations of treatment.
- New legal duties identified in the nurse-client relationship, such as the "duty to warn."
- The publicity given the sizable sums awarded in some psychiatric malpractice cases.

According to the American Psychiatric Association, the most frequent sources of claims (listed in order of decreasing frequency) for psychiatrists are:

1. Client suicide
2. Improper treatment
3. Ineffective or improper medication
4. Breach of confidentiality
5. Wrongful commitment
6. Injuries from electroconvulsive therapy
7. Sexual misconduct
8. Failure to obtain consent

The case of *Abille v U.S.* (482 F Supp 703 Calif) illustrates a breach of the ANA's Standards of Psychiatric–Mental Health Clinical Nursing Practice and emphasizes the importance of written communication between nurse and physician.

Aramul Abille was admitted to a U.S. Air Force base hospital after becoming increasingly depressed and suicidal secondary to the reserpine used to treat his hypertension. As a new client, he was not allowed to leave the unit. Four days later the nursing staff assumed without a verifying written medical order (later a verbal order would be claimed) that Mr. Abille was allowed to leave the unit with permission of the nurse on duty. Mr. Abille left the unit unescorted to attend Mass and returned without incident. The following morning he was allowed to go to breakfast unescorted. This time he committed suicide by jumping from a seventh floor window. The court ruled that the nurse involved with Mr. Abille's care breached the standard of care due under Alaska law. The nurse failed to exercise reasonable care to protect a suicidal client against foreseeable harm to himself.

Another case shows the importance of nursing observation and documentation, even though in this case it did not prevent a tragedy.

Distraught with problems and a pending divorce, Matthew Wassner was voluntarily admitted to a psychiatric hospital. During this admission he expressed thoughts of suicide and also thoughts of killing his wife and her mother. Three weeks after his discharge, he was readmitted again voluntarily after a suicide attempt. Nurses' notes revealed close observation of Mr. Wassner and his repeated homicidal threats. Three weeks after his second admission, he was given a pass. He subsequently secured a gun and shot and killed his wife and her friend. He was tried and convicted on two counts of murder. The children brought a wrongful death action against the hospital, seeking damages for the murder of their mother by their father. The court granted substantial damages to the children. No liability was attributed to the nurses involved, but the physician was judged negligent.

In another case, the court found that a nurse who forcibly administered medication to a competent adult client had committed an intentional tort.

The client was involuntarily committed to a mental hospital. She was a practicing Christian Scientist and refused medication. The court held that medication could be given over the client's religious objections only if she were harmful to herself or others. The court allowed her damages for assault and battery.

It is important to remember the nature and purpose of hospital records and to follow prudent, appropriate, and ethical procedures in record maintenance. Records that have been changed for whatever reason need to include the date, the reason for the change, and the signature of the person making the change. A dishonest change could result in the charge of fraud or misrepresentation, as in *Pisel v Stamford Hospital et al.* 430 A2d (Conn 1980).

A 23-year-old woman was admitted with a diagnosis of schizophrenia. She spent three days in a furnitureless quiet room for safety reasons. On the fourth day the bed was returned to the room, but no rationale was noted in the chart. A few days later, an order on the client's chart for an antipsychotic medication was not noted, and the client was without medication for three days. The client was later found in a semicomatose condition with her head lodged between the side rails and mattress. Subsequently, the nursing director ordered the nursing staff to "rewrite" the nursing notes. The substituted record clearly conflicted with other records and staff testimony. A $3.6 million verdict against the hospital has been upheld.

Many factors contribute to the initiation of a malpractice suit by a client. As long as a nurse is involved in practice, lawsuits are a possibility. The nurse may be sued without necessarily being singled out. A number of ways to protect against a successful lawsuit are to:

- Be aware of provisions in the state nurse practice act.
- Follow standards of care.
- Know the relevant law.
- Review hospital procedures and policies with both the standards of care and relevant law in mind, clarify any conflict with legal counsel if necessary, and then follow procedures.
- Document the nursing process, chart accurately and precisely, and chart any significant change as soon as possible. Remember that any omission is presumed not to have occurred.
- Chart objectively, avoiding phrases like "doing well" or "having a good day."
- Question the physician about any ambiguous orders before carrying them out.
- Be sure to adequately describe methods used in client education and evaluation of client comprehension.
- Make sure your nursing documentation reflects the precautions taken during intensive nursing actions such as one-to-one or the use of seclusion or restraints.
- Never alter a client's record after the fact.
- Have malpractice insurance.

The Client Advocacy Role of the Psychiatric Nurse

Gaps Between Theory and Practice

The rights clients have in theory and those in actual practice are often quite different. Richard Price and Bruce Denner aptly comment on this phenomenon: "Although Pinel was able to remove the chains from the inmates of the Bicêtre by declaring that they were mentally ill, today many people lose a substantial portion of their human and civil rights when the same declaration is made about them" (1973, p. 7). This discrepancy between rights in theory and practice is often cited but has received little systematic attention.

This discrepancy exists for two basic reasons: (1) the struggle between client and provider rights and authority, and (2) the "medical model" approach. For example, Szasz and others contend that within the medical model an individual is labeled "mentally ill" because of certain behavior or "symptoms." The label implies that sickness will prevent the client from knowing what is good in the way of treatment.

The gap between the rights clients have in theory and in practice may be the result of a knowledge deficit on the part of treatment providers. The remedy is simple: Educate the treatment providers so that they in turn can educate their clients. Another possibility that may not be so amenable to an easy solution is that direct care treatment providers are threatened by the expansion of client rights. When asked to comment on a California court's mandated review of psychoactive medication for involuntary clients, over 90% of nursing staff said the new regulation not only hampered treatment but made their job both more difficult and more dangerous (Hargreaves et al. 1987).

The federal government has encouraged states to develop ombudsmen or advocacy programs. These state advocacy programs have the authority to investigate reported incidents of neglect and abuse to the mentally ill in public or private hospitals, research facilities, and nursing homes.

Two recent pieces of federal legislation have implications for the rights of clients. In 1990, the Americans with Disabilities Act (ADA) extended federal protection to individuals with physical and/or mental health disabilities for access to public services, employment, and benefits. According to Zuckerman and Charmatz (1992), the ADA can be thought of as granting the same procedural and substantive protections to the disabled that the Civil Rights Act provides to minorities and women. In an effort to increase patient involvement in directing their own medical care, the Patient Self-Determination Act (PSDA) of 1991 was ratified by Congress as part of the Omnibus Budget Reconciliation Act. The PSDA was designed to inform competent patients at the time of their admission to a hospital of their rights to accept or reject aspects of their medical care.

Although laws can protect certain aspects of human rights, there is a far greater area that laws cannot protect. Laws rarely have a direct effect on a person's beliefs, values, and attitudes, which to a great extent determine whether the letter or the spirit of the law will be carried out. Psychiatric nurses practicing from a humanistic perspective are often in a position to advocate both the letter and the spirit of clients' rights.

Physical and Psychologic Abuse of Clients

Clients are particularly vulnerable to both physical and psychologic abuse and often do not have the ability or power to defend themselves. There is little actual information on how much client abuse exists in treatment settings. One advocate group ranked client abuse to be the most frequent rights violation complaint. Another ranked it third. These are the types of abuse reported to occur with some frequency:

- Supplying clients with drugs or alcohol in return for favors.
- Making privileges contingent on favors from clients.
- Slapping and kicking clients when staff members felt frustrated.
- Using restraints when other less intrusive alternatives were available.
- Verbal harassment, including threats, sarcasm, and other "put-downs."
- General threats of harm if clients do not behave "appropriately" or as they are told.
- Inhumane physical facilities.

Advocacy Strategies for Psychiatric Nurses

Psychiatric nursing intervention would be directed at some of the identifying causes that may lead to client abuse, including:

- Unsuitability of certain staff members who do not have the patience or understanding to work with clients having trouble with control.
- A buildup of stresses that have reduced both the staff's patience and ability to problem-solve (burnout).
- An actual lack of knowledge of other means of interacting with clients in a high-stress situation.

Other areas of advocacy include:

- Educating clients and their families about their legal rights.
- Monitoring treatment planning and delivery of service for the abuse of client rights.
- Evaluating policies and procedures regarding client rights infringement.
- Making sure clients have the necessary information to make an informed decision or give informed consent.
- Questioning other health care professionals when their care is based more on stereotypic ideas than an assessment of the client's needs.
- Speaking out for safe practice conditions when threatened by budget cutbacks.

Duty to Intervene

In medical-surgical nursing, it is often very easy to determine when and how to help clients. If a client has low blood sugar, you offer food to increase the blood sugar level. In mental health nursing, it is often difficult to determine when and how to intervene in particular situations. What is my responsibility? What should be done? Who should do it? What are the appropriate legal choices? What is an appropriate ethical response? Am I going to get sued for doing this? Am I going to get sued if I don't?

A contract for care implies that the client has a need for help and that the nurse has agreed to act in good faith for the interest of the client. Nurses form this contract when they accept the duty to care for a client during the process of working on a mental health unit. This contract focuses on the nurse's professional perception that there is an issue that requires management.

Notice that the client may not have asked for help. There are many times when the client is so ill that asking for help is not a reasonable expectation. When working with mental health clients, one general rule applies: Once a situation has come to your awareness, it is important that you take all reasonable and prudent actions to intervene to be helpful to the client.

The process of admission should prepare a client for the actions that the nurse will take given certain situations such as suicidal threats or acts of violence. Most mental health units have a list of client rights and administrative policies and procedures. For example, material that is confidential is explained and material that must be shared is discussed. At times, clients may attempt to use the mental health unit as a shield against facing legal charges, and the nurse must make relevant policies explicit to the client.

All interventions must follow a thorough assessment. The client must be informed that staff members will perform ongoing assessments to facilitate care, and if this is not clear, the client may become suspicious. When clients are not able to cooperate with assessments because of cognitive impairment, it is vital to obtain information from other sources including records from previous hospitalizations, family members, or community therapists (with client permission). The staff may need to review lab work to explore the level of reliability in the information presented by clients with respect to drug or alcohol use, for example.

Lying on the part of the client has several aspects with legal implications. Clients may deliberately mislead the staff member by telling stories that the client knows are not true. This is best dealt with through respectful confrontation. Clients may not actually lie but may frame a situation so that the client is viewed as a victim, without including details pertinent to a full understanding of the situation. In this case, it may be helpful to walk through the situation several times, with more than one interviewer, and ask for further details.

Some mental disorders affect the perception and memory of events so profoundly that only a third party such as a family member can offer an accurate view. Nurses must make a good faith effort to perform a full assessment of a client before intervening. This information must be recorded in the chart with statements not only related to information the nurse was able to obtain but also actions the nurse took to obtain information. Failure to assess the client and the situation may result in errors in judgment. It is essential to take time to collect information essential for decision making. This process requires expert communication skills not only with the client but with others involved in the client's care.

Responsibility to Communicate The duty to intervene requires that information be communicated clearly to others, particularly those who participate in the decision-making process. The nurse is responsible for informing all individuals involved in the care of a client of the results of the assessment and of the considerations for the intervention phase.

Providing optimal care to clients requires cooperation and collaboration with others. No one professional can make decisions without consultation with others. Each psychiatric nurse must be able to communicate effectively within the established protocols of the agency of employment. These policies and procedures are often called the chain of command. The chain of command is the expected pattern of communication surrounding the care of clients. Several aspects of the chain of command are important to remember.

1. Nurses are often responsible for the care provided by others. The nurse may work with several nurses' aides or mental health technicians. The nurse must make clear situations that demand immediate attention. The paraprofessionals working on a psychiatric nursing unit must be able to recognize situations that should be immediately reported.
2. The nurse often serves as a liaison to other departments. The nurse practice act in the state of employment will determine the dependent, independent, and interdependent roles of the nurse. Often these roles need to be explained to other professionals.
3. The ANA's Standards for Psychiatric–Mental Health Clinical Nursing Practice provide standards of care. Many professionals do not know that the psychiatric nurse must judge her practice based on these guidelines. The hospital or clinic will provide guidelines for notification and decision making that must be followed. It is vital to know the policies of the institution.

In an untoward situation, these three elements form a framework for actions that need to be taken. Once an event has occurred, the nurse must notify team members who may not be present on the unit. Usually, the nurse manager or supervisor, physician, psychologist, social worker, security department, and at times the family, a person who has been threatened, or the police must all be notified.

Formulating a Plan to Intervene It is vital to formulate a plan before making a decision to intervene. Nurses often complain of not having "think time," time to consider all options before acting. Many nurses indicate that they respond based on past experience or intuition. While this may work for many expert nurses, beginning nurses need to carefully think through options and learn to assess the clinical and legal implications of actions in a methodical fashion. Figures 11–1 and 11–2 illustrate two models that might be helpful in decision making.

Legal Aspects Involving Professionals At times, the nurse may notice that peers are engaging in illegal activities. While these unfortunate situations may occur, it is vital for each nurse to understand the legal mandate that requires a response from any professional who has knowledge of illegal, immoral, or unethical activities. Normally, this response will be to report the events to others in the agency using the chain of command. At other times, the nurse may need to seek the guidance of the State Board of Nursing or the American Nurses Association.

Nurse impairment is perhaps the most common situation encountered by professional staff. A nurse may be impaired through addiction to alcohol or narcotics, or through an event of personal experience with emotional illness. This impairment may be linked with other illegal acts such as theft of drugs or a client's personal property. Each nurse is first responsible to the client and must report such impairment in a reasonable, prudent, and timely manner. Although some nurses erroneously view this intervention as an invasion of privacy or "tattling," prompt efficient action may safeguard the client from harm while offering the impaired nurse a chance at recovery. Most hospitals have programs to assist impaired nurses to recover. Many state nursing boards or state professional associations have programs to assist the nurse addict or emotionally impaired nurse.

Legal Implications: Special Circumstances

Nurses offer care within legal guidelines defined by the nursing practice and prevailing state and local ordinances. Laws affecting mental health clients reflect the beliefs and struggles of the society that shapes such laws. There are sometimes areas in which legal issues and treatment issues are in conflict. One such area is in the treatment of clients who have addictive illnesses.

Addicts often exhibit poor judgment. For example, alcoholic clients may continue to drive while intoxicated. In most states, driving under the influence of alcohol or drugs is considered a crime for which the driver will face legal penalties. The law enforcement system may interact with the mental health system to force treatment on those found guilty of driving while intoxicated.

A mental health nurse may care for these clients who have been "mandated for treatment." Such clients may initially respond with minimal or superficial cooperation, although many clients do make positive changes as a result of mandated therapy. Clients mandated for treatment must be informed in writing of all policies inherent to the treatment process and the court mandate. Often this mandate will include written evidence of participation in one-to-one therapy, family therapy, educational programming, or attending 12-step meetings. At times, random drug testing may be court ordered.

Clients may attempt to manipulate you into withholding information from the court. To allow the client to manipulate you will jeopardize the treatment process. Successful manipulation may decrease the client's feeling of responsibility for recovery. At no time can you consider violating the court mandate. The law enforcement system has the right to file charges against a nurse who fails to cooperate fully with court mandates.

When the state laws clearly mandate a treatment course, you must work within legal mandates. It is much more difficult to decide what to do when public opinion and legal mandate are less clear, or when the mandates seem to interfere with prudent treatment. For example, pregnant women who suffer from substance addiction potentially face conflict between the legal system and basic prenatal care. States vary in approach to the pregnant addict. Some states seek to incarcerate pregnant women who continue to use illegal drugs, and others mandate that health care workers report all women who have tested positive for drugs, determining such behavior to be child abuse.

Women face special obstacles to treatment for addictions. Some obstacles seem rooted within the opposing beliefs about the nature of addiction: Is addiction a bad behavior that should result in punishment? Or is addiction an illness that should respond to treatment? In mental health settings, addiction is perceived as an illness. Participation in the treatment process is a central responsibility of each nurse.

At times, you may need to interact with the legal system during mandated treatment. You may serve as an advocate who will facilitate treatment for the addict and her baby. This process of intervention can be complex. For example, it is difficult to identify active addiction, secondary use, and recreational use. While any drug use is potentially hazardous, regular use seen in addiction may be more damaging to mother and baby.

Jason is a voluntary client hospitalized on an open unit who punched another client, fracturing his jaw. You assess Jason after he hit his peer and find him very calm. You place him on 1:1 supervision with staff until you can decide on a course of action. You review his record and discover that he has been in prison for assault and battery. While hospitalized he has not engaged in any violence before today. You call the doctor, the nursing supervisor, the social worker and security; you also call in extra staff to maintain safety.

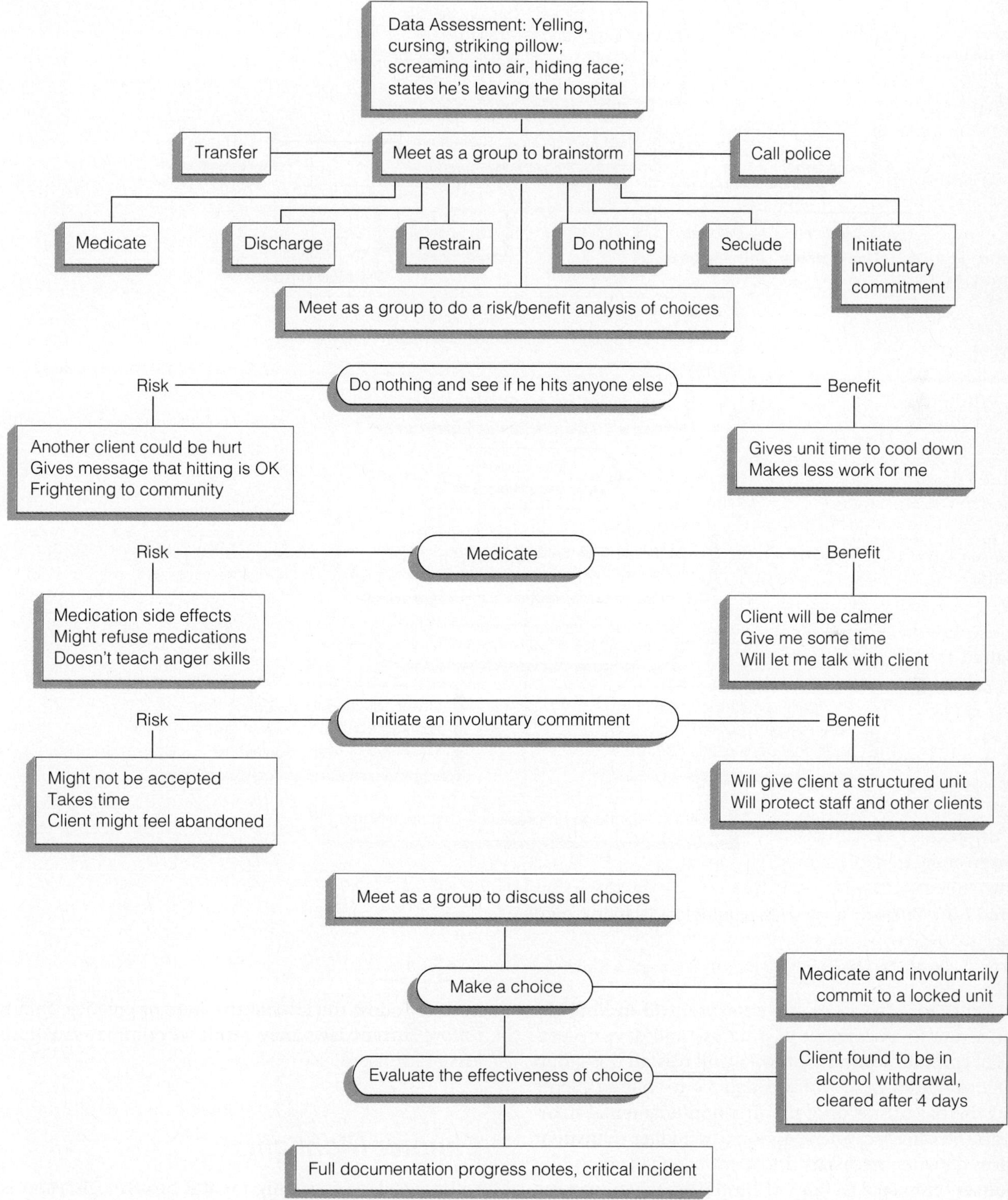

Figure 11-1 Risk/benefit analysis as a model for decision making.

A 34-year-old female client who is admitted with borderline personality disorder states that a male peer raped her. She alleges the incident occurred last night and insists that the male client be arrested. The unit has a "no sex policy" stating that each offending member must be transferred or discharged from the unit. You notify the nurse manager, the nursing supervisor, the physician, the therapist, the social worker, the risk manager and security. The hospital's legal counsel is called to help determine options for the client and the man identified as the rapist.

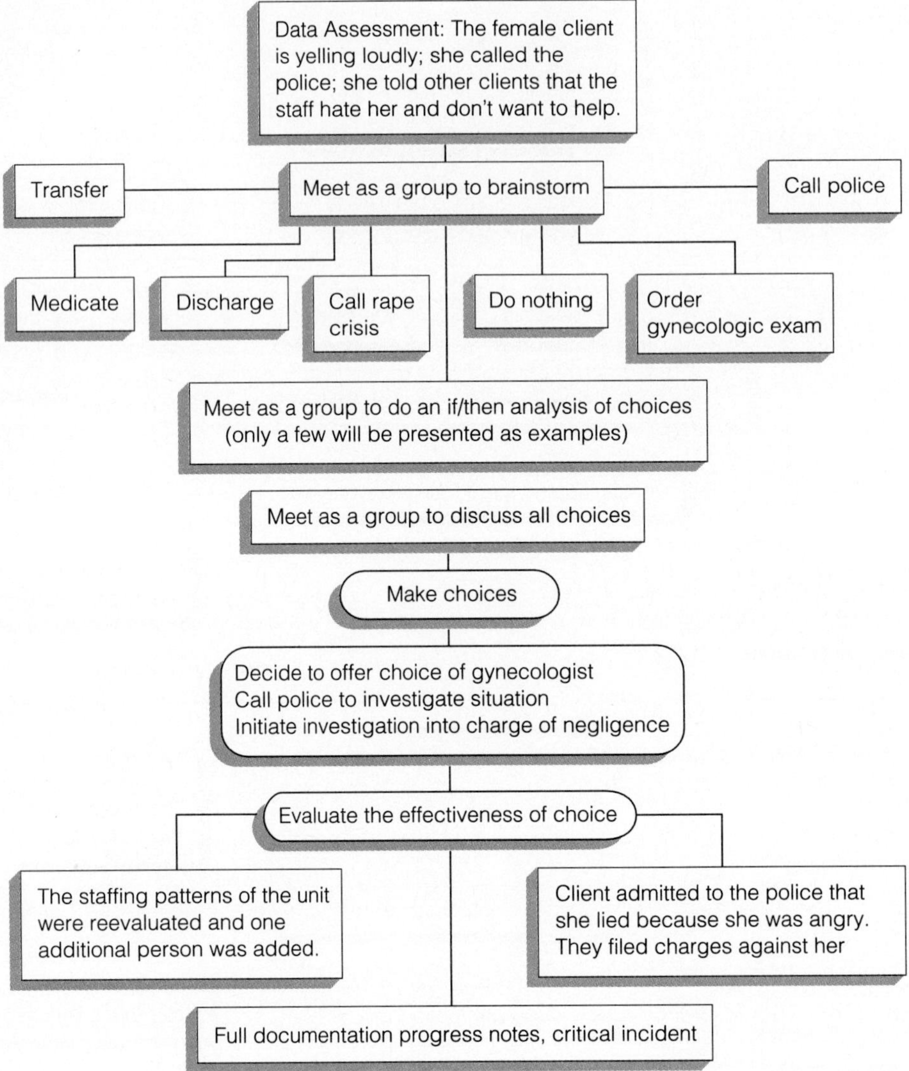

Figure 11-2 "If/then" analysis as a model in decision making.

In order to serve as an advocate, you will need to become astute in assessment of drug use and develop patterns of communication that will instill trust in this group of clients. Additionally, you are required to educate clients about the hazards of drug use in a nonjudgmental manner, and to offer treatment options, including outpatient services or, when necessary, inpatient hospitalization.

Nurses often face feelings of frustration when working with the disease of addiction, which is often characterized by relapse. Some nurses feel pulled between the rights of the fetus and the rights of the mother. Again, you will need to follow the laws of the state of practice. Failure to follow current laws may result in criminal sanctions or loss of licensure.

Chapter Highlights

- Knowledge of existing mental health legislation is essential for nurses to become politically active and protect the legal rights of individuals using mental health care services.

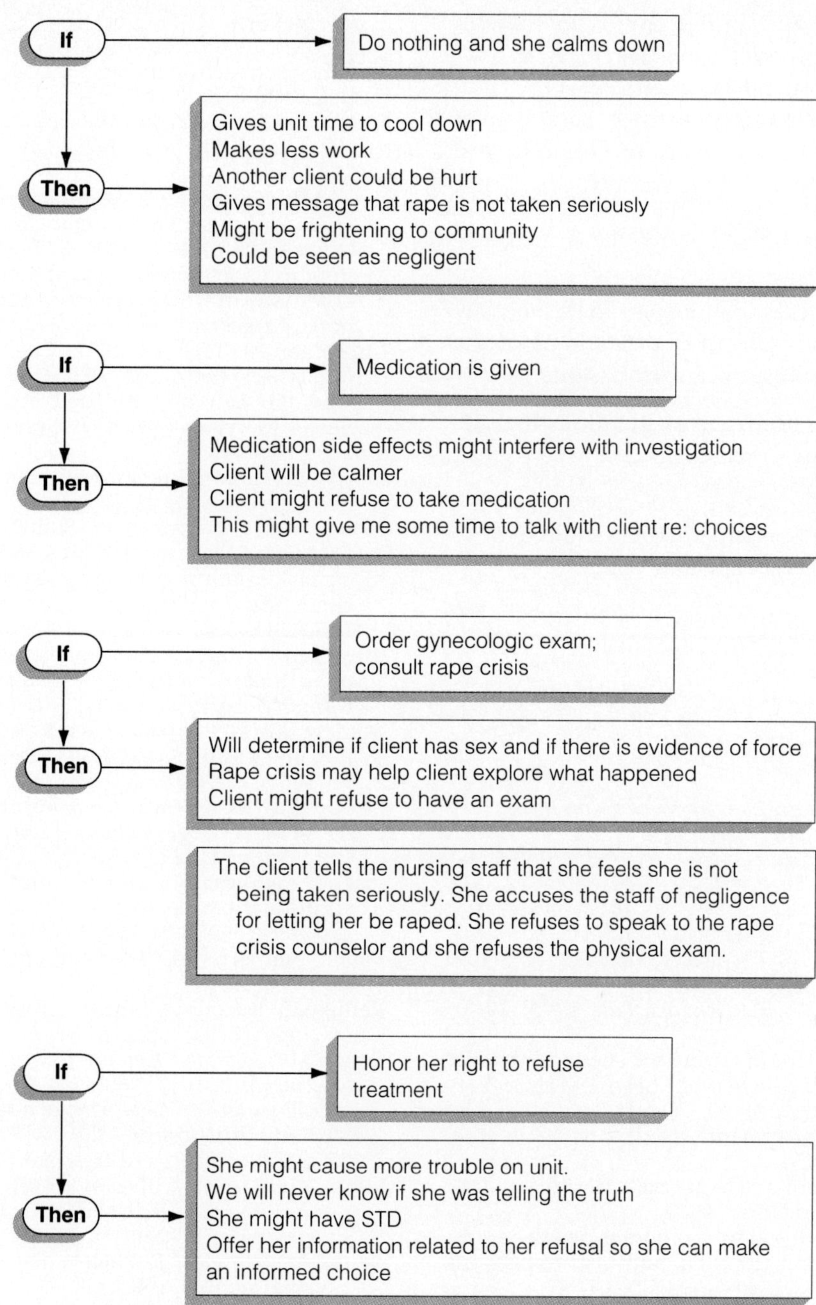

Figure 11-2 *(continued)*

- Mental health legislation varies considerably from state to state. In every state, mental hygiene laws identify procedures for admission to and discharge from mental hospitals, but only some states deal with the medical and legal rights of hospitalized people.
- Health care professionals are being held increasingly accountable for their behavior. They need to become familiar with the state laws that govern their responsibilities and actions.
- Contemporary legal issues important in humanistic psychiatric nursing practice include involuntary admission criteria, the right to treatment, the civil rights of hospitalized people, client-therapist relations, the controversial right to refuse treatment, and treatment in the least restrictive alternative.
- Theory about rights of mental health clients often is not reflected in practice.
- Effective implementation of client rights frequently depends on awareness, support, and advocacy by the psychiatric nurse.

- Mental health statutes and court decisions have an impact on the practice of psychiatry. Psychiatry also affects the resolution of such legal questions as the credibility of witnesses; competency to make a will or contract or to stand trial; custody of children; and most controversial, criminal responsibility.
- Risk/benefit analysis can facilitate the process of decision making.
- Informed consent requires that the person be mentally competent and demonstrate an understanding of the explanation offered by health care professionals.
- Nurses have a duty to intervene in situations that appear to denote a danger to self or others.
- Nurses have a duty to report any professionals who fail in duties to a client. The chain of command is used to report incidents involving clients or staff.
- Nurses who provide court-mandated treatment for addicts must act as advocates for clients while observing state and local laws.

References

American Nurses Association: *Code for Nurses with Interpretive Statements.* ANA, 1976.

American Nurses Association: *Standards of Psychiatric–Mental Health Clinical Nursing Practice.* ANA, 1994.

Americans with Disabilities Act of 1990, PL 101-336, Sec. 104.

Appelbaum P: Tarasoff and the clinician: Problems in fulfilling the duty to protect. *Am J Psychiatr* 1985; 142: 425–429.

Beck JC, Parry JW: Incompetence, treatment refusal and hospitalization. *Bull Am Acad Psychiatry Law* 1992; 20(3): 261–267.

Bender BM, Murphy D, Mark B: Caring for clients with legal charges on a voluntary psychiatric unit. *J Psychosoc Nurs* 1989;27(3):16–20.

Birnbaum M: The right to treatment. *American Bar Association Journal* 1960;46:499–505.

Brakel SJ, Parry JW, Weiner BA: *The Mentally Disabled and the Law.* American Bar Foundation, 1985.

Carstensen PC: The evolving duty of mental health professionals to third parties: A doctrinal and institutional examination. *Int. J Law Psychiatry* 1994;17(1):1–42.

Cohen LT: Psychiatric hospitalization as an experience of trauma. *Arch Psychiatr Nurs* 1994;8(2):78–81.

DeCoste B: The many faces of advocacy: Victory and peace. *Am J Nurs* 1990;90(1):80–81.

Donaldson K: *Insanity Inside Out.* Crown, 1976.

Douard W, Winslade WJ: Tarasoff and the moral duty to protect the vulnerable, in Monagle JF, Thomasma DC (eds): *Health Care Ethics—Critical Issues.* Aspen, 1994.

Galen KD: Assessing psychiatric patients' competency to agree to treatment plans. *Hosp Comm Psychiatry* 1993; 44(4): 361–363.

Garritson SH: Degrees of restrictiveness in psychosocial nursing. *J Psychosoc Nurs* 1983:21:9–16.

Geller JL: Clinical encounters with outpatient coercion at the CMHC: Questions of implementation and efficacy. *Community Ment Health J* 1992;28(2):81–93.

Hargreaves WA, et al.: Effects of the Jamison-Farabee consent decree: Due process protection for involuntary psychiatric patients treated with psychoactive medication. *Am J Psychiatr* 1987;144(2):188–192.

Hiday VA: Coercion in civil commitment: Process, preferences and outcome. *Int J Law Psychiatry* 1992; 15(4): 359–377.

Kapp MB: Treatment and refusal rights in mental health: Therapeutic justice and clinical accommodation. *Amer J Orthopsychiatry* 1994;64(2):223–233.

Kaufmann C: Reasonable accommodation to mental health disabilities at work: Legal constructs and practical applications. *J Psychiatr Law* 1993;21(2):153–174.

Kinzelman AJ, Taynor J, et al.: Clients' perceptions of involuntary hospitalization. *J Psychosoc Nurs* 1994;32(6):28–32.

LaFond JQ: Law and the delivery of involuntary mental health services. *Amer J Orthopsychiatry* 1994; 64(2): 209–221.

Lynch VA: Forensic nursing: Diversity in education and practice. *J Psychosoc Nurs* 1993;31(11):7–14.

Mental Health Systems Act: Summary and analysis. *Mental Disability Law Reporter* 1980;4:383–390.

Monahan J: Limiting therapist exposure to Tarasoff liability: Guidelines for risk containment. *Amer Psychologist* 1993; 48(4):241–250.

Mossman D, Hart KJ: How bad is civil commitment? A study of attitudes toward violence and involuntary hospitalization. *Bull Am Acad Psychiatry Law* 1993;21(2):181–194.

Munetz MR, Geller JL: The least restrictive alternative in the post-institutional era. *Hosp Comm Psychiatry* 1993; 44(10): 967–972.

National Mental Health Association NMHA, *Myth and Realities: A Report of the National Commission on the Insanity Defense.* March, 1982.

Parry J: Involuntary civil commitment in the 1990's: A constitutional perspective. *Mental and Physical Disability Law Reporter* 1994;18(3):320–338.

Patient Self-Determination Act, Omnibus Budget Reconciliation Act, 1991.

Perlin ML: Decoding right to refuse treatment law. *Int J Law Psychiatry* 1993;16(2):151–177.

Perlin ML: *Mental Disability Law: Civil and Criminal.* 3 vol. Michie Company, 1989.

Price R, Denner B: *The Making of a Mental Patient.* Holt, Rinehart and Winston, 1973.

Rachlin S: Retention and treatment issues on the psychiatric inpatient unit, in Bluestone H, Travin S, Marlow DB (eds): *Psychiatric-Legal Decision Making by the Mental Health Practitioner.* Wiley, 1994.

Simone RI: *Clinical Psychiatry and the Law*, ed 2. American Psychiatric, Inc., 1992.

Slobogin C: Involuntary community treatment of people who are violent and mentally ill: A legal analysis. *Hosp Comm Psychiatry* 1994;45(7):685–689.

Smith SR: Liability and mental health services. *Amer J Orthopsychiatry* 1994;62(2):235–251.

Szasz T: *Law, Liberty and Psychiatry.* Macmillan, 1963.

Weiss FS: The right to refuse: Informed consent and the psychosocial nurse. *J Psychosoc Nurs* 1990;28(8):25–30.

Winick BJ: The right to refuse mental health treatment. *Int J Law Psychiatry* 1994;17(1):99–117.

Zuckerman D, Charmatz M: *Mental Disability Law—A Primer,* ed 4. American Bar Association, 1992.

PART THREE

APPLYING THE NURSING PROCESS

CONTENTS

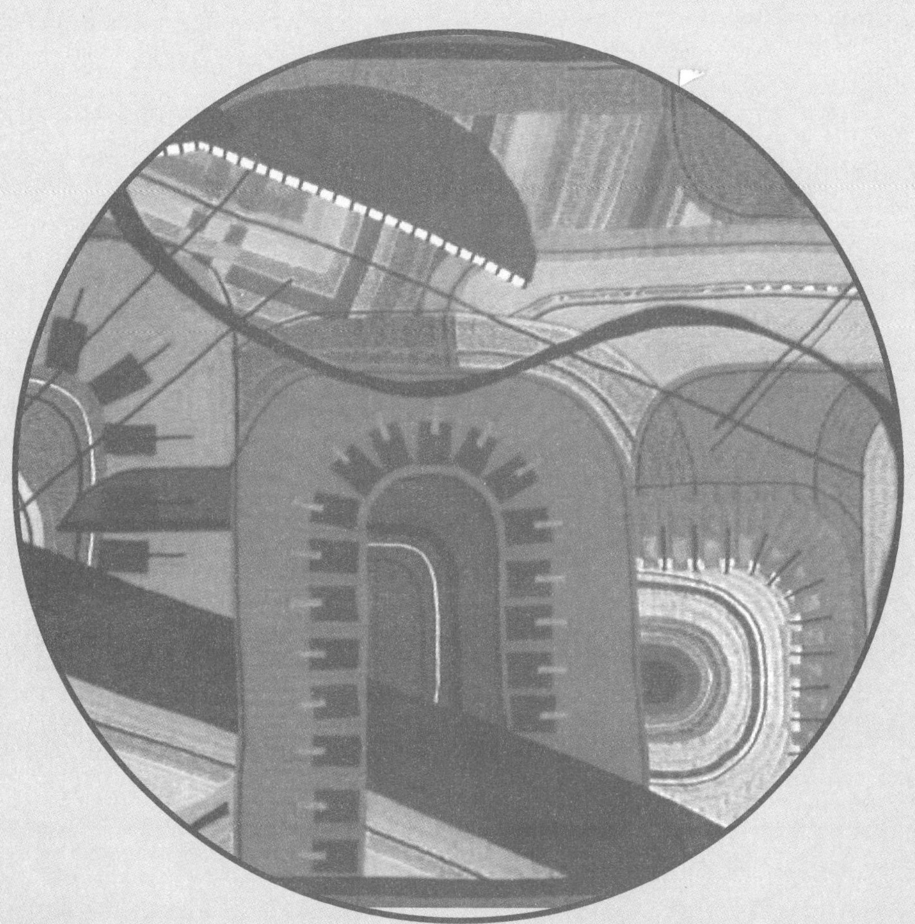

CHAPTER 12

CLIENTS WITH DELIRIUM, DEMENTIA, AMNESTIC DISORDER, AND OTHER COGNITIVE DISORDERS

Sally Hutchinson
Holly Skodol Wilson

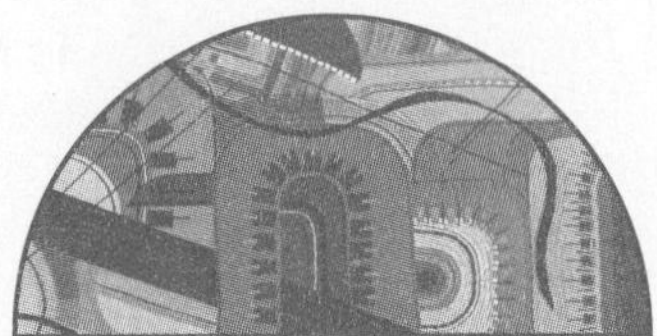

COMPETENCIES

- *Understand the biopsychosocial theories that explain delirium, dementia, amnestic disorder, and other cognitive disorders.*
- *Differentiate among the various types of cognitive disorders.*
- *Specify the DSM-IV diagnostic criteria for cognitive disorders.*
- *Assess relevant subjective and objective data for clients with cognitive disorders.*
- *Explain what causes you the most difficulty when caring for clients with cognitive disorders.*

Cross-References

Other topics relevant to this content are: Elderly, Chapter 38; Families, Chapter 32; Neuropsychiatric complications of AIDS, Chapter 27; Substance-related disorders, Chapter 13.

Critical Thinking Challenge

Psychiatrists and neurologists frequently advocate institutionalizing clients with Alzheimer's disease (AD). Family caregivers, however, often take offense at this suggestion in spite of the fact that they are mentally and physically exhausted. How would you handle this issue with the family? What suggestions or alternatives would you propose? At what point, if ever, should a professional exert pressure on family caregivers to institutionalize their loved one?

Now that we are living in "the Decade of the Brain" and the psychobiologic revolution is upon us, psychiatric nurses are becoming increasingly interested in clients with delirium, dementia, amnestic, and other cognitive disorders. Clients with these disorders provide a special challenge because they frequently cannot speak our language. Discovering how to reach these people, how to assess how they feel and how to care for them, are critical nursing tasks.

Ronch (1987) quoted eminent neuropsychologist A. R. Luria's poignant and insightful response to the frustrated Dr. Oliver Sacks' (1985) question about a patient with a cognitive disorder, "What is there to do to help Jimmy's memory?" Luria replied:

> Do whatever your ingenuity and your heart suggest . . . [but] a man does not consist of memory alone. He has feeling, will, sensibilities, moral being—matters of which neuropsychology cannot speak. And it is here,

> beyond the realm of an impersonal psychology, that you may find ways to touch him, and change him. And the circumstances of your work especially allows this for you work in a Home, which is like a little world, quite different from the clinics and institutions where I work. Neuropsychologically, there is little or nothing you can do; but in the realm of the individual, there may be much you can do.

Besides family caregivers, nurses are the most logical advocates for these clients. Frequently, nurses are in charge of day treatment centers or nursing homes, or they facilitate support groups. Families look to nurses for suggestions to ease their burdens, for strategies to cope with difficult behavioral symptoms, for education to explain unpredictable behavior, and for resources that might alleviate their situation.

Your knowledge of psychobiology and your holistic approach to client care are unique assets essential to providing quality care for clients with cognitive disorders.

Cognitive Disorders

Before the twentieth century, all organic brain disorders of the aged were categorized as *senile dementia.* Beginning at the turn of the century, neuropathologists doing autopsy work distinguished senile dementia from arteriosclerotic conditions and neurosyphilis (Butler and Lewis 1982). Arteriosclerotic brain disease was then considered the primary cause of confusional states in older adults. It was believed to be the result of diseased cerebral vessels (Wolanin and Fraelich-Philips 1981). By the middle of this century, a new category, *organic brain disease (OBD),* was added. This category was broader, allowing for both a defect in the vessels and in the brain itself. The category *organic brain syndrome (OBS)* then followed, which recognized the need for a diagnosis that included symptoms without a known cause. A few years ago, the term *organic mental syndrome (OMS)* referred to a group of psychologic or behavioral signs of unknown or unclear etiology, while *organic mental disorder (OMD)* referred to a particular syndrome whose etiology was known or presumed. Today, because of the recent reconceptualization of the *DSM-IV,* the diagnostic nomenclature includes *delirium, dementia, amnestic disorder,* and other *cognitive disorders.*

Delirium

The elderly, especially those with dementia, are prone to transient cognitive disorders, usually referred to as either *delirium* or *acute confusional state.* It is estimated that 30–50% of elderly medical-surgical clients will experience a life-threatening acute confusional state. One-fourth of these older adults with delirium die within one month of admission.

Delirium can be defined as a type of confusional state that is marked by a prominent disorder of perception, terrifying hallucinations and vivid dreams, a kaleidoscopic array of strange and absurd fantasies and delusions, inability to sleep, a tendency to convulse, and intense emotional disturbances (Adams and Victor 1993). Additional elements include disorientation, impaired attention and concentration, and diminution of all mental activity. Rage, depression, fear, apathy, and incontinence are common. Nurses and physicians fail to recognize 70% of delirium in clients who are in a delirious state (Foreman 1991). See the boxes on page 218 for DSM-IV diagnostic criteria and for a taxonomy of delirium.

Because delirium is usually caused by an underlying systemic illness, a prompt search is essential for treatable conditions like dehydration, diabetes, hyponatremia, hypercalcemia, thyroid crisis, infection, silent myocardial infarction, drug intoxication, or liver or renal failure. If the cause is removed, complete recovery can be achieved (Stern and Bernick 1987).

Signs of Delirium

Cognition The three components of cognition—perception, thinking, and memory—are all disrupted in delirium:

1. *Perception.* The person shows reduced ability to distinguish and integrate sensory information and to discriminate it from hallucinations, dreams, illusions, and imagery.
2. *Thinking.* The thinking process is fragmented and disorganized to the extent that the person is unable to reason, judge, abstract, or solve problems.
3. *Memory.* Memory is impaired in all three spheres; the person is unable to register, retain, or recall information.

Attention and Wakefulness Attention is impaired in all three spheres. The person has difficulty with

- Alertness or maintaining vigilance.
- Selectiveness, or the ability to focus on and selectively attend to stimuli at will.
- Directiveness, or the ability to direct and focus one's mental processes.

Wakefulness is usually reduced during the day, and the person experiences sleeplessness, restlessness, and agitation at night. Interestingly, delirium and dreaming are characterized by the same electroencephalographic (EEG) changes. The person is then caught between dreaming and hallucinating, sleep and wakefulness.

Diagnostic Criteria for 293.0 Delirium Due to . . . [Indicate the General Medical Condition]

A. Disturbance of consciousness (i.e., reduced clarity of awareness of the environment) with reduced ability to focus, sustain, or shift attention.

B. A change in cognition (such as memory deficit, disorientation, language disturbance) or the development of a perceptual disturbance that is not better accounted for by a preexisting, established, or evolving dementia.

C. The disturbance develops over a short period of time (usually hours to days) and tends to fluctuate during the course of the day.

D. There is evidence from the history, physical examination, or laboratory findings that the disturbance is caused by the direct physiological consequences of a general medical condition.

Coding note: If delirium is superimposed on a preexisting Dementia of the Alzheimer's Type or Vascular Dementia, indicate the delirium by coding the appropriate subtype of the dementia, e.g., 290.3 Dementia of the Alzheimer's Type, With Late Onset, With Delirium.

Coding note: Include the name of the general medical condition on Axis I, e.g., 293.0 Delirium Due to Hepatic Encephalopathy; also code the general medical condition on Axis III (see Appendix G in the *DSM-IV* for codes).

Source: American Psychiatric Association 1994, p. 129.

Types of Delirium

- Delirium Due to a General Medical Condition (Indicate the General Medical Condition)
- Substance-Induced Delirium (including medication side effects)

  Substance Intoxication Delirium

  Substance Withdrawal Delirium
- Delirium Due to Multiple Etiologies
- Delirium Not Otherwise Specified

Source: American Psychiatric Association 1994, p. 124.

Psychomotor Behavior The delirious client is either hyperactive or hypoactive, often alternating between. Speech may be slurred and disjointed, with aimless vocalizations and repetitions. Tremors and irregular spasmodic **(choreiform) movements** may be present.

WERNICKE-KORSAKOFF SYNDROME This neurological syndrome, which may result in delirium, is due to thiamine deficiency. It is often associated with alcoholism, and occasionally with malabsorption syndrome, severe anorexia, upper GI obstruction, prolonged intravenous feeding, thyrotoxicosis, or hemodialysis. It is a spectrum disease, meaning that the acute encephalopathy phase, called **Wernicke's encephalopathy**, may develop into a chronic condition, **Korsakoff's psychosis**, that includes both retrograde and anterograde amnesia (Franklin and Francis 1992).

Symptoms of Wernicke's encephalopathy include

- Confusion
- Oculomotor disturbances
- Cerebellar ataxia

It is a medical emergency that can be corrected with parenteral thiamine. In contrast, patients with Korsakoff's psychosis do not respond to thiamine replacement and often require institutionalization. In addition to the amnesia, confabulation in the early stages, apathy, inertia, and loss of insight are common (Franklin and Francis 1992).

Mr R, an 80-year-old bachelor with bilateral cataracts, lived alone in a small midwestern town with his pet cat, Suzy. Mr R was admitted to the community hospital for a hernia repair that he had been putting off for several months. Never hospitalized before, he was extremely anxious on admission and became more so with each preoperative procedure that day. By 10:00 that evening, Mr R was found wandering in the hallway looking and calling for Suzy. The nurse gave him a barbiturate sleeping preparation and returned him to his room. Three hours later he was again found wandering, this time nude and more disoriented than before. He was again sedated and confined to bed with a vest and soft wrist restraints. By morning, Mr R was so disoriented and agitated that the surgery was canceled. Mr R's physician then ordered Valium for sedation, and the client remained confined to bed. Within one week, Mr R's behavior had deteriorated to

the extent that he required institutionalization. He was transferred to a local nursing home for permanent care.

A 55-year-old man, Mr B, was involved with a difficult divorce and went drinking with his friends. He drank numerous "straight" drinks and shortly thereafter began screaming, crying, and acting aggressively toward others in the bar. At one point he tried to choke a man and later picked up a chair and threw it. The police took him to jail and, when he began to convulse, to the hospital.

Mrs W, a 65-year-old woman, was in the hospital with renal problems. Although previously alert, she rapidly became agitated and confused about where she was. She was unresponsive to the nurse's efforts to orient her and refused to cooperate during her morning care. Within hours after this extreme agitation, she lapsed into a stupor and then a coma.

Differentiating Delirium from Dementia

Several criteria distinguish delirium from dementia (Cook-Deegan et al. 1988):

- *State of consciousness.* People with delirium have fluctuating consciousness, whereas individuals with dementia are as attentive as they can be.
- *Stability.* In clients with delirium, the ability to pay attention and respond varies, whereas in clients with dementia, it is relatively stable.
- *Duration.* Delirium is short-lived; dementia is prolonged.
- *Rate of onset.* Delirium develops rapidly, whereas dementia is insidious.
- *Cause.* Delirium may be traced to a recent source, whereas dementia cannot be linked to another cause.

For a summary of the characteristics of delirium and dementia, see Table 12–1 on page 220.

PSEUDODELIRIUM In 5–20% of the cases of delirium, no organic cause can be identified. As in pseudodementia, the presence of inconsistencies in cognitive functioning (the client does not know where he or she is but can find the bathroom, bed, etc.) should raise the suspicion of a *pseudodelirium.* If the client also has a history of psychiatric illness, is grossly and consistently delusional, has marked manic or depressive features, or is unmotivated during cognitive testing, the diagnosis of this cognitive disorder may be appropriate.

Dementia

In the United States today, approximately 1.5 million people over age 65 suffer from dementia to the extent that they cannot care for themselves, and 1–5 million suffer from milder forms (Cook-Deegan et al. 1988). This number is ten times greater than at the turn of the century. Over 60% of people in nursing homes have been diagnosed with dementia. A now common clinical syndrome, **dementia** is marked by the following:

- Global cognitive impairment extending to the areas of abstract thinking, judgment, insight, complex capabilities (language, tasks, recognition), and personality change.
- Memory impairment.
- Decline in intellectual function.
- Altered judgment, in awake and alert states.
- Altered affect.
- Spatial disorientation.

Dementia is a mental disorder involving functional declines in multiple cognitive areas, including memory (Dickson and Ranseen 1990). Symptoms related to specific areas of brain damage are shown in Figure 12–1 on page 221. The *DSM-IV* further differentiates dementia as "sufficiently severe to cause impairment in occupational or social functioning. . ." (APA 1994, p. 134). See the box on page 222 for DSM-IV diagnostic criteria for dementia of the Alzheimer's type, and the box on page 223 for a taxonomy of dementia.

Dementias are classified according to causal agent or area of neurologic damage. The latter scheme distinguishes between cortical and subcortical dementias. Alzheimer's disease is the classic cortical dementia, whereas Huntington's disease and Parkinson's disease are common subcortical types. These categories are quite similar. People with subcortical dementias, however, have a higher order of functioning.

DEMENTIA OF THE ALZHEIMER'S TYPE **Alzheimer's disease (AD)**, a chronic progressive disorder, is the most common form of dementia seen in older adults. AD ravages the mind and robs the personality of about 4 million Americans (National Institute on Aging 1990). The most prevalent dementia, AD increases with age from 10% of individuals over 65 to 50% of those older than 85, the fastest growing segment of the population (Health Policy and Biomedical Research News of the Week 1990). AD accounts for some 20% of all clients in psychiatric hospitals (Adams and Victor 1993).

In 1991, AD cost the U.S. economy $536 billion (direct costs) and $1.75 trillion (total costs). AD costs approximately $47,000 per year per client, with the cost of long-term home and institutional care providing the major economic burden (Ernst and Hay 1994).

Alois Alzheimer first recognized AD in 1907 while conducting an autopsy on a 51-year-old woman with a 4½-year history of dementia. He discovered **senile plaques** in

Table 12–1 Impaired Cognitive Function

	Delirium	*Dementia*	*Depression*
Diagnostic Features	Disturbance of consciousness accompanied by a change in cognition unaccounted for by a preexisting or evolving dementia. Reduced clarity of awareness of the environment. Impaired ability to focus, sustain, or shift attention. Change in cognition may include memory impairment, disorientation to time and/or place, or language disturbance such as rambling, irrelevant or pressured and incoherent speech. Simple or complex perceptual disturbances may include misinterpretations, illusions, or hallucinations.	Multiple cognitive deficits including memory impairment and either aphasia, apraxia, or agnosia; or a disturbance in executive functioning (the ability to think abstractly, to plan, initiate, sequence, monitor, and stop complex behavior). Impairment in occupational or social functioning that represents a decline from earlier level of functioning.	Dysphoric mood, loss of interest or pleasure in usual activities and pastimes, appetite disturbance, change in weight, sleep disturbance, psychomotor agitation or retardation, decreased energy, feelings of worthlessness or guilt, difficulty concentrating or thinking, thoughts of death or suicide or suicide attempts.
Associated Features	Emotional disturbance: fear, anxiety, irritability, anger, euphoria, apathy. Disturbance in sleep-wake cycle with daytime sleepiness or nighttime agitation and difficulty falling asleep. Disturbed psychomotor behavior including groping or picking at bedclothes, sudden movements, or sluggishness and lethargy. Possible extremes of psychomotor activity during the day.	Spatial disorientation, poor judgment, poor insight, violence, suicidal behavior, disinhibited behavior, slurred speech, anxiety, mood and sleep disturbances, delusions, hallucinations, vulnerability to physical and psychosocial stressors.	Depressed appearance, tearfulness, feelings of anxiety, irritability, fear, brooding, excessive concern with physical health, panic attacks, phobias. Delusion or hallucinations may be present. In elderly, see symptoms suggesting dementia (e.g., disorientation, memory loss, distractibility, apathy, difficulty in concentration, inattentiveness).
Onset	May begin abruptly. Relatively rapid: over hours. Short period of time: a few days. Especially common in children and after the age of 60.	Depends on underlying etiology. May be rather sudden (e.g., head trauma) or insidious in onset and slow, but progress is relentless over several years (e.g., primary degenerative dementia).	Usually able to date onset with some precision. Onset is variable; symptoms usually developing over a period of days to weeks but may be sudden. In some instances, prodromal symptoms may occur over several months.
Course	Fluctuates; symptoms usually worse at night; lucid intervals usually in the morning.	Depends on underlying etiology. May be progressive, static, or remitting.	Often not recognized or misdiagnosed in the elderly. Need to differentiate from dementia.
Duration	May resolve in a few hours, or a few weeks.	May progress to death over several years. May be arrested or reversed.	Self-limiting. Median time period is 8 months; may last up to 2 years.
Outcome	Recovery if underlying disease is corrected or self-limiting. If disorder persists, shift to another more stable organic brain syndrome. May cause death.	Reversibility depends on underlying pathology, timely diagnosis, and treatment. The more widespread the structural damage to the brain, the less likely the clinical improvement.	Can be successfully treated. Spontaneous recovery is expected. Severe depression may end in suicide.
Etiologic Factors	Systemic infections. Metabolic disorders (hepatic or renal disease, hypoxia, hypercapnia, hypoglycemia, ionic imbalances, thiamine deficiency). Postoperative states. Substance intoxication and withdrawal. Head trauma. Lesions of the right parietal lobe and occipital lobe. Toxin exposure.	Primary degenerative dementia, Alzheimer type. Infections of central nervous system. Brain trauma. Virus (e.g., AIDS, Creutzfeldt-Jakob disease). Toxic metabolic disturbance. Vascular disease (e.g., multi-infarct dementia). Normal pressure hydrocephalus. Neurologic conditions such as Huntington's disease, multiple sclerosis, Parkinson's disease. Postanoxic or posthypoglycemic states.	Situational: bereavement, loss of health, major catastrophic event in person's life.

Sources: American Psychiatric Association 1994; Blazer, Hughes, and George 1987.

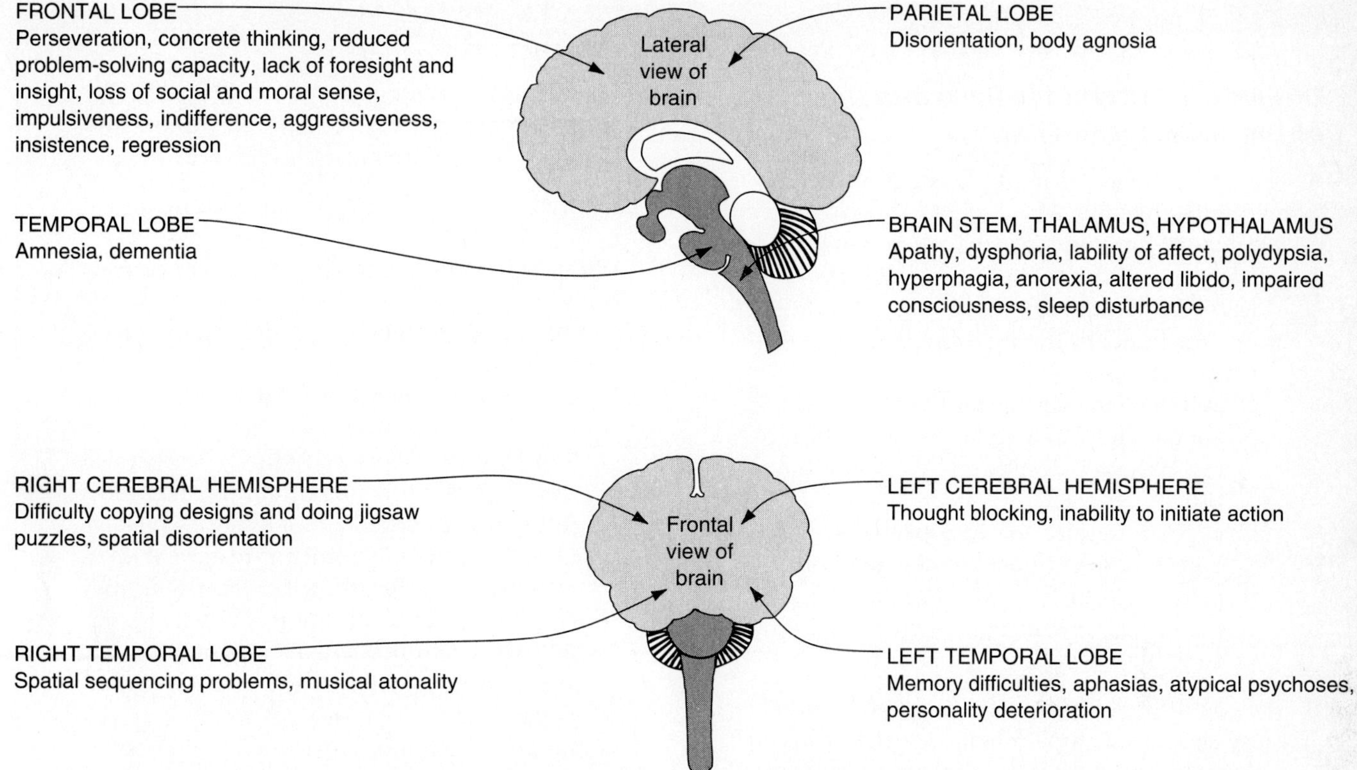

Figure 12–1 Behavioral changes related to specific areas of brain damage.

the brain and other pathologic lesions that he called **neurofibrillary tangles.** These are now referred to as Alzheimer-type changes. This disease may also destroy those neurons that secrete the neurotransmitter acetylcholine, which plays a role in memory and learning.

Signs of Alzheimer's Disease Signs of this disease include the following.

- **Aphasia** (the loss of language ability). Over time, the person experiences difficulty in finding words **(anomia)**, an inability to express thoughts in writing **(agraphia)**, and an inability to understand written language **(alexia)**. Eventually, the condition progresses to a loss of all verbal ability.
- **Apraxia** (the loss of purposeful movement without loss of muscle power or coordination in general). The ability to conceptualize or perform motor tasks deteriorates. People with apraxia may have difficulty carrying out complex tasks.
- **Agnosia** (the loss of sensory ability to recognize objects). Initially, the person has difficulty recognizing everyday objects. In the later stages, people with agnosia recognize neither loved ones nor their own body parts.
- **Mnemonic disturbances** (memory loss). The inability to remember recent events, especially in new or changing environments, extends to profound memory loss of both recent and past events (Adams and Victor 1993).

Progression of Alzheimer's Disease Reisberg et al. (1989) have compiled the most comprehensive profiles to date on clinically distinct global stages ranging from normal CNS (central nervous system) aging to severe AD. Their work, formalized in the Global Deterioration Scale (GDS), has been extended to 16 levels of functional disability corresponding to the 7 clinically identifiable global stages of CNS aging and AD and formalized as Functional Assessment Stages (FAST). Both the GDS and FAST stages are summarized in Table 12–2 on page 224. The GDS notes the cognitive decline, and the FAST stages specify corresponding levels of functional disability.

Vascular Dementia **Vascular dementia** accounts for about 17% of the dementias. Unlike Alzheimer's disease, vascular dementia is abrupt in onset and episodic, with multiple remissions. The client also demonstrates focal neurologic signs, such as one-sided weakness, emotional outbursts, a stepwise rather than progressive decline in intellectual functioning, and has a history of hypertension, diabetes, or cardiovascular disease affecting other organs.

In vascular dementia the brain tissue is destroyed by

Diagnostic Criteria for Dementia of the Alzheimer's Type

A. The development of multiple cognitive deficits manifested by both
   1. memory impairment (impaired ability to learn new information or to recall previously learned information)
   2. one (or more) of the following cognitive disturbances:
      a. aphasia (language disturbance)
      b. apraxia (impaired ability to carry out motor activities despite intact motor function)
      c. agnosia (failure to recognize or identify objects despite intact sensory function)
      d. disturbance in executive functioning (i.e., planning, organizing, sequencing, abstracting)

B. The cognitive deficits in Criteria A1 and A2 each cause significant impairment in social or occupational functioning and represent a significant decline from a previous level of functioning.

C. The course is characterized by gradual onset and continuing cognitive decline.

D. The cognitive deficits in Criteria A1 and A2 are not due to any of the following:
   1. other central nervous system conditions that cause progressive deficits in memory and cognition (e.g., cerebrovascular disease, Parkinson's disease, Huntington's disease, subdural hematoma, normal-pressure hydrocephalus, brain tumor)
   2. systemic conditions that are known to cause dementia (e.g., hypothyroidism, vitamin B_{12} or folic acid deficiency, niacin deficiency, hypercalcemia, neurosyphilis, HIV infection)
   3. substance-induced conditions

E. The deficits do not occur exclusively during the course of a delirium.

F. The disturbance is not better accounted for by another Axis I disorder (e.g., Major Depressive Disorder, Schizophrenia).

Code based on type of onset and predominant features:

With Early Onset: if onset is at age 65 years or below

290.11 With Delirium: if delirium is superimposed on the dementia

290.12 With Delusions: if delusions are the predominant feature

290.13 With Depressed Mood: if depressed mood (including presentations that meet full symptom criteria for a Major Depressive Episode) is the predominant feature. A separate diagnosis of Mood Disorder Due to a General Medical Condition is not given.

290.10 Uncomplicated: if none of the above predominates in the current clinical presentation

With Late Onset: if onset is after age 65 years

290.3 With Delirium: if delirium is superimposed on the dementia

290.20 With Delusions: if delusions are the predominant feature

290.21 With Depressed Mood: if depressed mood (including presentations that meet full symptom criteria for a Major Depressive Episode) is the predominant feature. A separate diagnosis of Mood Disorder Due to a General Medical Condition is not given.

290.0 Uncomplicated: if none of the above predominates in the current clinical presentation

Specify if:

With Behavioral Disturbance

Coding note: Also code 331.0 Alzheimer's disease on Axis III.

Source: American Psychiatric Association 1994, pp. 142–143.

intermittent emboli that can range from a few to over a dozen. Individual infarcts may vary by 1 cm in diameter, symptoms are commonly absent until 100–200 cc of brain tissue have been destroyed.

PARKINSON'S DISEASE Only recently has **Parkinson's disease** been associated with dementia. A minority of clients with dementia have Parkinson's disease. A subset of clients has both Parkinson's disease and Alzheimer's disease, and this diagnosis may be difficult. There are several different varieties of Parkinson's disease. The cause of classic Parkinson's disease is unknown. Another type, postencephalitic, has been linked to previous viral infection in the brain. An interesting feature of this type is the pres-

Types of Dementia

- Dementia of the Alzheimer's Type
- Vascular Dementia
- Dementia Due to HIV Disease
- Dementia Due to Head Trauma
- Dementia Due to Parkinson's Disease
- Dementia Due to Huntington's Disease
- Dementia Due to Pick's Disease
- Dementia Due to Creutzfelt-Jakob Disease
- Dementia Due to Other General Medical Conditions
- Substance-Induced Persisting Dementia
- Dementia Due to Multiple Etiologies
- Dementia Not Otherwise Specified

Source: American Psychiatric Association 1994, p. 133.

ence of neurofibrillary tangles similar to those found in clients with Alzheimer's disease (Whitehouse, Friedland, and Strauss 1992).

HUNTINGTON'S DISEASE **Huntington's disease** is a genetic progressive, degenerative disorder characterized by both motor and cognitive changes. This disease, one of the more frequently observed types of hereditary nervous system diseases, usually begins between the ages of 40 and 50. The movement disorder is thought to be caused by a loss of nerve cells in the brain. Mood disturbances, especially depression, are common early in the disease, followed by deterioration of cognitive function. Movement abnormalities slowly increase until all muscle groups are involved (Adams and Victor 1993). The motor dysfunction is characterized by **chorea:** quick, jerky, purposeless, involuntary movements. The average life span after an initial diagnosis is 15 years.

PICK'S DISEASE **Pick's disease** is a rare disorder in which cerebral atrophy is present in the frontal and/or temporal lobes. These circumscribed pathological changes are different from AD, in which atrophy is mild and diffuse.

The two patterns of behavior evident in Pick's disease, representative of the temporal and frontal types, respectively, include talkativeness, lightheartedness, gaiety, anxiety, and hyperattentiveness, or inertia, emotional dullness, and lack of initiative (Adams and Victor 1993). As the disease progresses, the deterioration becomes more global, affecting memory and language. The expected life span after the original diagnosis is 7 years. A higher incidence is seen in some families, suggesting a genetic predisposition.

CREUTZFELDT-JAKOB DISEASE **Creutzfeldt-Jakob disease** is a transmissible degenerative dementia affecting the cerebral cortex through cell destruction and overgrowth. It is marked clinically by a very rapid onset and involuntary movements. This profound dementia is evidenced by cerebellar ataxia, diffuse myoclonic jerks, and other visual and neurologic abnormalities. There may be a genetic susceptibility to infection; however, the only definitive spreading mechanism is iatrogenic, as seen after corneal transplantation, and after the injection of human growth hormone derived from the pituitary gland of cadavers (Adams and Victor 1993).

NORMAL PRESSURE HYDROCEPHALUS First recognized in 1965, **normal pressure hydrocephalus** is a relatively uncommon cause of dementia. Its importance is not frequency, but potential for correction. The classic description of findings is a combination of dementia with urinary incontinence; a slow, hesitant gait; and dilation of the fluid-filled spaces of the brain (Adams and Victor 1993). A history of head trauma, brain tumor, or bleeding in the brain may suggest normal pressure hydrocephalus.

Treatment is the implantation of a shunt to drain fluid from the brain to another body cavity (usually the abdomen). Successful relief of symptoms occurs in 40% of cases and brings rapid clinical improvement.

NEUROSYPHILIS **Neurosyphilis** or *dementia paralytica* is the direct result of untreated primary syphilis. The infecting organism (*Treponema pallidum,* a spirochete) produces cerebral atrophy in the frontal and anterior temporal lobes. Symptoms of this dementia may appear 1–12 years following the primary lesion (Adams and Victor 1993). The usual symptoms are paranoia, poor memory, faulty judgment, and disturbed emotional displays. Neurologic signs include fine and coarse tremors, abnormal reflexes, **dysarthia** (difficulty in speaking), and convulsions. Untreated, the disease is usually fatal within 3 years of onset.

PROGRESSIVE SUPRANUCLEAR PALSY **Progressive supranuclear palsy (PSP)** is a disorder similar to Parkinson's disease. It differs from Parkinson's in that the facial expression is a tonic grimace, rather than lack of movement; there is no tremor; posture is erect rather than stooped; oculomotor abnormalites are distinctive. PSP occurs

Table 12–2 Global Deterioration Scale (GDS) Stages and Functional Assessment Stages (FAST) in Alzheimer's Disease

Stage	GDS Characteristics	FAST Characteristics
1	No subjective complaints of memory deficit and no memory deficit in clinical interview	No decrement
2	Subjective complaints of memory deficits with no objective deficits in employment or social situations	Subjective deficit in word finding
3	Earliest clear-cut deficit with objective evidence of deficit on interview and decreased performance in demanding employment and social setting	Deficits in demanding employment
4	Clear-cut deficit on clinical interview as evidenced by decreased knowledge of current and recent events and concentration deficits on serial subtractions and other complex tasks such as managing finances or preparing dinner for guests	Requires help in complex tasks, e.g., handling finances, planning a dinner party
5	Deficit sufficient to interfere with independent community survival with inability to recall a major relevant aspect of current and past life such as address or phone number, names of close family members, etc.	Requires help choosing proper attire
6a	Deficit sufficient to require assistance with basic activities of daily life such as dressing and bathing, etc.	Requires help dressing in severe AD
6b		Requires help bathing properly
6c		Requires help with mechanics of toilet ing (e.g., flushing, wiping)
6d		Urinary incontinence
6e		Fecal incontinence
7a	Deficit sufficient to require help with toileting and feeding, urinary and fecal incontinence, etc.	Speech ability limited to about a half-dozen intelligible words
7b		Intelligible vocabulary limited to single word
7c		Ambulatory ability lost
7d		Ability to sit up lost
7e		Ability to smile lost
7f		Ability to hold up head lost

Source: Adapted from Reisberg et al. 1989.

between ages 45 and 73, usually in the sixties. Symptoms include balance difficulty, abrupt falls, visual and ocular disturbances, slurred speech, dysphagia, and personality changes including agitated depression (Adams and Victor 1993).

Pseudodementia Affective disorders, particularly depression, can be masked by symptoms suggestive of dementia. Clinical symptoms may include impaired attention and memory, apathy, self-neglect, and no complaints of depression. It is essential to detect pseudodementia in clients because, with appropriate treatment, they can recover. **Pseudodementia** should be suspected when the onset is abrupt, the clinical course is rapid, and the client complains about cognitive failures (Shimamura and Gershberg 1992). Clients with dementia often fail to perceive or attempt to cover up their deficits.

Ms S, a 57-year-old woman, complained she was having problems selecting the words she wanted to use and putting her thoughts on paper. She began to miss appointments and her scheduled workdays, and she could no longer handle her daily responsibilities.

Mr R, a 49-year-old male, had a stroke several years ago, diagnosed by a neurologist. Since then he has attended a day treatment center. Often he appears depressed, withdrawn, and confused, not knowing where he is, or who his family members are. He spends most of his day outside, staring at the garden or wandering back and forth. He talks slowly, frequently using the wrong words.

Mr J, a 45-year-old man, was in the hospital in the final stages of AIDS. He forgets what day it is and whether or not his family has visited. Occasionally he has visual hallucinations and on one occasion seemed to think he was at summer camp.

Mrs M, age 68, is in a nursing home. She spends all day socially withdrawn, unable to understand others or be understood. She walks back and forth for hours at a time, close to the wall. While walking, she has repetitive arm and leg movements, giving her gait an exaggerated appearance. Her head is down, she does not make eye contact, and she is incontinent.

Ms L was a 57-year-old widowed schoolteacher who had begun experiencing difficulties with her memory for the past year. Ms L was having problems selecting the words she wanted to use and putting her thoughts on paper. She began to miss appointments and scheduled workdays. Gradually, handling her own financial affairs became impossible.

She became incontinent as she wandered about the house, unable to find the bathroom. Increasingly anxious and paranoid, she began to see things crawling on the walls and mistook her own reflection in a mirror for a painting. When agitated, she was likely to walk out into the street.

Ms L was admitted to a long-term care facility when she became increasingly belligerent and aggressive with her daughter, wandered the house at night, and slept sporadically. After two years, Ms L was bedridden and unable to speak. She had to be tube fed. Ms L finally succumbed to pneumonia.

Amnestic Disorder

Amnestic disorder, a relatively uncommon cognitive disorder, is characterized by short- and long-term memory deficits, an inability to learn new material, confabulation, apathy, and a bland affect. Impairment may be moderate to severe. Possible causes include head trauma, hypoxia, encephalitis, thiamine deficiency, and substance abuse. See the accompanying box for a taxonomy of amnestic disorders.

Types of Amnestic Disorders

- Amnestic Disorder Due to a General Medical Condition (Indicate the General Medical Condition)
- Substance-Induced Persisting Amnestic Disorder
- Amnestic Disorder Not Otherwise Specified

Source: American Psychiatric Association 1994, p. 156.

Biopsychosocial Theories

Theories about the causes of cognitive disorders are as varied as the disorders themselves. Genetics, infection, and vascular insufficiency are all believed to be causative factors. Because delirium is usually caused by an underlying systemic illness, a prompt search is essential for treatable conditions like dehydration, diabetes, hyponatremia, hypercalcemia, thyroid crisis, infection, silent myocardial infarction, drug intoxication, or liver or renal failure. If the cause is removed, complete recovery from delirium can be achieved. For a description of the physiologic, psychologic, and environmental etiologies of acute confusional states in the hospitalized elderly, see the box on page 226.

The actual cause of Alzheimer's disease remains unknown, but several factors are believed to play a role. Alzheimer's disease has been correlated with the loss of specific groups of nerve cells and the disruption of communication between nerve cells (acetylcholine and serotonin deficits). Research is being done to identify a slow-acting viruslike causative agent. This work has been prompted by the findings of just such an agent in Creutzfeldt-Jakob disease.

To date, advanced age and family history are the only agreed upon risk factors for AD (Korten et al. 1993). People with AD have four times the family incidence of dementia. Yet in identical and fraternal twins, in only 40% of cases do both get AD, suggesting AD cannot be due to a single autosomal dominant gene. The disease also appears in twins and in varied family members at different times, making genetic studies difficult (Adams and Victor 1993).

Other possible risk factors are environmental toxins, past history of head trauma, stroke, thyroid disorder, lower educational status, and female gender (Butler 1994; Gorelik and Bozzola 1991). The link between aluminum and the development of AD is inconclusive.

Ongoing research focuses on causes and drug treatment that can either protect or restore neurons, thereby combatting memory loss. Additional drug studies focus on ameliorating behavioral symptoms. Vitamin B_{12} deficiency has been identified as a condition that mimics Alzheimer's disease, as explained in the box on page 227.

Physiologic, Psychologic, and Environmental Etiologies of Acute Confusional States in the Hospitalized Elderly

I. Physiologic
  A. Primary cerebral disease
    1. Nonstructural factors
      a. Vascular insufficiency—transient ischemic attacks, cerebral vascular accidents, thrombosis
      b. Central nervous system infection—acute and chronic meningitis, neurosyphilis, brain abscess
    2. Structural factors
      a. Trauma—subdural hematoma, concussion, contusion, intracranial hemorrhage
      b. Tumors—primary and metastatic
      c. Normal pressure hydrocephalus
  B. Extracranial disease
    1. Cardiovascular abnormalities
      a. Decreased cardiac output states—myocardial infarction, arrhythmias, congestive heart failure, cardiogenic shock
      b. Alterations in peripheral vascular resistance—increased and decreased states
      c. Vascular occlusion—disseminated intravascular coagulopathy, emboli
    2. Pulmonary abnormalities
      a. Inadequate gas exchange states—pulmonary disease, alveolar hypoventilation
      b. Infection—pneumonias
    3. Systemic infective processes—acute and chronic
      a. Viral
      b. Bacterial—endocarditis, pyelonephritis, cystitis
    4. Metabolic disturbances
      a. Electrolyte abnormalities—hypercalcemia, hyponatremia and hypernatremia, hypokalemia and hyperkalemia, hypochloremia and hyperchloremia, hyperphosphatemia
      b. Acidosis/alkalosis
      c. Hypoglycemia and hyperglycemia
      d. Acute and chronic renal failure
      e. Volume depletion—hemorrhage, inadequate fluid intake, diuretics
      f. Hepatic failure
      g. Porphyria
    5. Drug intoxication—therapeutic and substance abuse
      a. Misuse of prescribed medications
      b. Side-effects of therapeutic medications
      c. Drug-drug interactions
      d. Improper use of over-the-counter medications
      e. Ingestion of heavy metals and industrial poisons
    6. Endocrine disturbance
      a. Hypothyroidism and hyperthyroidism
      b. Diabetes mellitus
      c. Hypopituitarism
      d. Hypoparathyroidism and hyperparathyroidism
    7. Nutritional deficiencies
      a. B vitamins
      b. Vitamin C
      c. Hypoproteinemia
    8. Physiologic stress—pain, surgery
    9. Alterations in temperature regulation—hypothermia and hyperthermia
    10. Unknown physiologic abnormality—sometimes defined as pseudodelirium

II. Physiologic
  A. Severe emotional stress—postoperative states, relocation, hospitalization
  B. Depression
  C. Anxiety
  D. Pain—acute and chronic
  E. Fatigue
  F. Grief
  G. Sensory/perceptual deficits—noise, alteration in functioning of senses
  H. Mania
  I. Paranoia
  J. Situational disturbances

III. Environmental
  A. Unfamiliar environment creating a lack of meaning in the environment
  B. Sensory deprivation/environmental monotony creating a lack of meaning in the environment
  C. Sensory overload
  D. Immobilization—therapeutic, physical, pharmacologic
  E. Sleep deprivation
  F. Lack of temperospatial reference points

Source: Foreman 1986. Copyright © 1986 The American Journal of Nursing Company.

NUTRITION AND MENTAL HEALTH

Is It Alzheimer's Disease or Vitamin B_{12} Deficiency?

A deficiency of cobalamin, or vitamin B_{12}, can easily be mistaken for the dementia of Alzheimer's disease. Clinicians' ability to detect this common dietary disorder can prevent a great deal of misery among elderly clients.

Vitamin B_{12} depletion is common among older adults because of age-induced changes in the gastrointestinal tract. More specifically, they are prone to atrophic gastritis (Berkow 1987), which in turn reduces acid production and the secretion of digestive enzymes. Both are needed to separate B_{12} from other food components, thus freeing it for intestinal absorption (Herbert 1988). With time, gastric atrophy also reduces levels of intrinsic factor, a third substance required for cobalamin absorption.

Many nursing and medical textbooks state that a lack of vitamin B_{12} first causes pernicious anemia, and clinicians look for a drop in hemoglobin and a variety of other hematologic markers. The same texts explain that, with time, anemia is accompanied by neurologic signs and symptoms, including diminished vibration and position senses and dementia.

Unfortunately, it is rare for a clinician to suspect B_{12}-induced dementia when a client's complete blood count is normal. Recent research has shown that many older clients suffer the psychiatric effects of vitamin B_{12} deficiency *without* developing anemia.

For instance, Carmel (1988) found that among seventy patients with clear-cut vitamin B_{12} deficiency, 19% had no anemia and 33% had no evidence of macrocytosis: abnormally large red blood cells seen in pernicious anemia. Despite the normal blood profile, several clients had neurologic problems, including confusion, belligerence, disorientation, bizarre behavior, and numbness and weakness in the hands and feet. Sadly, many of these clients did not respond to vitamin therapy because irreversible nerve damage had already taken place. One way to prevent such needless tragedies is to perform routine serum B_{12} screening on all geriatric clients, thus increasing the likelihood of detecting a deficiency in an early, easily reversible stage.

A few words of caution, however, are in order about B_{12} screening: Recognizing a deficiency in its early stage is possible but requires astute assessment skills and a willingness to act as a strong client advocate, even in the face of resistance from other health professionals. Special effort is needed because some primary care physicians may not know how to interpret the diagnostic markers used to pinpoint the disorder.

Most reference works say serum B_{12} levels below 100–110 ng/L are consistent with B_{12} depletion. Thus, many clinicians ignore readings above that cutoff (Tietz 1985). Carmel (1988), however, has detected the disorder in clients with neuropsychiatric complaints and serum B_{12} readings between 100 and 299 ng/L. Others (Lindenbaum et al. 1988) have found similar symptoms in clients with readings of 100–200 ng/L. Of course, readings in this "subnormal" range—in the face of normal hematologic findings—do not prove conclusively that a client has B_{12} deficiency; some clients with "subnormal" serum levels have adequate cobalamin tissue levels. This finding should nevertheless prompt clinicians to investigate B_{12} status more thoroughly by performing either a Schilling test, which determines the ability to secrete intrinsic factor, or a serum methylmalonic acid test (Linderbaum, 1994), which can detect a subtle B_{12} deficit when the interpretation of serum B_{12} readings is questionable.

Once a B_{12} deficit is found, its origin must be determined. As mentioned earlier, older adults with this disorder are more likely than most to have gastric atrophy and poor absorption of the nutrient. Clients who have had a total gastrectomy and about 20% of those with partial gastrectomy will also develop a deficiency (Herbert and Colman 1988). Similarly, any disease or condition that severely damages the ileum—the site of B_{12} absorption—may induce a deficit. Among these are gluten intolerance, Crohn's disease, intestinal resection, and cancers of the small intestine. Likewise, certain drugs, including para-aminosalicylic acid, colchicine, and neomycin, can inhibit B_{12} absorption.

A B_{12} deficiency can result from poor eating habits alone, although this cause is less common among elderly clients. Those at greatest risk are strict vegetarians who avoid milk, eggs, and meats, virtually the only sources of the vitamin.

To correct a B_{12} deficiency, a clinician must first address the cause. In many malabsorption syndromes, including atrophic gastritis, the nutrient must be given intramuscularly, often for life. Among vegetarians, an oral supplement is adequate.

Paul L. Cerrato, BS, MA

The Nursing Process and Clients with Delirium, Dementia, Amnestic Disorder, and Other Cognitive Disorders

Assessment

SUBJECTIVE DATA It is often difficult to gather data about clients with delirium, dementia, amnestic disorder, and other cognitive disorders. Such clients are sometimes anxious and defensive; confused clients give unreliable histories; and often there is no reliable secondary source of information. All data should be gathered in a milieu that is free of distraction. The nurse should pace the questions slowly to allow the client time to answer comfortably. Aging people can normally process information after receiving it but may have difficulty taking in information. Placing the client in a situation that interferes with an already compromised sensory apparatus only heightens the client's anxiety and seriously compromises the nurse's attempts to evaluate effectively.

Health History When completing the client's health history, include all past and present medical conditions, paying special attention to chronic conditions for which

Assessment Instruments for Delirium

- Delirium Symptom Interview (DSI)
- Confusion Rating Scale
- Clinical Assessment of Confusion—A NEECHAM Confusion Scale
- Visual Analogue Scale for Confusion

Assessment Instruments for Dementia

Cognitive

- Blessed Dementia Rating Scale
- Brief Cognitive Rating Scale
- Clinical Dementia Rating Scale
- Clock Completion Test
- Hachinski Rating Scale
- Hamilton Depression Scale
- NINCDS/ADRDA Criteria (National Institute of Neurological and Communication Disorders and Stroke; Alzheimer's Disease and Related Disorders Association)
- SET Test
- Short Portable Mental Status Questionnaire
- Short Blessed Test
- Telephone Interview for Cognitive Status
- Wechsler Adult Intelligence Scale
- Mini-Mental State Exam (MMSE)

Memory

- Blessed Orientation, Memory Concentration Test
- The Story Retell
- Procedural Memory Task
- Wechsler Memory Scale

Language

- Modified Rey Figure
- Rey Verbal List
- Work Fluency
- Token Test
- Boston Naming
- Figural Fluency
- Proteus Mazes
- Verbal Fluency Task
- Wepman Aphasia Screening Test
- Western Aphasia Battery

Motor

- Manual Apraxia Battery
- Specific Activity Scale

Functional Level (Activities of Daily Living)

- Performance Test of Activities of Daily Living
- Physical Self-Maintenance Scale
- Refined ADL Assessment Scale (RADL)
- Schoulson's Scale of Dressing Ability

Table 12–3 Aids in the Evaluation of Clients with Possible Dementia

History	***Example***
Collateral source	Spouse, child, or friend
Premorbid function	Years of education, occupation(s)
Learning and memory	Recollection of recent events, repeating questions, misplacing important items
Functional capabilities	Financial affairs, shopping, travel arrangement, medications, hygiene
Behavioral disturbance	Dysphoria, crying, suicidal ideation, aggression, sleep disorder
Disease progression	Gradually progressive, abrupt recognition by family or true abrupt onset
Other conditions	Stroke, falling or gait disturbance, medications with potential to cause cognitive impairment
Level of consciousness	Awake and alert?
Mental status	
Orientation	Person, place, and time
Memory	Recall of three words, public figures, recent events
Attention	Recite months backward or serial sevens or threes, arithmetic
Language	Naming objects, word finding difficulty during conversation
Praxis	Draw a clock
Neurologic examination	
Focal findings	Asymmetric weakness or reflexes
Parkinsonism	Gait disturbance with impaired postural reflexes or stooped posture, slow movements, rigidity or tremor
Routine Tests	***Condition***
Vitamin B_{12}	B_{12} deficiency
T_4 or TSH	Hypothyroidism
RPR, FTA, MHA — TP	Syphilis
CT, MRI	Vascular disease (MRI more sensitive but less specific), mass lesions, hydrocephalus, demyelinating diseases and leukodystrophies (MRI superior)

Source: Bennett and Knopman 1994, p. 22.

the client is being treated and any recent changes in health status. Ask the client, "Are you seeing a physician at this time?" "Why did you seek medical help?" "What does the doctor say is the problem?" Infections may present as confusion and other symptoms of dementia before any change in temperature, pulse, and respirations is noted. See the boxes on page 228 listing assessment instruments for delirium and dementia. Table 12–3 suggests aids in the evaluation of people with possible dementia.

Sensory Impairment Older adults are particularly sensitive to the confusion associated with sensory deprivation. Physiologic changes in their sensory apparatus may be directly related to aging or to pathologic processes. Both diminish sensory receptive ability. The changes in sensory apparatus, however, are not clear-cut. The older adult may have difficulty hearing high-frequency sounds, such as consonants. Turning up the volume on the radio may help the person hear one range of sounds but may also cause sensory overload because the rest of the sounds are too loud. The overall result is deprivation and distortion.

Try to ascertain any possible sensory problems, especially in hearing and vision. To test hearing, stand so that the client can see your face, and ask a question in a normal tone of voice. The question should require more than a yes or no answer. Test vision with pictures the client will easily recognize.

Dietary History When possible, obtain an estimate of the client's food intake. "What do you eat for breakfast? Lunch? Dinner?" Make special note of protein and vitamin intake. Avitaminosis, pellagra, anemia, and hypoglycemia have all been associated with reversible brain syndromes. Hydration is also an important factor, easily noted in the client's physical state (a saliva pool below the tongue). Dehydration can also cause confusion.

Head Trauma Falls are common among elderly people. Cerebral contusions, midbrain hemorrhage, and subdural hematoma should all be considered. Confusion may be the primary result of such trauma.

Medication Older adults are prone to adverse drug reactions as a result of age-related bodily changes. These factors are compounded by high consumption of many different drugs: 45% of all prescriptions are written for elderly clients. The aged are particularly susceptible to drugs with anticholinergic properties (major tranquilizers, antidepressants, barbiturates, adrenal steroids, atropine, antiparkinsonians, antihistamines, antihypertensives, and diuretics). Question the client about both prescription and over-the-counter drugs: "Are you now taking any medicines that your doctor prescribed?" "Do you take laxatives, cold pills, or other medicines that you buy at your drug store without a prescription?"

Alcohol Consumption Ask the client about alcohol consumption. Alcohol is a CNS depressant, and intoxication may mimic symptoms of cognitive disorders. Alcohol also compromises nutritional status and may cause withdrawal effects. Ask questions such as "How much alcohol do you drink in one day/week?" and "Have you ever had periods of not remembering after you have been drinking?"

Cognitive Functioning Cognitive functioning includes memory, reasoning, abstraction, calculations, and judgment. Clients will not respond effectively unless they feel that the information requested is relevant, they see some purpose in the interview, and they are interested in the material. Choose testing materials carefully, and keep the endurance of the client in mind at all times. When assessing cognitive functioning, pay particular attention to the following list of clinical manifestations:

- *Appearance.* Clients who appear disheveled, dirty, or unkempt may be experiencing problems with poor memory or a shortened attention span. This deficit may not be apparent if the client has a caregiver who helps with grooming.
- *Manner.* Some clients may exaggerate mannerisms to compensate for a perceived decline in functioning. For example, compulsive clients may become more set in their ways.
- *Attitude.* An attitude of defensiveness, withdrawal, or paranoia may be a response to increasing anxiety about diminished abilities.
- *Communication.* The nurse assesses communication in the areas of speech, gestures, facial expression, and writing. Difficulty in finding words and naming objects may suggest **expressive aphasia.** Difficulty grasping complex concepts may suggest **receptive aphasia.** Assess the client's ability to use gestures and facial expressions to compensate for verbal aphasia. Not using facial expressions and gestures and speaking in a monotone may indicate depression. Also test written communication and reading ability, and assess the individual's language ability. Elderly individuals whose primary language is not English may revert to their native language.
- *Perception.* Perception is the client's ability to recognize and integrate sensory information, including the conscious recognition of oneself in relation to the environment. Clients with asymmetric brain involvement of Alzheimer's disease may neglect one side of their body. These clients may also have difficulty recognizing objects (agnosia).

  Clients with perceptual difficulty may distort sensory information, with resulting hallucinations and delusions.
- *Attention and wakefulness.* Attention refers to alertness and the ability to attend selectively to stimuli and to direct one's focus. Can the client sustain or pay attention to the interview process, or is he or she easily distracted by the environment? Attention can be assessed by asking the client to spell a word backward. Wakeful states range from hyperalertness to stupor. Stupor can be the result of medication intoxication or an acute systemic disease.
- *Motor activity.* Lethargy is often a symptom of depression, but it can also be the result of such medications as tranquilizers, antihypertensives, antidepressants, and antihistamines. Lethargy can also be caused by a number of disease processes, such as urinary tract infection, anemia, and meningitis. A shift between hypermotor and hypomotor activity is a sign of delirium. Agitation and physical striking out are occasionally demonstrated.

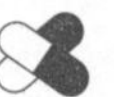

- *Mood and affect.* Depression may accompany the earlier stages of dementia. The more serious the dementia, however, the less depressed the client is. Clients with organic disease of the cerebral area are emotionally labile. Ask the client about any changes in eating or sleeping habits, and inquire about a recent loss of energy and interest in usual activities. If depression is suspected, evaluate the client for risk of suicide. Ask questions about suicide matter of factly, without hesitation, and record the findings carefully in the assessment notes.

- *Orientation.* Disorientation to time, place, and person must be measured in an environment where the client has easy access to the information. Days in a hospital are all the same to many of us. Acute disorientation in all spheres is commonly found in people having toxic states and traumatic brain disease. Disorientation to place and person usually indicates a degenerative disorder.
- *Memory.* At present there is no set of tests that can adequately measure the memory capacity of clients with dementia. Most tests measure *episodic memory:* the processing and storage of information, like recalling the events of the day. This type of memory is impaired in most clients with cognitive disorders, depression, and drug or alcohol intoxication. *Semantic memory,* or knowledge memory, is the ability to synthesize and think about events. It is used in language, abstraction, and logical operations. People with Alzheimer's disease have difficulty with semantic memory; however, depressed clients do not. Test episodic memory by asking the client to repeat a series of words or recall a recent event, such as a meal. Test semantic memory by asking the client to develop a scenario, such as describing the events from dinner until bedtime.

  Episodic memory is also tested in relation to time and is usually divided into three spheres: recent, remote, and past. People with dementias have difficulty acquiring recent memory or learning; this symptom may be a key to the early detection of dementia.
- *Abstract reasoning.* Proverbs are the most common way of testing abstract reasoning. "What does it mean when we say, 'People who live in glass houses shouldn't throw stones'?" "What does 'A stitch in time saves nine' mean to you?" Clients with Alzheimer's disease often interpret these proverbs quite literally.
- *Calculations.* The most common test of calculation ability is the serial sevens test: The person counts back from 100 in decrements of 7. This is a difficult process for the demented or delirious client. The test measures the client's ability to concentrate and focus thought. It may also be a measure of educational level.
- *Judgment.* The test for judgment should predict whether a person will behave in a socially accepted manner, including the planning and carrying out of activities that require the client to discriminate reality from unrealistic situations. You might ask the client, "If you needed help during the night, how would you get it?" "If you lost your wallet while doing errands, what would you do?"

Psychosocial History The psychosocial history should include an assessment of the client, the client's family, and their joint coping styles and level of intimacy. Some assessment of the client's function in the community should be included. Unlike cognitive testing, this assessment shows what clients are doing rather than what they might do.

Family History The families of impaired older adults can be a major source of information and support. In the United States, the majority of the elderly have seen one or more relatives the previous week, and many live within 30 minutes of their nearest child. Common living arrangements include living with a spouse, child, or sibling. Family assessment includes the following:

- Living arrangements.
- Care arrangements for the client (shopping assistance, daily visits, telephone calls).
- Family knowledge of the current illness.
- Family expectations for the future.
- Special family concerns about client care.
- Family style of coping with stress (death of a relative, illness).
- The identified spokesperson for the family.
- The family's perception of the client's coping abilities.

Throughout the interview, note the interactions between family members and the client. Do they support the client and respect what the client says? Do people listen to one another? What is the atmosphere in the group? What is the level of intimacy between family members? For a study about family caregiving demands of clients with AD, see the Research Note on the next page.

Activities of Daily Living Assess the client carefully for level of self-care. This is often called a *functional assessment.* What can the client do without help? For which activities is help required? What type of help is needed? As cognitive deficits increase, the client becomes more dependent on others for assistance.

Community Functioning The Comprehensive Functional Assessment (CFA) tool measures the ability to sustain oneself in the community. Assess not only the ability to live independently in the community but also the degree of social involvement. Does the client belong to any clubs or groups? Do friends visit the client at home? Does the client belong to a particular church or temple?

OBJECTIVE DATA Larson et al. (1984) have developed a three-step process for evaluating older adults with mental impairment.

1. *Physical assessment.* The client is given a thorough medical workup, including a complete neurologic exam (including evaluation of cranial nerves, motor and sensory systems, and reflexes) and a psychiatric consultation for possible psychiatric illness. Because

RESEARCH NOTE

Citation

Martinson I, Chesla C, Muwaswes M: Caregiving demands of patients with Alzheimer's disease. *Commun Health Nurs* 1993;10(4):225–232.

Study Problem/Purpose

This study describes the adaptive demands specific to the situation of caring for a family member with Alzheimer's disease. Adaptive demands are the qualities of the situation that require the caregivers to change how they relate to the ill person or adjust their own lives because of the caregiving necessities.

Methods

The sample, recruited from AD treatment centers and local lay support organizations, consisted of 18 family caregivers who were caring for the client at home at the beginning of the study. The caregiver was the spouse in 11 of the cases, and was an adult child in 7 cases. They had provided care to the client for 3–10 years. Client age averaged 74, while caregiver age averaged 57. Caregivers were interviewed at intake and every 6 months for 1.5 years.

Procedure

During interviews, caregivers described and gave specific examples of positive and negative incidents of caregiving that included the ways they managed the caregiving events. The interviews were tape recorded and transcribed for analysis and then subjected to Hermeneutical analysis, an interpretive method used with qualitative data. The three investigators looked for patterns and themes across the interviews as they read, reread, interpreted, and checked their interpretations against the data. Analysis was completed when there was consensual validation.

Findings

The investigators identified six illness qualities that comprise the central demands of caring for a person with AD: (1) The disease changes the client so dramatically that it creates a discontinuity of the self (boundaries of time and person become fluid), (2) the disease is constant and pervasive, (3) the disease introduces repetition into the caregiver's daily life, (4) the disease is unpredictable in its overall course, (5) the situation is perceived by the family members to be out of control, and (6) the disease always ends in death.

Implications

The investigators suggest that nurses use the six central demands of caring for a person with AD as a framework to help family members understand and anticipate the demands of caregiving during the course of the illness. It is hoped that this knowledge may help alleviate the stress of caregivers.

elderly people with organic illness frequently manifest confusion and depression, one works from the assumption that reversible illness is present. Chest X-ray films and an electrocardiogram are taken.

2. *Laboratory assessment.* The following tests are routinely ordered for elderly clients:
   - Complete blood count, including folic acid and vitamin B_{12} levels to detect anemia.
   - Erythrocyte sedimentation rate to detect infection.
   - SMA-12 to detect electrolyte imbalances.
   - Syphilis tests (VDRL).
   - Thyroid function studies.
   - Serum levels of barbiturates, bromides, and digitalis.
   - Liver function studies.
   - HIV.
   - Serology.
   - Heavy metals.
   - Toxicology.
   - Lumbar puncture studies.
   - Urinalysis.
3. *Computed tomographic brain scan (CT scan).* This test is ordered for clients at high risk, that is, those having acute deterioration in cognitive functioning of recent onset. This deterioration is often associated with focal lesions and hydrocephalus.

A number of elective procedures can also be used. However, their use should be limited unless indicated because of their cost. These are:

- Skull X-ray films.
- Lumbar puncture.
- Electroencephalography.

- Positron emission tomography (PET).
- Single-photon emission computed tomography (SPECT).
- Magnetic resonance imaging (MRI).
- Cerebral angiography.
- Isotope cisternography.

There are a number of brief rating scales for testing cognitive impairment, as listed in the Assessment Instruments boxes. None of these is perfect, and most need to be augmented by another test. The SET Test, developed in Scotland, is a tool for effective and quick nursing assessment (Hays and Borger 1985). The test measures mental function as a whole rather than its individual components. The test requires the person to count, name, and remember items, demonstrating motivation, alertness, concentration, short-term memory, and problem-solving ability.

The client is asked to list ten items from each of four groups: fruits, animals, colors, and towns/cities. The maximum score is 40; a score of 15 or below is positively correlated with dementia. Scores between 15 and 24 may not indicate dementia but may indicate mental changes caused by other factors. Mood disorders do not significantly affect the results of this test. For information about the assessment of early, middle, and late stages of AD, see the box below.

Nursing Diagnosis

A list of nursing diagnoses common to clients with cognitive disorders follows. These were developed by NANDA, the North American Nursing Diagnosis Association.

IMPAIRED PHYSICAL MOBILITY Gait changes due to neurologic involvement are seen in people with a number of

ASSESSMENT

Assessment of Early, Middle, and Late Stages of AD

Early Stage

Client complains of forgetfulness, as in remembering names and appointments.

Client covers up forgetfulness.

Client may blame others for forgetfulness.

Client acts confused, becomes irritable or quiet. Emotional lability is common.

Client begins to have problems in family, work, and social life.

Middle Stage

Memory problems become more pronounced. Recall of recent events is minimal.

Activities of daily living, including cooking, eating, bathing, and dressing, become increasingly problematic. Family and friends begin to take over for client.

Orientation and concentration are affected.

Client may become restless at night and may sleep only a few hours off and on throughout the day.

Client may become aggressive, even violent, when frustrated or when family attempts to help client.

Client may exhibit wandering and may call out and search for children or loved ones.

Client has increased aphasia, agnosia, and apraxia.

Hypertonia and unsteady gait are common.

Client may have insatiable appetite, yet lose weight.

Social habits are forgotten. Client may be socially inappropriate.

Late Stage

Client exhibits severe disorientation, including delusions, hallucinations, and paranoid ideation.

Client may lose all speech; may perseverate or echo sounds.

Client may touch self and objects frequently.

Client becomes bedridden, emaciated, and completely helpless.

the dementias. These include Alzheimer's disease, Huntington's disease, Parkinson's disease, Creutzfeldt-Jakob disease, normal pressure hydrocephalus, and progressive supranuclear palsy. Restlessness in the delirious client is reflected in hyperactive behavior. The client usually alternates between hyperactivity and hypoactivity.

Self-Care Deficit: Bathing/Hygiene, Dressing/Grooming, Feeding, Toileting Clients with delirium are unable to perceive, organize, or carry out the activities of daily living. They are far too distracted by stimuli and unable to focus. The Alzheimer's client has a distinct problem: apraxia, the loss of ability to perform formerly known skills. In the late stages of all the dementias, total care is a necessity as the client moves toward brain failure.

Sleep Pattern Disturbance *Sundowning*—confused behavior at night when environmental stimulation is low—is commonly seen in delirious clients. The client catnaps during the day and wanders at night. Poor sensory processing can also be seen in demented clients who also wander at night. The client with Alzheimer's disease may not sleep for several days, moving about in a confused state.

Altered Thought Processes (Agnosia) Agnosia, the failure to recognize familiar objects, is a progressive problem that eventually leaves the person without knowledge of loved ones. Overall, in both delirium and dementia, the client's ability to use information in making judgments may be seriously impaired.

Altered Thought Processes (Memory) Episodic short-term memory is affected by delirium, dementia, and mood disorders. Long-term memory is diminished in the later stages of Alzheimer's disease and acute delirium.

Altered Thought Processes (Orientation) Disorientation is seen in both demented and delirious clients. In the former it is related to progressive cerebral changes; in the latter, to an acute, usually identifiable causal agent.

Altered Thought Processes (Delusions) Delusions may be present in delirium and dementia. The client is prone to these cognitive processes as a result of reduced ability to distinguish and integrate sensory information. The problem is compounded by short- and long-term memory loss.

Impaired Verbal Communication Aphasia, both receptive and expressive, is one of the hallmarks of Alzheimer's disease. In the late stage of the illness, the client is completely mute. Confabulation is a common defense used by clients who cannot remember required information and therefore use fantasy to fill in the memory gaps.

High Risk for Violence: Self-Directed or Directed at Others In clients with Alzheimer's disease and most of the other dementias, there is a gradual decline in the social acceptability of their behavior. Hyperorality and touching all objects seen are a few of these impulsive and unpredictable behaviors. The client may also strike out at others while hallucinating or in a hyperactive phase. These behaviors are also seen in delirious clients, who are similarly unpredictable.

Altered Role Performance As the result of decreasing intellectual competence, the demented client moves from role of spouse, parent, employee, and community member to that of a dependent, regressed family member. The role loss and role change are anxiety-provoking and at times overwhelming for the client and family. Characteristically the family members experience a period of acute grief after receiving the diagnosis. Their level of depression should be assessed. Feelings of isolation and being overwhelmed are common.

Sensory/Perceptual Alterations The inability to attend and focus concentration is a hallmark of delirium. Decreased attention is also seen in the later stages of the dementias when the client loses the ability to encode. Delirium alters perception by reducing the client's ability to distinguish and integrate sensory information. As a result, the client has difficulty discriminating reality from hallucinations, dreams, illusions, and imagery. In the later stages of dementia, clients also experience hallucinations and delusions, which complicate delivery of care.

Self-Esteem Disturbance During the first stage of Alzheimer's disease and other dementias, the client is acutely aware of cognitive failure. This awareness and the resulting anxiety can be damaging to the self-esteem of a person living in a culture that does not tolerate or provide for dependence.

Functional Urinary Incontinence, Bowel Incontinence Incontinence of urine or feces is usually the result of confusion and failure to use the facilities. In the later stages of dementia, clients lose cortical control, but physiologic function remains. Incontinence of urine may also be an indication of normal pressure hydrocephalus.

Altered Nutrition, Less/More Than Body Requirements Poor nutrition and some metabolic disorders can be the direct cause of confusion in elderly clients. The reverse can also be true; confusion and cerebral change can cause nutritional deficits. Without supervision, many older clients are not capable of providing for or ingesting adequate amounts of food. Clients who are in the later stages of Alzheimer's disease have symptoms of bulimia followed by total loss of appetite.

Planning and Implementing Interventions

Nursing interventions for clients with cognitive disorders can be divided into two broad groups: interventions for clients with dementia and interventions for clients with delirium. Sample nursing care plans for these are presented in this chapter. With few exceptions, the interventions are similar, although the overall goals are different. The goal with the dementia is to minimize the client's loss of self-care capacity. Although functional loss is progressive, at every stage of the illness the nurse must assess and support the client's self-care capacity. Family members must also learn how to work with the client. See the Client/Family Teaching box below for suggestions for families. With delirious clients, the overall goal for nursing intervention is to support existing sensory perception until the cognition stage can return to previous levels of functioning. Of course in both diseases, keeping the client safe is the first priority.

PROMOTE NORMAL MOTOR BEHAVIOR Because of impaired coordination in dementia, falls become a safety concern. Living areas must be well lit and furniture left in the same place. Evaluate the client for visual and balance disturbances. Safety bars should be installed near toilets, showers, and tubs. Teach clients who need assistance the safe use of walkers and wheelchairs. Evaluate all clients using tranquilizers and antidepressants for postural hypotension. Blood pressure taken supine and standing is an indication. Restlessness and wandering can be dealt with by allowing the demented client to wander in a closed milieu. Avoid crowds or large open spaces without boundaries.

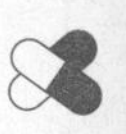

In clients with delirium, hyperactivity can be decreased by controlling environmental stimuli. If this does not help, medications can be used judiciously. Take vital signs one hour before and after the administration of any medication, and observe the client carefully for signs of stupor. Interrupt prolonged periods of hypoactivity with range-of-motion exercises, frequent turning, and having the client stand up at bedside, as tolerated. During periods of fluctuating motor behavior, there is always concern for the client's safety. A staff member should be present at all times, keep the bed lowered and the side rails up. In AD, wandering is a common and troublesome behavioral symptom. See the box on page 237 for guidelines for working with the wandering client.

MAINTAIN SELF-CARE Allow the client to do as much as possible unassisted. The more the client can effectively control the daily routine, the less anxiety the client will experience. Remind the client about daily grooming and personal hygiene, and repeat instructions. If the client resists oral hygiene, use mouth swabs with dilute hydrogen peroxide. If the client resists this as well, having the client eat an apple may help to clean the mouth. If the client resists any routine procedures, wait a few moments and try again. The client often forgets to offer new resistance. Clients who are acutely delirious or in the last stages of dementia need total bed care.

PROMOTE ADEQUATE SLEEP Clients with dementia and delirium respond poorly to hypnotics, which increase confusion and aggravate sundowning in older adults. A small amount of beer or wine at bedtime may produce enough relaxation without side effects. The most helpful measure may be to allow sleepless clients to wander in a confined area until they are tired. If the client is disorganized at night, make sure the room is light and without shadows. Possibly leave a radio on to provide more stimulation. Low doses of haloperidol or an antianxiety agent may be prescribed. (These medications should be used with caution and not on a nightly basis.) A Posey vest and soft restraints may have to be used if a staff member cannot sit with a delirious client or if the client attempts to remove IV tubing or bandages. (Use these according to established policy.) Reassure clients who have been restrained that they are safe and that the restraints are there to protect and help them.

CLIENT/FAMILY TEACHING

Suggestions for Families Who Have Just Had a Family Member Diagnosed with AD

- Have a family meeting and discuss strategies to care for the client at the present time and in the future, based on family responsibilities and resources.
- Contact the Alzheimer's Disease and Related Disorders Association (ADRDA) and request information. View their videotapes and read the available written material.
- Go to a support group for family caregivers.
- Contact an attorney and make decisions about power of attorney, and the control and distribution of client/family assets.
- Familiarize yourself with community resources such as day care treatment centers, nursing homes, and respite care for AD clients.
- Purchase a bracelet for the client identifying her/him as having AD.

CASE STUDY

A Client with Delirium

Identifying Information

Mr H is a 70-year-old married man who entered the hospital to have colon surgery. His wife stays with him and is extremely devoted.

Client's Description of the Problem

Mr H hallucinates and is delusional. He struck a nurse and lashed out at his wife. He ripped out an IV and a nasogastric tube. Twenty-four hours after surgery, Mr H became disoriented and delusional.

Psychiatric History

No prior psychiatric history.

Family History

Mr H has been married for 45 years. His two grown children live nearby. They and his wife are concerned, attentive, and willing to help with his care.

Social History

Mr H was a contractor and owned his own business. He retired 10 years ago. He and his wife live in a garden apartment and have many friends.

Health History

Mr H was diagnosed with a tumor of the colon and had a colon resection; path report was positive for cancer. Mr H has been healthy all his life until he noticed rectal bleeding a month ago.

Current Mental Status

Mr H is disoriented most of the time. He is often aggressive. He has frightening visual hallucinations, especially at night. He is delusional and acts as if people are trying to hurt him.

Other Subjective or Objective Clinical Data

He is on morphine for pain.

Diagnostic Impression

High risk for violence.

Nursing Diagnoses

Sensory/perceptual alterations

DSM-IV Multiaxial Diagnosis

Axis I: 780.09 Delirium
Axis II: V71.09 No Personality Disorder or Mental Retardation
Axis III: Cancer
Axis IV: Other psychosocial problems (colon surgery)
Axis V: GAF = 10 (current); GAF = 100 (highest level in past year)

NURSING CARE PLAN

Nursing Diagnosis

High Risk for Violence related to confusion, fear inherent in delirium.

Expected Outcome

Client will maintain appropriate impulse control.

Nursing Interventions

- Orient client when he or she seems confused.
- Move slowly, speak clearly, and explain all procedures.
- Depending on neurologic examination, medicate client with a low-dose antipsychotic.
- Restrain to protect client/self/others if emergency.

Outcome Met If

Client does not attempt to harm self or others.

Nursing Diagnosis

Sensory/Perceptual Alteration related to brain chemical imbalance inherent in delirium.

Expected Outcome

Patient will stop hallucinating and being delusional.

Nursing Interventions

- Reduce environmental stimuli; do only absolutely necessary procedures.
- Reduce the number of different people having contact with client.
- While working with client, move slowly, speak clearly, and provide information slowly.
- Orient the client often.
- Maintain adequate lighting.
- Begin orienting client to time, place, and person.
- Teach family members to orient client.
- Use touch, if effective, to calm and orient client.

Outcome Met If

- Client does not hallucinate.
- Client is not delusional.
- Client is oriented to time, place, and person.

INTERVENTION

Guidelines for Working with the Wandering Client

Strategy	Rationale
• Stay with the client, or be sure the client is in a safe, enclosed area.	• Wandering clients can get hurt. Safety is the first priority.
• Maintain a calm demeanor.	• Clients notice the feelings of others.
• Approach the client slowly and give her or him space. Use touch only if the client responds positively to it.	• The aim is to prevent aggressiveness, fear, and anxiety. Each client is different in response to touch, with specific people.
• Determine why the client is wandering. Is she or he upset? Thirsty? Hungry? Searching for family?	• When we understand why the client wanders, we can plan client-specific interventions.
• Meet the client's needs. If the client is searching, be supportive: "You are looking for X. . . . You must miss X. . . ."	• Support decreases anxiety, fear, and hostility.
• Attempt to engage the client in a repetitive activity such as rolling yarn or folding towels.	• Repetitive activities use energy and can be diversional.

Support Knowledge Processes The same interventions that are used to support memory and orientation are applied to the support of knowledge processes. Family education is imperative and can take the form of professional help or self-help groups.

Support Optimal Memory Functioning Gently orient the client. To allay anxiety, do not argue with the client about verbal discrepancies. Rather, direct the client toward areas of interest that are familiar and pleasurable. The environment should support whatever memory functions are still intact. Do not test the client for episodic memory unless it is absolutely necessary. If the client uses confabulation to fill in the memory gap, do not argue; note it as an ego-protective mechanism.

Because of their episodic memory loss, Alzheimer's clients do not respond well to reality orientation classes. But the nurse can trigger semantic memory by initiating a procedure the client can then complete. In this leading technique, a combination of words and nonverbal cues are used. For instance, while handing the client a toothbrush and pointing toward the mouth with a brushing motion, say, "Brush your teeth." Constant repetition in a kind, firm manner is often necessary. Music therapy may also trigger past associations, aid the client's long-term memory, and help a normally aphasic client participate in a group.

Drug therapy has also been proposed to assist the client in the early stages of Alzheimer's disease to maintain memory and orientation. Tacrine (Cognex), a potent anticholinesterase, is currently being studied in human trials. 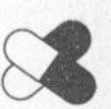 Clinical trials have resulted in both positive and negative results. The problems in demonstrating efficacy are believed to be due to methodological flaws, heterogeneity in AD clients, and the fact that tacrine provides only mild improvement. At present there is agreement on the required research design for conducting AD efficacy studies, so today's studies are methodologically sound. In one study, investigators noted that 3 months' treatment with tacrine resulted in a 6-month reversal of disease progression. However, 42% of clients who took tacrine dropped out, 25% because of negative side effects. The potential for hepatotoxicity requires clients to have their liver enzymes monitored frequently. Other side effects include nausea and vomiting, diarrhea, abdominal pain, and dyspepsia (Eggert and Crisman 1994).

Promote Optimal Orientation Structure the client's environment to support cognitive functions. The client should be wearing whatever aids (hearing, vision) are necessary to prevent sensory loss or distortion. Familiar objects from home, such as slippers, robe, and photographs, may also help orient the client. Easily read clocks, orientation boards, and a consistent daily routine that includes physical activity and socialization without sensory overload will also help orient the client. Verbally orient the client during conversation. Do not quiz the client about discrepancies.

CASE STUDY

A Client with Dementia

Identifying Information

Ms W is an 83-year-old widow living alone in an apartment. She was referred by her brother, who states: "She has been extremely forgetful recently." She lives on her husband's retirement and also receives Social Security.

Client's Description of the Problem

Ms W comes to the clinic this morning at the request of her brother, stating, "I had nothing to do with it. My brother's daughter must have a friend here." She states that she has been feeling "confused" and cannot remember things "from one moment to the next." She cannot remember how long this has been going on. She attributes this to getting old. Ms W states that nothing unusual has happened over the past year. She is able to provide limited information about her present problem. According to Ms W's 72-year-old brother, she has become increasingly disoriented over the last 6 months. On his own initiative, he brought her to her doctor, who was unable to find anything physically wrong. Her brother describes her as "forgetful and just not herself." On occasion, when he has gone to visit her, he has found her door unlocked and the burner on the stove left on.

Psychiatric History

No prior psychiatric history.

Family History

According to Ms W, her husband of 60 years "dropped dead two years ago while watching TV." She has one brother who is married with one daughter and lives nearby, and a daughter, 52 years old, married with three children and lives "in another state."

Social History

Ms W appears to have had a normal adulthood, passing through developmental milestones such as marriage, parenting, grandparenting, retirement, and widowhood without any problems. Ms W has no formal occupational training. She reminisces at length and with great detail about her work at the theater as a dresser. Ms W married when she was 21. When asked how long she had been married before her husband died, she replied, "Too many years." Her brother was able to report that she had been married for 60 years before her husband's death. Ms W described their relationship as "not very good." Ms W spends most of her days in her apartment.

Health History

There is no history of major illness or injuries. Ms W states that her appetite is "so-so," while her brother says she seems to have lost weight. When asked if she had any difficulty sleeping, she responded defensively, "No! No! No!"

Current Mental Status

Ms W is a cooperative elderly woman who appears somewhat unkempt with uncombed hair, wrinkled dress, and smelling of strong perfume. She is oriented to person and place, knows the year, but is unsure of the month and date. Her fund of general knowledge is poor, and she is unable to name the last five presidents. Ms. W is alert, labile, superficial, sporadically anxious, and irritable. She denies having illusions, hallucinations, or delusions. She shows loose associations but can be redirected easily. Her ability for abstract thought is impaired. She seems distractible and appears to have difficulty concentrating. She answers "I just don't know" frequently. Ms W becomes anxious and attempts to minimize cognitive defects. She tries to conceal them by circumstantiality, perseveration, and changing the topic. She has little insight into her current situation. She states, "I wish people would just leave me alone and get off my back. I don't know why everyone is so excited. I'm just getting old."

Other Subjective or Objective Clinical Data

She is not on any medications; suicide/violence potential minimal.

Diagnostic Impression

Nursing Diagnoses

Sleep Pattern Disturbance
Altered Nutrition
Altered Thought Processes

DSM-IV Multiaxial Diagnosis

Axis I: 290.0 Dementia of the Alzheimer's Type
Axis II: V71.09 No Personality Disorder or Mental Retardation
Axis III: Alzheimer's disease
Axis IV: Social isolation (family, friends, community)
Psychosocial stressors from severe memory loss
Axis V: GAF = 50 (current); GAF = 60 (highest level in past year)

This case study was adapted from the work of Kathleen Tomaselli while she was a graduate student in psychiatric nursing at the University of California, San Francisco.

NURSING CARE PLAN

A Client with Dementia

Nursing Diagnosis

Sleep Pattern Disturbance related to AD.

Expected Outcome

Client will sleep 8 hours at night.

Nursing Interventions

- Offer beer or wine at bedtime.
- Allow client to wander in a prescribed area until tired.
- Active daily schedule.

Outcome Met If

Client stays in bed at night for 8 hours and sleeps and/or rests.

Nursing Diagnosis

Altered Thought Processes related to memory loss in AD.

Expected Outcome

Client will maintain optimal cognitive functioning.

Nursing Interventions

- Structure environment to enhance memory (clocks, calendars, orientation board).
- Label objects.
- Use verbal and nonverbal communication to emphasize requests, repeating as necessary.
- Provide consistent daily routine that does not produce sensory overload.
- Do not argue with validity of delusions; try to understand and validate the feelings being indirectly expressed.
- Encourage physician to experiment with medication that will promote psychological comfort but not sedate client.
- Work with family to plan consistent daily routine.
- Teach family how to deal with delusions, client confusion, and anger. Explain reasons for this behavior.

Outcome Met If

Client is oriented to time, place, and person. Client appears less anxious; can sit for a period of time, does not look worried. Client does not express delusions.

Nursing Diagnosis

Altered Nutrition: less than body requirements related to loss of memory in AD (client forgets to eat).

Expected Outcome

Client will not lose weight, will take in adequate daily amounts of food and fluids.

Nursing Interventions

- Have family member and home health nurse monitor food and fluid intake.
- Supervise at mealtimes and assist as necessary.
- Give diet high in protein and carbohydrates in finger-food form with double portions.
- Weigh client weekly.
- Help family plan strategies to ensure client eats enough each day.

Outcome Met If

Client maintains or gains weight.

SUPPORT OPTIMAL VERBAL EXPRESSION As communication skills decrease, the client's nonverbal communications become more important. Clients respond physically to the environment, especially if they feel threatened. Call the client by name, approach in clear view, and give simple directions.

SUPPORT APPROPRIATE CONDUCT/IMPULSE CONTROL All measures used to support perception and orientation are imperative here. The client may strike out in response to hallucinations or delusions. The client functions best in an environment where stimulation is controlled and sensory overload prevented. All changes, whether environmental or personal, need to be made slowly. Always approach the client in full view, calling his or her name, and refrain from touching the client. Requests should be simple and nondemanding. A client with short-term memory loss can often be distracted. Restraints may be used to protect the client and others. They are, however, a last resort when the presence of staff members is no longer effective.

SUPPORT OPTIMAL ROLE PERFORMANCE To continue functioning in the family, the client must be viewed as an active member. Most clients with dementia remain at home until the caregiver can no longer manage the client's needs. The family needs support throughout this time such as home visits, day care, respite care, and support groups.

After the client is institutionalized, the family should be integral to the client's daily routine. Family members need extra emotional support as the rewards for maintaining involvement diminish. For the delirious client, role maintenance involves supporting the client's need to be oriented.

text continues on page 244

CRITICAL PATHWAY FOR A CLIENT EXPERIENCING DEMENTIA

Expected length of stay 8 days

	Date ________ Day 1	Date ________ Days 2–3	Date ________ Days 4–5
Daily outcomes	Client will: • Have stable vital signs. • Remain free of injury. • Consume 1500 cal and 2000 cc of fluid each day. • Verbalize thoughts and feelings. • Sleep 6–8 hr/night. • Participate in self-care to ability. • Demonstrate trust with caregivers and family.	Client will: • Have stable vital signs. • Remain free of injury. • Consume 1500 cal and 2000 cc of fluid each day. • Verbalize thoughts and feelings. • Sleep 6–8 hr/night. • Participate in self-care to ability. • Demonstrate trust with caregivers and family. • Maintain a stable weight. • Establish regular urine and bowel elimination patterns. • Spend short intervals with diversional activity. • Demonstrate increasing attention span.	Client will: • Have stable vital signs. • Remain free of injury. • Consume 1500 cal and 2000 cc of fluid each day. • Verbalize thoughts and feelings. • Sleep 6–8 hr/night. • Participate in self-care to ability. • Demonstrate trust with caregivers and family. • Maintain a stable weight. • Establish regular urine and bowel elimination patterns. • Spend short intervals with diversional activity. • Demonstrate increasing attention span. • Stay focused on simple task for 10 minutes.
Assessments, tests, and treatments	Mental status exam on admission and q shift. Vital signs q 4 hr if stable. Intake and output. CBC and urinalysis. Chemistry profile, electrolytes. Folate level. Chest X ray. EKG. PPD. Other diagnostic tests as indicated. Assess need for HIV testing. Weigh. Assess mood, affect, and behavior q 1–2 hr. Assess bowel and elimination patterns and sleep patterns. Initiate bowel protocol.	Mental status exam q 12 hr. Vital signs q 4 hr if stable. Intake and output. Assess mood, affect, and behavior q 1–2 hr. Monitor urine and bowel elimination and sleep patterns. Continue bowel protocol.	Mental status exam q 12 hr. Vital signs q shift and PRN. D/C intake and output if stable. Assess mood, affect, and behavior q 1–2 hr. Read PPD. Weigh on day 4. Monitor urine and bowel elimination and sleep patterns. Repeat laboratory studies as indicated.
Knowledge deficit	Orient client and family to room and routine. Use simple words and phrases. Include family in teaching. Review plan of care. Assess understanding of teaching.	Review plan of care with client and family. Use simple words and phrases. Include family in teaching. Assess understanding of teaching.	Review plan of care with client and family. Use simple words and phrases. Include family in teaching. Initiate discharge teaching regarding the need for ongoing outpatient care and medications. Assess understanding of teaching.

	Date ________ Day 1 *continued*	Date ________ Days 2–3 *continued*	Date ________ Days 4–5 *continued*
Diet	Encourage up to 2000 cc of fluids each day (unless contraindicated). Limit caffeine intake. Provide frequent, small, nutritious feedings, inclusive of all food groups. Nutrition assessment including calorie count if indicated.	Encourage up to 2000 cc of fluids each day (unless contraindicated). Limit caffeine. Dietary consult. Provide frequent, small, nutritious feedings, inclusive of all food groups.	Encourage up to 2000 cc of fluids each day (unless contraindicated). Limit caffeine. Provide frequent, small, nutritious feedings, inclusive of all food groups.
Activity	Assess safety needs and maintain appropriate precautions. Frequent observation. Activity as tolerated. PT evaluation if indicated. Toilet q 2–3 hr while awake and PRN. Assist with hygiene.	Maintain safety precautions. Frequent observation. Activity as tolerated. Prompt and assist with hygiene as needed. OT evaluation. Toilet q 2–3 hr while awake and PRN.	Maintain safety precautions. Frequent observations. Activity as tolerated. Prompt and assist with hygiene as needed. Toilet q 2–3 hr while awake and PRN.
Psychosocial	Assess level of anxiety. Provide information and ongoing support and encouragement to client and family. Use simple commands. Approach in calm, quiet manner. Assess sleep patterns and provide measures that promote rest and sleep. Encourage expression of thoughts and feelings. Approach in nonjudgmental manner. Explore availability of support system. Explore interests.	Assess level of anxiety. Encourage verbalization of concerns. Provide information and ongoing support and encouragement to client and family. Use simple commands. Approach in calm, quiet manner. Provide measures that promote rest and sleep. Encourage expression of thought and feelings. Approach in nonjudgmental manner. Explore availability of support system.	Assess level of anxiety. Encourage verbalization of concerns. Provide information and ongoing support and encouragement to client and family. Use simple commands. Approach in calm, quiet manner. Provide measures that promote rest and sleep. Encourage expression of thoughts and feelings. Approach in nonjudgmental manner. Explore availability of support system.
Medications	Routine meds as ordered. PRN meds for agitation.	Routine meds as ordered. PRN meds for agitation.	Routine meds as ordered. PRN meds for agitation.
Consults and discharge plan	Family assessment if not previously complete. Refer to neurologist and/or psychiatrist if indicated. Establish discharge objectives with client and family.	Review discharge objectives and anticipated discharge care with client and significant others. Refer to social service for discharge planning.	Review progress toward discharge objectives with client and significant others. Make appropriate referrals.

→

CRITICAL PATHWAY FOR A CLIENT EXPERIENCING DEMENTIA *(continued)*

	Date _________ Day 6	Date _________ Day 7	Date _________ Day 8 — Discharge
Daily outcomes	Client will: • Have stable vital signs. • Remain free of injury. • Consume 1500 cal and 2000 cc of fluid each day. • Verbalize thoughts and feelings. • Sleep 6–8 hr/night. • Participate in self-care to ability. • Demonstrate trust with caregiver and family. • Maintain a stable weight. • Maintain regular urine and bowel elimination patterns. • Spend increasing periods of time with diversional activities. • Demonstrate increasing attention span. • Stay focused on simple task for 15 minutes. • Establish sleep/rest routine to promote sleep.	Client will: • Have stable vital signs. • Remain free of injury. • Consume 1500 cal and 2000 cc of fluid each day. • Verbalize thoughts and feelings. • Sleep 6–8 hr/night. • Participate in self-care to ability. • Demonstrate trust with caregiver and family. • Maintain a stable weight. • Maintain regular urine and bowel elimination patterns. • Spend increasing periods of time with diversional activities. • Demonstrate increasing attention span. • Stay focused on a simple task for 15 minutes. • Establish sleep/rest routine to promote sleep.	Client is afebrile and has stable vital signs. Client remains free of injury. Client maintains adequate nutrition and fluid intake. Client's weight remains stable. Client has established a sleep/rest pattern and sleeps 6–8 hr/night. Client participates in self-care to ability. Client demonstrates trust with caregiver and family. Client maintains regular urine and bowel elimination patterns. Client spends increasing periods of time with diversional activities. Client demonstrates increasing attention span. Client stays focused on a simple task for 15 minutes. Client/family verbalizes discharge plans.
Assessments, tests, and treatments	Mental status q 12 hr. Vital signs BID if stable. Assess mood, affect, and behavior q 1–2 hr. Weigh. Monitor urine and bowel elimination and sleep patterns. Continue bowel protocol.	Mental status q 12 hr. Vital signs BID if stable. Assess mood, affect, and behavior q 1–2 hr. Monitor urine and bowel elimination and sleep patterns. Continue bowel protocol.	Mental status q 12 hr. Vital signs BID if stable. Assess mood, affect, and behavior q 1–2 hr. Weigh day 8. Monitor urine and bowel elimination and sleep patterns. Continue bowel protocol.
Knowledge deficit	Review plan of care. Use simple words and phrases. Include family in teaching. Continue discharge teaching regarding medications and activity. Assess understanding of teaching.	Review plan of care with client and family. Use simple words and phrases. Continue discharge teaching regarding medications, activity, and managing agitation. Assess understanding of teaching.	Client and/or significant other verbalizes understanding of discharge teaching, including exercise, diet, signs and symptoms to report, follow-up care, MD appointment, medications (name, purpose, dose, frequency, route, dietary interactions, and side effects), and home care arrangements. Assess understanding of teaching.
Diet	Encourage up to 2000 cc of fluids each day (unless contraindicated). Provide frequent, small, nutritious feedings, inclusive of all food groups.	Encourage up to 2000 cc of fluids each day (unless contraindicated). Provide frequent, small, nutritious feedings, inclusive of all food groups.	Encourage up to 2000 cc of fluids each day (unless contraindicated). Provide frequent, small nutritious feedings, inclusive of all food groups.

	Date ________ **Day 6** ***continued***	**Date ________** **Day 7** ***continued***	**Date ________** **Day 8 — Discharge** ***continued***
Activity	Maintain safety precautions. Frequent observation. Activity as tolerated. Prompt with self-care and hygiene.	Maintain safety precautions. Frequent observation. Activity as tolerated. Prompt with self-care and hygiene.	Maintain safety precautions. Frequent observation. Activity as tolerated. Prompt with self-care and hygiene.
Psychosocial	Assess level of anxiety. Encourage verbalization of concerns. Provide information and ongoing support and encouragement to client and family. Use simple commands. Approach in calm, quiet manner. Provide measures that promote rest and sleep. Encourage expression of thoughts and feelings. Approach in nonjudgmental manner. Encourage verbalization of concerns. Provide ongoing support and encouragement to client and family.	Assess level of anxiety. Encourage verbalization of concerns. Provide information and ongoing support and encouragement to client and family. Use simple commands. Approach in calm, quiet manner. Provide measures that promote rest and sleep. Encourage expression of thoughts and feelings. Approach in nonjudgmental manner. Encourage verbalization of concerns. Provide ongoing support and encouragement to client and family.	Assess level of anxiety. Encourage verbalization of concerns. Provide information and ongoing support and encouragement to client and family. Use simple commands. Approach in calm, quiet manner. Provide measures that promote rest and sleep. Encourage expression of thoughts and feelings. Approach in nonjudgmental manner. Explore availability of support system. Encourage verbalization of concerns. Provide ongoing support and encouragement to client and family.
Medications	Routine meds as ordered. PRN meds for agitation.	Routine meds as ordered. PRN meds for agitation.	Routine meds as ordered. PRN meds for agitation.
Transfer/ discharge plan	Review with client and significant others discharge objectives.	Review with client and significant others discharge objectives. Complete referrals for discharge.	Discharge with completed referrals.

NURSING SELF-AWARENESS

An Inventory for Nurses Who Care for Clients with Cognitive Disorders

- How do I feel about working with clients with cognitive disorders?
- What do I like about working with them?
- What frustrates me about working with them?
- What behavioral symptoms (wandering, agitation, hallucinations, delusion, hostility, eating problems, etc.) do I feel most competent to deal with? Least competent?
- What strategies have I used with clients that have been successful? Unsuccessful?
- Who are my favorite clients? Why? My least favorite clients? Why?
- What can I do to become more knowledgeable and/or skilled in dealing with clients with cognitive disorders?

Maintain Optimal Attention Span Repeat requests as needed. Speak in simple phrases, loud enough to be heard, and reinforce meaning with gestures. To decrease distractibility and hyperalertness, keep environmental stimulation at a minimum. Every effort should be made to lower the client's anxiety level by moving slowly, speaking clearly, and providing new information slowly.

Promote Optimal Self-Concept/Self-Esteem During the early stages of dementia, every effort should be made to maintain clients' self-esteem as they struggle with the personal awareness of cognitive loss. Encourage clients to express their fears and concerns, and listen attentively. Allow for the expression of anger and sadness.

Manipulate the environment to help the client with a failing memory. Helpful measures include labeling the bathroom and bedroom, posting notes to remind the client to turn off the stove and lock the door, and labeling the contents of drawers. Gently remind the client of forgotten events, and do not confront confabulations. Encourage the family to maintain the client as a productive member of this important group.

Support Optimal Perceptual Functioning A quiet environment with soft music prevents the client from experiencing sensory overload. When speaking with the client, stand or sit so that you are in direct view. First giving a verbal warning, touch the client's shoulder or hand, and slowly and clearly explain all procedures. Use touch with caution. Sometimes a very soothing touch can overexcite the client, who may respond by striking out. Make sure that the client is wearing hearing aids and eyeglasses if necessary.

In responding to hallucinations, simply state that you understand that these thoughts seem very real but that you do not experience the same thoughts. Do not argue or ask the client to elaborate. Give reassurance that these thoughts will go away. Say, "You are in a safe place." Do not leave the client alone or in an isolated room without some stimulation to help the client block out the hallucinations and support reality testing. The room should be well lit and without shadows or glare. If the client becomes combative, use physical restraints, but for as brief a period as possible. Then attempt to distract, reassuring the client, "You are in a safe place." Do not use restraints unless the client is a threat to others or self; restraints only frighten and aggravate perceptual problems.

Promote Optimal Patterns of Elimination A regular toileting schedule helps delirious clients control bowel and urine incontinence. Clients are often not able to let the nurse know when they have to use the toilet or have soiled themselves.

During the early stage of dementia, a toileting routine is essential. As the disease progresses, the client no longer recognizes a toilet or its purpose. Such a client may resist sitting on the toilet. Forcing the client will only produce agitation and combativeness. Distract and try again. If all efforts at maintaining a routine fail, use disposable pants or diapers. The use of catheters and external drains is not recommended because of the possibility of infection and their certain removal by a confused client.

Promote Optimal Nutritional Status Monitor the client's food and fluid intake. Give hyperactive clients a diet high in protein and carbohydrates, in finger-food form. Some clients may need double portions. Clients who chew constantly need to be reminded to swallow. Depending on the client's level of perception and motor activity, supervision and assistance at mealtimes may be necessary. Weigh the client routinely, and increase caloric intake as needed. In the final stages of the disease, the client loses all interest in food and must receive nasogastric, gastrostomy, or intravenous feedings.

Evaluation and Outcome Criteria

Specific outcomes for clients experiencing cognitive disorders are listed in the nursing care plans. Nurses should assess themselves as they work with clients with cognitive disorders; see the accompanying box above.

DELIRIUM EVALUATION CRITERIA The evaluation of nursing care for clients with delirium is based on the premise that clients are capable of returning to their previous level of functioning. During that process the goal is to help the client maintain optimal levels of sensory perception, participate in activities of daily living, and maintain physiologic homeostasis.

DEMENTIA EVALUATION CRITERIA Dementia entails progressive intellectual, behavioral, and physiologic deterioration. The goal of nursing care is not to effect a cure but rather to sustain the client at the optimal level of self-care. The nurse also helps the family sustain a personally rewarding relationship with their loved one throughout this terminal process.

Chapter Highlights

- Delirium is a cognitive disorder characterized by global cognitive impairment of abrupt onset and relatively brief duration in which perception, thinking, and memory are all disrupted.
- Delirium, common in older adults, is usually caused by an underlying systemic illness.
- Dementia is a condition marked by a loss of intellectual abilities of sufficient severity to interfere with social and occupational functioning.
- Alzheimer's disease, the most common form of dementia among the elderly, is a progressive, age-related chronic dysfunction marked by phases: early phases of forgetfulness, more advanced phases of disorientation and diminished concentration, and later and terminal phases of severe agitation, disorientation, psychosis, and complete helplessness.
- Age, decreased levels of acetylcholine and serotonin, genetic factors, viruslike substances, and environmental toxins are all under consideration as possible causes of Alzheimer's disease.
- Assessment for cognitive disorders is particularly challenging because confused clients are often poor historians; furthermore, the interview environment and procedure may increase the client's anxiety and seriously compromise the nurse's attempts to assess.
- Areas of subjective assessment include health history (including psychosocial lifestyle patterns), sensory impairment, dietary history, possibility of head trauma, medication use, cognitive functioning, and overall mental status.
- Objective data are obtained from physical examination, assessment of routine laboratory tests and scans, and objective reading scales of cognitive functioning.
- The overall goal of nursing interventions for clients with delirium is to support existing sensory perception until the client returns to previous levels of cognitive function.
- The goal of nursing interventions for clients with dementia is minimizing the loss of self-care capacity.

References

Adams R, Victor M: *Principles of Neurology.* McGraw-Hill, 1993.

American Psychiatric Association: *Diagnostic and Statistical Manual of Mental Disorders,* ed 4. APA, 1994.

Bennett D, Knopman D: Alzheimer's disease: A comprehensive approach to patient management. *Geriatrics* 1994;49(8):20–26.

Berkow R (ed): *Merck Manual of Diagnosis and Therapy,* ed 15. Merck, 1987.

Blazer D, Hughes D, George L: The epidemiology of depression in an elderly community population. *Gerontologist* 1987;27(3):281–287.

Butler R: ApoE: New risk factor for Alzheimer's. *Geriatrics* 1994;49(8):10–11.

Butler RN, Lewis MI: *Aging and Mental Health,* ed 3. Mosby, 1982.

Carmel R: The deoxyuridine suppression test identifies subtle cobalamin deficiency in patients without typical megaloblastic anemia. *JAMA* 1985;253(9):1284–1287.

Cook-Deegan RM, Mace N, Baily MA, Chavkin D, Hawes C: Confronting Alzheimer's disease and other dementias, in *Science Information Resource Center.* Lippincott, 1988.

Dickson LR, Ranseen JD: An update on selected organic mental syndromes. *Hosp Commun Psychiatr* 1990;41(3): 290–300.

Eggert A, Crisman M: Current concepts in understanding Alzheimer's disease. *Pharmacy* 1994;1(1):1–8.

Ernst R, Hay J: The U.S. economic and social costs of Alzheimer's disease revisited. *Am J Public Health* 1994;84:1261–1264.

Evans D, Funkenstein H, Albert M, Scherr P, Cook N, Chown M, Hebert L, Hennekens C, Taylor J: Prevalence of Alzheimer's disease in a community population of older persons. *JAMA* 1989:262(18):2551–2556.

Foreman MD: Acute confusional states in hospitalized elderly: A research dilemma. *Nurs Res* 1986;35:37–38.

Foreman M: The cognitive and behavioral nature of acute confusional states. *Scholarly Inquiry for Nurs Prac* 1991;5(1):3–16.

Franklin J, Francis R: Alcohol-induced organic mental disorders, in Yudofsky S, Hales R (eds): *Neuropsychiatry,* ed 2. American Psychiatric Press, 1992.

Gorelik P, Bozzola F: Alzheimer's disease. Clues to the cause. *Postgrad Med* 1991:89:231–239.

Hays A, Borger F: A test in time. *Am J Nurs* 1985;85: 1107–1111.

Health Policy and Biomedical Research News of the Week: *The blue sheet* 1990;33(15). Drug Research Reports.

Herbert V: Don't ignore low serum cobalamin (vitamin B_{12}) levels. *Arch Intern Med* 1988;148(8):1705–1707.

Herbert V, Colman N: Vitamin B_{12} and folic acid, in Shils M, Young V (eds): *Modern Nutrition in Health and Disease,* Lea and Febiger, 1988.

Korten A, Jorm M, Henderson A, Broe G, Creasey H, McCusker E: Assessing the risk of Alzheimer's disease in first-degree relatives of Alzheimer's disease cases. *Psycholog Med* 1993;23:915–923.

Larson E, Reifler B, Canfield C, Cohen G: Evaluating elderly outpatients with symptoms of dementia. *Hosp Commun Psychiatr* 1984;35:405–428.

Lindenbaum J, et al.: Neuropsychiatric disorders caused by cobalamin deficiency in the absence of anemia or macrocytosis. *N Eng J Med* 1988;318(26):1720–1728.

Lindenbaum J, et al.: Sensitivity of serum methylomalonic acid and total homocysteine determinations for diagnosing cobalamin and folate deficiencies. *Am J Med* 1994; 96(3):239–246.

Martinson I, Chesla C, Muwaswes M: Caregiving demands of patients with Alzheimer's disease. *J Commun Health Nurs* 1993;10(4):225–232.

National Institute on Aging: *Progress Report on Alzheimer's Disease: 1990.*

Reisberg B, et al.: The stage-specific temporal course of Alzheimer's disease: Functional and behavioral concomitants bases upon cross-sectional and longitudinal observation, in Kqbal K, Wisniewski H, Winbald B (eds): *Progress and Clinical and Biological Research: Alzheimer's Disease and Related Disorders.* Alan R. Liss, 1989.

Ronch J: Specialized Alzheimer's units in nursing homes: Pros and cons. *Am J Alzheimer's Care and Related Disorders and Res* July-August 1987:10–19.

Sacks O: *The Man Who Mistook His Wife for a Hat and Other Clinical Tales.* Summit Books, 1985.

Shimamura A, Gershberg F: Neuropsychiatric aspects of memory and amnesia, in Yudofsky S, Hales R (eds): *Neuropsychiatry* ed 2. American Psychiatric Press, 1992.

Tappen R: The effect of skill training on functional abilities of nursing home residents with dementia. *Res Nurs and Health* 1992;17:159–165.

Stern LZ, Bernick C: Mental disorders in the elderly. *Compr Ther* 1987;13(5):43–50.

Tietz N: Reference ranges and laboratory values of clinical importance, in Wyngaarden J, Smith L (eds): *Cecil Textbook of Medicine,* ed 17. Saunders, 1985.

Whitehouse P, Friedland R, Strauss M: Neuropsychiatric aspects of degenerative dementias associated with motor dysfunction, in Yudofsky S, Hales R (eds): *Neuropsychiatry* ed 2. American Psychiatric Press, 1992.

Wolanin MO, Fraelich-Philips LR: *Confusion, Prevention and Care.* Mosby, 1981.

CHAPTER 13

CLIENTS WITH SUBSTANCE-RELATED DISORDERS

Holly Skodol Wilson
Sally A. Hutchinson

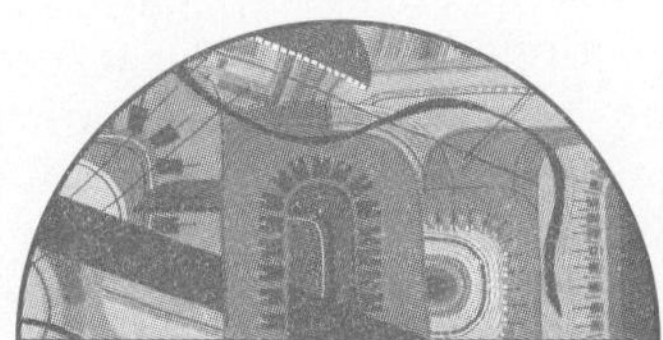

COMPETENCIES

- *Analyze the major theoretic explanations for substance-related disorders.*
- *Identify the groups at risk for substance-related disorders.*
- *Assess the physical, psychologic, and withdrawal effects of the major categories of substances.*
- *Formulate questions that are integral to a nursing assessment of clients who have substance-related disorders.*
- *Compare and contrast NANDA nursing diagnoses and DSM-IV diagnoses.*
- *Discuss a variety of short-term and long-term nursing intervention strategies for clients with substance-related disorders.*
- *Identify outcome criteria for clients who have substance-related disorders.*
- *Recognize your own feelings and attitudes about clients with substance-related disorders.*

Cross-References

Other topics related to this chapter are: Adolescents, Chapter 37; Depression, Chapter 15; Cognitive disorders, Chapter 12; Polydrug use among older adults, Chapter 38; Psychobiology, Chapter 3; Risk of AIDS for intravenous drug users, Chapter 27; Codependence, Chapter 25.

Critical Thinking Challenge

Billie is a 19-year-old homeless African-American woman pregnant with her third child and addicted to crack cocaine. When she appeared at your hospital's Family Practice Clinic for prenatal care one month before her delivery, she was referred to your team for assessment and treatment for her addiction. Billie is concerned about losing her children if she enters a drug treatment program, and she is fearful that her unborn baby is already damaged. She shuns AA and NA because admitting "powerlessness" and "turning her life over to God the Father" is unacceptable to her; as a marginalized poor black woman, she's had it with powerlessness and would rather empower her daughters so that they "don't turn their lives over to men." Others on your treatment team initially refuse to accept her as an outpatient because she will not promise complete abstinence and is reluctant to commit to attending one NA or AA meeting per day. What are your options for her care?

Drug and alcohol abuse, already a widespread problem, is rapidly escalating. Substance abuse is a psychosocial and a biologic problem. In the United States and Europe, television and radio advertisements entice viewers with the hope of relief from pain and problems. The values portrayed are clear: Discomfort should be erased; drinking is vital to a stress-free life; drugs are acceptable mediators of emotions.

Substance abuse is a complex public health issue with grave ramifications. It increases the crime rate, auto accident deaths, number of teenage pregnancies, and the suicide rate. Individuals and families are destroyed. Every part of a substance abuser's life—social life, family life, work productivity and relationships, physical health—is affected. Substance abuse in the work environment increases accidents, workers' compensation claims, absenteeism, and theft.

This chapter is a biopsychosocial exploration relevant to applying the nursing process with clients who have substance-related disorders. The significance of a knowledge base on this topic and the nurturing of caring attitudes as well as skills are underscored in the National Nurses Society on Addictions 1990 publication, *The Core Curriculum of Addictions Nursing* (Lynette 1990). The selection of information for this chapter was guided by that document.

Substance-Related Disorders

According to the *DSM-IV*, substance-related disorders are disorders that are: (1) a consequence of abusing a drug (such as alcohol); (2) the side effects of a medication (antihistamines, for example); or (3) related to exposure to a toxin (fuel, paint, or other inhalants). substance-related disorders are divided into two groups:

- Substance use disorders that include substance dependence and substance abuse.
- Substance-induced disorders (including substance intoxication and substance withdrawal as well as other substance-induced disorders such as substance-induced mood disorders and the like).

In keeping with the organizational scheme of *DSM-IV*, this chapter addresses the first group (substance depen-

Diagnostic Criteria for Substance Dependence

A maladaptive pattern of substance use, leading to clinically significant impairment or distress, as manifested by three (or more) of the following, occurring at any time in the same 12-month period:

1. tolerance, as defined by either of the following:
   a. a need for markedly increased amounts of the substance to achieve intoxication or desired effect
   b. markedly diminished effect with continued use of the same amount of the substance
2. withdrawal, as manifested by either of the following:
   a. the characteristic withdrawal syndrome for the substance (refer to Criteria A and B of the criteria sets for withdrawal from the specific substances)
   b. the same (or a closely related) substance is taken to relieve or avoid withdrawal symptoms
3. the substance is often taken in larger amounts or over a longer period than was intended
4. there is a persistent desire or unsuccessful efforts to cut down or control substance use
5. a great deal of time is spent in activities necessary to obtain the substance (e.g., visiting multiple doctors or driving long distances), use the substance (e.g., chain-smoking), or recover from its effects
6. important social, occupational, or recreational activities are given up or reduced because of substance use
7. the substance use is continued despite knowledge of having a persistent or recurrent physical or psychological problem that is likely to have been caused or exacerbated by the substance (e.g., current cocaine use despite recognition of cocaine-induced depression, or continued drinking despite recognition that an ulcer was made worse by alcohol consumption)

Specify if:

With Physiological Dependence: evidence of tolerance or withdrawal (i.e., either Item 1 or 2 is present)

Without Physiological Dependence: no evidence of tolerance or withdrawal (i.e., neither Item 1 nor 2 is present)

Course specifiers (see text for definitions)

Early Full Remission
Early Partial Remission
Sustained Full Remission
Sustained Partial Remission
On Agonist Therapy
In a Controlled Environment

Source: American Psychiatric Association 1994, p. 181.

dence and substance abuse), and intoxication and withdrawal for those classes of substances that have traditionally been called *psychoactive drugs*. The second group, substance-induced disorders, is addressed in appropriate chapters elsewhere in this text. (See, for example, Chapters 12, 15, and 16.)

Substance Dependence

Substance dependence is defined as a maladaptive pattern of substance use leading to clinically significant impairment or distress. The hallmarks of this pattern are: **tolerance**, the need for increased amounts of a substance to achieve the desired effect; **withdrawal**, uncomfortable and maladaptive physiologic and cognitive behavioral changes that are associated with lowered blood or tissue concentrations of a substance after an individual has been engaged in heavy use; **compulsive use**, the need for larger amounts of the substance than intended, making unsuccessful efforts to cut down or regulate substance use, devoting a great deal of time trying to obtain the substance, using the substance or recovering from the effects of the substance, and continuing to use the substance despite the recognition of associated adverse effects and difficulties. A summary of the DSM-IV diagnostic criteria for substance dependence appears in the box at left.

Substance Abuse

Substance Abuse is characterized by a pattern of repeated use of substances that is maladaptive in that significant adverse consequences occur. Examples include the failure to fulfill major role obligations, using substances in physically hazardous situations, and recurrent social and relationship problems. A summary of the DSM-IV diagnostic criteria appears in the box below.

Substance Intoxication

Substance intoxication refers to a reversible syndrome of maladaptive physiologic and behavioral changes that are due to the effects of a substance on a person's central nervous system (CNS). The syndrome includes disturbances of mood (such as belligerence or mood lability), perception, the sleep-wake cycle, attention, thinking, judgment, and psychomotor as well as interpersonal behavior. The box on page 250 summarizes the DSM-IV diagnostic criteria for substance intoxication.

Substance Withdrawal

Substance withdrawal refers to the development of maladaptive physiologic, behavioral, and cognitive changes that are due to reducing or stopping the heavy and regular use of a substance. Substance withdrawal syndrome is associated with distress and/or impairment in important areas of social functioning. See the box on page 250 presenting the DSM-IV diagnostic criteria for substance withdrawal.

Paul is a 40-year-old unemployed banker with a history of daily alcohol consumption that has gradually exceeded a quart per day of vodka for the past 25 years. He is estranged from his ex-wife and their two teenage children. He has tried

Diagnostic Criteria for Substance Abuse

A. A maladaptive pattern of substance use leading to clinically significant impairment or distress, as manifested by one (or more) of the following, occurring within a 12-month period:
   1. recurrent substance use resulting in a failure to fulfill major role obligations at work, school, or home (e.g., repeated absences or poor work performance related to substance use; substance-related absences, suspensions, or expulsions from school, neglect of children or household)
   2. recurrent substance use in situations in which it is physically hazardous (e.g., driving an automobile or operating a machine when impaired by substance use)
   3. recurrent substance-related legal problems (e.g., arrests for substance-related disorderly conduct)
   4. continued substance use despite having persistent or recurrent social or interpersonal problems caused or exacerbated by the effects of the substance (e.g., arguments with spouse about consequences of intoxication, physical fights)

B. The symptoms have never met the criteria for substance dependence for this class of substance.

Source: American Psychiatric Association 1994, p. 183.

Diagnostic Criteria for Substance Intoxication

A. The development of a reversible substance-specific syndrome due to recent ingestion of (or exposure to) a substance. **Note:** Different substances may produce similar or identical syndromes.

B. Clinically significant maladaptive behavioral or psychological changes that are due to the effect of the substance on the central nervous system (e.g., belligerence, mood lability, cognitive impairment, impaired judgment, impaired social or occupational functioning) and develop during or shortly after use of the substance.

C. The symptoms are not due to a general medical condition and are not better accounted for by another mental disorder.

Source: American Psychiatric Association 1994, p. 184.

Diagnostic Criteria for Substance Withdrawal

A. The development of a substance-specific syndrome due to the cessation of or reduction in substance use that has been heavy and prolonged.

B. The substance-specific syndrome causes clinically significant distress or impairment in social, occupational, or other important areas of functioning.

C. The symptoms are not due to a general medical condition and are not better accounted for by another mental disorder.

Source: American Psychiatric Association 1994, p. 185.

unsuccessfully to cut back on his drinking on numerous occasions, particularly when it became clear he would lose his job because of his declining performance, and when he received a second arrest for driving while intoxicated. He is brought into the community crisis unit for medical detoxification and referral to Alcoholics Anonymous (AA) meetings and a mandatory outpatient recovery group program. He smokes at least a pack of cigarettes each day and drinks six cups of strong coffee as well. His physical exam reveals hypertension that is not responsive to medication, elevated liver enzymes, and ascites. He complains of dull abdominal pain, dry skin, diarrhea, and indigestion. He is sweaty, shaking, and irritable. He has been requesting that the physician write a prescription for pain to ease his current discomfort.

Biopsychosocial Theories

Biologic Theories

The biologic explanation of alcoholism has assumed a great deal of importance in the last few years. Research to determine a genetic predisposition to alcoholism continues. Following are examples of research that is gaining respect in the scientific community.

- Classical research by Jellinek during the 1940s, 1950s, and 1960s, described as the Disease Model of Alcoholism, revealed that alcoholics proceed through phases, including the prealcoholic symptomatic phase, the prodromal phase, the crucial phase, and the chronic phase (Jellinek 1946). He recognized "loss of control" in addictive alcoholics and hypothesized that it may have a biochemical basis. Building on this early work, researchers have recently associated cocaine cravings with defects in dopamine (DA) neurotransmission in the brain (Hitre et al. 1994).
- In the late 1950s, researchers studied Scandinavian twins to determine whether alcoholism was inherited. The scientists studied twins of alcoholic parents who were reared by their own parents, foster parents, and different foster families. After 25 years, the records reveal that the degree of alcoholism in all three groups is almost identical. This finding suggests that a genetic factor predisposes some people to alcoholism (Mann 1983). Schuckit (1990) articulates the genetic theory but points out the absence of studies on drugs other than alcohol. Nurse expert Naegle (1988) contends that failure to control for other variables makes genetic predisposition an important but modest risk factor.
- Some people are born with a faulty hepatic enzyme system that may predispose them to alcohol addiction (Meyer 1994).
- Researchers have found that alcoholics metabolize ethanol more efficiently than nonalcoholics through the creation of alternative pathways and in response to chronic high blood alcohol levels. This phenomenon suggests an explanation for the abnormal increase in ethanol tolerance noted in the alcoholic population (Lieber and DeCarli 1970).
- P-450, an enzyme with opiatelike characteristics, has been found to develop in alcoholics, possibly creating the craving and compulsion to drink addictively.

- In animals, alcohol is metabolized into **tetrahydroisoquinolones (TIQs)**, opiatelike compounds that affect nerve receptors much as morphine and endorphins (the human body's naturally produced opiates) do. TIQ from alcohol has an opiate effect. In response, the body decreases or stops endorphin production. When the alcohol wears off, the endorphin level remains low, and the alcoholic cannot feel good without drinking. Some researchers believe alcoholics may be born with an endorphin deficiency, creating a low tolerance to pain and stress (Franks 1985).
- Animal research advances the notion that alcoholics have a metabolic anomaly that causes them to derive more pleasure from alcohol than other people do. When alcohol is absent from the body, the absence of this pleasure is felt as a deficiency (Franks 1985).
- Alcoholics may have neurophysiologic defects. They may be vulnerable to intense sensory input and use alcohol as a protection from this heightened sensitivity.
- Research demonstrates that children of alcoholics are at fourfold risk of becoming alcoholics. Even if they are adopted by different families at birth, identical twins of alcoholic parents have more than a 60% chance of becoming alcoholics; fraternal twins have less than a 30% chance. Children of nonalcoholics reared by alcoholics are not at increased risk for alcoholism (Schuckit 1985).
- When a control group of sons of nonalcoholics (a low-risk population) and an experimental group of sons of alcoholics (a high-risk population) were compared, three differences were found (Schuckit 1985):
  1. Sons of alcoholics appear to show a less-intense response to modest ethanol dosages, demonstrate lower amplitudes of a brain wave that might measure selective attention, and may have different brain alpha rhythms.
  2. Subjective and objective tests showed that sons of alcoholics were less affected by ethanol than sons of nonalcoholics.
  3. When both groups were given the same dosage of ethanol, controls showed poor performance on a number of cognitive and psychomotor tests and more intense changes in cortisol and prolactin, two hormones known to be affected by an injection of ethanol.

  Schuckit (1985) concludes that "there is consistent evidence that those in the high-risk group demonstrate significantly less-intense reactions to modest doses of ethanol than those in the low-risk group. It may be that they are feeling less ethanol effect at the blood alcohol concentrations at which most people make a decision to stop drinking."
- Postmortem neuropsychiatric studies indicate that clients with a history of cocaine use have both structural damage in the prefrontal cortex and neurochemical defects in their dopaminergic system (Hitre et al. 1994).
- Neurobiological studies are clearly attesting that biologic factors such as genetics underpin vulnerability to substance-related disorders and also result from them. Furthermore, medications with anxiolytic and antidepressant effects are being used in both detoxification and relapse-prevention treatment (Shaw et al. 1994).

Psychologic Theories

From the psychologic perspective, the substance abuser is viewed as regressed and fixated at pregenital, oral levels of psychosexual development. Some writers relate the pattern of drug taking to parental inconsistency, self-centeredness, and inner dishonesty. The following personality traits are often associated with disruptive drug abuse:

- Dominant and critical behavior with underlying self-doubts and passivity.
- Overt extroversion.
- Tendency to describe own parents as self-reliant and efficient but not emotionally warm.
- Personal insecurity, with low self-esteem and self criticism.
- Problems with sexual identification.
- Rebellious attitudes toward authority.
- Tendency to use defense mechanisms that are primarily escapist or sensation seeking.
- Difficulty with intimacy.
- Absence of a strong and efficient superego.
- Marked narcissistic trends.
- Difficulty with impulse control and feelings.

There is no real agreement about whether certain personality traits are sufficient to account for drug dependence, because the personality traits in question are studied after the diagnosis of substance abuse is made.

In a 1994 prospective study of personality tests as predictors of alcoholism, Schuckit et al. reported that except for antisocial personality disorder, it is difficult to identify a reliable personality profile associated with a person's risk of alcoholism. In their research, the men who went on to develop alcohol abuse did not differ on personality tests from those who did not develop alcoholism. This study's findings are often contradicted in twelve-step AA meetings, where references are made to a typical "alcoholic" personality. One characteristic presumed to be held in common is difficulty coping with feelings.

Sociocultural Theories

Sociocultural models of substance abuse emphasize social forces, role models, and adaptive responses to stress in the sociocultural environment. Life's harsh realities come in many forms: the hopelessness and defeat of urban slum dwellers, the academic and social pressures generated by upper middle class families, the adolescent's feeling of impotence and alienation, the peer group pressure to join in and share experiences, the social vacuum of unloving families, where meaningful attachments are dissolved or dissolving. All of these social conditions and contexts help create and sustain substance abuse. In addition, however, people who become addicts or alcoholics tend to live in environments where access to chemicals is easy and initiation into their use is widespread. Substance abusers describe in interviews how they learned to drink or use drugs at high school and college parties or at home by watching their families. They recognized chemicals as a remedy for psychic and physical pain.

Sociologist Howard Becker (1963) studied the process by which a person becomes a marijuana user. In this classic study, Becker emphasizes the role the subculture plays in teaching people to disengage from conventional social controls. The subculture also teaches them how to think about the experience and the techniques that ensure they will enjoy using the drug. Another sociologist, Alfred Lindesmith (1965), observes that people recognize they are addicted at the moment when the appearance of withdrawal symptoms makes voluntary abstinence impossible. At this point, they are ready to be assimilated into a genuine drug-dependent lifestyle, because they must begin planning how to make sure they have a future supply. They must learn the sources, devices, and customs they will use to solve their problems.

Gender researchers have suggested that in the case of abuse by the highly potent form of cocaine called crack, differences in how drug abuse begins and is maintained exist between women and men. Effective prevention and treatment programs depend on understanding such differences.

Studies clearly show that substance abuse is present in all cultures; however, which substance people abuse is often culturally determined. In Western culture, alcohol is the drug of choice. In Moslem countries, marijuana use is a problem because Islam prohibits alcohol use. Opium is used in China and other Eastern countries, whereas people in India and Africa use native herbs and chemicals. Native Americans use peyote and alcohol more than other drugs.

Family Systems Theories

A family systems explanation for substance abuse has gained increasing acceptance among health care professionals. Stanton and Todd's work (1982) is particularly useful because it proposes a theoretic framework, a treatment method, and evaluation methods based on family systems theory. Unlike social theorists who stress the power of the peer group, Stanton and Todd view adolescent drug abuse primarily as a family phenomenon. Adolescent drug addicts, they believe, are too close to their parents and consequently feel dependent, inadequate, and fearful of separation. The family is overly *enmeshed* or *entangled.*

Contrary to what one might expect, the adolescent drug abuser is striving to preserve the stability of the entangled family. The adolescent keeps the family in crisis and focused on the problems brought about by drug abuse. If the addict improves and begins to individuate and separate from the family, the underlying familial problems emerge. Thus, the entire family has a stake in maintaining the addiction. The drug use allows the addict to pseudoindividuate—to be both in and out of the family. Family characteristics and ways of relating are passed on to the next generation.

The family systems perspective also includes the phenomenon of **codependence.** A **codependent** is a person who allows another's behavior to affect him or her while being obsessed with controlling the other person's behavior. Codependents try to control events and people around them because they feel that everything around them and inside them is out of their control (Guy 1990). A codependent is a family member who alternately rescues and blames (persecutes) the addict.

Although **Alcoholics Anonymous (AA),** a support group for alcoholics, does not openly endorse the family systems theory, they do recognize clearly that alcoholism is a family disease. **Al-Anon** and **Al-Ateen** are groups for spouses, parents, and teenage children of alcoholics. The focus is on helping these nonalcoholics learn to live and work effectively with alcoholics. The underlying belief is that family members often assume the role of **enablers,** or coalcoholics, perpetuating the alcoholic's drinking patterns.

A cycle begins when the enablers do what they think is best in the situation. They begin to cover for the addict, such as by saying that he or she has a cold, is bruised because of stumbling in the dark, is asleep because of fatigue. Protected by the enabler, the addict is spared the consequences of his or her behavior and continues drinking or using drugs. The enabler, believing that the addict is coping with family, marital, or work problems "the best way he can," denies the disease of addiction. The addict blames the enabler; the enabler feels guilty and then attempts to control family life and the behaviors of the alcoholic/addict by throwing out liquor or taking the car keys. Of course this behavior does not work. The enabler has tried the roles of protector, rescuer, controller, and blamer, but none is effective in altering the course of the disease. Consequently, enablers feel worthless and helpless because they are unsuccessful in terminating the addiction. Intervention and confrontation are necessary to break the cycle.

Dysfunctional Family Roles When a family consists of one parent in the role of Addict, who is incapable of being emotionally present and fulfilling the parenting role adequately, and one parent in the role of Codependent or Enabler, who is trying to fix the Addict, children may be

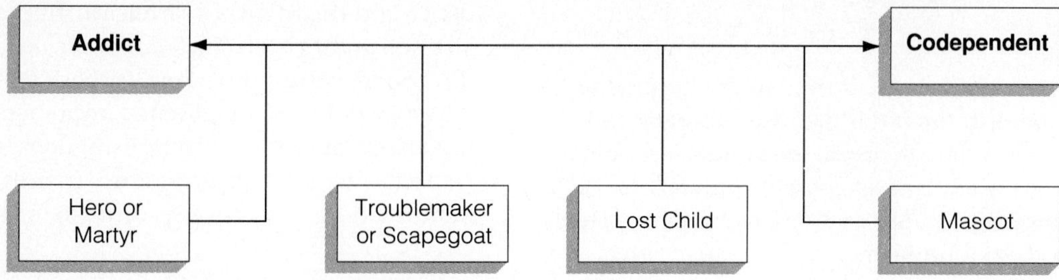

Figure 13–1 Dysfunctional family roles in the addict-codependent continuum.

Dysfunctional Family Roles

The Hero or Martyr

- Often the oldest girl or boy.
- Becomes the family caretaker (looking after younger children, making excuses for parents).
- Attempts to keep harmony.
- Is often an overachiever, seemingly very balanced.

The Troublemaker or Scapegoat

- Gets into trouble.
- Deflects attention from the dysfunctional family by becoming the focus of the family's problems.
- Acts out in school, in the community, and at home.
- Shows obvious pain.

The Lost Child

- Often the third or middle child.
- Less angry and more lonely.
- Hasn't learned to connect emotionally in the absence of role models.
- Is shy and afraid to speak up.
- Avoids confrontation and stress by withdrawing.
- Often shows misery by an inability to share and the development of health problems (allergies, headaches, bed-wetting, etc.).
- Sometimes become sexually active at a young age to meet intimacy needs.

The Mascot

- Often the baby of the family.
- May be in the dark about what is going on but feels tension and anxiety.
- Tends to develop phobias.
- Often has trouble concentrating; may be hyperactive.
- Teases and clowns around.
- Is often an underachiever.

forced into dysfunctional family roles (Figure 13–1). Such children are consumed with meeting family needs and miss out on nurturing. Children's roles may consist of:

The Hero or Martyr
The Troublemaker or Scapegoat
The Lost Child
The Mascot

These defensive personalities represent survival strategies for children living in what they perceive to be a frightening family environment. Behaviors associated with each of these dysfunctional family roles appear in the box above. Adult personalities are partially imprinted during childhood, and the roles that children take in order to cope in a family burdened by addiction can continue into adulthood if appropriate treatment is not provided.

Alcohol

Carol D, a 48-year-old woman, arrived at the hospital to be admitted for the fifth time. Her gait was unsteady and her speech slurred. Even though drunk, she avoided eye contact, appeared embarrassed, and apologized profusely for "getting into this mess again." She said "I really don't need to be here. I can handle this problem."

The accompanying box below presents key facts about alcohol. Several years ago, alcoholism was considered a neglected disease. Recently, because of its increasing incidence and the highway carnage attributed to alcohol use, alcoholism has been the focus of magazine articles and radio and television programs. Perhaps this media blitz is in part a response to heightened awareness of the devastating effects of chronic alcoholism: depression; loss of self-respect; alienation from family, friends, and coworkers; malnutrition; infections; and damaging physiologic effects to most body systems (see the box on page 255 concerning physical effects of chronic alcoholism).

Although alcoholism was historically viewed as a moral problem, increased awareness played a part in the redefinition of alcoholism as a disease. As research about

Key Facts About Alcohol (Ethyl Alcohol: C_2H_5OH or ETOH)

Examples

Liquor, wine, beer

Slang Terms

Hooch, booze, moonshine, sauce

Route of Administration

Oral (liquid)

Psychologic Symptoms

- Irritability*
- Mood swings*
- Short attention span*
- Loud and frequent talking*
- Decreased judgment
- Decreased inhibitions
- Interference with memory

Physical Symptoms

- Slurred speech*
- Lack of coordination*
- Unsteady gait*
- Blackouts
- Decreased REM sleep
- Nystagmus*
- Flushed face*
- Decreased psychomotor functions

Withdrawal Symptoms

- Nausea or vomiting
- Anxiety
- Depressed mood or irritability
- Malaise or weakness
- Autonomic hyperactivity
- Tachycardia
- Sweating; elevated blood pressure
- Orthostatic hypotension
- Coarse tremor of hands, tongue, eyelids

Time Frame for Withdrawal Symptoms

Mild withdrawal may begin within 12–24 hr following last drink. Symptoms may last 48–72 hr. Major withdrawal symptoms appear within 2–3 days following last drink and may last 3–5 days.

Dangers and Complications

Car accidents	Pancreatitis
Physical injury	GI bleeding
Malnutrition	Wernicke's encephalopathy
Hepatitis	Korsakoff's psychosis
Cirrhosis	Respiratory arrest
Gastritis	DTs
Suicide	
FAS (fetal alcohol syndrome)	

**Symptoms of intoxication noted in* DSM-IV.

its biochemical aspects became known, earlier beliefs were challenged. The social stigma attached to alcoholism is decreasing, and more people are seeking help. Professionals, laypeople, alcoholics, and nonalcoholics are attending workshops and seminars on alcoholism; college courses at the graduate and undergraduate levels are offered. Recovery programs are reported widely in the popular media.

The Effects of Alcohol

A sedative anesthetic (CNS depressant), alcohol is absorbed in the mouth, stomach, and small intestine. Approximately 95% is broken down by the liver; the rest is excreted through the lungs, kidneys, and skin. Generally, a person can metabolize 10 mL of alcohol (1 oz of whiskey) every 90 minutes. The rate of absorption varies based on many factors, such as weight, intake of food, and liver function. If taken in exceedingly high doses, alcohol can depress respiration and cause death. Intoxication occurs when a person's blood alcohol level is 0.10% or more. This blood alcohol level is the legal definition of inebriation in most states, although there is a trend toward lowering the level to 0.08 in some states. Simple intoxication lasts less than 12 hours and is usually followed by a hangover.

Physical Effects of Chronic Alcoholism

Hepatic System

- Alcoholic fatty liver syndrome
- Alcoholic hepatitis
- Laënnec's cirrhosis

Neurologic System

- Wernicke-Korsakoff syndrome (related to thiamine deficiency)
- Peripheral neuropathy (related to vitamin B deficiency)
- Marchiafava disease*
- Central pontine myelinosis*
- Cerebellar degeneration*
- Alcoholic amblyopia*

Cardiovascular System

- Alcoholic cardiomyopathy
- Hypokalemia
- Hypomagnesemia
- Hyperlipidemia
- Altered fluid balance
- Beriberi heart disease (related to thiamine deficiency)
- Hematologic abnormalities

Musculoskeletal System

- Acute alcoholic myopathy
- Subclinical alcoholic myopathy
- Chronic alcoholic myopathy

Gastrointestinal System

- Gastritis
- Esophagitis
- Mallory-Weiss syndrome
- Boerhaave's syndrome
- Pancreatitis
- Nutritional deficiency diseases
- Nausea
- Abdominal pain
- Erratic bowel function (constipation and diarrhea)
- Gastrointestinal hemorrhage
- Jaundice
- High incidence of digestive tract cancers
- Glucose intolerance

Reproductive System

- Impotence
- Sterility
- Gynecomastia
- Anorgasmic (women)
- FAS

**Very rare.*

Source: Adapted from Kneisl and Ames 1986.

Patterns of Use

Alcoholics manifest one of three patterns of use: regular daily intake of large amounts of alcohol, regular heavy drinking limited to weekends, or long periods of sobriety interspersed with binges of heavy drinking lasting for weeks or months. Regardless of the preferred pattern, people who drink excessively experience numerous negative physiologic and psychologic symptoms.

Alcohol Withdrawal Syndrome

Alcohol withdrawal often includes the symptoms described below.

HANGOVER The term *hangover* is used to describe the unpleasant symptoms occurring approximately 4–6 hours after alcohol ingestion. These symptoms include:

- Nausea and vomiting
- Gastritis
- Headache
- Fatigue
- Sweating and thirst
- Restlessness
- Irritability
- The "shakes"
- Vasomotor instability

The cause of the symptoms is unclear, but they are attributed to hypoglycemia and the accumulation of lactic acid and acetaldehyde in the blood.

ALCOHOLIC HALLUCINOSIS Alcoholic hallucinosis refers to auditory hallucinations reported by clients with alcohol dependence. The hallucinations occur approximately 24–48 hours after heavy drinking and may be vivid and frightening to the client.

GRAND MAL SEIZURES Grand mal seizures ("rum fits") may occur 2–3 days after the person stops drinking. They can be prevented in a good medically monitored withdrawal program.

DELIRIUM TREMENS **Delirium tremens (DTs)**, one symptom of withdrawal, is a condition of severe memory disturbance, agitation, anorexia, and hallucinations. Generally, DTs begin a few days after drinking stops and end within 1–5 days. They may, however, appear as late as the second week, especially when there is cross-addiction to other drugs. Additional medical illnesses may be present, such as pneumonia, pancreatitis, and hepatic decompensation.

Medical Detoxification

Medical treatment of alcoholism involves the management of withdrawal symptoms and the use of medication to deter the alcoholic from drinking. Alcohol withdrawal occurs after the addicted individual stops drinking. This syndrome is composed of a constellation of physiologic and behavioral symptoms that occur when the alcohol level drops. In the early 1950s, **alcohol withdrawal syndrome** was divided into four stages: tremor, hallucinations, seizures, and delirium tremens. Today, the syndrome is divided into two categories according to time of onset and severity of symptoms: early or minor withdrawal and late or major withdrawal (Kirk and Bradford 1987).

MINOR WITHDRAWAL **Minor withdrawal** occurs within 6–12 hours after the alcoholic's last drink. Early symptoms include anxiety, agitation, and irritability. As the syndrome progresses, other symptoms occur. These include tremor, tachycardia, hypertension, diaphoresis, and hallucinations. Gastrointestinal symptoms of nausea, vomiting, diarrhea, and anorexia may also be present. The appearance of hallucinations (visual, auditory, olfactory, or tactile) and seizures marks the onset of major withdrawal.

MAJOR WITHDRAWAL **Major withdrawal** is the most advanced, potentially life-threatening stage of alcohol withdrawal. Symptoms associated with DTs usually develop 72 hours after the last drink. Physical symptoms of impending DTs include elevated temperature, severe diaphoresis, hypertension, and tachycardia. Behavioral symptoms include confusion and disorientation, agitation, tremors, and alterations in sensory perception (auditory and visual hallucinations).

The best treatment for major alcohol withdrawal involves early detection. Medical treatment for withdrawal includes:

1. Monitoring the client's fluid status. Although some clients are overhydrated, many are dehydrated or have the potential for developing a fluid volume deficit. Fluids should be encouraged, up to 3000 mL/day if no evidence exists to contraindicate this. If the client is unable to take fluids by mouth, fluids may be administered intravenously. Many alcoholics suffer from a magnesium deficiency.
2. Administering magnesium sulfate to decrease the irritability caused by low magnesium levels and to prevent seizures.
3. Administering vitamins, especially thiamine (vitamin B_1) because alcohol interferes with the absorption of B vitamins.
4. Prescribing benzodiazepines, such as diazepam (Val-

ium) or chlordiazepoxide (Librium) to help prevent DTs. Seizures may be treated with IV diazepam, and the client may be placed on phenytoin (Dilantin).

5. Prescribing disulfiram (Antabuse, an agonist medication). Disulfiram may also be prescribed for alcoholic clients. Disulfiram inhibits acetaldehyde dehydrogenase, which normally metabolizes acetaldehyde. As a result, acetaldehyde accumulates if alcohol is consumed. Acetaldehyde is highly toxic, producing nausea and hypotension. Hypotension leads to shock and may be fatal. The dosage of disulfiram is usually 250 mg daily. Clients may stop taking the drug, and it may be useful to dispense it every 4 days during client visits to a clinic. If the client uses alcohol, a powerful disulfiram reaction may occur and last for up to 2 weeks. Reaction symptoms include nausea, vomiting, flushing, dizziness, and tachycardia. Because of the potential danger of disulfiram, instruct the client orally and in writing not to use alcohol in any form, including alcohol-based cough syrups or cold remedies. Clients with myocardial disease or those taking metronidazole (Flagyl) should not take Antabuse; in the latter case, a disulfiram reaction is possible.
6. Prescribing naltrexone (Trexan). Developed in 1984 for treatment of heroin abuse, this drug was approved in January 1994 for blocking the craving for alcohol and the pleasure derived from drinking it. It is the first new drug for alcoholism to be approved by the FDA in 47 years. Rather than making the alcoholic sick, it blocks the need and thus may help prevent relapse when it is combined with long-term support groups and individual counseling.

BLACKOUTS Having **blackouts** is frequently confused with passing out. In fact, passing out refers to unconsciousness, whereas a blackout is **anterograde amnesia:** loss of short-term memories with retention of remote memories. A person can function effectively for up to several days—talking on the telephone, working, and shopping—yet have absolutely no memory of doing so. To others, the alcoholic may appear normal or "high." Interestingly, alcoholics appear unconcerned by the blackouts and eventually learn to cover them up. This appearance of unconcern may, in part, be due to *euphoric recall:* The alcoholic recalls feeling good but does not recall behavior. Reality is distorted. Some clients find blackouts very disturbing and seek treatment.

Blackouts appearing later in the disease process may be indicative of physical dependence and are not related to the amount of alcohol consumed. They are unpredictable, and exactly how or why they occur is not clear. Some authorities believe blackouts are an acute syndrome caused by dehydration of brain tissue. When assessing an alcoholic client, determine whether blackouts are part of the symptoms.

Alcohol Amnestic Disorder (Korsakoff's Psychosis) and Alcoholic Encephalopathy (Wernicke's Enecephalopathy)

Alcohol amnestic disorder (Korsakoff's psychosis) is a disturbance of short-term memory that occurs in people who have been drinking alcohol heavily for many years. It is thought to be related to thiamine deficiency secondary to the malabsorption associated with heavy alcohol ingestion. It is irreversible. It often follows an acute episode of **alcoholic encephalopathy (Wernicke's encephalopathy)**, a neurological disease characterized by ataxia, sixth cranial nerve palsy, nystagmus, and confusion. Wernicke's syndrome may clear spontaneously in a few days or weeks and responds rapidly to large doses of parenteral thiamine in its acute, early stage. Once this disorder is established, however, it has a chronic course, and impairment can become severe.

Fetal Alcohol Syndrome

Nurses need to be aware of the harmful effects of alcohol on pregnant women and unborn children. **Fetal alcohol syndrome (FAS)** is found in children of women who engage in heavy drinking of alcohol during pregnancy. Physical and mental defects include severe growth deficiency, heart defects, malformed facial features, mental retardation, low birth weight, learning problems, and hyperactivity. If a child has one or two of these characteristics, the condition is called *fetal alcohol effects.* FAS affects 1 of every 750 babies born in the United States. A baby born to an alcoholic mother may need to be withdrawn gradually from alcohol.

Suicide and Alcoholism

Nurses must be alert to the possibility of suicide attempts by alcoholics. While 1% of the general population attempt suicide, 15% of alcoholics do. The nurse should watch for self-destructuve behavior and for events in a client's life that represent a loss, such as work, family, health, or legal problems. Such behavior and events put people in a high-risk category.

Barbiturates or Similarly Acting Sedatives or Hypnotics

Elizabeth W, a 45-year-old housewife, has been depressed and irritable over an impending divorce. Her physician prescribed Valium (5 mg) for sleep and for anxiety (every 6 hours as needed). Because this dosage was not helping decrease her anxiety as much as she wanted, Ms W increased

her dosage and began taking 50-100 mg a day over a period of a few weeks. This evening Ms W's estranged husband found her mumbling incoherently. Her speech was slurred, she was bumping into furniture, and she was quite drowsy.

The Effects of Barbiturates, Sedatives, or Hypnotics

The accompanying box presents the key facts about barbiturates. Barbiturates are highly addictive drugs that cause people to feel euphoric yet relaxed. They are frequently prescribed to relieve pain, reduce anxiety (sedative effects), and induce sleep (hypnotic effects). Barbiturates were the first drugs used to treat anxiety and insomnia. They were considered dangerous because of their ability to cause significant CNS depression and their lethality if used to overdose.

A new class of anxiolytic drugs, the benzodiazepines (BZDs), began to be widely used because of their ability to reduce anxiety without causing significant CNS depression. However, they also have the drawbacks of producing dependence and withdrawal syndromes in some clients (DeVane 1990). BZDs include many widely prescribed drugs, including diazepam (Valium), clorazepate (Tranxene), lorazepam (Ativan), and alprazolam (Xanax). These drugs are thought to modify anxiety by altering the balance of neurotransmitters, especially norepinephrine (NE) and gamma-aminobutyric acid (GABA) in the brain's limbic system. The limbic system is involved in the regulation of emotion. These drugs have a high risk for abuse and physical dependence. When the drug stops working and tolerance builds up, people tend to increase the dosage just "to cope."

Patterns of Use

In party situations, teenagers and young adults take high doses, often in combination with alcohol, to get "high." The resultant CNS depression makes this practice especially dangerous. *"Speed freaks"* (amphetamine abusers) use barbiturates to "come down" from a high. Dependence, tolerance, and cross-tolerance to other depressant drugs develop rapidly.

Action

Barbiturates are metabolized in phases by the liver. When taken orally, they are initially absorbed and partially metabolized. However, the unmetabolized parts become active metabolites that are stored in the fatty tissues. Consequently, taking these drugs over a period of time results in a cumulative effect, unsuspected dependence, and possible overdose.

More Americans die from barbiturate overdose than from opioid addiction. Many take alcohol and barbiturates together. While judgment is impaired, they take more pills, thereby unintentionally overdosing. Because alcohol and barbiturates are synergistic, an overdose can occur quickly. Barbiturates are often used in suicide attempts.

Withdrawal

Barbiturate withdrawal is unpleasant and life-threatening. A deep sleep is followed by decreased respiration, coma, and sometimes death. Babies born to mothers addicted to barbiturates are physically dependent and need to be helped through withdrawal.

Withdrawal from BZDs may produce symptoms similar to those of barbiturate withdrawal. The onset of withdrawal symptoms may occur within 24–72 hours of the last dose, depending on the half-life of the drug used. Symptoms include autonomic hyperactivity (alterations in vital signs and diaphoresis), marked anxiety, agitation, insomnia, depression, and seizures. Medical detox can prevent a potentially serious emergency during withdrawal.

Opioids

Steven Y, a 20-year-old male, arrived at the hospital in an ambulance. He was unconscious. His respiration was slow, and his pupils were pinpoints. "Tracks" were visible on his arms and behind his knees. A source said Steven had just "shot up" heroin.

The Effects of Opioids

The opioids include heroin and morphine, derived from the poppy plant, and synthetic drugs, such as meperidine (Demerol), codeine, methadone, and others. Opioids have analgesic qualities and are prescribed after surgery. Depending on the person, the drugs may produce a euphoric high, as in drug addicts, but they generally cause people to feel drowsy and out of touch with the world. See the box on page 260 for more facts about opioids.

Patterns of Use

In 1898, heroin became available and initially was not believed to be addictive. Within a short time, its addictive properties became known, and the government intervened (Harrison Narcotics Act of 1914). Addiction to opiates has increased through the years. Because most opioid abusers take the drugs intravenously, they are at high risk for AIDS and hepatitis. Overdose, malnutrition, and infections spread by dirty drugs and needles are dangers. Dealers often add impurities to "cut" heroin, thus increasing the quantity and their own profit. The impurities may cause poisoning and other problems.

Key Facts About Barbiturates or Similarly Acting Sedatives or Hypnotics

Examples

Lorazepam (Ativan), alprazolam (Xanax), diazepam (Valium), chlordiazepoxide (Librium), chloral hydrate, methaqualone (Quaalude), secobarbital (Seconal), phenobarbital, pentobarbital (Nembutal)

Slang Terms

Downers, ludes, sopors, 714s, yellow jackets, reds, blues, rainbows, trenks

Route of Administration

Oral (pills or capsules), intravenous

Psychologic Symptoms

Euphoria

Mood lability*

Intoxication

Talkativeness*

Impaired attention and memory*

Irritability*

Anxiety

Sexual aggressiveness*

Physical Symptoms

Drowsiness

Slurred speech*

Long periods of sleep

Fever

Vomiting

Postural hypotension

Lack of coordination*

Unsteady gait

Withdrawal Symptoms

Nausea and vomiting

Malaise or weakness

Autonomic hyperactivity

Tachycardia

Sweating; elevated blood pressure

Anxiety

Depression or irritability

Orthostatic hypotension

Coarse tremor of hands, tongue, eyelids

Painful muscle contractions

Seizures

Status epilepticus (major epileptic attacks succeeding each other with little or no intermission)

Hallucinations

Time Frame for Withdrawal Symptoms

Short-acting barbiturates and BZDs are associated with withdrawal symptoms within the first 24 hr after discontinuation. Longer-acting barbiturates and BZDs are associated with withdrawal symptoms within 48–72 hr of discontinuation. Seizures may occur for up to 2 weeks after withdrawal.

Dangers and Complications

CNS depression

Possible overdose and death, especially if mixed with alcohol

Typical Users

Middle-class, middle-aged females

Teenagers

Young adults

**Symptoms of intoxication noted in* DSM-IV.

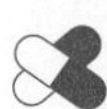

Opioid intoxication is indicated by constricted pupils, euphoria, psychomotor retardation, slurred speech, and/or drowsiness. If a client overdoses, naloxone (Narcan) (0.4–0.8 mg IV repeated in 5–15 minutes) is given. It is a fast-acting narcotic antagonist that counteracts respiratory depression. Abdominal cramps, rhinorrhea, and lacrimation may be treated with belladonna alkaloids or with phenobarbital.

Withdrawal

Because opioids are physically addictive, withdrawal is a threat. People who use high doses of a drug and who "shoot up" or "mainline" (use the drug intravenously) are at high risk for severe withdrawal symptoms. Withdrawal symptoms are usually evident within 12 hours after the last dose. The person experiences the most severe with-

Key Facts About Opioids

Examples

Heroin, morphine, hydromorphone (Dilaudid), codeine, methadone

Slang Terms

H, smack, junk, M, Miss Emma, Little D, School Boy, Horse

Route of Administration

Intravenous, oral, intramuscular, subcutaneous ("skin popping")

Psychologic Symptoms

Impaired attention/memory*

Euphoria*

Appearance of sedation ("nodding out")

Psychomotor retardation*

Insensitivity to pain

Agitation

Apathy*

Dysphoria*

Physical Symptoms

Pinpoint pupils

Drowsiness*

Slurred speech*

Nausea and vomiting

Hypothermia

Withdrawal Symptoms

(Presents like influenza)

Dilated pupils

Tearing

Runny nose

Piloerection

Sweating

Diarrhea

Fever

Yawning

Mild hypotension

Tachycardia

Insomnia

Restlessness and irritability

Muscle and joint pains

Increased respiration

Gastrointestinal symptoms

Loss of appetite

Time Frame for Withdrawal Symptoms

Withdrawal symptoms may appear within a few hours after the last dose of a short-acting opioid such as heroin. With longer acting opioids such as methadone, withdrawal symptoms may not appear for 2–3 days and may persist for 1–2 weeks.

Dangers and Complications

Death (especially if combined with barbiturates)

Pulmonary edema

Opioid poisoning (coma, shock, respiratory depression)

Malnutrition

Hepatitis; infections

AIDS

Typical Users

Teenagers

Young adults

**Symptoms of intoxication noted in* DSM-IV.

drawal within 36–48 hours, with the symptoms decreasing gradually over 2 weeks. During this stressful time, the person craves the drug. Clients in treatment may terminate against advice of health professionals as is evidenced in the Research Note on the next page. Babies who are born to addicted mothers must be treated for opioid withdrawal. These babies present with irritability, high-pitched crying, increased respirations, fever, sneezing, yawning, and tremors.

In 1964, methadone was introduced to treat opiate ad-

RESEARCH NOTE

Citation

Endicott P, Watson B: Interventions to improve the AMA discharge rate for opiate addicted patients. *J Psychosoc Nurs* 1994;32(8):36–40.

Study Purpose/Problem

This action-oriented evaluation project grew out of the recognition that almost half of the *against medical advice (AMA)* discharges in a 500-bed acute care center were occurring on the 14-bed chemical dependence unit. The study summarizes why opioid treatment failures are a significant concern, reviews treatment issues as well as ethical dilemmas, and describes a four-stage intervention strategy that resulted in a 61% improvement rate in the opioid AMA discharge rate.

Methods

The initiators of this demonstration project reviewed literature relevant to AMA treatment issues and ethical dilemmas. In addition, they implemented a four-stage treatment intervention on an adult chemical dependence unit of an acute care center in the midwestern U.S. The four stages included a treatment pledge, an appropriate medication regimen, use of the Endicott-Watson Subjective/Objective Opiate Withdrawal Scale, and the establishment of an enhanced community resource link. With the implementation of each of the four stages, AMA discharge rates were tracked.

Findings

While prior research had suggested that taking a pledge to "stick it out" in treatment enhanced a sense of self-efficacy, clients in this demonstration project generally felt unable to control their destiny, believing that nothing they could do would make a difference. Thus, AMA discharge rates did not alter with Stage 1 of the intervention. A new withdrawal medication regimen included Propoxyphene to ameliorate withdrawal symptoms; clonidine to decrease lacrimation, chills, rhinorrhea, diaphoresis, stomach cramps, and joint and muscle aches; temazepam (Restoril) to relieve the insomnia associated with opioid withdrawal; and chlordiazepoxide (Librium) for relief of restlessness and anxiety. Even with Stage 1 and Stage 2 of the intervention in place, a positive change had not yet occurred. Use of the Endicott-Watson Subjective/Objective Opiate Withdrawal Scale, implemented in the hope of enhancing the client's ownership of his or her withdrawal process and locus of control, and providing a culturally appropriate recovery mentor from the community resulted in a 61% improvement in the AMA discharge rate for these clients.

Implications

The United States is in the midst of a resurgence of opioid abuse. Easy availability and low cost are two of the factors contributing to the increased use of heroin. Opioid treatment failures are a significant concern because the population of IV drug users is one of the fastest growing subpopulations in the HIV epidemic. Other drug-related health problems abound. Typically when clients leave treatment against medical advice, staff members feel that they have failed, the therapeutic milieu is threatened, and costs escalate. This article describes a project that demonstrated a four-stage solution that resulted in a noteworthy drop in AMA discharge rates from their unit. Future studies under controlled conditions seem indicated.

diction. By the late 1960s and early 1970s, when the federal government allocated money for treatment, methadone maintenance programs mushroomed all over the United States. **Methadone**, a synthetic narcotic, was dispensed daily at clinics to narcotic addicts. Although addictive, methadone does not produce the "rush" (ecstatic feeling) associated with heroin. Methadone alleviates the addict's craving for narcotics and, therefore, was expected to decrease the illicit drug trafficking, theft, prostitution, and crime necessary to obtain money for the drugs, thereby allowing addicts to lead productive lives. Also, methadone therapy is far less expensive than residential programs or jail. Today, methadone maintenance programs remain a major treatment for opioid addicts.

Clients who are assessed to be not at risk for complications of the drug are first stabilized on methadone (3–5 days). Within 1–3 days after the methadone is discontinued, opiate withdrawal symptoms often appear. At this time, clonidine is begun and is given in increasing doses, until withdrawal symptoms are alleviated (up to 14 days). Clonidine blocks the withdrawal symptoms, making

Key Facts About Amphetamines

Examples

Dexedrine, methamphetamine

Slang Terms

Bennies, dexies, uppers, black beauties, pep pills, crank, speed, diet pills

Route of Administration

Oral, intravenous

Psychologic Symptoms

- Hypervigilance*
- Irritability
- Grandiosity*
- Talkativeness*
- Elation
- Impaired judgment
- Psychomotor agitation*
- Aggressive, violent behavior
- Paranoia
- Hallucinations, delusions
- Disorientation
- Increased libido
- Stereotypical compulsive behavior
- Visual/auditory hallucinations

Physical Symptoms

- Tachycardia*
- Increased blood pressure*
- Dilated pupils*
- Perspiration or chills*
- Nausea or vomiting*
- Diarrhea
- Headache
- Dizziness
- Cardiac arrhythmias
- Hyperthermia
- Decreased appetite
- Delirium

Withdrawal Symptoms

- Depression
- Fatigue
- Disturbed sleep
- Dreaming
- Restlessness
- Disorientation

Dangers and Complications

- Malnutrition
- Cerebrovascular accident
- Depression
- Hyperpyrexia
- Convulsions
- Suicide attempt

Typical Users

- Teenagers
- Young adults

**Symptoms of intoxication noted in* DSM-IV.

the detoxification process less painful and more rapid than with methadone. Psychologically, the client feels less anxious and depressed.

Recent clinical trials have shown that buprenorphine is an effective alternative to methadone (Strain et al. 1994). Buprenorphine is an opioid mixed agonist and potent analgesic. It is also being investigated for its effectiveness in treating cocaine abuse.

Amphetamines or Similarly Acting Sympathomimetics

Laura S, a 16-year-old high school girl, was on a diet so she could get into a favorite bathing suit. Her friend's brother, a pharmacist, gave her some Dexedrine "just until you lose the weight." Laura's mother initially noticed her rather unusual

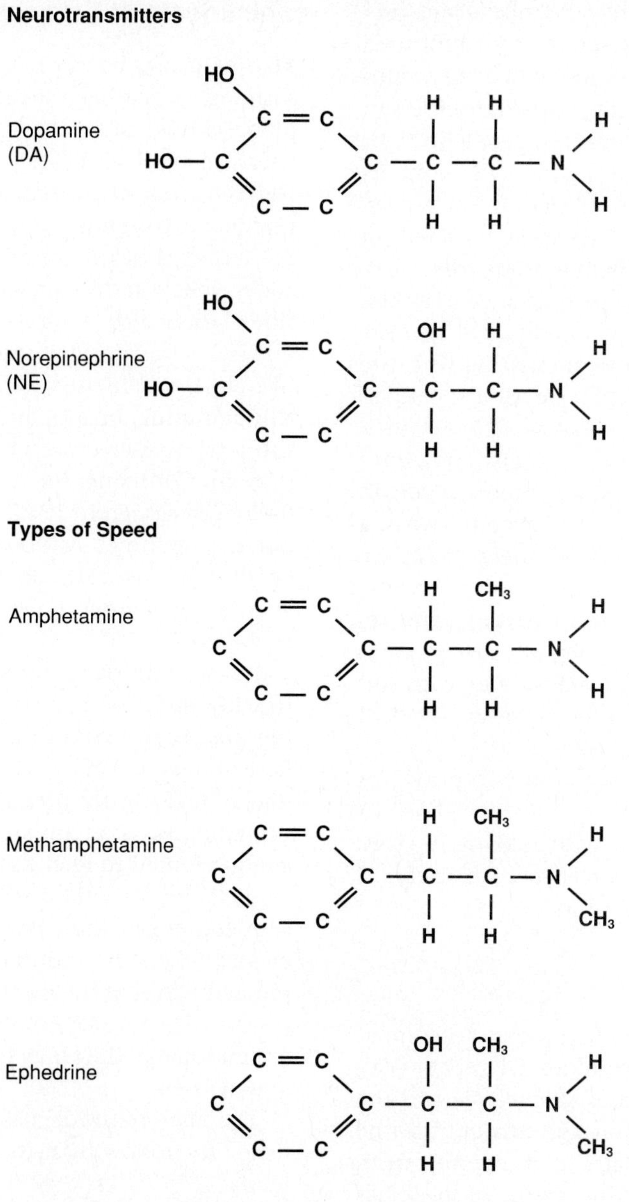

Neurotransmitters

Dopamine (DA)

Norepinephrine (NE)

Types of Speed

Amphetamine

Methamphetamine

Ephedrine

Figure 13–2 Chemical structures of neurotransmitters and speed.

hyperactivity, her euphoria, and the fact that she refused dinner. Over a period of a few weeks, Laura's behavior changed. She appeared suspicious and irritable and continued to speak and move rapidly.

The Effects of Amphetamines

The amphetamines/sympathomimetics ("speed") include groups of synthetic drugs derived from ephedrine that stimulate the release of adrenaline. In small doses, they cause a person to feel energetic, euphoric, and "turned on" to life. Users take these CNS stimulants to feel good. A growing number of people, who do uppers and downers in a cyclic fashion, take amphetamines to counteract the effects of barbiturates. Amphetamines are dangerous because they alter judgment and obscure feelings. Taken in high doses or intravenously, amphetamines can have dangerous side effects (see the accompanying box above).

Amphetamines act by mimicking the brain's most important neurotransmitters, dopamine (DA) and norepinephrine (NE). For the similarities in chemical structure between these neurotransmitters and speed, see Figure 13–2 above.

Patterns of Use

In the 1950s and 1960s, amphetamines were heralded as wonder drugs for depression and lassitude. By the 1970s, their dangers became known, and today physicians prescribe them less frequently. Amphetamines are still used to control appetite and treat depression, narcolepsy, minimal brain dysfunctions, and attention-deficit disorders in children. Abusers are usually teenagers or people in their early twenties who are looking for a good time. Abusers are also using different types of speed than in years past. Truck drivers may use amphetamines to stay awake on long trips, and students may use them to study for exams. Athletes, hoping to improve their performance, may use amphetamines. Tolerance develops rapidly, and chronic abusers may suffer a toxic psychosis presenting with the symptoms of paranoid schizophrenia. Delusions, hallucinations, stereotypic compulsive behavior, increased libido, panic, and violence may occur (Kneisl and Ames 1986). However, unlike a chronic schizophrenic, a person who abuses amphetamines does not present with a thought disorder or a flat affect. Instead, these clients are agitated and extremely anxious. Clients who are chronic amphetamine abusers begin to crave the drugs and require higher and higher dosages. They are rowdy, paranoid, and irritable. A "crash" (depression), often with suicidal symptoms, may last for several weeks. Cyclical patterns of abuse and crashing may occur.

The most hypercharged form of speed is "crystal" or methamphetamine. Sold in small chunks as "glass" or "ice," it is a maximum stimulant with maximum risks. "Crank" is another nickname for street speed. The effects are similar to those produced by "crystal."

Withdrawal

Chlorpromazine (Thorazine) may be ordered to combat the physiologic effects of amphetamines. Diazepam (Valium), given intravenously, decreases tachycardia and the chance of convulsions. Depression and anxiety are the most common psychologic pitfalls in recovering from the use of speed. Physiologically, the overuse of speed has been tied to stroke and even death.

Cannabis

Joe P, a 35-year-old captain of a rescue squad, was having trouble at his job. He paid less and less attention to the accuracy of his patient reports; he was often late for work; he forgot to repair and replace his equipment, causing his unit to be unsafe and ill-equipped. Joe told an emergency room nurse that he felt all the marijuana he was smoking was beginning to affect him. He revealed that he'd been a daily smoker for five years. At first, he felt there were no long-term effects, but lately he was concerned because "I never feel like doing anything." He has trouble concentrating, forgets what he is talking about in mid-sentence, and is unmotivated to make any positive changes in his life.

The Effects of Cannabis

Marijuana arrived in the United States in the early 1900s. Although it has been illegal in the U.S. since 1937, marijuana is used more than any other chemical except tobacco, alcohol, and caffeine (see the accompanying box). Derived from an Indian hemp plant *(Cannabis sativa),* marijuana contains the psychoactive substance delta 6-3,4-tetrahydrocannabinol (THC). THC is found in the sticky yellow resin secreted by the tops and leaves of the ripe plants.

THC is transformed into metabolites in the body. Unlike alcohol, which is water-soluble and leaves the body through urine, breath, and perspiration, THC is stored in the fatty tissues (especially the brain and reproductive system). Consequently, it can be detected in the body for up to 6 weeks. From 1984 to 1986, marijuana increased in potency ten times. Although marijuana contains over 400 chemicals, the THC content determines the potency. With an increase in potency comes an increase in health problems.

Researchers have found marijuana to be effective in treating epilepsy, glaucoma, asthma, hypertension, and the nausea and vomiting associated with chemotherapy. Researchers are currently studying the effects of marijuana smoking by pregnant women on the fetus. The cannabinoids of marijuana cross the placental barrier and are distributed to fetal tissues. The risk of fetal death and abnormalities—CNS disturbances, low birth weight, decreased length, and smaller head circumference—increases when the mother uses marijuana. A suppressed prolactin level in the mother makes nursing impossible. If people with a history of schizophrenia or mood disorders use marijuana, they may have a relapse or their symptoms may worsen.

The National Federation of Drug-Free Youth has published the following facts indicating the dangers of marijuana:

- Marijuana appears to lower testosterone levels in boys.
- In girls, hormone levels remain normal, but marijuana's chemicals may accumulate in the ovaries.
- Marijuana smoke has 50% more tar than regular cigarette smoke.
- Marijuana tar contains 70% more benzopyrene, a major cancer-causing chemical.
- Marijuana smoke produces greater cellular changes in the lungs than does tobacco smoke.
- Smoking two "joints" (marijuana cigarettes) can reduce lung capacity more than smoking one pack of tobacco cigarettes.
- Marijuana may cause emphysema twenty times faster than tobacco.
- Marijuana smoke increases airway resistance 25% under laboratory conditions in which a similar amount of

Key Facts About Cannabis

Examples

Marijuana, hashish, THC

Slang Terms

Pot, grass, bhang, hashish, ganja, joint, reefer, weed, "shit"

Route of Administration

Smoked in a pipe or cigarette, oral (mixed in food)

Psychologic Symptoms

Initial anxiety, then euphoria

Altered perceptions

Sensation of slowed time

Decreased concentration

Lack of motivation

Loss of short-term memory

Passivity

Abrupt mood changes

Paranoid ideation

Impaired judgment

Physical Symptoms

Dry mouth

Increased heart rate

Conjunctival irritation

Dilated pupils

Decreased coordination

Increased appetite, thirst

Craving for sweets

Fatigue

Impaired ovulation, impaired sperm count and motility, increase in abnormal sperm cells

Dangers and Complications

Lung damage

Psychologic dependence

Panic reaction

Impaired driving ability

Typical Users

Teenagers

Young adults

tobacco smoke produces no significant increase in airway resistance.

- Brain wave tests show that teenagers who get high twice a week or more often have evidence of diffuse brain impairment for up to 2 months after the last time they use the drug. They experience disruptions in learning, short-term memory loss, problems concentrating, and **amotivation syndrome** (confusion, declining performance, and difficulty finishing tasks).
- After a person smokes marijuana, THC can be found in the blood and urine for up to 2 weeks; if the THC is radioactively labeled, it can be detected for up to a month.

Patterns of Use

Because marijuana smoking is so prevalent among teenagers and because its dangers are becoming increasingly known, some health care professionals advocate a urine screening when teenagers have a checkup by a family doctor. In 1985, the American Academy of Pediatrics was challenged to confront the problem of substance abuse among teenagers. A key point was that chemical dependence takes 10–15 years to develop in adults and only a few years to develop in a child. Only 25% of kids in drug rehabilitation succeed, compared with 75% of adults who succeed. Because substance abuse is a "neglected disease," pediatricians should initiate educational and treatment programs on drug and alcohol abuse. Likewise, psychiatric nurses need to respond to this vital public health issue.

Marijuana use is endemic in the teenage culture. Therefore, nurses who work with teenagers must be knowledgeable about marijuana and its effects. When admitting a teenager to a psychiatric unit or interviewing a teenager as an outpatient, be aware of a variety of indicators of marijuana use. Parents should know these facts about marijuana and indications of its use:

- Marijuana smells like hemp or burning rope.
- Teenagers often burn incense or use perfumed sprays to mask its pungent odor.
- Teenagers may use eye drops (Murine) so that their eyes will not be red, and they may cough a lot.

Key Facts About Cocaine

Slang Terms

Coke, lady, blow, snow, rabbits, C, powder

Route of Administration

Intranasal (flakes or powder sniffed), subcutaneous or intravenous, smoked in a pipe (freebasing)

Psychologic Symptoms

- Psychomotor agitation*
- Anxiety
- Elation
- Talkativeness*
- Grandiosity*
- Hypervigilance*
- Impaired judgment
- Ideas of reference; paranoia
- Hallucinations
- Formication (sensation of insects crawling on the skin)
- Euphoria followed by depression and let-down (crash)
- Violence
- Insomnia
- Anorexia

Physical Symptoms

- Dilated pupils*
- Tachycardia*
- Elevated blood pressure*
- Perspiration or chills*
- Nausea or vomiting*
- Anorexia
- Dry mouth (characteristic bad breath)
- Weight loss
- Stuffy/runny nose
- Burns and sores of nasal membranes
- Tremors
- Muscle cramping
- Seizures

Withdrawal Symptoms

- Severe craving
- Fatigue
- Psychomotor agitation
- Hypersomnia
- Irritability

Time Frame for Withdrawal Symptoms

Symptoms may appear within 24 hr after use; peak in 2–4 days. Depression may persist for months.

Dangers and Complications

- Syncope
- Fever
- Chest pain
- Depression
- Death from convulsions
- Cardiac/respiratory arrest

Typical Users

- Teenagers
- College students
- Young urban professionals (yuppies)
- Rock and movie stars
- Executives

**Symptoms of intoxication noted in* DSM-IV.

- A teenager who uses marijuana may have smoking paraphernalia—plastic baggies filled with dried leaves, rolling paper, and "roach" clips, clips that hold the marijuana cigarette once it becomes too small to handle.

Cocaine

Will R, a 32-year-old male, was brought to the hospital by his father. Talkative and jumpy, his eyes darted around the examining room, and he repeatedly wiped his nose with his

finger and rubbed the bottom of his face. He acted suspicious and kept saying someone was after him. His family stated he had a $400 a day cocaine habit. He began casually snorting a few lines once in a while when he needed a sense of control over his full load of graduate school courses and full-time job. His use increased to every day, then every few hours.

Each year, 20 tons of cocaine enter the United States. After the cocaine is adulterated with sugar, quinine, amphetamine, ephedrine, or procaine, 80–160 tons are available on the streets. Since cocaine abuse has been recognized as a widespread problem, government agencies have spent much money trying to block cocaine shipments from South America. Planes, boats, and "mules" (people who transport cocaine) have been seized, and tons of cocaine have been confiscated and destroyed. Yet it is still plentiful and is purer today than ever before. The cocaine industry is a multibillion dollar enterprise involving bribery, corruption, and murder.

The Effects of Cocaine

Cocaine is a stimulant extracted from the leaves of the coca plant found in Bolivia and Peru. It has long been known and used. For hundreds of years, South American Indians have chewed coca leaves, enjoying the effects of decreased appetite and increased ability to work at high altitudes. Slaves became more productive when given cocaine. Freud experimented with cocaine. It was an ingredient in Coca Cola before federal regulations prohibited it in 1903. Today, cocaine is used as a local anesthetic in ear, nose, and throat surgery. When inhaled or injected, cocaine produces alertness and energy and makes users feel sociable, confident, and "in control." The drug blocks appetite and erases fatigue, which makes it appear to be the ideal performance booster for the 1990s.

Cocaine is no longer just the chic, expensive drug of choice (the champagne of drugs) of young upwardly mobile professionals and stars. In greater demand are smokable forms that have an effect similar to the injectable drug. Cocaine is now available to all cultural and socioeconomic groups; today, 50% of users are women. For some years, cocaine was believed to produce euphoria without addictive potential and without negative side effects. Lately the horrors of cocaine abuse have been described in both lay and professional literature. (See the box on page 269.)

It has not been proved that cocaine is physically addictive, but its ability to cause psychologic dependence is clear. Cocaine users crave the drug. After a brief postuse euphoria (lasting approximately 5–10 minutes), they experience a strong desire to repeat the high. This high is followed by a **crashing**, a terrible letdown called the "postcoke blues," or cocaine abstinence syndrome. Anxiety, depression, and fatigue are part of this syndrome. The **cocaine crash**, lasting for approximately 30–60 minutes, results from depletion of DA, the neurotransmitter responsible for feelings of pleasure and well-being. The addict responds to the crash by feeling irritable, depressed, and tired. Although the brain needs to synthesize more DA, resulting from the chemical misprogramming from the addiction, it craves more cocaine, which offers immediate relief. The crash intensity appears related to the amount of cocaine used. Addicts often use other drugs, such as alcohol, marijuana, or sleeping pills, during the crash.

One addict described these postcoke blues as "pure hell, the most painful depression I have ever felt. I wanted to die from the pain." This painful depression, along with the memory of the cocaine high, causes people to want to use cocaine again and again to recapture the momentary ecstasy. The period of agitation, anxiety, and insomnia usually ceases within 2 weeks.

Cocaine addicts develop a tolerance to the drug and use amounts that would have been lethal to them earlier. The euphoria diminishes. The development of new dendrites (branches of the nerve cells) to aid the uptake of the increased amount of DA accounts for the tolerance. Ultimately, the cocaine no longer produces pleasure, but not taking it feels even worse. Dopamine eventually becomes depleted, and the user becomes chronically fatigued, irritable, and anxious, even mentally confused, paranoid. Suicide attempts, accidents, and overdoses are common. The only effect of cocaine that is increased as tolerance develops is its ability to induce a convulsion or seizure. Nurses need to assess clients carefully to differentiate cocaine use from manic-depression and chronic anxiety. Figure 13–3, page 268, illustrates the cocaine use cycle.

Withdrawal

Detoxification for cocaine abusers is still in the experimental phase and may depend on the client's symptoms. Some hospitals use nothing; others administer diazepam (Valium) intravenously 1–20 mg at a slow rate (not more than 5 mg/min). In some hospitals, cocaine abusers are treated with a Valium protocol that lasts approximately 4 days; Valium is decreased from 10 mg q 4 hr PO/IM to 5 mg q 8 hr PO/IM, with additional doses as needed if the client has withdrawal symptoms. Other hospitals have PRN Valium orders only. Another protocol involves the use of phenobarbital in decreasing doses and imipramine hydrochloride (Tofranil). Because the depression is so great, Tofranil or other tricyclic antidepressants may be given for several weeks after detoxification. Tricyclics build up existing levels of neurotransmitters and make them available for transmission. Beta-adrenergic blockers such as propranolol (Inderal) may be used to counteract the tachycardia and hypertension that accompany acute

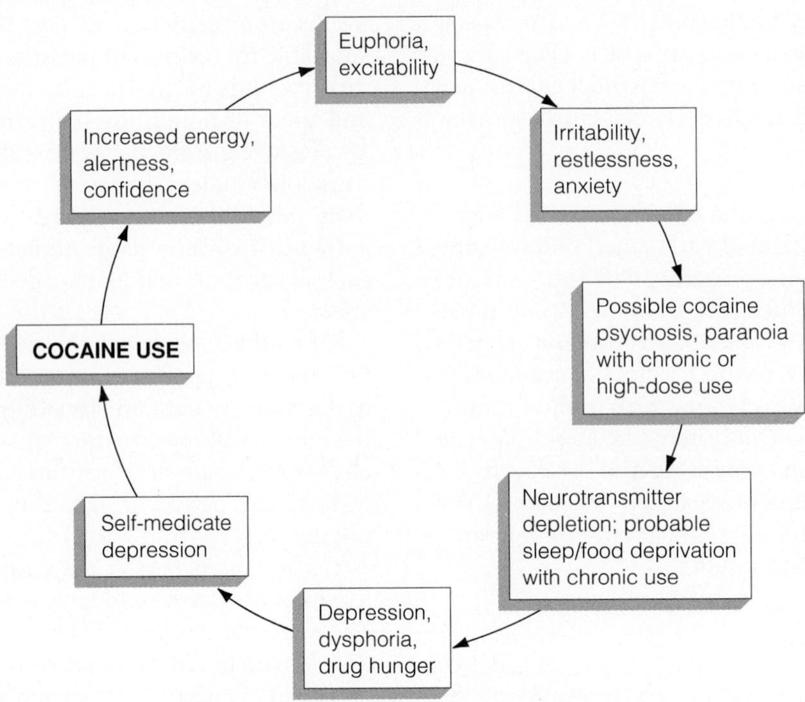

Figure 13–3 The cycle of cocaine use. *Source: Landry and Smith 1987, p. 13.*

cocaine intoxication, but their use may result in paroxysmal hypertension due to unopposed alpha-adrenergic stimulation. Therefore, they should be used cautiously and with constant blood pressure monitoring.

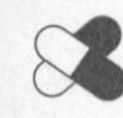

Use of tricyclic antidepressants to increase the number of neurotransmitters in the synapse is called *synaptic treatment.* Postsynaptic treatment for cocaine withdrawal and dependence includes the use of drugs such as bromocriptine (Parlodel) or amantadine (Amantadine), which increase dopaminergic activity in the synapse and enhance the effects of DA on the postsynaptic receptors. Presynaptic treatment with amino acids such as tryptophan was used until 1989, when tryptophan was removed from the market because of several deaths associated with its use. These amino acids were prescribed because the body converted them to neurotransmitters, which had been depleted by cocaine abuse.

Interestingly, low-level cocaine intoxication presents with symptoms similar to alcohol withdrawal: sweating, dilated pupils, psychomotor agitation, and increased blood pressure/heart rate. With higher doses of cocaine, a person becomes increasingly intoxicated. Symptoms include high fever, cardiac arrhythmia, seizures, hallucinations, and a paranoid schizophrenic syndrome. Hallucinations typically involve "cocaine bugs," which feel like bugs under the skin. The client may scratch furiously in an attempt to get rid of them. Haloperidol (Haldol) is used to combat the psychotic symptoms; phenothiazines should not be used because they may decrease the seizure threshold.

The strength of the physiologic effects of cocaine is revealed by animal research. Monkeys work harder at pressing a bar to receive cocaine intravenously than to get any other drug. Even when starving to death or when confronted with a sexually receptive female, monkeys continue pressing the bar. Receiving an electric shock every time they touch the bar does not alter their behavior. Research with cocaine users indicates that the drug bromocriptine mesylate (Parlodel), a DA receptor agonist, eliminates the craving that users feel after they stop using cocaine.

Cocaine initially increases DA neurotransmission. Over time, however, cocaine abuse depletes DA in the brain, and this depletion may be the basis for craving.

Crack

Crack, or "rock" cocaine, recently labeled "the most addictive drug known to man," is a potent form of hydrochloride cocaine that is mixed with baking soda

Key Facts About Crack (Hydrochloride Cocaine)

Slang Terms

Rock, crack

Route of Administration

Smoked

Psychologic Symptoms

- Paranoia
- Depression
- Insomnia
- Irritability
- Deterioration of mental function
- "Schizophrenia-like" psychosis
- Appetite suppression

Physical Symptoms

- Wheezing, shortness of breath
- Black phlegm
- Coughing blood
- Parched throat and lips
- Singed eyebrows and lashes
- Increased heart rate and blood pressure
- Weight loss

Withdrawal Symptoms

- Severe craving
- Depression
- Fatigue
- Hypersomnia
- Irritability

Time Frame for Withdrawal Symptoms

Severe craving within minutes to hours. Depression appears within 3–7 days; may persist for weeks.

Dangers and Complications

- Seizures
- Cardiac arrhythmias
- Respiratory paralysis
- Paranoid psychoses
- Pulmonary dysfunction

Typical Users

- Teenagers
- Young adults
- All socioeconomic and cultural groups

and water, heated, allowed to harden, and then broken or "cracked" into little pieces and smoked in cigarettes or glass water pipes. Crack is more insidious, addictive, and toxic than cocaine. One user said, "I am worse in three weeks of using crack than in six years of using cocaine."

Crack is cheap and easily bought on the street, or in special crack houses where people congregate to smoke. A crack high has a rapid onset and is intensely euphoric, followed by a dramatic crash. Within seconds after "coming down," users feel compelled to smoke more crack. Because addiction is so rapid, many people are "hooked" and seek help when they can no longer support their habit. Crack users are flooding treatment centers, many of which have long waiting lists. Recidivism is estimated by some experts at 90%.

Symptoms of crack use include irritability, paranoia, depression, and physical symptoms that go along with the smoking of a toxic chemical, such as wheezing and coughing blood and black phlegm (see the accompanying box). Cardiac arrhythmias caused by crack use may lead to death. There is an increase in the number of babies being born to mothers who use crack. These babies are more likely to be premature or have low birth weights. They present with irritability, tremors, and muscle rigidity.

Freebase

Freebase is a purified form of cocaine made by applying solvents to ordinary cocaine. The effects are brief but intense, and the short euphoria (3–5 minutes) immediately becomes a restless desire for more "base."

Phencyclidine (PCP)

Pete O, an 18-year-old college student, was offered marijuana at a fraternity party. After smoking several joints, he was driving home with a friend when he became severely agitated. He insisted his friend stop the car near a pay phone; he jumped out and attempted to call the police, believing someone was trying to kill him. When the police arrived because of the disturbance he was causing (by then he was shouting and hallucinating), he rushed them, kicking at passersby and shooting at them as if he had a gun. During an assessment interview, the friend confessed to putting PCP in the marijuana.

The Effects of PCP

PCP was originally used as an anesthetic for humans and as a tranquilizer for animals. Because of its dangerous side effects (see the accompanying box), it was removed from the market, except for veterinary use. However, by the mid-1960s, PCP was readily available as a street drug. PCP is inexpensive and easily synthesized by home chemists, making a supply always available.

People who use PCP frequently arrive at the emergency room in a psychotic, violent, and agitated state. Some fluctuate between coma and violence. Hallucinations are common. A differential diagnosis is important but difficult because the symptoms are similar to those of schizo-

Key Facts About Phencyclidine (PCP)

Slang Terms

PCP, angel dust, crystal, superjoint, hog, elephant tranquilizer, THC, rocket fuel, peace pill

Route of Administration

Oral, intravenous, smoked, inhaled

Psychologic Symptoms

- Euphoria*
- Psychomotor agitation*
- Anxiety*
- Grandiosity*
- Disorientation swings
- Emotional lability*
- Sensation of slowed time*
- Synesthesias (seeing sound or hearing colors)*
- Facial grimacing
- Muscle rigidity
- Hallucinations
- Paranoid ideation
- Violent or bizarre behavior
- Hostility, apathy
- Depersonalization, isolation

Physical Symptoms

- Vertical and horizontal nystagmus*
- Increased blood pressure or heart rate*
- Insensitivity to pain*
- Dysarthria*
- Ataxia*
- Perspiration
- Salivation
- Vomiting

Dangers and Complications

- Violence
- Hypertension
- Respiratory depression or arrest
- Stupor
- Coma
- Convulsions
- Death
- Suicide

Typical Users

- Adolescents
- Young adults

**Symptoms of intoxication noted in* DSM-IV.

phrenia. It is believed that schizophrenics are particularly sensitive to PCP and that PCP may aggravate schizophrenic symptoms.

A PCP high appears about 5 minutes after a person takes the drug and lasts 4–6 hours. Effects may last up to 48 hours. PCP may be recovered from the blood and urine for 7–10 days. While using PCP, a person experiences a wide variety of feelings ranging from euphoria and utter peace to violence, confusion, and disorganization. Distorted sensory perceptions are common. During a bad "trip," anxiety, fear, and paranoia predominate. The dramatic physical and emotional effects of PCP may last for several weeks. Users may suffer from depression, fatigue, memory loss, concentration difficulty, and poor impulse control.

Withdrawal

Treatment of acute PCP intoxication may include the use of diazepam for muscle spasms, seizures, and agitation. Haloperidol may be used for severe psychotic behavior, but phenothiazines should not be used because PCP is anticholinergic. Calcium channel blockers such as verapamil may be given. These drugs are thought to prevent or reverse PCP-induced vasospasm, thereby decreasing the hallucinogenic effects of PCP. This treatment is controversial, however, because some clinicians feel that the use of verapamil may potentiate the effects of PCP. Nursing care during this period should focus on protecting the client from injury and reorienting the person to reality. Providing a quiet, safe environment and addressing the person in a calm, reassuring manner are important.

A vital problem with PCP is the question of its purity and its concentration. Because it is generally manufactured illegally, users never really know what they are buying. Adulterants are often toxic to humans, causing a wide variety of responses, including death. Originally called the "peace pill," PCP is now recognized for its potential to cause violence, especially when the drug is taken in high dosages.

Hallucinogens

Two high school seniors decided to take LSD. After 8 hours, one student was enjoying music, describing the varied colors he saw as the music changed in tempo. The other student was sweating profusely. His pupils were dilated, and he was trembling. He saw brightly colored dogs with huge teeth and claws changing into cats, snakes, and lions. He said he felt his gallbladder working with his liver and stomach. He eventually became so out of control that the other student took him to the emergency room.

The Effects of Hallucinogens

Hallucinogens are synthetic and natural drugs that cause hallucinations and unusual sensory experiences. Developed in 1938 for scientific research, LSD became popular in the 1960s when Timothy Leary, a Harvard psychologist, described how it stimulated great insight and increased awareness. In the 1960s and 1970s, the U.S. Army secretly experimented with LSD by giving it to unsuspecting army employees. One dramatic and much publicized event concerned the army officer who leapt to his death from a window after unknowingly ingesting LSD. At this time the danger of LSD became publicized, as did the unethical research. Physician researchers also were interested in experimenting with the uses of LSD in the treatment of a variety of diseases; however, in 1966, LSD became illegal and could no longer be used in human research. Peyote, however, is still an integral part of religious rituals of Native Americans in the southwestern U.S. and Mexico.

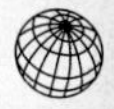

After a lull in use, LSD ("acid") is again being used by teenagers because it is cheap ($2–$5 a "hit") and causes an intense high that lasts 6–12 hours. Teenagers today are unacquainted with the horror stories of the 1960s. Today, people use LSD predominantly to get high rather than to expand consciousness. See the box on page 272 for additional information.

Withdrawal

The dangers of hallucinogens include "bad trips" and flashbacks. Users who experience bad trips may appear psychotic and extremely fearful. Reassuring the person and pointing out reality are helpful; occasionally, tranquilizers or antipsychotics are given. The symptoms usually disappear within 12 hours but may persist for months. People who are mentally ill or emotionally conflicted are more likely to have bad trips and flashbacks and to require hospitalization than are ordinary users.

Flashbacks are a spontaneous reliving of the experiences the person felt while under the influence of the drug, although the person is drug-free. The experience may involve perceptual distortions, a variety of physical feelings, and strong emotions such as fear and pleasure. Flashbacks are generally brief, and they occur less frequently over time. Flashbacks may be induced by stress, fatigue, and drug or alcohol ingestion.

Some authorities believe hallucinogens pose a particular danger to adolescents in that they may precipitate a psychosis. Because teenagers' egos and defenses are weak, they may be especially susceptible to the effects of hallucinogens.

Psychologic and physical dependence are unlikely because each experience with a hallucinogen is different. At the present time, researchers have demonstrated no rela-

Key Facts About Hallucinogens

Examples

LSD, psilocybin, DMT, psilocin, mescaline, peyote, MDA

Slang Terms

Acid

Route of Administration

Oral

Psychologic Symptoms

- Intensification of perceptions
- Depersonalization
- Derealization
- Illusions, pseudohallucinations
- Synesthesias (seeing sound or hearing colors)
- Anxiety
- Depression
- Intense emotions
- Body image changes
- Ideas of reference
- Paranoid ideation
- Impaired judgment
- Mood swings

Physical Symptoms

- Dilated pupils
- Tachycardia
- Sweating
- Palpitations
- Blurred vision
- Tremors
- Lack of coordination

Dangers and Complications

- Unpredictable behavior, resulting in harm to self or others
- Flashbacks

Typical Users

- Adolescents
- Young adults

tionship between hallucinogens and birth defects. Likewise, increased creativity and brilliant personality revelations, presumed effects of the drugs, are short-lived at best.

Inhalants

Carlos is an 11-year-old homeless child from Brazil living on the streets in Miami, Florida. He comes to the attention of the clinic because he has been arrested for purse snatching. He appears giddy, dirty, disheveled, confused, and belligerent. His speech is slurred, he has an unsteady gait, and he smells like glue. His eyes are red and tearing, he is coughing, and he is nauseated. He has avoided attending school and has received no health care.

The Effects of Inhalants

According to nurse expert Espeland (1993), the abuse of inhalants—glue, fuels, paints, aerosols, air fresheners, the substance used to resole shoes, and the propellants in canned whipped cream—is increasing at a frightening rate. It is estimated that 9 million Americans have experimented with inhalants and that at least 1 in every 6 eighth graders has used inhalants. Inhalants are inexpensive, easily available, and often legal. Their use causes euphoria, light-headedness, and excitement. Children, particularly Hispanic and Native American males, are the most frequent users. Adult users often have a long history of polydrug abuse.

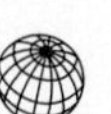

Patterns of Use

Inhalants are sniffed or inhaled through the mouth from a rag soaked with the inhalant and placed in a plastic bag. Gas is frequently inhaled directly from a tank. Most inhalant and solvent abusers seek out abandoned buildings, rooftops, and other isolated areas, although as Espeland (1993) points out, butyl nitrate can be easily concealed and passed around a classroom, and paint thinner can be concealed in a soft drink can. Use of these inhalants and solvents can cause ventricular fibrillation, decreased cardiac output, and sudden death.

Treatment

Although withdrawal must be managed as with the other substances covered in this chapter, careful assessment, early identification, detoxification, education, and prevention are particularly critical because so many inhalant abusers are children under 12. Nurses need to be aware of the programs and resources available and should support legislation to make it more difficult for minors to obtain glue and paint products.

Polydrug Use

Most substance abusers today are polydrug users. This fact complicates diagnosis and treatment and increases the hazards associated with abuse. *Synergistic* or *potentiating effects* are possible; the effects of two or more drugs taken together are greater than the singular effects of each drug. *Additive effects* occur when two drugs that have similar effects are used together. *Paradoxical effects* occur if a drug causes a reaction opposite to that expected. Paradoxical effects may occur when only one drug is taken or when several drugs are taken. A *pathologic reaction,* too, may result from the ingestion of only one or several drugs: It is an unexpected and dramatic response to the drug. For example, the combination of alcohol and marijuana is especially dangerous because THC suppresses the nausea that results from an overdose of alcohol. Consequently, the person may continue to drink, risking respiratory depression, coma, and even death. Cocaine and alcohol are frequently used together; the cocaine gives the user a brief high, and the alcohol masks the ensuing depression. When the cocaine wears off, the person is intoxicated and unable to drive safely. Prescription drugs and alcohol are also a common combination.

Designer Drugs

Designer drugs, a new threat on the drug scene, are chemical derivatives of controlled drugs. They are called analog drugs because they retain properties of controlled drugs, but one molecule is changed, making them initially not classifiable as controlled. According to the Controlled Substance Act of 1970, controlled substances (federally regulated substances) are classified from I (most regulated) through V, according to the potential for abuse and the current accepted medical use. As new information is made available, drugs may be reclassified.

Produced by underground chemists, analog drugs are initially legal until analyzed and researched by chemists. Once a dangerous pattern of use is determined (often 3–6 months after police discover the drug), the drug may be classified as a controlled substance. Fentanyl citrate (Sublimaze), a synthetic anesthetic used as an anesthetic agent, is similar chemically to some designer drugs. Fentanyl is 100 times as strong as morphine and 20–40 times as strong as heroin. It provides a fast rush and an extraordinary high. A person can become addicted after one shot of fentanyl (Gallagher 1986). *Ecstasy* (MDMA, Adam) was a designer drug; it has recently been classified as a Schedule I narcotic because research demonstrates that it causes structural damage to the brain. MTPT (China white), an analog of meperidine (Demerol), has an adverse reaction similar to the rigidity caused by Parkinson's disease.

Groups at Risk for Substance Abuse

Teenagers

Drug abuse among teenagers is pervasive in our society. Although many adolescents experiment with drugs for only a brief time, many more who do so become addicted. Susceptibility to addiction seems to depend on several variables: the form and potency of the drug, the dosage, the frequency of use, the pattern of use, stress, the personality and genetic makeup of the user, and the family culture. Straight, Inc., views drug abuse as a primary disease: an incurable chronic disease that is progressive and terminal. Newton (1981) describes drug use as a disease of feelings. Newton believes that psychoactive drugs affect the "old brain," the limbic system and center of feeling, and not the "new brain" (neocortex), the center of conceptualization. Consequently, a teenager's moods are affected not only at the moment of use but also over time. People use drugs that initially produce good feelings to escape from the stress and strain of life. A teenager who relies on a quick "fix" (a drug) to ease mental pain does not learn healthy coping processes. If teenagers do not learn healthy coping mechanisms or work through the pains and mood swings associated with living, they never complete a necessary developmental stage. As a consequence, they remain fixated at a dependent level of development. They enter a dangerous cycle that is unlikely to be interrupted without professional intervention. Drug use, regardless of what drug is used, inevitably affects all areas of a teenager's life: school, work, social and family relationships, and sense of self-worth (see the Assessment box on the next page).

Adolescent drug users manifest more psychopathologic conditions than nonusers do. Symptoms include feelings of depression, inadequacy, frustration, helplessness, and self-alienation. These teenagers also have ego structure deficiencies and poor impulse control. The earlier a child begins using a dependence-producing drug, the more likely the child is to use other dependence-producing drugs. Teenagers who use alcohol and drugs are likely to continue to use them in adulthood.

ASSESSMENT

Behavioral Changes Associated with Teenage Drug Abuse

- Unexplained periods or reactions of moodiness, depression, anxiety, irritability, oversensitivity, or hostility.
- Strongly inappropriate overreaction to mild criticism or simple requests.
- Lessening in accustomed family warmth; avoids interaction and communication with parents, withdraws from family activities.
- Preoccupation with self, less concern for the feelings of others.
- Loss of interest in previously important hobbies, sports, activities.
- Loss of motivation and enthusiasm (amotivational syndrome).
- Lethargy, lack of energy and vitality.
- Loss of ability for self-discipline and assuming responsibility.
- Need for instant gratification.
- Change in values, ideals, beliefs.
- Changes in friends, unwillingness to introduce friends.
- Secretive phone calls; callers refuse to identify themselves or hang up when you answer.
- Unexplained absences from home.
- Disappearance of money or items of value from home; handling of money becomes secretive.
- Desire for increased sensory stimuli.

Psychiatric Clients

Nurses need to be alert to possible substance abuse by psychiatric clients. Problems may occur if clients take a combination of substances, and treatment is hindered if clients are under the influence of drugs or alcohol. Close observation of teenagers and their visitors is useful, and the nurse should often ask clients directly if they are taking drugs. In most psychiatric hospitals, urine is routinely tested for the presence of drugs, if there are any indications of use. Drug screening is usually done on admission and when the client returns from a pass (see Chapter 25).

Women

Although alcoholism is a greater stigma for women than men, more women are drinking today. Many of these women are also using other drugs. Women respond to alcohol somewhat differently than men do because they metabolize alcohol less effectively than men.

Research on women and alcohol makes it clear that treatment programs should be geared to women's needs. Such programs might include women-only groups, lesbian-only groups, female therapists, meetings with recovered women alcoholics/addicts, and help for the client families. Kearney et al.'s (1994) nursing research urges the establishment of recovery centers for crack mothers that do not require that they give up their children. Hall's (1994) research urges creativity, flexibility, and cultural savvy on the part of health care providers when interacting with lesbians recovering from alcohol in both the initial health care and the later recovery phases.

General Hospital Clients

Nurses who work in the general hospital must be alert to the possibility that clients presenting with other illnesses may be substance abusers and may be in danger of withdrawal. Be alert and sensitive if physical assessment reveals any of the following:

- Debilitation out of proportion to the presenting health problem.
- Physical findings that do not correlate to the chief complaint.
- Unsteady gait, slurring of speech, dilated pupils, night sweats, chills, blackouts, tremors, skin tracks, abscesses, nasal septum perforation, jaundice.
- Weight loss, poor hygiene, and poor nutrition.

The nurse may want to alert the physician and suggest appropriate laboratory studies (such as liver function tests). A nursing assessment may include questions about a client's drinking habits. If alcoholism is suspected, a helpful, matter-of-fact but nonjudgmental stance will facilitate the client's acceptance of treatment for possible withdrawal symptoms. Even among obviously intoxicated clients, responses to such direct questions may be angry and defensive. Unfortunately, most problem drinkers go unrecognized in the medical-surgical population (Kitchens 1994).

The Elderly

Elderly clients who are being treated for several chronic illnesses by different physicians are at risk for drug problems from drug interactions and/or for drug dependence. For this reason, nurses should obtain a good history from the client, including a list of all the drugs taken, frequency of use, dosage, and duration of use. It is often useful to ask the family of an older client to bring all drugs to the hospital for review rather than relying on memory. Frequently, the confusion seen in elderly clients is a direct consequence of drug interaction or malabsorption.

In addition, substance abuse (especially alcoholism) is less likely to be detected and treated in older adults than in younger clients. It often goes unrecognized because the signs of substance abuse are difficult to distinguish from the changes associated with normal aging or degenerative brain disease. The difficulty in assessing drug abuse in older clients is further complicated by the paucity of elder-specific alcohol and drug treatment facilities, despite the fact that as much as 48% of the population over age 60 has an alcohol problem. This problem is only likely to increase with the future graying of America. Both early and late onset elderly alcoholics have reported loneliness, losses, depression, and meager social support networks as antecedents of their alcohol abuse.

Adult Children of Alcoholics

Adult children of alcoholics are at great risk of becoming alcoholics. If both parents are alcoholics, a child has a 70% chance of becoming an alcoholic; if one parent is an alcoholic, a child has a 40% chance. This type of alcoholism has been labeled *familial*. Research on familial alcoholism has shown that:

- A family history of alcoholism is present.
- Alcoholism develops early, usually by the time the person is in his or her late twenties.
- The alcoholism is generally severe and usually requires treatment.
- The risk of alcoholism is increased but not the risk of other psychiatric disorders.

Nurses

The issue of chemically dependent nurses has received attention in professional journals and lay literature. Many factors place nurses at risk for developing chemical dependence. A primary risk factor is codependence. Many codependents, whether adult children of substance abusers or products of other dysfunctional family systems, choose careers in the helping professions, such as nursing. Codependent nurses often give more of themselves than is necessary for effective client care. They seek perfection and tend to ignore or repress problems and difficulties. Codependent nurses are superb caretakers of everyone but themselves (Hall and Wray 1989).

Nurses also work under a great deal of stress and have easy access to drugs. Every day, they give people medication to decrease pain. It is an easy leap to begin to self-medicate (Figure 13–4). However, such behavior is a

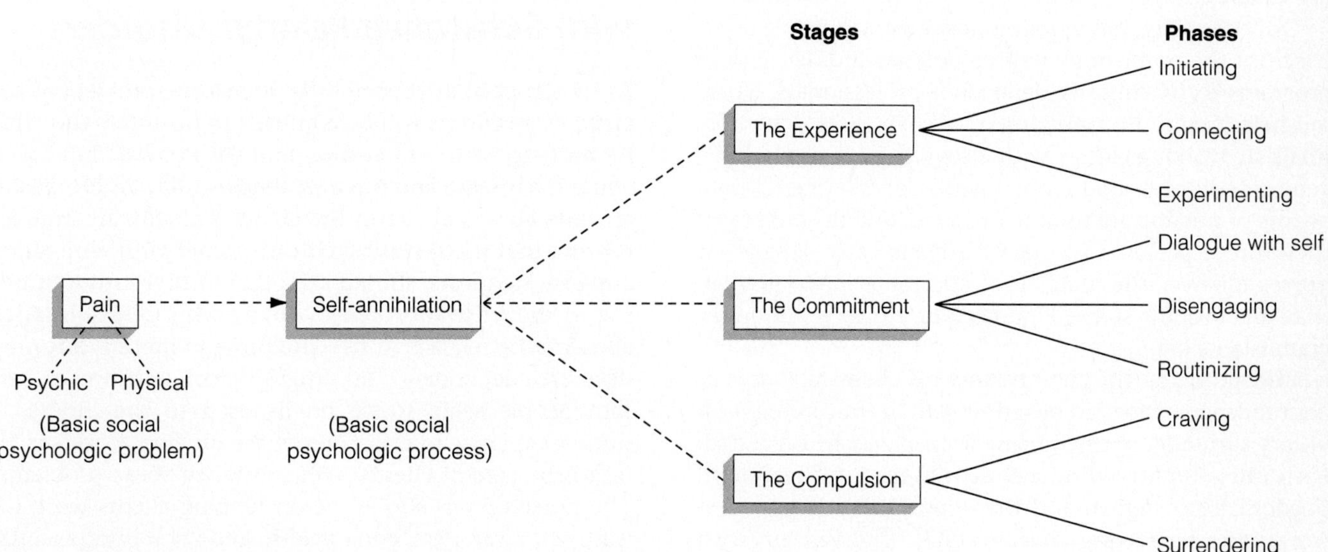

Figure 13–4 Chemically dependent nurses: the trajectory toward self-annihilation. *Source: Hutchinson 1986. Copyright ©1986, The American Journal of Nursing Company.*

NURSING SELF-AWARENESS

Warning Signs of Chemically Dependent Nurses

- Frequent absenteeism before and after days off; always working (for supply).
- Irritability.
- Abrupt mood changes; inappropriate affect.
- Sloppy charting and client care.
- Problems with drugs (missing drugs, frequent "wasting" of drugs, inaccurate records).
- Frequent errors of judgment.
- Alcohol (stale or fresh) on breath.
- Frequent disappearance from the unit.
- Offering to give medication to other nurses' clients.
- Frequent night shift work.
- The nurse's clients complain of little or no pain relief.

violation of state nurse practice acts and, depending on the drug and method of obtaining it, may be a criminal offense.

Colleagues of chemically dependent nurses need to be alert to behavior that suggests a problem (see the accompanying Nursing Self-Awareness box). They should attempt to talk with the nurse, who undoubtedly feels shame and guilt, before documenting and reporting such behavior to the head nurse or supervisor. It is very common to cover up the behavior. Shielding such a nurse puts clients, the nurse, and the nursing profession at risk and violates the nurse practice act, the nurse code of ethics, and the law in many states. Nurses, however, need to understand that their chemically dependent colleagues suffer from a disease, not a moral problem. This understanding enables nurses to work together to help each other.

Only recently has nursing administration begun to confront the problem by writing policies and developing programs for chemically dependent professionals. Nurse self-help groups are springing up all over, and some hospitals are working closely with recovering nurses on intervention strategies and requirements for treatment. State boards of nursing are usually involved, and in some cases they hire a person to work with chemically dependent nurses all over the state. Peer assistance programs are available in some states; Florida's Nurse Intervention Program is an example.

Depending on the circumstances, a chemically dependent nurse may need to be terminated or transferred. Voluntary surrender of the nursing license may be suggested. Each nurse is entitled to confidential medical treatment, freedom from stigma, and the opportunity to return to work upon recovering (Naegle 1985). Intervention with nurse substance abusers follows the pattern presented in the section entitled "Using Confrontation Strategies," later in this chapter. While in the process of recovery, chemically dependent nurses need regular drug screenings. Their work performance should be monitored, along with their attendance at a treatment program or group for a period of up to 2 years. With early intervention and continued support and treatment, chemically dependent nurses have a good prognosis.

Research in the area of chemically dependent nurses is just beginning. Hutchinson's seminal study (1986) describes the process by which nurses become chemically dependent. Researchers need to continue studying substance abusers and specific groups at risk.

The Nursing Process and Clients with Substance-Related Disorders

As substance abuse becomes an increasing problem in society, more clients will be admitted to hospitals and clinics for help with intoxication and withdrawal. Substance abuse is a disease and not a weakness or flaw. A moralistic attitude always alienates the client. Recognizing and accepting that the disease is chronic, often with remissions and exacerbations, should keep the nurse from succumbing to the frustration felt by many who treat substance abusers who relapse. At stressful times in life, anyone may develop a dependence on drugs or alcohol; however, certain people seem to be predisposed to the illness. A nurse's expertise in the stages of the nursing process is vital to the care of clients with substance abuse problems. The nurse's focus should be on helping clients work toward self-awareness, good health, and good interpersonal relationships so that they can lead productive, fulfilling, happy lives.

NURSING SELF-AWARENESS

A Guide to Analyzing Personal Responses Toward Substance Abusers

Analyze your responses to the following questions:

- What thoughts and feelings does the term *alcoholic* evoke in me?
- What thoughts and feelings does the term *addict* evoke in me?
- Do I believe that substance dependence occurs out of moral weakness?
- Do I believe that substance dependence is an illness that can be treated?
- Are people who abuse substances deliberately destroying their own lives and the lives of significant others?
- Who in my personal life has abused drugs, alcohol, or other chemicals?
- How does my experience with relatives, friends, colleagues, or clients who have abused substances affect my attitude toward caring for a substance-abusing client?
- Is substance abuse a social problem, an emotional-psychologic problem, or a physical abnormality?
- How do I view the family, spouse, or friends of the substance abuser? Do they encourage the abuse, or otherwise "enable" the person to continue their abuse? Or are they victims?
- How does my own personal use of nicotine, caffeine, drugs, or alcohol affect my attitude toward clients?

Source: Bittle, Feiginbaum, and Kneisl 1986, p. 254.

Drugs change rapidly, and nurses must keep up with the "drug scene" to assess and treat clients. Along with the knowledge acquired from reading, continuing education programs, and seminars, nurses need self-knowledge to be good therapists with substance abusers. Ongoing critical self-analysis of feelings, attitudes, and behavior toward clients is useful. See the box above for a list of questions to guide this self-analysis.

Assessment

The nurse must make an accurate assessment of the substances used and abused to anticipate potential toxic and withdrawal effects and to make nursing care plans as specific and relevant as possible. For example, a chronic alcoholic who is malnourished, exhausted, and depressed needs immediate diet regulation, rest, and gradual involvement in a treatment program. Cocaine or crack abusers are likely to be resistant to treatment and need active staff intervention and a structured program to involve them in treatment. They should not be left alone or purposefully isolated, as might be done with an alcoholic.

SUBJECTIVE DATA As part of the mental status exam and the psychiatric history, the nurse should conduct a thorough, nonjudgmental substance use assessment.

Interview Questions

1. How many packs of cigarettes do you smoke?
2. Do you take any prescription drugs now?
3. Do you drink alcohol each day? If yes, do you drink a pint or about a quart? (Let the client correct you on your overstatement rather than fear shocking you with the truth.)
4. Do you drink a pint or quart of alcohol or more on occasion? When was your last drink?
5. Do you have a drug habit? What drug do you use, and what's your daily cost?

Simply asking "How many drinks do you have at a time?" can be misleading and can minimize the problem if each drink exceeds standard bar amounts of about 2 oz. The CAGE questions discussed below are also helpful.

In an emergency situation the client may be unable to answer key questions like these:

- What did you take?
- How much did you take?
- When did you take it?
- What have you taken in the last 24 hours? In the last week?

text continues on page 280

CASE STUDY

A Client with Cocaine Intoxication

Identifying Information

Leigh S is a 25-year-old married woman who lives at 2205 Long Street. She was brought into the hospital by her husband. Leigh is an advertising executive with a large firm (Weeks, Bedde, and Law). She has a BA in business and an MBA in marketing. She is not and has never been under the care of a therapist.

Client's Description of the Problem

Leigh states she does not need to be in the hospital but rather needs to get back to work on her ideas for ads. She states that she is extremely creative and productive and needs "to get my ideas down on paper." She is incoherent occasionally during the interview. She does state that she is perspiring and "feels sick to my stomach." Leigh admits to "working very hard," but does not feel she needs care right now. She feels she can handle this herself. Leigh states she has been using cocaine intranasally for one year. She admits to spending most of her salary on cocaine and states that she has used cocaine four to five times a day for the last five days. Prior to this, she generally used cocaine once or twice a week. She has increased her use because "it helps me work harder and faster. I feel more productive." She is having trouble sitting still and sleeping. Leigh thinks that she has not slept more than an hour or two for several days. Leigh's husband and one woman colleague are her main support system.

Psychiatric History

No prior psychiatric history.

Family History

Leigh's parents are living and work in their own business, a shoe store. Leigh has one brother, 21 years old, a senior in college. She feels emotionally close to her family and brother, but because they live 2000 miles away, she sees them only on holidays. Leigh's father has a history of alcoholism, which has been under control for five years.

Social History

Leigh has always excelled, in both her academic work and her job. She is competitive and likes "being number one." She has a few close friends and socializes with numerous "acquaintances from work." She has smoked since age 17, drinks "moderately," but occasionally gets drunk on weekends. She has experimented with a variety of drugs but finds cocaine to be "what works for me." She describes herself as a "workaholic" but enjoys reading and tennis when time permits.

Health History

Leigh has no current or past medical problems. She states that she is in good health, but "feels horrible now." Assessment reveals a blood pressure reading of 140/90 and a pulse rate of 110.

Current Mental Status

Leigh is attractive, yet disheveled, agitated, hyperalert, alternately compliant and hostile, and occasionally incoherent. Her sensorium is impaired. She is oriented to time, place, and person; judgment is impaired. Her affect is labile (alternately hostile and compliant); mood swings are evident. She moves rapidly and frequently. Her thought content is grandiose. Delusions and illusions are present. She states that she wants to open her own advertising company very soon and says she is more efficient, intelligent, and productive than her boss. She reports seeing "signs" at work that are messages to her that she should "move onward and upward." Her thought processes reveal a thought disorder; she is occasionally incoherent and tangential. She is easily distracted and has difficulty concentrating. Presently she denies her problem and has little insight, stating, "I can take care of myself. I know what I'm doing."

Other Subjective or Objective Clinical Data

Leigh is not on any medications; suicide/violence potential minimal.

Diagnostic Impression

Nursing Diagnoses

Ineffective Individual Coping
Sleep Pattern Disturbance
Impaired Social Interaction
Altered Nutrition: Less than Body Requirements
Altered Thought Processes

DSM-IV Multiaxial Diagnosis

Axis I: 305.60 Cocaine Intoxication (primary diagnosis)
304.20 Cocaine Dependence
Axis II: V71.09 (no diagnosis; denial and rationalization)
Axis III: Hypertension
Axis IV: Occupational Problems
Axis V: GAF = 50 (current), serious symptoms in judgment; GAF = 60 (highest level in past year)

NURSING CARE PLAN

A Client with Cocaine Intoxication

Nursing Diagnosis

Ineffective Individual Coping related to Cocaine Abuse.

Expected Outcome

- Client will agree to become free from cocaine within 48 hr.
- Client will complete detox program.

Nursing Interventions

- Meet individually with client to discuss consequences of drug-using behavior. "You are having trouble at work, at home, and with friends. We will work with you on these problems."
- Assign client to a daily therapy group and to an individual counselor.
- Observe client every half hour; expect drug-seeking behavior. When you notice this, talk about client's feelings, explaining the anxiety and craving will disappear over time.

Outcome Met If

- Client's urine is "clean" 72 hr after last use.
- Client meets with counselor and attends group meetings according to schedule without prompting.
- Client talks about her feelings, including her anxiety and craving for cocaine.
- Discusses the problems cocaine has created for her.

Nursing Diagnosis

Sleep Pattern Disturbances related to Cocaine Abuse.

Expected Outcome

Client will sleep 5–6 hr a night after 1 week.

Nursing Interventions

- Record sleep activity every 24 hr.
- Administer medication as ordered.
- Teach relaxation skills.

Outcome Met If

- Client sleeps 5–6 hr a night.
- Client indicates satisfaction with sleep pattern.

Nursing Diagnosis

Impaired Social Interaction related to Cocaine Abuse.

Expected Outcome

Client will attend group meeting without leaving the room after 1 week.

Nursing Interventions

Record group meeting attendance and behavior.

Outcome Met If

- Client attends group therapy as scheduled and remains seated throughout.
- If agitated, client discusses her feelings.

Nursing Diagnosis

Altered Nutrition: Less than Body Requirements related to Cocaine Abuse.

Expected Outcome

Client will become physiologically stable and have no evidence of gastrointestinal distress.

Nursing Interventions

- Offer antacids PRN.
- Encourage diet as tolerated; monitor food intake.
- Weigh each week.

Outcome Met If

- Client is physiologically stable. No GI upset.
- Client eats three meals a day.
- Client maintains stable weight or gains weight.

Nursing Diagnosis

Altered Thought Process related to Cocaine Abuse.

Expected Outcome

- Client will speak clearly and sensibly within 72 hr.
- Client will not mention how wonderful she is, how she will start her own company, or other signs of grandiosity.
- Client will not evidence extreme anger or euphoria when in group or individual treatment or in conversations with others on the unit.

Nursing Interventions

- When client is incoherent, ask her to slow down and repeat what she was saying.
- Ask client to discuss some of the problems in her life that she feels are a result of cocaine.
- When she blames others, get client to focus on herself.
- When client is angry and agitated, say, "I know you have an idea that cocaine could help you now and I know you are suffering, but with hard work on your part, you will get better."

Outcome Met If

- Client repeats her statements when requested to do so by you.
- Client discusses her own feelings and anxieties and fears.
- Client's conversation is relevant, goal-directed.

When this happens, you must rely on family or friends as data sources, and then corroborate what you learn with the client once he or she is alert.

Common Defense Mechanisms in Client Responses Denial and projection are two defense mechanisms common to substance abusers. These mechanisms, along with other behaviors—conning, bargaining, feigning—complicate all phases of the nursing assessment of subjective data. Alcoholics and other drug abusers tend to deny they have a problem or minimize the problem: "I drink/use every day, but it rarely interferes with my work." Rationalization is common: "I know I shouldn't drink, and I'll stop as soon as I get through this problem. Drinking keeps me calm enough to function." A detailed assessment, along with family/coworker interviews, reveals that the problem is generally worse than the client says. Cocaine users tend to project and blame their difficulties on others, often a spouse. For instance, a man may bring up the issue of his wife's drinking and give a dozen reasons why he does not need treatment.

Substance abusers sometimes "con" (manipulate) people to get drugs. *DSB,* a term used in some treatment centers, refers to *drug-seeking behaviors,* such as feigning illness or an injury to get a drug. These people also bargain with themselves and staff members to get what they want. For example, an alcoholic/drug abuser is likely to think, "I know I shouldn't hang out with B and P since we all get loaded together, but I like them. I'll just be with them, I won't drink/use." Later on, the person may think, "I'll only use a gram of cocaine"; later, "I'll just do an eight-ball." This client might tell the nurse, "I'll be glad to go to group therapy next week; just let me rest for a few days. I'm really tired." Of course, substance abusers always con themselves first.

Motivation for Treatment Nurses need to consider some important psychosocial issues when clients come for treatment. Clients may enter a treatment program voluntarily. This situation is best, because they are internally motivated and therefore have a better chance of success. However, they may be coerced by family, friends, physicians, or the police to undergo treatment. Coerced treatment inevitably causes anger and resentment. These clients may lash out at people, blame them (including the nurse), and demonstrate resistant or arrogant behavior. In these difficult situations, the nurse must remain detached and nonjudgmental to avoid both power struggles and taking the role of persecutor or rescuer. At this time, the nurse functions as a data gatherer: "I know you are [uncomfortable, anxious, afraid, angry] now. To help you feel better, I need to ask you some questions about your drug use." A judgmental question is, "Don't you know that if you don't get help now you will only get worse?" Such questions prevent rapport and alienate the client.

The Importance of Language Knowing the language of the drug world is important in obtaining an accurate nursing assessment of a substance abuser. Drug users have a language all their own; to understand them and the extent and nature of their habit, a nurse needs to learn this language. For example, "basing and balling" refer to freebasing (using ether to purify cocaine and make it more potent) and speed-balling (combining heroin and cocaine); "copping an eight-ball" means acquiring one-eighth ounce of cocaine; a "mission" is several days' use of crack; "drug of choice" is the client's favorite drug. Often the clients themselves or a recovering addict can teach the nurse.

OBJECTIVE DATA In addition to assessing subjective data, you should include a thorough consideration of relevant objective data.

Physical Findings Less dramatic physical findings may include dry skin, hangnails, malnutrition, ascites, elevated blood pressure, and the smell of alcohol or an inhalant on the client's breath. As alcoholism progresses, the nurse should be alert to signs and symptoms of liver cirrhosis (see the accompanying box).

Standardized, Structured Questionnaires and Scales The list of standardized structured interviews, questionnaires, and scales used to assess substance abuse is long and includes the following, which are among the best known:

- The DSM-IV Structured Clinical Interview (SCID)
- The Addiction Severity Index
- The Chemical Use, Abuse, and Dependence Scale (CUAD)
- The Millon Clinical Multiaxial Inventory
- The Drinking Problems Index
- The CAGE Questionnaire

Of these, the CAGE is most frequently used for the detection of alcoholism in clinical settings. CAGE is a mnemonic for these four questions:

1. Have you ever felt like you should *cut down* on your drinking?
2. Have people *annoyed* you by criticizing your drinking?
3. Have you ever felt bad or *guilty* about your drinking?
4. Have you ever had a drink in the morning as an *eye-opener* to get rid of a hangover?

Accurate responses to these questions are most likely when they are part of an interview that includes general lifestyle inquiries about cigarette smoking, coffee consumption, and exercise habits. Experts agree that skillful

Signs and Symptoms of Liver Cirrhosis

- *Skin.* Extremely dry skin; severe pruritus; abnormal pigmentation; spider angiomas on the face, neck, arms, and trunk; telangiectasis on the cheeks; prominent abdominal vessels; ecchymosis; palmar erythema; jaundice.
- *Gastrointestinal.* Anorexia; indigestion; nausea and vomiting; diarrhea or constipation; hemorrhoids; dull, aching abdominal pain; musty breath; ascites.
- *Central nervous system.* Lethargy; slurred speech; asterixis (flapping tremor of the hands); peripheral neuritis; confusion; coma.
- *Hematologic.* Bleeding tendencies (frequent nosebleeds, easy bruising, bleeding gums); anemia.
- *Hepatic.* Hepatomegaly. In the early stages of cirrhosis, the liver will feel large and firm, with a sharp edge. Eventually it shrinks, and the edge feels nodular. There may also be pain in the right upper quadrant that intensifies when the client leans forward.

Source: Adapted from Meissner 1994.

assessment interviewing of clients and their family members remains the best source of data.

Laboratory Tests For years, researchers and clinicians have been searching for an objective biologic marker that will reflect problem drinking and make assessment less challenging. Common laboratory tests in which elevated values are associated with excessive alcohol intake are:

- Blood alcohol concentration
- Gamma-glutamyl transferase (GGT)
- Alanine aminotransferase (ALT, formerly SGPT)
- Aspartate aminotransferase (AST, formerly SGOT)
- Lactate dehydrogenase
- Alkaline phosphatase
- Total bilirubin
- Cholesterol
- Triglycerides
- Uric acid
- Mean corpuscular volume (MCV)

Table 13–1 A Sample Comparison of a DSM-IV Diagnosis and Nursing Diagnoses

DSM-IV Diagnosis	*NANDA Diagnoses*
305.30 Hallucinogen Abuse	Self-Care Deficits Sleep Pattern Disturbance Sensory/Perceptual Alterations Altered Thought Processes Ineffective Thermoregulation Ineffective Individual Coping Risk for Violence: Self-directed or directed at others

These elevated laboratory test values are only one of the alerting factors for problem drinking. No single test or combination of tests alone to date is appropriate for clinical screening. Confirmation of the excessive use of alcohol in a sensitively conducted assessment interview remains the preferred assessment approach and is considered a prerequisite for successful intervention.

Nursing Diagnosis

Because substance-related disorders are associated with biologic, psychosocial, and even spiritual distress, a wide variety of nursing diagnoses is likely to be fundamental to planning comprehensive care. A sample DSM-IV and related NANDA diagnoses are compared in Table 13–1.

Planning and Implementing Interventions

PROGRAMS Nurses may hold positions in any of the following settings. Their roles may be slightly different in each setting, depending on the client's stage of illness and presenting symptoms. Solari-Twadell (1983) describes five types of treatment programs where interventions can address the wide range of nursing diagnoses relevant to substance-related disorders.

General Hospital Care Substance abusers who are suicidal or acutely ill with DTs, hepatic coma, respiratory depression, or cardiac arrhythmias are often treated in a medical-surgical unit of a general hospital. Life-threatening physiologic symptoms are attended to first. When the client is out of danger, the alcoholism or drug addiction issues are addressed. In this setting, nurses:

- Monitor vital signs and respiratory and cardiovascular support.
- Administer prescribed medications.
- Apply ice packs for fever, such as fever caused by amphetamine intoxication.
- Decrease stimulation; provide a darkened quiet room.

- Point out reality: "I know you are seeing things, and I know you are frightened. You are in the hospital, and we are caring for you. There are no bugs or monsters here. You are safe and will feel better soon."
- Make sure clients get adequate nutrition and fluids (they are disoriented and generally forget to eat and drink).
- Assess changes in level of consciousness.
- Monitor fluid intake and output.
- Protect skin integrity.
- Offer emotional support and encouragement to the client and his or her family.
- Refer clients to community resources for recovery programs.

Specialty Hospital Care Specialty hospital care is given in inpatient hospital units that are geared specifically for the treatment of substance abuse. If the hospital is equipped with trained personnel and appropriate resources, acutely ill clients may be admitted. The physical environment is modified to handle problems with substance abusers. For example, padded seclusion rooms devoid of all but a mattress offer a quiet, unstimulating environment that prevents convulsions and decreases anxiety. A primary nurse may be assigned to decrease confusion and stimulation. Members of the staff are experts in detoxification, education, and treatment. Clients also receive treatment for coexisting medical and psychiatric problems. Staff efforts are geared toward stabilization.

Residential Rehabilitation Residential rehabilitation facilities offer inpatients expert care for substance abuse, but in some cases staff members are not skilled in treating medical or psychiatric problems.

Extended Residential Care Extended care facilities provide services for people with physical impairments and a home for recovering alcoholics or drug addicts who have been rejected by their families. Apartments for independent living, a relatively new concept, are useful for these clients.

Outpatient Care Outpatient care may consist of daily, weekly, or monthly individual, group, or family therapy in a variety of treatment centers. Daily care is usually given only in intensive programs of limited duration, usually one month. Employee assistance programs (EAP) are now common in many industries and are one example of outpatient care given not in a clinic but in the workplace. Substance abuse outreach counselors work with chemically dependent employees.

Nurses who work with clients who have substance-related disorders in any of these settings need to recognize that addiction is a chronic, progressive disease. Each treat-

The Twelve Steps of Alcoholics Anonymous

1. We admitted we were powerless over alcohol—that our lives had become unmanageable.
2. Came to believe that a Power greater than ourselves could restore us to sanity.
3. Made a decision to turn our will and our lives over to the care of God, as we understood Him.
4. Made a searching and fearless moral inventory of ourselves.
5. Admitted to God, to ourselves, and to another human being the exact nature of our wrongs.
6. Were entirely ready to have God remove all these defects of character.
7. Humbly asked Him to remove our shortcomings.
8. Made a list of all people we had harmed, and became willing to make amends to them all.
9. Made direct amends to such people wherever possible, except when to do so would injure them or others.
10. Continued to take personal inventory and when we were wrong, promptly admitted it.
11. Sought through prayer and meditation to improve our conscious contact with God, as we understood Him, praying only for knowledge of His will for us and the power to carry that out.
12. Having had a spiritual awakening as the result of these steps, we tried to carry this message to alcoholics, and to practice these principles in all our affairs.

Source: "The Twelve Steps" from Twelve Steps and Twelve Traditions, *reprinted with permission of Alcoholics Anonymous World Services, Inc.*

ment setting calls for different skills. For example, in general or specialty hospitals, nurses need psychosocial skills along with technical skills to assess and monitor the physiologic components of abuse and withdrawal. In residential rehabilitation and extended residential care centers, the nurse may educate clients about the disease, help clients reenter the community as much as possible, and facilitate or lead support groups. In an outpatient treatment center, the nurse functions as a counselor/therapist. In all cases, the nurse must have psychosocial, physiologic, and even spiritual skills. Such skills may include interviewing, teaching clients about the disease process and alternative coping strategies, referring clients to appropriate sources and community support systems, and knowing how to conduct individual, group, or family therapy. In all situations, the nurse cannot give quality care without an in-depth understanding of the disease process, from the varying theoretic explanations to the varying methods of treatment at different stages.

Self-Help Groups

Twelve-Step Programs: AA and NA In contrast to the previously described treatment programs, **Alcoholics Anonymous (AA)** and **Narcotics Anonymous (NA)** are not specifically treatment programs, but AA/NA community groups do hold meetings at various treatment facilities. Both are successful self-help groups that meet daily, or more often, in different parts of large cities and weekly in smaller towns. Anyone who has a desire to stop drinking or taking drugs is welcome. This belief pervades both organizations: "Once an alcoholic/addict, always an alcoholic/addict." Members admit they are powerless over chemicals, live "one day at a time," recite the serenity prayer, and believe in "a power greater than man." Members learn to turn their problems over to "the God of my understanding." Their philosophy is revealed in part through their key slogans, "First things first," "Easy does it," and "Let go and let God." Alcoholics learn the "Twelve Steps of AA" (see the accompanying box). Through AA/NA, people learn to change negative attitudes and behaviors into positive ones. A key concept of AA/NA is that total abstinence is essential to recovery. As members become sober or drug-free, they begin "sponsoring" (helping) other substance abusers. This offering of support is believed to be vital to recovery, as is regular attendance at AA/NA meetings. Twelve-step recovery programs also emphasize spirituality through meditation and prayer rather than will power as the means to recovery. See the Mind-Body-Spirit box on the next page. 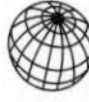 Recognizing that AA's twelve steps were written in the 1930s by and for white Christian males may require that the nurse adapt some of the language to a less patriarchal, less religious, and more generally spiritual and culturally relevant usage.

Women for Sobriety Women for Sobriety (WFS) is another self-help group. Unlike AA/NA, WFS is not based on a spiritual philosophy; instead, the program is based on abstinence. WFS's thirteen acceptance statements focus members on new ways of thinking. The women learn to cope and, over time, to change their daily lives. The group recognizes the differences of alcoholism in males and females.

Rational Recovery (RR) Alcoholics Anonymous is the most popular mutual-help recovery organization in the world. But it is not the only one. Alcoholics and addicts who failed to find a comfortable home in AA but were nevertheless determined to become sober have founded at least one other major organization to help others become clean and sober. This group, Rational Recovery (RR), rejects the spiritual approach of AA.

In some important ways, RR and AA are similar. Both set a goal of total abstinence for their members. And both recognize that life is not perfect and not always fair, but that the destructive consequences of alcohol and drug abuse are eminently avoidable with sobriety. Both groups specify that what happens at meetings is to be kept confidential. But in other ways, Rational Recovery is the very opposite of Alcoholics Anonymous. RR rejects the notion that alcoholics and addicts are powerless to stop their addictions, suggesting instead that until now they simply have not chosen to do so. Instead of reliance on a higher power (which RR considers another form of dependence), RR members are urged to build on strengths within themselves; the movement inspires independence whenever humanly possible. A constant theme is, "Think yourself sober."

Nor are there steps, sponsors, or moral inventories. RR asks that members learn to accept themselves as they are, to love themselves, drunk or sober, no matter what they do. There is no effort to try to become a better person; the goal is to stop ruining your life—because you are already worthwhile. Giving up alcohol and drugs may indeed be difficult, but in the end, it will make life better.

In RR, there is no making amends to others or even caring about what others think of you. According to rational emotive therapy, on which RR is based, human beings should feel good about themselves because they are human beings and not because others think well of them. The concept of staying sober one day at a time is rejected in favor of a decision to never drink or use again, period. Sobriety is not supposed to become the cornerstone of one's life. The goal is for members to wean themselves from dependence on alcohol, then from dependence on people, and finally from dependence on the group.

Meetings take place only twice a week, and most people attend for only one year, after which they may be pronounced "recovered." They can, however, return to meetings whenever the need arises. Discussions at meetings

MIND-BODY-SPIRIT CONNECTION

Twelve-Step Recovery

The twelve steps are grouped here into four categories: Surrender, Acceptance, Fellowship, and Bliss of Living. Each step is given a one-word description to indicate how the step works in the recovery process.

Surrender Steps

Step One: Honesty

Step Two: Hope

Step Three: Faith

Because many view surrender as a negative activity, using the words *honesty, hope,* and *faith* to describe each of the steps in the first category gives new meaning to the purpose of these steps. When seen from a patriarchal hierarchical view, the first step may appear to be a command. However, when it is a call to "get honest" with oneself, the step takes on new meaning without rewriting it or discounting the value it has had in helping others find recovery.

When seen as a way to expand one's spirituality through meditation and contemplation, the second step takes on new meaning as well. Hope comes from observation of others who have given up the need to control and be self-centered, who have found peace as a result of that action. The "came to believe" part of this step occurs over time as the client hears similar stories from multiple sources who share at twelve-step meetings. This is in part why a new member is urged to "Keep coming back . . . so more can be revealed."

The faith that results from taking the third step allows the client to move from ego-centered thinking to belief in a power greater than self, permitting that power to work on his or her behalf.

Acceptance Steps

Step Four: Courage

Step Five: Integrity

Step Six: Willingness

The next three steps follow from the change of attitude in the first three steps. These are action steps.

In the fourth step, clients uses newly discovered courage to examine the specific aspects of their character they need to nurture and develop, as well as those that need to be eliminated because they are responsible for current discomfort and distress.

The fifth step works to restore integrity to the client's life and may be responsible for the euphoria reported by many during early recovery. The client may feel a growing spiritual connection, and the nurse may be in a position to support the client's awareness of how the steps have contributed to his or her improved condition.

The sixth step is a willingness activity in which clients must decide how to convert their growing spirituality into a change of behavior.

Fellowship Steps

Step Seven: Humility

Step Eight: Forgiveness

Step Nine: Discipline

The fellowship steps help clients progress in their spiritual awareness and recovery by developing qualities of humility, forgiveness, and discipline in their personal relationships and public lives.

Bliss of Living Steps

Step Ten: Perseverance

Step Eleven: Love of self

Step Twelve: Gratitude

The bliss of living steps bring clients back to a life with meaning. By developing perseverance clients gain a freedom from worry about when the accumulation of undesirable behavior will be discovered and how it will lead back to the pain of the past. In the eleventh step, clients learn through prayer and meditation the love of self, love of others and love of life. They come to feel that they are not in charge of the world and that trusting in a higher power who is in charge is "OK." In the twelfth step recovering addicts and alcoholics express their gratitude for what they have achieved and learn to value reaching out to other sufferers to share the hope of step two, the courage of step four, and the love of step eleven.

Nurses have the opportunity to assist with the unfolding of the process of twelve-step recovery. Clients do the work supported by their spiritual beliefs, nurses can nourish the process of learning to live life in a new way.

Grace D. Dreyer, MSN, RN, CS

focus on the here and now rather than past history, and cross-discussion is encouraged. Like AA, the hat is usually passed at meetings to cover local costs. No money, except that raised from the sale of literature, goes to the national Rational Recovery Systems, a nonprofit organization.

Whereas AA relies totally on nonprofessionals helping one another, RR is run by professional coordinators, and each group has volunteer professional advisors available for advice and input. This is necessary because, unlike AA, there are no old timers around to help newcomers. Advisors attend meetings only occasionally. Rational Recovery, like AA, offers written materials, the core of which is *Rational Recovery from Alcoholism: The Small Book* (meant to contrast with the *Big Book of AA*).

RR spurns the concept of outside influences on individuals (a higher power, the group, family, friends, or even alcohol or drugs) playing a major role. "We may claim that we are angry or sad or irresponsible or drunk because of others, but this thinking is irrational. In reality we are the only ones responsible for the way we feel and the way we behave. We have a choice to drink or not to drink, and we are competent to make that choice" (an idea not foreign to AA).

RR suggests that we look within ourselves for strength and direction. We all have within us an inner voice, says RR, that challenges us to go wrong. It is this voice, nicknamed "Beast," that urges you to drink or use drugs, takes over during blackouts, gets you to do terrible things, and speaks louder than your rational self. It's the voice that tells you things like, "You can stop anytime (but not now)" or "You're not really addicted (you just like the taste)" and that tears angrily into those who criticize or try to help you.

Beast is an acronym used to help RR members avoid taking another drink or drug:

- *B is for Boozing Opportunities (weddings, parties, trips, and so on).* RR says to be aware of the pitfalls but do not necessarily avoid them. You are not powerless in the face of temptations, and you can choose not to succumb.
- *E is for Enemy Recognition.* Distinguish those thoughts from the Enemy (Beast) that are positive about booze or drugs.
- *A is for Accuse the Beast of Malice.* You can be angry at the Beast for its evil deeds (trying to tempt you), or you can laugh at it. Either way, make clear to the Beast that you have the upper hand and you won't relinquish it.
- *S is for Self-Control and Self-Worth Reminders.* Find ways of showing the Beast that you have self-control (like moving your hands in front of your face and holding them there, totally in your control, until the Beast backs down). Find ways of telling yourself that you are a worthwhile person. Choose not to drink for the same reason you drank: to feel good about yourself.
- *T is for Treasuring Your Sobriety.* Focus on the pleasures of life that are attainable only in sobriety (a concept similar to that in AA).

RELAPSE **Relapse** is common among substance abusers, and it seriously complicates treatment. Authorities in the field of alcoholism estimate that 60–75% of those who complete treatment programs drink again within the first 90 days. Data suggest that only 10–20% of alcoholics remain abstinent for one year following treatment, and that only 35% of these are abstinent five years later. In fact, recidivism rates are notoriously high across the spectrum of addictive behaviors.

Several attempts have been made to identify common stages of the relapse process:

1. Commitment to recovery and motivation for abstinence.
2. Initiating change.
3. Maintaining change. (Brownell et al. 1986)

As a result of a successful initial change, the person experiences perceived control while remaining abstinent. This feeling of perceived control continues until the person encounters a high-risk situation involving negative emotional states, interpersonal conflict, or social pressure. The person can avoid relapse by using effective coping responses in the high-risk situation. If, however, the individual cannot cope successfully, an initial "lapse" occurs in which he or she resorts to the use of a chemical to control stress. The person then feels less able to exert control and develops a tendency to "give in" to the situation ("It's no use, I can't handle this"). In subsequent high-risk situations, the individual again resorts to the use of chemicals to relieve stress. Repeated lapses set the stage for a return to uncontrolled use (relapse).

Many treatment centers are now incorporating the concept of relapse prevention into their treatment program. This program is designed to teach clients how to anticipate relapse. By learning skills to use in high-risk situations, clients gain confidence and the expectation of being able to cope successfully, thus decreasing the probability of relapse. The box on page 286 lists symptoms leading to relapse.

Research indicates that participation in a twelve-step program can help prevent relapse. These programs focus on the individual being "in recovery" and maintaining sobriety, as opposed to having recovered or being cured.

OTHER TREATMENT APPROACHES

Using Confrontation Strategies For many years, it was believed that alcoholics and drug abusers needed to "hit bottom" before they could accept their problem and request help. Today, most people believe that interven-

A Checklist of Symptoms Leading to Relapse

1. *Exhaustion.* Don't allow yourself to become overly tired or to have poor health. Many chemically dependent people are also prone to work addictions. Perhaps they are in a hurry to make up for lost time or are overworking to compensate for feelings of guilt or personal inadequacy. Good health and enough rest are essential to recovery. Good feelings of physical well-being are associated with a healthy, optimistic mental outlook. Fatigue and feelings of physical illness often induce negative thinking and a pessimistic attitude. You may begin to think a drug or drink would help you return to a positive frame of mind.
2. *Dishonesty.* This symptom begins with a pattern of unnecessary little lies and deceits with fellow workers, friends, and family. Then come important lies to yourself. This is called rationalizing—making excuses for not doing what you do not want to do, or for doing what you know you should not do.
3. *Impatience.* Things are not happening fast enough, others are not doing what they should or what you want them to.
4. *Argumentativeness.* Arguing about small and ridiculous points of view indicates a need to always be right. Chemically dependent people need to learn an attitude of acceptance of their disease and the value of the tools of recovery.
5. *Depression.* Unreasonable and unaccountable melancholy and despair may occur from time to time as a *natural part of recovering* from chemical dependence. Periods of depression are times when the risk of relapse is very high. Deal with your negative feelings; talk about them.
6. *Frustration.* Remember, everything is not going to be just the way you want it.
7. *Self-pity.* "Why do these things happen to me?" "Why must I be chemically dependent?" "Nobody appreciates what I'm doing for them."
8. *Cockiness.* "I've got this problem licked; I have nothing to fear from drugs or booze." This dangerous attitude may lead to going into situations where friends are drinking and using drugs to prove to others that you don't have a problem. Do this often enough and your defenses against relapse will wear down. Don't *test* your recovery. You may lose!
9. *Complacency.* It is dangerous to let up on disciplines because everything seems to be going so

tion can occur as soon as the problem is identified. Group intervention/confrontation is one strategy that aims to break down the substance abuser's denial. Nurses are often "intervention specialists" and leaders in the process.

Several family members, friends, employers, coworkers, and an alcohol/drug intervention specialist confront the substance abuser in a private meeting. They list the evidence by going around the group, one by one. For example:

> "You had slurred speech and didn't even respond when I told you I had to be hospitalized for surgery."
>
> "You have not made your daughter's dinner all week. And you forgot to pick her up from school."
>
> "You missed work for three days, and you have been late eight days in the past month."
>
> "You have alcohol on your breath (or needle marks on your arms)."
>
> "I found two bottles (a syringe and empty vial) hidden in the bathroom."

The family/friends/employer following the leader's cues, speak calmly and slowly with minimal emotion. They are presenting the facts, the objective evidence, to the alcoholic/drug abuser. Yelling, blaming, and haranguing are avoided because the alcoholic/drug abuser will inevitably respond by denying the behavior or making excuses. However, confrontation by several people who really care and who persistently present the facts breaks through the denial.

The next step in group intervention/confrontation requires the family/friends/employer to make clear and direct statements to the alcoholic/drug abuser about the consequences of their behavior:

> "Either you get help now or you will have to leave your job."
>
> "Either you enter a treatment program now or I will move out with the kids."

If the client agrees to treatment, the caring people agree to remain involved.

well. Always having a little fear is a good thing when it comes to maintaining abstinence. *More relapses occur when things are going well than when things are going badly.*

10. *Expecting too much from others.* "I've changed—why hasn't everybody else?" It's a plus if they do, but be prepared to deal with disappointment in your expectations of others. They may not trust you yet, may be looking for more evidence of your improved physical and mental health. You may be setting yourself up for a lot of frustration and other negative feelings if you expect others to change their lifestyle just because you have.
11. *Letting up on disciplines.* Continue with prayer, meditation, daily inventory, and twelve-step meeting attendance. This attitude may stem from complacency or from boredom. No chemically dependent person can afford to be bored with his or her recovery. The cost of relapse is too great.
12. *Use of mood-altering chemicals.* You may feel the need to ease things with a pill, and your doctor may agree with you. Perhaps you have had a problem only with alcohol or some other specific drug in the past. But you can easily lose hold of your recovery by starting to use mood changers. Different drugs may have unpredictable and treacherous reactions in chemically dependent people.
13. *Wanting too much.* Do not set goals you cannot reach with normal efforts.
14. *Forgetting gratitude.* You may be looking negatively on your life, concentrating on problems that still are not totally corrected. It is important to remember where you started from and how much better life is now.
15. *"It can't happen to me."* This kind of thinking is very dangerous. Almost anything can happen to you and is all the more likely to happen if you become careless with your recovery. Remember that you have a progressive disease and will be in even worse shape if you relapse.
16. *Omnipotence.* This is a feeling that results from a combination of many of the above attitudes. You may come to believe you have all the answers for yourself and for others. No one can tell you anything new. You may begin to ignore suggestions or advice from others. Relapse is probably imminent unless drastic change takes place.

Source: Anonymous

Educating Videotapes and talks by recovered substance abusers or experts in the effects of substance abuse are helpful. Education may take place in or out of the hospital, in one comprehensive session or several sessions over time. Nurse educators should focus on the types of abused substances and their physical, psychologic, and social effects. Families are often involved in these sessions because substance abuse is a family problem. The belief underlying such education is that knowledge and awareness may be useful in decreasing self-destructive behavior. But knowledge alone is never enough. Culturally sensitive and relevant educational resources should be used.

Referral and Self-Help Groups Support and self-help groups are extremely useful in helping clients feel better about themselves and acquire new attitudes and behaviors. Merely being with many people who are suffering in similar ways is beneficial. By observing people who have been sober or drug-free for long periods, clients can begin to learn similar behaviors. They can see that there is hope and that recovery is possible. Self-help groups also provide new friends, generally with healthy lifestyles. Clients may choose to attend support groups for the rest of their lives. Some clients who experiment with drugs or alcohol during one period of their lives and who succeed in stopping may attend only during the crisis.

Lifestyle Change An emphasis on the requirement for a total lifestyle change is necessary. Nurses can help clients discuss ways to alter their destructive habits by suggesting different coping strategies and by encouraging clients to discover new interests and capabilities within themselves. Nurses and clients can role-play new responses to old situations. Recognizing that relapse is always a threat, nurses may set up contracts with clients. For example, clients may agree to contact the nurse or an AA/NA sponsor if and when they feel the urge to drink or do drugs. This agreement represents new behaviors that are necessary for a lifestyle change.

Clients must realize that spending time with friends who are substance abusers or hanging out at places where

text continues on page 290

CASE STUDY

A Client with Chronic Alcoholism

Identifying Information

John Mills of 6950 Warden Road is a 54-year-old married civil servant. He is Catholic; has a high school education; and was referred from the Care Unit (a specialty hospital), where he has been for the last 30 days. His therapist's name is J. P. Allen, C.A.C.

Client's Description of the Problem

"I've had a drinking problem for 35 years. My wife and boss told me if I don't shape up, they'll kick me out of my home and my job. I want to feel better. It's been a living hell. But I'm not sure I can stop drinking. I've tried before." John describes drinking "to cope with my problems for most of my life." Wants to "stay dry." Fifteen years ago, John's social drinking escalated, and he began binge drinking on the weekends and later, drinking throughout the week. He drank daily for most of the last three years. He drank "enough to keep a buzz on" and occasionally enough "to pass out." John has long-term problems with work (showing up late, absenteeism, errors on the job). He also has long-term problems with his wife, who "either yells at me or takes care of me." John describes years of her pouring out his hidden liquor and her calling his boss to say John had the flu when he really was "hung over."

Psychiatric History

John has been in and out of AA groups and has seen three different psychiatrists. He has been hospitalized three times for car accidents and injuries due to drinking (a broken leg and ribs, contusions, and a concussion). After the last general hospital admission, he was admitted to the Care Unit for a 30-day alcohol treatment program.

Family History

Both of John's parents are deceased, and both were alcoholics. One female sibling, age 58, is a recovering alcoholic (has been "dry" for 10 years). The family has never been close. John feels he was never really "allowed to be a normal, active child." He reports that his sister cared for him when he was young and was "like my mother."

Social History

John developed normally but always "felt different." He worked every summer and took a full-time job after high school graduation. He enjoyed "drinking buddies" from work, but has never had a close friend he could depend on. John smokes one pack of cigarettes daily and uses no other drugs. He spends his leisure time watching TV and at bars with friends.

Health History

John has cirrhosis of the liver. He is malnourished from a history of chronic alcoholism, and has a long history of insomnia.

Current Mental Status

John is well-groomed, clean, and alert. His sensorium is within normal limits; affect is appropriate, yet apathetic. He appears depressed, and he expresses feelings of self-reproach and guilt for his years of drinking and their effect on others. He speaks slowly yet spontaneously. Motor behavior, thought content, and thought processes are within normal limits. Defenses are down in that he recognizes his alcoholism and expresses his fear of not being able to stop drinking. Insight is questionable. He recognizes his problem but is only beginning to be knowledgeable about alcoholism as a disease and about the stresses that cause him to drink.

Other Subjective or Objective Clinical Data

John is on multivitamins qd and Antabuse qd; no indication of suicide or violence potential.

Diagnostic Impression

Nursing Diagnoses

Altered Nutrition: Less than Body Requirements
Sleep Pattern Disturbance
Altered Thought Processes
Anxiety
Spiritual Distress
Social Isolation
Ineffective Family Coping: Disabling

DSM-IV Multiaxial Diagnosis

Axis I: 303.90 Alcohol Dependence
Axis II: No diagnosis
Axis III: Malnourished, chronic insomnia, alcoholic cirrhosis of liver
Axis IV: Occupational problems
Economic problems
Problems with primary support group
Axis V: GAF = 50 (current);
GAF = 50 (highest level in past year)

NURSING CARE PLAN

A Client with Chronic Alcoholism

Nursing Diagnosis

Altered Nutrition related to Alcohol' Abuse.

Expected Outcome

Client will eat three meals a day, plus snacks, and take vitamins as ordered.

Nursing Interventions

- Monitor intake of meals and snacks.
- Offer food/drink q 2 hr; initiate dietary consult to learn food preferences.
- During individual sessions, offer food and drink.
- In individual meetings and in orientation seminar, discuss the relationship between alcoholism and malnutrition; discuss resultant problems; discuss a well-balanced diet.

Outcome Met If

- Client gains 1 lb or more per week.
- Client discusses the relationship between alcoholism and malnutrition.
- Client discusses a well-balanced diet.

Nursing Diagnosis

Sleep Pattern Disturbances related to Alcohol Abuse.

Expected Outcome

Client will sleep a total of 6 hr a night.

Nursing Interventions

- Assess client's typical sleep pattern and what strategies aid sleep.
- If a client awakens after 2–3 hr of sleep, does reading or warm milk help client return to sleep? Once useful strategies are determined, have client put them into effect.

Outcome Met If

- Client sleeps 6 hr per night.
- Client uses sleep inducing strategies nightly.
- Client reports satisfaction with quality of sleep.

Nursing Diagnosis

Altered Thought Processes related to Alcohol Abuse.

Expected Outcome

- Client will not use alcohol.
- Client will attend individual counseling sessions and take Antabuse as ordered.
- Client will attend daily AA meetings.
- Client will call counselor or sponsor whenever he is anxious, fearful, depressed, or craving a drink.

Nursing Interventions

- Draw up a contract with client and have him agree to it and sign it. In the contract, client should agree to: attend AA meetings every night, see individual counselor from inpatient unit every week for the first month, and take Antabuse and return to physician as scheduled for refill.
- Discuss with client that ambivalent feelings are normal but to counteract them, he must call assigned counselor and/or sponsor from AA whenever he feels the urge to drink. Client may also write down feelings and experiences that increase the desire to drink.
- Plan with client other stress-reducing activities such as daily exercise, reading AA books, etc.
- Help condition client to call counselor and to execute strategies when feeling stressed.
- Teach client about the biochemical basis of alcoholism.

Outcome Met If

- Client remains alcohol- and drug-free.
- Client attends treatment program as contracted.
- Client takes Antabuse as prescribed.
- Client feels proud for each day of sobriety.
- Client repeats information learned about alcoholism as disease.

Nursing Diagnosis

Anxiety and Spiritual Distress related to Alcohol Abuse.

Expected Outcome

Client will discuss feelings at AA meeting and with counselor or sponsor.

Nursing Interventions

- Explain to client that all alcoholics experience these feelings and that they are worked on at AA meetings, where clients learn to surrender their problems to "a God of my understanding" and to confess their guilt and pray for help. They also learn to make amends to people after a rigorous moral inventory.
- Go over the twelve-step AA program with client; encourage client to participate in AA and to read AA books. Help client obtain copies of books.
- Each week, ask client if and how

NURSING CARE PLAN *(continued)*

guilt and self-reproach have changed.

Outcome Met If

- Client works the twelve-step program of AA.
- Guilt and self-reproach decrease over time.
- Client takes moral inventory and makes amends to selected people.

Nursing Diagnosis

Social Isolation related to Alcohol Abuse.

Expected Outcome

- Client will go to work where he will eat lunch with one or more people.
- Client will call a friend or acquaintance who does not drink at least once a week.

Nursing Interventions

- Discuss with client that it is important to stay away from people, places, and things that are associated with drinking: New friends can come from AA, and alcohol should not be available at new activities.
- Make it clear to the client that he must develop an entirely new lifestyle and that this will be difficult and take time. Encourage client to attend AA activities and educational programs.

Outcome Met If

- Client makes new friends who are in the AA program.
- Client feels better about socializing with people at work.
- Client begins to attend and enjoy social events with nondrinkers.

Nursing Diagnosis

Ineffective Family Coping related to Alcohol Abuse.

Expected Outcome

Understand alcoholism as a family disease.

Nursing Interventions

- Refer to family therapist or, if educationally prepared, work with alcoholic and wife and educate them about the typical alcoholic game (victim, rescuer/persecutor).
- Help client and wife see what games they have played and how these games serve only to perpetuate a dysfunctional family system.
- Teach client new coping strategies such as honesty about self and disease. Help client learn to accept that life is difficult and painful and there is no "quick fix."

Outcome Met If

- Wife attends Al-Anon.
- Client attends family therapy if prescribed.
- Client correctly recalls information about alcoholism as a family disease.
- Client begins to change coping mechanism (avoids role of victim, decreases conning and manipulating behaviors).
- Client accepts responsibility for self.

they used to take drugs or alcohol is not helpful. The mere sight or smell of paraphernalia or the desired substance is often enough to trigger a relapse. Old ties must be broken; new friends and activities must be pursued.

Nursing Care Plans The accompanying case studies and nursing care plans focus on cocaine and alcohol because they are such commonly abused drugs. Short- and long-term interventions are quite different, as the nursing care plans show. Nursing interventions with other types of substance abuse have differences and similarities. Differences in intervention tend to be medical (clonidine for opiates; haloperidol for PCP) and symptomatic (if a client hallucinates, decrease stimulation and point out reality). Similarities in intervention include confrontation strategies, therapeutic strategies, education, long-term self-help groups, and emphasis on a total lifestyle change.

Helping the Family Substance abuse affects not only the client but also the entire family system. Family members often engage in behaviors that enable clients to continue with their substance abuse by protecting them from the consequences of their substance abuse. Helping family members includes clarifying the problem and presenting possible solutions (treatment) and creating a support system for family members. Referring family members to Al-Anon can be a very helpful strategy.

In dysfunctional families, the substance abuser often becomes the "identified patient," focusing attention on that individual and away from the other problems in the family. Treatment for the substance abuser may require

CRITICAL PATHWAY FOR A CLIENT EXPERIENCING ALCOHOL WITHDRAWAL

Expected length of treatment 6 days

	Date ________ **Day 1**	**Date ________** **Day 2**	**Date ________** **Day 3**
Daily outcomes	Client will: • Have stable vital signs. • Remain oriented to time, place, and person. • Withdraw from alcohol without injury. • Consume 1500 cal and 2000 cc of fluid each day. • Verbalize thoughts and feelings. • Verbalize commitment to detox program. • Maintain a stable weight. • Demonstrate ability to cope.	Client will: • Have stable vital signs. • Remain oriented to time, place, and person. • Withdraw from alcohol without injury. • Consume 2000 cal and 3000 cc of fluid each day. • Verbalize thoughts and feelings. • Verbalize commitment to detox program. • Maintain a stable weight. • Demonstrate alternate coping mechanisms. • Attend AA daily. • Identify strategies to promote sleep/rest.	Client will: • Be afebrile with stable vital signs. • Remain oriented to time, place, and person. • Withdraw from alcohol without injury. • Remain free of signs and symptoms of delirium tremens. • Consume 2000 cal and 3000 cc of fluid each day. • Verbalize thoughts and feelings. • Begin to verbalize alcohol's negative effects on significant others and lifestyle. • Verbalize commitment to detox program. • Attend AA daily. • Maintain a stable weight. • Identify strategies to promote sleep/rest. • Demonstrate alternate coping mechanisms.
Assessments, tests, and treatments	Vital signs q 4 hr if stable. Intake and output. Blood alcohol level. CBC and urinalysis. Chemistry profile, electrolytes. Serum magnesium. Chest X ray. EKG. PPD. Assess need for HIV testing. Weigh. Assess q 1–2 hr for signs and symptoms of withdrawal, including anxiety, agitation, irritability, tremor, tachycardia, hypertension, diaphoresis, and hallucinations. Assess drinking history and patterns. Establish the date and time of last drink.	Vital signs q 4 hr if stable. Intake and output. Assess q 1–2 hr for signs and symptoms of withdrawal, including anxiety, agitation, irritability, tremor, tachycardia, hypertension, diaphoresis, and hallucinations.	Vital signs q shift and PRN. D/C intake and output if stable. Assess q 1–2 hr for signs and symptoms of withdrawal, including anxiety, agitation, irritability, tremor, tachycardia, hypertension, diaphoresis, and hallucinations. Monitor for delirium tremens. Read PPD. Repeat laboratory studies as indicated.
Knowledge deficit	Orient client and family to room and routine. Include family in teaching. Review plan of care. Assess understanding of teaching.	Review plan of care with client and family. Include family in teaching. Assess understanding of teaching.	Review plan of care with client and family. Include family in teaching. Initiate discharge teaching regarding the need for ongoing outpatient therapy and attending a self-help group. Assess understanding of teaching.

→

CRITICAL PATHWAY FOR A CLIENT EXPERIENCING ALCOHOL WITHDRAWAL *(continued)*

	Date ________ Day 1 *continued*	Date ________ Day 2 *continued*	Date ________ Day 3 *continued*
Diet	Encourage up to 3000 cc of fluids each day (unless contraindicated). Limit caffeine intake. Provide frequent, small, nutritious feedings, inclusive of all food groups. Nutrition assessment.	Encourage up to 3000 cc of fluids each day (unless contraindicated). Limit caffeine. Dietary consult. Provide frequent, small, nutritious feedings, inclusive of all food groups.	Encourage up to 3000 cc of fluids each day (unless contraindicated). Limit caffeine. Provide frequent, small, nutritious feedings, inclusive of all food groups.
Activity	Assess safety needs and maintain appropriate precautions. Activity as tolerated. Assist with hygiene.	Maintain safety precautions. Activity as tolerated. Prompt and assist with hygiene as needed.	Maintain safety precautions. Self-care/shower.
Psychosocial	Assess level of anxiety. Provide information and ongoing support and encouragement to client and family. Assess sleep patterns and provide measures that promote rest and sleep. Encourage expression of thoughts and feelings. Approach in nonjudgmental manner. Explore availability of support system. Encourage regular aerobic exercise. Explore interests and potential hobbies. Explore attending an AA meeting. Use gentle confrontation strategies. Provide education and set limits. Explore lifestyle changes.	Assess level of anxiety. Encourage verbalization of concerns. Provide information and ongoing support and encouragement to client and family. Provide measures that promote rest and sleep. Encourage expression of thoughts and feelings. Approach in nonjudgmental manner. Explore availability of support system. Choose and begin regular aerobic exercise. Explore interests and potential hobbies. Attend an AA meeting. Use gentle confrontation strategies. Provide education and set limits. Explore lifestyle changes.	Assess level of anxiety. Encourage verbalization of concerns. Provide information and ongoing support and encouragement to client and family. Provide measures that promote rest and sleep. Encourage expression of thoughts and feelings. Approach in nonjudgmental manner. Explore availability of support system. Choose and begin regular aerobic exercise. Explore interests and potential hobbies. Attend an AA meeting. Use gentle confrontation strategies. Provide education and set limits. Explore lifestyle changes.
Medications	Thiamine 100 mg IM or PO. Routine meds as ordered. Librium as ordered.	Thiamine 100 mg PO. Folic acid 1 mg PO. Multivitamin PO. Routine meds as ordered. Librium as ordered.	Thiamine 100 mg PO. Folic acid 1 mg PO. Multivitamin PO. Routine meds as ordered. Librium as ordered.
Consults and discharge plan	Family assessment if not previously completed. Consult with internist. Refer to neurologist if indicated. Discuss self-help groups. Establish discharge objectives with client and family.	Review discharge objectives and anticipated discharge care with client and significant others. Refer to self-help groups. Refer the family to self-help groups. Complete discharge planning.	Review progress toward discharge objectives with client and significant others. Make appropriate referrals.

	Date ________ Day 4	Date ________ Day 5	Date ________ Day 6–Discharge
Daily outcomes	Client will: • Be afebrile, have stable vital signs. • Remain oriented to time, place, and person. • Withdraw from alcohol without injury. • Remain free of signs and symptoms of delirium tremens. • Consume 2000 cal and 3000 cc of fluid each day. • Verbalize thoughts and feelings. • Verbalize alcohol's negative effects on lifestyle. • Verbalize commitment to detox program. • Attend AA daily. • Maintain a stable weight. • Establish sleep/rest routine to promote sleep. • Demonstrate alternate coping strategies.	Client will: • Be afebrile, have stable vital signs. • Remain oriented to time, place, and person. • Withdraw from alcohol without injury. • Remain free of signs and symptoms of delirium tremens. • Consume 2000 cal and 3000 cc of fluid each day. • Verbalize thoughts and feelings. • Verbalize alcohol's negative effects on lifestyle. • Verbalize commitment to detox program. • Attend AA daily. • Maintain a stable weight. • Establish sleep/rest routine to promote sleep. • Demonstrate alternate coping strategies.	Client is afebrile and has stable vital signs. Client is alert and oriented. Client has withdrawn from alcohol safely and without injury. Client maintains adequate nutrition and fluid intake. Client's weight remains stable. Client verbalizes understanding of hazards of alcohol. Client is independent in self-care. Client verbalizes times and places for AA meetings. Client verbalizes commitment to detox program and regular attendance at AA meetings. Client verbalizes home care instructions including the importance of ongoing counseling. Client has established a sleep/rest pattern and verbalizes understanding of sleep-promoting measures. Client demonstrates ability to cope with ongoing stressors.
Assessments, tests, and treatments	Vital signs BID if stable. Assess for signs and symptoms of withdrawal, including anxiety, agitation, irritability, tremor, tachycardia, hypertension, diaphoresis, and hallucinations. Monitor for delirium tremens.	Vital signs BID if stable. Assess for signs and symptoms of withdrawal, including anxiety, agitation, irritability, tremor, tachycardia, hypertension, diaphoresis, and hallucinations. Monitor for delirium tremens.	Vital signs BID if stable. Assess for signs and symptoms of withdrawal, including anxiety, agitation, irritability, tremor, tachycardia, hypertension, diaphoresis, and hallucinations. Monitor for delirium tremens.
Knowledge deficit	Review plan of care. Include family in teaching. Continue discharge teaching regarding detox program and need for ongoing counseling. Assess understanding of teaching.	Review plan of care with client and family. Continue discharge teaching regarding detox program and need for ongoing counseling. Assess understanding of teaching.	Client and/or significant other verbalizes understanding of discharge teaching including wound care, exercise program, strategies to prevent relapse, diet, signs and symptoms to report, follow-up care and MD appointment, medications: name, purpose, dose, frequency, route, dietary interactions, and side effects, and home care arrangements. Assess understanding of teaching.
Diet	Encourage up to 3000 cc of fluids each day (unless contraindicated). Provide frequent, small, nutritious feedings, inclusive of all food groups.	Encourage up to 3000 cc of fluids each day (unless contraindicated). Provide frequent, small, nutritious feedings, inclusive of all food groups.	Encourage up to 3000 cc of fluids each day (unless contraindicated). Provide frequent, small, nutritious feedings, inclusive of all food groups.

→

CRITICAL PATHWAY FOR A CLIENT EXPERIENCING ALCOHOL WITHDRAWAL (continued)

	Date _________ **Day 4 *continued***	**Date _________** **Day 5 *continued***	**Date _________** **Day 6–Discharge *continued***
Activity	Maintain safety precautions. Self-care/shower.	Maintain safety precautions. Self-care/shower.	Maintain safety precautions. Self-care/shower.
Psychosocial	Assess level of anxiety. Encourage verbalization of concerns. Provide information and ongoing support and encouragement to client and family. Provide measures that promote rest and sleep. Encourage expression of thoughts and feelings. Approach in nonjudgmental manner. Explore availability of support system. Continue regular aerobic exercise. Explore interests and potential hobbies. Attend an AA meeting. Use gentle confrontation strategies. Provide education and set limits. Explore lifestyle changes. Encourage verbalization of concerns. Provide ongoing support and encouragement to client and family.	Assess level of anxiety. Encourage verbalization of concerns. Provide information and ongoing support and encouragement to client and family. Provide measures that promote rest and sleep. Encourage expression of thoughts and feelings. Approach in nonjudgmental manner. Explore availability of support system. Continue regular aerobic exercise. Explore interests and potential hobbies. Attend an AA meeting. Use gentle confrontation strategies. Provide education and set limits. Explore lifestyle changes. Encourage verbalization of concerns. Provide ongoing support and encouragement to client and family.	Assess level of anxiety. Encourage verbalization of concerns. Provide information and ongoing support and encouragement to client and family. Provide measures that promote rest and sleep. Encourage expression of thoughts and feelings. Approach in nonjudgmental manner. Explore availability of support system. Continue regular aerobic exercise. Explore interests and potential hobbies. Attend an AA meeting. Use gentle confrontation strategies. Provide education and set limits. Explore lifestyle changes. Encourage verbalization of concerns. Provide ongoing support and encouragement to client and family.
Medications	Thiamine 100 mg PO. Folic acid 1 mg PO. Multivitamin PO. Routine meds as ordered. Librium as ordered. Routine meds as ordered.	Thiamine 100 mg PO. Folic acid 1 mg PO. Multivitamin PO. Routine meds as ordered. Librium as ordered. Routine meds as ordered.	Thiamine 100 mg PO. Folic acid 1 mg PO. Multivitamin PO. Routine meds as ordered. Librium as ordered. Routine meds as ordered.
Transfer/ discharge plan	Review with client and significant others discharge objectives regarding activity and home care.	Review with client and significant others discharge objectives regarding activity and home care. Complete referrals for home care.	Discharge with referrals for home health care.

including some type of family therapy. Family members may need treatment for codependence through group or individual therapy or involvement in a twelve-step program such as Al-Anon or Codependents Anonymous (CODA). The Adult Children of Alcoholics (ACOA) support groups are also helpful.

Evaluation and Outcome Criteria

Outcome criteria for substance abusers include sobriety (abstinence from drugs and alcohol, "being clean"); risk reduction; improvement of work, family, and social relationships; and lifestyle changes that may include a growing sense of spirituality. Clients become more effective in using new attitudes and behaviors. Better feelings about themselves result. Although the fear of relapse is always present, over time the craving for chemicals diminishes, and the client establishes a new, healthy lifestyle. Chychula (1984) lists ten client outcome criteria that continue to be useful in evaluating the recovery process:

1. Is the client beginning to take responsibility for his or her own actions?
2. Is the abuse pattern decreasing without a dependence on other substances?
3. Is there any indication of increased job stability?
4. Is there improvement in interpersonal relationships with others?
5. Are problem-solving techniques improving?
6. Is the client setting goals and following through?
7. Is the client less impulsive and compulsive?
8. Is the client able to delay gratification?
9. Are stress and anxiety decreasing without the use of chemicals?
10. Is there evidence of increased assertiveness?

These two additional questions are useful:

11. Is the client using community support systems?
12. Is the client engaging in social activities with people who are not substance abusers?

Improvement in these areas is a good indication that the client is well on the road to recovery. The Critical Pathway in this chapter outlines short-term steps to achieve this outcome.

Chapter Highlights

- Drug and alcohol abuse are serious problems in most developed countries.
- Contemporary explanations of substance abuse derive from biologic, psychologic, sociocultural, and family systems theories.
- Groups at risk for substance abuse include teenagers, psychiatric clients, women, general hospital clients, the elderly, adult children of alcoholics, and nurses.
- Substance abusers suffer from intoxication and physical and psychologic withdrawal effects.
- To arrive at an accurate nursing diagnosis and design effective nursing interventions, the nurse must make a comprehensive assessment of the substance abuser, focusing on types and amount of substances used and frequency of use.
- Nursing diagnoses for substance-abusing clients are diverse and wide-ranging.
- After the client is detoxified, effective nursing intervention strategies include education, support groups, writing a contract, and ultimately supporting a change in lifestyle.
- Evaluation and outcome criteria include substance abstinence or risk reduction; improvement in the areas of work, family, and social relationships; increased ability to solve problems and delay gratification; abstinence from all chemicals; increased feeling of well-being; the use of community services; and an enhanced sense of spirituality.

References

American Psychiatric Association: *Diagnostic and Statistical Manual of Mental Disorders,* ed 4. APA, 1994.

Becker H: *The Outsiders.* Free Press, 1963.

Bittle S, Feiginbaum J, Kneisl CR: Substance abuse, in Kneisl CR, Ames SA: *Adult Health Nursing: A Biopsychosocial Approach,* Addison-Wesley, 1986.

Brownell K, Marlatt G, Lichtenstein E, Wilson G: Understanding and preventing relapse. *Am Psychol* 1986; 41:765–782.

Chychula N: Screening for substance abuse in a primary-care setting. *Nurse Pract* 1984; 9:15–24.

DeVane C: *Fundamentals of Monitoring Psychoactive Drug Therapy.* Williams & Wilkins, 1990.

Endicott P, Watson B: Interventions to improve the AMA discharge rate for opiate addicted patients, *J Psychosoc Nurs* 1994;32(8):36–40.

Espeland K: Inhalant abuse: Assessment guidelines. *J Psychosoc Nurs* 1993;31(3):11–14.

Franks L: A new attack on alcoholism. *The New York Times Magazine* 1985;November:47–69.

Gallagher W: Pandora's pharmacy. *This World.* August 31, 1986;7–9.

Guy D: Co-Dependence. *Vim & Vigor* 1990;4(June):22–26.

Hall JM: Lesbians recovering from alcohol problems: An ethnographic study of health care experiences. *Nurs Res* July/August 1994;43(4):238–244.

Hall S, Wray L: Codependency: Nurses who give too much. *Am J Nurs* 1989;89:1456–1460.

Hitre A, et al.: Fewer dopamine transporter receptors in the prefrontal cortex of cocaine users. *Am J Psychiatr* 1994; 151:(7):1074–1076.

Hutchinson S: Chemically dependent nurses: The trajectory towards self-annihilation. *Nurs Res* 1986;35:196–201.

Increasing use of cocaine correlates with increased problems among users. *Drug Abuse Update* 1989;29(June):12–13.

Jellinek E: *Phases in the Drinking History of Alcoholics*. Hillhouse Press, 1946.

Kearney MH, et al.: Learning by losing: Sex and fertility on crack cocaine. *Qualitative Health Res* 1994;4(2):142–162.

Kirk E, Bradford L: Effects of alcohol on the central nervous system. *J Neurosci Nurs* 1987;19:326–335.

Kitchens JM: Does this patient have an alcohol problem? *JAMA* 1994;272(22):1782–1787.

Kneisl CR, Ames SA: *Adult Health Nursing*. Addison-Wesley, 1986.

Landry M, Smith DE: Crack: Anatomy of an addiction. *California Nurs Rev* 1987 (March/April):8–36.

Lieber C, DeCarli L: Hepatic microsomal ethanol oxidizing system. In vitro characteristics and adaptive properties in vivo. *J Biol Chem* 1970;245:2505–2512.

Lindesmith A: *Opiate Addiction:* University of Indiana Press, 1965.

Lynette J (ed): *The Core Curriculum of Addictions Nursing*. National Nurses Society on Addictions, 1990.

Mann G: *The Dynamics of Addiction*. Johnson Institute, 1983.

Meissner JE: Caring for patients with cirrhosis. *Nurs 94* September 1994:44–45.

Mello NK, et al.: Buprenopheno treatment of opiate and cocaine abuse: Clinical and preclinical studies. *Harvard Rev Psychiatry* 1993;1(3):168–182.

Meyer RE: What for, alcohol research? *Am J Psychiatr* 1994; 151(2):165–168.

Naegle MA: Creative management of impaired nursing practice. *Nurs Adm Q* 1985;9:16–26.

Naegle MA: Theoretical perspectives on the etiology of substance abuse. *Holistic Nurs Prac* 1988;2(4):1–13.

Newton M: *Gone Way Down*. American Studies Press, 1981.

Schuckit MA: Genetics and the risk for alcoholism. *JAMA* 1985;254:2614–2617.

Schuckit MA: Populations generally at high risk for developing alcohol abuse or dependence. *Current Opinion in Psychiatry* 1990;2:375–379.

Schuckit MA, et al.: Personality test scores as predictors of alcoholism almost a decade later. *British J Psychiatr* 1994; 165:515–523.

Shaw GK, et al.: Tiaprede in the prevention of relapse in recently detoxified alcoholics. *British J Psychiatr* 1994; 165:515–523.

Solari-Twadell P: *The Multiple Roles of a Nurse in a Comprehensive Level of Care System for Alcoholic Patients*. Gateway Community Services, 1983.

Stanton M, Todd T: *Family Therapy of Drug Abuse and Addiction*. Guilford Press, 1982.

Strain EC, et al.: Comparison of Buprenorphine and Methadone in the treatment of opioid dependence. *Am J Psychiatr* 1994;151(7):1025–1030.

CHAPTER 14

CLIENTS WITH SCHIZOPHRENIA AND OTHER PSYCHOTIC DISORDERS

Catherine A. Chesla

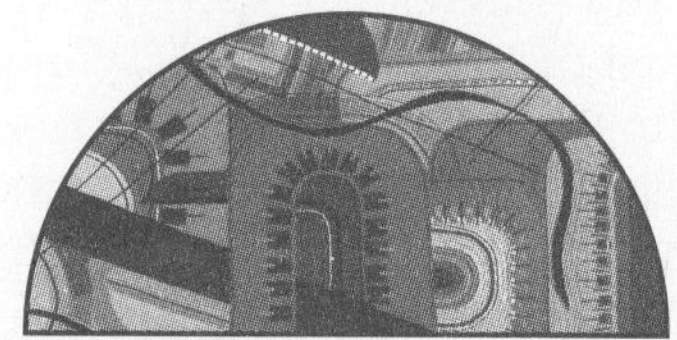

COMPETENCIES

- *Define the central features of schizophrenia.*
- *Recognize the DSM-IV diagnostic criteria for schizophrenia.*
- *Describe the neurologic dysfunctions of which at least two must be present for a diagnosis of schizophrenia.*
- *Identify psychologic and social pressures that influence the course of schizophrenia.*
- *Identify personal challenges in working with clients who have impaired relational capacities.*

Cross-References

Other topics relevant to this content are: Psychopharmacology, Chapter 33; Persistently mentally ill, Chapter 21; Therapeutic communication, Chapter 7; Community mental health, Chapter 35; Family, Chapter 32; Psychobiology, Chapter 3.

Critical Thinking Challenge

Individuals with schizophrenia are exquisitely sensitive to their environment. When stressed, they often run the risk of developing symptoms of further illness. Why do mental health care providers advocate that people with schizophrenia interact with the larger community, via treatment programs, jobs, and living in the community? Wouldn't they be better off in protected environments, like semistructured group homes?

People with schizophrenia are often feared and misunderstood, both by the general public and by health care professionals. Fear is generated by inaccurate and sensationalized depictions of schizophrenia sufferers as violent, aggressive, and evil. Misunderstandings arise because schizophrenia is confused with a rare yet dramatic dissociative disorder formerly called multiple personality disorder, which has been presented in stories like *Sybil* and *The Three Faces of Eve* in the popular media. People with schizophrenia may be further misunderstood because the symptoms of the disorder, while varied, generally set them apart from the general public. Their physical presentation, emotional responses to situations, unusual or bizarre thoughts, or altered capacity to relate with others may cause even health care professionals to distance themselves and fail to try to understand the person's experience and difficulties.

Individuals with schizophrenia are *people* who suffer from a complex, multifaceted, biologically based, environmentally sensitive disease that affects all areas of their life and functioning. Psychiatric nurses who work with schizophrenic clients are doubly challenged. The first challenge is to learn the spectrum of problems and combinations of problems that comprise the broad diagnostic category, schizophrenia. The second challenge is to understand and work with the broad variation in human responses to living with this difficult, chronic illness.

Schizophrenia

Schizophrenia is a complex disorder with an extremely varied presentation of cognitive and emotional and behavioral symptoms. Approximately 1% of the general population will have schizophrenia during their lifetime. The illness is diagnosed most frequently in the early twenties for men and late twenties for women. The progression of the disease is quite variable. In some cases, the disease progresses through exacerbations and remissions; in other cases, it takes a chronic, stable course; while in still others, a chronic, progressively deteriorating course evolves.

The diagnosis of schizophrenia requires not only the presence of distinct symptoms but the persistence of those symptoms over time. Symptoms must be present for at least 6 months, and active-phase symptoms (what are called Type A symptoms in the *DSM-IV*) must be present for at least 1 month during that time, before schizophrenia can be diagnosed. The diagnostic criteria for schizophrenia are presented in the accompanying box.

The symptoms of schizophrenia are conceptually separated into **positive symptoms,** which represent an excess or distortion of normal functioning, and **negative symptoms,** which represent a deficit in functioning. Positive symptoms include the two most pronounced outward signs of the disorder: hallucinations and delusions. Additional positive symptoms include disorganized speech and disturbances in behavior of two types: disorganized or catatonic behavior (American Psychiatric Association 1994).

Hallucinations are the most extreme and yet the most common perceptual disturbance in schizophrenia. A **hallucination** is a subjective perception of something that does not exist in the external environment. Hallucinations may be visual, olfactory (smell), gustatory (taste), tactile (touch), or auditory. The most common form of hallucination in schizophrenia is hearing voices that are distinct from the person's own thoughts. The voices may be friendly or hostile and threatening. Particularly significant symptoms are hearing two or more voices conversing with each other, or hearing a voice that provides continuous comments on the train of thought; reports of either of these symptoms have particular diagnostic significance.

Delusions are mistaken or false beliefs about the self or the environment that are firmly held even in the face of disconfirming evidence. Delusions may take many forms. In delusions of persecution, the person may think that others are following him, spying on him, or trying to torment him. In another common form, delusions of reference, the person thinks that public expressions, like a story on the radio or a newspaper article, are specifically addressed to him or her.

Other positive symptoms represent "excesses" of language or behavior. Disorganized speech is the outward sign of disordered thoughts and may range from less severe forms, where the person moves rapidly from one topic to another, to more severe forms, where the person's speech cannot be logically understood. Positive behavioral symptoms include disorganized behavior, which may present as agitated, nonpurposeful, or random movements, and as catatonia, in which there is a low level of behavioral response to the environment.

Negative symptoms of schizophrenia are less dramatic but just as debilitating as positive symptoms of the disorder. Negative symptoms include the "four As" of schizophrenia:

- Flattened affect
- Alogia
- Avolition
- Anhedonia

People with schizophrenia often appear to have nonemotional or restricted emotional responses to their experiences. **Flattened affect** describes this restricted range of facial and bodily expression of emotion, as well as poor eye contact. Brief, empty verbal responses are known as **alogia.** This poverty of speech is thought to be symptomatic of diminished thoughts and is different from a refusal to speak. A symptom that is frequently misunderstood by families and members of the larger community is **avolition,** an inability to pursue and persist in goal-directed activities. The schizophrenic person's experience of avolition is often misinterpreted as laziness or an unwillingness to support himself or herself, rather than as a symptom of this chronic disorder. **Anhedonia,** the inability to experience pleasure, does not define schizophrenia, but it is an important symptom that challenges many nurses. It is difficult to imagine, and painful to empathize with, someone who can't seem to enjoy even small aspects of life.

Negative symptoms of schizophrenia are difficult to assess because they differ in degree but not in form from everyday experience. While few of us have experienced true hallucinations, many know what it is like to have a day without energy to pursue goal-directed activities. Another difficulty in recognizing negative symptoms is that people with schizophrenia often live in difficult situations that may lead to restricted emotional expression and disturbed goal-directed activities. Living in poverty, or in unsettled circumstances like homelessness, can in-

DSM-IV Diagnostic Criteria for Schizophrenia

A. *Characteristic symptoms:* Two (or more) of the following, each present for a significant portion of time during a 1-month period (or less if successfully treated):
   1. delusions
   2. hallucinations
   3. disorganized speech (e.g., frequent derailment or incoherence)
   4. grossly disorganized or catatonic behavior
   5. negative symptoms, i.e., affective flattening, alogia, or avolition

   Note: Only one Criterion A symptom is required if delusions are bizarre or hallucinations consist of a voice keeping up a running commentary on the person's behavior or thoughts, or two or more voices conversing with each other.

B. *Social/occupational dysfunction:* For a significant portion of the time since the onset of the disturbance, one or more major areas of functioning such as work, interpersonal relations, or self-care are markedly below the level achieved prior to the onset (or when the onset is in childhood or adolescence, failure to achieve expected level of interpersonal, academic, or occupational achievement).

C. *Duration:* Continuous signs of the disturbance persist for at least 6 months. This 6-month period must include at least 1 month of symptoms (or less if successfully treated) that meet Criterion A (i.e., active-phase symptoms) and may include periods of prodromal or residual symptoms. During these prodromal or residual periods, the signs of the disturbance may be manifested by only negative symptoms or two or more symptoms listed in Criterion A present in an attenuated form (e.g., odd beliefs, unusual perceptual experiences).

D. *Schizoaffective and Mood Disorder exclusion:* Schizoaffective Disorder and Mood Disorder With Psychotic Features have been ruled out because either (1) no Major Depressive, Manic, or Mixed Episodes have occurred concurrently with the active-phase symptoms; or (2) if mood episodes have occurred during active-phase symptoms, their total duration has been brief relative to the duration of the active and residual periods.

E. *Substance/general medical condition exclusion:* The disturbance is not due to the direct physiological effects of a substance (e.g., a drug of abuse, a medication) or a general medical condition.

F. *Relationship to a Pervasive Developmental Disorder:* If there is a history of Autistic Disorder or another Pervasive Developmental Disorder, the additional diagnosis of Schizophrenia is made only if prominent delusions or hallucinations are also present for at least a month (or less if successfully treated).

Source: American Psychiatric Association 1994, pp. 285–286.

duce feelings of desperation or despair, which may mimic the negative symptoms of schizophrenia. It is important to try to separate environmental influences on experience from the disease process, and to note the persistence of the symptoms over time, across a variety of circumstances.

Another important criterion for recognizing schizophrenia is an impaired ability to perform and complete social and work obligations. It is diagnostic of schizophrenia that the person has difficulty performing in one or more areas of life including work, school, social relationships, and the maintenance of everyday activities such as dressing and providing food for oneself.

Subtypes of schizophrenia are used to designate which symptoms are prominent and should be included along with the diagnosis. The subtype should indicate symptoms that were prominent in the last reevaluation of the client, and that may change over time. For more information, see the box on the following page.

Paranoid Type

Prominent hallucinations and delusions are present in the **paranoid type** of schizophrenia. Delusions are often persecutory or grandiose, and they often connect into a somewhat organized story. Delusions may also be varied and include, for example, somatic or religious delusions. Hallucinations often link with the delusion, although this is not necessary. For example, a person who believes he is being monitored by the FBI may hear the voices of people

DSM-IV Diagnostic Criteria for Schizophrenia Subtypes

295.10 Disorganized Type

A type of Schizophrenia in which the following criteria are met:

A. All of the following are prominent:
   1. disorganized speech
   2. disorganized behavior
   3. flat or inappropriate affect

B. The criteria are not met for Catatonic Type.

295.20 Catatonic Type

A type of Schizophrenia in which the clinical picture is dominated by at least two of the following:

1. motoric immobility as evidenced by catalepsy (including waxy flexibility) or stupor
2. excessive motor activity (that is apparently purposeless and not influenced by external stimuli)
3. extreme negativism (an apparently motiveless resistance to all instructions or maintenance of a rigid posture against attempts to be moved) or mutism
4. peculiarities of voluntary movement as evidenced by posturing (voluntary assumption of inappropriate or bizarre postures), stereotyped movements, prominent mannerisms, or prominent grimacing
5. echolalia or echopraxia

295.30 Paranoid Type

A type of Schizophrenia in which the following criteria are met:

A. Preoccupation with one or more delusions or frequent auditory hallucinations.

B. None of the following is prominent: disorganized speech, disorganized or catatonic behavior, or flat or inappropriate affect.

295.90 Undifferentiated Type

A type of Schizophrenia in which symptoms that meet Criterion A are present, but the criteria are not met for the Paranoid, Disorganized, or Catatonic Type.

295.60 Residual Type

A type of Schizophrenia in which the following criteria are met:

A. Absence of prominent delusions, hallucinations, disorganized speech, and grossly disorganized or catatonic behavior.

B. There is continuing evidence of the disturbance, as indicated by the presence of negative symptoms or two or more symptoms listed in Criterion A for Schizophrenia, present in an attenuated form (e.g., odd beliefs, unusual perceptual experiences).

Source: American Psychiatric Association 1994, pp. 286–290.

he identifies as FBI agents laughing at him or talking with him when he goes out.

Disorganized Type

The central features present in the **disorganized type** of schizophrenia are disorganized speech and behavior, and flat or inappropriate affect. The client appears disorganized and unkempt because basic everyday tasks like dressing oneself cannot be accomplished. Emotional expression may be either inappropriate to the content of what the client is saying (such as laughing when discussing being kicked out of the house) or restricted and flat. To acquire this designation, the client should not display the signs of catatonic type, and hallucinations and delusions are typically more fragmentary and disorganized than in the paranoid type.

Catatonic Type

Although seen infrequently in the United States, the **catatonic type** of schizophrenia is characterized by extreme psychomotor disruption. The client may display substantially reduced movement accompanied by negativism and resistance to any intervention. Alternatively, extremely active and purposeless movement that is not influenced by what is going on around the person may be present. Additional signs of catatonic type are when a client repeats what others say or mimics their movements.

Undifferentiated Type

When a client presents in an active psychotic state, meaning that Type A criteria for schizophrenia are met, yet does not have prominent symptoms that match any of the prior subtypes, then **undifferentiated type** should be diagnosed.

Residual Type

Residual type of schizophrenia is reserved for a client who has had at least one documented episode of schizophrenia and who presents without prominent positive symptoms of the illness. Negative symptoms like flat affect and inability to work are present, but prominent hallucinations, delusions, and disorganized thoughts and behavior are not.

Besides variation in type, schizophrenia also varies in how it progresses over time. Along with a diagnosis of schizophrenia, illness course should be specified. The DSM-IV criteria for the various illness courses are described in the accompanying box.

DSM-IV Criteria for Specifying the Course of Schizophrenia

Episodic With Interepisode Residual Symptoms. Applies when the course is characterized by episodes in which Criterion A for Schizophrenia is met and there are clinically significant residual symptoms between the episodes. **With Prominent Negative Symptoms** can be added if prominent negative symptoms are present during residual periods.

Episodic With No Interepisode Residual Symptoms. Applies when the course is characterized by episodes in which Criterion A for Schizophrenia is met and there are no clinically significant residual symptoms between the episodes.

Continuous. Applies when characteristic symptoms of Criterion A are met throughout all (or most) of the course. **With Prominent Negative Symptoms** can be added if prominent negative symptoms are also present.

Single Episode in Partial Remission. Applies when there has been a single episode in which Criterion A for Schizophrenia is met and some clinically significant residual symptoms remain. **With Prominent Negative Symptoms** can be added if these residual symptoms include prominent negative symptoms.

Single Episode In Full Remission. Applies when there has been a single episode in which Criterion A for Schizophrenia has been met and no clinically significant residual symptoms remain.

Other or Unspecified Pattern. Used if another or an unspecified course pattern has been present.

Source: American Psychiatric Association 1994, pp. 278–279.

Other Psychotic Disorders

Schizophreniform Disorder

Schizophreniform disorder is very similar to schizophrenia except that the person has not been ill for very long. The diagnostic criteria for other psychotic disorders are the same as the Type A criteria for schizophrenia. The main difference is that the client has experienced the symptoms for at least 1 month and either recovered from the symptoms before 6 months, or 6 months have not yet elapsed since the original symptoms began. A second difference, besides duration, is that the client may show no impairment in social and work functioning. Some think that schizophreniform disorder may be prodromal to schizophrenia, yet approximately one-third of clients diagnosed with this disorder recover. The other two-thirds go on to have either schizophrenia or schizoaffective disorder.

Schizoaffective Disorder

In **schizoaffective disorder,** two sets of symptoms are present concurrently in the same illness episode, not just at some time in a client's life: Type A symptoms in schizophrenia, and symptoms of a mood disorder (either a major depressive or manic disorder). The specific symptoms signified in this disorder, and their required durations, are outlined in the *DSM-IV.* Schizoaffective disorder is less common than, and has a slightly better prognosis than, schizophrenia, but it has a worse prognosis than mood disorders. Subtypes of this disorder should also be specified, and the *DSM-IV* should be consulted for details about subtypes of all psychotic disorders.

Delusional Disorder

Delusional disorder is diagnosed when the client holds one or more nonbizarre delusions for a period of at least a month. The client must never have met the Type A criteria for schizophrenia. Although it is sometimes difficult to differentiate *bizarre* from *nonbizarre delusions,* the key is that the latter could conceivably arise in everyday life. People with delusional disorders may function quite well in areas of their life not affected by the delusion, yet behave oddly in activities touched by the delusion. For example, a gentleman holds the delusional belief that police are trying to entrap him. He goes to extremes to protect his home with surveillance and security equipment. At the same time, he believes that police won't bother him at work because his boss, with whom he works well, is the son of a policeman. Delusional disorders are not common and arise predominantly during middle and late adulthood.

Brief Psychotic Disorder

In a **brief psychotic disorder**, at least one of the Type A criteria for schizophrenia are present (hallucinations, delusions, disorganized speech or behavior) for at least one day, but for less than a month. Upon remission of symptoms, clients return to the level of functioning they had prior to the onset of the illness. This disorder may be brought on by a particular stressful event in the person's life, including the delivery of a baby. In other instances, a stressful life event cannot be identified.

Additional Disorders

Several other psychotic disorders are specified in *DSM-IV:*

- Shared psychotic disorder
- Psychotic disorder due to a medical condition
- Substance-induced psychotic disorder
- Psychotic disorder not otherwise specified (NOS)

Consult the *DSM-IV* for diagnostic criteria about these disorders. However, in diagnosing any psychotic disorder, the alternative explanation that the symptoms may be caused by an underlying medical disorder or by substance use *must* be explored.

Daryl, a 26-year-old with a diagnosis of paranoid schizophrenia, decided to stop taking his Haldol because it made him feel heavy and too tired to get up in the morning. Within a few days of stopping the medication, he was unable to leave the house for fear of someone harming him. Although he liked his unpaid job at the local cannery and knew that he had the chance to earn money in the near future, he refused to go to work for fear that he would be hit by a bus on his way there. He was eventually fired because of poor attendance. In this instance, a decrease in medication increased biologic vulnerability, with marked behavioral and eventually environmental consequences.

Jean, 22, had lived with her divorced mother and younger sister Mary since her release from the hospital after her second psychotic episode. She found living alone too frightening and was more comfortable staying in her old room at home. When Mary began preparing to leave home for college, Jean became increasingly anxious, demanding to sleep in Mary's room at night and hiding Mary's belongings. As Mary's departure grew near, Jean began actively hallucinating and withdrew to her room, refusing to talk to her mother or sister. In this case, the client did not have sufficient coping skills to deal with her sister's departure from the household, and the client retreated into psychosis.

Biopsychosocial Theories

Descriptive Psychiatry

The classic work of Kraepelin and Bleuler advanced the understanding of schizophrenia as a disease entity. Kraepelin began to describe the syndrome of schizophrenia, which he labeled **dementia praecox**, or early senility. He believed the syndrome was caused by an organic abnormality, was degenerative, and always ended in a state of disorganization that today would be called *psychosis.* Bleuler, who used the term *schizophrenia,* refined Kraepelin's descriptive picture of the illness. Bleuler attempted a psychologic explanation of schizophrenic symptoms but remained undecided about whether the illness was organic or psychologic. Unlike Kraepelin, Bleuler believed that there were many possible courses and outcomes of the disease.

Somatic treatments—insulin coma; drug or electrically induced shock treatments; and psychosurgery, including prefrontal lobotomies—were used in the 1930s. Many hoped these treatments were the long-sought-after cure for schizophrenia because they were relatively quick and inexpensive treatments compared to the analytic therapies. This hope was not realized.

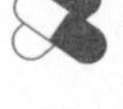

The introduction of psychoactive drugs in the 1950s provided new alternatives for the treatment of schizophrenia. Psychotropic medications, which influence the thoughts, mood, and behavior of clients, made previously uncontrolled symptoms manageable. In the period following the introduction of psychotropic medications, the use of seclusion and restraints declined dramatically, as did the duration of hospital stays and numbers of clients in state hospitals.

A new optimism arose regarding the possible outcomes of mental illness. Because they controlled the most difficult symptoms of psychosis, psychotropic medications made psychosocial or behavioral treatments possible for a much greater percentage of psychiatric clients. The major tranquilizers did not live up to their promise of providing a cure for schizophrenia and other chronic psychiatric illnesses. However, these drugs relieved the most debilitating symptoms for many clients and were the first step toward recovery or a higher level of functioning.

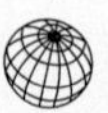

Diagnoses in Ethnically Diverse Populations In the United States, differences have been observed in the rates of diagnosis and treatment of psychiatric disorders in persons from different ethnic groups. Although studies are not conclusive, and factors other than race (such as age, socioeconomic status, gender) confound the findings, some differences have been observed consistently enough to warrant attention.

In a recent study of psychiatric inpatients and outpatients cared for in Los Angeles County (Flaskerud and Hu 1992) the chance of receiving a diagnosis of schizophrenia or other psychosis was significantly greater if the patient were African-American or Asian-American than if the patient were white. If the patient was Latino, she or he had a lesser chance of receiving a diagnosis of psychosis than if non-Hispanic white. These findings support many prior studies of how ethnicity affects diagnoses in psychiatric patients.

The factors that account for the differences in prevalence of diseases in ethnic groups are unclear but may include:

- Different patterns of use of the mental health system
- Stereotypical perceptions on the part of health care providers
- Biases against non-whites or non-English speakers in the diagnostic tools
- Misunderstanding expressions of cultural phenomenon as psychopathology
- Misunderstanding culturally specific expressions of psychopathology (Flaskerud and Hu 1992; Snowden and Holschuh 1992)

It is well documented that persons from Latino and Asian backgrounds underutilize mental health services, while African-Americans are overrepresented in the mental health system given their numbers in the population (Cheung and Snowden 1990).

Psychoanalytic Theories

Successful analytic work with schizophrenic clients by Sullivan and Fromm-Reichmann challenged earlier beliefs that schizophrenia could not be treated. By focusing on interpersonal relations, particularly from early childhood, these therapists attempted to understand and interpret the client's symptoms. Their work represented a departure from Freud's belief that people with schizophrenia could not form a therapeutic relationship and therefore could not be treated using analytic techniques. They claimed, as do their followers, that schizophrenic symptoms can be diminished though careful in-depth interpretive work. The effectiveness of insight-oriented therapies to treat schizophrenic clients continues to be debated today.

Biologic Theories of Schizophrenia

It is unlikely that schizophrenia is caused by a specific biologic abnormality. Scientists have searched unsuccessfully for a unique biologic marker consistently present in people with schizophrenia but absent in healthy people. At the same time, scientific evidence suggests that the disorder is not merely psychologic and that biologic alterations are present. Particularly convincing is the fact that the symptoms associated with schizophrenia, such as delusions or hallucinations, are found in healthy people only when they are in a state of metabolic imbalance or suffer from organic diseases. Individuals with brain tumors, or who have ingested certain drugs, for example, may experience hallucinations. See the box on food intolerance and schizophrenia.

GENETIC THEORIES Schizophrenia sufferers inherit a genetic predisposition to the disease rather than the disease itself. Evidence supporting this theory is the fact that relatives of schizophrenics have a greater chance of developing the disease than members of the general population do. While 1% of the population develops schizophrenia, 10% of the first-degree relatives (parents, siblings, children) of schizophrenics are diagnosed with the disease during their lifetimes. The risk of developing schizophrenia increases with the closeness of relation to a diagnosed person. Siblings have a greater risk of developing the disease than do half-siblings or grandchildren, and these have a greater risk than more distant relatives, such as cousins.

Twin studies indicate that both environmental and genetic factors are important in schizophrenia. Concordance rates (both twins either express or do not express the trait) for schizophrenia are consistently higher for monozygotic twins than for dizygotic twins. This finding supports the hypothesis of genetic transmission. However, concordance rates for monozygotic twins are in the range of 35–58%, indicating that environment plays a large part in the expression of the illness. If the disease were solely genetically determined, the concordance rates in this group would be close to 100%.

BRAIN STRUCTURE ABNORMALITIES As a group, people with schizophrenia have larger brain ventricles and smaller limbic structures than healthy control subjects (Cannon and Marco 1994). Although this finding is consistent over many studies, interpretations vary. The brain abnormalities may be a result of the disease and its treatment, because the degree of abnormality has at times correlated with illness duration. Alternatively, enlarged ventricles are thought to mark a subgroup of schizophrenic people who have more severe negative symptoms. Actual tests that measure negative symptoms and degree of structural abnormality have been equivocal. A third interpretation, which appears to account for more of the findings, is that altered brain structures are genetically based and represent a marker of vulnerability to schizophrenia that precedes any other symptomatology. Studies that have

NUTRITION AND MENTAL HEALTH

Can Food Intolerance Cause Schizophrenia?

Researchers have spent decades collecting the kind of data needed to establish a cause-and-effect relationship between food and psychosis. There is persuasive epidemiologic and clinical evidence for such a link.

Among 65,000 inland inhabitants of three Pacific islands who consumed little or no cereal grains, only two cases of overt schizophrenia were observed. A comparable survey of European populations—who rely heavily on grains such as wheat, oats, and rye—revealed a prevalence rate of 2 per 1000 adults. Similarly, among Pacific island peoples in more westernized coastal towns, in contrast to the inland groups, the number of cases of schizophrenia was sharply higher, as was the percentage of grain in the diet (Dohan et al. 1984).

Even stronger evidence comes from intervention trials in which gluten, the protein found in the above grains, was removed from the diets of psychotic clients. Of six controlled studies, three have found a significant improvement in those on a gluten-free regimen; three have not. However, the negative studies had a statistical power rating between 0.23 and 0.54. In practical terms, they could not rule out significant symptomatic improvement among those on a gluten-free diet because the studies contained too few subjects (King 1985).

A seventh double-blind trial in which twenty-four chronic schizophrenics received either gluten or a placebo demonstrated clear-cut benefits in two subjects. A 34-year-old psychotic with an 18-year history of the disease, for instance, improved markedly, showing less excitability, perceptual disorganization, grandiosity, and depressive mood. Investigators report that they were "impressed to see this almost continuously disturbed patient serving meals, helping staff with various jobs and talking much more rationally." Several psychiatric parameters deteriorated when gluten was reintroduced into the diet (Vlissides et al. 1986).

Although these reports point to food intolerances as a contributing cause of schizophrenia—at least for some clients—they do not shed any light on how to pinpoint the existence of an intolerance in individual clients. Unfortunately, there are no foolproof methods of doing so. Standard diagnostic procedures, such as the radioallergosorbent (RAST) or interdermal tests, detect the presence of only IgE antibodies, those produced during a true allergic reaction. But several researchers have found that many food sensitivities, although immunologic in nature, do not generate an IgE response. For

found enlarged ventricles in clients experiencing their first episode of psychosis support this interpretation. In addition, there is a positive relationship between the severity of the brain abnormality and illness severity. How the brain structure abnormalities influence the progress of the disease is not well understood and requires further study (Cannon and Marco 1994).

Biochemical Theories The biochemical basis of schizophrenia is captured in the **dopamine hypothesis,** which states that schizophrenic symptoms may be related to overactive neuronal activity that is dependent on dopamine. The hypothesis was supported by numerous studies demonstrating that medications that decrease DA activity alleviate symptoms. However, the relief of symptoms was not complete, and the negative symptoms of the disorder were much less responsive to DA blockers. Recent research suggests that the relationships between dopamine activity and schizophrenic symptoms are much more complex than originally hypothesized. It is now known that there are multiple types of DA receptors and that different types of receptors are concentrated in different regions of the brain (Davis et al. 1991). Original hypotheses that neuroleptics worked by blocking D_2 receptors have been challenged by clozapine tests. These tests demonstrate that clozapine, which binds poorly to D_2 receptors, positively affects schizophrenic symptoms in clients who were not responsive to traditional psychotropic medications.

Davis et al. (1991) propose a more complex story of dopamine action that results in the complex of symptoms in schizophrenia. They find that current studies suggest that DA disregulation in schizophrenia may occur at two levels. Hyperdopaminergia appears to occur in the mesolimbic neurons, while hypodopaminergia occurs in the mesocortical neurons. Investigation of how abnormalities in DA action at the cortical and subcortical levels of the brain are linked remains to be completed. However, this current interpretation of dopamine abnormalities holds promise, because it offers an explanation for the concurrence of positive and negative symptoms in schizophrenia.

NUTRITION AND MENTAL HEALTH *(continued)*

instance, some food sensitivities are accompanied by abnormal serum levels of IgA, IgG, or a series of proteins referred to collectively as complement (Breneman 1984, Crayton 1984).

Given this complex situation, the most practical way to detect a food intolerance, short of performing an array of expensive, highly sophisticated laboratory tests, is by either taking a careful food history or starting the client on an elimination diet. Clinical experience suggests that clients may crave the very foods they cannot tolerate, much as drug addicts crave the substance that causes their symptoms. A food history might reveal a diet that relies too heavily on the offending food. Someone who is sensitive to milk protein may consume large amounts of cheese, yogurt, and ice cream.

Because there are no controlled studies to confirm this addiction/allergy hypothesis, many clinicians turn to an elimination diet. The beginning diet consists of hypoallergenic foods, such as lamb, cabbage, cauliflower, pear, blueberry, rice, tapioca, olive oil, and milk-free margarine. To prevent nutritional deficiencies, vitamin and mineral supplements are added to the diet. See Golbert (1993) for details.

Although food sensitivities may contribute to schizophrenia, clinicians should also keep in mind that the disease, as well as other psychiatric disorders, can also affect the way clients view food, causing some to invent food allergies as an explanation for symptoms that may have strictly interpersonal or intrapsychic roots. One research team, for instance, was unable to confirm the presence of allergy-induced depression, anxiety, mood swings, sleep disturbance, and poor concentration in nineteen subjects who were tested by means of double-blind food challenges (Pearson and Rix 1983). A psychiatric evaluation, however, found that the subjects had neurotic depression, hypochondriacal neurosis, phobia, and several other conditions.

There is one other possibility to consider in clients who complain of psychiatric reactions to food: stress-induced food sensitivity. The physiologic stress induced by exercise, for instance, can precipitate anaphylaxis to foods in susceptible clients (Bell 1987). The stress generated by mental dysfunction may likewise generate an immune response, as is borne out by experiments that have found diminished lymphocyte function after the death of a loved one (Crayton 1986). Put another way, it seems likely that some clients become more allergy-prone when exposed to stress. The resulting food sensitivity in turn may trigger psychiatric symptoms.

Paul L. Cerrato, BS, MA

Psychologic Theories of Schizophrenia

Information Processing Many schizophrenic clients have information-processing deficits. Two central types of information processing have been identified: automatic and controlled or effortful processing. Automatic processing is the taking in of information unintentionally. Automatic processing can occur without the individual's being aware of it and it does not interfere with conscious thought processes occurring at the same time. Examples of automatic information processing are the initial awareness of physical features of a new environment.

People with schizophrenia are deficient in controlled information processing. Their ability to perform directed, conscious, sequential thinking—for example, making comparisons between two stimuli or organizing a set of stimuli—is consistently inferior to that of healthy people.

We do not know whether the schizophrenic person's inability to sustain conscious, directed thought is the primary problem or the result of a primary deficit in automatic thinking. If the primary deficit is in automatic processes, then the person is forced to complete automatic tasks at the conscious level, inhibiting and slowing controlled information processing. Sufficient evidence to resolve this question is not yet available.

Attention and Arousal Physiologic studies of attention and arousal in schizophrenic clients show promise of identifying clinically significant subgroups. Arousal and attention are measured by physiologic states and alterations, such as galvanic skin response, heart rate, blood pressure, skin temperature, and pupillary response. One subgroup of clients exhibits abnormally low response levels to novel stimuli. This finding suggests that these clients are less adept than healthy people at attending and responding to novel situations.

A second group of clients with schizophrenia demonstrates a state of hyperarousal evidenced by elevated electrodermal activity, heart rate, and blood pressure. Hyperarousal has been noted during both symptomatic and nonsymptomatic periods. These clients demonstrate

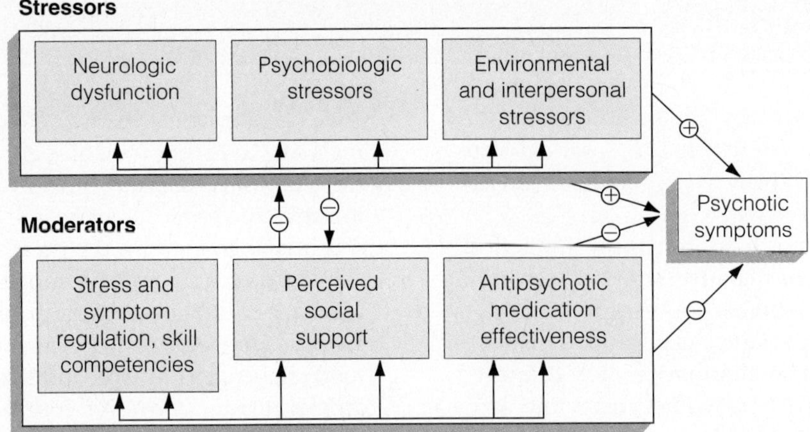

Figure 14–1 The effects of stressors and moderators on each other and on psychotic symptoms. Lines with + or – denote causal relationships; other lines denote correlations without specifying a causal direction. *Source: O'Connor 1994, p. 232.*

symptoms of irritability, excitement, and anxiety rather than apathy and withdrawal.

Family Theories of Schizophrenia

Numerous theories implicating family interaction as a cause of schizophrenia have been proposed. Terms that represent these theories include *schizophrenogenic mothers, double-binds,* and *pseudomutuality.* Research has failed to support the theory that dysfunctional family interaction causes the illness.

One theory suggests that disordered family communication (the inability to focus on and clearly share an observation or thought) causes schizophrenia only in the presence of a genetic predisposition to the disease. Living with this pattern of family communication during early development is thought to impair the schizophrenic person's ability to perceive the environment and communicate with others about it (Miklowitz 1994).

A second theory is that the family's emotional tone can influence the course of schizophrenia over time. Researchers found that schizophrenic individuals from families who are highly critical, hostile, or overinvolved tend to relapse more often than those from families who do not demonstrate these characteristics. Families exhibiting such characteristics have been described as having high **expressed emotion.** There is some evidence that family expressed emotion may be an influence on, rather than a response to, the illness, but this evidence is not definitive.

Humanistic-Interactional Theories of Schizophrenia

An interactional model of schizophrenia integrates many of the biologic and psychosocial theories already discussed. In this view, schizophrenia is due to the interaction of a genetic predisposition or biologic vulnerability, stress or change in the environment, and the individual's social skills and supports. In an interactional model, the influences are multidimensional. A biologic vulnerability may inhibit the individual's capacity to cope with even minor stressors such as the loss of a primary source of support. Similarly, schizophrenic people might grow worse upon entering an environment that demands coping skills they have not developed.

An interactional model for understanding schizophrenia that has received wide acceptance is the **stress-vulnerability model,** which suggests that people with schizophrenia have a genetically based, biologically mediated vulnerability, to personal, family, and environmental stress (Neuchterlein et al. 1992). O'Connor (1994) offers an application and extension of the stress-vulnerability model for understanding symptom production in schizophrenia (Figure 14–1). In this model, the interaction between stressors and stress moderators can result in a balanced or nonstressed system; or the stressors can overwhelm the resources, and symptoms result. Potential stressors include inherent neurologic dysfunction, including any abnormalities that may exist in brain structures or biochemical processes. Psychobiologic stressors include the stresses of living with schizophrenia itself. Altered attention and perception, as well as problems with motivation and energy, create stresses for people with schizophrenia. In addition, O'Connor (1994) notes the stress frequently encountered by young people with this disorder when combined with the use of drugs and alcohol. Environmental and interpersonal stressors include those that we all encounter, but a person with schizophrenia is particularly sensitive. These include stressful life events and environments that are highly demanding or stimulating. In addition, family or living environments that are highly negative present real stressors to those with schizophrenia.

Moderators of stress that are thought to affect the generation of symptoms in schizophrenia include:

- Skill in symptom regulation
- Social support
- Antipsychotic medication

The capacity to self-monitor the ebb and flow of schizophrenia and to develop coping strategies to influence symptoms at the first signs of trouble show promise in influencing the longer-term course of the illness. This capacity is a resource that may work to moderate stress that occurs in the person, family, or environment. Social support has proven helpful in moderating stress for general populations and for people with schizophrenia in particular. Supportive others who provide empathy, contact, financial aid, problem solving, and other forms of support moderate the difficulties of schizophrenia. Finally, antipsychotic medications have proven efficacy in moderating some symptoms of the disease, and thus some of the stressors induced by the disease (O'Connor 1994).

The Nursing Process and Clients with Schizophrenia

Assessment

Assessment of clients who have schizophrenia occurs at individual, family, and environmental levels. The nurse must be aware of the client's status and of changes in the client's personal life, family situation, and environment to plan care and intervene effectively. In addition, care that addresses multiple levels of the client's life is consistent with the interactional theory of schizophrenia because it is assumed that changes in any aspect of the client's environment influence all other aspects of the personal environmental balance.

SUBJECTIVE DATA

Perceptual Changes The perceptions of clients with schizophrenia may be either heightened or blunted. These changes may occur in all the senses, or in just one or two. For example, a client may see colors as brighter than normal or may be acutely sensitive to sounds. Another may have a heightened sense of touch and therefore be extremely sensitive to any physical contact.

Illusions occur when the client misperceives or exaggerates stimuli in the external environment. A schizophrenic client may mistake a chair for a person or perceive that the walls of a hallway are closing in. The perceptual changes are sufficient to cause the client to mistake the stimulus for something that it is not.

Hallucinations are the most extreme and yet the most common perceptual disturbance in schizophrenia. Auditory hallucinations are the most common form of hallucination. Although hallucinations are a hallmark of schizophrenia, their presence alone does not establish the presence of the disorder. Table 14–1 lists various types of hallucinations, along with a disease process commonly associated with the symptom.

Assess perceptual disturbances by asking the client about the experience and by observing for behaviors that indicate the client is frightened or attending to internal stimuli. Ask the client, "What are you seeing and hearing?" Note the degree to which this description differs from your perceptions of the environment.

Clients may be reluctant to discuss the extreme perceptual disturbance of hallucinations. A classic sign of auditory hallucinations is placing the hands over the ears. The client is frightened by the perception and tries to block it out. Less obvious signs of hallucinations are inappropriate laughing or smiling, difficulty following a conversation, and difficulty attending to what is happening

Table 14–1 Types of Hallucinations

Perceptual Disturbance	*Commonly Associated Disease Process*	*Example*
Auditory	Schizophrenia	Hearing voices of family members who aren't present.
Visual	Dementia	Seeing animals walking across the walls of the room.
Tactile	Acute alcohol withdrawal	Feeling bugs crawl on the skin.
Olfactory	Seizure disorders	Smelling foods that aren't present.
Gustatory	Seizure disorders	Tasting a sharp sweet taste on the tongue, in the absence of food.
Somatic	Schizophrenia	Sensing that one's head has a tunnel running through it.

ASSESSMENT

Hallucinations

A complete assessment of hallucinations should identify the following:

- Whether the hallucinations are solely auditory or include other senses.
- How long the client has experienced the hallucinations, what the initial hallucinations were like, and whether they have changed.
- Which situations are most likely to trigger hallucinations, and which times of day they occur most frequently.
- What the hallucinations are about. (Are they just sounds, or voices? If the client hears voices, what do they say?)
- How strongly the client believes in the reality of the hallucinations.
- Whether the hallucinations command the client to do something, and if so, how potentially destructive the commands are.
- Whether the client hears other voices contradicting commands received in hallucinations.
- How the client feels about the hallucinations.
- Which strategies the client has used to cope with the hallucinations and how effective the strategies were.

at the moment. Fleeting, rapid changes of expression that are not precipitated by events in the real world can be a further sign. Finally, clients may talk to themselves, presumably in answer to the voices they hear. For more information, see the Assessment box above.

OBJECTIVE DATA

Disturbances in Thought and Expression Clients with schizophrenia find that their thinking is muddled or unclear. Their thoughts are disconnected or disjointed, and the connections between one thought and another are vague.

The clarity of the client's communication often reflects the level of **thought disorganization.** Client responses may be simply inappropriate to the situation or conversation. They may have difficulty articulating a response or stop midsentence, as if they are stuck, a sign of **thought blocking.**

Note the rate and quality of the client's speech. Is it unusually loud, insistent, and continuous? Does the client wander from topic to topic (**tangential communication**) or bring up details that are irrelevant to the topic at hand (**circumstantial communication**)? Are the client's responses slow and hesitant, reflecting difficulty in taking in stimuli and responding?

Schizophrenic clients also have difficulty thinking abstractly. Their responses may be inappropriate because they interpret words literally rather than abstractly. For example, when told to prepare to have his blood drawn, a young man readied some paper and marking pens. Assess abstract thinking by asking clients the meaning of proverbs, a test requiring the client to abstract a general meaning from a specific or metaphysical statement, for example, "People who live in glass houses shouldn't throw stones."

Disruptions in Emotional Responses Tone of voice, rate of speech, content of speech, expressions, postures, and body movements indicate emotional tone. Disturbances in emotions commonly seen in schizophrenia are restricted or inappropriate expression of emotions. Assess the congruence between the content of the client's communication and the displayed emotion. For example, does the client laugh when describing a frightening or sad incident? The absence of emotion is also often indicative of schizophrenia.

Motor Behavior Changes Disruptions seen in schizophrenia include disorganized behavior and **catatonia.** Disorganized behavior lacks a coherent goal, is aimless, or is disruptive. Catatonic behavior is manifested by unusual body movement or lack of movement. This activity disturbance includes **catatonic excitement** (the client moves excitedly but not in response to environmental influences), **catatonic posturing** (the client holds bizarre postures for periods of time), and **stupor** (the client holds the body still and is unresponsive to the environment).

Changes in Role Functioning An important factor in predicting the course of schizophrenia is the client's level of functioning before the symptoms of the disease became pronounced. Assessment should therefore include a complete history of the client's success at completing developmental tasks. The prognosis is best if the client functioned at a high level prior to the onset of schizophrenic disturbance. Assess how well the client fulfilled role responsibilities in the family, in school, in relation to peers, and in work. Obtain a history of the rate of decline in these various roles. The onset of schizophrenia may be relatively acute, or degeneration may be slow.

Drug Use Clients with drug toxicity or withdrawal may present with behavior disturbances similar to those seen in schizophrenic clients. They may have auditory or visual hallucinations and may be confused, illogical, and highly anxious. For this reason, it is essential to obtain a detailed drug history. Assess both long-term and recent use of chemical substances. If the client is not a reliable historian, interview family or friends. In addition, both blood and urine should be tested for drugs if reliable information cannot be obtained.

Family Health History Part of assessment is noting any history of mental illness in the client's family. Of particular interest is a history of schizophrenia or any thought disorder, mood disorders (such as cyclical highs or depressions), or alcoholism in any family member. Note any report that family members had "nervous breakdowns" or any other colloquial descriptions of mental or emotional disorders.

Family Cohesion and Emotion A moderate level of family cohesion is optimal according to many family theorists. The two extremes—lack of cohesion, or **disengagement**, and too much cohesion, or **enmeshment**—signify problems in family functioning. In families of people with schizophrenia, enmeshment, combined with a negative emotional tone, is thought to be detrimental to the ill member's well-being. Schizophrenics from overinvolved families who criticize the client have a high relapse rate (Chesla 1994).

Much of the nursing assessment of families can be carried out unobtrusively. Assess levels of cohesion by noting who accompanies the client during admission. Is it the whole family or just one member? Does the client come in alone? Visits from family are a rich source of information. Who visits, how often, and for how long? How do family visitors behave with the client? Do the members spend time interacting and sharing activities, do they sit quietly together, or do they maintain physical and emotional distance from one another? Document these patterns of family interactions, and monitor the effect of family visits on the client.

Formal family assessment interviews can be arranged by the nursing staff, in conjunction with the interdisciplinary team. In this forum, family history and current functioning can be completely assessed. Do not overlook natural opportunities to assess families and their needs. During visits, join the family for a few minutes to learn about their understanding of the program, their concerns, and their questions. A trusting relationship with key members of the client's family is essential for establishing a flow of information and planning care.

Family Communication Problems Unclear or incomplete communication is frequent in families of people with schizophrenia. This area requires nursing assessment. Unclear communication may result from continual interaction with the ill member or may contribute to the disorder. Although research on this issue is inconclusive, clinicians evaluate how effectively the family communicates to determine the potential need for intervention.

Assess these aspects of family communication:

- Ability to focus on a topic
- Ability to discuss a topic in a meaningful way with other members
- Ability to maintain the discussion without wandering from the subject or becoming distracted
- Use of language and explanations that are generally understandable (not peculiar to that family alone)

Also note who in the family seems to do the talking, who talks to whom, and whether members talk for or interrupt one another.

Family Burden Most families of schizophrenic individuals report that caring for the ill member places a burden on the family unit. **Family burdens** reported most often are financial strain, disruption in family routines, worry about the future, and feeling overwhelmed or unable to cope. Families also report these needs:

- Information about the disorder
- Information about how to manage day-to-day problems due to schizophrenic symptoms
- Support for family members in their roles as caregivers

Environmental Assessment Assess the availability of support and services beyond the bounds of the family, including extended family and friends, as well as community groups and organizations that support schizophrenic clients. Mental health programs that address the specific needs of schizophrenic clients should be sought.

Nursing Diagnosis

Nursing diagnoses with schizophrenic clients focus on alterations in the patterns of activity, cognition, emotion processes, interpersonal processes, and perception. Alterations in ecologic, physiologic, and valuation processes are assessed as well, but the central nursing problems relate to the former five processes.

Impaired Communication

Verbal Schizophrenic clients communicate in a disorganized, sometimes incomprehensible fashion. Clients with less severe disorganization skip from topic to topic, making few if any logical links. When more severe thought disorganization is present, the client's statements may be totally incoherent. Some clients manifest thought disorganization by speaking very little, a characteristic labeled **poverty of speech.** Also note poverty of content in speech, in which the client converses but says very little.

Often clients with schizophrenia communicate in ways that are overly concrete (a sign of an inability to think and communicate abstractly) or overly symbolic (a sign of preoccupation with unreal or delusional material). The symbols are usually difficult to decipher because their meanings are idiosyncratic.

Nonverbal In schizophrenic clients, facial and body expressions that accompany verbal communication frequently do not match the content of the verbal message. This lack of congruence is primarily due to the blunting of emotions found in schizophrenia. Expected facial expressions—smiles, looks of concern or disgust—may not accompany the schizophrenic's statements. In addition, clients with motor or behavioral abnormalities—posturing, unusual movements, or grimacing—convey a confusing mix of verbal and nonverbal messages.

SELF-CARE DEFICITS People with schizophrenia frequently appear indifferent to their personal appearance. They may neglect to bathe, change clothes, or attend to minor grooming tasks such as combing their hair. Some show little awareness of current fashion styles, wearing clothing that makes them look out of place. Of greater concern are those who wear clothing that is inappropriate to the current season and weather conditions.

Lack of attention to grooming might be a simple annoyance to those who must live in close proximity to the person with schizophrenia. Health risks related to prolonged poor hygiene also arise. Assess immediate problems, such as inadequate nutrition, fluid intake, and elimination, as well as long-term problems, such as dental caries and increased susceptibility to infections.

Disregard for appearance and hygiene may extend to the client's environment. The client may fail to maintain a clean and safe living space. He or she may not take good care of personal belongings and may misplace them. Self-care deficiencies may result from consistently disturbed thought and perceptual processes. For example, a young man whose chronic hallucinations are only partly relieved by medication has difficulty concentrating for long periods and therefore demonstrates variable attention to grooming.

ACTIVITY INTOLERANCE The emotional disturbances of ambivalence and apathy, common in schizophrenic disorders, can result in lack of interest and inactivity. Inactivity induced by ambivalence is associated with higher levels of emotion. Anxious about choosing one course of action and rejecting another, the client is immobilized.

Jim is ambivalent about taking a pass out alone for the first time. He is undecided about taking the risk of leaving the hospital ward without a staff member yet yearns for the freedom of walking the streets alone. Indecision leaves him standing, immobilized, by the doorway to the unit.

Extreme ambivalence can manifest itself in even the most automatic of behaviors.

Mary cannot eat because of ambivalence about where to sit or what to eat. She stands in the center of the dining room, turning first to one chair and then another, unable to choose and thus begin eating.

Clients who are inactive because of apathy demonstrate little emotional tone. Such clients may spend long hours lying in bed staring into space or listening to music. Often, but not always, apathetic individuals prefer isolation. The nurse might find several clients sitting in the same room, engaged in no apparent activities and interacting with one another only when absolutely necessary.

SOCIAL ISOLATION Extreme anxiety about relating to others often leads schizophrenic clients to withdraw from interaction and to isolate themselves. Some clients tolerate only a few moments of direct communication, whereas others can manage extended periods of contact. Assess the client's tolerance of brief periods of contact with nurses and other clients. Document patterns of relating and withdrawal, also noting which activities the client engages in when in contact with others and when alone.

DECISIONAL CONFLICT Decisional conflict in schizophrenia is probably due to biochemical alterations in the brain that make it difficult for clients to take in, synthesize, and respond to information. Decisional conflict may be evident both in the mundane activities of daily life (selecting one's diet, for example) and in major life decisions.

Murray refuses to take medications, even though not taking them means that he will be evicted from the residential treatment program he likes.

SENSORY/PERCEPTUAL ALTERATIONS

Hallucinations Hallucinations are both a clinical diagnostic sign of schizophrenia and a focus for nursing care. You need to know the extent and nature of clients' hallucinations. Monitoring a client's hallucinations over time provides information on stressors that precipitate hallucinations, the client's response to psychotropic medications, and nursing actions that may diminish this symptom.

Document many aspects of the client's hallucinatory experience. Make note of situations or times of day that seem to trigger hallucinatory experiences. Record all sensory modes affected in the hallucination. The history of hallucinations and changes over time are important.

CASE STUDY

A Client with Schizophrenia

Identifying Information

Jack May is a 24-year-old single male who lives with his mother and supports himself with SSI. He is brought to the psychiatric emergency service by his mother. He currently attends a structured work program 5 days a week, but stopped attending 8 days ago.

Client's Definition of the Problem

Jack says that he does not need to be hospitalized, but that his mother is the one with the problem. He wants to be left alone to work on his computer projects. He admits that he has been hearing multiple voices in his head for the past week. For the past 2 weeks, Jack has been increasingly isolated working on his personal computer in his room. While he will not tell anyone what the work is about, his mother has seen printouts that suggest it is a plan to soundproof and secure his room. Jack stopped attending his work program a week ago, saying that he had "more important work" to do at home. He refuses to eat or talk with his mother. His mother believes he stopped taking his medications. An identifiable stressor is that 2 weeks ago his father announced plans to remarry in the near future.

Psychiatric History

Two years ago, Jack had a serious psychosis precipitated by his move to a college out of state. He was diagnosed with schizophrenia, paranoid type. He was hospitalized for 2 weeks, stabilized on Haldol, and discharged home. Persecutory delusions, which shift with news events, are always present at a low level. He has lived with his mother since diagnosis, attending day treatment and, for the last 8 months, a structured work program. He occasionally attends client support network meetings. His work attendance has been sporadic, and he has been on and off probation for nonattendance in this structured work environment. He receives medications and follow-up treatment at the community mental health center.

Family History

The Mays are both living and well. They were separated 3 years ago and divorced 2 years ago. Jack's father is an attorney, and Jack sees him approximately once a month. Their relationship is pleasant but not close. His mother runs her own crafts store and is agreeable to having Jack live with her. There are no other children.

Social History

Jack has completed high school and a few courses at the local community college. He was an above-average student and was always involved in school and extracurricular activities, until about 9 months before his first psychotic episode. Since that time, he has socialized primarily with his mother and rarely with a few acquaintances from the client support group. He smokes a pack of cigarettes a day and drinks beer occasionally. He denies any illicit drug use. Jack has a keen interest in computers. He took extensive coursework in computers in school and has collected considerable equipment and software, primarily gifts from his father. Other pastimes are listening to rock music and watching television.

Health History

No notable medical problems.

Current Mental Status

Jack is a healthy-looking 24-year-old who is anxious, somewhat guarded, but cooperative in the interview. He is oriented to person, time, and place, and demonstrates good memory and recall. Judgment is impaired. His affect is anxious. Speech is rapid, pressured, tangential. He is hyperalert to his environment and is notably startled by a siren outside. Persecutory delusions about people trying to take over his home and work are present, and he has hallucinations of unrecognizable voices and the voice of his father. No command hallucinations. Some loosening of associations present. Abstractions are concrete and self-referential. Insight poor; believes that his mother is "sick" and that she should not impede him in his important projects.

Other Subjective or Objective Clinical Data

Evidence that Jack may have stopped taking medications approximately 2 weeks ago. Suicide/violence potential minimal.

Diagnostic Impression

Nursing Diagnoses

Anxiety
Altered Thought Processes
Impaired Social Interaction

DSM-IV Multiaxial Diagnosis

Axis I: 295.30 Schizophrenia, Paranoid Type; Episodic, With Interepisode Residual Symptoms
Axis II: No diagnosis
Axis III: None
Axis IV: Problems with primary support group; father's impending remarriage
Axis V: GAF = 30 (current)

NURSING CARE PLAN

A Client with Schizophrenia

Nursing Diagnosis

Anxiety related to delusions.

Expected Outcome

Client will demonstrate decreased anxiety.

Nursing Interventions

- Give client a private room.
- Make frequent, supportive, brief contacts with client.
- Provide time alone in room to reduce anxiety.
- Provide prescribed medications and PRN medications for anxiety.

Outcome Met If

- Client describes subjective reduction of anxiety.
- Client participates in milieu.

Nursing Diagnosis

Altered Thought Processes.

Expected Outcome

Client will demonstrate reduced preoccupation with delusions of persecution.

Nursing Interventions

- Reassure client of safety in this environment.
- Allow client to describe delusions and acknowledge emotions that delusions cause.
- Avoid arguing with or contradicting the delusions.
- Highlight client's adaptive behaviors.
- Engage client in concrete interests, such as music.
- Give prescribed antipsychotic medication.

Outcome Met If

- Client can engage in conversations with nurse and peers without discussing delusions.
- Client is involved in activities other than computer work.

Nursing Diagnosis

Impaired Social Interaction due to negative symptoms of schizophrenia.

Expected Outcome

Client will express increased interest and involvement in peer relations.

Nursing Interventions

- Establish expectations for participation in program activities.
- Negotiate with client the level of involvement both short-term and long-term.
- Prompt client to attend activities at scheduled times.
- Construct opportunities for client to interact with similar age peers when staff can assist with introductions, transitions, finding similarities of experience.

Outcome Met If

- Client identifies commonalities in own and another client's illness experience.
- Client participates without prompting in some unit activities.

Look for major themes in the content of the hallucinations, particularly whether the hallucinations command the client to do something. The degree to which clients believe the experience is real and their ability to verify the reality of the experience by checking with others have important implications for interventions. Note the client's emotional response to hallucinations; some clients experience depression or despair about the continued presence of voices. Client coping strategies, and their effectiveness or ineffectiveness, are also an important aspect of the diagnosis.

Illusions Illusions make the client vulnerable to emotional and physical injury. The level of misperception may vary from day to day and even throughout the day. Misperceptions of the social environment make the client vulnerable to inappropriate responses and therefore ridicule. Misperceptions of the physical environment, such as misjudging the speed of an oncoming car, may lead to physical harm.

BODY IMAGE DISTURBANCE A body image disturbance is common in schizophrenic people. Clients may lose the sense of where their bodies leave off and where inanimate objects begin. They may become dissociated from various body parts and believe, for example, that their arms and legs belong to someone else. They may worry about the normalcy of their sexual organs. Clients often verbalize this altered sense of self directly, saying "I don't feel like myself" or "I feel like I am looking at my body from somewhere else in the room."

WATER INTOXICATION Water intoxication is a problem that is observed primarily in clients who reside in institutions such as state mental hospitals. This physiologic state is brought on by excessive drinking, characterized by hyponatremia, confusion, disorientation, and progresses to apathy and lethargy. In severe cases seizures and death may result. The cause of the polydipsia that precedes the water intoxication is unknown. For clients suspected to be at risk because of frequent drinking, preventative measures include regular measures of urine specific gravity, and regular weights designed to screen for increases in the body's fluid volume (Boyd 1990).

Altered Thought Processes

Delusions Clients express delusional thinking in direct interactions and, to a lesser extent, through behaviors. When asked, many clients willingly describe their delusional beliefs in detail. They seldom withhold this information because they believe firmly in the validity of the delusion, no matter how bizarre it seems to others. Clients' actions reflect the fixedness of their beliefs.

Gerry has the somatic delusion that her body is riddled with holes. She flatly refuses to drink, convinced that the fluid will flow directly out of the holes and soil her dress.

The content of delusions varies: delusions of persecution, reference, and so on (Table 14–2). Reality-based delusions may seem plausible because they could, under some circumstances, actually occur. Bizarre delusions, more common among schizophrenic clients, have no possible basis in reality. The false belief that one's husband is having an affair with a neighbor is a reality-based delusion. In contrast, the belief that one's thoughts are directed by a television announcer or that one's unspoken thoughts can be heard by others are bizarre delusions.

Delusions often reflect the client's fears, particularly about personal inadequacies. For example, a man's grandiose delusion that he is the mayor of New York City is a defense against feelings of inferiority. Similarly, persecutory delusions defend against the person's own feelings of aggression. Aggressive feelings are projected onto a person or organization—for example, the police, whom the client then fears.

Magical Thinking **Magical thinking** is the belief that events can happen simply because one wishes them to. Some people with schizophrenia claim they can exert their will to make people take certain actions or make specific events occur, like winning the lottery.

Thought Insertion, Withdrawal, and Broadcasting Hallmarks of schizophrenic thought are the beliefs that others can put ideas into one's head (**thought insertion**) or take thoughts out of one's head (**thought withdrawal**). In addition, some clients believe that their thoughts are transmitted to others via radio, television, or other means but not directly by the client. This belief is known as **thought broadcasting.**

Altered Emotional Responses*

Inappropriate Emotions Many individuals with schizophrenia demonstrate inappropriate affect—emotional responses that are inappropriate to the situation. For example, a client may smile or laugh while relating a history of having been abused as a child. Or a client may become angry and anxious when asked to join a group of other clients for dinner. The degree to which a client's emotions are inappropriate is a prognostic indicator. Clients whose emotional response is preserved and generally appropriate have a more favorable prognosis than clients who demonstrate inappropriate affect.

**Not a currently approved NANDA diagnosis.*

Table 14–2 Types of Delusions

Disturbances in Thinking	*Definition*	*Example*
Delusions of persecution	Belief that others are hostile or trying to harm the individual.	A woman notices a man looking at her and believes that he is trying to follow her.
Delusions of reference	False belief that public events or people are directly related to the individual.	A man hears a story on the evening news and believes it is about him.
Somatic delusions	Belief that one's body is altered from normal structure or function.	An elderly woman believes that her bowel is filled with cement and refuses to eat.
Thought broadcasting	Belief that one's unspoken thoughts can be heard.	A young client believes that everyone around him knows he's attracted to a nurse although he has said nothing.
Delusions of control	Belief that one's actions or thoughts are controlled by an external person or force.	A woman believes that her neighbor controls her thoughts by means of his home computer.

A marked decrease in the variation or intensity of emotional expression is called **blunted affect.** The client may express joy, sorrow, or anger, but with little intensity. In flattened affect, there is a total lack of emotional expression in verbal and nonverbal behavior; the face is impassive, and voice rate and tone are regular and monotonous.

Anhedonia As already mentioned early in the chapter, anhedonia is the inability to experience pleasure or to imagine a pleasurable emotion. This inability is very distressing to clients, who are aware of how they differ from other people. One young man lamented, "How can it be possible to feel so many awful things and *never* feel happy?"

ALTERED FAMILY PROCESSES

Family Overinvolvement and Negativity* At present there are no clear-cut clinical markers of what constitutes overinvolvement and negative emotions in families. Research criteria, which are too complex to apply in clinical settings, have been developed to identify families at risk. Nurses should note families who seem excessively bonded emotionally. Family members' inability to maintain emotional, social, or physical separateness is a clear sign of this problem. Also assess a high level of criticism among family members. Discuss with the treatment team families that seem seriously enmeshed or hypercritical.

Altered Family Functioning* Families burdened with the long-term responsibility of caring for a schizophrenic relative may suffer disruptions in their household routine, work, social interactions, and physical well-being. The household may be disrupted by the client's insistence that the family act on and accommodate delusional beliefs. The family may bend to the client's wish, fearing an increase in the client's anxiety and possible fighting or shouting if they do not comply.

The Walker family built an extra bathroom rather than fight with Tim, their schizophrenic son, who spends hours in the bath completing elaborate washing rituals. The Sherman family must eat out several times each week because Suzanne, their schizophrenic daughter, refuses to allow anyone in the room when she eats.

The family social life may be disrupted. For instance, the family may fear leaving the schizophrenic member home alone, or they may fear that the ill person will embarrass visitors if friends are invited in. Some families are willing to be open about the adjustments they make in living with a schizophrenic loved one, whereas others choose to live isolated lives.

Not a currently approved NANDA diagnosis.

Family members' work can suffer because of the emotional strain of living with an ill member. They must take time off to accompany the schizophrenic person to doctors' appointments, make hospital visits, and help during interviews with social agencies or the police. Family health may suffer because of general inattention or because of prolonged stresses within the home.

Planning and Implementing Interventions

When planning care for any client with a chronic illness, nurses must be careful to set realistic goals for client change. Particular care must be taken with schizophrenic clients because they are extremely sensitive to change and failure. Deterioration in all aspects of functioning is characteristic of the disease. Nurses must focus upon the most troublesome areas of client functioning and set incremental, short-term goals that pave the way for successes in achieving long-term goals. See the Self-Awareness box on the next page to increase your effectiveness in working with a psychotic client.

PROMOTING ADEQUATE COMMUNICATION Clients with schizophrenia try to communicate, even though their statements may be hard to understand. Close attention to what the client is saying and honest attempts to understand the real and symbolic aspects of the message are important. The client will perceive nuances of your behavior. Therefore, one of the most direct and successful ways to demonstrate caring and respect is to attend seriously to the client.

Clients make valid observations about their environment, needs, and concerns. A client may make observations about events or situations that are beyond your awareness. For example, take seriously a client's communications about another client's drug use or suicidal threats. If a client complains of a physical symptom such as stomach distress, consider the symptom as real until there is evidence otherwise. It is easy to dismiss a client's statements, particularly those of a delusional client. Doing so, however, shows lack of respect for the client's intact capacities to see and respond to what is happening in the environment.

PROMOTING COMPLIANCE WITH MEDICAL REGIMEN Psychotropic medications play an important part in the treatment of schizophrenic disorders. Drugs that diminish focal symptoms (hallucinations and delusions) and yet produce relatively few untoward effects are now available. You must recognize, however, that each individual responds to medications differently.

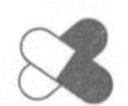

These interventions are nursing responsibilities:

1. Administer prescribed medication.
2. Observe client behavior for therapeutic effects.

NURSING SELF-AWARENESS

Working with Clients Who Have Schizophrenia

To increase self-awareness about working with active psychosis, ask yourself:

- How do I feel about approaching a person who is having hallucinations?
- How do I feel about talking to someone who has delusions that frighten him?
- Have I ever encountered someone in public that was psychotic?
- Do I fear that I might do something that might make the person's illness worse?
- What kinds of understanding and knowledge do I need to feel comfortable working with clients with psychosis?

To increase self-awareness about working with clients with disrupted ability to care for themselves, ask yourself:

- Do I react negatively when I think about someone my age who has never worked?
- What goes through my mind when I see someone who is disheveled, not well bathed or dressed?
- How can I find a point of connection between myself and someone whose life is so dramatically different from my own?

3. Monitor side effects of the medications.

4. Teach the client about the therapeutic and possible untoward effects of the medications prescribed.

5. Help the client take action to prevent untoward effects, such as maintaining fluid intake to avoid postural hypotension.

6. Evaluate the client's subjective response to the medication and attitude toward continued use.

Consistent compliance in taking medications as prescribed is not common among this client population. Researchers estimate that as few as 68% of psychiatric clients adhere to medication regimens while in the hospital. When these clients return to the community, 37% or fewer adhere to drug regimens. Clients may stop taking their medications for these reasons:

- They don't understand the administration instructions.
- They are too disorganized to follow the instructions.
- The side effects of major tranquilizers are too uncomfortable.
- They do not wish to be stigmatized as having schizophrenia and therefore reject treatment.

Clients who do not take medications are more vulnerable to stressors and risk more frequent relapse of symptoms than those who comply. Efforts to educate clients about their medications and to have them practice self-medication prior to discharge have increased the rate of compliance only marginally. Client attitudes toward the medications prescribed also influence their willingness to comply. You must be an active participant in assessing compliance and fostering a positive attitude toward medications. Commonly used antipsychotic medications are presented in Table 14–3 on the next page.

Clients are often ambivalent about taking medications. Maintaining adequate blood levels of therapeutic medications is important for schizophrenic clients. To help them overcome ambivalence, give them time to think about taking the medications. Set a time limit. If the client fails to comply, come back later and try again. Two useful strategies are reminding clients of the positive effects of the medication and framing the action as a way for them to help themselves get better.

ASSISTING WITH GROOMING AND HYGIENE Helping clients establish and maintain personal care habits is a complex process. If the client clearly lacks the skills, then teach the skills. If, however, the client has learned grooming skills but does not practice them, focus on ways to motivate the client. Intervention begins by establishing clear expectations about essential grooming habits. The frequency and timing of all aspects of grooming—including bathing, dressing, hair care, oral hygiene, and room care—should be specified in writing.

Formal training programs for helping chronically mentally ill clients improve their grooming skills can be applied in inpatient settings. These programs are well developed and tested. They systematically help clients in all steps of personal grooming, including collecting grooming supplies, moving to the grooming area (a bathroom or bedroom with sink and mirror), completing each grooming step, completing appropriate dressing, and storing grooming materials. Nursing interventions at each step can progress from simple verbal coaching, to modeling, to gentle physical guidance. Acknowledge client efforts during each phase with praise. The success of these programs probably depends on daily staff attention to the client's training, along with consistent, meaningful rewards. Avoid power struggles regarding the completion of tasks. If initial prompts don't work, leave the client alone for a short period.

Table 14–3 Action and Side Effects of Antipsychotic Medications

Generic and Trade Name	*Potency*	*Extrapyramidal Symptoms*	*Sedation*	*Anticholinergic*	*Hypotension*
Phenothiazines					
Chlorpromazine (Thorazine)	Low	++	+++	+++	+++
Thioridazine (Mellaril)	Low	+	+++	+++	+++
Perphenazine (Trilafon)	High	+++	+	++	+
Trifluoperazine (Stelazine)	High	+++	+	+	+
Fluphenazine HCl (Prolixin)	High	++++	+	+	+
Non-Phenothiazines					
Chlorprothixine (Taractan)	High	++	+++	++	++
Haloperidol (Haldol)	High	++++	+	+	+
Loxapine (Loxitane)	High	+++	++	+	++
Molindone (Moban)	High	+++	+	+	+
Clozapine (Clozaril)	Low	+	+++	+++	+++

Adapted from Davidson 1994.

PROMOTING ORGANIZED BEHAVIOR Clients whose behavior is disorganized require direction and limits to make their actions more effective and goal-directed. In working with a disorganized client, proceed slowly and remain calm. The client's perception of the environment may be distorted, but your calmness can help calm the client. Try to direct the client in simple, safe activities.

Examples of nursing goals and interventions for a disorganized client are given in the Intervention box on the next page. A case example of one such intervention follows.

George is moving quickly yet aimlessly from the refrigerator to the cupboard. He pulls a box of cereal from the cupboard, opens it, and then wanders away. Next he goes to the refrigerator, opens the door, peers in, and closes the door. Rummaging through all his pockets, he locates a cigarette, lights it, places it in an ashtray, and wanders back to the cupboard. This effortful yet unproductive behavior continues for several minutes when the nurse enters.

Nurse: **George, are you trying to get yourself some cereal?**

George: **Sort of. I was going to . . . smoke . . . no . . . eat something. Yeah, I wanted something to eat.**

Nurse: **Try to concentrate on one thing. First put out the cigarette. (He does so.) Now, come over here and get the cereal box. Here's a bowl. Here's a spoon. (She hands him the utensils.) Why don't you sit right here? (She seats him so that he has his back to the rest of the activity in the room.) Can you sit still for a bit?**

George: **I think so.**

Nurse: **Pour yourself some cereal. I'll get the milk for you. (She does so.)**

George begins to eat his cereal quietly. The nurse stays with him for a few minutes and directs him to continue eating when he becomes distracted by others who come into the room.

PROMOTING SOCIAL INTERACTION AND ACTIVITY The client's efforts to withdraw from social contact stem from past relationship failures and fear of rejection. Clients often find their internal world less risky and therefore more attractive than a world that requires interpersonal relating. When making efforts to help the client become less withdrawn, respect the client's overwhelming anxiety about human contact.

After establishing a basic level of trust, encourage the client to try out new behaviors within the relationship. The goal is to have the client experience success; therefore, encourage even small increments of change. If, for example, the client has difficulty initiating conversation, encourage the client to practice this skill once a day. Similarly, if the client avoids any activity in the environment because of fear of relating to groups, structure an activity involving the client, yourself, and one other client.

INTERVENTION

Promoting Behaviors That Contain or Manage Psychotic Symptoms

Client Behavior Encouraged	*Rationale*
Distraction • Talk with friends • Listen to music • Engage in physical activity	Client is actively engaged and thus symptoms are not reinforced.
Fighting back • Positive self-talk • Yell at voices • Ignore delusional thoughts	Actively working against symptoms; blocking voices by talking or turning attention away from delusions are effective in diminishing the symptoms.
Help-seeking • Go to the hospital • Talk with a health care professional • Seek support from family	A knowledgeable person can reinforce the person's perceptions and coach coping that has shown past success.
Attempting to feel better • Eat something • Take medication • Take a shower • Use relaxation	Bolstering self-esteem and self-comfort can cut off a cycle of self-criticism and decline.

Source: Adapted from Murphy and Moller 1993, p. 231.

SOCIAL SKILLS TRAINING **Social skills training** can be accomplished effectively in groups. Small groups provide structure and support, while you coach clients in simple yet essential social interactions. It is best to form groups of clients who function at similar levels. Provide structure by clearly setting times for group meetings, beginning and ending each session with a statement of goals, and recapping what the group has accomplished. Address social skills that are essential to functioning in the environment; introducing oneself, starting a conversation, ending a conversation, saying no, asking for assistance, and listening. Staff members can model these skills and help clients role-play each skill. Focus discussion on situations in which clients might need the skill. If they see its applicability to dilemmas in their personal lives, they will be motivated to learn the skill. Praise and, if available, material rewards can also motivate clients.

Schizophrenia can disturb a person's will and capacity to accomplish meaningful activity. Clients with distorted perceptions and thinking expend considerable energy merely taking in and interpreting their immediate worlds. In addition, major tranquilizers, which control the positive symptoms of the disease, can further inhibit a client's active involvement and interest in activities. You must be aware of how much work it takes to cope with schizophrenic symptoms. Do not assume that periods of quiet or inactivity are due to laziness or lack of interest. Rather, assess each individual's need for quiet periods in which to organize perceptions and thoughts.

At the same time, clients with schizophrenia live in a culture in which action and accomplishment are highly prized and rewarded. They are not immune to the pressure for personal productivity as a measure of personal worth. For this reason, they feel better about themselves when they are involved in meaningful activities. Your task is to help clients find activities that are intrinsically rewarding or that bring some social or tangible reward, yet are within their capacities.

Learning clients' personal interests is a first step. Providing opportunities for the client to actively engage in an activity of interest (by providing records, books, craft materials, or access to newspapers and television) is the next intervention. In addition, activities within the therapeutic milieu, such as attending groups and completing unit "jobs," can provide the external rewards of praise from staff and peers. These activities give clients confidence and develop their work habits. Success in these activities can lead to success in volunteer or paid work in the community after discharge.

PROMOTING REALITY-BASED PERCEPTIONS Illusions or hallucinations often frighten clients. Nurses can intervene by:

- Reassuring clients of their safety.
- Protecting them from physical harm as they respond to their altered perceptions.
- Validating reality.
- Helping clients distinguish reality from the hallucinatory experience.

Hallucinations are especially frightening if the client has never experienced them before or if their content is threatening or angry. Attempt to alleviate this anxiety by describing your perception of the frightened behavior and asking clients to discuss what they are experiencing. Make simple reassuring remarks, like "I know the voices are real to you, but no one else can hear them. No one means to harm you."

Protect clients from harm and reassure them about safety. A client may take impulsive action to escape the frightening experience or to obey voices in the hallucination. Prevent this by:

1. Closely observing client behavior during active hallucinations.
2. Intervening quickly by giving additional doses of psychotropic medications or placing the client in a quiet room.
3. If necessary, securing the unit so that the client cannot leave and take self-destructive or impulsive action.

Make every effort to help the client attend to real rather than internal stimuli, orient the client to the real situation, and encourage the client to focus on you rather than on the hallucination. "George, listen to me rather than to the sounds you say you hear. Remember you are in the hospital and I am your nurse. I will help you find your shoes. Come with me." Active involvement in some activity, such as finding shoes, will help the client maintain a focus on real events and perceptions.

INTERVENING WITH DELUSIONS General guidelines for working with delusional individuals are not to argue with their false beliefs, to focus on the reality-based aspects of their communications, and to protect them from acting on their delusions in a way that might harm themselves or others. See the Intervention box on the preceding page for suggested nursing interventions that contain or manage psychotic symptoms such as delusions.

PROMOTING CONGRUENT EMOTIONAL RESPONSES Working with clients who display blunted or flat affect can be confusing for nurses who are accustomed to reading emotional responses that fall within a more normal range. Be aware that these clients have feelings about events around them, including their interaction with you and other staff members, yet may have difficulty expressing those feelings.

Note any lack of congruence between the person's affect and the content of the message. If your relationship with the client is well established, you might comment on the incongruity and explore it with the client. ("George, what you are telling me is sad but you are laughing. What shall I pay attention to?") Modeling clear, congruent communications is helpful. Little can be done to change the client's anhedonia, yet empathic listening might comfort the client.

Ambivalence, the simultaneous experience of contradictory feelings about a person, object, or action, can trouble schizophrenic clients. Ambivalence can even become great enough to immobilize a client. Such clients cannot express one emotion or the other, or choose one action over the other. You may be able to partially alleviate the client's unease by identifying aloud the emotions the client may be experiencing. ("John, I think you might be feeling both very happy to see your father and at the same time very angry.") Naming the conflicting emotions gives the client the opportunity to talk about them, although many times he or she may not be able to do so.

Immobility due to ambivalence is extremely uncomfortable. One way of intervening is to limit the number of choices the indecisive client has to make. For example, a man may be immobilized by his inability to decide whether to go out alone for the first time. You can help by telling him that it seems too soon for him to go out alone and that, for today, he must be accompanied. Another example is a young woman who is undecided about where to sit. You can remove extra chairs at the table in the dining room so that she has only one choice.

PROMOTING FAMILY UNDERSTANDING AND INVOLVEMENT When a schizophrenic client is hospitalized, encourage the family and help them remain involved in the client's care. Except in unusual circumstances, share information on the client's status, treatment program, and future treatment plans, including discharge plans. Of course, nurses need to comply with the client's wishes and with the laws governing disclosure of information, which vary by state and by institution.

Some mental health care professionals have a bias against family involvement. This bias is a remnant of now-discredited theories that family interaction patterns cause schizophrenia. The Research Note in this chapter suggests quite the opposite. Nurses may need to be active advocates for families' rights to information about, and involvement in, the care of the schizophrenic member. This question is a useful way to check one's bias against the family's rights: Am I responding to this family any differently than I would to the family of a client with a medical condition? The family who has cared for the client with schizophrenia has an in-depth understanding of the client's illness, history, and ability to function in the community. Include the family's insights in the assessment phase, and, if appropriate, use them in the planning of care, particularly care after discharge.

If assessment suggests that the family needs information about the disease and treatment, refer the family to education programs, if they are available. Family psychoeducation programs are preferable to direct teaching because they often combine education with mutual support. In such groups, families can meet others who share their life difficulties. These peers can provide informal support and information to help the family deal with the tasks that lie ahead. Nurses can reinforce the formal teaching that occurs in such programs when they meet with individual families. See the Client/Family Teaching box on page 320.

Without exception, families should know about a national family support group with many local and state affiliates. The **National Alliance for the Mentally Ill (NAMI)** serves families through educational programs, local support groups, and political activism. Most local or-

RESEARCH NOTE

Citation

Howard PB: Lifelong maternal caregiving for children with schizophrenia. *Arch Psychiatr Nurs* 1994; 8(2):107–114.

Study Problem/Purpose

Research on caregiving for people with serious mental illness continues to suggest that care presents demands and sets up risks for the caregiver. However, the body of research to date has been cross-sectional and has lacked a historical perspective. This study used a life-span perspective to document the problems and adaptations that mothers of people with schizophrenia recalled from the time of diagnosis to the present.

Methods

A naturalistic grounded-theory study was designed. Ten women were selected (theoretically and purposively) from a core of 34 members who volunteered after solicitation by a local National Alliance for the Mentally Ill. Care had been provided from 1.5 to 28 years. In-depth interviews that lasted a average of 4 hours were conducted and transcribed. In addition, diaries and field notes served as data for interpretation. Data analysis consisted of constant comparative analysis of study themes and verification of themes.

Findings

An overriding theme was maternal care that involved watching, working, and waiting. Watching entailed vigilance about the child and his or her needs. Working encompassed the cognitive and practical tasks of providing care for a vulnerable person. Waiting referred to the emotional work of standing by and anticipating what might be needed, even though no action is ongoing. In addition, four phases of maternal caregiving were identified. (1) *Perceiving the problem.* This phase consists of the early struggle to make sense of the child's differences and cope with the realization and shock over the severity of the difficulties. (2) *Searching for solutions.* This phase involved acknowledging the diagnosis but searching, often unsuccessfully, for help in understanding the illness process. (3) *Enduring the situation.* This phase entailed continuing the persistent work of supporting the vulnerable child, but making progress at truly understanding the illness as biologic and chronic. (4) *Surviving the experience.* This final phase marked the mothers' acceptance of the illness, although with intense sorrow, and at the same time finding ways to care for themselves and their children.

Implications

This longitudinal examination of mothers' experience in caring for children with schizophrenia documents the continued struggle and commitment that these mothers had in their work and waiting. Repeatedly documented are the difficulties mothers experience in trying to learn about the disorder. The stories underscore the essential nature of careful but comprehensive education for families about the disease and its appropriate treatment.

ganizations are listed in telephone directories or can be reached through the local community mental health agency responsible for information and referral.

The Oddstads were worried about their daughter's failing grades at college for the last semester and were surprised to learn that she ended a relationship with her boyfriend. When she came home for spring break, she seemed disinterested and noncommunicative and wouldn't eat or socialize with the family. Her parents found her burning incense and chanting to herself in the mirror at 3:00 AM. In a panic, they took her to the local emergency room. After a complete workup, they were shocked to learn that the probable diagnosis was schizophrenia. Furthermore, the physician wanted their daughter to start on medication.

The rapidity of the decline in their daughter's functioning, and the fact that she had hidden many of her symptoms from them, left the Oddstads feeling guilty, sad, and yet disbelieving. They could not fathom how this had happened to their beautiful daughter. A nurse at the emergency room had given them the number of a local NAMI support group and Hotline. In their anguish, they called and were able to speak with other parents who helped them begin to deal with their emotions, and directed them to helpful books that explained schizophrenia and its treatment.

Promoting Community Contacts An awareness of a client's community supports and potential treatment programs can guide nurses in preparing clients for discharge. For example, the client's most important peer support

CLIENT/FAMILY TEACHING

Supporting Families of Clients with Schizophrenia

To assist families, you need to evaluate the family's current responses to living with and caring for a family member with schizophrenia. The following suggestions apply to the time period shortly after the disease has been diagnosed.

Suggestions	***Rationale***
Discuss the basic nature of the disorder: Schizophrenia is a disease of the brain, like any other biologic disease.	Families misunderstand mental illness to be a personal failing and are comforted by the fact that it has a biologic basis.
Help families identify their responses to the early ambiguous signs of the illness and notice how their responses have changed now that the diagnosis has been made.	Families often misinterpret early signs of the disorder to be acting-out or developmentally appropriate behavior. On learning that these signs are part of the illness, they feel guilty for not seeking help sooner.
Reinforce families for supporting the ill member in seeking treatment.	Stigma about mental illness persists, and families need support for taking action and engaging with treatment systems.
Refer families to structured educational or psychoeducational programs in which they can learn about the disease and its treatment, as well as receive support.	Schizophrenia is extremely complex, and its treatment is multifaceted. Families can benefit by structured classes. Programs that offer support to families in addition to education have proven efficacy in improving the illness course for the ill member.
Inform families about how to reach the local National Alliance for the Mentally Ill. Hand out fliers that provide telephone numbers and people to contact.	NAMI is a nationwide family support organization that provides peer support, education, and advocacy for the seriously mentally ill and their families.
Provide families with access to information and recommend manuals such as Torrey's (1983) *Surviving Schizophrenia: A Family Manual* and Walsh's (1985) *Schizophrenia: Straight Talk for Family and Friends.*	

group might be the clientele at a local day treatment program. If so, several visits to the program prior to discharge will help the client make the transition back to the community.

Preparing clients for the residence they will enter after hospital discharge is a central nursing task. Often, placement depends on how the client functions in the hospital. If the client is able to manage medications, participate in a variety of groups, and live cooperatively with other clients, then placement in a residential care facility that supports independent functioning is appropriate. In contrast, clients who need assistance with structuring free time, resist taking medications, or cannot be responsible for self-care require a more structured environment.

Nurses work with clients to help them achieve their highest level of functioning. They document clients' abilities to perform various tasks and make recommendations to the treatment team about appropriate placements.

Evaluation and Outcome Criteria

To complete the nursing process, nurses evaluate changes in client status and behavior in response to nursing interventions. Evaluation criteria are linked to nursing goals and reflect an understanding of the limitations of schizophrenic clients.

COMMUNICATION Clients will, with greater regularity, express their thoughts clearly and congruently. They will feel sufficient trust to talk to the nurse about troublesome symptoms or experiences. Because clients will probably continue to experience some symptoms even after medications have taken effect, this trust allows the client to express what has changed and what is still troublesome.

SELF-CARE Clients will consistently appear clean and well-groomed and will independently manage personal grooming and hygiene. Clients will have clean and reasonably appropriate clothes, in terms of both fashion and season. Individual styles of dress, which are the client's way of expressing or presenting the self, will remain and be supported by nurses. The means for maintaining self-care after discharge from acute care are identified.

ACTIVITY INTOLERANCES Clients will participate in goal-directed activities with minimal intervention. Clients will complete the activities they begin. Clients will demonstrate a broader range of interest and activities than they did on admission.

SOCIAL ISOLATION Clients will demonstrate the capacity to interact, for at least brief periods, with nursing staff, with other clients, and in small groups. They will consistently demonstrate socially required interactions, such as greeting and starting a conversation with a stranger, asking for assistance, saying no, and listening to another's conversation. Clients will be inactive for shorter periods and spend more time engaged in interesting or meaningful activity. They will demonstrate the capacity to function outside the protective environment of acute or sheltered care.

SENSORY/PERCEPTUAL ALTERATIONS Clients will have fewer episodes of attending to internal stimuli. If hallucinations persist, clients will begin to identify stressors or situations that precipitate them. Clients will identify and practice personal coping strategies that decrease the hallucination or its effects, such as going to a quiet room, engaging in social activities, and performing activities that demand concentration.

THOUGHT PROCESSES Clients will engage in reality-based discussions. If delusions persist, clients will not act on delusions in ways that are harmful or detrimental to themselves or others. They will also identify significant others in their current living environment who can help them limit their hallucinations via distraction or social contact.

EMOTIONAL RESPONSES Clients will have increased awareness that their emotional expressions at times do not match their verbal communications. They will monitor other's responses to them to learn cues about how they are varying their emotional expressions. Clients will experience fewer episodes of extreme discomfort due to ambivalence about people, events, or actions.

FAMILY FUNCTIONING Families will be involved in all aspects of client care, including assessment, planning interventions, inpatient treatment choices, and planning for discharge. Family understanding of the illness trajectory and client capacities and limits will improve. Family difficulties with caring for clients will be considered in treatment and discharge planning, and adequate resources will be identified to support family needs. Families will report that their questions about the schizophrenic disease process, and about varying modes of treatment for the disorder, have been answered.

Chapter Highlights

- People with schizophrenia experience disturbances in perception, thought, affect, and activity.
- The biologic, psychologic, and family theories of schizophrenia can be largely incorporated into one stress-vulnerability model of the disorder.
- Care of schizophrenic clients requires an awareness of the client's multiple functional deficits and of the nurse's personal response to working with this population.
- Nursing assessment of individual problems in schizophrenia focuses on changes in clients' perceptions, thoughts, expressions, and role functioning.
- Nursing assessment of family problems in schizophrenia focuses on family communication, cohesiveness, emotions, and burdens.
- Nursing diagnoses for clients with schizophrenia identify the communication, conduct, judgment, perceptual, and emotional alterations commonly found in this disorder.
- Nursing planning for clients with schizophrenia involves setting realistic goals and continually reevaluating expectations based on clients' current status.
- Nursing interventions promote adequate communication, compliance with medical regimen, activity, social interaction, grooming, and perception in clients with schizophrenia.
- Nurses evaluate the effectiveness of their interventions with individual schizophrenic clients and their families.

References

American Psychiatric Association: *Diagnostic and Statistical Manual of Mental Disorders,* ed 4. American Psychiatric Association, 1994.

Boyd MA: Polydipsia in the chronically mentally ill: A review. *Arch Psychiatr Nurs* 1990; 5(3):166–175.

Cannon TD, Marco E: Structural brain abnormalities as indicators of vulnerability to schizophrenia. *Schizophrenia Bull* 1994; 20(1):89–102.

Chesla CA: Parents' caring practices with schizophrenic offspring, in Benner P (ed): *Interpretive Phenomenology.* Sage, 1994.

Cheung FK, Snowden LR: Community mental health and ethnic minority populations. *Commun Ment Health,* 1990; 26: 277–291.

Davidson MA, Kuhn MA: *Pharmacotherapeutics: A Nursing Process Approach,* ed 3. FA Davis, 1994.

Davis KL, Kahn RS, Ko G, Davidson M: Dopamine in schizophrenia: A review and reconceptualization. *A J Psychiatr* 1991; 148(11):1474–1486.

Flaskerud JH, Hu Li-Tze: Relationship of ethnicity to psychiatric diagnosis. *Nervous and Ment Dis* 1992; 180(5):296–303.

Holmes H, Ziemba J, Evans T, Williams CA: Nursing model of psychoeducation for the seriously mentally ill patient. *Issues Ment Health Nurs* 1994; 15:85–104.

Howard PB: Lifelong maternal caregiving for children with schizophrenia. *Arch Psychiatr Nurs* 1994; 8(2):107–114.

Kales A, Stefanis CN, Talbot J (eds): *Recent Advances in Schizophrenia.* Springer-Verlag, 1993.

Miklowitz D: Family risk indicators in schizophrenia. *Schizophrenia Bull* 1994; 20(1):137–149.

Murphy MF, Moller MD: Relapse management in neurobiological disorders: The Moller-Murphy Symptom Management Assessment Tool. *Arch Psychiatr Nurs* 1993; 8(4):226–235.

Neuchterlein KH, Dawson ME, Gitlin M, Ventura J, Goldstein MJ, Snyder K, Yee CM, Mintz J: Developmental processes in schizophrenic disorders: Longitudinal studies of vulnerability and stress. *Schizophrenia Bull* 1992; 18:387–425.

O'Connor FW: A vulnerability-stress framework for evaluating clinical interventions in schizophrenia. *Image.* 1994; 26(3):231–237.

Reinhard S: Living with mental illness: Effects of professional support and personal control on caregiver burden. *Res Nurs and Health* 1994; 17:79–88.

Selzer MA, Sullivan TB, Carsky M, Terkelsen KG: *Working with the Person with Schizophrenia.* New York University Press, 1989.

Snowden LR, Holschuh J: Ethnic differences in emergency psychiatric care and hospitalization in a program for the severely mentally ill. *Commun Ment Health,* 1992; 28(4), 281–291.

Torrey EF: *Surviving Schizophrenia: A Family Manual.* Harper & Row, 1983.

Walsh ME: *Schizophrenia: Straight Talk for Family and Friends.* Warner Books, 1985.

Weiden P, Havens L: Psychotherapeutic management techniques in the treatment of outpatients with schizophrenia. *Hosp Commun Psychiatr* 1994; 45(6):549–555.

Nutrition Box References

Bell I: Effects of food allergy on the central nervous system, in Brostoff J, Challacombe S: *Food Allergy and Intolerance.* London: Bailliere Tindall, 1987, p. 710.

Breneman JC: *Basics of Food Allergy,* ed 2. Springfield, Ill.: Charles C. Thomas, 1984, pp. 212–255.

Crayton JW: Adverse reactions to foods: Relevance to psychiatric disorders. *J Allergy Clin Immunol* 1986;78(Suppl 1, Pt 2):244.

Crayton JW: Effects of food challenges on complement in "food sensitive" psychiatric patients. *J Allergy Clin Immunol* 1984;73(Suppl Pt 2):134.

Dohan F et al.: Is schizophrenia rare if grain is rare? *Biol Psychiatry* 1984;19(3):385–399.

Golbert I: Food allergy and immunologic disease of the gastrointestinal tract, in Patterson R, et al. (eds): *Allergic Diseases: Diagnosis and Management.* Philadelphia, JB Lippincott 1993.

King D: Statistical power of the controlled research on wheat gluten and schizophrenia. *Biol Psychiatry* 1985;20: 785–787.

Pearson DJ, Rix KJ: Food allergy: How much in the mind? A clinical and psychiatric study of suspected food hypersensitivity. *Lancet* 1983;2:1259–1261.

Vlissides D et al.: A double-blind gluten-free/gluten-load controlled trial in a secure ward population. *Br J Psychiatry* 1986;148:447–452.

CHAPTER 15

CLIENTS WITH MOOD DISORDERS

Kay K. Chitty

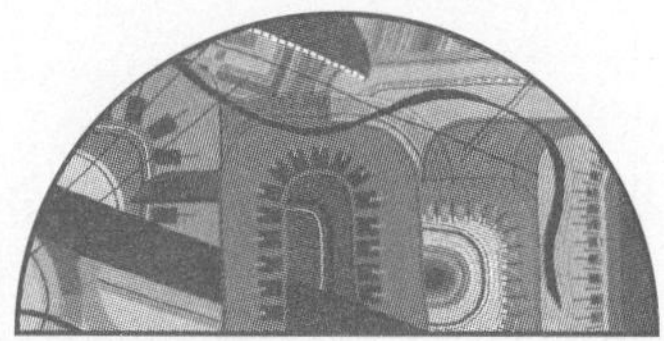

COMPETENCIES

- *Define major depressive disorder, dysthymic disorder, and bipolar disorder.*
- *Describe the biopsychosocial theories contributing to the understanding of mood disorders.*
- *Recognize the DSM-IV diagnostic criteria for mood disorders.*
- *Conduct a nursing assessment of clients with mood disorders.*
- *Identify nursing diagnoses for clients with mood disorders.*
- *Describe your role in appropriate nursing and biopsychologic therapies for clients with mood disorders.*
- *Evaluate the effectiveness of nursing interventions with clients with mood disorders.*
- *Discuss the nursing challenges associated with caring for clients with mood disorders.*

Cross-References

Other topics related to this chapter are: Psychobiology, Chapter 3; Sleep disorders, Chapter 19; Suicide, Chapter 24; Psychopharmacology, Chapter 33.

Critical Thinking Challenge

In some treatment settings, electroconvulsive therapy (ECT) is recommended for severely depressed, dangerously manic, acutely suicidal, and other clients who have not responded to less invasive psychopharmacologic interventions. While this practice is ostensibly in the client's best interest, clients themselves are often quite fearful of this procedure and have many misconceptions about its effects. What are the rights of severely ill psychiatric clients in determining their own treatment? Do they differ from other clients with physiologic disorders who now enjoy almost complete self-determination if they choose to exercise it? At what point does a client's right to autonomy and self-determination end? How might a treatment facility's philosophy on this issue be implemented to ensure consistency of care?

Depression affects 11 million Americans and costs $43.7 billion or more every year. Yet depression, the most common of the mood disorders, is a frequently overlooked mental disorder. Because health care policy makers often consider insurance coverage for mental illness to be a luxury, nearly two-thirds of the depressed people in this country go undiagnosed and untreated.

According to Dr. Frederick Goodwin, director of the National Institute of Mental Health, "Major depression is far more disabling than many medical disorders, including chronic lung disease, arthritis, and diabetes." (Goleman 1994, p. 1). In 1990, it was estimated that 88 million working days were lost because people were so severely depressed that they were unable to work. The symptoms of mood disorders—poor memory and concentration, fatigue, apathy, indecisiveness, and loss of self-confidence in those who are depressed and grandiosity and unrealistic overconfidence in those with mania—all reduce the capacity to work.

Mood disorders are a group of psychiatric diagnoses characterized by disturbances in physical, emotional, and behavioral response patterns. These patterns of **affect** (mood) range from extreme elation and agitation to extreme depression with a serious potential for suicide. They are the most common of all mental disorders, largely due to the prevalence of depression. Other mood disorders that occur far less frequently than depression but can be severely incapacitating include dysthymic disorder and the bipolar disorders.

Many people with mood disorders are never seen in psychiatric settings. This is because the symptoms of depression are often masked by physical complaints for which the client seeks help from primary care providers. Nurses are often in an excellent position to identify early signs of mood disorders and initiate treatment or action leading to early treatment.

Major Depressive Disorder

Major depressive disorder is characterized by one or more episodes of depressed mood or loss of interest lasting at least two weeks and accompanied by at least four additional symptoms of depression (American Psychiatric Association 1994). Individuals with a history of a manic or hypomanic episode may not be classified under major depressive disorder but instead are diagnosed under bipolar disorders. Major depressive disorder may consist of a single episode or may recur at various points in life. The depression is not warranted by real circumstances in the individual's life and is different from the normal sadness and grief resulting from a personal loss or tragedy.

Major depressive episodes can begin at any age, but the average age of onset is the mid-twenties. It seems to be occurring in younger and younger people, however. The risk of developing a major depressive disorder during a lifetime varies from 10% to 25% for females and from 5% to 12% for males, making depression twice as likely for women as for men. First-degree biologic relatives (parent or sibling) of people with major depressive disorder are up to three times as likely to develop depression as are members of the general population (APA 1994).

Symptoms of Major Depressive Disorder

Symptoms usually develop over a period of time. The person may experience anxiety and mild depression for several days, weeks, or months before the onset of a full major depressive episode. Untreated, major depression lasts 6 or more months. In about 20–30% of cases, some depressive symptoms persist for longer periods, ranging from months to years. When this occurs, it is considered a partial remission and is thought to be predictive of later depressive episodes and the development of chronic depression.

To be diagnosed with a major depressive disorder, the person must also experience at least four of the following symptoms accompanied by depressed mood and loss of interest or pleasure:

- Changes in appetite or weight, sleep, and psychomotor activity
- Decreased energy
- Feelings of worthlessness or guilt
- Difficulty thinking, concentrating, or making decisions
- Recurrent thoughts of death or suicidal ideation, plans, or attempts

The symptoms should be new or clearly worse than before the episode. Symptoms must be present for most of each day for at least two consecutive weeks and be accompanied by significant distress or impairment of activities of daily functioning.

Clients do not always describe their mood as "depressed." Instead, they may say that they are sad, discouraged, "down in the dumps," or feel helpless. Or they may complain of having no feelings or feeling "blah." In other cases, vague somatic complaints such as aches and pains are reported, while others report increased anger, frustration, and irritability, with uncharacteristic outbursts over minor matters.

When a person experiences a major depressive disorder, activities that previously gave pleasure, such as socializing, hobbies, sports, and sexual activities, often are no longer enjoyed. This condition is known as **anhedonia.**

Changes in physiologic functioning during depression are called **vegetative symptoms.** Changes in appetite, usually experienced as a reduction or loss of interest in food, is often seen, although increased appetite and cravings are also reported. Sleep disturbances are also common, particularly **insomnia.** Two types of insomnia are most often experienced by people having a major depressive episode. *Middle insomnia* refers to waking up during the night and having difficulty falling asleep again. *Terminal insomnia* refers to waking at the end of the night and being unable to return to sleep. Also reported is **hypersomnia**, in which the person sleeps for prolonged nighttime periods as well as during the day.

Fatigue and decreased energy are characteristic symptoms of depression, a condition known as **anergy.** Individuals report being tired upon awakening, regardless of how long they have slept. Even the smallest task seems insurmountable, and routine activities require substantial effort and take longer to accomplish. Decreased energy may be manifested in **psychomotor retardation,** in which thinking and body movements are noticeably slowed and speech is slowed or absent. Psychomotor agitation also may occur in which the person cannot sit still, paces, wrings hands, and picks at the fingernails, skin, clothing, bedclothes, or other objects.

Other common symptoms in significantly depressed individuals include guilt or a sense of worthlessness, self-blame, impaired concentration and decision making ability, even about trivial things, and suicidal ideation.

Becky is a 26-year-old insurance underwriter who was seen by the family planning nurse in a local Planned Parenthood clinic for a yearly checkup and Pap test. During the examination, she asked whether she might be anemic because she was "just exhausted all the time." Becky revealed that for the past month she had had difficulty getting out of bed in the morning. Getting dressed and ready for work left her drained. She described standing in front of her closet for long periods, unable to decide what to wear. She was also having extreme difficulty calling on potential clients. Whereas she was normally an assertive salesperson who called on perfect strangers with ease, she now described sitting at her desk for hours, trying to work up the motivation to pick up the phone. Coworkers, including her boss, had commented on her 7-lb weight gain, and these comments precipitated several uncharacteristic angry and tearful outbursts at work.

See the box on the next page for the DSM-IV criteria for a major depressive episode.

Dysthymic Disorder

A diagnosis of **dysthymic disorder** requires a chronically depressed mood for the majority of most days for at least 2 years (1 year for children and adolescents). There should have been no symptom-free interval of longer than 2 months. Symptoms in dysthymic disorder tend to be less severe than those in major depressive disorder, and there are fewer physiologic symptoms (disturbed sleep, problems with appetite, weight loss or gain, and psychomotor retardation and agitation).

Dysthymic disorder tends to predispose people to the development of major depressive disorder. According to the *DSM-IV,* 10% of individuals diagnosed with dysthymic disorder will develop major depressive disorder within the next year.

Dysthymic disorder often occurs in childhood, adolescence, or early adulthood and tends toward a chronic course. While both females and males are equally affected as children, in adults there are two to three times as many females as males with dysthymic disorder. The lifetime risk of developing dysthymic disorder is approximately 6% in the general population.

The symptoms of dysthymic disorder are similar to those of chronic major depressive disorder. This makes it difficult, even for experienced clinicians, to make an accurate differential diagnosis. Dysthymic disorder is mentioned here because you may read or hear of this diagnosis and should know what it means. In clinical practice, however, nursing care of the dysthymic client is similar to that of any depressed client.

Gregory G is a 14-year-old who was brought to a nurse psychotherapist by his mother upon the suggestion of the guidance counselor in his private school. In the letter of referral, the counselor stated that she was concerned because of Gregory's "persistent pessimistic outlook on life."

According to Mrs G, who interviewed alone, Gregory has always been a cranky and irritable child. Since starting kindergarten, he has had difficulty relating to other children and is often left out of activities and social invitations. At home, he stays in his room much of the time, where he plays computer games and writes poetry. He does not do well in school, although testing has shown him to be far above average in intelligence. Despite their best efforts, his parents have never been able to interest him in scouting, sports, or other activities they deem appropriate for a boy his age. His parents reported that Gregory's weight, eating habits, and sleeping patterns were unchanged.

When Gregory was interviewed, he responded in monosyllables, made poor eye contact with the therapist, and sat slumped in his chair with no facial expression. He stated that he knew his parents were "disappointed" in him.

Bipolar Disorders

The **bipolar disorders** are a group of mood disorders that include manic episodes, mixed episodes, depressed episodes, and cyclothymic disorder. Bipolar disorders tend to be recurrent, decreasing in frequency as the individual ages. Most clients return to normal functioning during remissions, but approximately 20–30% have chronic mood and interpersonal difficulties.

Manic Episodes

Mania is characterized by an abnormal and persistently elevated, expansive, or irritable mood lasting at least one week, significantly impairing social or occupational functioning, and generally requiring hospitalization. This disturbance in mood must be accompanied by at least three additional symptoms such as "inflated self-esteem or **grandiosity**, decreased need for sleep, pressure of speech, **flight of ideas**, distractibility, increased involvement in goal-directed activities or psychomotor agitation, and

Diagnostic Criteria for Major Depressive Episode

A. Five (or more) of the following symptoms have been present during the same 2-week period and represent a change from previous functioning; at least one of the symptoms is either (1) depressed mood or (2) loss of interest or pleasure. **Note:** Do not include symptoms that are clearly due to a general medical condition, or mood-incongruent delusions or hallucinations.

1. depressed mood most of the day, nearly every day, as indicated by either subjective report (e.g., feels sad or empty) or observation made by others (e.g., appears tearful). **Note:** in children and adolescents, can be irritable mood.
2. markedly diminished interest or pleasure in all, or almost all, activities most of the day, nearly every day (as indicated by either subjective account or observation made by others)
3. significant weight loss when not dieting or weight gain (e.g., a change or more than 5% of body weight in a month), or decrease or increase in appetite nearly every day. **Note:** In children, consider failure to make expected weight gains.
4. insomnia or hypersomnia nearly every day
5. psychomotor agitation or retardation nearly every day (observable by others, not merely subjective feelings of restlessness or being slowed down)
6. fatigue or loss of energy nearly every day
7. feelings of worthlessness or excessive or inappropriate guilt (which may be delusional) nearly every day (not merely self-reproach or guilt about being sick)
8. diminished ability to think or concentrate, or indecisiveness, nearly every day (either by subjective account or as observed by others)
9. recurrent thoughts of death (not just fear of dying), recurrent suicidal ideation without a specific plan, or a suicide attempt or a specific plan for committing suicide

B. The symptoms do not meet criteria for a Mixed Episode.

C. The symptoms cause clinically significant distress or impairment in social, occupational, or other important areas of functioning.

D. The symptoms are not due to the direct physiological effects of a substance (e.g., a drug abuse, a medication) or a general medical condition (e.g., hypothyroidism).

E. The symptoms are not better accounted for by Bereavement, i.e., after the loss of a loved one, the symptoms persist for longer than 2 months or are characterized by marked functional impairment, morbid preoccupation with worthlessness, suicidal ideation, psychotic symptoms, or psychomotor retardation.

Source: American Psychiatric Association 1994, p. 327.

excessive involvement in pleasurable activities with a high potential for painful consequences" (APA 1994, p. 328). Psychotic symptoms, such as delusions or hallucinations, may be a feature of severe mania.

Hypomania is a less extreme form of mania that is not severe enough to markedly impair functioning or require hospitalization. Individuals experiencing hypomania will feel wonderful, "on top of the world," and will not recognize changes in themselves. Those who know the person well, however, will be aware of the changes in mood and behavior. There are no psychotic features in hypomania.

The onset of manic episodes is usually in the early twenties but may begin at any time. It often follows a severe disappointment, embarrassment, or other psychic stressor.

The mood of clients experiencing a manic episode is euphoric or "high." Their behavior is excessive and out of bounds. It is characterized by overly enthusiastic involvement in projects of an interpersonal, political, religious, or occupational nature. When thwarted, they become irritable, and their moods alternate between euphoria and irritability. Increased sexual behaviors are often seen. Woman may dress in an uncharacteristically flashy or seductive manner and wear garish makeup. Speech is pressured, and racing thoughts or flight of ideas are often present. Grandiosity can reach delusional proportions. These clients rarely believe they are sick, even when they get into financial or legal trouble, and may vehemently protest treatment.

Mr. Gray, a 52-year-old engineer, was brought to the emergency psychiatric clinic by two adult sons at 2:00 AM. Their mother had called them to come help with their father, who had not slept in three days. When they arrived at their parents'

home, they found their father working in the backyard on a large landscaping project involving stonework, a waterfall, fishpond, and extensive plantings of trees, shrubs, and flowers. According to the sons, Mr. Gray had three prior episodes of manic behavior, beginning when he was in the Army many years earlier. He was stabilized on lithium carbonate for years, but stopped taking it about a year ago because he felt so good. The current episode began about one week ago after he was passed over for a promotion at work. He then took a leave of absence from his job to create what he called "the world's first home-based theme park." Any attempt by his wife to talk him out of the project was met with anger and renewed resolve. Mr. Gray angrily told the admitting nurse, "I don't know why these boys brought me here. I need to get back to work! I'm going to get millions for this franchise."

See the accompanying box below for the DSM-IV criteria for manic episode.

Mixed Episodes

In a **mixed episode**, symptoms of both mania and depression are present nearly every day in rapidly alternating succession over a period of at least a week. These clients are often agitated, suffering from insomnia and appetite disturbances, and may exhibit suicidal and psychotic thinking. They may have recently had a manic episode or a major depressive episode, although this is not always the case. Because the depressive symptoms are part of the clinical picture, they suffer more psychic pain than do individuals who are in a state of mania and may seek help more readily.

Mrs. Kent is a 32-year-old high school teacher who was readmitted to the psychiatric unit 2 weeks after she was discharged following 3 weeks of treatment for a major depressive episode. Her husband described her recent behavior as being extremely unstable, with rapidly alternating moods. "She is driving herself and me crazy, crying and talking about killing herself one day and out shopping for a new, glitzy wardrobe the next. She tried to go back to work right after she got out of the hospital the first time, but the principal put her on a leave of absence until the end of the year. He said she made a pass at him and was behaving flirtatiously toward the coaches and even some of her students."

Depressed Episodes

A diagnosis of bipolar disorder does not always mean that manic or hypomanic behaviors will be manifested in the

Diagnostic Criteria for Manic Episode

A. A distinct period of abnormally and persistently elevated, expansive, or irritable mood, lasting at least 1 week (or any duration if hospitalization is necessary).

B. During the period of mood disturbance, three (or more) of the following symptoms have persisted (four if the mood is only irritable) and have been present to a significant degree:
   1. inflated self-esteem or grandiosity
   2. decreased need for sleep (e.g., feels rested after only 3 hours of sleep)
   3. more talkative than usual or pressure to keep talking
   4. flight of ideas or subjective experience that thoughts are racing
   5. distractibility (i.e., attention too easily drawn to unimportant or irrelevant external stimuli)
   6. increase in goal-directed activity (either socially, at work or school, or sexually) or psychomotor agitation
   7. excessive involvement in pleasurable activities that have a high potential for painful consequences (e.g., engaging in unrestrained buying sprees, sexual indiscretions, or foolish business investments)

C. The symptoms do not meet criteria for a Mixed Episode.

D. The mood disturbance is sufficiently severe to cause marked impairment in occupational functioning or in usual social activities or relationships with others, or to necessitate hospitalization to prevent harm to self or others, or there are psychotic features.

E. The symptoms are not due to the direct physiological effects of a substance (e.g., a drug of abuse, a medication, or other treatment) or a general medical condition (e.g., hyperthyroidism)

Note: Manic-like episodes that are clearly caused by somatic antidepressant treatment (e.g., medication, electroconvulsive therapy, light therapy) should not count toward a diagnosis of Bipolar I Disorder.

Source: American Psychiatric Association 1994, p. 332.

current illness. There are several types of bipolar disorders in which manic or hypomanic episodes have occurred in the past, but the features of the current episode are purely depressive. Treatment of these depressed bipolar disorders is similar to treatment of any depression, with the possible exception of pharmacologic treatment.

Cyclothymic Disorder

When clients have suffered for at least 2 years from "chronic, fluctuating mood disturbances involving numerous periods of hypomanic symptoms and numerous periods of depressive symptoms," they are diagnosed with **cyclothymic disorder** (APA 1994, p. 363). They must be free of severe symptoms that qualify for the diagnosis of manic disorder or major depressive disorder. These individuals are often considered to be moody, unpredictable, or temperamental, and they may go on to develop an overlay of symptoms that are of major depressive or manic intensity.

Cyclothymic disorder begins early, usually in adolescence or early adulthood. Although not common, with a lifetime risk of only 0.4–1% of the general population, it is thought to predispose the person to other mood disorders. The incidence is approximately equal between males and females.

Other Mood Disorders

It is widely recognized that mood disorders may be manifestations of physiologic conditions, such as hepatitis or thyrotoxicosis. Mood disorders may also be induced by substance abuse, such as cocaine or amphetamines, prescribed medications, such as antihypertensives or oral contraceptives, or toxins, such as lead or carbon monoxide. Practitioners should carefully evaluate the general medical condition of clients before making a diagnosis of mood disorder.

Biopsychosocial Theories

People with certain personality types or temperaments are more prone than others to develop depressive and elated behaviors. Significant efforts have been devoted to identifying a single psychologic factor, trait, or mechanism that is unique to the development of mood disorders.

Research exploring the causative factors of mood disorders has focused on reactions to early separation from parents or parental loss, early mother-child relationships, and other aspects of human development and experience. To date, no single personality type, trait, or constellation of experiences has been established to account for all forms of mood disorders. In attempting to understand the major mood disorders, nurses must consider a variety of hypotheses dealing with the multiple complex factors contributing to their development.

Psychoanalytic Theory

The psychoanalytic theory of depression was originally formulated by Freud and later refined by others. It focuses on an unsatisfactory early mother-infant relationship as the primary factor predisposing individuals to later depression. If an infant's needs go unmet, a sense of loss occurs. Unresolved grief over the loss results in anger turned inward and the development of self-hate. The child's ego development is thereby adversely affected, resulting in a weak ego and an overdeveloped, punitive superego.

The psychoanalytic school of thought suggests a different etiology for bipolar disorder. This theory holds that the mother/primary caregiver derives pleasure from the infant's early dependence but feels threatened by increasing autonomy as the child develops. Independent behaviors are considered "bad," and the child must suppress his or her needs in order to sustain parental affection. Ambivalence resulting from the coexisting desires to please the parents and become more autonomous causes resentment and leads to a love-hate relationship with the parenting figures. Again, a weak ego and punitive superego create depression. Mania is seen as the denial of depression taken to the extreme (Kaplan and Sadock 1989).

Cognitive Theory

Cognitive theorists, such as Beck et al. (1961), believe that depression results from impaired cognition, or thinking processes. People who think negative thoughts evaluate themselves critically. They feel inadequate and hopeless about the future. Beck and his colleagues designed the Beck Depression Inventory, a clinical assessment tool. It asks clients to rate themselves on 21 groups of questions designed to detect negative thinking. Cognitive therapy seeks to teach individuals how to stop negative thinking and replace it with more positive self-appraisals.

Bowen's Family Systems Theory

Dr. Murray Bowen (1978) was a pioneer in the family movement, which seeks to understand human behavior through understanding the entire family as a system. A key feature of family systems theory is the multigenerational nature of family patterns and processes. In other words, it is necessary to understand the "emotional baggage" carried by husband and wife from their own families of origin in order to begin to understand their current patterns of relating to each other and their children.

In Bowen's family systems theory, anxiety is seen as the response of an organism to stress. If anxiety is too great for an individual's usual anxiety-management techniques to work, it may become chronic. When anxiety is chronic, tension builds in the individual or in the individual's relationships. Tension precipitates symptoms, such as those seen in mood disorders.

Learning Theory

Seligman (1974) proposed that learning plays an instrumental role in the development of depression. His theory of **learned helplessness** holds that depression is based on the person's belief that he or she has no control over life situations. This conclusion is drawn from repeated failures, either real or perceived, to control life events. The result is that the individual gives up, stops trying to control, becomes dependent on others, and is predisposed to depression.

Object Loss Theory

In Bowlby's (1973) **object loss theory** of depression, the forced, often traumatic separation from, or abandonment of an infant by, the primary caregiver during the first 6 months of life plays a major role. Separation interrupts the bonding process that is so essential to the later development of relationships, and the child withdraws from other people and the environment. This establishes a pattern of anxiety, grief, helplessness, and hopelessness. Once the pattern is established, the individual uses these behaviors to deal with all subsequent losses, whether of major or minor magnitude. Such people feel helpless in coping effectively with the normal ups and downs of life and assume a hopeless, depressed attitude.

Biologic Theories

The most promising findings about the causes of mood disorders today are emerging from studies of biologic factors. Research on the physiologic basis for depression has been under way for more than 30 years and has generated a variety of hypotheses.

GENETIC THEORIES Numerous studies have concentrated on the role heredity plays in depressive illness. Interest in this field of research was stimulated by the observation that the incidence of depression is higher among relatives of depressed individuals than in the general population. Studies of illness rates within and between generations of families, of monozygotic and dizygotic twins, of the general population, and those using known genetic markers such as blood type or color blindness all support the genetic transmission of depression.

Studies have demonstrated that bipolar disorder is also increased among first-degree relatives of individuals with that disorder. Kolata's 1987 study of identical twins reported an 80% concordance rate in bipolar disorder. This means that if one twin has the disorder, there is an 80% chance that the other twin will also develop it.

The role of genetics in the development of major mood disorders is complicated by the familiar question: Which plays the more important role, genes or environment? People who are biologically related tend to spend time together and influence one another's thinking. It is therefore difficult to determine the relative weight of genetics, thinking patterns, family relationships, and learning in the development of mood disorders.

BIOCHEMICAL THEORIES More than 30 years ago, Gibbons (1960) established that an error in metabolism results in an electrolyte imbalance that seems to play a role in depression. He established that sodium and potassium were transposed in the neurons of depressed individuals. This transposition alters the sensitivity of the neuronal cell membranes. Alterations in sensitivity of neuronal receptors is likely to lead to alterations in behavior. This may account for the efficacy of drugs, such as **lithium carbonate** and antidepressants, in the treatment of mood disorders.

Scientific research has focused on the role of certain chemicals, the neurotransmitters in the central nervous system. They are responsible for the transmission of nervous impulses. Levels of these biogenic amines—norepinephrine (NE), serotonin (5-HT), acetylcholine (Ach), and dopamine (DA)—are deficient in depressed people (Janowsky 1988) and elevated in individuals experiencing manic episodes.

The metabolism of the neurotransmitter serotonin (5-HT) has been studied extensively in recent years. Dysfunction of certain serotonergic neurons has been linked with depression. This finding led to the development of antidepressant drugs.

Psychoendocrinology is the study of the relationship between endocrine function and psychological state. It has long been observed that increases and decreases in hormone levels affect mood. Many women, for example, report a worsening of their depressive symptoms in the days before the onset of menstruation. Other biologic factors, such as neurophysiologic alterations and autonomic nervous system impairments, have also been studied extensively.

Biochemical theories are inconclusive and controversial. The difficulty is determining whether biochemical changes *cause* depression or *result from* depression. Although researchers have yet to resolve this chicken-or-egg question, they are optimistic about advancing the accuracy and effectiveness of diagnosis and treatment of mood disorders through biochemical research.

BIOLOGICAL RHYTHMS It is widely recognized that we have self-sustained internal physiological cycles that occur every 24 hours. These **circadian rhythms**, which include body temperature, sleep, and appetite, are activated, controlled, and integrated by the hypothalamus in the brain. The central controlling pacemaker is commonly known as the biological clock.

Researchers have described diurnal variations in mood, rest and activity cycles, EEG patterns, and neuroendocrine secretions. Circadian rhythm dysfunction can explain a number of mood disorder symptoms, such as insomnia, hypersomnia, early morning awakening, and variations in appetite, rest, and activity cycles.

Animal studies have demonstrated that alcohol and antimanic drugs, such as lithium, slow the biological clock, while estrogen and tricyclic antidepressants accelerate it or restore normal rhythms. Observations of animals and humans in carefully controlled environments have led to a hypothesis that bipolar disorder is a disorder of the kinetics of bodily functioning (Wehr 1977).

SEASONAL AFFECTIVE DISORDER Natural light is frequently taken for granted, but it influences the human experience in ways of which most people are unaware. As early as the days of Hippocrates, observers of human behavior noticed that some people suffer mood changes as the seasons change.

The relationships between light, biological rhythms, and mood are the subject of a great deal of current scientific study. This research focuses on the use of light in the treatment of **Seasonal Affective Disorder (SAD)**, a depressive disorder that occurs in relation to the seasons, usually during winter months. Natural light may help modulate daily rhythms that influence sleep and activity patterns, neuroendocrine functions, and brain chemical systems.

Research studies have explored the application of different forms of ultraviolet light to the skin and eyes at different times of day with mixed results. The exact relationship between light, biological rhythms, and events at the cellular level have yet to be determined.

Psychologic Factors

All people, regardless of personality patterns, can and do become depressed. Mild depression is widely acknowledged as a part of the human experience.

Although most of us have had "the blues" from time to time, it is widely believed that certain people are more prone to developing true depression than others. Individuals who exhibit certain traits—such as low self-esteem; lack of personal goals and direction; dependence and passivity in interpersonal relationships; a limited ability to form enduring, mature relationships; and internalization of blame—are thought to be at risk for the development of depressive disorders (Kaplan and Sadock 1989).

Sociocultural Factors

Most clinical investigators believe that life events and environmental stress play a role in mood disorders. There is less agreement, however, as to whether life events play a primary role or merely contribute to the onset of an inevitable episode of a mood disorder. Certain events, such as the death of a loved one, divorce, and other losses are widely recognized by both mental health professionals and the general public as precipitating events in depression. The unremitting stresses of living in poverty, and society's devaluation of the disadvantaged, also seem to predispose people to developing depression (Warren 1994).

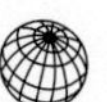

Culture exerts a powerful influence on how individuals experience and communicate psychic distress. Some cultures experience depression largely in somatic terms. Nurses should be alert to complaints of headaches or "nerves" in Hispanic clients, of weakness or "imbalance" in Asian clients, and of bodily metaphors involving the heart in Middle Eastern and certain Native American clients. These may be culturally determined ways of expressing depression.

Be aware of the unique needs of clients who are likely to perceive the meaning and severity of psychiatric symptoms in relation to the norms of their cultural reference group. They include new immigrants to this country, individuals who are still heavily involved in the culture of origin, those who do not speak English, and those whose entire network of social and religious support remains embedded in the culture of origin.

Differences in culture and social status of clients and caregivers can create problems in diagnosis and treatment. Language differences, for example, create barriers in forming therapeutic relationships, while cultural differences in the expression of symptoms make it difficult to determine whether a behavior is normal or pathological (Pachter 1994).

The Nursing Process and Clients with Major Depressive Disorder

Nursing care of clients with mood disorders follows a problem solving model you are already accustomed to using, the nursing process.

Assessment

As already discussed, depression is characterized by low mood, often related to a loss. The loss may be concrete, such as the loss of a loved one or a job, or perceived, such as the loss of a cherished wish or disillusionment with a respected role model.

SUBJECTIVE DATA Clients with depressive disorders may express some of the following:

- Feelings of sadness
- Fatigue
- Lack of interest in relationships and activities that were previously pleasurable
- Feelings of worthlessness
- Impaired concentration
- Impaired decision-making ability
- Sleep disturbances
- Loss of appetite; weight loss
- Excessive sleep
- Increased appetite; weight gain

Clients will often describe how long it takes them to complete activities that formerly were easily accomplished, such as preparing a simple meal. Tearfulness and emotional outbursts may also be a part of their description of the problem. They may or may not mention a loss or disappointment that they relate to the feelings.

Somatic Concerns Somatic concerns are often the presenting complaint. Depressed clients may complain of abdominal pains, headaches, and vague bodily aches. A problem with sexual functioning or lack of desire may also be a presenting complaint. Constipation is a common result of the general slowing of metabolism due to inactivity.

Suicide Assessment All clients who describe depressive symptoms should be assessed for suicide risk by direct questioning. Nurses should inquire about suicidal thinking, history of suicide attempts, and whether the client has a specific suicide plan. This aspect of assessment is reassuring, not alarming, to clients. Ask clients direct questions about suicidal thinking, history of suicide attempts, and whether they have specific suicide plans. You might ask, for example, "Tell me how you plan to kill yourself. Do you have the gun/pills/poison?" It is important to know whether the client has actually planned the suicide or if it is a vaguely formed thought. The more organized the plan is the more concern it generates, particularly if the client has access to a lethal weapon, chemical, or other means of self-injury.

Other aspects of suicide will be discussed more fully later in this chapter under the heading "Promoting Client Safety."

OBJECTIVE DATA Depressed clients are most likely to be females under the age of 40. They often have had prior episodes of depression and a family history of depression or bipolar disorder. A history of a recent stressful event and the lack of social support are also common features.

Objective signs and symptoms of depression are few. Psychomotor agitation or retardation may be observable if it is profound or if the nurse is familiar with the client's usual level of functioning. Family members may report observations of the client's agitation or apathy and lack of pleasure in usual activities. They may describe a pattern of social withdrawal and lack of social participation, combined with an intense preoccupation with the client's own feelings.

During assessment, many clinicians find it useful to provide a list of symptoms and ask clients to check the ones they are experiencing. Examples of self-reporting instruments designed to assess mood state include the Beck Depression Inventory (Beck et al. 1961), the Zung scale (Zung 1965), and the AUSSI scale (Parker et al. 1994), which measures both mood state and social impairment.

Other objective information to obtain during the nursing assessment includes concurrent general medical illnesses and concurrent substance use and abuse. Autoimmune, neurologic, metabolic, oncologic, and endocrine disorders often trigger depression. For example, hypothyroidism may be accompanied by depressive symptoms due to the underlying medical disease, while a client with AIDS or cancer may become depressed as a result of the diagnosis, prognosis, or disability connected with the disease.

Alcohol, which is a CNS depressant, and certain legal and illegal drugs can cause or complicate depression. A complete list of all substances and medications used by the client should be obtained through matter-of-fact questioning. A few prescription medications have depression as a side effect, and these should not be overlooked in the complete assessment. Birth control pills, sedatives, reserpine, glucocorticoids, and anabolic steroids have all been associated with the development of depression.

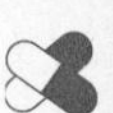

There are currently no laboratory tests specific for depression, but abnormal findings on several tests have been noted in depressed clients. Sleep EEG abnormalities are found in 40–60% of outpatients with major depressive episode and in up to 90% of inpatients. Neurotransmitter levels in blood, cerebrospinal fluid, or urine are often abnormal, as are **dexamethasone suppression tests** and other neuroendocrine challenges. Some of these findings precede the development of clinical depression and persist following remission (APA 1994).

Nursing Diagnosis

The following sections discuss the implications of several nursing diagnoses commonly seen in depressed clients.

RISK FOR SELF-DIRECTED VIOLENCE As mentioned earlier, depressed clients often experience thoughts about or impulses toward self-harm. These thoughts and impulses are related to feelings of worthlessness, feelings of guilt, repeated failure experiences, feelings of helplessness and hopelessness, or psychotic thinking.

Suicidal clients should be hospitalized on either a general or a specialized hospital unit. Regardless of setting, whenever a client is at high risk for self-harm, that becomes *the* priority nursing diagnosis, and client safety becomes the most important aspect of nursing care.

SELF-ESTEEM DISTURBANCE Depressed clients often express, either directly or indirectly, negative feelings about themselves and their abilities. Reduced self-esteem may be related to a variety of factors, including feeling abandoned by loved ones, experiencing repeated failures or losses, lacking positive feedback from others, thinking negative thoughts, engaging in negative "self-talk," or feeling guilty over real or perceived transgressions.

Evidence of low self-esteem is seen in clients who withdraw from social interaction; have difficulty accepting compliments or positive feedback; are harshly critical of themselves or others; are reluctant to try new activities because of fear of failure; express feelings of inferiority, worthlessness, and pessimism about the future; are overly sensitive to criticism; see social slights where none are intended; or set unrealistic goals and engage in grandiose thinking (denial of low self-esteem).

POWERLESSNESS Individuals who have led lives characterized by helplessness believe that their own actions cannot significantly influence an outcome. This is related to their consistent dependence on others to meet their needs and a resulting perception of lack of control. They come to doubt their own abilities and may be criticized by others for their passivity.

Evidence of powerlessness is seen in the behavior of clients who refuse to engage in self-care, do not participate in decision making, verbally express a lack of control and doubts about their abilities, and are reluctant to express feelings because they fear being rejected by caregivers.

SOCIAL ISOLATION Low self-esteem and doubts about abilities lead many depressed clients to withdraw socially. Because inadequate social skills and self-absorption create impediments to positive interpersonal relationships, clients with low self-esteem frequently *are* avoided by others. This further reinforces their fears of undesirability and increases their social isolation. Evidence of social isolation and impaired social interaction is seen in behaviors such as spending inordinate amounts of time in bed, lack of verbalization, lack of eye contact, dull or monosyllabic responses to others' attempts at conversation, a preference for being alone, turning away or closing the eyes, and exhibiting discomfort in the presence of others.

Planning and Implementing Interventions

When planning and implementing interventions designed to help clients suffering from depression, keep two general principles in mind. First, it is impossible to make depressed people feel better by being cheerful. In fact, an overly cheerful attitude tends to make them feel even worse because it belittles their feelings. Try to adopt a more emotionally neutral attitude while maintaining confidence that they will feel better. Second, recognize that working with depressed people may eventually make you feel depressed yourself. Stay in touch with your own feelings. If you find yourself getting down, assert yourself by asking to be assigned to a different type of client for a time.

PROMOTING CLIENT SAFETY There are few times when "always" and "never" apply. Client safety, however, *always* takes priority over other nursing care concerns. When the risk for self-directed violence is high, a number of actions call for immediate intervention. Evaluate suicide level of intent regularly, and institute the appropriate level of staff supervision.

Suicidal clients need to know that the environment is safe for them. Reassure them by removing sharp objects, razors, breakable glass items, mirrors, matches, and straps or belts. Explain why these objects are being removed. Place suicidal clients in a centrally located room near the nurses' station to facilitate ease of observation. Avoid establishing a predictable pattern of observation during the day and especially at night. Be particularly alert during change of shifts, on holidays or other times when staffing is limited, and during times of distraction, such as mealtimes and visiting hours.

The no-suicide contract is a useful intervention, and it is discussed in detail in Chapter 24. Encourage clients to seek you or another staff member when bothered by suicidal thoughts or impulses. Discussing these thoughts and impulses may be sufficient to diminish them and prevent a suicidal crisis from occurring. Avoid discussing suicidal ruminations in repetitious detail, however, since this may reinforce maladaptive behavior.

Encourage discussing all feelings. Clients need to know that all feelings are valid and that it benefits them to express their emotions, particularly anger and hopelessness, rather than acting them out through maladaptive behaviors. Assist in the transition from hospital to home by helping clients identify people in their usual environments to whom they can express feelings candidly without being judged.

Collaborate with clients to identify community resources to which they can turn if suicidal thoughts recur outside the hospital. Almost all communities have access to hotlines that are staffed around the clock with trained volunteers or professionals who are available to discuss feelings before they reach crisis proportions. Be aware that the risk of suicide increases as the severest stage of depression is alleviated, because clients then have sufficient energy and cognitive ability to plan and successfully implement a suicide plan.

Promoting Improved Self-Esteem While low self-esteem is a chronic problem, there are a number of things nurses can do to reduce negative thinking, thereby promoting improved self-esteem.

- Provide distraction from self-absorption by involving the client in recreational activities and pleasant pastimes. Simple conversation with a staff member or another client helps interrupt the pattern of negative thoughts. Use care to select activities that are not too complex for the client's current level of functioning. Experiences of success, not more failures, are needed. Increase complexity of activities as the client progresses.
- Dispel the notion clients often have that when they feel better, they will want to engage in activities. Explain that they must begin doing things *in order* to feel better. Be sure to acknowledge that it takes self-discipline and energy to do something when one doesn't really feel like it.
- Recognize accomplishment; do not use flattery or excessive praise. Give positive, matter-of-fact reinforcement, like "I notice that you have combed your hair," rather than overly enthusiastic insincerity, such as "What a great hairstyle!" Appropriate recognition will increase the likelihood that the client will continue the positive behavior, while insincerity can be perceived as ridicule.
- Help clients identify their personal strengths. It may be useful to write these down. Recognize that it often takes some time for clients with low self-esteem to realize that they even have strengths. Avoid the temptation to point out characteristics you have noticed. It is far more useful for you to be supportively expectant of their ability to recognize their own positive qualities.
- Be accepting of clients' negative feelings, but set limits on the amount of time you will listen to accounts of past failures. Be alert for opportunities to interrupt the negative conversational patterns with more neutral ones.
- Teach assertiveness techniques, such as the ability to say "No" to protect one's own rights while respecting the rights of others. Clients with low self-esteem often allow others to take advantage of them. Defining passive, aggressive, and assertive behavior and giving examples of each are also helpful when teaching assertiveness (see the Client/Family Teaching box on page 334). Encourage clients and their family members to practice the new techniques in their relationship with you, so you can give feedback on how it feels to the recipient.

Promoting Feelings of Control Clients who feel they lack control over important aspects of their lives tend to form dependent relationships. Be aware of this tendency, and work from the first contact to minimize the likelihood that maladaptive dependence occurs in the nurse-client relationship. Emphasizing the short-term nature of the relationship is essential. If the client singles out one staff member exclusively and refuses to relate to others, this is a clue that undue dependence is developing.

Avoid giving dependent clients the hope that the nurse-client relationship can continue after the end of therapy. Kindly but firmly refuse requests for your address or telephone number, and remind clients that contact following discharge will not be allowed. If you find yourself wanting to continue relationships with certain clients, discuss these feelings with your instructor, a respected peer, or supervisor. It is essential to separate your professional life from your social life.

Provide clients with responsibility and choices in the planning of their own care. For example, allow a client to choose whether to bathe in the morning or at night, or to choose from a short list of activities to attend.

Engage clients in setting goals they hope to achieve during hospitalization or outpatient therapy. Remember that unrealistically optimistic goals will ensure another failure experience and reinforce the client's sense of powerlessness. Make sure goals are attainable.

Clients who feel powerless also need help in identifying ways to gain a sense of control in their relationships and lives outside the hospital. Collaborate with clients to identify changes they wish to make and action steps toward achieving them. Make the steps small and manageable. Accomplishment of even small steps leads to a sense of mastery and control.

Teach clients problem-solving techniques, and encourage them to use them when confronting life situations. For example, if a client has difficulty paying rent, help him or her identify options, such as moving to a less expensive apartment or taking in a roommate. Explore the pros and cons of each option and the possible consequences. Emphasize confidence in the client's ability to identify, select, and carry out problem-solving activities that will result in a greater sense of control in his or her life.

Equally important is to help clients identify the aspects of their lives that are not within their control. The ability to accept what *cannot* be changed is just as essential as developing the ability to bring about positive change.

Planning for discharge should begin with the first client contact and is particularly important with powerless, dependent clients. Help them to identify resources in the community and to build support systems. Support

CLIENT/FAMILY TEACHING

Assertive Communication

Assertiveness is learned behavior. Everyone has assertiveness potential, but we aren't born knowing how to be assertive. Children learn patterns of communicating from the adults around them. You can unlearn communication patterns if they aren't working and learn new ones and that is what assertiveness training is all about. The goal is helping people express themselves without fear of disapproval from others. Being assertive does not guarantee that others will always agree with you, but you do have the satisfaction of giving your opinion.

Definitions

Aggressive behavior is directed toward getting what one wants without considering the feelings of others. Aggressive communicators want to get their own way at any cost. They want others to "back off" and use intimidation to convey this message. An example of aggressive behavior is insisting on going to a certain movie even though you know your companion does not enjoy that type of movie. The outcome of aggressive behavior is that although you may get what you want in the short run, others feel discredited and tend to avoid you.

Passive behavior consists of avoiding conflict at any cost, even at the expense of one's own happiness. An example of passive behavior is agreeing to go to a movie you don't want to see because your friend pressures you to go. Passive communicators hold their feelings in and allow anger to build up. Anger can come out suddenly in an explosion or can be expressed in what is known as passive-aggressive behavior. An example of passive-aggressive behavior is taking a long time to get ready to go out while your friend is waiting because you are angry at him for insisting on seeing a movie you don't want to see. The outcome is that the passive person gives up control and is left with resentment, which usually emerges in other ways that damage relationships.

Assertive behavior consists of expressing one's wishes and opinions, or taking care of oneself, but not at the expense of others. An example of assertive communication is saying, "I really don't care for violent movies. Let's look at the movie listings and see if there is something playing that we can both enjoy." The outcome of assertive behavior is self-confidence and self-esteem.

Ways of Becoming More Assertive

1. Recognize your usual patterns. Are you passive, aggressive, or assertive in dealing with others?

2. Deliberately work on changing your pattern of thinking. Assertive people do not respond automatically; they take time to look at the situation and plan their responses. Don't be pressured into a quick decision. Instead say, "I want some time to think about it."

groups, therapy groups, and social groups, such as Parents Without Partners, can all help clients separate from caregivers more readily when the time comes to end therapy (see the Research Note on page 336).

Promoting Social Interaction When designing interventions for promoting social interactions, realize that both the quality and the quantity of a client's social behavior may be impaired. Early in the nurse-client relationship, make brief but frequent contacts with withdrawn clients, without making any demands. Your interest can increase a client's self-worth.

With extremely uncommunicative clients, simply spending time sitting quietly without any demand for interaction may be helpful. This approach communicates your belief that they are worth the investment of time. Nurses often find it difficult to be comfortable with silence, and they communicate that discomfort to clients. Remember that silence conveys acceptance and is a useful therapeutic communication technique.

When clients express feelings or cry, be nonjudgmental. Avoid showing surprise or disapproval. Recognize that ventilating feelings may provide temporary relief, particularly if anger is expressed. If clients are unable to verbalize feelings, they sometimes can act them out in safe and appropriate ways, such as tearing up an old magazine or beating on a pillow or bed. Provide privacy during these times.

Encourage both verbal and nonverbal expressions of feelings by teaching clients that these are healthy behaviors. This intervention reinforces your acceptance of clients as unique and valuable individuals. Avoid disagreeing with, or otherwise belittling, a client's feelings by using overly cheerful reassurances like, "Now, now Mrs. Hamilton. You're feeling down right now but you'll feel better after a good night's sleep."

CLIENT/FAMILY TEACHING *(continued)*

3. Don't feel guilty about your assertive behavior. Choose not to be responsible for others' feelings when you know your actions were reasonable.
4. Stand firm without precipitating an argument by using the "broken record" technique. This involves calmly repeating an assertive statement over and over. For example, you might say, "I really don't like violent movies," until your friend hears you.
5. Don't expect others to read your mind. This is an unrealistic expectation that ultimately will be destructive to your relationships. Instead, use assertive statements of feeling, such as, "Something is bothering me. I am feeling like my movie preferences don't matter."
6. Focus on remaining relaxed and calm. Breathe deeply, consciously relax your muscles, and speak in an even tone of voice. Make eye contact, and choose to remain in control of yourself.
7. Use "I" statements such as, "I am feeling on the spot. I want to have a nice evening with you, but I also want to see a movie I can enjoy." This expression of your own feelings and opinions helps the other person be nondefensive and listen to what you are saying instead of planning his response.
8. Use the "fogging" technique to respond to manipulative criticism. For example, if your friend says, "You're certainly being difficult tonight!" respond with, "I suppose I am." This sends a clear signal, "I'm not going to fight, and I'm not going to cave in, either."

Things to Keep in Mind

1. Don't expect too much too soon. Change comes slowly, with repeated practice. Be patient, and give yourself a chance.
2. Begin with small steps. What you need is a few successes to give you confidence. Go slowly and build a solid foundation.
3. Remember to give yourself credit when assertive behavior succeeds.
4. Ask for help when you need it. Seek qualified help, and state assertively what help you want. This may be an assertive friend, a teacher, or a counselor.
5. Remember that being assertive doesn't always work. Don't let setbacks stop you from trying.
6. Continue to learn about assertiveness. These books can be obtained through your local library: *Stand Up, Speak Out, Talk Back* by Robert E. Alberti and Michael L. Emmons; *When I Say No, I Feel Guilty* by Manuel J. Smith; and *Don't Say "Yes" When You Want To Say "No"* by Herbert Fensterheim and Jean Baer.

Once clients are comfortable interacting with one person, encourage group activities. Although this step may be difficult and frightening for clients, you can minimize their discomfort by attending activities with them at first. If their anxiety gets too uncomfortable, let them know that they can leave the situation without losing your approval. Give recognition for even small steps, gradually removing yourself and allowing them to stay in groups on their own.

Sometimes clients avoid social situations because they lack social skills and the self-confidence that they provide. Create opportunities for clients to learn social skills and practice them in a protected environment. For example, teach them to read the newspaper and select several items of interest to use in making "small talk." Demonstrate making small talk, and encourage them to practice with you. Give feedback on their progress. Make sure this is an enjoyable and nonthreatening activity.

Individuals who are either extremely passive or too aggressive in their social interactions are often avoided by others. Teaching such clients how to use assertive behavior can improve their interpersonal relationships. Use roleplaying to help them become comfortable with new skills. (Refer again to the Client/Family Teaching box).

Evaluation and Outcome Criteria

Specific client behaviors indicate that nursing interventions have been successful. Evaluation and outcome criteria answer the question, "How do we know that the depressed client's condition has improved?" Refer to the Critical Pathways on pages 337 and 342.

Safety The risk of self-directed violence is decreased when the client verbalizes no suicidal thoughts and commits no acts of self-violence. Clients who are not suicidal

RESEARCH NOTE

Citation

Maynard, CK: Comparison of effectiveness of group interventions for depression in women. *Arch Psychiatr Nurs* 1993; 7(5):277–283.

Study Problem/Purpose

Depression affects twice as many women as men. Treatment models that are cost-effective and available to more women are needed. The efficacy of a structured cognitive-behavioral group intervention designed by V. Gordon to reduce depression among women was tested.

Methods

Thirty-four women age 18–65 were enrolled in the study. All were able to read and speak English, not chronically ill or physically handicapped, and not seeing a mental health therapist. All participants were white, middle-class, and well-educated. The study used an experimental three-group pretest-posttest design. One group received an intervention based on Gordon's structured approach, one group received a supportive group approach, and the third group was untreated.

Findings

The participants in Gordon's structured, nurse-facilitated group had significant reductions in depression, hopelessness, and anxiety, as well as a significant increase in self-esteem. No significant changes occurred in any of these variables in the support or untreated groups. Further research involving women from different cultural and socioeconomic backgrounds is needed.

Implications

Women are more likely than men to be economically disadvantaged and may not be able to afford psychiatric care. It is therefore incumbent upon nurses to find ways of offering widely available, effective, and cost-conscious treatment modes to women seeking care. Although findings are preliminary and require further research and clarification, the results of this study deserve the attention of psychiatric nurses working with depressed women for several reasons. First, substantial savings can be realized by working with clients in groups rather than in individual therapy, and cost-effectiveness is an essential criterion in choosing treatment modalities in today's cost-conscious climate. Second, the use of a structured cognitive approach may prove more acceptable to potential clients than either a support group or a therapeutic group approach. Third, if this nurse-led treatment modality can be demonstrated as effective in reducing women's depression, hopelessness, and anxiety and in increasing their self-esteem in only 12 weeks, it can become a model that is far less expensive than either inpatient care or traditional one-to-one psychotherapy.

demonstrate the use of alternative ways of dealing with stress and emotional problems. They can verbalize names of resources where help is available if suicidal thoughts return following discharge.

Self-Esteem Clients who have improved levels of self-esteem can verbalize positive aspects of themselves and speak about increased feelings of self-worth. Their behaviors are consistent with increased self-esteem; for example, they groom and dress themselves with some care. They are able to express feelings directly and openly and to communicate assertively with others. They will express some optimism and hope for the future. Clients demonstrate self-esteem when they evaluate their own strengths realistically, set realistic goals for themselves, and work toward reaching them.

Control An increase in feelings of control is evidenced when clients verbalize elements of plans to attain control over life situations. They will also verbalize feelings about situations over which they have no control. They are able to describe a problem-solving system that they have successfully used and will use in the future when confronted with problem situations.

Social Interaction Improved social interactions are apparent when clients communicate and socialize with others. Voluntarily attending group activities is a measure of success. They can initiate interaction with another person appropriately and assume responsibility for dealing with feelings, including finding others with whom to talk. They plan for discharge by establishing or maintaining relationships, a social life, and a support system outside the hospital.

text continues on page 347

CRITICAL PATHWAY FOR A CLIENT WITH DEPRESSION WITHOUT PSYCHOTIC FEATURES OR AGITATION

Expected length of stay: 8 days

	Date ________ Day 1	Date ________ Days 2–3	Date ________ Day 4
Daily outcomes	Client will: • Remain free of self-inflicted injury. • Communicate suicidal ideation. • Contract for safety. • Identify initial goals for hospitalization. • Verbalize need for medications. • Remain oriented to time, place and person with prompting. • Participate in assessment. • Identify current dietary pattern and food preferences. • Identify current elimination pattern. • Identify recreation and leisure interest and capabilities. • Identify current self-care patterns including sleep, physical activity, and hygiene.	Client will: • Remain free of self-inflicted injury. • Communicate feelings related to depressed mood. • Maintain contract for safety. • Participate in development of transdisciplinary treatment plan. • Identify name, dose, and major side effects of medications. • Demonstrate orientation to time, place, and person. • Participate in menu plan for balanced meal. • Identify need for laxative if no BM in 3 days. • Attend 25% of leisure activities as scheduled with prompting and support.	Client will: • Remain free of self-inflicted injury. • Identify at least one reason for living. • Identify 3 positive attributes of self. • Identify one false perception or misbelief. • Communicate feelings related to managing loss and stress. • Participate in transdisciplinary plan: Identify changes in symptoms as a result of medications; remain oriented to time, place, and person; consume diet as per menu plan; attend 50% of scheduled activities independently; identify need for laxative; perform self-care activities independently 50% of time.
Assessments, tests, and treatments	Complete psychosocial assessment to include mental status, mood, affect, behavior, and communication q shift and PRN. Assess suicidal ideation, gestures, threats, plans and means. Contract for safety. Observe for safety per protocol. Complete nursing database assessment. Weight. Initiate suicide precautions as indicated. CBC, urinalysis. Chemistry profile. Thyroid profile. RPR. Other laboratory as ordered. Vital signs BID.	Psychosocial assessment q shift and PRN. Observe for safety per protocol. Monitor dietary intake, sleep pattern, and bowel elimination pattern. Continue suicide assessment. Reinforce safety contract. Suicide precautions as indicated. Monitor effects of and compliance with medications. Routine vital signs.	Daily psychosocial assessment. Observe for safety per protocol. Monitor dietary intake, sleep pattern, and bowel elimination pattern. Continue suicide assessment. Reinforce safety contract. Suicide precautions as indicated. Monitor effects of and compliance with medications. Routine vital signs.

→

CRITICAL PATHWAY FOR A CLIENT WITH DEPRESSION WITHOUT PSYCHOTIC FEATURES OR AGITATION *(continued)*

	Date ________ Day 1 *continued*	Date ________ Days 2–3 *continued*	Date ________ Day 4 *continued*
Knowledge deficit	Orient client and family to patients, staff, and program. Review initial plan of care. Assess learning needs of client and family. Initiate medication teaching. Assess understanding of teaching.	Review unit orientation with emphasis on program. Continue medication teaching. Assess understanding of teaching.	Review plan of care. Include family in teaching. Initiate teaching regarding anxiety, depression, treatment modalities, and preventive techniques. Assess medication teaching response and need for additional teaching. Assess understanding of teaching.
Diet	Monitor dietary intake. Diet as tolerated; encourage small, frequent feedings from all food groups. Provide preferred snacks and foods. Provide adequate time for meals and snacks. Encourage fluids. Low tyramine diet if on MAOIs.	Monitor dietary intake. Diet per menu plan; encourage fluids; encourage small, frequent feedings from all food groups. Provide preferred snacks and foods. Provide adequate time for meals and snacks. Encourage fluids. Low tyramine diet if on MAOIs.	Monitor dietary intake. Diet per menu plan; encourage small, frequent feedings from all food groups. Provide preferred snacks and foods. Provide adequate time for meals and snacks. Encourage fluids. Low tyramine diet if on MAOIs.
Activity	Assess safety needs and maintain appropriate precautions. Encourage client to be in milieu 10 hr/day. Encourage brief periods of activity and interaction. Provide sleep-enhancing atmosphere for 45 min prior to sleep.	Maintain safety precautions. Encourage activities during the day; prompt client to attend 25% of activities. Prompt and assist with hygiene as necessary. Encourage to participate in simple exercise. Prompt to engage in simple structured activities. Provide sleep-enhancing atmosphere 45 min prior to sleep.	Maintain safety precautions. Encourage involvement in 50–75% of activities. Prompt with hygiene as necessary. Prompt to participate in exercise.
Psychosocial	Observe behavior. Assess level of anxiety. Encourage verbalization of feelings and thoughts. Listen attentively, giving adequate time to respond. Approach with nonjudgmental and accepting manner. Formulate initial plan of care with client and family. Offer realistic hope to client and family. Identify current support system. Encourage structured activities. Provide information regarding illness and treatment. Provide ongoing support and encouragement to client and family. Meet with client 4 times each shift for 5-min periods focused on establishing relationship.	Observe behavior. Assess level of anxiety. Encourage verbalization of concerns and feelings. Provide information and ongoing support and encouragement to client and family. Provide simple structured activities. Identify potential support system and strategies to access additional supports. Prompt to attend group therapy. Acknowledge accomplishments. Meet with client 10–15 min twice a shift during waking hours and focus on working on initial goals.	Observe behavior. Assess level of anxiety. Encourage verbalization of concerns and feelings. Provide information and ongoing support and encouragement to client and family. Provide increasingly complex structured activities. Initiate cognitive restructuring. Review strategies to access support system using problem-solving strategies. Encourage group therapy independent attendance with spontaneous involvement x 1. Acknowledge accomplishments. Meet with client 15 min every shift waking hours to work on therapeutic goals.

	Date ________ Day 1 *continued*	Date ________ Days 2–3 *continued*	Date ________ Day 4 *continued*
Medications	Identify target symptoms. Antidepressants as ordered. Routine meds as ordered.	Identify target symptoms. Antidepressants as ordered. Routine meds as ordered. Colace/Metamucil if indicated. PRN laxative if no BM in 3 days.	Assess target symptoms. Antidepressants as ordered. Routine meds as ordered. Colace/Metamucil if indicated. PRN laxative if no BM in 3 days.
Consults and discharge plan	Family assessment. Establish discharge objectives with client and family. Occupational and recreational therapist.	Review discharge objectives with client and significant others. Initiate referrals for discharge care.	Review progress toward discharge objectives with client and significant others. Make appropriate referrals to support groups.

	Date ________ Day 5	Date ________ Day 6	Date ________ Days 7–8 to Discharge
Daily outcomes	Client will: • Remain free of self-inflicted injury. • Verbalize at least one reason for living. • Communicate feelings spontaneously and appropriately in 1:1 and group activities. • Identify method in which strengths can be used to improve coping skills. • Describe how distorted perceptions affect coping. • Begin to reframe false beliefs. • Participate in transdisciplinary plan: consume diet as per menu plan; perform self-care independently 75% of the time; attend 75% of scheduled activities independently; identify need for laxative; identify changes in symptoms as a result of medications; verbalize awareness of long-term medication needs for depression; identify discharge activity pattern; remain oriented to time, place, and person.	Client will: • Remain free of self-inflicted injury. • Verbalize at least one reason for living. • Communicate feelings spontaneously and appropriately. • Spontaneously and appropriately participate in 1:1 and group activities. • Identify methods in which strengths can be used to improve coping skills. • Describe how distorted perceptions affect coping. • Reframe distorted beliefs. • Verbalize plan to use strengths to enhance coping skills. • Participate in transdisciplinary plan: consume diet as per menu plan; perform self-care independently 100% of the time; attend 100% of scheduled activities independently; identify need for laxative; identify changes in symptoms as a result of medications; demonstrate self-administration of medication safely and correctly; verbalize awareness of and commitment to long-term medication needs for depression; remain oriented to time, place, and person.	Client is free of self-inflicted injury and verbalizes reasons for living. Client expresses a positive self-perception and self-esteem. Client communicates feelings honestly and openly. Client participates in activities that promote physical health. Client identifies cues to increasing depression. Client develops sustaining relationships with friends and family members. Client utilizes strengths and skills in managing current and ongoing stressors. Client is alert and oriented. Client verbalizes/demonstrates home care instructions including the importance of ongoing mental health care. Client attains maximum independence in self-care. Client demonstrates ability to adaptively cope with ongoing stressors.

→

CRITICAL PATHWAY FOR A CLIENT WITH DEPRESSION WITHOUT PSYCHOTIC FEATURES OR AGITATION (continued)

	Date ________ Day 5 *continued*	Date ________ Day 6 *continued*	Date ________ Days 7–8 to Discharge *cont.*
Assessments, tests, and treatments	Daily psychosocial assessment. Observe for safety. Monitor dietary intake, sleep pattern, and bowel elimination pattern. Weight. Continue suicide assessment. Reinforce safety contract. Suicide precautions as indicated. Monitor effects of and compliance with medications. Routine vital signs.	Daily psychosocial assessment. Observe for safety. Monitor dietary intake, sleep pattern, and bowel elimination pattern. Continue suicide assessment. Reinforce safety contract. Suicide precautions as indicated. Monitor effects of and compliance with medications.	Psychosocial assessment. Monitor dietary intake, sleep pattern, and bowel elimination pattern. Suicide assessment. Suicide precautions as indicated. Monitor effects of and compliance with medications.
Knowledge deficit	Review plan of care. Include family in teaching. Review teaching regarding anxiety. Initiate teaching regarding coping strategies utilizing client strengths. Review current level of knowledge regarding medications, treatments, symptom management and follow-up care. Assess understanding of teaching.	Review plan of care with client and family. Reinforce current level of knowledge regarding medications, treatments, symptom management and follow-up care. Assess understanding of teaching.	Client and/or significant other verbalizes understanding of discharge teaching including activity level and exercise program, safety measures, diet, signs and symptoms to report, follow-up care and MD appointment, medications (name, purpose, dose, frequency, route, dietary interactions, and side effects) and follow-up care arrangements. Assess understanding of teaching. Make referrals to community caregivers for any knowledge deficits regarding medications, treatments, symptoms management, and follow-up care.
Diet	Diet as tolerated; encourage small, frequent feedings from all food groups. Encourage fluids. Provide preferred snacks and foods. Provide adequate time for meals and snacks. Monitor dietary intake. Low tyramine diet if on MAOIs.	Diet as tolerated; encourage small, frequent feedings from all food groups. Encourage fluids. Provide preferred snacks and foods. Provide adequate time for meals and snacks. Monitor dietary intake. Low tyramine diet if on MAOIs.	Diet as tolerated; encourage small, frequent feedings from all food groups. Encourage fluids. Provide preferred snacks and foods. Provide adequate time for meals and snacks. Monitor dietary intake. Low tyramine diet if on MAOIs.
Activity	Maintain safety precautions. Encourage involvement in 75–100% of activities. Prompt with self-care. Provide sleep-enhancing atmosphere for 45-min period before sleep. Engage client and family in identifying reasonable activity plan following discharge.	Maintain safety precautions. Encourage involvement in 100% of activities. Encourage independence in self-care. Provide sleep-enhancing atmosphere for 45-min period prior to sleep. Identify plan to create sleep-enhancing environment in after-discharge setting.	Maintain safety precautions. Independently involved in 100% of activities. Independent in self-care. Provide sleep-enhancing atmosphere for 45-min period prior to sleep.

	Date ________ Day 5 *continued*	Date ________ Day 6 *continued*	Date ________ Days 7–8–Discharge *cont.*
Psychosocial	Assess level of anxiety. Support client in implementing stress and anxiety reduction strategies. Provide information and ongoing support and encouragement to client and family. Reinforce and utilize role playing strategies as approach to developing support system. Client attends scheduled group therapy sessions independently. Reinforce skills learned in group therapy. Identify progress with cognitive restructuring and reinforce learning. Acknowledge accomplishments. Encourage verbalization of feelings and concerns. Meet with client 15 min every shift waking hours to discuss progress in terms of therapeutic goals. Encourage client to acknowledge accomplishments. Provide ongoing support and encouragement to client and family.	Assess level of anxiety. Reinforce stress and anxiety reduction strategies. Encourage verbalization of concerns and feelings. Provide information and ongoing support and encouragement to client and family. Cliengt attends group therapy independently. Provide specific, realistic feedback. Encourage constructive expression of feelings. Meet with client 15 min every shift waking hours to discuss progress in terms of therapeutic goals. Reinforce strategies for cognitive restructuring and reinforce learning. Encourage client to acknowledge accomplishments. Provide ongoing support and encouragement to client and family.	Assess level of anxiety. Reinforce stress and anxiety reduction strategies. Encourage verbalization of concerns and feelings. Provide information and ongoing support and encouragement to client and family. Client attends group therapy independently. Meet with client 15 min every shift waking hours to discuss progress in terms of therapeutic goals. Acknowledge accomplishments. Reinforce progress with and strategies for cognitive restructuring and reinforce learning. Provide ongoing support and encouragement to client and family.
Medications	Assess target symptoms. Antidepressants as ordered. Routine meds as ordered. Colace/Metamucil as indicated. PRN laxative if no BM in 3 days.	Assess target symptoms. Antidepressants as ordered. Routine meds as ordered. Colace/Metamucil as indicated. PRN laxative if no BM in 3 days.	Assess target symptoms. Antidepressants as ordered. Routine meds as ordered. Colace/Metamucil as indicated. PRN laxative if no BM in 3 days.
Transfer/ discharge plan	Review discharge objectives with client and family.	Review discharge objectives with client and significant others. Complete referrals for discharge care.	Review progress toward discharge objectives. Review need for any discharge referrals. Discharge with referrals.

→

CRITICAL PATHWAY FOR A CLIENT WITH BIPOLAR DISORDER, MANIC PHASE

Expected length of stay: 14 days

	Date ________ Day 1	Date ________ Days 2–4	Date ________ Days 5–7
Daily outcomes	Client will: • Remain free of injury to self or others. • Identify initial goals for hospitalization. • Contract for management of intrusive behaviors. • Participate in transdisciplinary treatment plan: participate in assessment; identify most recent medication regime; drink 2000 cc of fluids each day; identify current dietary pattern and food preferences. • Remain oriented to time, place and person.	Client will: • Remain free of injury to self or others. • Identify initial goals for hospitalization. • Maintain contract for management of intrusive behaviors. • Participate in transdiciplinary treatment plan: participate in assessment; begin to verbalize need for medications; participate in menu planning; drink 2000 cc of fluids each day; participate in physical activity groups as scheduled; respond to redirection while participating in physical activity groups; establish rest/sleep promoting environment. • If sleep period less than 4 hr, client will increase sleep period by 5%. • Remain oriented to time, place, and person.	Client will: • Remain free of injury to self or others. • Identify initial goals for hospitalization. • Maintain contract for management of intrusive behaviors. • Participate in transdiciplinary treatment plan: verbalize reasons for medications; consume diet per menu plan; drink 2000 cc of fluids each day; listen and respond to topic for a few minutes; increase sleep period by 5%; participate in physical activity groups as scheduled; respond to redirection while participating in physical activity groups; perform self-care activities independently 50% of time; establish rest/sleep promoting environment; stay focused on simple task for a few minutes. • Remain oriented to time, place, and person.
Assessments, tests, and treatments	Psychosocial assessment to include mental status, mood, affect, behavior, and communication q shift and PRN. Complete nursing database assessment. Observe behavior and activity level. Weight. Monitor fluid intake. CBC, urinalysis. Thyroid profile. Chemistry profile. Drug screen. RPR. Electrolytes. Lithium level. Other laboratory as ordered. Vital signs BID and PRN.	Psychosocial assessment q shift and PRN. Observe for safety per protocol. Monitor behavior and activity level. Monitor effects and compliance with medication. Monitor fluid intake. Assess sleep pattern. Lithium level day 3. Routine vital signs.	Psychosocial assessment q shift and PRN. Observe for safety per protocol. Monitor behavior and activity level. Monitor effects and compliance with medication. Monitor fluid intake. Assess sleep pattern. Lithium level day 7. Routine vital signs.

	Date ________ Day 1 *continued*	Date ________ Days 2–4 *continued*	Date ________ Days 5–7 *continued*
Knowledge deficit	Orient client/family to unit and program. Assess learning needs of client and family. Review initial plan of care. Initiate medication teaching. Assess understanding of teaching.	Review unit orientation with emphasis on program. Continue medication teaching. Assess understanding of teaching.	Review plan of care. Include family in teaching. Initiate teaching regarding treatment modalities and preventive techniques. Assess medication teaching response and need for additional teaching. Assess understanding of teaching.
Diet	Monitor dietary intake. Diet as tolerated; encourage small, frequent feedings from all food groups. Provide preferred snacks and foods. Encourage fluids and finger foods, making them accessible throughout the day.	Monitor dietary intake. Diet as tolerated; encourage small, frequent feedings from all food groups. Provide preferred snacks and foods. Encourage fluids and finger foods, making them accessible throughout the day.	Monitor dietary intake. Diet as tolerated; encourage small, frequent feedings from all food groups. Provide preferred snacks and foods. Encourage fluids and finger foods, making them accessible throughout the day.
Activity	Assess safety needs and maintain appropriate precautions. Observe activity level. Develop schedule for stimulus titration (quiet time and periods in the milieu). Manage agitation with periods of physical activity. Provide sleep-enhancing atmosphere for 45 min prior to sleep.	Maintain safety precautions. Observe activity level. Maintain schedule for stimulus titration. Manage agitation with periods of physical activity. Prompt to attend physical activity groups. Prompt and assist with hygiene as necessary. Provide sleep-enhancing atmosphere for 45 min prior to sleep.	Maintain safety precautions. Observe activity level. Maintain schedule for stimulus titration. Manage agitation with periods of physical activity. Prompt to attend physical activity groups. Encourage to attend small group activities. Prompt with hygiene as necessary. Provide sleep-enhancing atmosphere for 45 min prior to sleep.
Psychosocial	Approach with nonjudgmental and accepting manner. Observe and monitor behavior. Provide structured activities and contracts. Direct to structured activities as per contract. Minimize environmental stimuli and provide a safe environment. Redirect intrusive behaviors: sexual, aggressive, and/or manipulative. Provide information regarding illness and treatment to client and family. Avoid power struggles by maintaining kind but consistent approach. Redirect frequent requests and attempt to meet demands in effective manner. Maintain scheduled contacts.	Approach with nonjudgmental and accepting manner. Observe and monitor behavior. Provide structured activities and contracts. Direct to structured activities as per contract. Minimize environmental stimuli and provide a safe environment. Redirect intrusive behaviors: sexual, aggressive, and/or manipulative. Provide information regarding illness and treatment to client and family. Avoid power struggles by maintaining kind but consistent approach. Redirect frequent requests and attempt to meet demands in effective manner. Maintain scheduled contacts.	Approach with nonjudgmental and accepting manner. Observe and monitor behavior. Provide structured activities and contracts. Direct to structured activities as per contract. Minimize environmental stimuli and provide a safe environment. Redirect intrusive behaviors: sexual, aggressive, and/or manipulative. Provide information regarding illness and treatment to client and family. Avoid power struggles by maintaining kind but consistent approach. Redirect frequent requests and attempt to meet demands in effective manner. Maintain scheduled contacts.

→

CRITICAL PATHWAY FOR A CLIENT WITH BIPOLAR DISORDER, MANIC PHASE *(continued)*

	Date __________ Day 1 *continued*	Date __________ Days 2–4 *continued*	Date __________ Days 5–7 *continued*
Medications	Identify target symptoms. Lithium as ordered. Carbamazepine or valproic acid as ordered. Antipsychotics as ordered. Routine meds as ordered.	Assess target symptoms. Lithium as ordered. Carbamazepine or valproic acid as ordered. Antipsychotics as ordered. Routine meds as ordered.	Assess target symptoms. Lithium as ordered. Carbamazepine or valproic acid as ordered. Antipsychotics as ordered. Routine meds as ordered.
Consults and discharge plan	Family assessment. Consult with internist if ordered. Occupational and recreational therapist. Establish discharge objectives with client and family.	Review with client and significant others discharge objectives. Complete discharge planning.	Review with client and significant others progress toward discharge objectives. Make appropriate referrals to support groups.

	Date __________ Days 8–9	Date __________ Days 10–12	Date __________ Days 13–14 to Discharge
Daily outcomes	Client will: • Remain free of injury to self or others. • Discuss goals for hospitalization. • Maintain management of intrusive behaviors. • Participate in transdisciplinary treatment plan. • Verbalize reasons for medications and understanding of side effects of medication. • Consume diet per menu plan. • Participate in physical activity groups as scheduled. • Listen and respond to topic. • Increase sleep period by 5%. • Begin to identify consequences of manic behavior. • Respond to redirection when participating in physical activity groups. • Perform self-care activities independently 75% of time. • Establish sleep/rest promoting environment. • Stay focused on simple task for 10-min period. • Maintain usual elimination patterns. • Remain oriented to time, place, and person.	Client will: • Remain free of injury to self or others. • Discuss goals for hospitalization. • Maintain management of intrusive behaviors. • Participate in transdisciplinary treatment plan. • Verbalize reasons for medications and need for long-term therapy. • Consume diet per menu plan. • Participate in physical activity groups as scheduled. • Adaptively use listening skills. • Respond to redirection when participating in physical activity groups. • Perform self-care activities independently 100% of time. • Establish sleep/rest promoting environment. • Stay focused on simple task for 15-min period. • Maintain usual elimination patterns. • Remain oriented to time, place, and person.	Client is free of injury to self or others. Client is alert and oriented. Client communicates feelings of self-worth. Client's weight is stable. Client achieves maximum independence in self-care. Client adaptively uses listening skills. Client enjoys 6 hr. of uninterrupted sleep. Client identifies plan if symptoms recur. Client eats a well-balanced diet inclusive of all food groups. Client drinks 2000 cc of fluids each day. Client has resumed preadmission urine and bowel elimination pattern. Client verbalizes/demonstrates home care instructions including the importance of ongoing mental health care. Client participates in regular exercise program. Client demonstrates ability to adaptively cope with ongoing stressors.

	Date ________ Days 8–9 *continued*	**Date ________ Days 10–12 *continued***	**Date ________ Days 13–14 to Discharge *cont.***
Assessments, tests, and treatments	Psychosocial assessment BID and PRN. Observe for safety per protocol. Monitor behavior and activity pattern. Monitor effects and compliance with medication. Monitor fluid intake. Assess sleep pattern.	Psychosocial assessment QD PRN. Observe for safety per protocol. Monitor behavior and activity pattern. Monitor effects and compliance with medication. Monitor fluid intake. Assess sleep pattern. Lithium level day 12.	Psychosocial assessment. Observe for safety per protocol. Monitor behavior and activity pattern. Monitor effects and compliance with medication. Monitor fluid intake. Assess sleep pattern.
Knowledge deficit	Review plan of care. Include family in teaching. Review current level of knowledge regarding medications, treatments, symptom management, and follow-up care. Assess understanding of teaching.	Review plan of care with client and family. Reinforce current level of knowledge regarding medications, treatments, symptom management, and follow-up care. Assess understanding of teaching.	Client and/or significant other verbalizes understanding of discharge teaching including activity level and exercise program, safety measures, diet, signs and symptoms to report, follow-up care and MD appointment, medications (name, purpose, dose, frequency, route, dietary interactions, and side effects) and follow-up care arrangements. Assess understanding of teaching. Make referrals to community caregivers for any knowledge deficits regarding medications, treatments, symptom management, and follow-up care.
Diet	Monitor dietary intake. Diet as tolerated; encourage small frequent feedings from all food groups. Provide preferred snacks and foods. Encourage fluids and finger foods, making them accessible throughout the day.	Monitor dietary intake. Diet as tolerated; encourage small frequent feedings from all food groups. Provide preferred snacks and foods. Encourage fluids and finger foods, making them accessible throughout the day.	Monitor dietary intake. Diet as tolerated; encourage small frequent feedings from all food groups. Provide preferred snacks and foods. Encourage fluids and finger foods, making them accessible throughout the day.
Activity	Maintain safety precautions. Observe activity level. Maintain schedule for stimulus titration. Encourage working at activities until completion. Manage agitation with periods of physical activity. Encourage to eat meals in dining room. Prompt with hygiene as necessary. Provide sleep-enhancing atmosphere for 45 min prior to sleep.	Maintain safety precautions. Observe activity level. Maintain schedule for stimulus titration. Manage agitation with periods of physical activity. Encourage independent attendence at physical activity groups. Encourage independence in self-care. Provide sleep-enhancing atmosphere for 45 min prior to sleep.	Maintain safety precautions. Observe activity level. Maintain schedule for stimulus titration. Manage agitation with periods of physical activity. Prompt to attend physical activity groups. Client is independent in self-care. Provide sleep-enhancing atmosphere for 45 min prior to sleep.

→

CRITICAL PATHWAY FOR A CLIENT WITH BIPOLAR DISORDER, MANIC PHASE *(continued)*

	Date ________ Days 8–9 *continued*	Date ________ Days 10–12 *continued*	Date ________ Days 13–14 to Discharge *cont.*
Psychosocial	Approach with nonjudgmental and accepting manner. Observe and monitor behavior. Provide structured activities and contracts. Direct to structured activities as per contract. Minimize environmental stimuli and provide a safe environment. Redirect intrusive behaviors: sexual, aggressive, and/or manipulative. Provide information regarding illness and treatment to client and family. Avoid power struggles by maintaining kind but consistent approach. Redirect frequent requests and attempt to meet needs in effective manner. Prompt to attend physical activity groups. Client independently attends short, small group activities. Prompt to start attending group therapy as tolerated. Meet with client 2 times each shift for 5-min periods focused on activities of daily living and behavior. Maintain scheduled contacts.	Approach with nonjudgmental and accepting manner. Observe and monitor behavior. Provide structured activities and contracts. Direct to structured activities as per contract. Minimize environmental stimuli and provide a safe environment. Redirect intrusive behaviors: sexual, aggressive, and/or manipulative. Provide information regarding illness and treatment to client and family. Avoid power struggles by maintaining kind but consistent approach. Redirect frequent requests and attempt to meet needs in effective manner. Client eats meals in dining room without prompting. Client independently attends group therapy for increasingly longer period. Client independently attends short, small group activities. Client attends discharge planning group. Meet with client 2 times each shift for 5-min periods to work on discharge goals. Maintain scheduled contacts.	Approach with nonjudgmental and accepting manner. Observe and monitor behavior. Provide structured activities and contracts. Direct to structured activities as per contract. Minimize environmental stimuli and provide a safe environment. Redirect intrusive behaviors: sexual, aggressive, and/or manipulative. Provide information regarding illness and treatment to client and family. Avoid power struggles by maintaining kind but consistent approach. Redirect frequent requests and attempt to meet needs in effective manner. Meet with client 2 times each shift for 5-min periods to discuss after-discharge care and management. Maintain scheduled contacts.
Medications	Monitor target symptoms. Lithium as ordered. Carbamazepine or valproic acid as ordered. Antipsychotics as ordered. Routine meds as ordered.	Monitor target symptoms. Lithium as ordered. Carbamazepine or valproic acid as ordered. Antipsychotics as ordered. Routine meds as ordered.	Monitor target symptoms. Lithium as ordered. Carbamazepine or valproic acid as ordered. Antipsychotics as ordered. Routine meds as ordered.
Transfer/ discharge plan	Review discharge objectives with client and significant others.	Review progress toward discharge objectives with client and significant others. Complete referrals for discharge care.	Discharge with referrals.

The Nursing Process and Clients with Bipolar Disorders

Because the nursing care of clients experiencing depressive symptoms is the same whether the diagnosis is major depressive disorder, dysthymic disorder, or depressed episode bipolar disorder, this section will focus on hypomania and mania, which constitute the other half of the bipolar continuum of behaviors.

Assessment

The onset of a hypomanic or manic episode may be gradual or dramatic. Affect is euphoric or elated, but can change quickly to irritability or hostility if the person is confronted with limits or is otherwise frustrated. The signs and symptoms range in severity from mild in hypomania to extreme in a frank manic episode.

Subjective Data Manic clients experience changes in their thought processes, sometimes stating that their "thoughts are racing." They often experience inflated self-esteem, sometimes to the extent of having delusions of grandeur. Delusions of persecution also may be a feature. They ignore fatigue and hunger, being too involved in activity to focus on physiologic sensations. Suffering from an inability to concentrate, they are easily distracted by the slightest stimulus in the environment. They may experience hallucinations. Hypomanic individuals and those early in manic episodes feel wonderful and do not understand why anyone is upset with their behavior.

Objective Data Manic clients are most likely to be young people in their twenties, although adolescents are sometimes affected. Although bipolar disorder appears to have little gender specificity, the initial episode is likely to be manic in males and depressive in females (APA 1994). To date there is no documented evidence of the effect of race or ethnicity on bipolar disorder.

The hallmark of manic clients is constant motor activity. During a manic episode, they will not stop to eat. They do not rest, have disordered sleep patterns, and may go for days without sleep. Bruises and other injuries sometimes result from the constantly agitated behavior.

Flight of ideas is manifested in the manic client's communications, and pressured speech is an obvious symptom. Family members often report that they exhibit poor judgment, such as going on spending sprees and committing sexual and other indiscretions that are completely out of character with their usual behavior. Appearance may be unusual, such as inappropriate dress and garish makeup.

Impairment in occupational functioning may result in work layoff or being placed on a leave of absence because the behavior is disruptive in the workplace. Manic people cause interpersonal chaos by their manipulative behavior, testing limits and playing off one person against another. If their manipulation attempts fail, they become irritable or hostile, and naturally such behavior alienates others.

Just as they fail to settle down long enough to eat and sleep, they also neglect bathing. In time, the absence of personal hygiene further alienates them from other people.

There are no laboratory findings specific for the diagnosis of mania. Individuals experiencing manic episodes have been noted to have abnormal cortisol levels as well as abnormalities in neurotransmitter systems. But it is not known whether these abnormalities are causative of or result from the disorder.

Manic clients are not usually able to cooperate fully in the nursing assessment process. In many cases, nurses will find it necessary to rely on their own assessment skills and secondary sources, such as family members, in obtaining essential assessment data. Family members can often provide detailed information about the onset and progression of symptoms, as well as information about previous episodes, if any.

Nursing Diagnosis

The following sections discuss the implications of several nursing diagnoses commonly seen in manic clients.

Risk for Injury Manic individuals are at risk for injury because their usual adaptive and defensive abilities are impaired. Because of their hyperactivity and agitation, they often lose control of their movements and bump into objects, fall, and otherwise injure themselves.

Their impulsivity, poor judgment, and propensity toward hostile outbursts also place them at risk for injury. Other clients are often extremely annoyed by inappropriate or unacceptable social behavior and may attack manic clients. As with self-directed violence, preventing injury becomes the nursing priority.

Altered Thought Processes Manic clients experience disruption of their usual cognitive processes. This may be related to a variety of factors, including biochemical alteration, genetic predisposition, sleep deprivation, a severe blow to self-esteem, or massive denial of depression.

Evidence of altered thought processes is seen in clients who cannot concentrate, have short attention spans, are easily distracted, and have impaired problem-solving abilities. They exhibit unwarranted optimism and poor judgment due to inaccurate interpretations of the environment. Delusional belief systems held by clients indicate a severe impairment of thought processes, as do hallucinations. Pressured speech, tangentiality, and flight of ideas are ample evidence of disrupted cognitive operations.

Impaired Social Interaction Unlike depressed clients who may isolate themselves and avoid social interaction, most manic clients are extremely gregarious and excessively social. But their social interactions are highly dysfunctional. Manipulating other people to meet their own wishes and needs is a major impediment to positive social interactions. Egocentrism, impulsiveness, lack of interest in the needs and concerns of others, and an unwillingness to accept responsibility for the impact of behavior on others all make manic clients difficult to tolerate. Poor personal hygiene aggravates the situation.

Nurses often have difficulty dealing with the unreasonable behavior of manic clients. The Nursing Self-Awareness box will help you determine how you may be affected by these behaviors.

Self-Care Deficit Clients experiencing a manic episode have an impaired ability to perform the self-care activities of feeding, bathing, toileting, dressing, and grooming. This is related to hyperactivity, the inability to make accurate judgments about personal needs, alterations in thought processes, lack of awareness of personal needs, and fatigue. Self-Care Deficit is evidenced by inadequate food and fluid intake, an inability or refusal to bathe, a lack of interest in grooming and appropriateness of appearance, and an inability or unwillingness to toilet without assistance.

Sleep Pattern Disturbance The sleep pattern of manic clients is so disrupted that exhaustion and even death can result. Disrupted sleep is related to hyperactivity, agitation, and possibly to biochemical alterations. Sleep Pattern Disturbance includes the inability to fall asleep, roaming or pacing the halls during the night, awakening frequently during the night, and sleeping only for short naps with long periods of hyperactive, restless behavior in between.

Planning and Implementing Interventions

With manic clients, your demeanor should be calm and relaxed but firm and matter-of-fact, particularly when communicating limits. Your own self-behavior serves as a model and is reassuring to out-of-control clients. As with all clients, building a trusting relationship is important. Therefore, make promises only when you are certain you can keep them.

Promoting Client Safety Provide a safe environment for manic clients by reducing environmental stimuli. This means providing a simply furnished private room that has had all unnecessary items removed. It should be in a quiet location to reduce noise stimulation. Low lighting can also be calming to the hyperactive client. Some hospitals have "quiet units." From there, clients can be transferred to milieu units when they are more able to deal with the distractions of community living.

Because manic clients have difficulty interacting appropriately with others, limit their participation in group activities until they are less agitated. Group settings tend to overstimulate these clients, which causes them to antagonize others.

Smoking materials are particularly hazardous in the hands of agitated clients. They may burn themselves or

NURSING SELF-AWARENESS

Potential Reactions to Working with Manic Clients

Working with manic clients will challenge your maturity, self-control, and professionalism. Listed below are some common reactions. When you work with manic clients, you may experience some of these feelings. Think about and discuss with classmates and your instructor how you might handle each of these reactions in order to maintain a positive nurse-client relationship.

- I feel annoyed by the client's demanding behavior.
- I feel outsmarted and outmaneuvered; I question whether my judgments and actions are appropriate.
- I develop rescue fantasies in response to a client's flattery and think I am the only one who understands this client.
- I become defensive and angry when colleagues point out a client's manipulative behavior.
- I feel anxious and insecure when a client turns on me, saying, "I'm not progressing because you're cold and mean."
- I have difficulty being objective about manic clients.
- I disagree emphatically with colleagues about how to handle a client's manipulative behavior; the client sits back and watches nurses fight with each other.
- I become angry and unsure of my judgment when a client consistently exceeds established limits.
- I withdraw and avoid manic clients to prevent embarrassment and self-doubt.

leave burning cigarettes lying around when they become distracted by other stimuli. Allow them to smoke only under supervision.

Scheduling a program of appropriate activity, interspersed with rest periods, helps provide an outlet for tension while protecting clients from exhaustion. Appropriate activities include walks, exercising or dancing with the supervision of an activity therapist, and supervised vacuuming or sweeping chores. Avoid highly competitive activities that bring out hostility and overly aggressive behaviors.

Set and enforce limits on unsafe or socially inappropriate behavior with clients who are unable to control their impulses. Matter-of-fact intervention rather than angry scolding is the most effective approach. These clients may respond to verbal reminders, or you can use their distractibility to redirect them into safer and more appropriate activities. Remember to reward appropriate behavior with positive reinforcement such as, "I enjoyed our walk today because you were able to walk with me rather than running ahead."

Medications Hyperactive and agitated behavior usually responds to antipsychotics such as chlorpromazine (Thorazine) or haloperidol (Haldol). These medications are often used to help manage manic clients who have started on lithium carbonate therapy, since lithium takes 1–3 weeks to become effective.

Nursing interventions include monitoring clients for adverse side effects of antipsychotic medications. Side effects include postural hypotension, dizziness, dry mouth, blurry vision, urinary retention, pseudoparkinsonism, and tardive dyskinesia. (See Chapter 33.)

PROMOTING REALITY-BASED THINKING Present reality by spending time with clients; identify yourself, the time and day, location, and other orienting information as needed. Engage clients in reality-based, concrete activities, such as discussing a current event.

Consistency is reassuring to clients with altered thought processes. Establish consistency by having a schedule so clients understand what is expected of them. Consistency is also enhanced by assigning the same caregivers to work with the client whenever possible.

When dealing with delusional or hallucinating clients, communicate your acceptance of their need for false beliefs, while clearly stating that you do not share their perceptions. A statement such as, "I understand that you believe you are the Princess Anastasia, but I do not see it that way," conveys acceptance without supporting delusional thinking.

It is fruitless to argue or try to reason with delusional clients. This often serves to harden the belief system and can impair the development of trust. Instead, use statements such as, "I find that hard to believe" or "That is extremely unusual," to instill reasonable doubt as a therapeutic intervention.

When clients communicate altered reality perceptions, reflect their statements back to them for validation. For example, "Are you saying that your husband is trying to poison you with monosodium glutamate?" can help a client understand how her perceptions sound to others. You will recognize that clients are becoming less delusional when they make statements such as, "I know this sounds bizarre, but . . . ." Remember to give positive reinforcement when clients begin to focus on reality.

PROMOTING ADAPTIVE SOCIAL INTERACTION The major maladaptive behavior of manic clients that significantly impairs social interactions is manipulativeness. This may take a simple form, such as borrowing cigarettes from other clients rather than buying their own. Or it may be highly complex, such as pitting staff members against one another by giving them false information about each other.

Manipulativeness serves the purpose of increasing a client's sense of control and interpersonal power. Nursing interventions that promote client security often enable clients to curb their manipulative behavior or give it up entirely. Be aware of your own control needs, and provide opportunities for clients to be in control when appropriate.

Setting Limits Out-of-control, manipulative behavior requires setting limits. All staff members must agree upon the established limits and must enforce them consistently. Violations of limits must have established consequences, also agreed upon by all staff. Clients must know what behaviors are expected and what consequences will result if limits are exceeded. Inconsistent application of consequences will cause failure in the efforts to decrease manipulative behavior.

You can expect clients to give charming explanations of why they had to exceed this or that limit, but do not be disarmed by these explanations. They are another form of manipulative behavior. Matter-of-fact limit enforcement and the consistent application of consequences are essential in promoting adaptive behaviors. The Intervention box on the next page provides an overview of how to effectively set and enforce limits.

PROMOTING IMPROVED SELF-CARE A minimal level of personal hygiene is needed to ensure self-esteem and healthy social interactions. Hyperactive clients who are unwilling or unable to bathe, brush their teeth, shave, wash their hair, change clothes, or use the toilet must be assisted. Autonomy is desirable, so allow clients to do as much for themselves as possible with verbal encouragement. Reinforce any attempts at self-care with recognition, for example, "I see you shaved, Mr. Adams."

INTERVENTION

Setting and Enforcing Limits

Effective limit setting requires that all members of the mental health team participate in establishing limits and determining and enforcing the consequences for exceeding them.

1. Establish limits only when and where there is a clear need. Limits must help client growth.
2. Establish reasonable and enforceable consequences for exceeding limits.
3. Explain the limits and consequences to clients in language they can understand. Explain why the limits are necessary, and allow clients to express their feelings about them.
4. Enforce the limits consistently. Written care plans help assure consistency.
5. Evaluate the continued need for limits frequently. Turn control over to clients as soon as behavior indicates the ability to exercise self-control.
6. Keep the client's dignity in mind at all times. Limit setting is not a punishment but a part of therapy.

Incontinence of urine or feces is occasionally seen in severely regressed manic clients. This can be very disturbing to other clients and to members of the nursing staff. Intervention requires establishing a schedule of frequent toileting. Accompany the client to the bathroom every hour or half hour until "accidents" no longer occur.

A more common elimination problem is constipation. Clients suppress the urge to defecate and may become severely constipated. The anticholinergic effect of antipsychotic medications may exacerbate constipation. Frequent fluid intake and a high-fiber diet can reduce constipation.

Well-being is compromised when clients do not receive sufficient nourishment and fluids for extended periods of time, particularly during periods of hyperactivity. Monitoring intake and output is an important part of nursing care. Frequent small snacks that can be eaten "on the go" are most likely to be consumed by the hyperactive client. Work with the dietitian to ensure that high-calorie finger foods and nutritious liquids are available on the nursing unit until the client is able to attend regular meals.

Promoting Rest and Sleep Clients in the manic phase of bipolar disorder appear deceptively energetic when they may actually be nearing the point of exhaustion. Monitor them closely for signs of fatigue, and make provisions for rest periods. Promote nighttime sleeping by limiting extended daytime naps. Preliminary research findings indicate that sleep may promote the rapid resolution of first episodes of mania (Nowlin-Finch et al. 1994).

Prior to bedtime, decrease light and noise and encourage quiet activities, such as listening to soothing music. A warm bath and snack may aid relaxation, as may a backrub. Administer sleeping medications as ordered.

If clients experience extended nighttime wakefulness, avoid engaging in long conversations or otherwise stimulating or giving extra attention during the night. Firmly encourage clients to stay in their darkened rooms with the expectation that they will fall asleep. If they will not stay in their rooms, assign a monotonous, repetitive task, such as folding towels or sorting papers to encourage drowsiness.

Evaluation and Outcome Criteria

Specific client behaviors indicate that nursing interventions have been successful. Evaluation and outcome criteria answer the question, "How do we know that the manic client's condition has improved?"

Safety If nursing interventions have been successful in promoting safety, clients will be free of accidental injuries. They will not engage in agitated or impulsive behaviors that can endanger them. Their social behaviors will no longer irritate or enrage other people, so they will no longer risk attacks from others. Clients will be able to enumerate safe ways of relieving excess tension when it occurs, such as verbal expression of feelings, writing feelings down in a diary or journal, or other adaptive methods. Clients will name their medications, understand the proper dosages, describe adverse effects, and explain lab monitoring needed, if any.

Reality-Based Thinking Clients who base their thinking on reality will be oriented to time, place, and person. They will no longer experience delusional thinking or hallucinations. They will be able to establish trust relationships. Their attention spans will be increased. Their speech will be less pressured and will reflect diminished flight of ideas and tangentiality. Clients will recognize and verbalize errors in perception when they occur. Their thought processes and perceptions of environmental stimuli will be accurate and can be validated by others.

Social Interaction Improvements in social interactions will be demonstrated when clients can recognize and describe which of their interactions are successful and which are unsuccessful. The absence of, or dramatic decrease in, the use of manipulation as a method of meeting their own needs also will signal improvement in social interaction. They now accept responsibility for their own behavior.

Other signs of improved social interaction include nondisruptive participation in activities, reestablishment of a social life outside the hospital, and identification of individuals outside the hospital with whom they can develop a social and support network.

SELF-CARE Clients who have reestablished self-care will demonstrate this ability by performing the activities of daily living autonomously and willingly. This includes adequately bathing and grooming themselves, selecting appropriate clothing and makeup, establishing and maintaining adequate nutrition and fluid intake, and establishing and maintaining patterns of elimination without reminders or assistance.

REST AND SLEEP The need for uninterrupted sleep varies from person to person depending on age, activity level, and usual pattern of sleep. Generally, clients who are able to sleep 6 or more hours per night without sleeping medication and awaken refreshed will have successfully reestablished healthy sleep patterns. Being able to fall asleep within 30 minutes or less is another indicator. Recognizing fatigue and voluntarily resting also indicates that clients are attending to their bodily sensations once again.

Biopsychologic Therapies for Mood Disorders

A number of psychotropic drugs are effective in mood disorders. **Electroconvulsive therapy (ECT)** is also effective with both profoundly depressed and severely manic clients.

Psychopharmacology in the Treatment of Depression

The three main types of antidepressants in popular use today are tricyclic antidepressants (TCAs), monoamine oxidase inhibitors (MAOIs), and the atypical antidepressants such as selective serotonin reuptake inhibitors (SSRIs). All antidepressants exert positive effects on mood and behavior. As some are sedating and others are energizing, the individual client's symptoms guide the choice of drug. None of the antidepressants is recommended for use during pregnancy.

Antidepressants are effective in alleviating symptoms and are helpful adjuncts to treatment. Because they do nothing to affect underlying psychosocial conflicts, they should not be used as a single treatment modality for depressed clients but should be used in conjunction with individual, family, and/or group therapy.

TRICYCLIC ANTIDEPRESSANTS **Tricyclic antidepressants (TCAs)** are first-line agents widely used and effective in the treatment of depression. Commonly used TCAs include amitriptyline (Elavil), amoxapine (Asendin), desipramine (Norpramin), imipramine (Tofranil), and nortriptyline (Aventyl; Pamelor). They cause an elevation of mood, stimulate activity and appetite, and promote the normalization of sleep patterns. They are not useful in clients suffering from agitated depression. It takes 2–4 weeks for the maximum benefit to be achieved with TCAs.

Tricyclics increase the action of neurotransmitters, causing an excited effect. Because they are rapidly absorbed through the gastrointestinal mucosa, they are administered orally. Single bedtime doses are effective, but divided doses are also administered. If insomnia results from the stimulant effect, the dose can be given early in the day. Initial doses are low, then gradually increased until a threapeutic response is achieved.

If improvement is achieved with a TCA regimen, it should be maintained for a period of 3–6 months. If satisfactory relief results, the medication can be discontinued gradually, to prevent withdrawal symptoms. If improvement is not seen in 4 weeks, another TCA can be tried.

Adverse effects of TCAs caused by their anticholinergic action are experienced by most clients. These include dry mouth, blurred vision, constipation, headaches, and urinary retention. Postural hypotension, tachycardia, dizziness, and palpitations are cardiovascular effects often seen, especially in elderly clients. Caution is imperative when administering TCAs to older clients or those with cardiac disease.

Larger doses sometimes cause serious reactions, such as confusion, disorientation, nightmares, tremor, and numbness, again particularly in elderly clients. Allergic reactions, such as skin rashes, photosensitivity, petechiae, and edema may occur, as well as nausea, vomiting, diarrhea, anorexia, and epigastric discomfort.

Blood dyscrasias may result from long-term use. Endocrine effects, such as testicular swelling, gynecomastia, and impotence in men and swollen breasts and galactorrhea in women may occur. Changes in sexual responsiveness and blood sugar levels occur in both males and females and are thought to be due to endocrine changes.

Drug interactions occur with TCAs when given with the following preparations: MAOIs, CNS depressants, thyroid preparations, phenothiazines, barbiturates, alcohol, methylphenidate, guanethidine, and anticholinergic agents. Serious reactions may occur.

Because the risk of suicide is always present with de-

INTERVENTION

Guidelines for Working with Clients on Antidepressant Therapy

Proper client education enhances the effectiveness of drug therapy. Good education can make the difference between client compliance and noncompliance with the drug regimen. It begins when drug therapy begins and is repeated during the course of the client's hospitalization. Give instructions orally and in writing. Include family members or significant others if they will supervise home administration.

Initiating Antidepressant Therapy

- Make sure the client knows the name and dose of the drug(s) being taken. *(Rationale: This is basic information every client should know.)*
- Advise the client to arise slowly from a sitting or lying position, and to sit on the side of the bed before standing up. *(Rationale: This allows the body time to compensate for postural hypotension.)*
- Encourage the use of ice chips, gum, hard candy, and increased fluids. *(Rationale: To alleviate dryness of mouth.)*
- Advise both client and family that it will take 2–4 weeks to see a therapeutic response to antidepressant therapy. *(Rationale: To prevent discouragement and impatience.)*
- Monitor for urinary retention or constipation, and take necessary actions. *(Rationale: These conditions may result from the anticholinergic effects of antidepressants.)*
- Give medication early in the day if insomnia occurs. *(Rationale: Some antidepressants have a stimulating effect.)*
- Monitor and record sleep patterns. *(Rationale: Normalization of sleep patterns should occur.)*
- Avoid giving TCAs and MAOIs concurrently. *(Rationale: To avoid hypertensive crisis, give 2–3 weeks apart.)*
- Observe the client for skin rashes, photosensitivity, weight gain, and signs of infection. *(Rationale: These are adverse side effects and should be evaluated.)*
- Advise the client that drowsiness, blurred vision, dry mouth, and jittery feelings will diminish after a few days on the drug. *(Rationale: Sedation and anticholinergic effects [except dry mouth] usually diminish over time. They will recur when dosage is raised, however.)*
- Monitor the client for suicide risk, particularly as depression begins to lift. *(Rationale: Profoundly depressed clients lack the energy to plan and implement suicide. As they begin to improve, risk increases.)*

pressed clients, large doses of medication should not be prescribed, and clients should be observed for increased suicidal risk as the depression improves. For more information, see the accompanying Intervention box.

MONOAMINE OXIDASE INHIBITORS **Monoamine oxidase inhibitors (MAOIs)** are second-line agents usually used when TCA therapy has been unsuccessful. They include phenelzine (Nardil), isocarboxazid (Marplan), and tranylcypromine (Parnate). Because these drugs can have serious, even potentially fatal, adverse reactions, they must be used with great care. Clients and their families must be reliable, cooperative, and willing to be taught how to use these agents safely.

Monoamine oxidase (MAO) is a naturally occurring enzyme that destroys monoamines such as the neurotransmitters epinephrine, norepinephrine, and serotonin. When these chemicals build up in the brain, psychomotor activity is increased.

MAOIs elevate mood and stimulate psychomotor activity and appetite. Symptom relief is not usually seen for 1–4 weeks following the initiation of therapy. The effect lasts until the enzyme is regenerated, which takes weeks. As with TCAs, MAOIs are easily and rapidly absorbed when given orally. Initial doses are small with gradual increases. Single or divided daily doses may be used. They should be taken for several months and withdrawn gradually.

MAOI side effects are similar to those of TCAs. Postural hypotension and anticholinergic effects of dry mouth, blurred vision, urinary retention, and confusion are reported. Delayed ejaculation has been reported in some males taking MAOIs.

The greatest danger to clients taking MAOIs is the toxic reaction that occurs when the pressor amine, tyramine, is ingested. Tyramine is found in certain foods, some beverages, and some over-the-counter diet, cold, and cough preparations. It interacts with MAOIs to increase the NE

INTERVENTION *(continued)*

- For clients on high doses of TCAs, observe closely for seizures. *(Rationale: High-dose tricyclics lower the seizure threshold.)*

Clients on MAOIs

- Supervise the client's intake, and make sure no tyramine-rich agents are offered. *(Rationale: Tyramine may precipitate hypertensive crisis.)*
- Monitor the client closely for headaches and elevated blood pressure. Withhold medication, and report these signs to the prescribing professional immediately. *(Rationale: These may be early signs of hypertensive crisis.)*
- Keep phentolamine mesylate (Regitine) on hand for treating hypertensive crisis. *(Rationale: This is an alpha-adrenergic blocker and potent antihypertensive agent.)*
- Observe diabetic clients closely for hypoglycemia. *(Rationale: MAOIs promote hypoglycemia.)*

Prior to Discharge

- In collaboration with the client, work out a time schedule that fits the client's lifestyle. *(Rationale: This will increase the likelihood that the client will actually take the medication.)*
- Advise the client to take the medication as ordered and to avoid using alcohol or other CNS depressants during therapy. *(Rationale: Varying the dosage impairs the maintenance of therapeutic blood levels. Alcohol and other CNS depressants have a potentiating effect on antidepressants and may cause stupor or coma.)*
- Teach the client and family about possible adverse reactions and measures to initiate if they occur. *(Rationale: To ensure maximum comfort and safety.)*
- Caution the client not to operate dangerous equipment, drive a car, or engage in tasks requiring mental alertness if drowsiness persists. *(Rationale: To ensure safety.)*
- Teach the client not to discontinue the drug abruptly. *(Rationale: Antidepressant dosage should be gradually decreased to avoid withdrawal symptoms of nausea, dizziness, insomnia, and headache.)*
- For clients on MAOIs, provide a list of tyramine-containing substances, and make sure the client and family understand the consequences of consuming tyramine. *(Rationale: To ensure client safety.)*
- Record accurately and completely what drug education the client and family have received. *(Rationale: Documenting client education provides legal protection for the nurse and institution in the event of an adverse reaction.)*

level in the blood. Because NE is a vasoconstrictor, high levels cause a rise in blood pressure. A rapid, marked rise in blood pressure causes hypertensive crisis, which can be fatal. Common agents that cause interactions with MAOIs are listed in the box on the following page.

The symptoms of hypertensive crisis are dramatic and include severe occipital headache, nausea, vomiting, fever, pallor, sweating, pain and rigidity in the neck, elevated blood pressure, photophobia, dilated pupils, and tachycardia or bradycardia (Spencer et al. 1993). Intracranial bleeding may occur. The drug must be discontinued immediately and an alpha-adrenergic blocker, such as phentolamine mesylate (Regitine), administered intravenously.

ATYPICAL ANTIDEPRESSANTS A new class of antidepressant drugs has recently been marketed: **selective serotonin reuptake inhibitors (SRRIs).** Their onset of action is reportedly faster, they have fewer disturbing side effects, and their cardiotoxic effects are said to be less than the TCAs and MAOIs. Fluoxetine (Prozac) and paroxetine (Paxil), the best known of the SSRIs, have been hailed as miracle drugs and have been used to treat everything from depression to eating disorders and premenstrual syndrome.

SSRIs block the reuptake of serotonin, thereby increasing its concentration at postsynaptic cells and facilitating the transmission of nerve impulses. As their name implies, they are specific for serotonin and tend to have fewer anticholinergic effects than TCAs. Their sedating effect is also reportedly lower. Side effects of SSRIs include nausea, anorexia, insomnia, edginess, nervousness, and sexual dysfunctions.

Although they have fewer adverse side effects than other antidepressants, SSRIs may not be as effective in alleviating depression. Longer clinical use and further research will reveal whether or not these are truly the new wonder drugs they have initially seemed to be.

Tyramine-Containing Agents Interacting with MAOIs

Medications

- Appetite suppressants (diet pills, amphetamines, cocaine)
- Cold remedies (sinus, hay fever, cough, or cold tablets and liquids)
- Antihypertensives (methylodopa, guanethidine, reserpine)
- Antiparkinsonian agents (levodopa)
- Sedatives, CNS depressants (meperidine, morphine, codeine, barbiturates, alcohol)
- Systemic anesthetics

Foods and Beverages

Aged cheeses (cheddar, Camembert, Gruyère)

Red wines (Chianti, burgundy, cabernet)

Beers and ales

Chicken and beef livers

Avocados

Bananas

Fava beans

Pickled herring

Preserved meats and sausages

Yogurt

Soy sauce

Caffeine (coffee, tea, colas, chocolate)

Other agents that are used to treat depression and can be termed atypical antidepressants include sertraline (Zoloft), bupropion (Wellbutrin), and trazodone (Desyrel). Even lithium, long thought to be effective only in manic disorders, has been used successfully in the treatment of both unipolar and bipolar depression.

Psychopharmacology in the Treatment of Mania

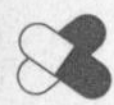

Several psychopharmocologic agents have proven effective in the treatment of mania. The most effective and widely used of these agents is lithium carbonate.

Lithium Carbonate Lithium carbonate is a potentially dangerous alkali metal that has been used in the treatment and prevention of acute manic episodes since the 1960s. It is now used in preventing the recurrence of bipolar disorder as well. Current research focuses on improvement in lithium's effectiveness when used in conjunction with other psychoactive drugs (Peselow et al. 1994).

Lithium alters neurotransmission in the central nervous system. It is thought to interfere with the ionic pump mechanism in brain cells, but its exact mode of action is unknown. Its use is not recommended during pregnancy, breast-feeding, or in clients with "impaired renal function, congestive heart failure, sodium-restricted diets, organic brain disease, and impaired CNS functioning" (Spencer et al. 1993, p. 523).

Administered orally, the onset of action ranges from 1 to 3 weeks. The dosage is gradually increased until the recommended therapeutic blood level of 1.0–1.5 mEq/L are achieved. When the desired effect is achieved, the dosage is adjusted downward to the maintenance blood level of 0.6–1.2 mEq/L.

Toxic symptoms begin appearing at blood levels above 1.5 mEq/L. Because there is such a narrow margin between therapeutic and toxic levels of lithium, serum concentrations must be closely monitored until stabilized. Symptoms of early lithium toxicity include: nausea, vomiting, diarrhea, polyuria, muscle weakness, fine hand tremors, and headache. Symptoms progress to blurred vision, slurred speech, dizziness, sluggishness, abdominal cramping, and tinnitus. Major adverse reactions include marked lethargy, confusion, coarse tremors, muscular twitching, ataxia, convulsions, coma, and circulatory failure.

Because of the need for close monitoring, clients are usually hospitalized when lithium therapy is initiated. Before they are discharged, both clients and families need to learn how to safely continue lithium therapy at home.

Instructions given to the client and family should include the following:

- The diet must include adequate salt and fluid intake, and the client should not take diuretics at any time.
- Regular testing of serum levels must be done, and the client's physician should be notified of any illness, especially if vomiting and diarrhea occur.
- The client should not vary the dosage and should continue to take the medicine even when feeling well, because discontinuing lithium therapy often precipitates a manic episode.
- If symptoms of lithium toxicity occur, the client should immediately discontinue the drug and contact the physician.

Alternative Mania Therapy The use of the anticonvulsants carbamazepine (Tegretol) and valproic acid (Dalpro, Depakene) is under study. These agents seem to be beneficial to the 30% of manic clients who do not respond to lithium carbonate therapy. Use in the prevention of unipolar depression is also being studied.

Electroconvulsive Therapy

Electroconvulsive therapy (ECT) is useful in clients with severe depression, acute mania, some psychotic conditions, and those who are acutely suicidal. It is usually given several times a week until a course of 12 treatments is completed. Caution is advised when ECT is administered to clients with increased intracranial pressure, pregnant clients, and those who have had recent myocardial infarctions.

A separate consent for treatment must be signed because ECT requires the administration of anesthesia. While informing clients and obtaining consent forms is legally a medical responsibility, in practice it is often shared by nurses. Preparation includes explaining the procedure to clients and answering all questions as fully as possible.

Clients are prepared for anesthesia by being NPO for at least 4 hours before treatment. Just prior to treatment they should void and also remove contact lenses, earrings, necklaces, hairpins, and dentures. Pretreatment vital signs are obtained.

Procedures vary slightly from facility to facility, but generally an atropinelike drug, such as glycopyrrolate (Robinul), is given to decrease secretions and block cardiac vagal reflexes during seizure. A short-acting anesthetic, such as methohexital sodium (Brevital), is administered intravenously. Following induction, a skeletal muscle relaxant, such as succinylcholine chloride (Anectine), is administered to prevent injuries during the seizure. The client must be artificially ventilated until the muscle relaxant is fully metabolized, usually in 2–3 minutes. Oxygen is administered by positive pressure with a rubber bite block in place.

An electrical current is passed through the brain by means of unilateral or bilateral electrodes placed on the temples. This causes a **grand mal seizure**, the effects of which are masked by the muscle relaxant. Often the only observable signs of seizure are a fluttering of the eyelids and carpopedal spasms.

Clients are recovered in the lateral recumbent position to facilitate drainage and prevent aspiration. Upon awakening they will be confused and somewhat disoriented. After they are fully recovered and have been reoriented by the nurse, they may eat breakfast.

During a course of ECT, short-term memory loss is expected. This is distressing to some clients, and they need to be reassured that memory is usually completely restored. Since ECT is not curative, ongoing psychotherapy and pharmacotherapy are often continued to prevent relapse.

text continues on page 358

CASE STUDY

A Client with Depression

Identifying Information

Margaret is a 59-year-old, unmarried legal assistant who was admitted to the psychiatric unit following a gastric lavage in the emergency department. She had ingested 30 imipramine tablets. She is employed in a large metropolitan law firm.

Client's Description of the Problem

Margaret stated that she had been at home alone for two days, became convinced that no one would care if she died, and took the imipramine that her family doctor had prescribed for depression. She became frightened almost immediately, was unable to make herself vomit, and called 911.

Margaret reports that she has been concerned about her impending retirement at age 65 and her elderly mother's declining health. She states that she has built her life around her work and cannot imagine what she would do without it. Because she works around the clock, she has virtually no social life and except for a few coworkers, she has no friends. She has stopped going to church in recent months, stating, "I just don't fit in anywhere and I never have."

About a month ago, Margaret's 84-year-old mother, who lives in a small town about 3 hours away, began to experience a deterioration in her health. Margaret now fears that she will have to go care for her mother, with whom she has never gotten along. Her siblings are pressuring her, as the "family caretaker," to move back home. She feels she will eventually have to go.

For the past 3 weeks she has been "exhausted," has not slept well, has lost weight, had crying spells, been irritable with coworkers, and had difficulty concentrating at work. She had suicidal thoughts but did not have a specific plan. Two days ago the firm's senior partner told her to take a few days off to "get yourself together." Margaret stated, "I have always been unattractive and nobody has ever loved me. If I died, all my family would lose is a nursemaid for Mama."

→

CASE STUDY *(continued)*

A Client with Depression

Psychiatric History

Although she reports occasional "blue spells," Margaret has no previous psychiatric history. For the past 30 years, she has had a close relationship with her family doctor, who helps her through her "blue spells" with support and antidepressant therapy. He prescribed the imipramine about 10 days ago, but it had not helped.

Family History

Margaret is the oldest of five children. She grew up in a small town where her father was "the town character." His manic-depressive behavior was an embarrassment to the family on many occasions. She describes her mother as "totally ineffectual. She couldn't even do her own hair. I ran the house." Her father died about 20 years ago, and her mother has lived alone ever since.

Two of Margaret's siblings live in the same town as her mother, but they do not seem to feel responsible for her care. She describes a very troubled relationship with her youngest sister, Mary, "who I raised." She has had no contact with Mary in several years and this grieves her very much. One of her brothers is an alcoholic. She is unaware of any depressive or other psychiatric problems in the family.

Social History

At age 16, Margaret was forced to drop out of school to help her mother care for the younger children and her father. She never felt like she was loved or appreciated for anything. "What I wanted to do never mattered. I just did what they wanted me to do."

She remained at home, keeping house for the family, until all her siblings were grown. At age 28 she was befriended by a woman who sent her to a special school, where she completed her high school education. This benefactor then paid her tuition to a legal assistant program where, for the first time in her life, Margaret found something she excelled at and enjoyed. Upon graduation she began work at the law firm, and has worked her way up through the ranks for the past 27 years. She states, "The law is my life."

Health History

Margaret suffers from osteoarthritis, obesity, and hypertension. Vital signs: T, 98.6; P, 77; R, 16; Ht, 5′4″; Wt, 190 lb; BP, 148/98.

Current Mental Status

Margaret is overweight, disheveled, and wearing mismatched, dirty clothing. She slumps in her seat and avoids eye contact. She is cooperative but slow to respond to questions. She is oriented to time, place, and person. Her judgment is good and ability to think abstractly is slow but unimpaired. Her affect is depressed, and she wept frequently throughout the interview. There are no delusions, illusions, hallucinations, or other signs of thought disorder. She is distressed that law firm employees will know her "personal business" and that this hospitalization will further endanger her continued employment.

Other Subjective or Objective Clinical Data

Margaret does not use alcohol or any CNS depressants. She takes nonsteroidal anti-inflammatory drugs (NSAIDS) for arthritis and is on a low-fat, low-sodium diet for hypertension. She has been taking imipramine for 10 days without noticeable effect.

Diagnostic Impression

Nursing Diagnosis

Risk for Self-Directed Violence related to recent suicide attempt
Self-Esteem Disturbance related to impaired cognition fostering negative view of self
Powerlessness related to lack of positive feedback
Social Isolation related to fear of rejection

DSM-IV Multiaxial Diagnoses

Axis I: 296.23 Major Depressive Disorder, Single Episode, Severe Without Psychotic Features (primary diagnosis)
Axis II: V71.09 No diagnosis
Axis III: Osteoarthritis, obesity, hypertension
Axis IV: Primary support group problems (health problems in family; discord with siblings); problems related to the social environment (inadequate social support; adjustment to impending retirement); occupational problems (unable to function at work)
Axis V: GAF = 20 (current); some danger of hurting self; GAF = 60 (highest level in past year)

NURSING CARE PLAN

A Client with Depression

Nursing Diagnosis

Risk for Self-Directed Violence related to recent suicide attempt.

Expected Outcome

- Client will approach nurse and discuss any suicidal urges.
- Client will make no-suicide contract with nurse.

Nursing Interventions

- Remove all dangerous articles from client's environment.
- Observe client closely, using irregular schedule.
- Adopt neutral, matter-of-fact attitude.
- Evaluate suicidal intention at every shift and institute appropriate level of supervision.
- Establish no-suicide contract.
- Encourage client to seek nurse out when bothered by suicidal thoughts or impulses.
- Limit repetitive discussion of suicidal ruminations.
- Encourage the expression of feelings.
- Help client identify alternative ways of dealing with stress.
- Help client identify community resources and supports.
- Teach client safe use of antidepressant medication.

Outcome Met If

- Client does not harm self during hospitalization.
- Client demonstrates alternative ways of dealing with stress, such as talking, exercise, relaxation techniques.
- Client verbalizes resources where she can seek help if suicidal thoughts recur following discharge, such as crisis line, minister.
- Client verbalizes safe uses of antidepressant medication; describes potential drug interactions.

Nursing Diagnosis

Self-Esteem Disturbance related to impaired cognition fostering negative view of self.

Expected Outcome

- Client will participate in unit activities.
- Client will verbalize positive aspect of self.
- Client will verbalize increased feelings of self-worth.
- Client will express feelings directly.

Nursing Interventions

- Teach client that activity helps decrease depression.
- Help client with hygiene and grooming as needed.
- Involve client in simple recreational activities.
- Increase the complexity of activities as client progresses.
- Give positive recognition when progress is shown.
- Help client enumerate personal strengths.
- Set limits on time spent reviewing past failures.
- Teach client assertiveness techniques.

Outcome Met If

- Client expresses some hope for the future. Plans for retirement.
- Client sets realistic goals for self and works toward them; plans to return to work within 1 week of discharge.
- Client communicates assertively with others; explains to siblings that she will not give up her career to come home to care for her mother.
- Client's posture and grooming are consistent with increased self-esteem; sits and walks erectly, combs hair neatly, wears clean, matching clothes.

Nursing Diagnosis

Powerlessness related to lack of positive feedback.

Expected Outcome

- Client will establish nondependent nurse-client relationships.
- Client will identify situations over which she has no control.
- Client will identify situations over which she can attain control.

Nursing Interventions

- Emphasize the short-term nature of client's relationship with nurses.
- Provide choices when possible.
- Explore problem-solving models and practice using them with small daily problems.
- Engage client in goal setting for self.
- Assist client to identify supports available in the community.

Outcome Met If

- Client verbalizes plans to attain control over life situations; works with siblings to find appropriate caretaker for mother.
- Client verbalizes feelings about situations over which she has no control; realizes that siblings' expectations do not control her responses.
- Client demonstrates a problem-solving system that she has used successfully.

→

NURSING CARE PLAN *(continued)*

A Client with Depression

- Client successfully terminates nurse-client relationships; makes transition to identified community resources and does not attempt to stay in touch following discharge.

Nursing Diagnosis

Social Isolation related to fear of rejection.

Expected Outcome

- Client will communicate with members of the nursing staff.
- Client will socialize with other clients on the unit.
- Client voluntarily attends group activities.
- Client can initiate interaction as desired without undue fear of rejection.

Nursing Interventions

- Make brief, frequent contacts.
- Spend time sitting with client with no demands.
- Use nonjudgmental attitude.
- Encourage client to ventilate feelings verbally or through activity.
- Accompany client to group activities initially, withdrawing as tolerated.
- Teach social skills, and encourage practice.
- Teach assertive communication, and encourage role playing.
- Give positive feedback for all signs of progress.

Outcome Met If

- Client assumes responsibility for dealing with feelings, including seeking others out; identifies key individuals outside hospital and initiates contact to renew relationships.
- Client plans for discharge by establishing a social life and support system outside the hospital; begins attending church again; contacts old acquaintances and plans for lunch meetings; joins AARP (American Association of Retired Persons) and attends local chapter meetings.

Chapter Highlights

- Mood disorders are extreme emotional states. They are characterized by disturbances of cognitive, behavioral, and physical response patterns.
- Depression is the most common mood disorder, affecting 11 million Americans annually.
- A variety of causative theories have been postulated, including biologic and psychologic ones. The study of biologic factors that influence mood disorders holds promise for greater understanding in the future.
- Major depressive disorder includes symptoms of depressed mood; loss of interest or pleasure in activities; changes in appetite, weight, sleep, and psychomotor activity; decreased energy; feelings of worthlessness and guilt; difficulty thinking, concentrating, and making decisions; and suicidal thoughts, plans, or attempts.
- Symptoms of depression are often masked by somatic complaints of headache, abdominal pain, and vague bodily aches and pains.
- Mania includes symptoms of elevated or euphoric mood, inflated self-esteem, decreased need for sleep, pressured speech, flight of ideas, uncharacteristic excessive behaviors, and psychomotor hyperactivity or agitation.
- Bipolar disorder is characterized by one or more manic episodes and one or more major depressive episodes. There are six subtypes of bipolar disorder.
- Mood disorders may be manifestations of physiologic conditions, so a thorough general medical evaluation should be completed before making a diagnosis of mood disorder.
- Culture plays a role in how individuals express emotions and must be taken into consideration when working with clients from different ethnic and racial backgrounds.
- Nurses collaborate with other mental health care professionals, clients, and their families in providing individualized nursing care to clients with mood disorders.

- Client safety is a primary nursing concern in working with clients with mood disorders.
- Nurses will find challenges in working with clients with mood disorders. Self-awareness is the key to dealing with these challenges.
- Psychopharmacologic and electroconvulsant therapy are frequently used in the treatment of severe mood disorders.

References

American Psychiatric Association: *Diagnostic and Statistical Manual of Mental Disorders,* ed 4. American Psychiatric Association, 1994.

Beck AT, Ward CH, Mendelson M, Mock J, and Erbaugh J: An inventory for measuring depression. *Arch Gen Psychiatr* 1961;4:561–571.

Blazer DG, Kessler RC, McGonagle KA, Swartz MS: The prevalence and distribution of major depression in a national community sample: The national comorbidity survey. *Am J Psychiatr* 1994;151(7):979–986.

Bowen M: *Family Therapy in Clinical Practice.* Jason Aronson, 1978.

Bowlby J: *Attachment and Loss: Separation, Anxiety, and Anger.* Basic Books, 1973.

Carpenito LJ: *Nursing Diagnosis: Application to Clinical Practice,* ed 5. Lippincott, 1993.

Devanand DP, Dwork AJ, Hutchinson ER, Bolwig TG, Sackeim HA: Does ECT alter brain structure? *Am J Psychiatr* 1994;151(7):957–970.

Freud S: Mourning and melancholia, in *Standard Edition of the Complete Psychological Works of Sigmund Freud,* vol. 4. Hogarth Press, 1957.

Gibbons JL: Total body sodium and potassium in depressive illness. *Clin Sci* 1960;19:133–141.

Goleman D: Depression's personal, fiscal toll high. *The Chattanooga Times* 1994;124 (303):1.

Harris B: Biological and hormonal aspects of postpartum depressed mood: Working towards strategies for prophylaxis and treatment. *Brit J Psychiatr* 1994;164(3):288–292.

Janowsky DS: Neurochemistry of depression and mania, in Georgotas A, Cancro R (eds): *Depression and Mania.* Elsevier, 1988.

Kaplan HI, Sadock, BJ: *Comprehensive Textbook of Psychiatry,* ed 5. Williams & Wilkins, 1989.

Klein M: A contribution to the psychogenesis of manic-depressive states, in *Contributions to Psychoanalysis.* Hogarth Press, 1934.

Kolata G: Manic-depressive gene tied to chromosome 11. *Sci* 1987;235:1139.

Maynard C: Comparison of effectiveness of group interventions for depression in women. *Arch Psychiatr Nurs* 1993;7(5):277–283.

McEnany GW: Psychobiological indices of bipolar mood disorder: Future trends in nursing care. *Arch Psychiatr Nurs* 1990;4(1):29–38.

Nowlin-Finch NL, Altshuler LL, Szuba MP, Mintz J: Rapid resolution of first episodes of mania: Sleep related? *J Clin Psychiatr* 1994;55(1):26–29.

Pachter LM: Culture and clinical care. *JAMA* 1994;271(9): 690–694.

Parker G, Hadzi-Pavlovic D, Sengoz A, Boyce P, Mitchell P, Wilhelm K, Hickie I, Brodaty H: A brief self-report depression measure assessing mood state and social impairment. *J Aff Dis* 1994;30(2):133–142.

Peselow ED, Fieve RR, Difiglia D, Sanfilipo MP: Lithium prophylaxis of bipolar illness: The value of combination treatment. *Brit J Psychiatr* 1994;164:208–214.

Schultz JM, Videbeck SD: *Manual of Psychiatric Nursing Care Plans,* ed 4. Lippincott, 1994.

Seligman M: Depression and learned helplessness, in Friedman R, Katz M (eds) : *The Psychology of Depression: Contemporary Theory and Research.* VH Winston & Sons, 1974.

Spencer RT, Nichols LW, Lipkin GB, Henderson HS, West FM: *Clinical Pharmacology and Nursing Management,* ed 4. Lippincott, 1993.

Suppes T, Baldessarini RJ, Faedda GL, Tondo L, Tohen M: Discontinuation of maintenance treatment in bipolar disorder: Risks and implications. *Harvard Rev Psychiatr* 1993;1:131–144.

Tinkleberg M: Shift work and circadia rhythm. *Healthwatch: The Nurse's Newspaper,* January 7, 1991.

Townsend MC: *Nursing Diagnoses in Psychiatric Nursing,* ed 3. FA Davis, 1994.

U.S. Department of Health and Human Services, Public Health Service, Agency for Health Care Policy and Research (ACHPR): Depression in primary care: detection, diagnosis, and treatment. *J Psychosoc Nurs* 1993;31(6): 19–28.

Warren BJ: Depression in African-American women. *J Psychosoc Nurs* 1994;32(3):29–33.

Wehr TA: Phase and biorhythm studies of affective illness. *Ann Intern Med* 1977;87:321–333.

Zung WWK: A self-rating depression scale. *Arch Gen Psychiatr* 1965;12:63–70.

CHAPTER 16

CLIENTS WITH ANXIETY, SOMATOFORM, AND DISSOCIATIVE DISORDERS

Sue C. DeLaune

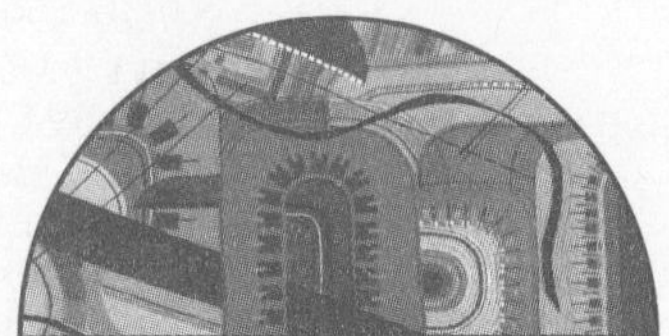

COMPETENCIES

- *Describe the theoretic foundations related to anxiety disorders, somatoform disorders, and dissociative disorders.*
- *Differentiate clinical features characteristic of each of these disorders as defined in the* DSM-IV.
- *Relate the concept of anxiety to anxiety disorders, somatoform disorders, and dissociative disorders.*
- *Develop appropriate nursing diagnoses for clients experiencing anxiety disorders, somatoform disorders, and dissociative disorders.*
- *Apply the nursing process for clients with anxiety disorders, somatoform disorders, and dissociative disorders.*

Cross-References

Other topics relevant to this content are: Psychobiology, Chapter 3; Basics related to anxiety, stress, and coping, Chapter 4; Crisis intervention for the acute stage of posttraumatic stress disorder, Chapter 30; Dissociative problems in victims of childhood sexual abuse, Chapter 23; Guidelines for teaching clients and families about antianxiety drugs, Chapter 33; Psychopharmacologic treatment of anxiety (the antianxiety drugs), Chapter 33; Relaxation and stress-management techniques, Chapter 29.

Portions of the material in this chapter were contributed to the fourth edition by Marilynn Petit.

Critical Thinking Challenge

Some health care providers think that clients experiencing the disorders discussed in this chapter are "faking it," perhaps in order to gain attention or for financial gain. They may think that multiple personalities are not possible, they are skeptical of bizarre symptoms, and they may believe that people with conversion disorder or hypochondriasis have nothing really *wrong with them. What do you think?*

Although anxiety is a universal experience, people vary in their ability to tolerate anxiety and anxiety-producing situations. This chapter explores the experience of individuals with anxiety disorders, somatoform disorders, and dissociative disorders. People with these disorders all have one thing in common: The degree of anxiety is so disabling that they are unable to function. The functional disabilities may affect all dimensions of life:

- Physical
- Emotional
- Cognitive
- Sociocultural
- Spiritual

Anxiety Disorders

Anxiety disorders are characterized by a mixture of physiologic, psychologic, behavioral, and cognitive symptoms. The *DSM-IV* classifies anxiety disorders into the following types:

- Panic disorder
- Social phobia
- Special phobia
- Generalized anxiety disorder
- Obsessive-compulsive disorder
- Posttraumatic stress disorder
- Acute stress disorder

In this group of disorders, anxiety is either the predominant disturbance, as in generalized anxiety disorder; or anxiety is experienced as avoidance behavior when the person attempts to master the symptoms, as in confronting the dreaded object or situation in a phobic disorder. When anxiety is not tied to a specific stimulus, it may be called *free-floating anxiety.*

People in anxiety states experience anxiety both as a subjective emotion and as a variety of physical symptoms resulting from muscular tension and autonomic nervous system activity. (See Chapter 4 for a discussion of the symptoms of anxiety.) When acute, the anxiety rapidly drives the individual to seek help. When subacute or chronic, anxiety can lead to a number of somatic discomforts or disabilities. Heartburn, epigastric distress, diarrhea, and constipation may occur. Chronic muscular tension can lead to a variety of musculosketetal aches and pains.

Onset may be sudden or gradual. Some people experience an unexpected, incapacitating outbreak of acute anxiety, as in panic disorder. In others, anxiety may express itself through relatively mild somatic symptoms in which the existence of basic anxiety is missed unless specifically inquired about, as in generalized anxiety disorder.

Panic Disorder

An apparently common disorder, **panic disorder** is characterized by recurrent attacks of severe anxiety lasting a few moments to an hour. These attacks are not associated with a stimulus but instead seem to occur suddenly and spontaneously. They may, however, become associated with certain situations, such as going into a shopping mall or driving a car. The person usually experiences such physical symptoms as palpitations, rapid pulse, nausea, diarrhea, dyspnea, and a feeling of choking or suffocation. The pupils are dilated, and the face is flushed. The person may feel dizzy or faint and often has a sense of impending doom or death. It is not uncommon to fear going crazy or doing something uncontrolled. Restlessness is acute, and the person may make pleading, apprehensive appeals for help.

In its most advanced state, panic creates a symptom constellation totally mimicking myocardial infarction and mitral valve prolapse. This symptom complex, seen most frequently in young adults, is called **cardiac neurosis.** Symptoms include palpitations, tachycardia, chest pain, dyspnea, easy fatigability, dizziness, sweating, irritability, faintness, and a feeling of impending doom.

Panic attacks may occur on occasion in normal, healthy individuals, leaving little or no residual disability. Panic-related symptoms are common and felt by approximately 10% of adults at one time or another (Laraia 1991). When the attacks occur frequently and when they interfere with the person's social functioning at work, school, or in the family, the condition is called panic disorder. A panic attack generally last for several minutes. People who have repeated attacks, or persistently worry about having another attack, are diagnosed with panic disorder.

Anticipatory fear of helplessness or of losing control during a panic attack is a common complication of the disorder. The individual frequently avoids situations that induce the fear, sometimes developing a phobic avoidance reaction. The *DSM-IV* states that a diagnosis of **panic disorder with agoraphobia** is appropriate for an individual who experiences panic attacks and has phobic avoidance. In the absence of phobic avoidance, the condition is termed **panic disorder without agoraphobia. Agoraphobia,** the marked fear of being alone or in public places from which escape might be difficult or in which help might not be available, is secondary to panic attacks. Agoraphobia without panic attacks is uncommon. Agoraphobia with symptoms of panic attack is now treatable with some drugs. DSM-IV criteria for both forms of panic disorder are listed in the box on the next page.

Panic disorder is often first noted in late adolescence or early adulthood. It may be limited to a single brief period lasting several weeks or months, recur several times, or become chronic. Though it is rarely incapacitating, the disorder can be severe. When complicated by agoraphobia, it can interfere greatly with individual functioning. Panic disorder is diagnosed much more frequently in women than in men, and some clinicians believe that sudden object loss and separation anxiety in childhood are predisposing factors. Such physical disorders as hypoglycemia, hyperthyroidism, and amphetamine or caffeine intoxication must be ruled out before a diagnosis of panic disorder can be made. The ways in which hypoglycemia mimics a panic attack are discussed in the Nutrition box on page 363.

Phobic Disorders

Like the other anxiety disorders discussed in this chapter, a phobic disorder is a response to experienced anxiety. Unlike people whose anxiety is free-floating, people with phobias fear specific places or things. A **phobia** is a persistent and irrational fear of a specific object, activity, or situation that results in a compelling desire to avoid the

Diagnostic Criteria for 300.01 Panic Disorder Without Agoraphobia and 300.21 Panic Disorder With Agoraphobia

A. Both 1 and 2:
   1. recurrent unexpected Panic Attacks
   2. at least one of the attacks has been followed by 1 month (or more) of one (or more) of the following:
      a. persistent concern about having additional attacks
      b. worry about the implications of the attack or its consequences (e.g., losing control, having a heart attack, "going crazy")
      c. a significant change in behavior related to the attacks

B. The presence of Agoraphobia (for 300.21 Panic Disorder With Agoraphobia)
   OR
   The absence of Agoraphobia (for 300.01 Panic Disorder Without Agoraphobia)

C. The Panic Attacks are not due to the direct physiological effects of a substance (e.g., a drug of abuse, a medication) or a general medical condition (e.g., hyperthyroidism).

D. The Panic Attacks are not better accounted for by another mental disorder, such as Social Phobia (e.g., occurring on exposure to feared social situations), Specific Phobia (e.g., on exposure to a specific phobic situation), Obsessive-Compulsive Disorder (e.g., on exposure to dirt in someone with an obsession about contamination), Posttraumatic Stress Disorder (e.g., in response to stimuli associated with a severe stressor), or Separation Anxiety Disorder (e.g., in response to being away from home or close relatives).

Source: American Psychiatric Association 1994, pp. 402–403.

dreaded object or situation. Nearly all phobic individuals panic when in contact with the phobic situation. The fear is recognized by adults or adolescents as unreasonable in proportion to the actual danger. However, children do not always identify their fears as being unrealistic.

The usual explanation of the development of phobia is that fear arises through a process of displacing an unconscious conflict to an external object symbolically related to the conflict. Thus, in becoming phobic, the individual fears a specific external object rather than an unknown internal source of distress. The phobic person can then control the intensity of the anxiety by avoiding the object with which the anxiety is associated.

A diagnosis of a phobic disorder is generally made when the avoidance behavior becomes so extreme or the problem so pervasive that it interferes with the person's normal functioning at home, work, or school. The *DSM-IV* divides the phobic disorders into three main types:

1. *Agoraphobia:* fear of being alone or in public places from which escape might be difficult or help might not be available.
2. *Social phobia:* fear of situations in which an individual may be exposed to scrutiny by others or that may be humiliating or embarrassing.
3. *Specific phobia:* fear of specific things.

AGORAPHOBIA Agoraphobic individuals often fear leaving the safety of home, worrying that they might develop an incapacitating symptom, such as dizziness, loss of bowel or bladder control, or cardiac distress. Normal activities are increasingly curtailed as the fears dominate the person's life. Agoraphobic people often limit travel and need a companion when away from home. Those who endure the phobic situation experience intense anxiety. Other phobias associated with agoraphobia are listed in Table 16–1 on page 364.

Agoraphobia without panic attacks is relatively rare. More commonly, people with agoraphobia have spontaneous panic attacks.

Most agoraphobics have a history of generalized anxiety or anxiety attacks at the onset of the phobic behavior. Onset of this disorder usually occurs in the middle to late twenties. Agoraphobia is more frequently diagnosed in women than in men. Separation anxiety in childhood and sudden object loss appear to be predisposing factors. Depression, anxiety, rituals, minor "checking" compulsions, and rumination are frequently associated features of agoraphobia.

The prognosis is variable. Some less severely disturbed individuals experience intermittent symptoms and sometimes have periods of remission. The more severely impaired may suffer lifelong disability.

NUTRITION AND MENTAL HEALTH

Can Hypoglycemia Mimic an Anxiety Attack?

Much has been written in the lay press about the dangers of low blood sugar. Some popular authors claim it is a major scourge that afflicts millions of Americans, causing severe psychologic harm. Although there is little controlled clinical research to support that view, psychiatric nurses should not dismiss hypoglycemia as a hypochondriac's invention.

Postprandial hypoglycemia is a drop in plasma glucose following a carbohydrate load. It can occur after gastric surgery or in the very early stages of diabetes. However, when it has no clear-cut organic cause, it is called functional hypoglycemia.

Functional low blood sugar presents in two major ways: Epinephrinelike signs and symptoms include nervousness, faintness, weakness, tremulousness, palpitations, sweating, and hunger. Central nervous system signs and symptoms include headache, confusion, visual disturbances, muscle weakness, ataxia, and marked personality changes (Berkow 1987).

No one challenges the existence of the syndrome or its signs and symptoms. Its prevalence, however, is open to debate. Studies suggest that between 3 and 23 percent of subjects complaining of hypoglycemialike problems actually meet standard diagnostic criteria (Betteridge 1987, Foster and Rubenstein 1985).

Most clinicians use the five-hour glucose tolerance test to detect the condition. The three diagnostic markers are a drop in blood glucose to below 50–60 mg/dL, symptoms of hypoglycemia during the test, and symptomatic relief upon eating sugar. Although it is reasonable to conclude that clients who meet all three criteria have hypoglycemia, one cannot always rule out the condition among those who do not.

Researchers have found that clients with blood glucose readings above 60 mg/dL may still have functional hypoglycemia, apparently because their normal blood glucose range is significantly higher than that of the population mean (Chalew et al. 1986). Clients with blood glucose readings below 50 mg/dL who experience no symptoms during the test most probably do not have hypoglycemia. Apparently their normal range is *below* the average.

The five-hour glucose tolerance test may not be the gold standard for detecting functional hypoglycemia. Some specialists have challenged its validity on the grounds that it does not simulate everyday eating patterns. Very few people consume 75 or 100 grams of pure glucose at one sitting, and clients' glycemic and symptomatic response to that much sugar may not reflect real-world conditions. With that in mind, some clinicians recommend that clients consume a normal diet and that blood glucose levels be measured throughout the day with a portable glucose monitor. A drop in readings during a hypoglycemialike episode strongly suggests the presence of the disorder (Palardy et al. 1989).

If a client does meet the criteria for hypoglycemia, and the possibility of an insulin-secreting tumor of the pancreas has been ruled out as the cause of hypoglycemic symptoms, how should they be managed? Before recommending or adopting a dietary regimen, both nurse and client must understand its rationale. Functional hypoglycemia is brought on by an oversensitivity to carbohydrates. Whereas a normal person secretes just enough insulin in response to a heavy carbohydrate meal to lower blood glucose levels to physiologic levels, someone with functional hypoglycemia secretes too much, causing blood glucose levels to drop too low and depleting the brain of its primary fuel.

To compensate for this abnormality, the diet must allow a slow, steady absorption of sugars, thus preventing the pancreas from overreacting. That is accomplished by reducing intake of simple carbohydrates such as table sugar (sucrose), jams, honey, and corn syrup, replacing them with starches (complex carbohydrates) and proteins. Complex carbohydrates include breads, cereals, potatoes, rice, and corn. Whole-grain versions of these foods are preferable because the fiber they contain helps moderate intestinal absorption. These foods are then combined with protein-rich foods such as meat, fish, beans, and milk to further control sugar utilization. As a rule, between-meal snacks are also encouraged to prevent blood glucose levels from dropping too low two to three hours after main meals.

Paul L. Cerrato, BS, MA

Table 16–1 Common Phobias

Fear of	*Name of Phobia*
High places	Acrophobia
Open places	Agoraphobia
Closed places	Claustrophobia
Water	Hydrophobia
Dead bodies	Necrophobia
Strangers	Xenophobia
Animals	Zoophobia

SOCIAL PHOBIA The main characteristic of **social phobia** is persistent fear and avoidance of situations in which the person may be exposed to scrutiny by others. The person especially fears he or she will act in an embarrassing or humiliating manner. Examples of social phobias are extreme fear of performing or speaking in public, making complaints, or writing or eating in front of others. Others include fear of interacting with members of the opposite sex, superiors, or aggressive individuals. Usually a person has only one social phobia.

According to the *DSM-IV,* 10–20% of those who have anxiety disorders are also affected by social phobias. Often appearing in late childhood or early adolescence, social phobia usually progresses to a chronic course. Some lessening of symptoms may occur in middle age, but the disorder is usually lifelong with only occasional remissions.

Sex ratio, familial pattern, and predisposing factors are unknown, although some investigators believe that the incidence is evenly distributed between men and women. Generalized anxiety, agoraphobia, or specific phobia may coexist with social phobia.

SPECIFIC PHOBIA More common than any other type of phobic disorder, **specific phobias** are isolated fears focused on one situation or object, such as darkness, heights, or reptiles. This category of phobic disorders encompasses all phobias not included in agoraphobia or social phobia.

Many specific phobias begin in childhood and subsequently disappear. Those that persist into adulthood rarely go away without treatment. Specific phobia is more often diagnosed in females than in males.

Specific phobias generally cause minimal impairment if the phobic object is rarely encountered and easily avoided; for example, a fear of snakes does not seriously impair an individual living in a high-rise condominium. The phobia can, however, be incapacitating if the phobic situation is frequently encountered and not easily avoided. A fear of heights or elevators would seriously incapacitate a person living in a high-rise condominium, for instance.

A specific phobia may lead to lifestyle restrictions varying in severity according to the degree of anxiety.

The object or situation avoided determines the subtype of specific phobia. The *DSM-IV* identifies these subtypes:

- *Animal type:* fear precipitated by animals, birds, or insects.
- *Natural environment type:* fear triggered by elements of nature, such as water, or weather.
- *Blood-injection-injury type:* fear caused by the sight of blood or an injury, or by receiving invasive medical procedures, such as an injection. The vasovagal response often occurs with this type of phobic reaction. There is a strong familial pattern with this subtype.
- *Situational type:* fear resulting from contact with enclosed places, bridges, and/or public transportation.

Generalized Anxiety Disorder

Generalized anxiety disorder (GAD) is considered less specific and less debilitating than panic disorder and Phobic disorder. GAD is characterized by pervasive, persistent anxiety of at least 6 months' duration but without phobias, panic attacks, or obsessions and compulsions. The person experiences chronic feelings of nervousness and apprehension "for no reason" and is unable to control the worry. The worry is greatly exaggerated in relation to the probability that the event will actually occur. The frequency, duration, and intensity of the anxiety are disproportionate to the source of worry. Autonomic symptoms may be less frequent or less severe than in panic attacks.

There is little generally accepted information about age of onset, predisposing factors, cause of illness, prevalence, sex ratio, or familial pattern, although there appears to be a more equal sex ratio than in panic disorder. Associated mild depressive symptoms are not uncommon in individuals with Generalized anxiety disorder. Although impairment in social or occupational functioning is rarely more than mild, the abuse of alcohol or other drugs may be a serious complication and may interfere with effective motivation.

Obsessive-Compulsive Disorder

Obsessive-compulsive disorder (OCD) is classified with the anxiety disorders because of the anxiety symptoms that develop when an individual tries to resist an obsession or compulsion. Although compulsions are attempts to reduce tension, they eventually increase tension because the individual becomes increasingly agitated, unable to decide whether to stop or to continue their compulsive actions.

Obsessive-compulsive people usually fear that they will harm someone or something. They rely heavily on avoidance and are best understood in terms of their control needs. Individuals who develop obsessive-compulsive symptoms have a great need to control themselves, others, and their environment.

An **obsession** is a recurring thought that cannot be dismissed from consciousness. These intrusive thoughts are sometimes trivial or ridiculous, often morbid or fearful, and always distressing and anxiety-provoking. An example of a strange but trivial obsession is that of a young man who could not get the rhyme "Snips and snails and puppydog tails" out of his mind. An example of a much more ominous obsession is that of a woman who could not stop thinking that she must kill her children to prevent a worldwide race war. Other common obsessive thoughts have to do with violence or contamination.

A **compulsion** is an uncontrollable, persistent urge to perform certain acts or behaviors to relieve an otherwise unbearable tension. Most compulsive acts are attempts to control or modify obsessions because compulsive people either fear the consequences or are afraid that they will not be able to control the primary impulse.

Typical compulsive acts are endless hand washing, checking and rechecking doors to see if they have been locked, and elaborate dressing and undressing rituals. Such defensive compulsive acts are used to contain, neutralize, or ward off the anxiety related to the primary impulse. The young man who could not dismiss the rhyme from his mind developed a compulsion that involved ritualistic washing of his genitals to ward off the anxiety generated by his apparently silly obsession. The woman obsessed with thoughts about killing her children engaged in symbolic rituals of touching religious objects to repel evil influences through magical interventions by the saints. Such compulsive acts as counting and elaborately checking routine duties are frequently associated with the fear of failing or making a mistake, or with the need to be perfect.

Table 16–2 lists some common obsessions and compulsions. Obsessions and compulsions occur together in 75% of cases and usually follow a chronic course with fluctuations in the severity of symptoms. In severe cases, extreme preoccupation or compulsive activity disrupts daily life. Obsessions and compulsions have the following features in common:

- An idea or impulse insistently, persistently, and impellingly intrudes itself into the person's awareness.
- A feeling of anxious dread accompanies the primary manifestation and often leads the person to take countermeasures against the forbidden thought or impulse.
- Both the obsessions and the compulsion are ego-alien—foreign to one's self-perception.
- No matter how compelling the obsession or compulsion is, the person has enough insight to recognize it as irrational and experience it as a significant source of distress.
- Many of the personality traits associated with obsession and compulsion are highly valued in American culture. Success in many professions and occupations demands cautiousness, deliberateness, and rationality. These traits are usually associated with the tendency toward obsession or compulsion. When these personality traits are carried to an extreme, or when the balance between control and impulse expression leads to paralysis, they become a liability.

Table 16–2 Common Obsessive-Compulsive Behaviors

Behavior	*Related Compulsion*	*Related Obsession*
Repetitious hand washing	Urge to wash, scrub, or clean	Fear of disease or contamination
Returning home often to make sure appliances are turned off.	Need to recheck related to self-doubt	Fear of disaster
Hoarding junk mail, receipts, and all types of papers	Need to keep everything	Fear of losing things
Ritualistic counting of number of stairs climbed	Urge to count repeatedly	Belief that counting will yield control and thus prevent making mistakes

OCD is equally common in both men and women. The usual age of onset is the late teens to mid-twenties, though it has been diagnosed as early as childhood. For many years, it was believed that OCD was extremely rare. However, a study by the National Institute of Mental Health discovered that obsessive-compulsive disorder may affect as many as 2% of the population, making it even more common than schizophrenia (NIMH 1991). DSM-IV diagnostic criteria for this disorder are listed in the box on page 366.

Posttraumatic Stress Disorder

Posttraumatic stress disorder (PTSD) may be defined as the experience of a significant, recognizable stressor or trauma, outside the range of usual experience, that is followed by recurrent subjective reexperiencing of the trauma. PTSD includes traumatic stress reactions to military combat, and to civilian and natural catastrophes such as assault or rape, incest, skyjacking, and earthquake. For a discussion of PTSD as it relates to the experience of rape or incest, see Chapter 23.

Diagnostic Criteria for 300.3 Obsessive-Compulsive Disorder

A. Either obsessions or compulsions:

Obsessions as defined by 1, 2, 3, and 4:

1. recurrent and persistent thoughts, impulses, or images that are experienced, at some time during the disturbance, as intrusive and inappropriate and that cause marked anxiety or distress
2. the thoughts, impulses, or images are not simply excessive worries about real-life problems
3. the person attempts to ignore or suppress such thoughts, impulses, or images, or to neutralize them with some other thought or action
4. the person recognizes that the obsessional thoughts, impulses, or images are a product of his or her own mind (not imposed from without as in thought insertion)

Compulsions as defined by 1 and 2:

1. repetitive behaviors (e.g., hand washing, ordering, checking) or mental acts (e.g., praying, counting, repeating words silently) that the person feels driven to perform in response to an obsession, or according to rules that must be applied rigidly
2. the behaviors or mental acts are aimed at preventing or reducing distress or preventing some dreaded event or situation; however, these behaviors or mental acts either are not connected in a realistic way with what they are designed to neutralize or prevent or are clearly excessive

B. At some point during the course of the disorder, the person has recognized that the obsessions or compulsions are excessive or unreasonable. **Note:** This does not apply to children.

C. The obsessions or compulsions cause marked distress, are time consuming (take more than 1 hour a day); or significantly interfere with the person's normal routine, occupational (or academic) functioning, or usual social activities or relationships.

D. If another Axis I disorder is present, the content of the obsessions or compulsions is not restricted to it (e.g., preoccupation with food in the presence of an Eating Disorder; hair pulling in the presence of Trichotillomania; concern with appearance in the presence of Body Dysmorphic Disorder; preoccupation with drugs in the presence of a Substance Use Disorder; preoccupation with having a serious illness in the presence of Hypochondriasis; preoccupation with sexual urges or fantasies in the presence of a Paraphilia; or guilty ruminations in the presence of Major Depressive Disorder).

E. The disturbance is not due to the direct physiological effects of a substance (e.g., a drug of abuse, a medication) or a general medical condition.

Specify if:

With Poor Insight: if, for most of the time during the current episode, the person does not recognize that the obsessions and compulsions are excessive or unreasonable

Source: American Psychiatric Association 1994, pp. 422–423.

The course of the disorder is variable. Most people who have suffered a significant stressor tend to have an acute reaction from which they recover spontaneously. In others, however, the reaction may be delayed or prolonged and eventually become chronic.

PTSD is divided into categories according to onset and duration of symptoms:

- Acute: symptoms last less than 3 months.
- Chronic: symptoms last 3 months or more.
- Delayed onset: at least 6 months have lapsed between the trauma and the occurrence of symptoms.

Many veterans of the armed forces have experienced PTSD. Upon returning home from combat, they essentially relived their experience through recurrent nightmares. Other sleep disturbances, including insomnia, often occurred. Psychic numbing—emotional anesthesia in relation to other people and to previously enjoyed activities—was common. Some veterans have reported difficulty in concentrating and remembering. Many veterans feel guilty about having survived when others did not, or about actions they took to survive. When veterans were exposed to situations or events that resembled or symbolized the traumatic event, their symptoms often increased, and they felt even greater distress. Reactions such as these continue to disturb some Vietnam and Persian Gulf war veterans even today.

PTSD can occur in people of any age, even children. Associated symptoms of depression, anxiety, and increased irritability are common, sometimes leading to unpredictable explosions of hostility with little or no provocation.

People with PTSD avoid the stimuli associated with the traumatic event. For example, a woman who is raped in an elevator may very likely avoid using any elevator. This example shows how PTSD can restrict daily functioning. A significant complicating problem is the use of alcohol or other substances to maintain control and soothe emotions. The DSM-IV diagnostic criteria for PTSD are listed in the box below.

Diagnostic Criteria for 309.81 Posttraumatic Stress Disorder

A. The person has been exposed to a traumatic event in which both the following were present:
   1. the person experienced, witnessed, or was confronted with an event or events that involved actual or threatened death or serious injury, or a threat to the physical integrity of self or others
   2. the person's response involved intense fear, helplessness, or horror. **Note:** In children, this may be expressed instead by disorganized or agitated behavior

B. The traumatic event is persistently reexperienced in one (or more) of the following ways:
   1. recurrent and intrusive distressing recollections of the event, including images, thoughts, or perceptions. **Note:** In young children, repetitive play may occur in which themes or aspects of the trauma are expressed.
   2. recurrent distressing dreams of the event. **Note:** In children, there may be frightening dreams without recognizable content.
   3. acting or feeling as if the traumatic event were recurring (includes a sense of reliving the experience, illusions, hallucinations, and dissociative flashback episodes, including those that occur on awakening or when intoxicated). **Note:** In young children, trauma-specific reenactment may occur.
   4. intense psychological distress at exposure to internal or external cues that symbolize or resemble an aspect of the traumatic event
   5. physiological reactivity on exposure to internal or external cues that symbolize or resemble an aspect of the traumatic event

C. Persistent avoidance of stimuli associated with the trauma and numbing of general responsiveness (not present before the trauma), as indicated by three (or more) of the following:
   1. efforts to avoid thoughts, feelings, or conversations associated with the trauma
   2. efforts to avoid activities, places, or people that arouse recollections of the trauma
   3. inability to recall an important aspect of the trauma
   4. markedly diminished interest or participation in significant activities
   5. feeling of detachment or estrangement from others
   6. restricted range of affect (e.g., unable to have loving feelings)
   7. sense of a foreshortened future (e.g., does not expect to have a career, marriage, children, or a normal life span)

D. Persistent symptoms of increased arousal (not present before the trauma), as indicated by two (or more) of the following:
   1. difficulty falling or staying asleep
   2. irritability or outbursts of anger
   3. difficulty concentrating
   4. hypervigilance
   5. exaggerated startle response

E. Duration of the disturbance (symptoms in Criteria B, C, and D) is more than 1 month.

F. The disturbance causes clinically significant distress or impairment in social, occupational, or other important areas of functioning.

Specify if:

Acute: if duration of symptoms is less than 3 months

Chronic: if duration of symptoms is 3 months or more

Specify if:

With Delayed Onset: if onset of symptoms is at least 6 months after the stressor

Source: American Psychiatric Association 1994, pp. 427–429.

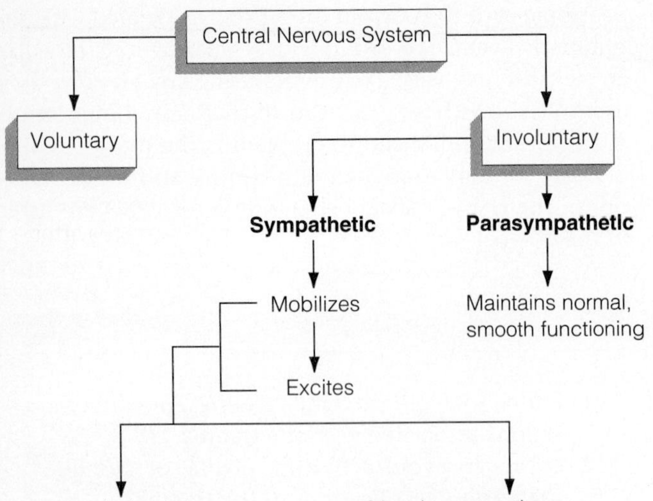

Figure 16–1 Physiologic responses to anxiety disorders.

Individuals with acute stress disorder may experience depression accompanied by despair and helplessness. Thus, there is a very real danger of suicide. They may feel they are responsible for the outcome of the trauma. For example, if another person was killed in the traumatic event, survival guilt frequently occurs. They often neglect safety precautions and basic needs for daily living.

Biopsychosocial Theories

Biologic Factors

There are several different schools of thought regarding possible physiologic causes of anxiety disorders. To understand the biologic basis of anxiety disorders, see Figure 16–1, which summarizes the physiologic responses. Notice that they are the same as the fight-or-flight response described in Chapter 4. However, a person experiencing an anxiety disorder is in a state of hyperarousal characterized by physiologic imbalances. A major research question that remains unanswered is: Are the physiologic imbalances a *cause* or a *result* of the anxiety disorder?

Following are some psychobiologic factors:

- The noradrenergic system in the brain is especially sensitive to the neurotransmitter norepinephrine (NE). One section of the noradrenergic system, called the locus ceruleus (located in the brain stem), appears to be involved in precipitating panic attacks. Drugs that increase the activity of the locus ceruleus have been found to cause panic attacks; drugs that inhibit the activity of the locus ceruleus block panic attacks. Tricyclic antidepressant medications stabilize the locus ceruleus and noradrenergic system; thus, they are sometimes useful in alleviating the symptoms associated with panic attack (Kaplan and Sadock 1991).

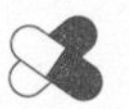

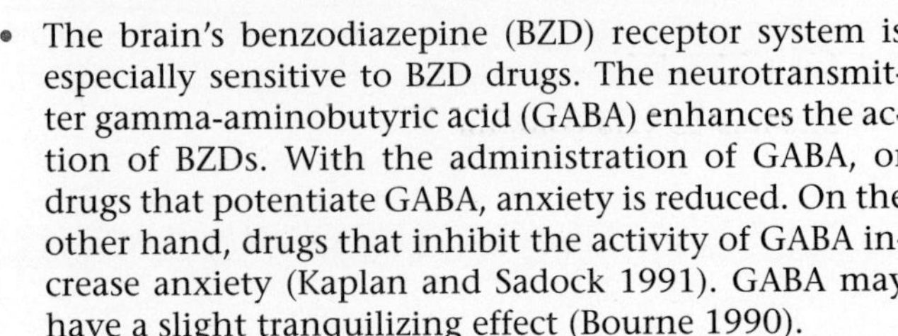

- The brain's benzodiazepine (BZD) receptor system is especially sensitive to BZD drugs. The neurotransmitter gamma-aminobutyric acid (GABA) enhances the action of BZDs. With the administration of GABA, or drugs that potentiate GABA, anxiety is reduced. On the other hand, drugs that inhibit the activity of GABA increase anxiety (Kaplan and Sadock 1991). GABA may have a slight tranquilizing effect (Bourne 1990).

- Simoni (1991) reports that clomipramine (Anafranil, a tricyclic antidepressant) reduced the amount of serotonin and is therefore useful in decreasing the symptoms of OCD in some people. Serotonin is thought to exert a major influence on the existence of OCD (Casey 1992).
- OCD is believed by some researchers to be linked with Tourette's disorder and learning disabilities (see Chapter 36). OCD is closely related to other psychiatric disorders that have biologic components (Casey 1992).
- Lactic acid levels are higher in some individuals experiencing panic attack. Lactic acid may actually precipitate anxiety in some people (Bourne 1990).
- Many substances increase anxiety levels. Caffeine stimulates the central nervous system (CNS) and increases NE production. In fact, caffeine produces the same physiologic arousal response experienced with exposure to stress. The result is increased sympathetic nervous system activity and a release of adrenalin. Caffeine causes some people to remain in a chronically tense, aroused condition. Some researchers state that caffeine actually triggers panic attacks. If caffeine consumption is stopped abruptly, withdrawal symptoms may occur (see Chapter 13).
- Nicotine is another substance that is a suspected trigger for panic attacks. Nicotine, which is a strong stimulant, results in increased physiologic arousal, vasoconstriction, and increased blood pressure. Nicotine consumers tend to sleep less well than nonsmokers.

Acute Stress Disorder

A disorder newly defined in the *DSM-IV*, **acute stress disorder** is the development of anxiety and dissociative symptoms occurring within 1 month of an extremely traumatic event. The precipitating stressors are similar to those of PTSD. They include:

- Exposure to a traumatic event in which the individual experienced or witnessed event(s) that involved actual or threatened injury or death.
- A response involving intense helplessness, fear, or horror.

text continues on page 372

CASE STUDY

A Client with Panic Disorder with Agoraphobia

Identifying Information

Mrs R is 43 years old, married, Irish Catholic, and mother of four daughters in their late teens or early twenties. Until very recently she had been employed as a secretary at a local pediatrician's office. She has a high school education and recently attempted attending community college, hoping to fulfill a lifelong dream of getting a college degree. She was referred to the psychiatric outpatient clinic for follow-up counseling by the emergency department of the local general hospital, where she had been rushed in acute distress the prior evening with symptoms of a panic attack.

Client's Description of the Problem

At the time of the panic attack, Mrs R believed she was having a heart attack and feared she was dying. She reported racing heartbeat, sweating, and feeling faint. She could not identify any events, thoughts, or feelings that precipitated the incident; it seemed to her to occur "out of the blue." She wanted relief from her fears of a medical emergency and felt unable to cope with the severity of the symptoms of the attack: "I tried to talk myself out of it; to tell myself it would go away, but it only got worse."

Mrs R reported she had had similar attacks over the years and that she had always been reassured of her medical and cardiac health, but when these attacks occurred, she "feared the worst" and "lost all perspective." The attacks could last from 2 minutes to 2 hours. Her daily routine had become quite restricted, as she now sought to have one of her daughters or her husband with her when she went out of the home due to fear of an attack. She sometimes could make it to school on her own but only with great effort, forcing herself to go. She did not feel comfortable when alone in her home and could not go to sleep if the other family members were not home. As an aside, she wondered what she would do when all the girls were off in college and she had no "sidekick." She felt ashamed and angry about her growing disability and often tried to cover up her fears to friends and family.

By interviewing the family, the nurse was able to gather information about a number of significant recent life events preceding the panic episode:

- Recent major surgery. A hysterectomy occurred 4 weeks earlier.
- Loss of her employment due to her hospitalization. She was abruptly terminated from her position at a new job due to too many absences.
- A recent discovery that her oldest daughter was taking birth control pills.
- The upcoming anniversary date of her father's sudden death from a heart attack.

Psychiatric History

Mrs R had never been hospitalized before for a psychiatric condition, although she had been to the emergency room on three prior occasions with symptoms of panic attack. She had seen a therapist years ago when the attacks first occurred, "about the time I left home to marry." She did not follow up with the therapist, however, saying she felt ashamed ("I've always been a strong and effective person!"), that the episodes were not so severe then, and that she found relief from panic attacks after she had the children.

Family History

Both Mrs R's parents died within the past 6 years. She was especially close to her father, and the second anniversary of his death was approaching. Mrs R's mother was considered a "homebody"; she rarely left the house and took part in social activities only if they occurred at the family home. Mrs R suddenly wondered if her mother had "these fears" too. She did not feel close to her mother in her adolescence, and there were many conflicts over her growing independence. She remembered feeling hurt that her father would not stand up to her mother and "protect me" when she felt her mother was in the wrong or especially harsh. Mrs R had four older sisters and one older brother. They were "always around," and she realized only after she married "how important that was" to her feelings of security.

Social History

Mrs R had always been considered a "doer" and an achiever, "someone people came to for help with problems, not the other way around!" She liked her new position as secretary for a pediatrician's office but felt angry at being terminated from the position. In addition to her absences for gynecologic problems, she acknowledged that her fears she would have a panic attack at work were interfering with her attendance as well.

She reported she had begun to curtail social and recreational activities, preferring to stay at home

→

CASE STUDY *(continued)*

A Client with Panic Disorder with Agoraphobia

where she was most comfortable. She noticed she was "living through the kids" rather than participating actively in golf and church activities, as she had previously done with her husband.

She described her relationship to her husband as emotionally warm and supportive. Although she sometimes resented his being away from her, she recognized this as part of her "problem" with being alone. Her primary relationships had been with her husband and children. She talked of facing the "empty nest" as her daughters, one by one, left for work or college. She "was shocked" to discover that her oldest daughter was using birth control pills but had "gotten over it," concluding that she was being old-fashioned and judgmental "like my mother."

Health History

With the exception of chronic gynecologic problems leading to the recent hysterectomy, Mrs R reported a history of good health. She had no allergies or other chronic illnesses. Her only other hospitalizations were to have her children. The recent hospitalization had been more physically taxing than she expected, and the fact that she was not allowed to return to work after her recovery came as a blow: "Going back to work would have been good for me. I felt discarded."

Current Mental Status

Mrs R is an attractive, carefully groomed woman who looks her stated age. She sits erect in the office chair, appearing somewhat tense. She answers questions cooperatively, but at times with some hesitation and as if expectant of criticism or judgment from the interviewer. She said, for example, "Well how would *you* feel?" in response to an inquiry about her emotional reaction to a significant event.

She is oriented to time, place, and person. She exhibits a good fund of knowledge, appropriate for her education and experience. Her memory is intact and recall good. She has no difficulty with calculations. Her judgment is unimpaired. During times of panic, however, sensory and perceptive awareness are greatly impaired.

Affect appears normal, with occasional evidence of anger in the form of irritability and light sarcasm. Mood is within normal limits. Speech is normal in flow and volume. It appears pressured at times when she attempts to correct an impression she believes the interviewer holds. Posture is at times rigid, but she relaxes as she becomes more comfortable with the interview. There are no delusions, ideas of reference, or hallucinations. Obsessive worry about the occurrence of panic episodes and of her safety are present. Embarrassment and shame over her symptoms are apparent. Suicidal or homicidal thoughts are denied. Associations and abstractions are appropriate, and there is no evidence of thought process disorder or difficulty in concentration, except during acute panic, at which times concentration is impaired and thought processes are disorganized. Some guardedness toward the interviewer is noted. Rationalization, overintellectualization, and avoidance are other coping and defense mechanisms used. Insight into the meaning of the current situation is minimal.

Other Subjective or Objective Clinical Data

Mrs R is considering the use of a trial of antipanic medication, despite "hating the idea" of medication.

Diagnostic Impression

Nursing Diagnoses

Altered Role Performance
Sensory/Perceptual Alterations
Altered Thought Processes
Anxiety
Fear
Ineffective Individual Coping
Altered Health Maintenance
Social Isolation

DSM-IV Multiaxial Diagnosis

Axis I: 300.21 Panic Disorder with Agoraphobia
Axis II: None
Axis III: Gynecologic disorder, under treatment
Axis IV: Psychosocial stressors; recent hysterectomy, acute event; loss of employment, acute event; recent knowledge of daughter's use of birth control, acute event; upcoming anniversary of father's sudden death, acute event
Severity: 3-moderate
Axis V: GAF = 42 (current); GAF = 76 (highest level in past year)

NURSING CARE PLAN

A Client with Panic Disorder with Agoraphobia

Nursing Diagnosis

Altered Role Performance related to fear and anxiety level.

Expected Outcome

Client will expand activities of daily living.

Nursing Interventions

- Maintain a calm manner.
- Stay with the client
- Acknowledge that client will not die.
- Use short, simple sentences and firm, authoritative voice.
- Direct client's attention to repetitive or physically exhausting task.
- Consider administration of antianxiety medication; should be done in combination with other therapeutic approaches.

Outcome Met If

- Client no longer has altered lifestyle.
- Client conducts normal activities at home, work, and/or school.

Nursing Diagnosis

Sensory/Perceptual Alterations related to psychological stress.

Expected Outcome

Client will gain mastery over incidents of panic.

Nursing Interventions

- Maintain a calm manner.
- Stay with the client
- Acknowledge that client will not die.
- Use short, simple sentences and firm, authoritative voice.
- Direct client's attention to repetitive or physically exhausting task.
- Consider administration of antianxiety medication; should be done in combination with other therapeutic approaches.

Outcome Met If

- Client reports feeling able to manage incidents of anxiety.
- Client demonstrates use of relaxation techniques.

Nursing Diagnosis

Altered Thought Processes related to high level of anxiety.

Expected Outcome

Client will be better able to concentrate.

Nursing Interventions

Teach client relaxation exercises.

Outcome Met If

- Client reports that she can concentrate better.
- Client demonstrates improved ability to concentrate at home, work, and/or school.

Nursing Diagnosis

Anxiety/Fear related to inability to relax.

Expected Outcomes

- Client will experience less discomfort, including dyspnea, tachycardia, sweating, fear, and anxiety.
- Client will gain mastery over incidents of panic.

Nursing Interventions

- Maintain a calm manner.
- Stay with the client.
- Acknowledge that client will not die.
- Use short, simple sentences and firm, authoritative voice.
- Direct client's attention to repetitive or physically exhausting task.
- Consider administration of antianxiety medication; should be done in combination with other therapeutic approaches.

Outcome Met If

- Client has reduced symptoms of dyspnea, tachycardia, sweating, fear, or anxiety.
- Client reports no fear of dying.

Nursing Diagnosis

Ineffective Individual Coping related to situational crisis.

Expected Outcome

Client will develop effective coping strategies.

Nursing Interventions

- Help client identify and use own resources (including social supports).
- Teach client relaxation techniques.

Outcome Met If

- Client reports and demonstrates use of effective coping strategies.
- Client no longer uses excessive avoidance.
- Client has expanded activities outside home environment.

- Dissociative symptoms and avoidance of specific stimuli.
- Symptoms of hyperarousal.

Genetic Theories

Recent research indicates that a familial predisposition for anxiety disorders may exist:

- Children of parents with an anxiety disorder are at risk for developing an anxiety disorder (Barloon 1993).
- First-degree relatives of people with panic disorder are 4–7 times more likely to develop panic disorder (APA 1994).
- In one study, as many as 25% of children with OCD had close relatives with the disorder (Casey 1992).
- In approximately 25% of individuals with GAD, there is a family history of the disorder (Kaplan and Sadock 1991).

Psychosocial Theories

In psychoanalytic approaches, anxiety is seen as a sign of psychologic conflict resulting from the threatened emergence into consciousness of forbidden or repressed ideas or emotions. The individual fears expressing and discharging the forbidden impulses, which occur in four forms, according to the nature of their consequences:

1. Superego anxiety, in which people suffer from anxious expectation of guilt if they break their inner code of ethics and standards.
2. Castration anxiety, or fear of fantasized danger or injuries to the body or genitals.
3. Separation anxiety, or fear of losing the love, esteem, and caring of significant people.
4. Id or impulse anxiety, or fear of the complete annihilation of self.

Other analytic views, sometimes referred to as neo-Freudian, evolved from the work of Freud and differ about the nature of anxiety. Rank (1952) believed that anxiety can be traced back to birth trauma. Sullivan (1953) stressed the importance of the early relationship between the mother and the child and the transmission of the mother's anxiety to the child. Existential analysts viewed anxiety as the central feature of the human condition, and the fear of nonbeing as a primary human fear.

Today analysts view the intrapsychic conflict around the following issues:

- Obedience versus defiance.
- Hostility due to giving up one's desires and submitting to authority.
- Fear of bearing caught and punished for transgressions (Zetin and Kramer 1992).

According to this model, the unconscious conflict must be brought into consciousness so that the real source of anxiety can be discovered and dealt with. Treatment takes the form of analysis or the less time-consuming psychodynamic psychotherapy.

It has also found that individuals who are agoraphobic have a significantly higher incidence of negative life events that occurred prior to the development of the phobic disorder (Laraia 1991).

One sociocultural factor that influences PTSD is homelessness. Recent studies document a very high rate of PTSD among homeless individuals (North and Smith 1992). The inevitable question remains: Is homelessness the precipitating factor or the result of PTSD? (Homelessness is discussed in Chapter 21.)

Currently, researchers are examining the relationship between battered woman syndrome and PTSD. Battered woman syndrome is a complex collection of manifestations including continued exposure to violence and/or threat of future violence, reexperiencing the traumatic event, and numbness and avoidance. Frequently, battered women shut off all emotion and appear to be unfeeling and indifferent (Woods and Campbell 1993). (For more information concerning the effects of family violence on individuals, see Chapter 23.)

Behavioral Theories

Behaviorists (learning theorists) view anxiety as a learned response that can be unlearned. For example, behaviorists believe that the cause of phobias is traumatic exposure to the avoided object, situation, or activity. According to learning theory on the development of obsessions, an original neutral obsessive thought evokes anxiety because it becomes associated with an anxiety-provoking stimulus. In compulsions, a person discovers that a certain action relieves anxiety associated with the obsessive thought. The person repeats the action to achieve relief until eventually the act becomes fixed into a learned pattern of behavior. Behaviorists see compulsive behavior as a maladaptive attempt to alleviate anxiety (Zetin and Kramer 1992).

Behavior modification is treatment that teaches clients new ways to modify their behavior. "Conditioning" techniques—using positive and negative reinforcements—are examples of modification techniques. Another usual method of treatment is **systematic desensitization**, in which a client builds up tolerance to anxiety through exposure to a series of anxiety-provoking stimuli.

Behavioral approaches have been most effective in treating behavior disorders and disorders of impulse control such as overeating, excessive alcohol use, and nicotine dependence. However, behavioral approaches are also frequently effective in the treatment of anxiety and are widely used for modifying symptoms in phobic disorder and obsessive-compulsive disorder. Behavioral therapists believe it is unnecessary to use analysis to induce clients to struggle with the anxiety. Instead, clients need only face the anxiety repeatedly until it becomes manageable. Behavioral treatment approaches are often used in treating phobic individuals because the methods are more efficient, less costly, and less time-consuming than other forms of insight-oriented psychotherapy treatment. Like some psychodynamically and psychoanalytically oriented therapists, behavioral therapists tend to avoid the use of medication because they believe it may interfere with the client's ability to learn behaviors.

Humanistic Theories

The nurse must consider the external situation, the brain, and the mind when assessing, diagnosing, and planning interventions for anxious clients. This nursing perspective identifies biologic, sociocultural, and intrapersonal factors as important.

The humanistic perspective is particularly important in understanding the anxiety disorders. Environmental stressors, biologic factors, and intrapsychic fears or conflicts cannot be adequately dealt with separately but only as they interact with one another. For example, clients suffering from a phobic disorder experience shame and helplessness as they attempt to cope with fears of annihilation in the presence of the dreaded object or situation. The result may be interpersonal and functional withdrawal, creating long-lasting disability.

This recognition has given rise to a multifaceted approach to the care of clients with these conditions. Humanistic treatment approaches are integrative and may include the range of psychotherapeutic interventions, including psychotherapy (cognitive, behavioral, and/or dynamic), measures to develop or ensure effective social support systems, measures to reduce environmental stress, and psychopharmacologic treatment.

The Nursing Process and Clients with Anxiety Disorders

Chapter 4 covers concepts of anxiety, stress, and coping that are relevant to the care of clients with anxiety disorders; it also covers the general anxiety continuum and the need to identify the level of anxiety. The subject of this section is the nurse's role with clients whose anxiety is severe enough to be classified as an anxiety disorder.

Assessment

Clients with anxiety disorders have impaired psychosocial and physiologic function. The emotional disturbances and physical and intellectual changes that take place as a result of extreme or chronic anxiety affect the client's work, school, and social functioning and frequently impair or threaten previously meaningful interpersonal relationships. These signs and symptoms are listed in the Assessment box on page 374.

The occurrence of acute anxiety and its related symptoms is common to a number of other physical conditions and acute medical emergencies. Therefore, a careful evaluation should always be conducted. A history and physical examination should rule out such conditions as hyperthyroidism and other endocrine problems, Ménière's syndrome, brain disorders, caffeine intoxication, mitral valve prolapse, and medical emergencies (such as myocardial infarction). (See the Research Note on page 375.)

Differentiation from other psychiatric diagnoses is difficult when anxiety and depression are mixed. The question of which one predominates can puzzle many practitioners and demands continued careful evaluation. Anxiety is part of many other clinical syndromes, such as schizophrenia and mood disorders. The medical diagnosis may be made on the basis of the dominant, most debilitating symptom.

In the assessment phase, determine not only whether the client is anxious (and, if so, how anxious) but also what the source of the anxiety might be. Knowing the source will help you plan and implement effective care. These two steps can be useful:

1. Help the client recognize and name the experience as anxiety: "You're trembling. How are you feeling?" Some clients can immediately connect their behavior with feeling anxious. For clients who cannot, it is helpful to make the connection: "Often people tremble because they're feeling anxious (or nervous, uncomfortable, or worried). I was wondering if you could be feeling anxious (or nervous, uncomfortable, or worried) right now."
2. Help clients discuss the experience more fully by moving into the cognitive dimension. It is premature to ask clients why they feel anxious. Encouraging them to discuss their thoughts will more likely bring their concerns out into the open. Then determine the source of the anxiety and gather data relevant to appropriate nursing diagnoses.

ASSESSMENT

Common Features of Anxiety

Physiologic	*Emotional*	*Cognitive*
Increased heart rate	Irritability	Forgetfulness
Elevated blood pressure	Angry outbursts	Preoccupation
Tightness in chest	Feelings of worthlessness	Rumination
Breathing difficulty	Depression	Mathematical and grammatical errors
Sweaty palms	Suspiciousness	Errors in judging distance
Trembling, tics, or twitching	Jealousy	Blocking
Tightness in neck or back muscles	Restlessness	Diminished fantasy life
Headache	Helplessness	Lack of concentration
Urinary frequency	Withdrawal	Lack of attention to details
Diarrhea	Diminished initiative	Past rather than present or future orientation
Nausea and/or vomiting	Tendency to cry	Lack of awareness of external stimuli
Sleep disturbance	Sobbing without tears	Reduced creativity
Anorexia	Reduced personal involvement with others	Diminished productivity
Sneezing	Tendency to blame others	Reduced interest
Constant state of fatigue	Excessive criticism of self and others	
Accident-proneness	Self-deprecation	
Susceptibility to minor illness	Lack of interest	
Slumped posture		

Panicked or extremely anxious clients are an exception; in this case do not use this general strategy. For these clients, suspend formal data gathering in favor of immediate, direct action to reduce anxiety. Common features of panic attack are listed in the box on page 375.

SUBJECTIVE DATA Clients with an anxiety disorder may report a variety of physical and emotional symptoms. It is important to encourage clients to describe symptoms in their own words and to explain how the symptoms affect their daily activities. They may report emotional distress, cognitive and perceptual changes, somatic discomforts, and/or role impairments.

Emotional Distress Clients with anxiety disorders may reveal a number of distressing emotional feelings:

"I have a sense of impending doom—as if something terrible is going to happen."

"I feel helpless; vulnerable for no reason at all!"

"I just can't seem to enjoy life—everything bothers me."

Anger, guilt, feelings of worthlessness, and anguish frequently accompany anxiety. When the anxiety is acute or extreme, as in panic disorder or PTSD, the client feels in immediate danger and may seek protection and reassurance from others. If the anxiety is too severe, however, clients may become immobilized and unable to report their terrifying feelings at all, or they may refuse assistance and attempt to flee.

Sometimes clients with anxiety disorders may deny the existence of anxious feelings. They try to protect themselves by dissociating these feelings. It is important to recognize clients' anxiety despite their denials. In such instances, assessment requires an especially careful observation of objective data.

Cognitive and Perceptual Changes Clients frequently have difficulty concentrating and making decisions. Some clients report feeling as if they are "going in circles," unable to think through a problem to make a confident decision. They may worry about their effectiveness at work and fear losing their job as a result of these attention and judgment problems.

In the clinical situation, clients may ask staff members to make decisions for them or to give directions. At the same time, however, they may express difficulty following through with suggestions, finding many loopholes or possible problems with the plan of action. Other clients become forgetful or misinterpret what they hear.

In extreme anxiety, as in a panic attack, the client is unable to assess a situation accurately and realistically.

RESEARCH NOTE

Citation

Shear K, Maser J: Standardized assessment for panic disorder research: A conference report. *Arch Gen Psychiatr* 1994;51:346–354.

Study Problem/Purpose

This investigation was conducted in order to develop a standard assessment package. The purpose was to establish a comprehensive assessment battery appropriate for clients experiencing panic disorders.

Methods

The investigators (who represented panic disorder research facilities in the United States and Canada) convened at a 2-day conference to identify techniques essential in assessing panic disorder. The group of 26 investigators were divided into subcommittees that examined specifically assigned topics related to the assessment of panic disorder. The topics were: structured diagnostic assessment; panic attacks and limited-symptom episodes; anticipatory anxiety; phobic symptoms; overall functional impairment, global severity, and improvement; comorbidity and coexisting symptoms; definitions of responder, remission, and relapse; and follow-up. The subcommittees used questionnaires and discussion to facilitate investigation of the topics.

Findings

A structured diagnostic interview is essential for ensuring conformity of assessment results. A comprehensive assessment of the client experiencing panic disorder must consider comorbidity.

Implications

Use of a structured format can be time-consuming. If the structured assessment is performed by someone with inadequate training, significant error could occur. Thus, it was recommended that an experienced clinician have input into the final diagnostic decision.

ASSESSMENT

Common Features of Panic Attack

Psychic	*Somatic*
Sudden onset of:	Sudden onset of:
Intense nervousness or apprehension	Tachycardia or palpitations
Feeling of impending doom or death	Chest discomfort
Mental confusion	Dyspnea
Feelings of unreality	Unsteadiness, dizziness, vertigo
Fear of going crazy or doing something uncontrolled during an attack	Sweating
	Choking or smothering sensations
	Faintness
	Hot and cold flashes
	Paresthesias
	Trembling or shaking

Such a client needs immediate attention from and orientation by the nurse. The client may later report having had a frightening feeling of personality disintegration.

Somatic Discomfort Clients with anxiety disorders may complain of nausea, indigestion, headache, lack of appetite, a constant feeling of fatigue, or other psychophysiologic conditions. They may relate these somatic disturbances to having "bad nerves," or they may be unaware of any psychologic component of their discomfort.

Clients with OCD who engage in repetitive activity, like compulsive hand washing or hair pulling, may report special health problems (tissue breakdown or hair loss) as a result. Clients with PTSD may report fitful sleep, terrifying nightmares, and a fear of returning to sleep. Common features of PTSD are listed in the box on page 376.

Role Impairment Clients may be aware of the impact that the emotional, cognitive/perceptual, and somatic changes have on their social, family, and work roles. They report worry about losing their job or being unable to continue caring for their families.

A young mother despairs that she is unable to take her daughter out to the playground because her phobias prevent her leaving the house.

A middle-aged accountant, obsessed about tallying his firm's financial data, is unable to put his job aside for the weekend and misses his son's football game. He experiences anger, guilt, and self-recrimination as a result.

ASSESSMENT

Common Features of PTSD

Aggressive behavior	Intrusive memories
Avoidance behavior	Memory impairment
Constricted affect	Nightmares
Depression	Panic attacks
Detachment	Phobic responses
Guilty rumination	Poor concentration
Hyperalertness	Repetitive dreams
Impulsiveness	Startle reactions
Insomnia	

OBJECTIVE DATA In addition to noting general signs and symptoms of anxiety as discussed in Chapter 4, other specific physical, emotional, and intellectual changes may be observed in very anxious clients.

Physical Findings Clients with acute or extreme anxiety—clients with PTSD or panic disorder, and clients with phobic disorder who cannot avoid the phobic situation—may experience a panic reaction and show extreme discomfort and the desire to flee. Look for acute physical changes, such as breathing difficulty, sweating, trembling, and/or vomiting, during these incidents. The client may be unable to verbalize, or verbalizations may be confused and incoherent. During a panic episode, clients may be so frightened that they may refuse help at the moment and may require firm reassurance and protection until the episode subsides.

The client with an anxiety disorder may develop long-term physiologic effects, such as a susceptibility to viral infections or the development of ulcers, hypertension, or asthma. Alcohol or other substance abuse may develop into a serious complicating problem when clients try to alleviate anxiety through chemical means. Substance abuse, which frequently occurs in individuals experiencing PTSD, may be the client's attempt to avoid traumatic memories. Other physical findings may be the effects of ritualistic or compulsive activity—skin lesions in a client who obsessively picks at the skin, for example.

Emotional Changes Family and friends of a client with PTSD may report personality changes in the client: increased irritability, suspiciousness, angry outbursts, and a tendency to blame others and to withdraw from them emotionally. Remember to pay attention to your own feelings when interacting with highly anxious clients. Because anxiety can be transmitted interpersonally, use self-awareness to determine the source of your own anxiety.

Individuals with phobic disorder and obsessive-compulsive disorder show a lack of emotional distress as long as the phobic object or situation is avoided or eclipsed by activity. There may be little spontaneity or active involvement by the client during assessment. Rigid, stereotyped behavior patterns are common.

Cognitive Deficits Unrealistic or distorted perception of a situation is common in anxiety states. During panic attacks, clients may distort or exaggerate details. They may complain about some seemingly insignificant detail. Clients may lose their ability to take in other pertinent data, and thus make errors in judgment. In assessment interviews, clients with an anxiety disorder are forgetful and unable to concentrate or pay attention to details. Errors in calculation and grammar are common.

Impact on Role Function The symptoms of anxiety disorder affect social, work, and family relationships (Figure 16–2). It is important to understand the possible effects of anxiety symptoms on interpersonal relationships. Obsessive-compulsive acts, for instance, may become so pervasive that they take the place of relating to other people. In other cases, clients may use obsessions and compulsions to negotiate social interactions and social roles. It is not unusual for people to establish a reciprocal pattern of interaction based on obsessions. Nurses who plan intervention strategies for obsessive-compulsive clients and those with an anxiety disorder should first assess the impact on the family system of intervening in one member's coping style.

Client or family member reports that the client is having trouble at work are additional evidence of role impairment. The client may be in jeopardy of losing a job because of poor performance. A person with PTSD, for example, may be fired for absences, drug or alcohol abuse, or for outbursts of temper.

Many clients with panic disorder report that fear of having a panic attack prevents them from seeking employment or from traveling to job interviews. For these people, as for many with severe phobic fears, normal activity may be greatly restricted.

Nursing Diagnosis

The following sections discuss the implications of nursing diagnoses for the client and the nurse.

ANXIETY/FEAR/HOPELESSNESS Apprehension, tension, and fright are emotional experiences common to clients with anxiety disorders. Anger and rage may accompany excessive anxiety. A client with PTSD, for example, may "fly off

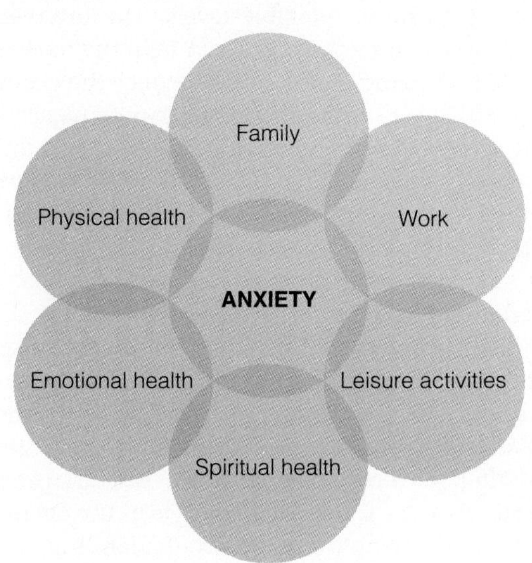

Figure 16–2 The holistic impact of anxiety.

the handle" without apparent warning or provocation, reacting to an inner stimulus.

Feelings of distress, anguish, fear, hopelessness, and guilt may also accompany anxiety disorders. The focus of emotional expression may be impaired; clients may worry excessively, ruminating about what might go wrong in the future. They may express anxiety through worry about their physical well-being; somatic preoccupation or hypochondriasis may develop. The potential for substance abuse is high, and suicidal potential is increased. Sexual drive or behavior may be inhibited as well.

Ineffective Individual Coping Excessive anxiety can cause alterations in conduct and impulse control. Some clients, such as those with PTSD or panic disorder, manifest unpredictable behaviors in an attempt to cope with their overwhelming fears. Individuals with an obsessive-compulsive disorder are unable to alter behavior, even though they may recognize it as harmful or unnecessary.

Clients with anxiety may turn to substance abuse, which in turn results in disordered conduct and impaired impulse control.

Altered Role Performance Anxiety disorders impair performance in the family, at school, and at work. Anxious clients may become less efficient and accurate at work or school because of distractibility or other perceptual and cognitive difficulties. Clients may withdraw emotionally from formerly important and meaningful relationships, or they may become overly dependent on help from others. They may isolate themselves and avoid previously enjoyed activities and recreation. Excessive need for reassurance, decreased productivity, reduced creativity, impaired hygiene, and impaired home maintenance are all possible outcomes for the client with anxiety disorder.

A particularly debilitating consequence of a phobia is the incredible restriction it may impose. People who have several phobias concurrently, as is often the case, may become walled off and isolated from many normal activities. A housewife who is afraid of crowds and vehicles becomes gradually less able to carry out her responsibilities of grocery shopping, car pooling, and so on. Highly anxious people often acknowledge the irrationality of their fears but cannot help experiencing them intensely.

Impaired Verbal Communication Clients with anxiety disorders often have difficulty communicating. They may speak too quickly or too loudly and may overelaborate or talk about too many subjects at once. Easily distracted, they may have trouble understanding explanations or retaining information. A client with severe anxiety may be incoherent, making verbal communication impossible. Written communication may also be impaired.

Risk for Trauma Impairments in motor behavior are often related to hyperactivity and restlessness and place the client at risk for accidental injury. Wringing of the hands, poor coordination, and the appearance of a startle reaction are motor behaviors associated with anxiety disorders. Clients with OCD may perform bizarre repetitive acts, such as repeatedly washing the hands or counting, checking, and rechecking activity. These ritualistic acts often result in self-injury.

Altered Thought Processes and Sensory/Perceptual Alterations Anxiety disorders affect perception and thinking and reduce the client's ability to solve problems. Judgment, concentration, abstract thinking, and attention are impaired. The client is indecisive but at the same time may make decisions impulsively to relieve tension. In panic disorder, the client may become disoriented, misinterpret reality, and distort the meaning of situations or events. Loss of self-esteem and a lowered self-concept often result as the client loses previous skills and capacities.

Altered Tissue Perfusion/Diarrhea/Functional Incontinence Alterations in circulation and elimination may occur as a result of stimulation of the autonomic nervous system. The client may experience increased blood pressure, rapid heart rate, dizziness, and palpitations as well as dry mouth, cold or clammy hands, sweating, shortness of breath, and a bad taste in the mouth. Diarrhea, enuresis, and slowed digestion may occur.

With extreme anxiety or panic, these symptoms are intensified, and the client may faint or vomit. A medical emergency may arise if the client has an additional major health problem such as cardiac illness.

Sleep Pattern Disturbance Insomnia is a frequent response to anxiety. Nearly all clients with anxiety disorders complain of trouble sleeping. Sleep may be further disturbed by nightmares or night terrors.

Planning and Implementing Interventions

Planning and implementing the nursing process with anxious clients depend on a thorough assessment of the level of anxiety and determining the appropriate nursing diagnoses. It is important for planning and implementation to take place as soon as possible. Anxiety, which is communicated interpersonally, often affects the client's family and friends, other clients, and staff members as well.

Most mental health care professionals believe that clients who cope with the stress of anxiety disorders can grow and change with therapeutic intervention. Nursing interventions for clients with anxiety disorders should be geared toward resolution. Outpatient treatment for a client with panic disorder is summarized in the Critical Pathway on page 384. Also refer to the Case Study and Nursing Care Plan earlier in this chapter.

Reducing Anxiety To help clients who are anxious, nurses must understand the operational definition of anxiety. This is the classic definition by Manaser and Werner (1964):

- Expectations or needs are present.
- Expectations or needs are not met.
- Unexpected discomfort (anxiety) is felt.
- Anxiety is controlled and power is restored through some automatic behavior (anger, withdrawal, somatization) that has been effective in restoring control in the past.
- The relief behavior is rationalized or justified rather than explained or understood.

Because anxiety is such an uncomfortable feeling, we learn early in life to reduce it or diminish its effects as soon as possible. Although individuals use a variety of behaviors, the most common automatic responses to anxiety are anger, withdrawal, and somatization. Automatic responses are limiting, rigid, and inflexible. Because they are automatic, these responses prevent a creative response to the threat and inhibit learning.

Intervening with Panicked Clients Clients who are extremely anxious or in panic require more immediate, direct, and structured intervention. During an acute panic attack, perception and personality are disrupted to such a degree that the client cannot solve problems or discuss the source of anxiety. The first priority is to reduce the anxiety to more tolerable levels. The interventions listed in the accompanying box can help the nurse alleviate the client's panic. The goal is to reduce the client's immediate anxiety to more moderate and manageable levels. The family of the distressed person needs counseling about how to respond therapeutically in such events because they are often involved in or present during a panic episode.

Intervening in Cases of Less Severe Anxiety A nurse can frequently detect subtle indications of mounting anxiety and intervene to prevent escalation. Some clients are adept at covering up their anxiety, even though their behavior usually transmits something to the sensitive observer. Often your own feelings of increased tension are a useful cue that the source of anxiety is in the client. Anxiety may make people excessively demanding. Your response to the demands must take into account the consequences for the course of the client's anxiety. In some cases, it may be reassuring to set limits and deny the request. In other cases, such a response may place further stress on the client.

You must know how to treat clients who suffer from prolonged anxiety. The intervention strategies are intended to help clients use their anxiety to learn about themselves and their coping strategies. This requires that the client endure the anxiety while searching out its causes. The client must then develop more effective and satisfying coping strategies to replace the old ones. To help clients learn to cope more effectively with anxiety, first detect the anxiety and then make thoughtful observations and responses that facilitate learning. Hildegard Peplau's five-step plan of action, which includes the interventions listed in the box on page 380, is now considered a classic model for nursing intervention with anxious clients.

In working through this step-by-step intervention approach, avoid getting bogged down in clients' justifications of their usual ways of coping. Often clients try to give plausible explanations for their ineffective anger, withdrawal, or somatization (automatic responses to anxiety; see Chapter 4). However, these rationalizations do not explain the relief in terms of the factors that caused the anxiety. The relief afforded by the usual coping patterns does not last long because the needs or expectations that originally caused the symptoms still exist. The needs may even become more intense. Clients can begin to alter disturbed coping patterns only when they understand what their unmet needs are, what they did instead of fulfilling these needs, and their subsequent feelings.

Anxious clients have two alternatives. They can reduce or change their hopes and expectations, or they can try

INTERVENTION

Guidelines for Working with Panicked Clients

Strategy	*Rationale*
Stay with the client.	Being left alone may further increase the anxiety.
Maintain a calm, serene manner.	Knowing that the nurse is calm and in control may be calming to the client.
Use short, simple sentences.	Because the client's perceptual field is disrupted, the client will experience difficulty focusing.
Use a firm and authoritative voice.	Conveys the nurse's ability to provide external controls.
Move the client to a quieter, smaller, and less stimulating environment.	Prevents further disruption of the perceptual field by sensory stimuli.
Focus the client's diffuse energy on a repetitive or physically tiring task.	Repetitive tasks or physical exercise can help drain off excess energy.
Administer antianxiety medications if ordered.	Antianxiety medications may help reduce anxiety.

new tactics or resources to get their needs met. Discuss these options with the client, and negotiate a contract to work on one or both goals. Realizing either option often involves problem solving. You and the client must find ways to alter structural features of the client's environment to reduce or meet the need.

Simple physical activities often help reduce anxiety to more tolerable levels. Encourage adaptive coping mechanisms that work. Here are a few:

- Soaking in a warm bath.
- Listening to soothing music.
- Taking a walk or doing other exercise.
- Having a massage or back rub.
- Drinking a warm nonalcoholic beverage.
- Engaging in whatever activity is relaxing.
- Taking slow, deep breaths to counteract the effects of hyperventilation.

You can use a variety of psychotherapeutic techniques and skills in intervening with clients who experience states of anxiety. Progressive relaxation, meditation, "thought-stopping" techniques, autogenic training, and guided imagery may help clients learn new ways to reduce the disturbing affect (see Chapter 29). Other methods include helping clients test reality, because their sense of danger is often out of proportion to actual danger. Developing goal-oriented contracts may help reduce a client's sense of inner chaos by providing structure and direction. The use of contracts also actively involves clients in their own healing process. This involvement increases their sense of control, thereby alleviating some of their feelings of powerlessness.

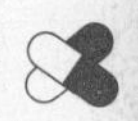

Teaching Clients About Their Medications Educating clients about the use of medications is one of your essential responsibilities. Clients should be aware of the major drugs used to manage acute anxiety and their limitations and possible side effects. Anxiety that is secondary to major medical illness or acute trauma (such as the death of a child) requires a different dosage than that prescribed for the treatment of primary anxiety.

Short-term use of higher-dosage antidepressants has been found to help control panic attacks. Benzodiazepines have proved effective and relatively safe in controlling situational anxiety for periods of 4–8 weeks. Antianxiety agents such as meprobamate (Equanil), diazepam (Valium), alprazolam (Xanax), and chlordiazepoxide (Librium) or adrenergic blocking agents such as propranolol (Inderal) may be used.

The last decade has seen significant progress in pharmacologic treatments for agoraphobia with associated panic attacks. Pharmacologic agents have been found to reduce or eliminate panic episodes associated with agoraphobia, most notably tricyclic antidepressents (TCAs), such as imipramine (Tofranil); monoamine oxidase inhibitors (MAOIs), such as phenelzine (Nardil); and second-generation benzodiazepines (BZDs), such as alprazolam (Xanax). Performance anxiety, a type of social phobia, is sometimes treated with beta-blockers (such as propranolol HCl). It is recommended that the client also be treated with nonpharmacologic methods, such as behavioral approaches (Daroff et al. 1993).

INTERVENTION

Guidelines for Working with Anxious Clients

Step of Plan	Nursing Intervention
1. Observe the client for increased psychomotor activity, anger or withdrawal, excessive demands, and tearfulness.	Verbalizations intended to help client recognize and name his experience as anxiety. "Are you feeling uncomfortable?" "Are you anxious or nervous now?" When client says "Yes," he is ready for step 2.
2. Connect the feeling of anxiety with relief behavior. The client acknowledges, describes, and names feelings of nervousness or anxiety.	Ask client what he does to feel more comfortable when he feels anxious. When client understands that when he feels anxious he gets angry, withdraws, or somatizes, he is ready for step 3.
3. Investigate the situation that immediately preceded the feeling of anxiety.	Encourage client to recall and describe what he was experiencing immediately before he got anxious (including thoughts, actions, and other feelings).

4. Help the client observe, describe, and analyze connections between what led to the anxiety and what happened after. Only through seeing all parts of this experience can the client understand why the anxiety occurred.
5. Formulate the causes of the anxiety. Help the client state the causes. Help the client observe and recall similar instances of anxiety. Through such extensive discussions, the client will eventually be able to recognize and perhaps alter his or her pattern of handling anxiety.

Source: Peplau H: Interpersonal techniques: The crux of nursing. Copyright © 1962. The American Journal of Nursing Company. Adapted with permission from the American Journal of Nursing, June, Vol. 62, No. 6.

Although the antipanic drugs are primarily antidepressants, the existing evidence suggests that clients with panic disorder with agoraphobia do respond to these drugs. The therapeutic effect is thought to be the result of the side effects on the vagal system. Phobic states not associated with panic episodes do not respond well to antianxiety or antidepressant medication.

Antianxiety medication should be used cautiously and sparingly. Certain antianxiety medications (diazepam, for one) are among the most overprescribed and abused drugs in the United States and Canada. Diazepam overreliance is a serious medical problem that has prompted the formation of a self-help group, Valium Anonymous, to help addicted people get off the drug. Older adults are particularly sensitive to the effects of CNS depression associated with diazepam.

Although medications may alleviate the symptoms of anxiety, they do nothing to help clients understand its source or manage their own lives in more comfortable ways. At best, these drugs should be used for the short-term treatment of anxiety—days or even weeks, not months or years.

PROMOTING EFFECTIVE COPING

In Obsessive-Compulsive disorders Clients with OCD avoid anxiety by engaging in compulsive acts and rigid thinking. Nurses working in all practice areas will probably encounter an obsessive-compulsive client whose problem is severe enough to require hospitalization. Form a therapeutic alliance with your clients. One way to foster the bond is letting clients know that although their thoughts are irrational, they are rational beings. Differentiate the irrational thoughts from the person having the irrational thoughts (Greist et al. 1990).

Clients use compulsive rituals to control anxiety. Therefore, carefully consider and time any intervention to avoid increasing the client's anxiety. For example, clients with washing compulsions may completely remove the skin from their hands, and nurses have successfully intervened by suggesting surgical gloves. However, it is not usually fruitful, and may be harmful, to interfere prematurely with a ritual unless it threatens the client's or another person's life or health. Generally, the client needs plenty of time to complete the ritual. When the client is prohibited from, or interrupted when, carrying out the compulsive behavior, anxiety escalates. These clients often have a strong tendency toward negativism, which may cause them to become more firmly entrenched in their defenses if modifications are introduced prematurely or hurriedly. Attempt to develop an affirming, dependable relationship before suggesting that clients change their behavior patterns, gradually introducing a substitute behavior. Balance the value of intervening in behavior that protects clients from mental anguish against the need to prevent physical deterioration caused by the behavior. It is best to time therapeutic activities to occur immediately following the ritual because the client's anxiety level is lowered by performing the ritual.

In Posttraumatic Stress Disorder Clients with PTSD frequently experience behavioral disturbances as a result of the intense anxiety triggered by reexperiencing the trauma. Alcohol or other drugs, when used to relieve anxiety, may contribute to destructive and impulsive acts. In the acute stage, crisis counseling is essential. Because of the chronic course of PTSD and the many psychosocial problems associated with it, a comprehensive treatment approach is needed. Clients often experience disordered family relationships, physical disability, social and recreational disruptions, and impaired ability to work or attend school. They may experience symptoms and attitudes of demoralization that further hamper their functioning.

When planning care for the client with PTSD, determine the type and duration of trauma experienced. Was the trauma a single, brief incident? Several, ongoing incidents? A human trauma (combat or rape)? A natural trauma (hurricane or earthquake)? Natural disasters and human-induced traumatic events can have different effects. For example, a survivor of human-induced trauma (such as rape) frequently experiences more guilt and humiliation. After a natural disaster, a person may discuss feelings of survivor guilt. Clients with PTSD verbalize feelings of no longer being safe and will often exhibit passive and dependent behaviors.

The goal of therapy in treating clients with PTSD is to desensitize them to the memories of the traumatic event so that the ego, or coping functions, can gain mastery over the anxiety. The following interventions or techniques may be used singly or in combination:

- *Education/explanation.* Explaining the dynamics of the disability and giving a rationale for the treatment help engage the client's ego in treatment.
- *Relaxation training.* Typical training programs may include muscle relaxation and imagery. The emphasis is on providing new "tools" or skills that the person may use when faced with memories of the traumatic event (see Chapter 29). Teaching clients about these self-management approaches encourages self-care and provides the clients with tools to use at home, at school, and on the job as well as in the health care setting.
- *Hypnosis or narcoanalyses* (the injection of barbiturates or other drugs to induce partial anesthesia). Some therapists use these techniques to bring to consciousness repressed and suppressed material so that it can be integrated into the ego structure, where it will have a less powerful influence. (Self-hypnosis is discussed in Chapter 29.)
- *Cognitive skill therapies.* These include techniques such as thought stopping, thought substitution, and providing the client with positive reinforcing statements. Cognitive restructuring of events giving new, less noxious interpretations may be used.
- *Abreaction/systematic desensitization.* The client may derive a therapeutic effect through emotional release, or **abreaction**, after recalling the painful repressed experience. Systematic desensitization in which the dreaded object, thought, or situation is introduced to the client in gradual amounts may be used as well. Systematic desensitization is discussed in the next section on phobic disorders.
- *Family conferences.* Efforts are frequently needed to engage the family in working to resolve the many psychosocial effects caused by the trauma. If successful, the family may provide a crucial supportive function.
- *Group treatment.* The benefits of group membership have been clearly demonstrated in recent years. Vietnam Veterans, Alcoholics Anonymous, Mothers Against Drunk Drivers, and Women Against Violence Against Women are just a few of the growing number of self-help groups organizing to assist and support victims of trauma and violence.
- *Exercise and nutrition.* Maintaining a healthy physical state as an adjunct to other therapies strengthens the body's adaptive efforts following trauma.
- *Individual therapy.* Individual psychotherapy can provide important ego-supportive and/or cathartic benefits.

Recent advances in psychopharmacology have led to the use of medication as an adjunct to the psychologic treatment of PTSD. As is true for the other anxiety disorders, however, you must be aware of the heightened potential for drug abuse among clients who suffer disorders of acute distress. The desire for immediate, total relief is powerful and may foster drug dependence and abuse.

BZDs, TCAs, MAOIs, lithium, beta-blockers, alpha-adrenergic antagonists, and neuroleptics have all been reported to relieve PTSD symptoms, either partially or totally (Elledgrie and Bridges 1985). During the initial stage (4–8 weeks), the use of benzodiazepines may be helpful in the treatment of anxiety, insomnia, and nightmares. Most recently, preliminary investigations are being conducted using the beta-adrenegic blocker propranolol (Inderal) and the anticonvulsant clonazepam (Clonopin) in an effort to avoid the side effects of BZDs.

When depression is a major factor, one of the cyclic antidepressants or an MAOI may be used. Sleeplessness, another common feature, is best treated with a behavioral approach first, such as relaxation techniques, guided imagery, muscle relaxation, and exclusion of daytime naps. Sedatives are discouraged except for very brief use. Your goal is to help the client reestablish the ability to sleep naturally and cope with stress without the use of drugs.

In Phobic Disorders Clients with phobic disorders attempt to avoid anxiety by binding it to a specific object or situation. Many people manage to lead successful, productive lives by binding their anxiety up in this way. For others, though, the phobia severely limits their activities, and their performance at work, home, or school may be greatly compromised. It is essential to recognize that forcing clients to come into contact with the feared object or the basic source of their anxiety can create in them an intense, disorganizing flood of panic.

Many clinicians agree that clients with phobic coping patterns are highly resistant to most insight-oriented therapies. These therapies require clients to confront and at least temporarily experience some of their originating anxiety. It is not surprising that they are ineffective with phobic clients, since the phobic's style is basically one of *avoidance*. In recent years, however, some symptomatic improvements have been made using techniques derived from behaviorist learning theory. The most commonly used interventions are desensitization and reciprocal inhibition.

In *systematic desensitization* (introduced earlier), the client is exposed to a series of increasingly anxiety-provoking situations that the client has graded in a hierarchy from the least to the most frightening. Through techniques of progressive relaxation, the person becomes desensitized to each stimulus in the series and then moves up to the next most frightening stimulus. Eventually, the stimulus that originally induced the most anxiety no longer elicits the same painful response. For example, a man who is irrationally afraid of earthworms might first talk about earthworms until the topic no longer evokes the same anxiety. Then he might be shown pictures of earthworms until he masters that level of closeness, and so on, increasing contact until he can actually hold a live earthworm in his hand.

In *reciprocal inhibition,* the anxiety-provoking stimulus is paired with another stimulus associated with an opposite feeling strong enough to suppress the anxiety. Through the use of antianxiety medications, hypnosis, meditation, yoga, or biofeedback training, clients are taught how to induce in themselves both psychologic and physical calm. Once they have mastered these techniques, they are taught to use them when faced with the anxiety-provoking hierarchy of stimuli.

Two other behavior-based interventions may also be used. In *cognitive restructuring* or *relabeling,* the client is encouraged to relabel a frightening situation, object, or activity. Closely linked to learning theory, this intervention is based on the belief that anxiety stems from erroneous interpretations of situations. In *exposure* or *flooding,* the client is repeatedly brought in prolonged contact with those situations that usually evoke distress until discomfort in their presence subsides.

Using behavioral conditioning techniques to rid the client of a phobia merely eliminates the symptom without removing the original stressor or conflict. If clients give up a phobic reaction without learning a more effective coping strategy, they can usually expect some alternative and equally troublesome disturbed pattern to emerge.

Promoting Effective Communication Nursing interventions that reduce anxiety are important general measures that promote more effective communication and behavior (see the two Intervention boxes earlier in this chapter). Many times, simply offering the opportunity to acknowledge and discuss feelings of anxiety helps the client regain control. At this point, clients are more likely to share their concerns because you have already taken the first steps in demonstrating genuine interest and concern in the client's experiences.

After encouraging the client to express feelings, listen. Clients may express fear, anger, sadness, disappointment, or alienation, and it may be difficult to hear about the client's pain. Some nurses feel helpless in the face of their client's catharsis and think they should be able to provide ready answers. Instead, ready answers are more likely to interfere with and thwart the client's communication. Genuine, concerned listening without judgments is an effective intervention in itself.

Explanations should be simple, clear, and concise. Be careful not to overload severely anxious people with more information than they can handle. If anxiety has contributed to knowledge deficit, reduce the anxiety before trying to teach about health or provide information. If the client's perceptual field (see Chapter 4) is narrow or disrupted, the client will be unable to assimilate information.

Clients with OCD require patience and an unhurried attitude, especially in regard to details and ruminations. It is frustrating to try to communicate with people who cope by developing an obsessive-compulsive reaction. If you use the customary techniques of paraphrasing and reflecting, these clients will say you did not get the details right. They will then go on to correct, qualify, and clarify. This striving for accuracy produces greater vagueness and confusion. It is as if parallel conversations are going on. Clients hear only themselves repeating and correcting insignificant details and completely lose the overall meaning of the message. Developing patience in listening and skill in providing well-timed, simple direction is crucial to working effectively with clients with OCD.

PROMOTING SAFETY Lack of coordination or tremors make anxious clients prone to accidents. Counsel clients not to perform potentially dangerous activities, such as driving a car, when anxiety is high. Advise them to move more slowly or to go over instructions carefully when they undertake new tasks or use tools.

PROMOTING OPTIMUM TISSUE PERFUSION AND ELIMINATION Like communication, circulation and elimination improve when anxiety is reduced. Pay attention to proper nutrition and adequate activity, because clients with anxiety frequently overlook their self-care and health needs. Walking, participating in sports, and/or developing new hobbies and interests promote healthy physiologic functioning and should be part of a comprehensive nursing treatment plan.

PROMOTING EFFECTIVE SENSORY PERCEPTION AND THOUGHT PROCESSES To function more effectively and independently, the client needs to know about normal anxiety and anxiety disorders. Providing accurate information at the right time and in an appropriate manner is an essential nursing responsibility. Other strategies to promote effective perception and cognition include the following:

- Use adjuncts to verbal communication, such as visual aids or role playing, to stimulate the retention of information.
- Practice problem-solving vignettes to improve judgment and insight.
- Identify misperceptions that clients hold as a result of a narrowed perceptual field. Begin with comments such as "I wonder if you've considered this possibility?" or "Perhaps if we tried this tack?"
- Help clients reality-test, that is, explore their opinions in the light of validated experience rather than emotional needs that block accurate perception.

PROMOTING SLEEP Nonpharmacologic nursing measures to promote sleep should be used before medications. These may include any of a variety of relaxation techniques. A currently popular method is the use of audio tapes. Like guided imagery, they provide a relaxing atmosphere; listening to the sounds of a beach or of birds in a wooded forest is soothing and sleep-promoting to some people.

Suggest that the client read a boring book in bed, drink warm liquids, or take a warm tub bath before retiring. A client with PTSD may fear going to sleep because of nightmares. Having another member of the family nearby and aware of the client's fear may be reassuring. (Chapter 19 more fully discusses ways of promoting sleep.)

Evaluation and Outcome Criteria

ANXIETY Clients will show no evidence of acute or intense anxiety and be able to perform activities of daily living independently when appropriate. Clients will verbalize feeling less anxious, and they will have fewer somatic complaints. They will state they feel more comfortable.

Clients will have fewer symptoms of physiologic distress, such as racing pulse, diaphoresis, and/or hyperventilation. Clients will be without signs of increased psychomotor activity. They will no longer complain of tearfulness, feelings of rage, or impatience. When appropriate, they will more readily engage in interactions with others. Phobic clients will tolerate the presence of the feared object, activity, or situation without experiencing panic or the need to flee.

INDIVIDUAL AND FAMILY COPING The obsessive-compulsive client will limit or cease performing compulsive rituals; for example, a client with a hand-washing compulsion will wash the hands no more than four times a day.

Clients will demonstrate the ability to continue with necessary activities even though some anxiety is present. They will be less likely to panic or flee. Family members will report that the client is "more like himself/herself" and appears less agitated, driven, or explosive in conduct.

ROLE PERFORMANCE The client will attend work or school on a regular basis. Family members will report that relationships at home have improved and that the client is once again taking responsibility for family activities.

Clients will report engaging in recreational or social activity and independently performing self-care. They will express feeling more comfortable about their performance at home, work, or school. Phobic clients will perform daily activities with less restriction or interference from any feared object, activity, or situation.

COMMUNICATION AND SAFETY Clients will state satisfaction with their communication; they feel heard and understood. There will be open lines of communication between client and nurse and client and family. Clients will report no tremors and will not have accidents due to poor motor coordination. They will report being able to perform usual small motor tasks, such as writing, in a competent manner.

CRITICAL PATHWAY FOR A CLIENT WITH PANIC DISORDER: OUTPATIENT TREATMENT

Expected length of treatment: 8 weeks

	Date ________ Weeks 1–2	Date ________ Weeks 3–6	Date ________ Weeks 7–8
Weekly outcomes	Client will: • Identify initial goals for therapy. • Contract for ongoing treatment. • Participate in treatment plan. • Begin to identify sources of anxiety/panic.	Client will: • Identify ongoing goals for therapy. • Maintain contract for ongoing therapy. • Participate in treatment plan. • Identify strategies to manage anxiety and panic.	Client will describe ongoing strategies to manage panic disorder. Client will demonstrate ability to cope with ongoing feelings of panic. Client will describe strategies to cope with an inability to cope with stressors.
Assessments, tests, and treatments	Psychosocial assessment to include mental status, mood, affect, behavior, and communication. Assist client to explore factors that precipitate panic attacks.	Psychosocial assessment. Assess recent history of anxiety and panic attacks. Explore contributing factors. Discuss effectiveness of cognitive restructuring strategies.	Psychosocial assessment. Assess recent history of anxiety and panic attacks. Explore contributing factors. Discuss effectiveness of cognitive restructuring strategies.
Knowledge deficit	Orient client to therapy program. Assess learning needs of client. Review initial plan of care. Assess understanding of teaching. Discuss the etiology and management of anxiety and panic disorders. Discuss the physical symptoms of panic and the importance of understanding the meaning of anxiety and panic disorders. Instruct client to maintain journal of anxiety and panic attacks.	Review therapy program and treatment objectives. Review journal of recent panic attacks. Assist client to identify the early signs of anxiety and panic attacks. Discuss strategies to cope with early signs and symptoms of panic attacks, including talking or activity. Discuss additional strategies to cope with panic attacks including expressing anger, positive self-talk, or guided imagery. Teach principles of cognitive restructuring and practice during session. Teach relaxation techniques and practice during session. Discuss use of exercise to alleviate anxiety/panic. Assist client to explore problem-solving strategies. Assess understanding of teaching.	Review plan of care. Review principles of cognitive restructuring. Assess understanding of teaching.
Diet	Nutritional assessment. Encourage well-balanced diet from all food groups. Contract with client to avoid stimulants.	Encourage a well-balanced diet from all food groups. Encourage the avoidance of stimulants.	Encourage a well-balanced diet from all food groups. Encourage the avoidance of stimulants.
Activity	Discuss the importance of regular aerobic exercise. Contract for regular exercise program. Sleep pattern assessment. Discuss strategies to provide sleep-enhancing atmosphere for 45 min prior to sleep.	Review ability to begin and continue exercise program. Maintain contract for regular exercise programs. Encourage client to practice relaxation response. Discuss effectiveness of sleep-enhancing strategies.	Review ability to continue exercise program. Maintain contract for regular exercise programs. Discuss effectiveness of sleep-enhancing strategies.

	Date ________ Weeks 1–2 *continued*	Date ________ Weeks 3–6 *continued*	Date ________ Weeks 7–8 *continued*
Psychosocial	Approach with nonjudgmental and accepting manner. Observe and monitor behavior. Assist client to understand relationship of unexpressed feelings to anxiety and panic experience. Encourage client to express feelings, thoughts, ideas, and beliefs.	Approach with nonjudgmental and accepting manner. Observe and monitor behavior. Encourage client to express feelings, thoughts, ideas, and beliefs. Provide positive feedback for efforts to incorporate coping strategies into daily life. Assist client to understand relationship of feelings to panic. Assist client to realistically identify strengths and limitations. Explore ways of reframing limitations in a positive manner. Assist client to practice and implement effective coping strategies. Assist client to identify potentially stressful situations and role-play coping strategies.	Approach with nonjudgmental and accepting manner. Encourage client to review strategies to manage anxiety and panic.
Medications	Identify target symptoms.	Assess target symptoms. Assess need for medications and refer as indicated. Routine meds as ordered.	Assess target symptoms. Routine meds as ordered.
Consults and discharge plan	Family assessment. Establish objectives of therapy with client.	Review with client progress toward therapy objectives.	Review with client progress toward therapy objectives. Make appropriate referrals to support groups.

Tissue Perfusion and Elimination Clients will report feeling energetic. Somatic complaints will decrease, and clients will report engaging in daily physical activity. Vital signs will be normal, and weight will be stable.

Thought Processes and Perception Clients will recall information taught by the nurse. They will begin to make decisions about their health care and ask questions about the anxiety process.

Clients will describe what led to their anxiety and what happened after they felt anxious. They will state the cause of their anxiety and recall similar instances. They will verbalize techniques to reduce anxiety.

Clients will correctly verbalize the use, side effects, and limitations of their medications. They will verbalize increased awareness of their environment.

Sleep Clients will sleep through the night without medication or with appropriately prescribed medication. They will have fewer nightmares or wake less frequently during the night.

Somatoform Disorders

The essential features of **somatoform disorders** are physical symptoms suggesting physical disorders for which there is no evidence of organic or physiologic causes. Somatoform disorders are sometimes confused with physical disorders.

Somatoform disorders may also be confused with **factitious disorders**, which are not genuine or natural. The *DSM-IV* includes in this category disorders in which clients consciously produce physical or psychologic symptoms. For example, a client may take anticoagulants to produce blood in the urine or dislocate a shoulder on purpose for no other reason than to assume a dependent role. **Malingering** is a term that refers to deliberately faking symptoms in order to benefit. Malingering, like factitious disorder, is consciously motivated and usually results in secondary gain. The distinctions between somatoform disorder, factitious disorder, and malingering are listed in Table 16–3 on the following page.

Table 16–3 Somatoform Disorder, Factitious Disorder, and Malingering Compared

Somatoform Disorder	*Factitious Disorder*	*Malingering*
Symptoms are not under voluntary control	Symptoms are intentionally produced	Symptoms are feigned (consciously produced)
Unconscious motivation	Motivated to assume sick role in order to obtain medical treatment	Motivations are varied: avoiding duties, monetary gain, obtaining drugs
Primary gain: anxiety reduction	No obvious secondary gain	Obvious secondary gain(s) or payoffs

Somatization Disorder

The diagnosis of **somatization disorder** applies to clients who have sought medical attention for recurrent and multiple somatic complaints of several years' duration and seemingly without physiologic causes. Historically, somatization disorder has been referred to as "hysteria," "hysterical reaction," and "Briquet's syndrome." This problem usually begins before the age of 30, has a chronic course, and is often accompanied by anxiety and depressed mood. Clients believe they have been sickly for a good part of their lives and report lengthy lists of symptoms, including blindness, paralysis, convulsions, nausea and other gastrointestinal difficulties, and painful menstruation. These symptoms are not caused intentionally, nor are they feigned. The pain experienced by individuals with somatization disorder is real. Psychogenic pain hurts just as intensely as pain with a biologic basis.

Even though somatization is common in children, somatization disorder is rarely diagnosed in children and adolescents. Common childhood complaints include headache, recurrent abdominal ache, chest pain, limb pain, and aching muscles—the so-called growing pains (Campo and Fritsch 1994). Children who are diagnosed with somatization disorder tend to have a caregiver who consistently overreacts to the somatic complaints. (Saarmann 1992).

Conversion Disorder

In **conversion disorder,** clients report loss or alteration of physical function that suggests a physical disorder but in fact is related to the expression of a psychologic conflict. Two mechanisms are thought to explain what a person "gets" from having a conversion disorder. (But remember that symptoms in conversion disorder are not consciously produced.) The first, **primary gain,** helps the person keep the psychologic need or conflict out of awareness. For example, a woman may become "blind" to avoid acknowledging a traumatic event she has seen. In this instance, the symptom is a partial solution to the underlying conflict (not having to acknowledge witnessing the traumatic event because she has suddenly been struck blind). The second mechanism, **secondary gain,** helps the person avoid a distressing, uncomfortable, or repugnant activity while at the same time receiving support from others. For example, a soldier with a paralyzed arm could hardly be expected to fire a gun and is also likely to receive sympathy for his paralyzed condition.

The problem usually begins in adolescence or early adulthood, although a conversion disorder may appear at any time of life. Regardless of the time of onset, a conversion disorder can seriously impede normal life activities.

Pain Disorder

In **pain disorder,** clients experience pain in the absence of physiologic findings and the presence of possible psychologic factors. The pain is usually severe enough to disrupt several functional areas. As a result of this dysfunction, the client often experiences unemployment, disability, and/or family problems. A person with Pain disorder is often convinced that somewhere there is a health care provider who can "cure" the pain. In this situation, the person may spend much time, money, and energy needlessly in pursuit of a "cure." The pain becomes the central issue of one's life; pain takes control of one's ability to function.

Hypochondriasis

Clients with **hypochondriasis** are preoccupied with the fear or belief that they have a serious disease, which on physical evaluation is not present. The preoccupation may be built around any of the following:

- Bodily functions (peristalsis, heartbeat).
- Minor physical problems (an occasional headache, a slight cough).
- Ambiguous, vague physical feelings ("tired ovaries" or "aching veins").

The unrealistic fear or belief persists for a period of at least 6 months despite medical reassurance. This fear impairs the social or occupational functioning of the client.

Body Dysmorphic Disorder

Clients with **body dysmorphic disorder** are preoccupied with some imagined defect in physical appearance. The preoccupation is out of proportion to any actual abnormality. The belief is overvalued but it is not of delusional proportion.

People with body dysmorphic disorder often use avoidance to cope with their perceived defect(s). The avoidance may result in extreme social isolation. For example, a man who tries to camouflage his "defect" of imaginary hair loss may leave his home only at night, and then only with a hat covering the "defective" part. The preoccupation with one's appearance is very time-consuming; thus, it restricts activities.

Undifferentiated Somatoform Disorder

In **undifferentiated somatoform disorder,** clients have multiple physical complaints lasting at least 6 months, and extensive evaluation reveals no organic problem. When there is related organic disease, the complaints or impairments are grossly excessive. Remember that the symptoms experienced by an individual with this disorder are not intentionally produced. The pain, which is psychogenic in nature, is real to the client.

Biopsychosocial Theories

Biologic Factors

In somatoform disorders, physical symptoms are present but evidence of physiologic disorder is not. The symptoms are thought to be linked to psychologic factors or emotional conflict. However, there is some evidence that brain abnormalities may lead to altered pain perception (Bourne 1990; Kaplan and Sadock 1991). Biochemical imbalances, such as decreased amounts of endorphins and serotonin, may cause some people to experience pain more intensely than people with normal brain chemistry.

Genetic Theories

Somatization disorder occurs in 10–20% of female first-degree biologic relatives of women with somatization disorder (APA 1994). The results of adoption studies indicate that both genetic and environmental factors contribute to the risk for somatization disorder (APA 1994). Other studies with identical twins have shown an increased occurrence of hypochondriasis (Kaplan and Sadock 1991).

Psychosocial Theories

Some communication theorists believe that manifestations of somatization are really nonverbal body language intended to communicate a message to significant others. Sometimes the message is as general as "pay attention to me" or "take care of me." At other times the *conversion of anxiety* actually symbolizes the nature of the specific underlying conflict. For example, a woman who wants to strike her children may develop a paralysis of her arm. A

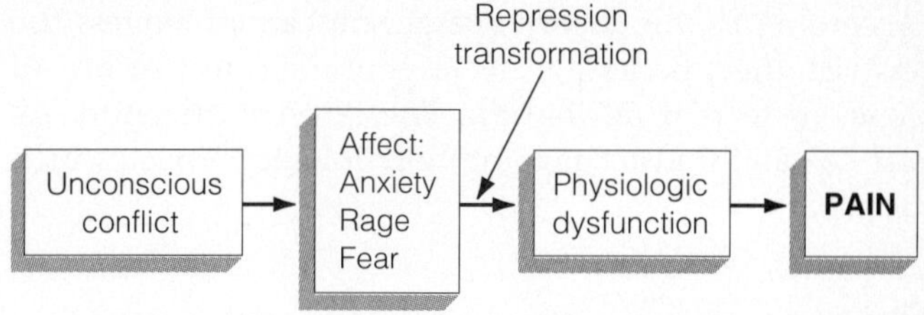

Figure 16–3 The mechanism of idiopathic pain.

girl who feels guilty about reading erotic books may become blind. Both realize the primary gain of protection from the anxiety-provoking impulses, and both get secondary gains of attention and sympathy as well. These patterns are most likely to occur among clients who do not have more aggressive alternatives.

Many somatizing individuals were reared in chaotic families. The family dysfunction was usually marital discord, substance abuse, and/or character disorders. Many somatizing people suffered physical or sexual abuse as children. For whatever reason, the child received inadequate nurturing. Adults with somatization disorder typically tend to marry an abusive spouse (Ford et al. 1993).

Clients who deal with anxiety by converting it to physical symptoms usually show no other psychologic symptoms, such as disturbed thoughts or depressed moods. However, they often exhibit subtler behavior patterns. Characteristics that have come to be associated with conversion disorder clients are self-dramatization, exhibitionism, narcissism, emotionalism, seductiveness, dependence, manipulativeness, childishness, and suggestibility. It is interesting to note, however, that these characteristics have usually been attributed to female clients by male psychiatrists.

Pain is associated with a great many disease processes, including many of the organ-specific somatoform disorders. Pain can be an adaptive or a maladaptive response. It often indicates real danger to the organism, but sometimes it interferes with functioning.

Consciousness, attention, perception, and cognition are all necessary for the experience of pain. According to modern theories of pain perception, humans have a control system over pain that operates as a "gate." Pain stimuli can be "allowed in" to or "shut out" from the cerebral cortex, depending essentially on the meaning the person attaches to the stimulus. This underscores the importance of meaning, symbol, and affect in the experience of pain sensation.

Figure 16–3 shows the basic mechanism for so-called idiopathic pain (pain of unknown origin). In psychoanalytic concepts, the unconscious conflicts are a result of traumatic or frustrating childhood experiences that are reawakened in adult life by a similar stress or frustration.

According to this theory, the person cannot express the evoked affect because of feelings of guilt, fear of loss of love, or fear of retribution. The affect is therefore repressed and transformed into physiologic correlates such as pain.

The Nursing Process and Clients with Somatoform Disorders

Assessment

Assessment of clients with somatoform disorders is complex because of the many psychobiologic factors involved.

Subjective Data Clients with somatoform disorders report physical symptoms for which there is no positive evidence of organic or physiologic cause. Clients with hypochondriasis, for example, may return many times to the outpatient clinic or emergency department, demanding to be reexamined or retested. They feel sure that they are suffering from some major illness that has been undetected. They are not reassured by the lack of physical findings and may go from doctor to doctor hoping to find someone who will validate their fears. This "doctor shopping" may lead to overmedication. Because the person is usually a poor historian, a complete medical history (including medications taken) is not always obtained. Although individuals with somatoform disorder usually describe their condition with colorful, exaggerated words, it is difficult to obtain specific facts about previous medical and surgical treatments.

In conversion disorder, the individual has loss of function or an alteration in function. A client may be unable to walk, for instance, complaining, "I woke up this morning with no feeling in my legs; for some reason they won't move." Examination reveals normal sensitivity, however, and no reason for the apparent loss of function. Interestingly, however, the client with conversion disorder seems unconcerned about the presenting problem despite its apparent severity. An inappropriate lack of concern about their disabilities—**la belle indifférence**—is characteristic of such clients. This nonchalant attitude toward physical problems indicates that the symptom is providing primary gain; that is, the anxiety is alleviated through the conversion process. The person is calmer as a result.

Clients with somatization disorder or hypochondriasis, in contrast, are overly dramatic and emotional in telling about their symptoms and pain. They report the history in vivid detail and colorful language but often pay more attention to how the symptoms have affected relationships in their lives than in giving careful description of the nature, character, location, onset, and duration of the symptoms.

Clients with body dysmorphic disorder may request unnecessary operations—for example, demanding cosmetic surgery for an imagined or greatly magnified defect in appearance.

Careful interviewing frequently uncovers a stressful life situation with which the client is not coping, suggesting that the preoccupation with somatic disorder is a way of avoiding underlying conflict. Helping the client identify and talk about this is a crucial beginning to psychotherapeutic intervention.

Objective Data Physical examination reveals no evidence for the physical symptoms of the client. Laboratory findings likewise do not substantiate organic or physiologic disorder. Despite this, the client may have undergone many exploratory procedures without relief or diagnosis.

Family members often report that the client is moody, self-centered, or demanding. They feel alienated from the client and are frustrated with the client's chronic preoccupation with physical symptoms. In a hospital setting, these clients often create scenes that bring them the attention they need without regard for the needs of either fellow clients or staff. Nurses frequently find it difficult to be kind, understanding, and nonjudgmental with these clients. Nurses who cannot cope with their own reactions to these clients cannot work with them effectively. It may help to remember that these clients do not intentionally produce their symptoms, nor do they appreciate the effects of their behavior on other people. Nurses who appreciate the whole story can sometimes feel more empathy for a client's coping style.

Nursing Diagnosis

Impaired Communication Clients with somatoform disorders have an impaired ability to communicate their needs. Though they may be highly verbal, careful listening reveals many gaps, oversimplifications, overdramatizations, and overgeneralizations in their communications. Somatoform disorders are considered nonverbal substitutes for the expression of underlying conflicts.

Consider the nonverbal communication function of the symptom itself. Symptoms of blindness, deafness, pain, numbness, itching, swelling, vomiting, paralysis, and so forth may be communicating something as general as "take care of me," "pay attention to me," or "I want out of these responsibilities." Specific symptoms may have more exact or symbolic meanings. The "blind" person may be saying, "I don't want to see something, because not having to see it allows me to escape my feelings about it." The client about to be married may suddenly develop acute pain in the genital area as a way of saying "I'm afraid of becoming sexually involved."

Altered Role Performance and Altered Family Processes The manipulative and dependent traits of the client with a somatoform disorder lead to impairment in social, work, and family relationships and to diminished performance in these roles. Friends and relatives eventually tire of the demands and become less available for support. Clients become emotionally isolated because their self-absorption makes them unable to respond appropriately to the needs of others.

Work performance suffers from frequent absences due to imagined illness. Preoccupation with their health uses up creative energy that could otherwise be directed toward work.

Ineffective Individual Coping Clients with somatoform disorders experience anxiety, anger, and feelings of helplessness. They may feel these emotions acutely and demonstrate these feelings excessively, as in somatization disorder and hypochondriasis. Paradoxically, they may show an uncanny lack of feeling where more would be expected, as in the blithe reaction to loss of physical function in conversion disorder.

The emotional life of the client becomes increasingly constricted. The focus of emotional experience becomes somatic concerns, and clients no longer experience meaningful emotional connections with other people, activities, and events. Range of expression of emotion may be limited to making demands, manipulation, and symbolic manifestation of anxiety.

Altered Thought Processes and Sensory/Perceptual Alterations These clients show selective inattention; that is, they filter out stimuli as a response to anxiety. Because they must keep ideas and events out of awareness, their judgment is often impaired. In a further effort to prove their ideas, they distort reality and tend to ramble. It is evident to the nurse that their conclusions are not logical. They may distort memory or show selective memory as well.

Clients with somatoform disorders have a body image disturbance; they sense that they are weak or vulnerable physically. They perceive sensory data incorrectly. For example, they may perceive abdominal discomfort as cancer rather than common indigestion.

Planning and Implementing Interventions

Effective intervention involves the following:

1. Recognizing and understanding the life problem or adjustment the client is facing.
2. Recognizing and understanding the client's self-perception as being unable to cope.
3. Helping the client identify and learn more effective ways of adapting.

These steps may be accomplished by insight-oriented or supportive psychotherapy, behavior modification, hypnosis, or any of several other psychologic, as well as some physical, therapies. None can claim superior effectiveness, and new approaches and techniques are indicated when traditional ones prove inadequate.

It is important to recognize that many clients with somatoform disorders are highly resistant to change. Progress may be slow and recovery partial.

Promoting Effective Communication After assessing the meaning behind the client's communication patterns, plan intervention strategies that enhance the client's verbal communication and self-esteem to the point where the client feels ready to face problems.

It is usually necessary to help these clients tone down their characteristic extravagances. Express respectful skepticism regarding their oversimplifications and overdramatizations. A communication and feelings group gives clients the opportunity to receive feedback about the effect of their behavior on others. Establishing a trusting relationship is key to effective therapy with a somatizing client.

Promoting Improved Role Performance and Family Processes Working with the family is especially important for clients with somatoform disorders. Educate the family and the client about the disorder, stressing the importance of avoiding unnecessary surgical or medical procedures. Support self-sufficiency, encourage independent functioning, and reduce the possibility of secondary gain by not focusing on physical symptoms. Assume a matter-of-fact, supportive attitude, with the optimistic expectation that the client will return to functioning in work, family, and social roles.

Promoting Effective Individual Coping The goal of counseling clients with somatoform disorders is to help them express their conflicts verbally rather than acting them out in symptomatic behaviors. The aim of long-term (insight) therapy is to promote effective emotional expression by exploring the sources of anxiety. It is a real challenge for nurses to help clients with somatoform disorders acknowledge the effects of psychosocial stress on symptoms. Supportive therapy seeks to improve self-esteem, perhaps through such measures as expanding clients' interest in their environment.

In general, try to avoid reinforcing the client's symptoms. A well-known psychiatric axiom that applies to clients in this general category is: Ignore the symptoms but never the client. Concentrating on the physical symptom by trying to get a "paralyzed" client to walk or a "blind" client to see again is giving the symptom more importance than it merits, thus increasing the secondary gain associated with it. Ultimately, this merely makes it harder for the client to relinquish the symptom.

Promoting Improved Perception and Thought Processes Help clients improve their capacity for perception and thinking by supporting general measures to reduce anxiety and improve the communication of needs. In addition, maintain a calm, unhurried attitude toward the client, listen carefully, and maintain an objective and undistorted view of reality. Avoid a premature challenge to the client's symptoms and complaints.

As clients gradually relinquish their defenses, propose other ways of understanding the condition, such as by suggesting a psychologic explanation for a physical complaint.

Evaluation and Outcome Criteria

Communication Clients will more regularly express feelings and conflicts verbally. They will have fewer physical complaints and fewer somatic symptoms. Conversation with the client will "flow," with fewer monologues by the client and more natural dialogue between client and nurse. In other words, the client's communication will be spontaneous.

Role Performance and Family Processes Clients will attend work regularly without frequent absences due to illness or interference due to worry about physical health. They will be more interested in outside activities and may begin to engage in socialization and recreation. Family and friends will report being more satisfied with their relationship with the client and will be more willing to interact with the client socially.

Individual Coping Clients will be less demanding, manipulative, and attention-seeking in interaction with others. They will appear less anxious and will talk about subjects other than their current physical status. They will appear less helpless and more able to participate in and make responsible decisions about their health care. For example, they may carry out a plan of treatment without voicing innumerable objections or worries.

They will appear more interested and involved in the activities and attitudes of others and be more aware of the impact of their own behavior.

Perception and Thought Processes The client will distort and misinterpret reality less frequently. Judgment, insight, and memory will improve as a result of reduced defensiveness in perception and cognition. Clients may report feeling more positive about their bodies. They will be more assertive in physical activities because they no longer tend to feel so vulnerable.

Dissociative Disorders

Dissociative disorders have, as their common denominator, the defense mechanism of dissociation, in which the client strips an idea, object, or situation of its emotional significance and affective content. Dissociative disorders are complex and are usually difficult to distinguish from one another. They share another characteristic: In any dissociative disorder, a cluster of related mental events is beyond the client's power of recall but can return spontaneously to conscious awareness. Dissociative disorders are not attributable to mental disorders that have an organic basis.

Dissociative disorders are commonly identified in adult survivors of childhood sexual abuse (McElroy 1992). See the Mind-Body-Spirit Connection box in Chapter 4 for a discussion of dissociation and recovered memory in childhood sexual abuse.

Dissociative Identity Disorder

Formerly known as multiple personality disorder, **dissociative identity disorder (DID)** is the presence of two or more distinct personalities within one individual. Each personality, at some time, takes full control of the person's behavior. There is much controversy about dissociative identity disorder. Many professionals are skeptical that such a phenomenon exists. However, clinical evidence of the existence of DID abounds.

Dissociative Fugue

A person with **dissociative fugue** wanders, usually far from home and for days a a time. During this period, clients completely forget their past life and associations; but unlike people with amnesia, they are unaware of having forgotten anything. When they return to their former consciousness, they do not remember the period of fugue. Clients experiencing dissociative fugue are generally reclusive and quiet, so their behavior rarely attracts attention. They may assume a completely new and apparently well-integrated identity during the fugue state.

Dissociative Amnesia

People with **dissociative amnesia** have one or more episodes of memory loss of important personal information due to psychologic reasons. They suddenly become aware that they have a total loss of memory for events that occurred during a period that may range from a few hours to a whole lifetime. In *localized amnesia,* the most common form, a person forgets only specific and related past times, usually surrounding a disturbing event. *Selective amnesia* for some, but not all, of the events is less common. Least common are *generalized amnesia,* which encompasses the person's entire life, and *continuous amnesia,* in which the person cannot recall events up to a specific time, including the present. *Systematized amnesia* is the loss of memory for certain categories of information, such as all memories related to one's occupation, or all memories that are related to one's family members.

Depersonalization Disorder

The essential feature of **depersonalization disorder** is one or more episodes of feeling detached from one's self so that the usual sense of personal reality is temporarily lost or changed. All the dissociated feelings are ego-dystonic. Individuals often describe their experience as similar to living in a dream or a movie: "I don't feel real any more." "I'm not feeling like myself." Frequently they have an out-of-body experience in which their own life is observed. They fear going "crazy" and/or losing control.

Dissociative Disorder, Not Otherwise Specified (NOS)

This is a residual category to be used for disorders in which the predominant feature is a dissociative reaction that does not meet the diagnostic criteria for any other specific dissociative disorder. An example is a person who enters a dissociated state following a period of brainwashing or thought reform.

Biopsychosocial Theories

Biologic Factors

At present, there is little documented evidence of a physiologic cause of dissociative disorders. However, certain physical illnesses (such as brain tumors and epilepsy) may lead to symptoms indicative of depersonalization disorder. Also, certain drugs may cause some people to experience depersonalization symptoms. These drugs include alcohol, scopolamine, barbiturates, benzodiazepines, and hallucinogens (Kaplan and Sadock 1991).

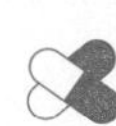

Genetic Theories

According to the *DSM-IV,* dissociative identity disorder occurs more often in first-degree biologic relatives of people with the disorder.

Psychosocial Theories

Pierre Janet (1859–1947) was the first to develop the concept of the "splitting off," or dissociation, of a part of consciousness. He believed that the individual needed to have a normal amount of "mental energy" to maintain integrative mental processes. When the level of energy was high, integration was maintained. When it became low, however, the personality might cease to function as a

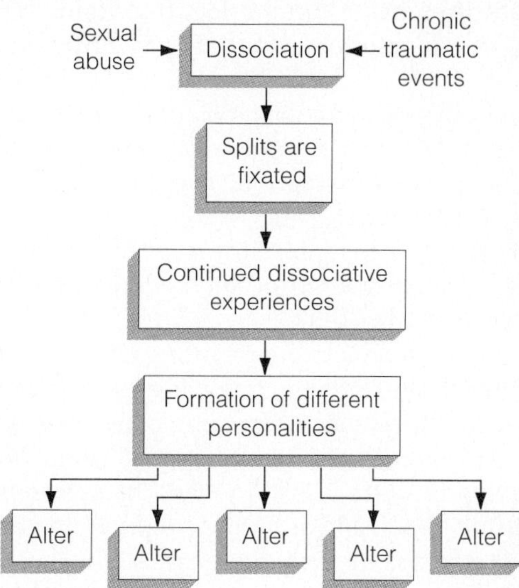

Figure 16–4 The development of dissociative identity disorder.

unit and split or dissociate. Nearly any type of emotional illness could result, he thought.

Freud, in contrast, proposed the concept of repression to explain the loss of conscious awareness in dissociation. He then introduced the notion of the *dynamic unconscious,* a part of the mind in which affects or ideas that were unacceptable to a person were pushed from awareness or recall. Freud and other early analytic theorists accepted the basic concept of psychologic dissociation.

Current explanations of dissociation are based on Freud's dynamic concepts. The repression of ideas that leads to amnesia and other forms of dissociation is conceived as a way of protecting the individual from emotional pain. External circumstances or internal psychologic conflicts are viewed as precipitating factors. A dissociative reaction may be viewed as a flight from crisis or danger—a major psychologic route of escape from anxiety. Sometimes, as in states of dissociative fugue and dissociative identity disorder, the dissociated area takes over temporary direction and control of the entire personality. During such times, the person may even appear to be functioning well.

Dissociative identity disorder originates in childhood as a result of chronic, unpredictable trauma. The trauma may be physical, psychologic, or both. The major form of child abuse which contributes to the development of DID is sexual abuse. In attempts to cope with the horror of reality, the child's ego splits through the dissociative process. Each trauma-induced dissociative experience shapes the development of alternate (alter) personalities. Each **alter** has a unique identity, holds different feelings and memories and performs different functions.

Chronic abuse leads to a fixation of the dissociated ego splits. Figure 16–4 on the previous page illustrates this process. Through dissociation, the child may see the abuse as if it were occurring to someone else, like in a movie. This ability to remove the self from the abuse is a protective mechanism. Dissociation is the escape that allows survival (Curtin 1993).

Additional dynamic considerations relevant to dissociative disorders include the following ideas. In Dissociative amnesia, the pattern is similar to conversion disorder except that the individual does not avoid some unpleasant situation by getting sick. Instead, the person does so by forgetting (repressing or suppressing) certain traumatic events or stresses. In DID, there appears to be a deep-seated conflict between contradictory impulses and beliefs. A resolution is achieved by separating the conflicting parts and developing each into an autonomous personality.

ASSESSMENT

Differentiation of Postconcussional Amnesia and Dissociative Amnesia

Properties of Postconcussional Amnesia

History of a head injury.

Retrograde amnesia does not extend beyond a week into the past.

Amnesia disappears slowly, and memory for events that occurred during the amnesic period is not completely restored.

Properties of Dissociative Amnesia

No history of head injury.

Retrograde amnesia extends indefinitely into the past.

Client can recover suddenly with total restoration of memory.

The Nursing Process and Clients with Dissociative Disorders

Assessment

The major areas to focus on during assessment are identity, memory, and consciousness.

SUBJECTIVE DATA Clients with dissociative disorders often report a sudden loss of memory of events. Clients may report, for example, that they cannot recall certain important personal events or information. They may not recall aspects of their own identity, such as how old they are and where they reside.

Sometimes amnesia is only partial, and clients remain conscious of what happened, although they report that they feel no control over it. In cases of complete or nearly complete amnesia, the "lost" memories can be recovered under certain therapeutic circumstances, or they may return spontaneously. Clients who have sustained a loss of their own reality may have adopted a new identity.

If motor behavior is affected in dissociative disorders, clients or their families may report episodes during which clients physically traveled away from home. Clients with depersonalization disorder may report fears that they are going crazy and have great secondary anxiety. In clients with DID, the original personality typically is not aware of the existence of the secondary ones. However, the secondary personalities may be aware of the original personality as well as of each other and may report this awareness to the nurse.

OBJECTIVE DATA The nurse conducts a careful assessment of the client's physical condition because of the possibility of organic causes, such as a brain tumor. Many of the behaviors of clients with dissociative disorders resemble behaviors associated with organic conditions, including postconcussional amnesia and temporal lobe epilepsy. The accompanying box summarizes the major differentiating points of postconcussional amnesia and disassociative amnesia.

The nurse's observations of the character, duration, frequency, and context of the dissociative disorder are crucial data. Physical examinations are not continued as part of the long-term intervention program, however, because they reinforce the symptoms and provide secondary gain. Therefore, the completeness and accuracy of the initial physical assessment are of the utmost importance.

A psychosocial assessment is conducted to discover the fundamental source of the anxiety as early as possible. Although many episodes of dissociation appear to occur spontaneously, there may be a history of a specific, shocking emotional trauma or a situation charged with painful emotions and psychologic conflict. Family or friends may provide clues to the client's conflict and should be included in the psychosocial data gathering.

When assessing someone with DID, you may note some of the following:

- Amnesia, loss of time, time distortion.
- Confabulation.
- Multiple somatic complaints, including severe headaches.
- Client's report of "hearing voices."
- Reports by others of uncharacteristic behavior that the client does not recall.
- Client's discovery of unfamiliar objects, clothing, or writings in one's possession for which the client cannot account.
- Client's use of "we" when speaking.
- History of childhood abuse or trauma.
- Frequent nightmares, insomnia (Stafford 1993).

Events associated with the trauma can trigger memories that had been repressed. These stimuli can trigger a switch of alters.

When interacting with the client, be alert for:

- Fluctuations of voice tone, speech, and mannerisms.
- Evidence of forgetfulness.

Notice from session to session if there are uncharacteristic changes in behavior. Are there differences in hairstyles or dress?

To assess for amnesia, ask if the client has ever had blackouts, blank spells, lost time, or memory gaps.

To assess for dissociation, question whether the client ever "spaces out."

Nursing Diagnosis

Sensory/Perceptual Alterations and Altered Thought Processes Clients with dissociative disorders may experience sudden memory loss, disorientation, loss of personal identity, and alteration in state of consciousness. Clients with dissociative amnesia have a partial or total inability to recall or identify past experiences. In clients with depersonalization disorder, feelings of unreality and estrangement can be severe and painful. These can affect their perception of the physical and psychologic self and of the world around them. Parts of the body or the entire body may seem foreign. Dizziness, anxiety, and distortion of time and space are common.

Altered Role Performance Unexplained disappearances, absences from work, unreliability, and unpredictability are common manifestations of dissociative disorders. Thus, the social or occupational functioning of the client is adversely affected.

Symptoms of depersonalization lead to limited or superficial involvement with others and to withdrawal or disengagement in work or social pursuits. As expected, relationships become highly complicated and disorganized when a client has multiple personalities.

Ineffective Individual Coping In addition to amnesia, a fugue state may occur in clients with dissociative disorders. In this state, clients defend against perceived danger by active flight. They may wander away from home. Days, weeks, or sometimes even years later they may suddenly find themselves in a strange place, not knowing how they got there. There is complete amnesia for the period of the fugue. Clients experiencing dissociative fugue may adopt a new identity and life pattern.

Planning and Implementing Interventions

In choosing intervention strategies for clients with dissociative disorders, the treatment team must decide whether to alleviate the troublesome symptoms or reintegrate the anxiety-producing conflict. Some teams emphasize the disruptions in day-to-day functioning precipitated by dissociative disorders. These include unexplained disappearances, absences from work, unreliability, and unpredictability. The dread associated with them justifies intervention strategies designed to change the disruptive behavior pattern. Others believe that new problems are created by removing the so-called symptoms without considering how they help the client control internal anxiety and maintain some balance in external social life.

Keep in mind that although clients may complain about the difficulties associated with their symptoms, the symptoms often form the basis of relationships with other significant people in their lives. These clients' roles in social groups are likewise built around their coping styles. Anyone who alters these coping styles must offer clients more effective and satisfying ways to handle anxiety and get support in their social network. Such a learning task usually requires long-term psychotherapy. However, behavior modification strategies can alleviate symptoms.

When planning care for a client with DID, you must remember that trust is a major issue. The basic building blocks of therapy with the dissociative individual are:

- Trust
- Safety
- Acceptance

Mapping is helpful in working with the client experiencing DID. A map is a diagram or chart that lists each alter's name, age, function, and degree of power.

For many individuals, receiving a diagnosis of DID is a relief. For years, they have been misdiagnosed and treated incorrectly. In addition to a sense of relief, another common reaction to the diagnosis is disbelief. The diagnosis itself may trigger the switching of alters. Thus, a safe, supportive environment is essential. The focus of treatment is to form a therapeutic alliance and work through the issues of each alternate identity.

The goal of integrating the alternate identities into one fused identity is difficult to achieve—but it is feasible. Integration occurs when there is no further need for separateness between identities. The integration process can be very painful for the client, as memories of previous trauma surface. It is important for the client to recall painful memories in order to work through the unresolved conflicts.

When planning care for the dissociative client, remember to:

- Trust the client to express his or her needs.
- Listen to each identity.
- Help the client accept the diagnosis.
- Provide support.
- Allow time.

Promoting Improved Sensory Perception and Thought Processes Strategies for identifying the underlying source of anxiety include those for recovering unconscious content, such as free association or dream description. At times, more active strategies are used. These may include projective psychometric tests (Rorschach, Thematic Apperception Test) and hypnosis, with or without intravenous administration of thiopental sodium (Pentothal).

Supportive insight therapy may be used with the goal of surfacing and integrating traumatic experiences in order to learn new ways of coping with future anxiety. This is especially relevant for those clients in whom the dissociative phenomena arise primarily against a background of intrapsychic conflict.

Promoting Effective Role Performance and Family Processes Including family members in a therapeutic counseling relationship helps them learn new ways of dealing with the client. As stated earlier, considerable secondary gain is often associated with dissociative behavior: The client can use the illness to escape responsibility and get special treatment. Families often need support in learning to avoid reinforcing dissociative behavior by acting as the source of secondary gain.

Environmental manipulation may be an indicated intervention. For example, it may be necessary to assist the client in problem solving with the goal of minimizing other stressful aspects of the environment. In learning to confront and become desensitized to the underlying conflict, the client will experience some anxiety and discomfort. This anxiety must be kept within manageable limits. Therefore, more obvious and alterable sources of stress and anxiety should be minimized.

Promoting Effective Individual and Family Coping The nurse may use measures such as psychotherapy (if prepared as a clinical specialist), environmental manipulation, and behavior modification to help the client with a dissociative disorder cope more effectively with impairments of conduct and impulse, such as unpredictable and bizarre behavior. Treatment may prove to be long-term, and progress may be slow. Establishing a supportive therapeutic alliance with the client and the family is crucial for helping the family and client understand the periodic occurrence of symptoms and in supporting improved behaviors.

Evaluation and Outcome Criteria

Sensory Perception and Thought Processes Clients will no longer experience sudden memory loss, disorientation, loss of identity, or alteration in state of consciousness, or they will experience it less frequently. They will correctly recall and identify past experiences.

Role Performance and Family Processes Clients will experience increased satisfaction with family and work relationships. Involvement with others will occur more often and will be more fulfilling. They will be more successful at work or school. They will attend work or school regularly, without unexplained absences due to dissociative episodes.

Individual Coping Clients will no longer exhibit bizarre or unpredictable behaviors, or they will experience them less frequently. For example, incidents of being missing from home without explanation will occur less frequently or not at all.

Chapter Highlights

- Anxiety is a universal experience. However, when successful adaptation does not occur, an individual may experience an anxiety disorder, somatoform disorder, or dissociative disorder.
- The development of these disorders involves the interaction of physiologic, psychosocial, and behavioral factors.
- Obsessions are intrusive, ego-alien thoughts that cannot be controlled even though the individual recognizes that the thoughts are irrational.

- Compulsions are repetitive behaviors performed in a ritualistic manner to reduce the anxiety resulting from obsessions.
- Posttraumatic stress disorder occurs as a result of exposure to extremely traumatic events. Flashbacks and a state of hyperarousal are characteristic of people with PTSD.
- Somatoform disorders are a response to high levels of anxiety and involve the conversion of psychologic pain into physical symptoms.
- The pain experienced by people with somatoform disorders is real even though there is no evidence of organic involvement.
- Dissociative disorders involve the process of separating the emotions from traumatic events. Amnesia is a classic symptom in the dissociative disorders.
- Dissociative identity disorder (formerly called multiple personality disorder) is a result of chronic exposure to trauma. Separate psychologic identities develop to handle various functions, which the host identity is unable to perform.

References

American Psychiatric Association: *Diagnostic and Statistical Manual of Mental Disorders,* ed 4. American Psychiatric Association, 1994.

Barloon DE: Effects on children of having lived with a parent who has an anxiety disorder. *Issues Ment Health Nurs* 1993;14(2):189–199.

Beck A, Emery G: *Anxiety Disorders and Phobias: A Cognitive Perspective.* Basic Books, 1985.

Blake D, et al: *Clinician-Administered PTSD Scale (CAPS).* National Center for Posttraumatic Stress Disorder, 1990.

Bourne EJ: *The Anxiety and /9 Workbook.* New Harbinger Publications, 1990.

Braun BG: *The Treatment of Multiple Personality Disorder.* American Psychiatric Press, 1986.

Breur J, Freud S: *Studies in Hysteria.* Avon Books, 1966.

Campo JN, Fritsch SL: Somatization in children and adolescents. *J Am Acad Child Adolescent Psychiatr* 1994;33(9): 1223–1235.

Casey DA; Obsessive-compulsive disorder: Characteristic features, pharmacologic management. *Postgraduate Medicine* 1992;91(2):171–174.

Curtin SL: Recognizing multiple personality disorder. *J Psychosoc Nurs* 1993;31(2):29–33.

Daroff RB, Frishman WH, Lederman RJ, Stewart WC: Beta-blockers: Beyond cardiology. *Patient Care* 1993;27(1): 47–70.

Elledgrie E, Bridges M: Posttraumatic stress disorder. Symposium on Anxiety Disorders. *Psychiatr Clin North Am* 1985;8(1):89–103.

Forchuk C, Brown B: Establishing a nurse-client relationship. *J Psychosoc Nurs* 1989;27(2):30–36.

Ford CV, Katon WJ, Lipkin M: Managing somatization and hypochondriasis. *Patient Care* 1993;27(1):44.

Greist JH, Jefferson JW: *Obsessive-Compulsive Disorder Casebook.* American Psychiatric Association, 1995.

Greist JH, Rappoport J, Rasmussen SA. Spotting the obsessive-compulsive. *Patient Care* 1990;24(9):47–73.

Hickey J, Baer P: Psychological approaches to assessment and treatment of anxiety and depression. *Med Clin North Am* 1988;74(4):911–927.

Kaplan HI, Sadock BJ: Synopsis of psychiatry, ed 6. Williams & Wilkins, 1991.

Laraia MT, Stuart GW, Best CL: Behavioral treatment of panic-related disorders: A review. *Arch Psychiatr Nurs* 1989;3:125–133.

Laraia MT: Biological correlates of panic disorder with agoraphobia: Practice perspectives for nurses. *Arch Psychiatr Nurs* 1991;5(6):373–381.

Manaser JC, Werner AM: *Instruments for the Study of Nurse-Patient Interaction.* Macmillan, 1964.

McElroy LP: Early indicators of pathological dissociation in sexually abused children. *Child Abuse and Neglect* 1992;16: 833–846.

Murburg MM: *Catecholamine Function in Posttraumatic Stress Disorder: Emerging Concepts.* American Psychiatric Association, 1994.

National Institute of Mental Health. Obsessive-Compulsive Disorder, ed 3. U.S. Department of Health and Human Services, 1991.

North CS, Smith EM: Posttraumatic stress disorder among homeless men and women. *Hosp Commun Psychiatr* 1992; 43(10):1010–1016.

Olson M: The out-of-body experience and other states of consciousness. *Arch Psychiatr Nurs* 1987;1(3):201–207.

Peplau H: Interpersonal techniques: The crux of nursing. *Am J Nurs* 1962;62(6).

Rank O: *The Trauma of Birth.* Robert Brunner, 1952.

Rapoport J: *The Boy Who Couldn't Stop Washing.* Dutton, 1989.

Rogers B, Nickolaus J: Vietnam nurses. *J Psychosoc Nurs* 1987; 25(4):11–15.

Ross C: Epidemiology of multiple personality disorder and dissociation. *Psychiatr Clin N Am* 1991;14:504–517.

Saarmann L: Is it live or is it Memorex? Dealing with patients with somatoform or factitious disorders in the emergency department. *Topics in Emergency Medicine* 1992;14(4): 43–57.

Shear K, Maser J: Standardized assessment for panic disorder research: A conference report. *Arch Gen Psychiatr* 1994;51: 346–354.

Simoni PS: Obsessive-compulsive disorder: The effect of research on nursing care. *J Psychosoc Nurs* 1991;29:19.

Spiegel D: *Dissociation: Culture, Mind, and Body.* American Psychiatric Association, 1994.

Stafford LL: Dissociation and multiple personality disorder: A challenge for psychosocial nurses. *J Psychosoc Nurs* 1993;31(1):15–20.

Steinberg M: *Handbook for the Assessment of Dissociation: A Clinical Guide.* American Psychiatric Association, 1995.

Sullivan HS: *The Interpersonal Theory of Psychiatry.* Norton, 1953.

van der Kolk BA; The body keeps the score: Memory and the evolving psychobiology of posttraumatic stress. *Harvard Rev Psychiatr* 1994;1:253–265.

Whitley G: Anxiety: Defining the diagnosis. *J Psychosoc Nurs* 1989;27(10):7–12.

Woods SJ, Campbell JC: Posttraumatic stress in battered women: Does the diagnosis fit? *Issues Ment Health Nurs* 1993;14(2):173–186.

Zetin M, Kramer MA: Obsessive-compulsive disorder. *Hosp Commun Psychiatr* 1992;43(7):689–699.

References for Nutrition Box

Berkow R (ed): *Merck Manual of Diagnosis and Therapy,* ed 15. Merck and Co., 1987.

Betteridge DJ: Reactive hypoglycemia. *Br Med J* 1987;295:286.

Chalew S, et al.: Diagnosis of reactive hypoglycemia: Pitfalls in the use of the oral glucose tolerance test. *South Med J* 1986;79:285–287.

Foster D, Rubenstein A: Hypoglycemia, insulinoma, and other hormone-secreting tumors of the pancreas, in Wyngaarden J, Smith L (eds): *Cecil's Textbook of Medicine,* ed 17. Saunders, 1985.

Palardy, J et al.: Blood glucose measurements during symptomatic episodes in patients with suspected postprandial hypoglycemia. *N Engl J Med* 1989;321(21):1421–1425.

CHAPTER 17

CLIENTS WITH GENDER IDENTITY AND SEXUAL DISORDERS

Karen Lee Fontaine

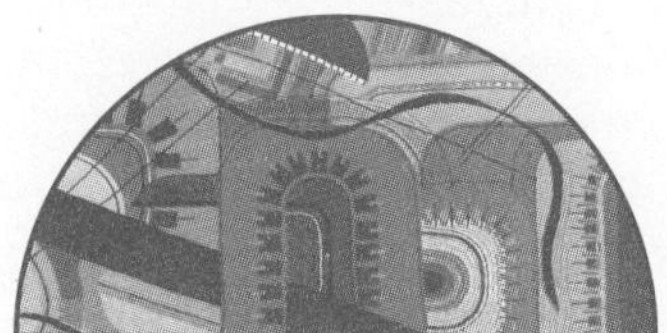

COMPETENCIES

- *Identify the DSM-IV diagnostic criteria for sexual problems.*
- *Describe biopsychosocial etiologies of various gender identity and sexual disorders.*
- *Identify principles common to most treatment plans for gender identity and sexual disorders.*
- *Assess your personal values regarding sexuality.*
- *Demonstrate a sensitivity to the diversity of sexual values that exist in the world.*

Cross-References

Other topics relevant to this content are: Family dynamics, Chapter 32; HIV and high-risk sexual behaviors, Chapter 27; Incest and rape, Chapter 23.

Critical Thinking Challenge

When clients are admitted to inpatient settings for treatment of mental disorders, their sexual needs are very rarely addressed. Clients and their partners/spouses are expected to remain celibate throughout the hospital stay. There is no privacy provided for clients and their loved ones. In fact, visiting is often restricted to public areas. Do you agree with this practice? Are professionals imposing their values on clients? When clients are admitted, do they lose their right to consensual sexual activity with their partner?

All humans are sexual beings. Regardless of gender, age, race, socioeconomic status, religious beliefs, physical and mental health, or other demographic factors, we express our sexuality in a variety of ways throughout our lives.

Human sexuality is difficult to define. "Maleness, femaleness, sensuality, sense of self, ego, perception of self in relationship to the world and others, the quality or state of being sexual, the condition of having sexual activity or intercourse, the expression of receiving and expressing sexual interest are all connotative of human sexuality" (Monat 1982, p. 1). Sexuality is an individually expressed and highly personal phenomenon whose meaning evolves from objective and subjective experiences. Physiologic, psychosocial, and cultural factors influence a person's sexuality and lead to the wide range of attitudes and behaviors seen in humans. There are no normal, universal sexual behaviors. Satisfying or "normal" sexual expression can best be described as whatever behaviors give pleasure and satisfaction to those involved, without threat of coercion or injury to others.

Sexual health is an individual and constantly changing

phenomenon falling within the wide range of human sexual thoughts, feelings, needs, and desires. A person's degree of sexual health is best determined by that individual, sometimes with the assistance of a qualified professional.

Sexual health care is a relatively new area of involvement for psychiatric nurses. Until recently, sexuality has not been viewed as falling within the scope of treatment. Currently, sexuality is increasingly recognized as an important component of a holistic approach to our overall health status. Sexual health care is a legitimate and appropriate nursing concern. The close and often extended relationships that psychiatric nurses have with clients and families foster the rapport necessary to discuss this private area of clients' health status.

Nursing roles in the area of human sexuality are evolving gradually. Psychiatric nurses involved in nursing activities related to human sexual functioning need to have the following:

- Concrete and comprehensive knowledge about sexual function and dysfunction.
- Skill in communication techniques.
- Acceptance of, and comfort with, their own sexual values and expressions.
- A willingness to explore and separate personal values and attitudes from those of clients.
- Proficiency in using the nursing process to assess, diagnose, intervene, and evaluate care to promote optimal sexual health.

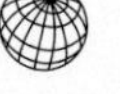

Historically, human sexuality has been shrouded in myth and controversy. This history has hindered both the delivery and the receipt of services that promote sexual health and well-being. Although scientific knowledge has expanded immensely during the past decade, modern North Americans continue to view sex and sexuality with discomfort. Our confusion is complicated by our traditional religious and social values. Nurses may hold some of these negative attitudes and biases. Psychiatric nurses must confront these negative, inappropriate, or stereotyped ideas and opinions before they can meet professional standards of care in helping clients attain optimal sexual health.

NURSING SELF-AWARENESS

Check Your Knowledge and Attitudes About Sex

Use this checklist periodically to assess changes in your knowledge and attitudes.

Knowledge

Circle True or False for each statement.

T F Women can and do have orgasms while sleeping.
T F It is dangerous to engage in intercourse during menstruation.
T F Sex drive usually diminishes after a vasectomy.
T F The older male may actually have some advantages over the younger male in sexual activity.
T F Masturbation is a relatively common practice of both women and men.
T F Females have two kinds of orgasm: clitoral and vaginal.
T F Children raised by homosexual couples are very likely to become homosexual.
T F An adult male who has been castrated immediately loses his sex drive.
T F Intercourse should always be avoided during the last trimester of pregnancy.
T F Oral-genital stimulation is unhygienic.

Attitudes

Circle the letter corresponding to your level of agreement with each statement.
A: Strongly agree; B: Agree; C: Uncertain;
D: Disagree; E: Strongly disagree

A B C D E Sex education has caused a rise in premarital intercourse.
A B C D E Extramarital relations are almost always harmful to a marriage.
A B C D E Relieving tension by masturbation is a healthy practice.
A B C D E Premarital intercourse is morally undesirable.
A B C D E Parents should stop their children from masturbating.
A B C D E Women should have sexual experience before marriage.
A B C D E Homosexual and bisexual behavior should be against the law.
A B C D E Seeing family members nude arouses undue curiosity in children.
A B C D E Promiscuity is widespread on college campuses today.
A B C D E Men should have sexual experience before marriage.

Basic to nursing is the notion that the nurse's personal beliefs should not influence the quality of care given a client. It is easier for nurses to live up to this standard if they engage in values clarification before providing sexual health care. Giving nonjudgmental nursing care does not mean that the nurse has to agree with others' beliefs and values about sexuality. However, self-awareness can help psychiatric nurses respect their clients' sexual rights and needs. Use the accompanying Nursing Self-Awareness box to check your sexual knowledge and attitudes.

Gender Identity Disorder

Gender identity is an individual's personal or private sense of identity as female or male. Gender identity develops from an interaction of biology, identity imposed by others, and self-identity. A newborn is assigned a gender (identity imposed by others) according to the appearance of the external genitals (biology); by 3 years of age, the child says "I am a girl" or "I am a boy" (self-identity). Gender identity can be viewed as a continuum. At one end of the continuum are those whose gender identity is congruent with their anatomic sex. In the middle are transvestites, who have both a male and female gender identity. At the other end of the continuum are transsexuals, whose gender identity conflicts with their anatomic sex.

Gender role is the role a person is expected to perform as a result of being male or female in a particular culture. In American culture, gender roles are more strictly enforced for males than for females, and males are socially punished for female behavior. In many Western countries, however, there is a growing appreciation of **androgyny**, or flexibility in gender roles. Proponents of androgyny view most characteristics and behaviors as human qualities that should not be limited to one specific gender or the other. In an increasingly complex world, adults who can behave flexibly fare better than those who adopt rigid stereotyped gender roles.

Gender Identity Disorder of Childhood, Adolescence, and Adulthood

Gender identity disorders occur in children who feel persistent and intense distress about their biologic gender and state an intense desire to be of the other sex. A girl may insist that she is a boy, has a penis, and will not grow breasts or menstruate. She may demand to wear boys' underwear and clothing and wish to urinate in a standing position. Similarly, a boy may demand to wear girls' underwear and clothing, express intense dislike of his penis, and voice the desire to grow breasts. This classification by the *DSM-IV* refers only to children who have not reached puberty and who express these symptoms persistently (APA 1994).

Gender identity disorder may also occur for the first time in adolescence or adulthood. In addition to feeling persistent discomfort and a sense of inappropriateness about one's assigned sex, the person engages in *cross-dressing*. Cross-dressing behavior ranges from the occasional wearing of a single item of clothing to dressing entirely as a member of the other sex. (See the box on the next page for the DSM-IV criteria for gender identity disorder.)

The *nonfetish transvestite* is typically a married heterosexual male who cross-dresses to express the feminine side of his personality. (Transvestic fetishism is discussed in the section on paraphilias.) Most transvestites exhibit stereotypic masculine identity and behavior in their public and professional lives. Cross-dressing is a conscious choice and usually occurs at home or in a setting where discovery is unlikely. It is not unusual for nonfetish transvestites to have a female name to go with the female personality and wardrobe. This type of transvestism occurs more frequently in cultures where males are expected to be strong, independent, and unemotional protectors. In a climate of rigid gender roles, it is understandable that some men can express their gentleness and dependence only by creating a separate world and female persona (Bullough and Bullough 1993).

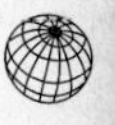

Often these individuals do not tell their spouses about the cross-dressing before their marriage. Some are embarrassed and do not know how to bring up the subject. Others view the need to cross-dress as a problem and hope that it will disappear after the marriage. Most wives eventually find out. For some women, the discovery raises doubts about their own sexuality and self-worth, and they may decide to terminate the relationship. Other women are not threatened by the cross-dressing but fear it will become public knowledge.

Paraphilias

The *DSM-IV* classifies **paraphilias** as a group of psychosexual disorders characterized by unconventional sexual behaviors. The person, usually a male, has learned to associate sexual arousal with some environmental stimulus, which triggers the unusual behavior. Paraphilias are not by definition pathologic. Many people engage in mild forms of the noncoercive behaviors and consider them simply love play. The behavior becomes pathologic when it is severe, insistent, coercive, and harmful to the self or others.

Paraphilias can be divided into noncoercive and coercive types. Coercive paraphilias (those that are forced upon nonconsenting persons) are described in the legal code, and the sexual behavior is considered a criminal act (Schwartz and Masters 1994).

Paraphilias have a strong obsessive-compulsive component. Affected individuals are often preoccupied with, and feel compelled to engage in, their particular sexual

DSM-IV Diagnostic Criteria for Gender Identity Disorder

A. A strong and persistent cross-gender identification (not merely a desire for any perceived cultural advantages of being the other sex).

In children, the disturbance is manifested by four (or more) of the following:

1. repeatedly stated desire to be, or insistence that he or she is, the other sex
2. in boys, preference for cross-dressing or simulating female attire; in girls, insistence on wearing only stereotypical masculine clothing
3. strong and persistent preferences for cross-sex roles in make-believe play or persistent fantasies of being the other sex
4. intense desire to participate in the stereotypical games and pastimes of the other sex
5. strong preference for playmates of the other sex

In adolescents and adults, the disturbance is manifested by symptoms such as a stated desire to be the other sex, frequent passing as the other sex, desire to live or be treated as the other sex, or the conviction that he or she has the typical feelings and reactions of the other sex.

B. Persistent discomfort with his or her sex or sense of inappropriateness in the gender role of that sex.

In children, the disturbance is manifested by any of the following: in boys, assertion that his penis or testes are disgusting or will disappear or assertion that it would be better not to have a penis, or aversion toward rough-and-tumble play and rejection of male stereotypical toys, games, and activities; in girls, rejection of urinating in a sitting position, assertion that she has or will grow a penis, or assertion that she does not want to grow breasts or menstruate, or marked aversion toward normative feminine clothing.

In adolescents and adults, the disturbance is manifested by symptoms such as preoccupation with getting rid of primary and secondary sex characteristics (e.g., request for hormones, surgery, or other procedures to physically alter sexual characteristics to simulate the other sex) or belief that he or she was born the wrong sex.

C. The disturbance is not concurrent with a physical intersex condition.

D. The disturbance causes clinically significant distress or impairment in social, occupational, or other important areas of functioning.

Code based on current age:

302.6 Gender Identity Disorder in Children

302.85 Gender Identity Disorder in Adolescents or Adults

Specify if (for sexually mature individuals):

Sexually Attracted to Males

Sexually Attracted to Females

Sexually Attracted to Both

Sexually Attracted to Neither

Source: American Psychiatric Association: 1994 pp. 537–538.

behaviors. One of the distinguishing characteristics of paraphilias is the person's inability to control or stop the behavior.

Fetishism

Humans respond to a wealth of sexual stimuli. Some people are aroused by the strident beat of rock music, while others are aroused by romantic music. Some people prefer making love in a brightly lit room; others, by candlelight; still others, in the dark. Everyone associates sexual arousal with an individual set of stimuli. An association or stimulus that is not typical for the culture is called a **fetish.** A fetish is the sexualization of a body part, such as feet or hair, or an inanimate object, such as shoes, leather, or rubber. In **fetishism,** early associations of a particular object or body part with sexual arousal condition the person to respond sexually to that stimulus. Once the initial association is made, repeated viewing or use (fantasized or actual) of the part or object during sexual activity (usually masturbation) reinforces its arousing nature. For instance, a boy may get an erection after trying on his mother's panties. The erection is pleasurable. The next time the boy masturbates, he puts the panties on or fantasizes about them. With repeated experiences, seeing the panties or putting them on becomes a sexual stimulus.

DSM-IV Diagnostic Criteria for 302.81 Fetishism

A. Over a period of at least 6 months, recurrent, intense sexually arousing fantasies, sexual urges, or behaviors involving the use of nonliving objects (e.g., female undergarments).

B. The fantasies, sexual urges, or behaviors cause clinically significant distress or impairment in social, occupational, or other important areas of functioning.

C. The fetish objects are not limited to articles of female clothing used in cross-dressing (as in Transvestic Fetishism) or devices designed for the purpose of tactile genital stimulation (e.g., a vibrator).

Source: American Psychiatric Association 1994, p. 526.

Ken, a 24-year-old college graduate with a major in accounting, was unable to hold a job because of his foot fetish. Ken spent a considerable amount of time fantasizing about feet—bare feet, pretty feet, long feet—and how they looked, they felt, they tasted, and they smelled. He fantasized at work, at the grocery store, and at the library (where he even went under tables to look at women's feet). Ken's fantasies made it impossible for him to work effectively or to maintain satisfactory interpersonal relationships with others. Ken refused therapy, preferring instead to pray that he would "get over it."

The DSM-IV diagnostic criteria for fetishism are in the accompanying box above. As with all people, fetishists' responses are highly individual. Fetishism is not considered a problem as long as it is not harmful and occurs in the context of consenting adult partners (Strong and DeVault 1994).

Transvestic Fetishism

In contrast with nonfetish transvestites, men who become sexually aroused by dressing in women's clothing are considered **transvestic fetishists.** They are typically heterosexual males and may wear female underclothes or may cross-dress completely. Like other fetishists, they have often undergone conditioning, and female clothing is an intense sexual stimulus. Many report great emotional stress if they try to resist the urge to cross-dress. Like other fetishists, cross-dressing is not considered a problem among consenting adult partners (Bullough and Bullough 1993).

Consistently strong feelings of being trapped in the body of the wrong sex is called **transsexualism.** For transsexuals, anatomy is not consistent with gender identity. Most transsexuals report that they have had these feelings since earliest childhood, and their families report that transsexuals insisted since childhood that they were of the other sex. Psychologic gender identity is stronger than anatomy, and most transsexuals develop an aversion to their genitals. They may hide their problem from family and friends from fear of being considered "crazy." As self-understanding and acceptance increase, many transsexuals live part time or full time as members of the other sex. Cross-dressing not only makes their outward appearance consistent with their inner identity and gender role but also increases their comfort with themselves. Sexually, they are attracted to people of the same biologic sex but consider themselves heterosexual because of their gender identity.

Sexual Sadism and Sexual Masochism

Sexual sadism and sexual masochism (S/M) is highly stigmatized in North American culture, and few people admit to being sexually aroused by receiving or inflicting emotional or physical pain. As much as 10% of the population may participate in some form of S/M activity, and all groups—heterosexual, bisexual, homosexual—are represented. Physical behaviors include intense stimulation (scratching, biting, use of ice), discipline (slapping, spanking, whipping), bondage (holding down, tying down), or sensory deprivation (use of blindfolds, hoods, ear plugs). Psychologic behaviors include humiliation or degradation, such as verbally berating others or requiring them to perform menial acts. S/M behavior varies in intensity and in its significance in the lives of couples. Some couples engage in the behavior only during sex. Some integrate the roles throughout the relationship, but not at all times. Other couples attempt to live out the dominant/submissive roles continuously. Thus, S/M may be only a part of foreplay, or it may be a significant component of lifestyle. Most sadomasochists do not engage in S/M behavior unless the partner is willing. Typically, both participants agree to safety "rules," and seldom is the behavior dangerous. Sadomasochists do not see the behavior as a problem and therefore do not wish to change (Strong and DeVault 1994).

Exhibitionism, Voyeurism, and Frotteurism

Coercive paraphiliacs become sexually aroused by including nonconsenting persons in their sexual acts. **Exhibitionists** and **voyeurs,** who are almost exclusively men, have powerful urges to display their genitals to strangers or peep at unsuspecting women involved in intimate behaviors. **Frotteurs** rub up against others, as in a crowded train or elevator, to achieve sexual arousal. The frotteur does not attempt to engage in sex with the victim and has no desire to form a relationship. Many describe the urge to peep, expose themselves, or rub themselves against others as something that just "happens" to them and thus have difficulty assuming responsibility for their behavior (Strong and DeVault 1994).

Pedophilia

A **pedophile** is an adult who is sexually aroused by, and engages in sexual activity with, children. All sexual relationships between adults and children are viewed as criminal in the United States. The courts consider these acts as nonconsensual because minors are presumed to have insufficient knowledge of the consequences of their acts to give meaningful consent. Pedophiliac activity can include exposure, voyeurism, explicit sex talk, touching, oral sex, intercourse, and anal sex. The child usually knows the pedophile, who may be a family member, neighbor, or friend. For a thorough discussion of the dynamics and consequences of the sexual abuse of children, see Chapter 23.

Sexual Dysfunctions

The *DSM-IV* classifies problems or difficulties with sexual expression, referred to as **sexual dysfunctions,** according to the phase of the sexual response cycle that is affected. Not mentioned are dissatisfaction problems, which account for a significant group of individuals seeking sex therapy. Sexual dysfunctions are generally acquired at some point in a relationship but may be lifelong. They may be generalized to all sexual interactions and settings, or they may be situational, occurring in a specific setting or with specific types of sexual activity.

It is often difficult to sort out the multiple factors contributing to an individual's or a couple's sexual problems. Generally, a number of past and current factors are involved. Negative events or situations in the past include lack of sex education, internalization of the teaching that sex is dirty or sinful, parental punishment for normally exploring one's genitals; or severe trauma, such as rape or childhood sexual abuse. Current situations or events contributing to sexual dysfunctions may include negative feelings, such as guilt, anxiety, or anger, that interfere with the ability to experience pleasure and joy. Fear of failure in sexual performance often becomes a vicious cycle; that is, fear of failure creates actual failure, which in turn produces more fear. *Spectatoring* is the detached appraisal of sexual performance or the body during a sexual act: "Am I going to lose my erection?" "Am I going to have an orgasm this time?" "My stomach is too fat." "When did his thighs get that fat?"

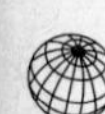

Table 17–1 Factors Contributing to Sexual Dysfunctions

Type	*Past Factors*	*Current Factors*
Psychologic	Taught that sex is dirty Childhood sexual abuse	Performance anxiety Spectatoring Fear of failure Guilt Negative thoughts
Spiritual	Taught that sex is sinful Childhood sexual abuse	Not feeling connected to partner Lack of intimacy Fear of intimacy
Sociologic	Punished as child for normal sex play Lack of sex education	Failure to communicate Relationship conflict
Physical	Trauma: abuse, rape	Illness/injuries Organic disorders Medications Substance abuse Failure to engage in effective sexual behavior

Lack of intimacy and feeling like a sex object inhibit the feeling of communion and connection that is an important part of making love. Fear of intimacy prevents some people from truly entering into a trusting and loving relationship. Another factor in dysfunction is expecting one's partner to read one's mind about one's sexual needs. Lack of sex education and failure to communicate may result in one or both partners not knowing how to please the other.

Sexual dysfunction may also be symptomatic of relationship conflict. Until relationship issues are resolved, sex therapy is largely inappropriate. Even when couples are functioning well in all of these areas, physical changes brought on by illness, injury, or surgery may inhibit full sexual expression.

Sexual fulfillment is the result of the positive interaction of psychologic, spiritual, sociologic, and physical factors, and dysfunctions are the result of a negative interaction. For an overview of past and current factors that may contribute to sexual dysfunctions, see Table 17–1.

Sexual Desire Disorders

HYPOACTIVE SEXUAL DESIRE DISORDER For most people, sexual desire varies from day to day as well as over the years. Some people, however, report a deficiency in or absence of sexual fantasies and persistently low interest or a total lack of interest in sexual activity; these clients suffer from **hypoactive sexual desire disorder.** If both individuals in a relationship are similarly uninterested in sex, there really is no problem. More typically, there is a disparity of sexual needs, and the person with the greater desire becomes dissatisfied with the sexual relationship and often initiates seeking help. The key issue in the relationship is not frequency but rather the dovetailing of partners' needs.

Physiologic factors associated with lack of desire are fatigue, illness, pain, the use of medications, and substance abuse. Intrapersonal factors may contribute to this dysfunction. Because vulnerability and intimacy are inherent in most sexual relationships, fear of these may lead to an avoidance of sex. Some people fear that if they allow themselves to experience sexual desire and pleasure, they will lose all control and continually act out sexually. Thus, these individuals may prefer to deny all desires rather than to try to fulfill them.

Relationship problems may be the source of inhibited sexual desire. Conflict and anger with one's partner are not conducive to positive sexual interaction. Some no longer feel physically attracted to one another or feel more attracted to someone else. Unless the partners experiment, sex may, in time, become boring. If there is a power imbalance in the relationship, the less powerful partner may lose interest in sex as a passive-aggressive way to achieve covert control. Typically, clients have little insight into the association between their lack of sexual desire and their negative feelings and relationship problems. The DSM-IV diagnostic criteria are in the accompanying box.

DSM-IV Diagnostic Criteria for 302.71 Hypoactive Sexual Desire Disorder

A. Persistently or recurrently deficient (or absent) sexual fantasies and desire for sexual activity. The judgment of deficiency or absence is made by the clinician, taking into account factors that affect sexual functioning, such as age and the context of the person's life.

B. The disturbance causes marked distress or interpersonal difficulty.

C. The sexual dysfunction is not better accounted for by another Axis I disorder (except another Sexual Dysfunction) and is not due exclusively to the direct physiological effects of a substance (e.g., a drug of abuse, a medication) or a general medical condition.

Specify type:

Lifelong Type

Acquired Type

Specify type:

Generalized Type

Situational Type

Specify:

Due to Psychological Factors

Due to Combined Factors

Source: American Psychiatric Association 1994, p. 498.

SEXUAL AVERSION DISORDER **Sexual aversion disorder** is a severe distaste for sexual activity or the thought of sexual activity, which then leads to a phobic avoidance of sex. It occurs in both women and men. Intense emotional dread of an impending sexual interaction also can trigger the physiologic symptoms of anxiety: sweating, increased heart rate, extreme muscle tension. The client then stops the sexual interaction or prevents it from even beginning. The most common cause of sexual aversion disorder is childhood sexual abuse or adult rape. This severe trauma can lead to a phobic response to sexual activity (Strong and DeVault 1994).

Linda and Mike, each of whom is 32 years of age, dated all through high school and have been married for 12 years. Linda has a strong aversion to body secretions. She spends hours in the bathtub before she and Mike have sex. Although Mike wears a condom, Linda jumps up and out of bed before he has finished ejaculating, and runs to the bathtub.

Linda can't identify any reasons for her feelings of disgust about body secretions and denies a history of sexual abuse. She does however, talk about feeling violated by Mike when he "talked me into sex" at age 18. Sometimes she refers to this first sexual experience as date rape.

Despite this problem, Linda and Mike refer to themselves as best friends. Linda has suggested that their marriage be conducted as a platonic relationship. Mike's not sure he wants to live that way the rest of his life. They are in counseling and want to learn how to enjoy one another sexually. Currently they are learning how to be less genitally focused and to spend more time cuddling, stroking, and touching.

Sexual Arousal Disorders

Sexual arousal refers to the physiologic responses and subjective sense of excitement experienced during sexual activity. Lack of lubrication and failure to attain or maintain an erection are the major disorders of the arousal phase. In **female sexual arousal disorder**, the lack of vaginal lubrication causes discomfort during sexual

CASE STUDY

A Client with Low Sexual Desire and Orgasmic Disorder

Identifying Information

Maria is a 46-year-old married woman who has come with her 48-year-old husband, John, to the local mental health outpatient clinic. Neither of them has received mental health services prior to this time.

Client's Description of the Problem

Both Maria and John agree that there is a disparity of sexual needs. Maria is satisfied to have sex once a month, and John wants to have sex several times a week. Maria has never been orgasmic with John but does admit to achieving orgasms during masturbation, a fact she has never been able to tell John. Maria states that she would probably like to have sex more often if she would enjoy it. Her fear is that she will not become orgasmic. John thinks that entering therapy is the first big step, and he is hopeful that their sexual relationship will improve.

They both describe their sex life at the beginning of their marriage as fine for the first several years, although Maria states that she was never orgasmic during that time. They never talked about their sex life. Some years ago, after reading a "sex book," Maria experimented with masturbation for the first time and began to experience orgasms. She was never able to share this information with John because she felt guilty about touching herself when she was alone. They are verbally and physically affectionate with one another, but, they say, not as much as they used to be. Very seldom do they express their anger to one another, and they manage most relationship conflicts by avoiding the issue.

Psychiatric History

No prior psychiatric history.

Family History

Both Maria and John are second-generation Americans of Eastern European descent. Both describe their parents as very modest and noncommunicative about any sexual issues. No sex education was given in the family. Maria and John have been married 25 years and have two children: a daughter, 19; and a son, 14. John has a good position in sales, and Maria is employed as a bookkeeper.

Sexual History

They both agree that John initiates sexual activity, primarily nonverbally. Sex typically occurs in the bedroom, after midnight, when they are both tired. Maria determines the length of foreplay, which usually lasts 5–10 minutes. The only position they use is man-on-top, but both agree they would like to try other positions. John has minimal verbal communication during sex, and Maria says she is too shy to say anything while they are making love. They both have difficulty talking about their sex life with one another. Maria states she is somewhat uncomfortable when John touches her body, except for her genitals and breasts. She is comfortable touching John's genitals but not touching her own genitals in front of him. She likes to receive oral sex but is uncomfortable giving it because she is afraid John will ejaculate in her mouth. Their mutual goals in therapy are to have sex more often, to feel freer to experiment, to discuss sex openly, and to have Maria experience pleasure and orgasms.

Health History

John has no current or past medical problems. Maria had a hysterectomy 5 years ago for endometriosis and is on hormone replacement therapy.

Current Mental Status

They are both quiet-spoken but articulate individuals. Eye contact is appropriate, mood is stable and appropriate, thought processes are logical, and there are no obvious symptoms of stress. Although they were both uncomfortable discussing sex, it became easier during a 2-hour history-taking time.

Diagnostic Impression

Nursing Diagnoses

Knowledge Deficit related to lack of sex education and lack of communication with one another

Altered Sexuality Patterns related to disparity of needs

Ineffective Individual Coping related to masturbatory guilt (Maria)

Sexual Dysfunction related to situational nonorgasmic response (Maria)

DSM-IV Multiaxial Diagnosis

Axis I:	302.71 Hypoactive sexual desire disorder 302.73 Female orgasmic disorder
Axis II:	None
Axis III:	Surgical menopause
Axis IV:	Avoidance of conflict; ineffective communication patterns Severity: 3-mild
Axis V:	Current GAF = 81; GAF = 81 (highest level in past year)

NURSING CARE PLAN

A Client with Low Sexual Desire and Orgasmic Disorder

Nursing Diagnosis

Knowledge Deficit related to lack of sex education and lack of communication.

Expected Outcome

- Both will state understanding of sexual anatomy and physiology.
- They will openly communicate with each other about sex.

Nursing Interventions

- Give reading assignments.
- Discuss with both their own responses.
- Give homework assignment of listing all the sexual words they know. Have them decide on acceptable words.
- Discuss how they can verbally seduce each other.
- Encourage them to talk about what they like while they are making love.

Outcome Met If

- Clients verbalize an increase in knowledge.
- Clients come in with a list of words; starred items indicate acceptable words.
- Clients agree on verbal signals to indicate sexual interest.
- Clients report an increase in verbal sharing that was sexually stimulating for both.

Nursing Diagnosis

Altered Sexuality Patterns related to disparity of needs.

Expected Outcome

- Both will state expectations about frequency of sexual activity.
- They will agree on an average frequency of sex.

Nursing Interventions

- Analyze the way unspoken expectations lead to disappointments and hurt feelings.
- Discuss meaning of and methods of compromise.
- Discuss alternate behaviors such as masturbation.

Outcome Met If

- Clients state they shared expectations prior to sexual interactions.
- Clients agree to do home play exercises three times a week.
- John acknowledges he is comfortable with masturbation when Maria is not interested in sex.

Nursing Diagnosis

Ineffective Individual Coping related to masturbation.

Expected Outcome

Maria will verbalize less guilt.

Nursing Interventions

- Discuss source of guilt.
- Assign readings on the normalcy of masturbation throughout life.
- Assign them the task of sharing with each other their feelings about masturbation.
- Encourage them to decide if this is acceptable to try when they are together.

Outcome Met If

- Clients identify family values/beliefs.
- Maria states she enjoys masturbation now and is able to touch herself with John present.

Nursing Diagnosis

Sexual Dysfunction related to situational nonorgasmic responses.

Expected Outcome

Maria will report achieving orgasms when sexually active with John.

Nursing Interventions

- Encourage Maria to demonstrate to John how she achieves orgasms with masturbation.
- Encourage John to try these techniques with verbal and nonverbal direction from Maria.
- Suggest they might wish to incorporate the use of a vibrator.

Outcome Met If

- Maria stimulates herself while John watches.
- John stimulates Maria; within 3 weeks she begins to achieve orgasm with manual and oral stimulation.
- They state they are considering buying a vibrator.

intercourse. The diagnosis of **male erectile disorder** is usually made when the man has erection problems during 25% or more of his sexual interactions. Some men cannot attain a full erection, and others lose their erection prior to orgasm. The pejorative term commonly applied to this condition, *impotence,* implies that the man is feeble, inadequate, and incompetent. The accurate term is *erectile inhibition,* which is objectively descriptive and not judgmental. Arousal disorder may also be diagnosed even when lubrication and erection are adequate if individuals report a persistent or recurring lack of subjective sexual excitement or pleasure.

Both male and female arousal can be inhibited by physiologic factors interfering with the vasocongestion necessary for lubrication or erection to occur. The absence of vasocongestion may result from disruption of the genital blood supply, from interference with innervation of the genitals, or, in women, from insufficient estrogen levels. Researchers estimate that 50% of erectile problems are predominantly organic, although the emotional reaction to the disorder must not be underestimated (Ackerman, Montague, and Morganstern 1994; Rosen and Leiblum 1992).

Psychologic factors may also be the primary cause of arousal disorders. They include all the previously mentioned factors, such as fear of failure, anxiety, anger, spectatoring, poor communication, and relationship conflict. Insufficient vaginal lubrication is less likely than erectile inhibition to create severe distress for couples, because using saliva or a water-based lubricant such as KY Jelly can correct the immediate problem. Erectile problems may be threatening because the man often feels his whole sense of masculinity is at stake. Men tend to be dominated by a genital focus more than women are. Thus, any difficulty in getting the penis to "perform" results in feelings of humiliation and despair.

Maria and Jorge, both 45 years of age, sought counseling when Jorge found it impossible to achieve an erection. The first time Jorge was unable to achieve an erection was 6 years ago. This was an emotionally traumatic experience for Jorge, who spent a considerable amount of time worrying that it would happen again. Eventually, it did, and Jorge found that he could not attain an erection more and more often. About 6 months ago he consulted a urologist. Nighttime penile tumescence studies showed normal functioning.

The couple was referred to a nurse sex therapist who discovered that Jorge had believed, from an early age, that sexual functioning stopped once the man reached age 49. In working with the couple, the nurse focused on providing sex education and sensate focus work. Once it didn't matter whether Jorge achieved an erection, his performance anxiety was decreased and he was able to do so.

Orgasmic Disorders

FEMALE ORGASMIC DISORDER The pejorative term commonly applied in the past to women who did not experience orgasm, *frigid,* implies that the woman is totally incapable of responding sexually. The more accurate and objective term is **female orgasmic disorder**, which simply means that the sexual response stops before orgasm occurs. *Preorgasmic* women have never experienced an orgasm; *secondarily nonorgasmic* women have had orgasms in the past but do not currently experience them; and *situationally nonorgasmic* women have orgasms in some situations but not in others. Studies indicate that 10% of women are preorgasmic, and another 20% report irregular orgasms (Strong and DeVault 1994). Compounding the orgasmic difficulty is the associated anxiety. In the preoccupation with orgasm, the real goal of being sexual—mutual pleasuring and intimacy—is lost, and the interchange becomes one of anxiety, frustration, and anger.

Physiologic factors related to inhibited female orgasm include fatigue, illness, neurologic or vascular damage, and drugs interfering with sexual response. In the physically healthy woman, lack of information or negative attitudes about female sexual response often contribute to orgasm disorder. Women who were taught that masturbation is sinful may not have explored their own bodies. If so, they cannot teach a partner where, how, and when to touch.

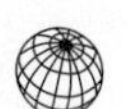

PREMATURE EJACULATION **Premature ejaculation** is one of the most common sexual dysfunctions among men. There are many definitions, with descriptions ranging from ejaculating before being touched, ejaculating before penetration, ejaculating with one internal thrust, to ejaculating within a minute or two of penetration. A more helpful description is the absence of voluntary control of ejaculation. The problem is best self-defined: A man is concerned about his ejaculatory control, or the couple agrees that ejaculation is too rapid for mutual satisfaction.

There is very little information about the mechanisms causing rapid ejaculation. Possible influences include the man's inability to perceive his arousal level accurately, a lowered sensory threshold due to infrequent sexual activity, early conditioning resulting from hurried masturbation or hurried sexual intercourse, and/or extreme anxiety during the sexual interaction, resulting in ejaculation triggered by sympathetic nervous system activity.

MALE ORGASMIC DISORDER The opposite problem is **male orgasmic disorder.** Men with this disorder can maintain an erection for long periods (an hour or more) but have extreme difficulty ejaculating. In heterosexual intercourse, the difficulty may be limited to ejaculation in the vagina. Some men ejaculate after self-stimulation or manual or oral stimulation by the partner, whereas others have great difficulty ejaculating with any type of stimulation. This disorder is much less common than rapid ejaculation.

Organic causes inhibiting orgasm include spinal cord injuries, multiple sclerosis, Parkinson's disease, and use of certain medications. Psychogenic factors include fear of pregnancy, performance pressure, fear of losing control, and anxiety and guilt about engaging in sexual activity. As with other dysfunctions, the difficulty can adversely affect the sexual relationship.

Sexual Pain Disorders

VAGINISMUS **Vaginismus** is an involuntary spasm of the outer one-third of the vaginal muscles, making penetration of the vagina painful and sometimes impossible. The woman often experiences desire, excitement, and orgasm with stimulation of the external sexual structures. Attempts at intercourse, however, elicit the involuntary spasm. She may have similar difficulty undergoing pelvic exams and inserting tampons or a diaphragm.

The partner often becomes fearful and anxious about hurting her or may become resentful and believe she is having the spasms on purpose. The partner may then develop secondary dysfunctions as a result of these negative feelings and interpretations of rejection.

Causes of vaginismus are thought to be psychophysiologic. The vaginismic response may develop initially as a protection against real or anticipated pain. It is often associated with sexual trauma, such as childhood sexual abuse or adult rape. Emotional conflict, such as extreme fear of pregnancy or intense guilt about engaging in sexual activity, may be additional contributing factors.

DYSPAREUNIA Both women and men can experience **dyspareunia**, pain during or immediately after intercourse. It is associated with many physiologic causes, especially those that inhibit lubrication. Thus, skin irritations, vaginal infections, estrogen deficiencies, and use of medications that dry vaginal secretions can cause women to experience discomfort with intercourse. Pelvic disorders, such as infections, small lesions, endometriosis, scar tissue, or tumors, can result in painful intercourse. Engaging in painful intercourse can lead to vaginismus because the body reflexively becomes guarded and tense. Similarly, in males, infection or inflammation of the glans penis or other genitourinary organs can cause pain with coitus. Also, some contraceptive foams, creams, or sponges can irritate either the vagina or the penis, causing pain. For both women and men, fear and anxiety in anticipation of pain can undermine the person's ability to feel pleasurable sexual responses and may lead to an avoidance of sexual activity.

Other Sexual Concerns and Problems

There are several other sexual concerns and problems, not identified in *DSM-IV*, that are important to understand in order to provide effective sexual health care.

Problems with Satisfaction

Some people experience sexual desire, arousal, and orgasm and yet feel dissatisfied with their sexual relationships. These sexual problems are more related to the emotional tone of the relationship than the physiologic response. Since the giving and receiving of pleasure in a mutually intimate relationship are the primary goals of sex for most people, dissatisfaction problems may be more disturbing than other types of sexual dysfunctions.

At times, satisfaction problems may be *situational*. For example, one partner may choose an inconvenient time, or a partner may feel anxious and therefore cannot experience much pleasure or joy. Some people describe their problems as related to *lack of extragenital satisfaction*. These people describe how much they miss and continue to need all the touching and caressing of their earlier lovemaking experiences. Unfortunately, people who have been relating sexually for a long time often become genitally focused and neglect the rest of the body. One or both partners may feel touch-starved, long for more extragenital loving, and become dissatisfied with sex.

Often satisfaction problems are related to *relationship difficulties*. The inability to communicate effectively in other relationship areas frequently results in sexual frustration. Partners who are angry at each other and make love without resolving the conflict may feel unhappy about the relationship in spite of having experienced arousal and orgasm. Couples who define their relationship in terms of rigid, unequal power and gender roles may have difficulty negotiating and compromising about sexual issues. Not infrequently, the person with the least amount of power feels helpless and dissatisfied with the sexual interchanges.

Lack of intimacy or a feeling of connectedness is understandably related to satisfaction problems. If one has sex with a stranger, the body may function well, but there is often a sense of something missing after the sexual experience. Making love to one person while feeling more attracted to or in love with another person can result in feelings of emptiness or disconnection. Even couples in a committed relationship may complain of lack of intimacy. Dissatisfaction issues include lack of romance, love, tenderness, and nurturance. Fulfillment of sexuality, then, depends on the ability to relate with a partner in an intimate and mutually pleasing manner that is compatible with values and chosen lifestyle (Morokoff 1993).

Increased Sexual Interest

Symptomatic of the manic phase of bipolar disorder is an increased interest in sex and sexual activity. Mood elevation is accompanied by a corresponding rise in sexual activity, variety of activity, and often, number of partners. This behavior occurs despite contrary values and isout of the client's control. The end of the manic episode signals a return to the person's usual level of sexual interest and activity. Since memory is not impaired, the person may feel embarrassment and shame about the uncontrolled sexual behavior during the manic episode.

Some adult survivors of childhood sexual abuse may go through periods of high sexual activity. This is often a desperate attempt to obtain the nurturance, love, care, and power they were denied in childhood. Having been sexualized at an inappropriately early age, some have learned to survive in a hostile environment by using their sexual availability to make contact with or control others.

Sexual Addiction

Frequency of sexual activity can be viewed on a continuum, with most people falling in the middle range. Some people have sex frequently in a way that enhances their lives; others have sex infrequently and report contentment and satisfaction. A sexual pattern that falls at either extreme of the continuum, however, can signal problems. At the low extreme are individuals who have great difficulty in choosing to be sexual; such people may have a sexual dysfunction. At the high extreme are people who have lost their ability to choose or control their sexual behavior; these people are sexual addicts. *Sexual addiction* is a disorder in which the central focus of life is sex. People with this addiction spend 50% or more of all waking hours dealing with sex, from fantasy to acting-out behavior. Acting-out behavior is often victimless, as in having affairs; overindulging in masturbation, fetishism, pornography use, or commercial telephone sex; or visiting prostitutes. Victimizing behaviors (those with a nonconsenting partner) are less frequent and include obscene phone calls, frotteurism, voyeurism, exhibitionism, child sexual abuse, and rape.

The incidence of sexual addiction is difficult to determine because of secrecy and shame, but it is estimated that 3–6% of the population may be affected. Of individuals in treatment, 75–80% are males (Shaffer 1994).

It is unethical to label as sexual addicts people who do not conform to conventional moral codes. Sexual addiction is not simply the frequent enjoyment of sexual behaviors. Many people engage in those behaviors without becoming sexual addicts. Rather, sexual addiction is a progressive disorder in which sex is used to numb pain. The payoff is the same as in any other addiction: an intensely pleasurable high, a short-lived release from pain, and an escape from the problems of daily life. The consequences are also the same in that the addict's life eventually becomes unmanageable.

The components of sexual addiction have the hallmarks of obsessive-compulsive behavior.

- The first component is *preoccupation:* The person spends hours thinking or obsessing about sex. Preoccupation, in itself, gives a sexual high and is so time-consuming that the person cannot fulfill work, school, or family responsibilities.
- The second component is *ritualization:* The individual engages in specific behaviors done just the "right" way and in the same sequence each time. Ritual behaviors include wearing certain clothing, taking certain steps to get ready, driving certain routes, or looking for partners only in a certain area. The ritual seems to control anxiety; once addicts begin a ritual, they cannot stop until the cycle is completed.
- The third component is *compulsivity:* The person cannot control sexual behavior, and this behavior becomes the most important aspect of life. Some demonstrate sexually compulsive behavior in a regular pattern; others resist for a time and then have a binge cycle.
- The fourth component is *shame and despair.* At the end of the cycle, the person experiences guilt and shame at the loss of control. The pain of despair creates the need to begin the cycle all over again, because the addict seeks to relieve pain by getting high. Like other addicts, these individuals want to stop their behavior, promise to stop, try to stop, and are unable to stop without treatment (Schwartz and Masters 1994; Shaffer 1994).

Until their lives become totally unmanageable, sexual addicts may successfully live a double life. They work very hard to appear normal, moral, and responsible individuals. Many of them grew up in homes where they were emotionally, physically, or sexually abused. Most of them suffer from low self-esteem and believe themselves to be unlovable. Having a desperate need for love, they equate sex with proof of love. They are so fearful of rejection that they establish only superficial relationships, thus avoiding intimacy and potential abandonment. Often, there is a codependent in the family who is essentially addicted to the addict. The codependent enables the addict by denying the disease or obsessively trying to reform the addict. Codependents also suffer from low self-esteem, inability to express feelings, fear of abandonment, and resistance to change (Shaffer 1994). Codependency is discussed in depth in Chapter 26.

Sexual Dysfunction Among Gay Men and Lesbians

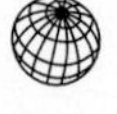

Gay men and lesbians may have the same sexual dysfunctions that occur in the heterosexual population. However, living in a culture that has fairly strict gender role expectations and is highly homophobic, gays and lesbians experience additional pressures, which may contribute to sexual dysfunctions.

Men, whether gay or straight, may accept stereotyped male gender roles that can lead to ambivalence about intimacy and dependence. Because social norms require that men be unemotional, competitive, and in control, two men in an intimate relationship are likely to experience conflict if both try to be "macho men." The success of the relationship often depends on the partners' ability to negotiate and compromise on issues of power, control, dependence, tenderness, and nurturance. Some gay men find it difficult to develop a positive sexual self-concept in a culture that does not positively model or reinforce a homosexual identity. Gays who internalize society's negative attitudes about homosexuality have low self-esteem and may have sexual problems as a result. It is not uncommon for gay men to interpret sexual problems in relationships as a sign that the relationship is over, as opposed to seeing the dysfunction as a problem to be solved (Wood 1994).

Not surprisingly, the reality of HIV infection and AIDS has increased the incidence of sexual dysfunctions in the gay community. Anxiety about past exposure and/or fear of future exposure to HIV is not conducive to pleasurable and joyful sexual relations. Adapting sexual behavior to safer sex practices may be a source of temporary dysfunction for some gay men. Not to be overlooked is the role of grief for gay men. A normal aspect of grief for all humans is a period of decreased sexual desire. With lovers and friends dying from AIDS, gay men begin to see the grief process as never-ending, and some wonder if they will ever again be able to experience sexual desire. (For further discussion of HIV and AIDS, see Chapter 27.)

The most common sexual problem for lesbians in a committed relationship is one of low desire or low frequency of sexual activity. It is highly unusual for lesbian couples to have difficulty with arousal, orgasm, or satisfaction. The pattern of low desire is typically secondary; that is, it develops at a later point in an ongoing relationship. When sexual activity does occur, both partners feel a general sense of satisfaction.

There are several differences between lesbian couples and heterosexual couples experiencing low sexual desire. Unlike heterosexual couples, lesbian couples do not typically withdraw from sex because of a lack of intimacy, a power imbalance, or rigid gender roles in the relationship. A lesbian couple is more likely to report that the nonsexual areas of their relationship are pleasing and agreeable and that there is minimal conflict about sex. Decreasing sex drive may be related to the socialization of women as passive recipients rather than assertive initiators. Both lesbian and heterosexual women have been taught many sex-negative attitudes, experience more conflict about sex than men do, and may fail to develop their full potential as sexual beings. When two women in an intimate relationship each wait for the other to initiate sex, the result may be low frequency of activity. Thus, many lesbian couples must often make a conscious effort to make love regularly (Rothblum and Brehony 1993; Wood 1994).

Obscene Phone Calling

Most women and many men have been victims of an *obscene phone caller.* The caller typically does not know the victim and becomes aroused when the victim reacts with upset, disgust, or shock. Some obscene callers breathe heavily, some make sexual noises, and some utter profanities. The caller may tell the victim that he is masturbating or may suggest they get together for sexual activity. Some pretend to have legitimate reasons for talking about sex (posing as researchers conducting a survey, for example) and continue until the victim is offended. The caller is sexually aroused by the combination of proximity (intimate conversation) and anonymity (Matek 1988).

Autoerotic Asphyxia

A noncoercive but often fatal sexual behavior is *autoerotic asphyxia.* At present, it is not categorized as a paraphilia in the *DSM-IV,* but, like paraphilias, it is a compulsive and unconventional sexual behavior. Called head-rushing or scarfing, this behavior typically begins in adolescence and is primarily a male affliction. The person fashions a tourniquet-like device that constricts the neck, decreasing the blood and oxygen supply to the brain. The person masturbates and, at the point of orgasm, releases the bonds to enhance the sensation or sexual high. Tragically, this practice causes many deaths. The vagal nerve complex in the carotid artery is stimulated by pressure around the neck, slowing the heart rate and decreasing oxygen flow to the brain even further. The person becomes unconscious, slumps forward, and accidentally hangs himself. Many believe the cause of death is suicide, but family and friends cannot understand the reason for the suicide, since these young men are not mentally ill or even troubled. It is often helpful to the family to explain that the death was a tragic accident.

Biopsychosocial Theories

Human sexual behavior has been studied from various theoretic perspectives. The most significant are intrapersonal, behavioral, sociocultural, and biologic theories.

A review of the various theoretic perspectives shows that human sexuality has been historically characterized by judgments and controversy that have inhibited sexual health care services. It is important for health care professionals to remember that *all* people to some extent deviate from some physical, social, behavioral, or emotional norm. Some are left-handed, some stutter, some are disabled, some are loners, and some are filled with fears. To achieve the highest level of professional practice, nurses must look beyond the characteristics and respond to the whole person. Workshops, such

RESEARCH NOTE

Citation

Cohen G, Byrne C, Hay J, Schmuck ML: Assessing the impact of an interdisciplinary workshop in human sexuality. *J Sex Ed and Therapy* 1994; 20(1):56–68.

Study Problem/Purpose

Previous research has demonstrated that it is important for health care professionals to clarify their personal sexual values prior to learning knowledge and skills because personal attitudes can interfere with learning. Even though educators in the health care professions recognize the importance of interdisciplinary education, this is seldom accomplished. The purposes of this two-day intensive workshop in human sexuality were to increase students' self-awareness, develop an acceptance of the values of others, increase their comfort level in openly discussing sexuality, and provide an overview of knowledge about the biopsychosocial aspects of human sexuality.

Methods

This interprofessional workshop was offered to students from nursing, medicine, physiotherapy, and occupational therapy. The study used a matched pretest and posttest design to evaluate the impact of the workshop. The questionnaire included anonymous data on gender, age, field of study, attitudes toward sexuality, comfort in working with clients posing a variety of sexual concerns, and knowledge about sexuality.

Findings

Overall, the significantly positive shift in sexual attitude and the increase in comfort over the course of the workshop for the total group suggest a willingness by students to explore their own sexual values and attitudes and to acknowledge the range of others' values, attitudes, and behaviors. The study showed no significant interdisciplinary differences in the attitude, comfort, or knowledge scales either before or after the workshop.

Implications

Some educators might argue that students from each discipline are different and have very specific educational needs. Since this study found no significant interdisciplinary differences there should be no major curricular problems specific to any particular discipline or program. A positive effect of the workshop was student benefit from the professional socialization facilitated by the combined format.

as the one described in the Research Note above, will help to meet this goal.

Only in the past 30 years has human sexuality been scientifically studied from a multidisciplinary approach. With this knowledge came the beginnings of planned interventions for individuals suffering from a variety of sexual problems and disorders. Nursing has been an active participant in the evolution of treatment approaches and programs to provide sexual health care.

Intrapersonal Theory

Intrapersonal theorists view gender identity disorders, paraphilias, and sexual dysfunctions as problems occurring within the individual. Some view them as expressions of arrested psychosexual development, some seek an explanation in sexual guilt, and others see the issue as being one of self-punishment. People who grew up with rigid family and religious taboos about sex often experience guilt and anxiety about their adult sexual roles and behaviors. Performance anxiety, negative self-concept, and negative body image are all seen as contributing to sexual problems. Problems to be solved during the treatment process include fears of intimacy, losing control, pain, pregnancy, and sexually transmitted diseases.

Behavioral Theory

Behaviorists believe that gender identity disorders arise from social learning; that is, that the child was rewarded in some way for adopting behaviors of the other sex. They believe paraphilias are learned responses; the person is conditioned to respond erotically to nonsexual objects or particular sexual acts. In the area of sexual dysfunctions, contributing factors include poor communication skills, lack of sexual experience with oneself or a partner, concern with sexual performance, and ineffective stimulation. The dysfunctions, too, are seen as learned responses.

Sociocultural Theory

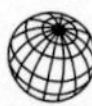

Ideas about sexuality and sexual behavior are based on cultural values and understanding. What is considered normal or abnormal depends on each group's specific viewpoint. The same behavior may be seen as positive in one culture and pathologic in another. Each culture tends to incorporate **ethnocentrism** in its beliefs; that is, its members believe their particular sexual values and behaviors are superior and preferable to those of any other culture. Ethnocentrism encourages people to view the sexual behavior of other people as eccentric, exotic, and bizarre.

Consider the diversity of sexual values throughout the world. The Mangaia of Polynesia believe that young adolescents of both genders have high sexual drives. However, as they leave young adulthood, they expect their desire to rapidly decline. In contrast, the Dani of New Guinea believe that neither women nor men have high sexual drives and that the primary purpose of sex is for reproduction. Following the birth of a child, the husband and wife remain celibate for the next five years. Among the Sambrans of New Guinea, young boys around age 7 or 8 have sex with older boys. It is believed that the ingestion of semen is required for physical growth. This pattern of behavior changes to heterosexual interaction as the young men become adults. Cultures in some parts of Africa and the Middle East practice ritual mutilation of the clitoris as a rite of initiation into womanhood. Because of serious medical complications and psychologic trauma, the practice has been outlawed in many countries, although the laws are rarely enforced. Among many cultures throughout the world, there is a third gender. Among the Zuni of New Mexico, this person is called a berdache, a male who assumes female dress, gender role, and status. Individuals with this third gender are often considered to have great spiritual power (Strong and DeVault 1994).

The sexual ethics of a culture reflect the culture's assumptions about the purpose of sex. In American culture, sexual practices have been strongly influenced by the Judeo-Christian tradition, which historically considered procreation to be the primary purpose of sex. As a result, even modern American culture is fairly sexually intolerant and harshly critical of those whose gender identity or sexual behavior is not in the mainstream.

How people communicate about sexuality is culturally determined. In general, American culture reflects European-American values, which include a negative view of public sexual communication, as evidenced by censorship and sex as a taboo topic for general discussion. However, there are ethnic differences in communication patterns. African Americans tend to be very expressive and communicate directly about sexual topics. Latinos from the Caribbean and Central American cultures tend to use restraint in expressing their feelings while those from Argentina and some other Latin American countries are emotionally expressive. Asian Americans are often less verbally expressive, so nonverbal communication assumes even more importance. The gay and lesbian subculture has developed private words and expressions in reaction to the homophobia of the dominant culture (Hecht, Collier, and Ribeau 1993; Strong and Devault 1994; Ting-Toomey and Korzenny 1991).

People with little tolerance for cross-gender behavior view transsexuals and transvestites as deviants within the American culture. The sexual acts of paraphiliacs conflict with the traditional value of sex for procreation, and they, too, are made to feel like outcasts. Sociocultural theories regarding sexual dysfunctions focus on disturbed relationships between partners, negative early learning, and past or present traumatic events.

Biologic Theory

Those who take a biologic approach are concerned with the physiologic aspects of gender identity and sexual behavior. Some believe there is a neurologic basis for gender differences and look to fetal exposure to sex hormones and adult levels of sex hormones as an explanation of gender identity disorders. They explore sexual dysfunctions to discover factors (such as organic disease, injury, medications, pain, and/or depression) that interfere with the physiologic reflexes during the sexual response cycle.

At this time there is no clear understanding of the etiology of transsexualism. Biologic theory is based on animal studies because experimental research cannot be conducted with humans. When exposed prenatally to increased male hormones, experimental animals exhibit increased male behavior. Decreasing the levels of male hormones prenatally increases female behavior in animals. In humans, the male gonads develop and begin secreting androgen during weeks 8–12 of gestation. Differentiation of the hypothalamus to a male pattern, which occurs in months 4–5 of gestation, requires high androgen levels. Thus, one explanation of transsexualism is that prenatal androgen levels were sufficient for the development of male anatomy but insufficient for differentiation in the brain. In transsexuals who are anatomically female, the androgenic influences may have been high at the critical time of hypothalamic development, although not at the time of genital formation (Benn 1993).

The Nursing Process and Clients with Gender Identity and Sexual Disorders

Assessment

The psychiatric nurse finds numerous opportunities to apply the nursing process to the promotion of sexual health. Assessment of sexual status is part of a thorough and comprehensive assessment of a client's general health.

Subjective Data The sexual history provides subjective assessment data needed for formulating nursing diagnoses. Elicit sexual information much as you elicit a general nursing history. However, pay special attention to planning a setting where privacy and uninterrupted time are available. Such a setting helps clients feel comfortable discussing these private aspects of their lives. It is helpful to begin the interview by explaining why you are asking about sexuality, for example: "Sexuality is a part of people's lives. People often have questions about sexual activity when they have changes in their health. I'd like to take this time to talk with you about your sex life."

Move from general to specific questions. This gradual focus on specific sexual behavior promotes trust and rapport. Initially, questions can relate sexuality to health status. Open-ended questions encourage clients to expand on their sexual experiences and concerns. Reassure clients that it is normal to have sexual concerns and questions, for instance: "It is common for many people to feel concerned about. . . . Do you have any questions?" Restate clients' responses to encourage them to expand on feelings. The accompanying Assessment box lists questions that can be part of a general nursing history. If clients do identify a sexual problem or if they take medications that affect sexual desire or sexual behavior, you can use the information in Table 17–2 to formulate your questions.

Objective Data Objective data include observed nonverbal behaviors, laboratory data, test results, medical diagnoses, physical examination results, and other documented sources, such as the chart.

Objective data may also include results of physiologic assessment of sexual function. The nocturnal penile tumescence (NPT) procedure provides a direct measure of erectile capacity. The device measures penile engorgement that occurs during sleep. NPT measurement is considered the best available method to determine if a man's erectile difficulties are physiologic. If so, there is minimal penile engorgement during sleep. Men whose erection difficulties appear to be psychologic in origin have

ASSESSMENT

Sexual History: The ABCs

Affective Assessment

To whom do you feel most intimate and connected?

Describe the type of love and affection in this relationship.

In what way do you experience anxiety about sex?

In what way do you experience guilt about sex?

How depressed are you feeling?

In what way does anger interfere with your sexual functioning?

Do you dislike or feel an aversion to any parts of your body?

Behavioral Assessment

Describe your level of satisfaction with the frequency of your sexual activity.

Describe the positive aspects of your own sexual functioning.

Describe the negative aspects of your own sexual functioning.

What concerns do you have about your future sexual functioning?

What are your partner's concerns about current or future sexual functioning?

Cognitive Assessment

When you were growing up, how did you learn about sex?

How has your religion influenced your sexual values and behaviors?

What "shoulds/should nots," "musts/must nots" do you believe about your sexual behavior/relationships?

How rigidly were gender roles enforced in your family of origin?

How are gender roles enacted in your present relationship/family?

Describe the negative thoughts you have about sex.

Does the use of fantasy increase or decrease your sexual desire?

Sensation Assessment

Describe any physical discomfort you feel during sexual activity.

To what degree do you experience pleasure during sexual activity?

Table 17–2 Drugs and Related Sexual Side Effects

DRUG	**SEXUAL SIDE EFFECTS**						
	Increased Sex Drive	***Decreased Sex Drive***	***Decreased Arousal***	***Retrograde Ejaculation***	***Inhibited Ejaculation***	***Painful Ejaculation***	***Orgasm Problems***
Alcohol	small amts	large amts	yes		yes		
Amphetamines	yes		may		yes		yes
Antihypertensives		yes	yes		yes		
Antipsychotics		yes	yes	may	may		yes
Anxiolytics (very few side effects)							
Beta-blockers		yes	yes				
Cocaine	yes				yes		yes
Diuretics		yes	yes				
Hallucinogens (unpredictable side effects)		may	may				may
Heroin		yes	yes		yes		yes
MAO inhibitors		may	may				may
Marijuana	small amts	large amts	chronic use				
Mood stabilizers		yes	yes				yes
Steroids		yes	yes				
Tricyclic antidepressants		yes	yes		yes	may	yes

normal engorgement during sleep. Although the NPT procedure is an important source of objective data, its results are not always reliable. Research findings report 28–42% error in accuracy (Rosen and Leiblum 1992).

Physiologic assessment of female sexual function is accomplished by the use of vaginal plethysmographs or probes. These devices are inserted into the vagina and measure vasocongestion of the vaginal wall tissue.

Several sophisticated and expensive laboratory tests are designed to assess sexual function. For instance, testosterone and estrogen blood levels may be measured. However, laboratory data must be interpreted with caution because test results are not always reliable indicators of actual sexual behavior. Thus, clients' self-reports of sexual performance, feelings, and values (the subjective data) are of prime importance in assessment.

Nursing Diagnosis

The following sections discuss the most likely nursing diagnoses and their implications for clients and nurses.

ANXIETY AND FEAR Anxiety and fear inhibit the physiologic sexual response as well as the ability to experience pleasure and joy. People who grow up learning that sex is dirty and sinful often experience anxiety in an adult relationship or are so fearful that they develop a phobic avoidance of sex. Adults who have been emotionally, physically, or sexually abused as children often fear intimacy and find they cannot have a trusting relationship with another person. Even individuals with a positive sexual history may at some time feel anxious about their sexual performance and develop a secondary fear of failure as a sex partner.

SPIRITUAL DISTRESS Lack of fulfillment in a sexual relationship may be related to a temporary feeling of distance from one's partner or an ongoing lack of intimacy in the relationship. Factors relating to lack of intimacy are relationship conflict, multiple fears, adult sexual abuse, or childhood sexual abuse.

INEFFECTIVE FAMILY COPING: COMPROMISED It is difficult to experience sexual fulfillment when the relationship is in trouble in nonsexual spheres. The difficulty may be as straightforward as poor communication or as complex as conflict, anger, and unequal power. Other socioeconomic stressors include underemployment, unemployment, and lack of social network support. When one of the partners is a transvestite, the other partner must come to terms with the behavior if a healthy relationship is to be maintained. Being part of a family with a transsexual means finding ways to reintegrate the person as a member of the other sex, or else reject the transsexual and distance the family from this particular member.

Personal Identity Disturbance In cultures with rigid gender roles, transsexuals and transvestites suffer a great deal of pain as they struggle with their gender identity. Transsexuals completely reject their anatomic sex, and transvestites alternate between their male and their female personas.

Altered Role Performance Sexual addicts often cannot maintain work, family, and social roles. The addiction is so time-consuming that the addict cannot devote time or energy to work or relationships.

Altered Sexuality Patterns Some people cannot achieve sexual arousal and orgasm without the stimulation of an unusual object or situation. These individuals are considered to have one of the paraphilias, which may be coercive or noncoercive. Most often they are preoccupied with, and feel compelled to engage in, their particular sexual behaviors.

Risk for Violence: Self-Directed or Directed at Others Autoerotic asphyxia is noncoercive but often fatal. People with this sexual behavior are not suicidal and have no intention of harming themselves but often accidentally kill themselves during sexual activity. Coercive paraphilias are considered violence against others because the victim is nonconsenting and offended or hurt by the paraphiliac's sexual behavior.

Pain A nursing diagnosis of Pain applies to women who experience vaginismus. The origin may be past sexual trauma or current emotional conflict. The pain of dyspareunia may occur in both women and men and is typically related to organic factors.

Knowledge Deficit People who grow up with no or very limited sex education may have difficulties in their adult sexual functioning. For people who don't know what to expect or how to touch themselves or their partners, sexual interactions can be frustrating rather than pleasurable. Lack of knowledge can contribute to ineffective sexual techniques and sexual dysfunctions.

Sexual Dysfunction Many of the above nursing diagnoses may be contributing factors to the development of sexual dysfunctions. In addition, illness, injury, surgery, medications, or substance abuse may contribute to sexual dysfunction. Problems with satisfaction may be described under either of these diagnoses: Sexual Dysfunction or Spiritual Distress.

Planning and Implementing Interventions

Nurses play several roles in promoting sexual health. The Mims-Swensen Sexual Health Model (1980) identifies four levels at which nurses can intervene, consistent with their comfort and knowledge.

1. *Life experience level.* This level of intervention is the minimal level of practice. Interventions are based solely on the nurse's own personal experiences. Interventions may be appropriate for clients who share similar life experiences. However, clients having different values or demonstrating different behaviors may perceive interventions based on the nurse's life experiences as irrelevant.

   Despite increased openness regarding homosexuality, many nurses remain biased and unqualified to intervene with gay and lesbian clients. Much of their bias can be attributed to the heterosexist and homophobic attitudes of the society in which we live. *Heterosexism* is a value system that assumes that heterosexuality is the only appropriate form of sexual interaction and thereby devalues homosexuality and bisexuality. *Homophobia* is discrimination, oppression, and violence against homosexuals and bisexuals. In order to be effective, nurses must learn to move beyond the life experience level of intervention.
2. *Basic level.* This intervention level is grounded in the nurse's self-awareness combined with a nonjudgmental respect for others' sexual beliefs, practices, and concerns. Nurses at this level have some knowledge about human sexual function. The knowledgeable and nonjudgmental nurse can intervene as a facilitator for clients needing to talk about their sexuality.
3. *Intermediate level.* Nurses practicing at this level of intervention synthesize knowledge, self-awareness, communication skills, and the use of the nursing process. Nurses are validators of normal sexual behavior and accept the range of sexual expression in our society. Teaching about sexual response is another intervention to resolve client concerns. Teaching is often directed at helping clients understand their stage of sexual development. For instance, teenagers and young adults frequently require accurate information regarding anatomy and physiology, sexual desire, and contraception.

   Counseling interventions are also implemented in the intermediate level. Counseling is not merely giving advice. The nurse counselor helps clients clarify their sexual problems and decide on alternatives to resolve the problems. Some specific sexual counseling strategies are listed in the accompanying Intervention box.
4. *Advanced level.* At this level of intervention, nurses must have specialized preparation and knowledge of

sexual and gender identity disorders. Nurses at the advanced level practice sex therapy, develop and present formal education programs, and do sex research.

Most nurses refer clients who require sex therapy. Nurses who do function in the sex therapist role should meet the qualifications for practice identified by the American Association of Sex Educators, Counselors, and Therapists (AASECT), which differentiate sex counseling from sex therapy. *Sex counseling* helps clients incorporate their sexual knowledge into satisfying lifestyles and socially responsible behavior. *Sex therapy* is a highly specialized, in-depth treatment to help clients resolve serious sexual problems, especially some sexual disorders. AASECT publishes a national directory of professionals certified to provide sex education, counseling, or therapy. This directory is a sex therapy resource for nurses.

Reducing Anxiety and Fear Accurate identification of feelings is the first step in the problem-solving process, and clients may need help labeling the feelings they are experiencing. Following this step, help clients identify one anxiety-producing situation within their sexual interactions. At this stage, it is productive to focus diffuse anxiety on a manageable single situation or event. With the client, analyze the situation or event to discover negative anticipatory thoughts that may be the source of the

INTERVENTION

Guidelines for Working with Clients with Sexual Difficulties

Male Orgasmic Disorder

Reestablish a climate of comfort and acceptance for sexual interaction.

Encourage the client to masturbate and enjoy touch and body stimulation in general.

Premature Ejaculation

Instruct the client to stimulate the erect penis until the premonitory sensations of impending orgasm are felt. Then penile stimulation is abruptly stopped. This process is repeated to lower the threshold of excitability and make the client more tolerant of the stimuli. Sometimes the client uses the squeeze technique: At the point of orgasm, she squeezes the head of the penis with thumb and first two fingers for 3–4 seconds. This stops the urge to ejaculate.

The couple is also instructed in ways to reduce friction in the vagina by limiting the frequency of thrusts or the movement within the vagina.

Female Orgasmic Disorder

Instruct the client to avoid intercourse. Nongenital caressing exercises begin, with man and woman alternating as the initiator of a session of caressing, thus sharing responsibility for sexual interaction.

Next, genital stimulation is added to provide positive sexual experiences without intercourse. When intercourse is attempted, the woman is instructed to assume the superior position and insert the man's penis into her vagina. When setbacks occur, the couple is advised to rely on sexual techniques that do not involve intercourse. The woman is to place her hand lightly on her partner's to indicate her preference for contact. The emphasis is not on achieving orgasm but on learning erotic preferences.

The couple is instructed to use the side-by-side position, which enables both partners to move freely with emphasis on slow, exploratory thrusting. The goal is to develop an ability to enjoy pelvic play with the penis inside the vagina.

Vaginismus

Begin with a physical demonstration to the woman of her involuntary vaginal spasm by inserting an examining finger into her vagina. Then Hegar dilators in graduated sizes are inserted by the man into the woman's vagina. At first she manually controls his insertion of the smallest dilator. Later he can insert larger dilators following her verbal instructions. After larger dilators are successfully inserted, she is instructed to retain the dilator for several hours each night. Most involuntary spasms can be relieved in 3–5 days with the daily use of dilators.

In addition to physical relief from spastic constriction, therapy is directed toward alleviating the fear that led to the onset of symptoms.

Sexual Acting-Out

After identifying increased levels of anxiety with clients, openly discuss the meanings of behaviors. Give feedback about inappropriate behavior, and discuss appropriate ways to meet sexual needs. Reassure clients that you are not rejecting them, but the behavior.

anxiety. Together, review how the client has handled anxiety in the past and evaluate the range and effectiveness of this past coping behavior. It may be appropriate to help the client redefine the sensations of anxiety as sensations of sexual excitement, which is more likely to result in positive expectations. Together, explore alternative coping behaviors, and have the client evaluate their effectiveness after implementing them.

Many adult survivors of childhood sexual abuse are periodically overwhelmed by anxiety, fear, and panic (see Chapter 16). Refer adult survivors to support groups such as Incest Survivors Anonymous or VOICES, as well as individual therapy with a therapist who specializes in this field.

Decreasing Spiritual Distress Because the origin of spiritual distress is a lack of intimacy or connection, the goal of nursing intervention is to help clients achieve and maintain a level of intimacy each partner finds comfortable. In the context of therapy, couples discuss their individual needs for closeness and identify barriers to intimacy. They are instructed to make three or four half-hour "dates" each week, during which they share warmth and intimacy. They spend some of the time discussing specific sexual issues; during other "dates," the couple explores intimate, nonsexual topics, such as hopes and expectations for the future. Couples should give these dates top priority, because a common way of avoiding intimacy is by not setting time aside for each other.

Promoting More Effective Family Coping Good communication is an important part of a sexually fulfilling relationship. Apart from setting specific times to share feelings and beliefs, some couples need training in more effective communication skills. If they give ambiguous signals to indicate sexual interest, they need to learn how to state their interest clearly. Some people expect their partners to "read their minds" about sexual needs and desires; these people need encouragement to assert their needs tactfully. Teach couples to avoid "you" language, which evokes a defensive response and results in arguments, and to use "I" language, which expresses personal thoughts, feelings, and needs. Following are some examples of accusatory "you" statements and accountable "I" statements:

- *"You" language*

  "You only have sex on your mind. You're a pervert."

  "You keep grabbing at me like I'm always ready to go to bed with you."

  "You never pay attention to what turns me on. Are you dumb or hard of hearing?"

- *"I" language*

  "I'm concerned because we seem to have different expectations of how often we would like to make love."

  "I miss all the hugging and caressing we used to do even when we couldn't make love afterward."

  "I feel frustrated and hurt when it seems like I'm repeating myself. Maybe I'm not communicating my needs very clearly."

If the relationship is in significant trouble, refer the couple for relationship or sex therapy.

If cross-dressing is a newly divulged secret, offer education and support. If the relationship is to continue, both partners need to agree on where and how cross-dressing will take place. Some couples compromise; for instance, a husband may agree never to cross-dress in front of his wife, and she may agree to give him privacy. Some agree to limit cross-dressing to the home; others are comfortable going out in public with the partner cross-dressed. Some transvestites join a transvestite club where they can express their female personality in a safe social situation. The long-term success of the relationship depends on the couple's ability to negotiate these issues.

Promoting Comfort with Personal Identity Many adult transsexuals seek hormonal therapy or sex-change surgery to make their bodies congruent with their gender identity. Surgical intervention has been a source of controversy and at this time appears to be decreasing in frequency. This trend may be associated with the cost and practical difficulties of the complex procedures involved, or it may reflect a cultural denial of the reality of the problem. The success rate of hormonal or surgical reassignment appears to be correlated with the degree of gender identity disorder prior to treatment as well as the overall emotional stability of the individual.

Refer transsexuals to therapists who specialize in this area or to gender identity disorder clinics. Because gender identity is stable and nonchangeable, the goal of treatment with transsexuals is to help them live and function in society in the cross-gender role. They need a great deal of support and assistance as they establish themselves in their new role. If the present job is not gender-role stereotyped, they may be able to remain in the same or similar position. Others may need retraining programs to find acceptable employment. A multidisciplinary approach is most effective in helping transsexuals adjust to their situation. Family and friends need support and counseling to reintegrate this person into their lives as a person of the other sex (Devor 1993).

Promoting Effective Role Performance Like other addicts, sexual addicts often do not seek help until they literally cannot manage their lives. They may lose job, home, and relationships before admitting the consequences of the addiction. When that occurs, they may become severely depressed and even suicidal. Refer sexual addicts to self-help groups and specialized professional therapy. Recovery is a long-term process facilitated by individual, group, couple, family, and family-of-origin therapy. The cornerstone of recovery is a twelve-step program modeled on the Alcoholics Anonymous program. Partners and codependents are also referred to appropriate self-help groups. A variety of groups, such as Sexaholics Anonymous, Sex Addicts Anonymous, Sex and Love Addicts Anonymous, S-Anon, and Co-Dependents of Sexual Addicts, have been formed throughout the country.

PROMOTING NONCOERCIVE SEXUALITY PATTERNS Once paraphilias are a programmed part of arousal, they are very difficult to deprogram. The response to certain sexual or erotic stimuli tends to persist through life. A noncoercive, nonharmful paraphilia practiced with an adult consenting partner requires no nursing intervention other than client and partner education and possible couple negotiation about the behavior.

DECREASING VIOLENCE AGAINST THE SELF AND OTHERS The most important nursing intervention regarding autoerotic asphyxia is community education. Warnings about autoerotic asphyxia should be routinely included in adolescent sex-education programs. Teenagers who practice it must be encouraged to seek immediate professional help. Parents should be taught to look for physical signs of trauma to the neck, such as bruising, abrasions, pressure marks, or rope burns. Ropes, knotted sheets, knotted T-shirts, or the like hidden in the bedroom may be warning signs.

Individuals who practice coercive paraphilias typically end up in the criminal justice system. The court may or may not mandate therapy. Therapy for sex offenders is a specialized area that should not be undertaken lightly. Although behavior-modification techniques, group therapy, and hypnosis are used, they are generally unsuccessful. In severe cases, male sex offenders are treated with the antiandrogen drug medroxyprogesterone acetate (Provera or Depo-Provera), which induces a reversible chemical castration. The drug reduces the male sex drive, erections, ejaculation, and decreases the obsessional focus on sex.

DECREASING PAIN Whenever pain is associated with intercourse a thorough physical examination is necessary to find and treat the organic cause of the pain. During vaginal exams, careful attention must be paid to tiny tears in the vaginal wall, which are often overlooked. Even very small tears can cause great pain during intercourse. Vaginismus is treated with education, dilators, and supportive psychotherapy. (See the Intervention box, page 415.)

INCREASING KNOWLEDGE The lack of sex education is not unusual among people with sexual dysfunctions. Nurses can intervene by teaching clients sexual anatomy and the sexual response cycle. Encourage couples to talk with one another about their individual responses. Some people may be very uncomfortable with sexual language and need help learning sexual vocabulary and identifying which words are acceptable for intimate use. Part of the learning and desensitization process is having them repeat the words aloud to one another until they feel comfortable using them.

MANAGING SEXUAL DYSFUNCTIONS: SEX THERAPY There are many approaches to the treatment of sexual dysfunctions, including individual, couple, and group treatment with one or two sex therapists. The duration of treatment programs varies. Treatment programs may be for heterosexual or homosexual individuals or couples. The effectiveness of these programs depends on the client's needs and the therapists' skill.

Sex therapy programs have these components in common:

- *Information and education about sexual functions.* The therapist gives clients specific information about their particular needs. The therapist may assign books to read or discuss the information.
- *Experiential/sensory awareness.* The therapist helps clients recognize feelings of anxiety, anger, and pleasure by tuning into bodily cues. Clients focus on and describe feelings both in therapy sessions and at home. If they believe their genitals are ugly and unclean, the therapist assigns desensitization exercises at home for clients to explore and become familiar with their own bodies. Some clients need fantasy training if nonsexual thoughts interfere with sexual arousal.
- *Insight.* The therapist attempts to learn and understand what is causing and perpetuating the sexual problem. The goal is for clients to assume responsibility for their own behavior and recognize that change is possible.
- *Cognitive restructuring.* Clients identify and reevaluate their fears about sexual interaction. The therapist encourages them to identify and eliminate negative self-statements and irrational expectations.
- *Behavioral interventions.* Focus is on changing nonsexual behavior that contributes to sexual problems. The therapist may assign assertiveness training, communication training, stress-reduction exercises, and problem-solving techniques. Behavioral interventions include assigned pleasuring sessions to discover what is arousing and pleasing to the self and partner (see the Interventions box).

Evaluation and Outcome Criteria

ANXIETY AND FEAR Clients will be able to use the problem-solving process as one tool for decreasing anxiety and fear. They will implement effective coping measures and verbalize a decrease in anxiety. Adult survivors of childhood sexual abuse will participate in support groups and engage in psychotherapy to manage the fears and trauma of the past.

Spiritual Distress Couples will report an acceptable and meaningful level of intimacy in their relationships. They will continue to set aside time for each other and engage in meaningful intimate time.

Family Coping Couples will increase the use of "I" language and decrease the use of blaming "you" language. They will express their sexual desires, needs, and preferences directly. If the relationship is in significant trouble, they will report a willingness to seek therapy. If one partner is a transvestite, the couple will negotiate the cross-dressing behavior, and both partners will report satisfaction with their relationship.

Gender Identity Clients will report increasing comfort and satisfaction in their new gender role, which will be congruent with their gender identity. Each will be able to function socially and economically as a person of that gender. Family and friends will be supportive and accepting of these clients.

Role Performance Clients will participate actively in self-help groups as well as professional therapy. They will be able to manage their addiction in such a way that they can maintain intimate relationships and be financially responsible. Family members will participate actively in the appropriate self-help groups.

Noncoercive Sexuality Patterns Clients and partners will verbalize an understanding that noncoercive paraphilias are lifelong patterns. Couples will be able to negotiate the behavior in a way that is mutually satisfying.

Violence Community and family education programs will be established about the danger of autoerotic asphyxia. Victims of this disorder will be identified and referred for immediate treatment. Clients with this disorder will remain safe. Coercive paraphiliacs will curb their behavior, or society will set strict limits to protect potential victims.

Pain Individuals will report less pain or no pain during intercourse. Clients suffering from vaginismus will report success in using conscious control to relax vaginal muscles, allowing for pain-free intercourse.

Knowledge Clients will describe sexual anatomy and the phases of the sexual response cycle. Couples will report increased communication about individual responses and preferences using a selected sexual vocabulary.

Sexual Dysfunction Clients will report a satisfying and fulfilling sex life. They will experience minimal difficulty with desire, arousal, or orgasm. They will be able to identify and label feelings and acknowledge responsibility for their own behavior. They will implement a chosen variety of sexual techniques.

Chapter Highlights

- Nurses must be able to accept and respect the client's sexual beliefs, attitudes, and behaviors as equal in value to, although possibly different from, their own personal beliefs, attitudes, and behaviors.
- Gender identity disorders have multiple causes. Biologic, environmental, cultural, and learning influences determine the severity and intensity of the disorders.
- Noncoercive paraphilias typically are not harmful, are practiced between consenting adults, and do not require nursing intervention.
- Coercive paraphilias are described in the legal code and are considered criminal acts.
- Sexual dysfunctions have psychophysiologic causes. Classification is according to the phase of the sexual response cycle primarily affected.
- Sexual addiction is a progressive condition in which sex is used to numb pain.
- Nurses are appropriate promoters of sexual health by virtue of self-awareness, communication skills, theoretic knowledge, use of the nursing process, and the unique characteristics of the nurse-client relationship.
- Nurses are responsible and accountable for the delivery of care that promotes sexual health, including accurate assessment, diagnosis, education, counseling, and referral.
- Nurses should take a sexual history to assess general sexual health and, if indicated, gather detailed information about specific sexual problems.
- To gauge the effectiveness of nursing interventions for sexual problems, the nurse can evaluate how well the client has understood education and what changes the client reports or the nurse observes.

References

Ackerman MD, Montague DK, Morganstern S: Impotence: Help for erectile dysfunction. *Patient Care* (March 15) 1994;28(5):22–56.

American Psychiatric Association: *Diagnostic and Statistical Manual of Mental Disorders,* ed 4. American Psychiatric Association, 1994.

Benn SL: *The Lenses of Gender.* Yale University Press, 1993.

Bullough VL, Bullough B: *Cross-Dressing, Sex, and Gender.* University of Pennsylvania Press, 1993.

Cohen G, Byrne C, Hay J, Schmuck ML: Assessing the impact of an interdisciplinary workshop in human sexuality. *J Sex Ed and Therapy* 1994;20(1):56–68.

Devor H: Sexual orientation identities, attractions, and practices of female-to-male transsexuals. *J Sex Res* 1993; 30(4):303–315.

Hecht M, Collier MJ, Ribeau S: *African American Communication*. Sage, 1993.

Matek O: Obscene phone callers, in Dalley DM (ed): *The Sexually Unusual: Guide to Understanding and Helping*. Haworth Press, 1988.

Mims FH, Swensen M: *Sexuality: A Nursing Perspective*. McGraw-Hill, 1980.

Monat KK: *Sexuality and the Mentally Retarded*. College Hill Press, 1982.

Morokoff PJ: Stress, sexual functioning and marital satisfaction. *J Sex Res* 1993;30(1):43–53.

Rosen RC, Leiblum SR: *Erectile Disorders*. Guilford Press, 1992.

Rothblum ED, Brehony KA: *Boston Marriages*. University of Massachusetts Press, 1993.

Schwartz MF, Masters WH: Integration of trauma-based, cognitive, behavioral, systemic and addiction approaches for treatment of hypersexual pair-bonding disorder. *Sexual Addiction & Compulsivity* 1994;1(1):57–76.

Shaffer HJ: Considering two models of excessive sexual behaviors: Addiction and obsessive-compulsive disorder. *Sexual Addiction & Compulsivity* 1994;1(1):6–18.

Strong B, DeVault C: *Human Sexuality*. Mayfield, 1994.

Ting-Toomey S, Korzenny F: *Cross-Cultural Interpersonal Communication*. Sage, 1991.

Wood JT: Gender and relationship crises: Contrasting reasons, responses, and relational orientations, in Ringer RJ (ed): *Queer Words, Queer Images*. New York University Press, 1994.

CHAPTER 18

CLIENTS WITH EATING DISORDERS

Kay K. Chitty

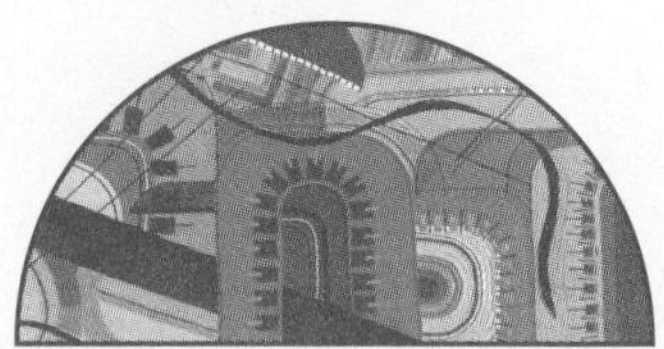

COMPETENCIES

- *Define anorexia nervosa, bulimia nervosa, and compulsive overeating.*
- *Describe the biopsychosocial theories contributing to the understanding of eating disorders.*
- *Recognize the DSM-IV diagnostic criteria for eating disorders.*
- *Assess individual and family problems of clients with eating disorders.*
- *Identify nursing diagnoses for clients with eating disorders.*
- *Describe the nurse's role and appropriate nursing interventions for clients with eating disorders, and their families.*
- *Evaluate the effectiveness of nursing interventions with clients with eating disorders, and their families.*
- *Explain why you may feel frustrated caring for clients with eating disorders.*

Cross-References

Other topics relevant to this content are: Adolescents, Chapter 37; Codependence, Chapter 26; Eating disorders in infancy or childhood, Chapter 36; Mood disorders, Chapter 15; Personality disorders, Chapter 20; Psychophysiologic conditions, Chapter 22; Stress, anxiety, and coping, Chapter 4; Stress management, Chapter 29.

Critical Thinking Challenge

Because eating is closely bound up with emotions, disorders of eating indicate emotional difficulties that fall within the scope of psychiatric nursing. In your opinion, what is the responsibility of nurses in educating the public about prevention of eating disorders? What kinds of information do people, particularly parents, teachers, and coaches, need to communicate about eating and health? What messages have you received that have helped or hindered you in developing healthy eating attitudes and behaviors?

Over the past 25 years, developed countries have experienced what has been described as an epidemic of eating disorders. The emphasis on slimness has made increasing numbers of adolescents and young adults obsessively concerned about eating, weight, and body shape, size, and appearance. In a desperate attempt to achieve perfection, the need for which is often psychologically obscure, some individuals go to extreme lengths to achieve thinness. While they starve themselves, sometimes to death, others apparently reject the cultural norms, overeat, and become obese.

For many, eating symbolizes parental nurturing—the love and care that are the prototype of and basis for all future intimate relationships. For some, however, eating creates anxiety because of its association with unsatisfactory and unpleasant parent-child interactions. Clearly, food and eating have greater individual and cultural meaning and importance than merely an activity undertaken to sustain life.

The three major eating disorders discussed in this chapter—anorexia nervosa, bulimia nervosa, and compulsive overeating—create biologic, psychologic, and social imbalances that interfere with the individual's normal functioning. Changes in biochemistry, metabolic rate, emotional state, family relationships, and social status brought about by eating disorders can create depression, isolation, and sometimes self-destructive behavior. The degree of hopelessness and anguish experienced by clients with these disorders is extreme and may be underestimated by caregivers.

Anorexia Nervosa

Anorexia nervosa is a potentially life-threatening disorder characterized by extreme weight loss, intense fear of gaining weight, body image disturbances, strenuous exercising, and peculiar food-handling patterns. Hilde Bruch (1978) has called it "the relentless pursuit of thinness." Unchecked, the course of anorexia nervosa results in a mortality rate of 5–21%, depending on time elapsed since onset (Halmi 1985). It is estimated that 95% of anorexia nervosa clients are female, usually between the ages of 12 and the mid-thirties (Herzog 1988). The onset of the disorder is sometimes associated with a stressful life event.

Simone is a tall, quiet girl who was considered polite, well-liked, and a good student. She was given responsibility beyond her years at both school and home because of her quiet competence and maturity. When she was 15, she entered a beauty contest at a local amusement park as a lark but did not win. She became convinced that she lost because her legs were too large and her abdomen protruded. She decided to diet. To radically control her own intake without arousing the family's suspicions, she began preparing all the family's meals. She did not eat herself, but played with her food during mealtimes.

Simone spent long hours alone in her room studying, dancing, and exercising vigorously. She began weighing herself several times daily, and if the scales showed an unacceptable number, she exercised even more frenziedly.

As she lost weight, Simone disguised her gauntness with loose clothes. One day, when she and her mother were shopping, her mother saw her without her blouse and was dismayed. She insisted that Simone see the family physician, who encouraged her to eat more and prescribed nutritional supplements.

When Simone collapsed at a shopping mall a few weeks later, her parents prevailed on the family doctor to admit her to the psychiatric unit of the community hospital. As an IV was started in the emergency room, Simone asked the nurse, "How many calories are in that bag? It won't make me gain weight, will it?"

For the DSM-IV diagnostic criteria for anorexia nervosa, see the accompanying box.

DSM-IV Diagnostic Criteria for Anorexia Nervosa

A. Refusal to maintain body weight at or above a minimally normal weight for age and height (e.g., weight loss leading to maintenance of body weight less than 85% of that expected; or failure to make expected weight gain during period of growth, leading to body weight less than 85% of that expected).

B. Intense fear of gaining weight or becoming fat, even though underweight.

C. Disturbance in the way in which one's body image or shape is experienced, undue influence of body weight or shape on self-evaluation, or denial of the seriousness of the current low body weight.

D. In postmenarcheal females, amenorrhea, i.e., the absence of at least three consecutive menstrual cycles. (A woman is considered to have amenorrhea if her periods occur only following hormone, e.g., estrogen, administration.)

Restricting Type

During the current episode of Anorexia Nervosa, the person has not regularly engaged in binge-eating or purging behavior (i.e., self-induced vomiting or the misuse of laxatives, diuretics, or enemas).

Binge-Eating/Purging Type

During the current episode of Anorexia Nervosa, the person has regularly engaged in binge-eating or purging behavior (i.e., self-induced vomiting or the misuse of laxatives, diuretics, or enemas).

Source: American Psychiatric Association 1994, pp. 544–545.

Bulimia Nervosa

Bulimia nervosa is a disorder characterized by **binge eating**, the frequent compulsion to eat large quantities of food in a short period of time. These periods of overeating are usually followed by **purging**, self-induced vomiting and/or use of large doses of laxatives and diuretics. Enemas may also be used to rid the body of all traces of food consumed during a binge. Many anorexia nervosa clients also indulge in binge eating and purging. There must be a minimum average of two binge-eating episodes per week for at least 3 months to warrant this DSM-IV diagnosis. Most bulimics are young females of high school or college age of normal or slightly above-average weight. Recent statistics show bulimia is escalating among older women and young men as well. Like anorexics, bulimics are preoccupied with body shape and size.

Beth, a 17-year-old student, came to the mental health center because of binge eating. She complained that although she was very concerned with her weight and very invested in her physical image, she regularly went on gluttonous eating binges for one to two days. These would leave her nauseated, exhausted, and disgusted with herself. Her inability to control the behavior voluntarily was making her depressed.

In the course of her therapy, it became apparent that although Beth consciously wanted to make certain improvements in her academic and social life and her appearance, she had subtle ways of sabotaging any movement in that direction. Binge eating destroyed any attempts to control her weight and thus feel positive about her body image.

Movement in a self-interested direction had become attached in Beth's mind to repudiation of her depressed mother, with whom she felt very close. Individual successes, she felt, were antagonistic toward her mother because they might lead to her own greater independence. Although she wished such independence for herself, she also feared losing her mother's support, which she needed. Thus, she developed ways of undermining her own efforts.

Psychotherapeutic work with Beth involved discovering these meanings, bringing her concerns to the surface for discussion, and attempting to resolve issues of dependence and fear of separation. When these subjects were directly discussed, Beth had less need for indirect expression of conflict, and the binge-eating behavior subsided.

For the DSM-IV diagnostic criteria for bulimia nervosa, see the accompanying box.

DSM-IV Diagnostic Criteria for Bulimia Nervosa

A. Recurrent episodes of binge eating. An episode of binge eating is characterized by both of the following:
   1. Eating, in a discrete period of time (e.g., within any 2-hour period), an amount of food that is definitely larger than most people would eat during a similar period of time and under similar circumstances.
   2. A sense of lack of control over eating during the episode (e.g., a feeling that one cannot stop eating or control what or how much one is eating).

B. Recurrent inappropriate compensatory behavior in order to prevent weight gain, such as self-induced vomiting; misuse of laxatives, diuretics, enemas, or other medications; fasting; or excessive exercise.

C. The binge eating and inappropriate compensatory behaviors both occur, on average, at least twice a week for 3 months.

D. Self-evaluation is unduly influenced by body shape and weight.

E. The disturbance does not occur exclusively during episodes of Anorexia Nervosa.

Purging Type

During the current episode of Bulimia Nervosa, the person has regularly engaged in self-induced vomiting or the misuse of laxatives, diuretics, or enemas.

Nonpurging Type

During the current episode of Bulimia Nervosa, the person has used other inappropriate compensatory behaviors, such as fasting or excessive exercise, but has not regularly engaged in self-induced vomiting or the misuse of laxatives, diuretics, or enemas.

Source: American Psychiatric Association 1994, pp. 549–550.

Compulsive Overeating

Compulsive overeating is "a process of responding to an emotional need or experience with an inappropriate behavior that attempts to address it but cannot" (Miller 1991). People who overeat compulsively do so when they are not physically hungry and continue to eat even after they have had enough. They ignore their bodies' **satiety** cues, the sensation of being full after a meal, because they are eating for emotional rather than physical reasons. Compulsive overeaters choose food as a means of calming or nurturing themselves. They attempt to compensate for the love and nurturing they desire and to relieve stress by numbing themselves with food. Consequently, they often become obese.

Obesity can be defined as the "excessive storage of energy in the form of fat" (Wurtman and Wurtman 1987). Although obesity has adverse effects on both longevity and health, it also may adversely affect mental health. There is considerable controversy as to whether obesity by itself should be classified as an eating disorder. It is not included under that category in the *DSM-IV,* and many obese individuals are apparently quite well adjusted. Many others, however, experience anxiety, depression, low self-esteem, and poor body image. Obesity and compulsive overeating, therefore, are included in this chapter on eating disorders. Compulsive overeating can be diagnosed under the *DSM-IV* category "psychological factors affecting physical condition."

Joan, an obese 45-year-old secretary, is 5′3″ tall and weighs 167 lb. She came to the outpatient department of a private psychiatric hospital because of depression over her weight. She reported that her weight problem began about 10 years ago when her husband left her on the day of her parents' twenty-fifth wedding anniversary. She and her 10-year-old son moved back in with her parents, and the family had many long discussions concerning what Joan should do. At about the same time, she lost her job. It took Joan nearly 6 months to find a comparable job, and she suffered severe financial stresses. Again, her parents helped. She felt trapped by, yet dependent on, her parents.

Joan described herself during that period as "tense and angry all the time." Her weight gradually crept up. She tried to diet, but the problems remained, and eating seemed to be the only way to dull the pain. "When I'd look at myself in the mirror, I would be so discouraged that I'd eat a whole pan of brownies, just to feel better."

Psychotherapy with Joan involved exploring the meaning of her obesity and focused on her concerns about her attractiveness to men. Her relationship with her parents, particularly dependence/independence issues, were also explored. Joan, who has been in therapy for only 4 months, now says, "My behavior is destructive; I am using food as an escape from emotional stress and pain. I still wish I were thinner."

Biopsychosocial Theories

Although many clinical studies have been published, the literature on eating disorders shows no theoretic consensus on etiology and treatment. Psychoanalytic theory, cultural theory, family systems theory, behavioral theory, feminist theory, and biologic theories all contribute to an understanding of the development and dynamics of eating disorders.

Psychoanalytic Theory

Since Freud first identified it as such, food ingestion has been regarded as a critical aspect in the psychologic growth and development of infants, children, and adults. It is widely recognized that the infant at the breast already is beginning to internalize certain primitive knowledge about life through the quality of the feeding experience.

Psychoanalytic theory considers eating disorders symptoms of unconscious conflicts that the person resolves by gaining insight into the nature and meaning of the conflicts. Little attention is given to the biologic or cultural domains. Aspects of psychoanalytic theory related to eating disorders include the concept of regression to prepubertal phases of development and repudiation of developing sexuality. In psychoanalytic thinking, compulsive overeating represents overcompensation for unmet oral needs during infancy. Obesity is also thought to represent a defense against intimacy with the opposite sex.

The basic treatment modality in the psychoanalytic model is long-term individual psychotherapy, sometimes accompanied by group therapy. The goal of therapy is the development of insight and subsequent "working through" of underlying issues to resolve the unconscious conflicts manifested by the eating disorder.

Cultural Theory

Culture profoundly affects food choices, attitudes toward food, food rituals, preferences, and taboos. Eating behaviors are learned in the family and reflect the ethnic background of the family group. Culture also affects perceptions of beauty, which include cultural norms regarding body size and shape.

The cultural approach to eating disorders assumes that Western society's current emphasis on thinness plays a pivotal role in the development of eating disorders. People in Western cultures are preoccupied with the importance of creating a body that "fits" contemporary norms of size and shape exemplified by fashion models, dancers, and Hollywood stars. Gourmet cooking, "designer foods," and the sensual pleasures of preparing and consuming foods are emphasized simultaneously, creating confusion and conflict. The cultural emphasis on sexual freedom is also a problem, particularly to the female adolescent most likely to be affected by eating disorders. There is increasing evidence in psychiatric literature that anorexia nervosa is also prevalent in non-Western cultures. Clinical patterns may differ across cultures, however.

Family Systems Theory

Hilde Bruch (1978) was a pioneer in the application of family systems theory in her work with individuals with anorexia nervosa. Other therapists have incorporated family systems theory into their work with people who have other eating disorders as well. According to Bruch, the eating disorder itself expresses unconscious intrapersonal and interpersonal conflicts of the client and the family. The symptom stabilizes the family by allowing them to focus on the client, thus ignoring their own unresolved conflicts.

Bruch described the anorexic family as consisting of parents with overly rigid expectations of an overly compliant child. The child's conflict is between enslavement to parental expectations and the drive for autonomy. Anorexic adolescents sometimes see controlling their own body size as the only way to assert control in their lives.

Treatment in the family systems model focuses on defining the family conflicts for which the eating disorder compensates. Through both individual and family therapy, indirectly expressed conflicts are resolved. Healthier and more direct means of expressing family conflicts are learned. An interesting aspect of Bruch's therapeutic orientation is her insistence on the client's "physiological restoration." She refuses to work with families until the psychologic effects of starvation have been ameliorated through weight gain.

The family systems approach to compulsive overeating includes a working theory that ambivalence of a parent or parents toward a child sets the stage for the child's obesity. Conflict between parents and subsequent scapegoating of a child also are seen as contributing factors.

Behavioral Theory

Behavioral theory views eating disorders as learned behaviors. It focuses on changing cognitive and behavioral responses to physiologic, psychologic, and social stimuli. Insight into the nature of the maladaptive behavior (the eating disorder) is integrated with new and healthier responses to emotional stimuli. Because food cannot be entirely avoided, education about the psychology of compulsive behavior and the physiologic effects of starvation and purging behaviors is usually incorporated into the therapeutic process. Cognitive approaches include correction of perceptual disturbances and elimination of irrational thoughts and beliefs such as, "Eating any food is too much," "Eating makes me feel better when I'm anxious or insecure," and "I have always been fat and I will always be fat."

Both individual and group therapy are useful in the behavioral treatment of eating disorders. Group support over the long term is helpful in reinforcing and solidifying new behaviors as they are adopted.

Feminist Theory

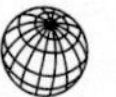

With few exceptions, throughout history, women were considered desirable when they had plump breasts, hips, and thighs. Plumpness was fashionable, demonstrated that the male was a good provider, and symbolized sensuality. The female form has always been an object of pleasure for men, and this emphasis has powerfully affected each woman's relationship with her body. Viewed in historical context, eating disorders can be interpreted as an understandable, although extreme, response to disturbances in that relationship. The rapid and sweeping societal changes of the last 50 years have created the right climate for the proliferation of eating disorders in Western society.

In her feminist model of the etiology and treatment of eating disorders, Orbach (1978) emphasizes female issues and resulting conflicts that contribute to abnormal eating patterns. In addition to sexuality, the issues include nurturance, individuality and boundaries, and societal limitations on the power of women. Orbach asserts that women select abnormal eating patterns as a means of coping with these conflicts when healthier and more direct means of coping are not available. Overeating is thought to reflect a need to fill oneself "up and out" to attain the stereotypic, all-giving, nurturing role that women have been encouraged to assume. Anorexia, by contrast, can be interpreted as a rejection of that stereotype.

For Orbach, the goals of therapy include differentiating between the desire to eat and the physiologic need for food, understanding the meaning of food and eating to the individual, and developing an understanding of the meaning of "being fat" and "being thin." Psychologic, cognitive, and cultural insights are the goals of therapy, which may combine individual sessions with either therapy or self-help groups, or both.

Biologic Theories

The biologic forces that shape the behavior of people with eating disorders have received relatively little attention. Because the neurochemical control of eating is the result of complex interactions between neurotransmitters and the brain, it has been much simpler to explain eating disorders as based on cultural, family, and intrapsychic phenomena. (For a discussion of neurotransmitters, see Chapter 3.) These explanations are incomplete, however, without further examination of the biologic factors influencing disordered eating behaviors.

Some research has focused on the hypothalamic sites that control feeding and has led to speculation about the exact nature of the physiologic bases of eating disorders. A neurochemical model has been proposed for anorexia nervosa (Morley et al. 1986), but it is clearly not useful for bulimia nervosa. Heredity is thought to be a factor in obesity, but environmental factors may be equally or more important (Wurtman and Wurtman 1987).

Both extreme weight loss and excessive weight gain can be caused by physical conditions. Certain conditions must be ruled out before an eating disorder diagnosis can be made. Such wasting conditions as advanced cancer, tuberculosis, AIDS, hyperthyroidism, pyloric obstruction, and drug abuse must be considered when weight loss is a feature. Rapid weight gain can result from a brain tumor or an endocrine disorder. A good history and physical examination usually provide enough information to eliminate the possibility of a physical basis for sudden weight loss or gain.

Currently there is renewed research interest in the possible physiologic bases of eating disorders. Further investigation will undoubtedly reveal new knowledge about the biology of these disorders. For now, an understanding of the relationship between physiologic processes and eating disorders is just emerging.

Biologic factors, sociocultural pressures to overeat or undereat, and intrapsychic or interpersonal fears and conflicts cannot—and should not—be dealt with separately. The interaction of these factors creates a cyclical pattern. For example, clients suffering from severe obesity may experience shame and helplessness as they attempt to cope with fears of rejection and loss of love. These feelings can lead to compensatory overeating behaviors, which in turn may create interpersonal conflict with family members. The client may withdraw from others, thus reinforcing the feelings of rejection and increasing social disability. Only by understanding the interrelated factors leading to eating disorders can psychiatric nurses take a holistic approach to the care of affected individuals and their families.

Why do some people develop eating disorders while others do not? Despite research efforts, no satisfactory answer has been found.

Caloric Intake and Metabolic Requirements Even in today's calorie-conscious society, the quality of care a mother gives to her infant is measured, at least in part, by the infant's "healthy" appearance. A chubby baby is considered by some to be a healthy baby who outwardly embodies the nurturing and love of the mother. Some mothers encourage food intake exceeding the infant's metabolic requirements. The resulting fat cells, once in existence, remain throughout life.

During childhood, activity level is high. Children learn to consume an abundance of food, often snack foods rich in carbohydrates and fat, daily. They are also encouraged to eat larger portions at meals as they grow.

Over time, obesity results from the imbalance between caloric intake and energy expenditure. During adolescence, both boys and girls experience growth spurts that require additional energy. Because boys continue to increase in muscle mass well beyond puberty, they need additional calories. By the age of 16, a girl's energy requirements have fallen off considerably. If she continues to eat as she did during childhood and early adolescence, she is bound to gain weight at a time when she is most concerned about appearance and attractiveness to members of the opposite sex.

Neurochemical Abnormalities and Genetic Factors Anorexic and bulimic clients have various neurochemical abnormalities. Whether these changes are a result of the starvation state or a cause of it has not been determined, but nearly all the abnormalities disappear with weight restoration (Herzog 1988).

Studies of bulimia suggest possible CNS abnormalities of the serotonergic and noradrenergic systems. Serotonin studies in animals have linked satiety to serotonin levels. Bulimics appear to have low levels of serotonin, which may predispose them to binge-eating behavior. Studies of twins support the hypothesis that genetic factors predispose to eating disorders, even when environmental factors are different (Holland et al. 1984).

Psychologic Factors

Some studies have suggested that people with eating disorders are more neurotic and obsessive than normal eaters. The idea that people eat to compensate for the emptiness of their lives has been hypothesized as a causative factor in obesity. Anorexics are thought to fear sexual maturity; the anorexia is seen as a rejection of the feminine form and a desperate attempt to regain the contours and dimensions of a prepubertal child. Study results are so mixed, however, that clear-cut personality traits predisposing to these disorders are difficult to validate.

Although personality traits are difficult to identify, it is possible to identify common feelings and experiences. Some 25–50% of people with eating disorders are thought to have major depressive disturbances. Controversy surrounds the chicken-or-egg relationship between depression and eating disorders, and research continues.

It is commonly recognized that people with eating disorders almost universally have distorted attitudes about food, eating, and the size of their bodies. Early developmental failure is common, as is family dysfunction. Anorexics in particular are excessively concerned about achieving perfection and avoiding self-indulgence. They

RESEARCH NOTE

Citation

Welch SL, Fairburn CG: Sexual abuse and bulimia nervosa: Three integrated case control comparisons. *Am J Psychiatr* 1994; 151(3):402–407.

Study Problem/Purpose

The purposes of this study were to determine whether sexual abuse increases the risk of developing bulimia nervosa, to determine if the increased risk was specific to bulimia nervosa, and to compare clients being treated for bulimia nervosa with a control group in terms of exposure to childhood sexual abuse.

Methods

Fifty community-based female subjects with bulimia nervosa, but not in treatment, were compared with 100 comparison subjects without an eating disorder, 50 subjects with other psychiatric disorders, and 50 clients with bulimia nervosa and in active treatment. The subjects were matched for gender, age, and parental socioeconomic class. An investigator-based interview was used to assess sexual abuse.

Findings

A significantly higher number of the community-based subjects with bulimia nervosa (26%) reported sexual abuse involving physical contact than did the matched normal comparison subjects (10%). There was no significant difference between the community-based subjects with bulimia nervosa and either the subjects with general psychiatric disorders or the clinic clients with bulimia nervosa. Surprisingly, the community-based group not in treatment reported higher rates of sexual abuse than the clients in active treatment for bulimia nervosa.

Implications

While there has been increasing interest in recent years in the prevalence of childhood sexual abuse and its relationship to bulimia nervosa, sexual abuse alone does not appear to be a specific predisposing factor for bulimia nervosa. It appears to be a risk factor for psychiatric disorders in general, including bulimia nervosa. The multiple risk factors for bulimia nervosa require further study to determine what role, if any, childhood sexual abuse plays in predisposing women to this disorder.

equate weight gain with being "bad" or "out of control." Some bulimics report childhood sexual abuse (see the Research Note above).

Common feelings reported by anorexic, bulimic, and obese individuals include a sense of ineffectiveness and preoccupation with food and eating. Most have perceptual disturbances, such as not feeling satiated even after a large meal.

Sociocultural Factors

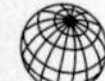

The incidence of anorexia nervosa in the United States has doubled over the past 25–30 years. Reports on the frequency of bulimia nervosa vary. Between 4% and 10% of the female high school and college students in one study were bulimic. A survey of medical students revealed that 12% of the female students reported lifelong history of bulimia (Herzog 1988). Estimates of obesity range as high as 80 million North Americans, depending on criteria used (Stunkard 1980).

In the past, most anorexics were from middle-class or upper-middle-class families. Recent studies show greater representation of all classes. Obesity, by contrast, is clearly related to social class, with a higher incidence among socioeconomically disadvantaged groups than others.

Women are at greater risk than men for developing eating disorders, partly because of the cultural bias that large size is acceptable for men but not for women. In television and magazine ads, women portrayed as successful, attractive, healthy, and popular are invariably slim. Becoming slim is a major pursuit in this country. The diet and exercise industry is based on the desire to achieve that cultural norm. Some populations at higher risk for the development of weight-loss eating disorders are dancers, long-distance runners, flight attendants, high school and college wrestlers, and fashion models. Housewives, mothers of young children, professional cooks, and people who prepare family meals are at high risk for obesity.

A 1992 study of Miss America contestants from the years 1979–1985 showed a steady downward trend in their weights and body measurements (Davis et al. 1994). While the rest of the population was growing heavier, women who wished to be perceived as beautiful were receiving strong messages to be thinner than ever. Society has thus created the potential for tremendous secondary gains for anorexic behaviors.

Coexisting with the emphasis on thinness is a renewed interest in preparing and consuming food. Gourmet food stores and kitchen supply firms have burgeoned in response to the emphasis on cooking and entertaining at home. In women's magazines, photographs of beautifully prepared foods are shown side by side with the latest diet information and tips on effortless weight loss. Women thus receive the conflicting messages "Food is love," "Eat what you are given," and "Stay slim so that you will be attractive to men." It is hardly surprising that these conflicting messages confuse the young who, because they are just beginning to develop their own sexual identities, are at high risk for developing eating disorders.

The Nursing Process and Clients with Anorexia Nervosa

The following section discusses the specific steps of the nursing process for clients with anorexia nervosa. Also see the Critical Pathway on the next page.

Assessment

The nurse assessing clients with anorexia nervosa must take into consideration the multiple biopsychosocial factors involved in this complex disorder. Although anorexia nervosa and bulimia nervosa are discussed separately in this chapter, the two disorders often coexist. The first decision to be made is whether to hospitalize the client or treat the client in the community. Indications for hospitalization include deteriorating physical condition, increasing parental discord leading to either scapegoating of the client or unhealthy coalition between client and one parent, or a request by the client for hospitalization. Inpatient treatment within the therapeutic milieu, in conjunction with behavior therapy, generally yields positive results. With the increasing emphasis on health care reform and managed care, however, the number of anorexic clients treated in community settings is expected to increase. The same principles of treatment and nursing care can be applied, regardless of setting.

Subjective Data Clients with anorexia nervosa perceive themselves as overweight, no matter how thin they may be. However emaciated their bodies, they can always find some body part they believe is fat.

They are preoccupied with thoughts of food and simultaneously obsessed with rigidly controlling their own intake. They often collect cookbooks, cook prodigious amounts of food, and insist that others eat while not taking a morsel for themselves. They are fearful of even the slightest weight gain and view with suspicion anyone who encourages them to eat.

Another preoccupation is with exercise. It is not uncommon for anorexics to engage in extremely lengthy sessions of aerobics or calisthenics, or to run, bike, or walk to excess, even when in an emaciated condition. They push themselves to greater and greater levels of endurance and deprive themselves of sleep as a measure of self-control.

Anorexics frequently deny that they have a weight problem. They insist that they have never felt better and simply wish to be left alone about food. They report feeling strong, powerful, and good as a result of self-denial. They therefore resist treatment, although they may admit to feeling isolated and lonely and may even describe themselves as exhausted with the effort it takes to achieve the perfection they seek. They tend to have difficulty accepting nurturing behavior from others and therefore have difficulty forming therapeutic alliances (Deering 1987). They report a loss of interest in sex but do not perceive this as a problem.

Objective Data Anorexic clients are most often well-educated teenage females from middle-class and upper-middle-class families (Herzog 1988). There is evidence of extreme and/or rapid weight loss of at least 15% of original body weight. In women, amenorrhea is a cardinal sign. The client has extensive knowledge of the nutritional and caloric value of foods.

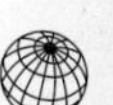

The anorexic client appears emaciated, with a sunken-eyed, skeletonlike look. In very young clients, growth failure may be present. Lanugo growth (babylike, fine hair) on the face, extremities, and trunk may occur. Other physical symptoms include bradycardia, hypotension, arrhythmias, delayed gastric motility, and a hypothyroid-like state manifested by dry skin, listlessness, and dry, falling hair. Peripheral edema may be a feature in advanced starvation.

Laboratory tests may reveal leukopenia, mild anemia, low serum potassium, and elevated blood urea nitrogen (BUN). High serum calcium levels indicate osteoporosis is occurring, and there is an increased risk of fracture (Kotler et al. 1994).

Nursing Diagnosis

Altered Nutrition: Less Than Body Requirements By the time anorexic clients are hospitalized, their physical condition is often so deteriorated from self-imposed starvation that it becomes the priority for nursing care. Life-threatening malnourishment is seen in 5–20% of these clients. Death may occur from malnutrition, infection, or cardiac abnormalities related to electrolyte imbalances. Intravenous therapy, tube feedings, and hyperalimentation are required in cases of medical emergency.

text continues on page 432

CRITICAL PATHWAY FOR A CLIENT WITH ANOREXIA NERVOSA

Expected length of stay: 24–32 days

	Date ________ Days 1–3	Date ________ Days 4–7	Date ________ Days 8–14
Daily outcomes	Client will: • Remain free of malnutrition, infection, electrolyte and cardiac abnormalities. • Identify initial goals for hospitalization. • Remain oriented to time, place, and person with prompting. • Participate in assessment. • Identify current dietary pattern and food preferences. • Identify current elimination pattern. • Identify current self-care patterns, including sleep, physical activity, and hygiene. • Remain free of dehydration. • Maintain oral intake of 1000 cc/day. • Ingest food provided as per contract. • Remain free of self-induced vomiting.	Client will: • Remain free of malnutrition, infection, electrolyte and cardiac abnormalities. • Participate in development of transdisciplinary treatment plan. • Participate in menu plan for balanced meal. • Remain free of dehydration evidenced by moist mucous membranes and urine output > 30 cc/hr. • Maintain oral intake of 1000 cc/day. • Ingest food provided as per contract. • Gain 1/2 lb each day. • Remain free of self-induced vomiting.	Client will: • Remain free of malnutrition, infection, electrolyte and cardiac abnormalities. • Identify two positive attributes of self. • Participate in transdisciplinary plan. • Remain oriented to time, place, and person. • Consume diet as per menu plan. • Remain free of dehydration evidenced by moist mucous membranes and urine output > 30 cc/hr. • Maintain oral intake of 1200 cc/day. • Ingest food provided as per contract. • Make dietary choices consistent with a well-balanced diet. • Gain 1/2 lb each day. • Remain free of self-induced vomiting.
Assessments, tests, and treatments	Complete psychosocial assessment to include mental status, mood, affect, behavior, and communication q shift and PRN. Contract for safety. Observe for safety per protocol. Complete nursing database assessment. Weight. CBC, urinalysis. Chemistry profile. Thyroid profile. EKG. Other laboratory studies as ordered. Vital signs BID.	Psychosocial assessment q shift and PRN. Observe for safety per protocol. Monitor dietary intake, sleep pattern, and bowel elimination pattern. Monitor effects of and compliance with medications. Routine vital signs.	Daily psychosocial assessment. Observe for safety per protocol. Monitor dietary intake, sleep pattern, and bowel elimination pattern. Monitor effects of and compliance with medications. Routine vital signs. Repeat laboratory studies if indicated.
Knowledge deficit	Orient client and family to clients, staff, and program. Review initial plan of care. Assess learning needs of client and family. Instruct client and family regarding behavior-modification program. Assess understanding of teaching.	Review unit orientation with emphasis on program. Reinforce behavior-modification program. Assess understanding of teaching.	Review plan of care. Include family in teaching. Continue behavior-modification program. Assess understanding of teaching.

	Date ________ Days 1–3 *continued*	Date ________ Days 4–7 *continued*	Date ________ Days 8–14 *continued*
Diet	Nutritional assessment. Dietary consultation. Monitor dietary intake. Diet as tolerated; encourage small, frequent feedings from all food groups. Provide preferred snacks and foods. Encourage fluids. Provide pleasant mealtime environment.	Monitor dietary intake. Diet per menu plan. Encourage fluids; encourage small, frequent feedings from all food groups. Provide preferred snacks and foods. Provide pleasant mealtime environment.	Monitor dietary intake. Diet per menu plan; encourage small, frequent feedings from all food groups. Provide preferred snacks and foods. Provide pleasant mealtime environment.
Activity	Assess safety needs and maintain appropriate precautions. Encourage brief periods of activity and interaction. Engage client in identifying reasonable activity/exercise plan.	Maintain safety precautions. Encourage activities during the day. Client will participate in exercise program of moderate intensity and duration.	Maintain safety precautions. Encourage involvement in 50–75% of activities. Client will participate in exercise program of moderate intensity and duration.
Psychosocial	Observe behavior. Assess level of anxiety. Encourage verbalization of feelings and thoughts. Listen attentively, giving adequate time to respond. Approach with nonjudgmental and accepting, calm, matter-of-fact attitude and positive expectation. Formulate initial plan of care with client and family. Identify current support system. Provide information regarding illness and treatment. Provide ongoing support and encouragement to client and family. Meet with client 4 times each shift for 5–10 min periods focused on establishing relationship.	Observe behavior. Assess level of anxiety. Encourage verbalization of concerns and feelings. Approach with nonjudgmental and accepting, calm, matter-of-fact attitude and positive expectation. Provide information and ongoing support and encouragement to client and family. Provide simple structured activities. Identify potential support system and strategies to access additional supports. Prompt to attend group therapy. Acknowledge accomplishments. Meet with client 10–15 min twice a shift during waking hours and focus on working on initial goals. Avoid discussion of food and eating habits. Discuss problem-solving strategies.	Observe behavior. Assess level of anxiety. Encourage verbalization of concerns and feelings. Approach with nonjudgmental and accepting, calm, matter-of-fact attitude and positive expectation. Provide information and ongoing support and encouragement to client and family. Review strategies to access support system using problem-solving strategies. Attend group therapy independently with spontaneous involvement × 1. Acknowledge accomplishments. Meet with client 15 min every shift during waking hours to work on therapeutic goals. Explore effective coping strategies. Explore fears related to sexuality and weight gain. Practice problem-solving strategies.
Medications	Routine meds as ordered.	Routine meds as ordered.	Routine meds as ordered.
Referrals and discharge plan	Family assessment. Establish discharge objectives with client and family.	Review discharge objectives with client and significant others. Initiate referrals for discharge care.	Review progress toward discharge objectives with client and significant others. Make appropriate referrals to support groups.

→

CRITICAL PATHWAY FOR A CLIENT WITH ANOREXIA NERVOSA *(continued)*

	Date _________ Days 15–21	**Date _________ Days 22–26**	**Date _________ Days 27–Discharge Day**
Daily outcomes	Client will: • Remain free of malnutrition, infection, electrolyte and cardiac abnormalities. • Communicate feelings spontaneously and appropriately in 1:1 and group activities. • Identify method in which strengths can be used to improve coping skills. • Participate in transdisciplinary plan. • Begin to explore issues of body image and self-esteem. • Maintain oral intake of 1200 cc/day. • Ingest food provided as per contract. • Make dietary choices consistent with a well-balanced diet. • Begin to verbalize accurate assessment of body size and nutritional needs.	Client will: • Remain free of malnutrition, infection, electrolyte and cardiac abnormalities. • Communicate feelings spontaneously and appropriately. • Spontaneously and appropriately participate in 1:1 and group activities. • Identify methods in which strengths can be used to improve coping skills. • Verbalize plan to use strengths to enhance coping skills. • Participate in transdisciplinary plan. • Realistically discuss issues related to body image and self-esteem. • Maintain oral intake of 1200 cc/day. • Ingest food provided as per contract. • Make dietary choices consistent with a well-balanced diet. • Continue to verbalize accurate assessment of body size and nutritional needs. • Participate in discharge planning.	Client remains free of malnutrition, infection, electrolyte and cardiac abnormalities. Client expresses a positive self-perception and self-esteem. Client expresses less anxiety about weight gain. Client verbalizes accurate assessment of body size and nutritional needs. Client communicates feelings honestly and openly. Client participates in activities that promote physical health. Client develops sustaining relationships with friends and family members. Client verbalizes/demonstrates home care instructions including the importance of ongoing mental health care. Client demonstrates ability to adaptively cope with ongoing stressors. Client verbalizes positive attributes regarding self. Client accepts positive feedback.
Assessments, tests, and treatments	Daily psychosocial assessment. Observe for safety. Monitor dietary intake, sleep pattern, and bowel elimination pattern. Weigh. Monitor effects of and compliance with medications. Routine vital signs.	Daily psychosocial assessment. Observe for safety. Monitor dietary intake, sleep pattern, and bowel elimination pattern. Monitor effects of and compliance with medications.	Psychosocial assessment. Monitor dietary intake, sleep pattern, and bowel elimination pattern. Monitor effects of and compliance with medications.
Knowledge deficit	Review plan of care. Include family in teaching. Initiate teaching regarding coping strategies utilizing client strengths. Review current level of knowledge regarding medications, treatments, symptom management, and follow-up care. Assess understanding of teaching.	Review plan of care with client and family. Reinforce current level of knowledge regarding medications, treatments, symptom management, and follow-up care. Assess understanding of teaching.	Client and/or significant other verbalizes understanding of discharge teaching including activity level and exercise program, safety measures, diet, signs and symptoms to report, follow-up care and MD appointment, medications: name, purpose, dose, frequency, route, dietary interactions, and side effects, and follow-up care arrangements. Assess understanding of teaching. Make referrals to community caregivers for any knowledge deficits regarding medications, treatments, symptoms management, and follow-up care.

	Date __________ Days 15–21 ***continued***	**Date __________ Days 22–26** ***continued***	**Date __________ Day 27–Discharge** ***continued***
Diet	Diet as tolerated; encourage small, frequent feedings from all food groups. Encourage fluids. Provide preferred snacks and foods. Provide adequate time for meals and snacks. Monitor dietary intake. Provide pleasant mealtime environment.	Diet as tolerated; encourage small, frequent feedings from all food groups. Encourage fluids. Provide preferred snacks and foods. Provide adequate time for meals and snacks. Monitor dietary intake. Provide pleasant mealtime environment.	Diet as tolerated; encourage small, frequent feedings from all food groups. Encourage fluids. Provide preferred snacks and foods. Provide adequate time for meals and snacks. Monitor dietary intake. Provide pleasant mealtime environment.
Activity	Maintain safety precautions. Encourage involvement in 75–100% of activities. Engage client and family in identifying reasonable activity plan following discharge. Client will participate in exercise program of moderate intensity and duration.	Maintain safety precautions. Encourage involvement in 100% of activities. Client will participate in exercise program of moderate intensity and duration.	Maintain safety precautions. Client is independently involved in 100% of activities. Client will participate in exercise program of moderate intensity and duration.
Psychosocial	Assess level of anxiety. Support client in implementing stress- and anxiety-reduction strategies. Provide information and ongoing support and encouragement to client and family. Attend scheduled group therapy sessions independently. Reinforce skills learned in group therapy. Identify progress with cognitive restructuring and reinforce learning. Acknowledge accomplishments. Encourage verbalization of feelings and concerns. Meet with client 15 min every shift during waking hours to discuss progress in terms of therapeutic goals. Encourage client to discuss body image and self-esteem as well as role in family. Encourage client to acknowledge accomplishments. Provide ongoing support and encouragement to client and family.	Assess level of anxiety. Reinforce stress- and anxiety-reduction strategies. Encourage verbalization of concerns and feelings. Provide information and ongoing support and encouragement to client and family. Attend group therapy independently. Provide specific, realistic feedback. Encourage constructive expression of feelings. Provide ongoing support and encouragement to client and family. Meet with client 15 min every shift during waking hours to discuss progress in terms of therapeutic goals. Encourage client to discuss relationship to others in family. Encourage realistic discussion of body image. Encourage client to acknowledge accomplishments.	Assess level of anxiety. Reinforce stress- and anxiety-reduction strategies. Encourage verbalization of concerns and feelings. Provide information and ongoing support and encouragement to client and family. Client will attend group therapy independently. Meet with client 15 min every shift during waking hours to discuss progress in terms of therapeutic goals. Acknowledge accomplishments. Provide ongoing support and encouragement to client and family.
Medications	Routine meds as ordered.	Routine meds as ordered.	Routine meds as ordered.
Consults and discharge plan	Review discharge objectives with client and family.	Review discharge objectives with client and significant others. Complete referrals for discharge care.	Refer to support group and ongoing mental health care. Review need for any discharge referrals. Discharge with referrals.

The client's preoccupation with food, evidenced by reading recipes, discussing food, and preparing food for others, is due to suppression and sublimation of the client's own hunger. Over exercising creates even more extreme nutritional deficits. In those anorexic clients who also purge by vomiting or using laxatives, nutritional status is further endangered.

Clients in a state of starvation experience hormonal, metabolic, and emotional changes. Some of those changes are manifested in amenorrhea or delay of onset of menses, ketosis, severe vitamin deficiencies, depressed immune response, lethargy, weakness, and irritability (Miner 1988), conditions that vitally affect nurse-client relationships.

Ineffective Individual Coping Clients experiencing anorexia nervosa demonstrate impairment of adaptive behaviors, such as self-care in activities of daily living. They have difficulty meeting daily demands, and role performance may be affected. Their preoccupation with the pursuit of thinness deprives them of the energy necessary for adaptive behavior and distracts them from interest in role fulfillment. The quest for thinness is the entire focus of their lives.

In addition, developmental issues such as the desire for independence and the longing for dependence combine with traditionally adolescent resentment of authority to influence the quality and character of the nurse-client relationship. Family overprotectiveness and unwillingness to allow the client to separate contribute to self-doubt and the inability to accept responsibility for self.

Body Image Disturbance Clients with anorexia nervosa are unable to make realistic appraisals of their own body size, although they can accurately evaluate the size of others. They drastically underestimate their own bodily needs, even in the face of overwhelming evidence of malnutrition. Profound disturbances in accurate perception of size and intense client denial indicate a poor prognosis. The client's body image disturbance is often the source of conflict in family and therapeutic relationships.

Self-Esteem Disturbance Anorexic clients' lack of confidence in themselves and feelings of inferiority are main factors in the disorder. Their self-deprivation and self-denial make them feel powerful and superior to others who cannot muster such profound self-control. The quest for perfection is never-ending, but they can never achieve a level of thinness that is satisfying; there are always a few more pounds to shed. They often present the picture of "model clients," in contrast to seemingly more disturbed clients in inpatient settings. As a result, novice nurses may have difficulty assessing the severity of the illness accurately.

The low self-esteem of anorexic clients stems from unrealistic expectations by self and others, complicated by unmet dependence needs. The clinical picture is further complicated because cultural norms of thinness reinforce

NURSING SELF-AWARENESS

Possible Reactions to Working with Clients with Eating Disorders

- You feel exhausted and defeated by the structured demands of the client's care plan.
- You feel resentment at the client's efforts to manipulate and attempts at "staff splitting."
- You identify with the client because of your own personal body image concerns.
- You feel overprotective of the client and allow a coalition between yourself and the client to form.
- You feel annoyance and anger toward the client and are unnecessarily rough during physical care.
- You have difficulty recognizing that the client's symptoms are as serious as those of a hallucinating or delusional client.
- You fail to monitor the client's mealtime and after-meal behaviors, allowing the client to continue maladaptive patterns of coping.
- You allow the client to reenact power struggles from home, such as those about food, weight, and exercising.
- You believe that the client is deliberately engaging in maladaptive coping behaviors to upset the staff and family.
- You feel repelled by the client's eating habits or the appearance of the client's body.
- You feel hopeless and are affected by the client's despondency.

maladaptive behavior. The nurse-client relationship is affected by the extreme difficulty these clients have in accepting positive feedback and by their nonparticipation in self-care and therapeutic activities. Their preoccupation with their appearance and with others' perceptions of them may be irritating to other clients. The nurse-client relationship is also affected by the client's need to control, which often leads to manipulative behaviors. (See the Nursing Self-Awareness box on page 432 for possible reactions of nurses working with clients with eating disorders.) Self-aware nurses recognize their own emotional reactions to clients and view clients' self-absorption and manipulativeness as symptoms of the disorder.

Planning and Implementing Interventions

When a client's behavior meets the criteria for a diagnosis of anorexia nervosa, effective nursing intervention is directed toward ensuring that the client will not die and helping the client learn more effective ways of coping with the demands of life. A variety of approaches, including behavioral, insight-oriented, and cognitive therapies may be useful; pharmacologic therapy may be used also. You must recognize that many, if not most, anorexic clients are extremely resistant to change. Progress may be slow, and recovery may be defined as the lessening of symptoms. In severely debilitated clients, inpatient treatment is indicated (see the accompanying box at right).

Criteria for Inpatient Admission

- Clients who are suicidal or severely out of control (self-mutilative; abusing large amounts of laxatives, emetics, and diuretics or street drugs).
- Severely emaciated clients (more than 30% below normal weight).
- Clients who have demonstrated a rapid, dramatic weight loss (in less than a 3-month period).
- Clients who have body temperature less than 96.8F (36C) from hypothermia due to loss of subcutaneous tissue.
- Clients who demonstrate fluid and electrolyte imbalance (K < 2.5 mEq/L).
- Clients who need extensive diagnostic evaluation to rule out comorbidities.
- Clients who develop somatic illnesses and are already compromised (as with infection).
- Clients who repeatedly fail to gain weight with outpatient treatment.

Source: Adapted from Love and Seaton 1991, p. 687.

Promoting Improved Nutrition To establish adequate eating patterns and fluid and electrolyte balance, assume a calm, matter-of-fact attitude and a positive expectation of the client. Meeting minimal nutritional goals, with the overall goal of gradual weight restoration, is nonnegotiable. A caloric intake of 1200–1500 cal/day is the usual range (see the Intervention box on page 434).

Nursing interventions may include tube feedings or intravenous therapy, which are administered in a nonjudgmental manner. Weighing the client daily, recording intake and output, observing the client during meals, and observing bathroom behavior may be necessary if the nurse suspects the client is discarding food or inducing vomiting. Avoid discussing food, recipes, restaurants, and eating with the client because these conversations reinforce maladaptive behaviors. Providing a pleasant mealtime environment and adopting realistic expectations of how much the client will eat are critically important aspects of nursing care. Clients find frequent, small meals more acceptable than three large meals. Setting a time limit of about a half hour is a good way to forestall mealtime "marathons"—protracted meals during which the client eats little.

Acknowledge and recognize the efforts of clients who meet weight gain goals but avoid praise or flattery. Education about adequate eating patterns is a necessary part of discharge planning.

Consistency and coordination among hospital staff members are essential to avoid manipulation by clients. Interdisciplinary planning conferences and adherence to written care plans promote effective care. Behavior-modification programs, which base privileges on weight gain, may be useful for focusing on emotional issues, not just eating behaviors. You and the client may engage in a contract for weight gain, such as the one in Figure 18–1 on page 435.

A target weight is usually chosen by the treatment team in collaboration with a dietitian. Target weight for hospital discharge is usually 90% of average for age and height (Rock and Curran-Celentano 1994). Discharge planning can include referral to self-help groups such as the American Anorexia/Bulimia Association, Anorexia Nervosa and Related Eating Disorders, and Anorexia Nervosa and Associated Disorders.

Promoting Effective Individual Coping The best way to promote individual coping is by involving clients in their own treatment planning while they are hospitalized.

INTERVENTION

Guidelines for Refeeding

Strategy	Rationale
• Validate the client's fears of weight gain.	• Reassures the client that fears are expected and not unique.
• Collaborate with the client and dietitian to plan a flexible refeeding program for gradual weight gain.	• Enlists the client as an active participant in treatment.
• Adopt a matter-of-fact, consistent, and nonjudgmental attitude.	• Conveys your confidence and acceptance of the client.
• Contract with the client for food and fluid intake adequate to meet the weight-restoration goal.	• Meets the client need for structure and control.
• Support the client during refeeding sensations of fullness and bloating; teach that these are normal and transient feelings.	• The gastrointestinal tract must readjust to unaccustomed intake.
• Encourage the expression of feelings of loss of control.	• Upon resuming adequate intake, clients fear "losing control" and "becoming fat."
• Monitor fluid and electrolyte intake and output, vital signs, body temperature, and mood.	• Refeeding may precipitate both psychologic and metabolic emergencies. Monitor both physiologic and psychologic effects.

Source: Adapted from Love and Seaton 1991, p. 687.

Self-determination fosters adaptive coping mechanisms in clients' day-to-day hospital experiences; this process carries over to daily life outside the hospital setting and helps clients meet its demands.

Although trust is difficult to establish with anorexic clients, it is the basis for all therapeutic relationships. Being honest, available, and matter-of-fact helps establish trust and encourages clients to express their feelings. If necessary, allow clients to assume a dependent role at first, but as trust is developed and physical condition improves, encourage them to take more responsibility for themselves. Participating in the planning of care gives clients opportunities to practice making decisions. Letting clients have input into their treatment plans also fosters compliance. Provide flexibility in activities of daily living, type and timing of exercise, and choice of occupational and recreational therapy activities. This autonomy increases clients' sense of responsibility for themselves.

Giving clients the opportunity to practice problem solving may lead to power struggles if you disagree with clients' choices. Demonstrate positive belief in their ability to regain healthy functioning and a willingness to tolerate "mistakes." The treatment team must set firm and clear limits, however, to provide the secure environment clients need to learn more effective coping behaviors. Also help clients identify ways to feel in control by other than anorexic and manipulative behaviors.

Clients need to explore their extreme fears of gaining weight before they can relinquish maladaptive behaviors. It is helpful to explore client feelings about their family, their role in the family, and their autonomy within the family system. This process often helps heal the hurt inner child. Bradshaw (1990) believes that a child whose development is arrested by having to repress feelings, especially feelings of anger and hurt, grows to be an adult with an angry, hurt child inside. Psychotherapeutic strategies directed toward healing the hurt inner child can help clients with various types of eating disorders begin to understand their unmet needs, a neccesary step in the path toward recovery (Kneisl 1991). Because this type of therapeutic work is insight-oriented, you will need exceptional clinical skill and advanced preparation.

Client's Name: ______________________ Weight: ______________

Date of Birth: ______________ Age: ______________ Height: ______________

Goal Weight Range: ______________

You will be weighed daily in the morning after voiding, wearing a hospital gown and no jewelry. Nothing is to be consumed prior to being weighed.

No exercising, jogging, etc. is to be done.

Ensure or Ensure Plus is given as a medication. It must be taken within 15 minutes while sitting at the nurses' station. No conversations, reading, knitting, other activity while drinking Ensure.

Must drink ____ cans of Ensure per day if weight gain is $\frac{1}{4}$ pound or more over your last highest weight.
Ensure will be dispensed at: ______ ______ ______ ______ ______ ______

Must drink ____ cans of Ensure per day if weight gain is less than $\frac{1}{4}$ pound over your last highest weight.
Ensure will be dispensed at: ______ ______ ______ ______ ______ ______

Weights to be attained for status change/privileges:

Independent Status: ______________ pounds
Monitor Status: ______________ pounds for ________ consecutive days
Buddy Status: ______________ pounds
Passes: ______________ pounds for ________ consecutive days

Ensure can be made optional, at the discretion of your primary clinician, once you reach Buddy Status weight.

To use Buddy Status or take passes, a weight gain of $\frac{1}{4}$ pound above your last highest weight must be attained on that day.

Participation in dance therapy and walks: at Monitor Status weight and/or with staff permission.

Participation in gym: At Buddy Status weight and/or with staff permission.

Additional comments/issues:

Signature of Client ______________________________

Signature of Primary Clinician ______________________________

Date: ______________________

Figure 18–1 A sample client contract for weight gain.
SOURCE: *Courtesy Patricia Worthy, Head Nurse, and the nursing staff of the Adolescent and Young Adult Treatment Unit, Yale-New Haven Hospital, New Haven, Connecticut.*

Promoting Improved Perception of Body Image To help clients regain an accurate perception of their body size and nutritional needs, first encourage clients to express feelings about body size. Reframe clients' misperceptions by using language that emphasizes health, strength, and evaluation. For example, if the client says "My thighs are huge," reply "Your thighs are becoming stronger now that you're gaining weight. Healthy muscles are rounded and firm, like yours." With practice, clients can replace negative thinking with positive self-talk. Teach and reinforce this skill, and help them practice it. For example, ask clients to make three positive statements (positive affirmations) about their bodies each day.

For clients who are unable or unwilling to discuss their feelings about body size, Miller (1991) recommends asking them to draw themselves as they are now and as they desire to be. These drawings not only focus the discussion of body size and nutritional needs but also help the nurse understand how clients view their bodies. Because clients with bulimia nervosa and compulsive overeating also have distorted body images, this activity can be incorporated into their plans of care as well.

When clients share feelings honestly, show improvement in accurate perception of body image, or demonstrate healthier eating behaviors, reinforce their efforts through verbal recognition. It is also useful to examine with clients the ways in which the fashion and advertising industries support unrealistic cultural norms of excessive thinness incompatible with healthy functioning.

Promoting Improved Self-Esteem Help clients reexamine negative feelings about themselves and identify their positive attributes. Encourage clients to record in a diary thoughts that are difficult to share directly. Essential elements are nonjudgmental acceptance of negative feelings and positive reinforcement of the honest expression of all feelings. Encouragement is particularly important when clients experiment with independently made decisions, even when outcomes are not entirely positive. The client needs to interpret each experience as worthwhile. Emphasize the feeling of control gained through independent decision making.

Together, you and the client explore the client's attempt to achieve perfection by controlling weight. The idea is for the client to realize that perfection is an unrealistic goal. You are a role model of the person who accepts imperfection yet retains self-esteem. One way to model strong self-esteem is to admit errors willingly. Also model appropriate expressions of anger and teach clients the destructive effects of unexpressed anger.

Evaluation and Outcome Criteria

Nutrition Clients will regain and maintain at least 90% of normal weight for their height and age. Clients will follow eating patterns that demonstrate they recognize the importance of adequate nutrition. They will regain and maintain normal elimination patterns, vital signs, fluid and electrolyte balance, and muscle tone. Female clients will have normal menstrual cycles.

Individual Coping Clients will participate actively in treatment planning and discharge planning using problem-solving skills. They will demonstrate interest and competence in self-care activities such as hygiene, sleep, activity, rest, diversional activities, and nutrition. They will accurately identify both maladaptive coping behaviors and adaptive coping behaviors that can be integrated into daily routines. Clients will express less anxiety about weight gain and will verbalize other means of feeling in control of their lives.

Body Image Clients will accurately assess their own body size and nutritional needs. They will use criteria such as strength and health, rather than appearance alone, to evaluate body size. They will verbalize less preoccupation with body size. They will easily verbalize positive statements about their own bodies.

Self-Esteem Clients will verbalize their own positive attributes. They will demonstrate less preoccupation with their own appearance and will focus increasingly on others. They will accept compliments and positive feedback and show greater interest in activities around them. The will verbalize that perfection is an unrealis-tic life goal. Clients will express anger appropriately without experiencing incapacitating guilt. They will demonstrate interpersonal relationships substantially free of manipulation.

The Nursing Process and Clients with Bulimia Nervosa

Assessment

Although the two disorders are described separately, the boundary between anorexia and bulimia is blurred. Many bulimics were formerly anorexic, while others may become anorexic in the future. As many as half of all anorexics are estimated to binge and purge at some time during their illnesses. During the assessment phase of the nursing process, keep in mind that these two conditions, although distinctly different, often coexist.

Subjective Data Clients with bulimia nervosa have feelings of low self-esteem, worthlessness, inadequacy, and guilt. They experience shame and embarrassment over their secret binges (eating several quarts of ice cream, buckets of popcorn, or eight or more candy bars is not unusual) and subsequent purging activities. This shame

text continues on page 439

CASE STUDY

A Client with Bulimia Nervosa

Identifying Information

Lauren, a 28-year-old married woman, was admitted to the psychiatric unit from the emergency department where she was taken after collapsing during a marathon. She is a master's prepared social worker who works in a drug abuse prevention program.

Client's Description of the Problem

Lauren reports that she has been training for the marathon for about a year, running at least 35 miles a week. She believes that she had to be hospitalized because she did not ingest sufficient carbohydrates and fluids before the race.

Lauren states that she has been binge eating and purging for about 3 years, ever since she read about ballet dancers' and gymnasts' use of purging for weight control. On a typical day she arises at 5:00 AM, runs at least 5 miles, then gets ready for work. On the way to work she buys and consumes a dozen doughnuts. She arrives at work before anyone else and vomits in the employee's bathroom. She eats no lunch unless she can be sure of access to a "good" bathroom, which she describes as one with a single toilet and an outside door that locks. In the evening while preparing dinner she consumes a can of salted peanuts and four or five glasses of wine. She denies ever getting "high." After a large dinner she showers, vomiting while the shower is running. Her husband of 4 years is unaware of her "problem" but worries about her drinking and wonders how she can eat so much and never gain weight.

Psychiatric History

No prior psychiatric history.

Family History

Lauren is the oldest of three children and the only girl. Her parents, both retired schoolteachers, live in a nearby town. She sees them infrequently because "they still treat me like I'm a little girl." She rarely sees her younger brothers and feels closer to her husband's family. There is no family history of eating disorders or substance abuse.

Social History

As the daughter of two schoolteachers, Lauren was expected to be the top student in her school. She had few friends because she was "the class geek." In college she excelled academically but was a "social failure." She has never smoked and only began drinking after she married. She states that she can drink an entire bottle of wine, vomit, and "sober up instantly." She has few friends or interests except running. She describes her job as "not fulfilling."

Health History

Lauren has no significant health problems. Vital signs: T, 98.2; P, 68; R, 14; Ht, 5′7″; Wt, 110 lb; BP, 108/68.

Current Mental Status

Lauren is slim, neatly groomed, and cooperative, but reluctant. She is alert and oriented to time, place, and person. Her judgment is good and her ability to think abstractly is unimpaired. She is articulate; affect is appropriate to verbal content; no delusions, illusions, hallucinations, or other signs of thought disorder. She fidgets in her seat but makes good eye contact. She expresses embarrassment about hospitalization and shame about her behavior. She emphatically does not want her husband or office informed of the extent and details of her "problem." She maintains that she does not need to be hospitalized and can handle this herself.

Other Subjective or Objective Clinical Data

Lauren reports that she has not had a menstrual period in over 1 year. She takes no medications.

Diagnostic Impression

Nursing Diagnoses

Anxiety
Potential Fluid Volume Deficit
Ineffective Individual Coping

DSM-IV Multiaxial Diagnoses

Axis I: 307.51 Bulimia nervosa, purging type (primary diagnosis)
305.00 Alcohol abuse
Axis II: V71.09 No diagnosis (denial)
Axis III: Amenorrhea
Axis IV: Inadequate social support; job dissatisfaction
Axis V: GAF = 53 (current); moderate difficulty in social functioning; GAF = 60 (highest level in past year)

NURSING CARE PLAN

A Client with Bulimia Nervosa

Nursing Diagnosis

Anxiety related to low self-esteem.

Expected Outcome

- Client will identify at least three sources of anxiety.
- Client will demonstrate the use of relaxation techniques to manage anxiety.

Nursing Interventions

- Adopt a calm, reassuring attitude.
- Provide a quiet, nonstimulating environment.
- Teach progressive relaxation techniques and meditation.
- Help client recognize situations and events that create anxiety.
- Encourage client to identify previously used, successful coping behaviors.
- Encourage client to identify alternatives to alcohol abuse, binge eating, and purging in response to anxiety.
- Limit overexercising.
- Negotiate a client contract to limit hoarding, vomiting, and other problem behaviors.

Outcome Met If

- Client verbalizes anxiety-provoking situations and events.
- Client identifies ways of structuring her environment to prevent feeling out of control, such as planning a new route to work that doesn't go by the doughnut shop.
- Client verbalizes her understanding of the role alcohol abuse plays in her out-of-control behavior.
- Client demonstrates alternative ways of dealing with anxiety, such as relaxation techniques and meditation.
- Client verbalizes acceptance of normal body weight without intense anxiety.

Nursing Diagnosis

Potential Fluid Volume Deficit related to abnormal fluid loss due to self-induced vomiting and excessive exercising.

Expected Outcome

- Client will drink a minimum of 2 oz of fluids per hour.
- Client will not vomit following meals.

Nursing Interventions

- Teach client the importance of adequate fluid intake.
- Offer client her favorite beverages frequently during the day.
- Weigh client daily to evaluate rehydration.
- Keep accurate intake and output records.
- Assess skin turgor and condition of mucous membranes daily and record.
- Give positive recognition when progress is shown.
- Monitor laboratory values, reporting significant alterations to the physician.
- Observe client for at least 1 hour after meals to prevent purging.
- Encourage frequent mouth care to promote comfort.

Outcome Met If

- Oral mucosa is moist, skin turgor is restored, and urine output is sufficient.
- Client's vital signs and laboratory values are within normal limits.
- Client verbalizes her understanding of the relationship between dehydration, self-induced vomiting, and overexercising.
- Client verbalizes her understanding of the dehydrating effect of alcohol.

Nursing Diagnosis

Ineffective Individual Coping related to feelings of helplessness and lack of control in life situation.

Expected Outcome

- Client will eat regularly within 1 week.
- Client will refrain from discussing food and body image within 1 week.

Nursing Interventions

- Help client establish a trust relationship with you.
- Help client plan for and practice how to deal with daily demands.
- Help client identify events preceding binge/purge episodes.
- Encourage client to identify ways of nurturing herself without using food or alcohol.
- Engage client in a process of identifying, naming, and expressing negative feelings.
- Help client identify alternative ways of expressing negative feelings.
- Teach client assertiveness techniques, and encourage her to practice their use.
- Refer client to eating disorders support group.

Outcome Met If

- Client lists maladaptive coping behaviors.
- Client demonstrates adaptive ways of dealing with anxiety and negative feelings.
- Client identifies situations that place her at risk for binge/purge behavior and verbalizes alternative self-nurturing behaviors.
- Client demonstrates assertive communication techniques.
- Client prepares for discharge by attending support group meetings regularly and following up with therapy.

may be manifested in self-deprecating remarks. Clients report feeling out of control, but at the same time they feel an excessive need to control. Unlike anorexics, clients with bulimia nervosa recognize that their eating behaviors are abnormal and bizarre.

Anxiety and unsatisfactory interpersonal relationships are features of this disorder. Anxiety is intensified when others see the bulimic as successful and in control, and they often appear so to others. They are impulsive and cannot delay gratification. Preoccupation with food, weight, and dieting is a prominent feature. Bulimic clients may report feeling weak and lethargic.

OBJECTIVE DATA Like anorexic clients, bulimic clients tend to be young females. Bulimia first manifests itself later than anorexia, typically during late adolescence or young adulthood. Clients are likely to be white, middle-class females with a history of weight-control problems. They are usually of normal or slightly above-average weight. Appearance does not provide diagnostic clues, hence the term *normal-weight bulimic.* Weight tends to fluctuate but does not get dangerously low unless anorexia occurs concurrently (Herzog 1988).

Clients with bulimia nervosa are more outgoing than anorexics and tend to be more comfortable with sexual relationships. They sometimes manifest impulsive behaviors such as substance abuse, shoplifting, and self-inflicted injury (Herzog 1988). In inpatient settings, they may steal others' food and hoard food in their rooms.

Physical signs of bulimia nervosa include hoarseness and esophagitis, dental enamel erosion, enlarged parotid glands, abrasions or calluses on knuckles from inducing vomiting, and amenorrhea in about 40% of cases (Herzog 1988). The client may also have symptoms of fluid volume deficit: concentrated urine, decreased urine output, hypotension, elevated temperature, poor skin turgor, and weakness.

Laboratory tests may reveal electrolyte abnormalities, particularly low serum potassium. Potentially fatal cardiac arrythmias may result. The overuse of syrup of ipecac, an emetic agent, can create cumulative systemic toxicity affecting the gastrointestinal, neuromuscular, and cardiovascular systems, potentially leading to death from cardiotoxicity (Parks and Fischer 1987).

Another concern is the fact that the frequency of bulimia in diabetics is increasing, particularly among young women. This is a potentially deadly combination because binge eating and purging increase the risk for both hypoglycemic episodes and diabetic ketoacidosis (DKA) (Krakoff 1991). Closely monitoring blood glucose levels is indicated for these clients.

Nursing Diagnosis

ANXIETY Clients with bulimia nervosa experience anxiety: vague, uneasy feelings of moderate to intense severity and unknown cause (see Chapter 4). A rise in the client's anxiety level is usually a forerunner of binge/purge behaviors and may lead to purchasing or hoarding food in preparation for a binge.

FLUID VOLUME DEFICIT Depletion of body fluids in clients with bulimia nervosa is usually due to self-induced vomiting and the excessive use of laxatives and diuretics, combined with decreased fluid intake. Extreme dehydration may lead to changes in mental status such as lethargy and confusion.

INEFFECTIVE INDIVIDUAL COPING Binge and purge behaviors are ineffective ways to cope with the stresses of life. Other impulse control problems, such as alcohol abuse, drug abuse, and shoplifting, are equally ineffective ways to reduce stress. The bulimic client is often dealing with adolescent issues such as independence/dependence, identity, and self-determination. Ineffective coping is manifested in the bulimic client's preoccupation with body size, poor self-esteem, distorted body image, and excessive overeating followed by purging.

INEFFECTIVE FAMILY COPING The families of clients with bulimia nervosa perceive themselves as unable to deal effectively with the client's eating disorder. They, too, may have distorted perceptions of the problem. Parents may have difficulty allowing the client to grow up and may be overprotective; at the same time, they may have overly high expectations of the client. The bulimic client's behavior may become the family's focus, preventing the fulfillment of essential family roles. If disruption is extreme, the family may not be able to interact effectively with the larger community. Usual problem-solving methods are only partially adequate to deal with the stress of having a bulimic family member.

Planning and Implementing Interventions

In addition to the nursing interventions discussed below, pharmacologic therapy has been somewhat useful in treating bulimia nervosa. Treatment is directed at symptoms or predisposing factors, particularly depression. Both anticonvulsant and antidepressant agents have been used. Some success has been reported with the tricyclic antidepressants (TCAs), such as amitriptyline (Elavil), imipramine (Tofranil), nortriptyline (Pamelor), desipramine (Norpramin), and amoxapine (Asendin). Although not a TCA, trazodone (Desyrel) has also been used.

Caution must be used when TCAs are given to clients with cardiac conditions because these medications may interfere with the conduction of electrical impulses in the heart. A baseline EKG and EKG monitoring until therapeutic blood levels are reached are safeguards. Teach clients to expect a delay of 2–5 weeks before seeing improvement of symptoms. They can also expect some unpleasant but temporary side effects, such as orthostatic hypotension, dry mouth, blurry vision, urinary retention, tachycardia, and palpitations.

Not all researchers are fully convinced of the value of TCAs in the treatment of bulimia nervosa. Leitenberg et al. (1994) terminated their study early because of a lack of positive response in the group being treated with desipramine (Norpramin), compared to the group being treated with cognitive-behavioral therapy.

Recent research on the effectiveness of fluoxetine hydrochloride (Prozac), a selective serotonin reuptake inhibitor (SSRI), has demonstrated some effectiveness in treating bulimia. Ongoing research on the association between bulimia nervosa and abnormalities of vasopressin secretion also offers hope for more effective pharmacologic treatment in the future (Taylor et al. 1992).

Promoting Effective Coping with Anxiety The goal of nursing interventions with anxious bulimic clients is to help them recognize events that create anxiety and to avoid binge eating and purging in response to anxiety. Initially, being available to the anxious client is useful. Project a calm, reassuring attitude, and provide a quiet, nonstimulating environment. After trust is established, help the client identify anxiety-producing situations. Clients experience anxiety as occurring "out of the blue" and are often unaware that it is related to emotional issues and situations. Help clients identify previously used coping behaviors to determine whether they might be useful in current situations. How did the client handle anxiety before starting to binge and purge? Help bulimic clients identify feelings that precede binge/purge episodes, and explore healthier ways of dealing with those feelings.

Teach clients to recognize anxiety early, before it is severe, and to manage increasing anxiety. Energy-consuming activities, such as walking, running, and exercising, are useful but must be used very judiciously if the client's prehospital behaviors included overexercising. Clients can benefit from being taught progressive relaxation techniques and meditation. Administer antianxiety medications as ordered, but use caution because of the tendency to habituation.

Client contracts are useful with bulimic clients. The contract is jointly developed by the client and the nurse and renegotiated at periodic intervals, depending on the client's goals, severity of symptoms, and compliance with the contract. Such a contract might include agreements about binge eating, vomiting, or hoarding food, such as these:

> I will sit at the nurses' station for a half hour following my meals.
>
> I will not vomit after my meals.
>
> I will not hoard food.
>
> I will not take laxatives or diuretics.
>
> I will not bring any such substances onto the unit.
>
> I will tell the nursing staff if I feel like binge eating.
>
> I will stay away from the kitchen if I feel like going on a binge.
>
> Client ____________________
>
> Nurse ____________________
>
> Date ____________________

Using a contract encourages clients to assume responsibility for themselves.

Promoting Improved Fluid Volume The importance of accurate intake and output records cannot be overstated. Daily consumption of 2000–3000 mL of liquid promotes rehydration. Accurate daily weights are needed. Always weigh the client at the same time of day (immediately upon arising is preferred) and on the same scale. Assess and document the condition of the skin and oral mucous membranes daily, and monitor laboratory values, reporting significant alterations to the physician. Observe clients for at least an hour after meals to prevent purging. To promote comfort in the dehydrated client, give frequent mouth care.

Promoting Effective Individual Coping Clients with bulimia nervosa can learn adaptive coping mechanisms to replace the out-of-control, binge/purge cycle. During hospitalization, once trust is developed, help the client plan and practice strategies for dealing effectively with intense feelings and the demands of daily living. It is important for clients to identify situations and patterns of events that precede binge/purge episodes. Clients learn to identify, name, and express feelings that they formerly perceived only as "bad." Once this is accomplished, explore alternative ways for clients to express those feelings.

Help clients identify times when they are at risk for binge eating and lack impulse control, such as times when they are bored, frustrated, angry, lonely, or feeling unloved. Teach clients ways to nurture themselves during these times other than eating and purging. Suggest taking a warm bath, calling or visiting an old friend, or a hobby not involving food.

Clients with bulimia nervosa often perceive feelings of guilt and underlying resentment as overwhelming. They need to learn effective ways of expressing these feelings and assertiveness techniques to diminish guilty interactions in the future. Role playing with the nurse is a good way to practice assertiveness.

The worsening of both mood and bulimic symptoms during the winter has been reported in eating disorder literature with increasing frequency. Lam et al. (1994) reported that bright white light treatment has proven effective in treating bulimics with seasonal mood and symptom patterns.

Involve the client in discharge planning. Topics covered in discharge planning include the productive use of time, identification of diversional activities not related to food, and participation in support groups.

PROMOTING EFFECTIVE FAMILY COPING Certain family dynamics reinforce maladaptive eating behaviors; therefore, families must also develop effective coping mechanisms to support the client's healthier coping behaviors. Assess the family's feelings and perceptions of the client's bulimia, listening carefully for what is most stressful and threatening to family members. Correct misperceptions about the disorder. Encourage family members to explore together their usual coping strategies, and determine if any previously used strategies can be useful in the present situation.

Help the family identify their strengths and weaknesses. Encourage family members to share their thoughts and feelings, including feelings of guilt, blame, and resentment, with one another and with the client. Teach family members to use "I" statements, thereby acknowledging their feelings.

If the client's disorder impairs family functioning, help the family reorganize roles to reduce stress and ensure that members' needs continue to be met during the client's recovery. Help the family understand that two normal developmental needs of adolescents and young adults are to develop autonomy and to establish identities outside the family. Make appropriate referrals to community resources, such as the American Anorexia/Bulimia Association, Anorexia Nervosa and Related Eating Disorders, and Anorexia Nervosa and Associated Disorders groups.

Home visits for an evening or weekend can help both the client and the family learn to use their new coping behaviors. Planning before visits and evaluating the success of visits afterward are essential parts of nurse-client and nurse-family interventions.

Evaluation and Outcome Criteria

ANXIETY Clients will verbally identify situations and events that evoke anxiety. They will identify ways of structuring the environment to prevent feeling out of control. Clients will eliminate binge/purge behaviors and demonstrate the use of anxiety-reduction strategies unrelated to eating. They will verbalize their acceptance of normal body weight without intense anxiety.

FLUID VOLUME Dryness of oral mucosa and skin will not be evident. Skin turgor will be normal. Clients' vital signs and results of laboratory studies will be within normal limits. Clients will verbalize their understanding of the relationship between dehydration and self-induced vomiting, laxative abuse, and diuretic abuse. Clients will verbalize understanding the physiologic and psychologic consequences of dehydration.

INDIVIDUAL COPING Clients will accurately assess maladaptive coping behaviors. They will demonstrate healthier ways to deal with stress and intense feelings. They will identify times of risk and verbalize alternative self-nurturing behaviors. They will demonstrate assertive communication techniques. Clients will demonstrate self-control in eating behaviors. They will verbalize increased self-confidence in the ability to handle the demands of daily life. They will follow through with recommended self-help or support groups and therapy following discharge.

FAMILY COPING Families will verbalize accurate perceptions of their situation. They will verbalize their feelings about having a family member with an eating disorder. They will identify useful strategies for coping with the impact of bulimia nervosa on the family. They will use "I" statements during communication with one another, the client, and the nurse. They will verbalize an understanding of the developmental needs of adolescents and young adults. The family will reorganize family roles as necessary. They will identify community resources available to them and will follow through on referrals.

The Nursing Process and Clients with Compulsive Overeating

Assessment

The assessment of compulsive overeating is not as straightforward as it might seem. Many obese individuals are apparently content and well adjusted. The nurse must not assume that all obese people are emotionally distressed. There is considerable disagreement in the psychiatric literature regarding the nature of obesity and psychopathology (Telch and Agras 1994). For example, Ross (1994) found that the only social group in which being overweight caused depression was the well-educated group with college educations or advanced degrees. This finding is at odds with conventional psychiatric wisdom that a high proportion of obese clients are depressed, regardless of educational level. The following discussion pertains to those clients who suffer psychologically from their excessive weight and who seek treatment for the resulting psychologic pain.

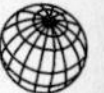

Subjective Data Being overweight in a culture that equates attractiveness with thinness can cause depression, anxiety, low self-esteem, anger, and isolation. These psychologic stresses in turn create the desire to eat, and a pathologic cycle begins. Most obese individuals report a lifelong inability to maintain normal weight. They tend to use food as a substitute for other forms of gratification, such as companionship, attention from others, and emotional nurturing. They may also eat when happy or to reward themselves.

When obesity has its onset in childhood, the child may have a permanently distorted body image (Stunkard 1980). These people view themselves as fat, even following weight loss. The resulting negative feelings impair social functioning and may lead to withdrawal and isolation. Isolation intensifies the obsessive preoccupation with food.

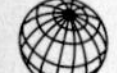

Attitudes toward food and eating are strongly influenced by cultural and ethnic background. These attitudes are firmly established by adulthood and are difficult to change. Family traditions and beliefs about food are influential. Parents' use of food to punish or reward a child or to deal with negative feelings teaches children to do the same. They learn that they need not deal with feelings directly as long as they can eat. Obesity is thought to be related to ambivalence in the parent-child relationship (Orbach 1986). In homes where there is marital conflict, children may become scapegoats, and they may seek protection by becoming obese (Orbach 1986). In some families, children are punished unless they eat everything they are served. This teaches them to disregard satiety messages and contributes to overeating in later life. Because the tendency toward obesity may be hereditary, a family history is useful (Wurtman and Wurtman 1987).

Be sure to obtain a medication history. A number of medications, including birth-control pills, some antipsychotics, the cortisones, some antidepressants, and antacids, may contribute to weight gain. Some postmenopausal women attribute increased appetite to hormone replacement therapy.

Objective Data In our culture, obesity is generally defined as body weight that exceeds by 20% the recommended weights on standard height and weight tables. Although obesity is more common among women of all ages, many men are obese. Obesity is most prevalent in people between the ages of 20 and 50.

Obese people tend to be inactive, which further widens the gap between calorie intake and expenditure of energy. Obesity-related disorders include hypertension, shortness of breath, and palpitations upon exertion.

Nursing Diagnosis

Knowledge Deficit Despite their preoccupation with food and eating, clients often lack sufficient information about nutrition to make healthy decisions about diet. This knowledge deficit may be related to lack of interest, anxiety, denial of the need for information, or other factors.

Evidence of nutritional knowledge deficit includes a history of noncompliance with dietary regimens, statements indicating a lack of knowledge, misconceptions about the diet plan, and requests for information.

Altered Nutrition: More Than Body Requirements The obese client consumes more calories than required while expending few calories in exercise and activity. A sedentary lifestyle and occupation are common. Unhealthy eating patterns, such as night eating and binge eating, complicate the picture.

Recognize that the client's negative self-concept reinforces the desire for nurturance—that is, food—and that all negative feelings may be identified as hunger. These clients often ignore internal cues to hunger and eat in response to external cues, such as the time of day or stressful situations.

Obese clients are vulnerable to a variety of weight-loss fads such as appetite suppressants, fad diets, and expensive "get-thin-quick" programs at diet centers. Some 95% of dieters are unsuccessful, and in general, only 5% of obese individuals maintain a weight loss of at least 20 lb for 2 years or more (Miller 1991). The failure of these efforts leads to guilt and a sense of hopelessness about ever losing weight. Depression and loss of faith in self are common in obese clients.

Hopelessness Clients who compulsively overeat frequently feel hopeless about their repeated failure to lose weight or to control their eating behavior. The inability to feel positive about the present life situation is manifested in a despondent and passive approach to living. Any effort seems too extreme; every task is too great. "What's the use?" is a question characteristically posed by hopeless clients.

Hopelessness is debilitating because clients cannot mobilize energy on their own behalf; nor do they believe that anyone else can help. Hopelessness is demonstrated by apathy and a lack of involvement in activities that profoundly affect the nurse-client relationship. Clients may lose interest in self-care activities, and oversleeping, decreased affect, and decreased response to stimuli are associated features. The speech of hopeless clients is filled with despondency. They may verbalize a loss of faith in God or another higher power.

Social Isolation Obese clients are sometimes rejected by others or choose to withdraw from social interaction because of self-consciousness and fear of rejection. Regardless of the cause of social isolation, the resulting alienation and loneliness increase the client's depression and preoccupation with food. Obese clients want to participate in social situations, but their negative past experiences have conditioned them to expect ridicule and rejection.

Planning and Implementing Interventions

PROMOTING KNOWLEDGE OF NUTRITION Providing basic nutritional education is the goal of interventions with clients who have a knowledge deficit in this area. First determine what knowledge or misconceptions the client has, and begin teaching at that level. Asking obese clients to write down and share with you the history of their numerous attempts to lose weight may be helpful. This provides an opportunity to establish rapport by demonstrating empathy for the anguish, helplessness, and hopelessness experienced by these clients. The goal of the exercise is for the client to realize that dieting has not created a lasting change or sustained weight loss. If the client's information base of normal nutrition is minimal, begin by showing pictures of the basic food groups. Provide lists of foods in each group, and encourage the client to select favorite foods in each group. Discuss the body's need for proteins, carbohydrates, fats, vitamins, and minerals. Help the client plan a day's menus, keeping the client's food preferences in mind. Teach the client to analyze labels on prepared foods to determine foods with high nutrient value and reasonable caloric content. Supplement educational sessions with written materials the client can keep for later reference. Opportunities for teaching clients about nutrition can be used as a trust-building strategy.

PROMOTING IMPROVED NUTRITION In planning interventions to help obese clients improve their nutritional status, collaborative goal setting is essential. The client must set a personal goal of controlling eating behaviors and establish a realistic weight-loss goal. Help the client explore measures for changing eating habits. For instance, clients can keep a food diary to monitor the types and amounts of foods they eat. Slowing the rate of eating by chewing more thoroughly, placing implements on the plate between bites, conversing with table companions, and avoiding eating alone are helpful. Establishing a program of gradually increasing physical activity helps narrow the gap between caloric intake and energy expenditures.

Encourage clients to voice their feelings, maintaining a calm and accepting attitude as they do. Help clients develop new, nonfood-related coping strategies for dealing with troublesome feelings.

Cognitive restructuring techniques, such as correcting clients' irrational beliefs, are helpful. Help the client practice replacing negative self-talk with positive self-talk.

Give positive reinforcement and recognition when clients achieve any small weight loss. Do not allow small "slips" to assume major importance or to impede steady progress. Teach the client how to select balanced, nutritionally sound meals when dining outside the home.

Provide information about community resources for exercise, such as the YMCA and YWCA. Make referrals to support groups and self-help groups, such as Overeaters Anonymous, Weight Watchers, and the National Association to Aid Fat Americans. Some support groups, such as Overeaters Anonymous, make use of sponsors for new members. Sponsors are individuals who are successfully coping with eating disorders and who can provide encouragement and support at difficult points in the recovery process. These individuals are a particularly valuable resource to people struggling to overcome reliance on compulsive overeating behaviors.

PROMOTING HOPEFULNESS Personal hygiene and good grooming promote a sense of well-being. Spending time conversing with obese clients at mealtimes can slow the eating process and demonstrate that change is possible. Assume an unhurried and caring attitude.

Unresponsive, apathetic clients become more responsive when exercise becomes part of their daily routine (Parent and Whall 1984). Encourage daily exercise or activity for obese clients.

Also encourage clients to express both positive and negative feelings as an important step toward accepting their feelings as valid. Adopt an empathic, nonjudgmental attitude, and over time, help clients move from expressing feelings to exploring ways of coping other than by eating.

Attaining an intellectual understanding of one's condition promotes hope and a sense of control. Helping compulsive overeaters learn to feel and respond to their internal body cues, particularly cues to hunger and satisfaction, is essential. This is a lengthy process that requires external support and inward self-examination. The purpose of the extra weight also must be explored. What protective function does being fat provide? The advantages and disadvantages of being both overweight and normal weight should be examined. Keeping a diary or journal may be helpful to clients as they struggle to experience and express their feelings without the numbing effect of overeating.

Visualization and guided imagery are useful with hopeless clients (see Chapter 29). Encourage them to focus on happy experiences from the past and to envision themselves as they wish to be—healthy, energetic, and filled with vitality. Reinforce any expression of hopefulness, no matter how tentative.

PROMOTING SOCIAL INTERACTION For the socially isolated obese client, the goal of nursing interventions is to increase time voluntarily spent in group settings. The first step is to offer companionship; just sitting quietly with the client while making no demands for interaction signifies your acceptance. Frequent, brief contacts indicate interest and foster the development of a therapeutic nurse-client relationship. Next, engage the socially isolated client in a noncompetitive one-to-one activity, such as working on a jigsaw puzzle. After the client feels comfortable during one-to-one activities, offer to accompany the client to a group activity. Help the client plan ahead, making sure the client realizes that leaving is OK if anxiety becomes too high. Positively reinforce any amount of time in groups, however brief.

As the client becomes more comfortable in groups, withdraw gradually, but remain available. Role playing social skills helps clients increase their repertoires of socially acceptable behaviors. Teach assertiveness techniques, because passivity and aggressiveness both invite rejection by others.

Evaluation and Outcome Criteria

NUTRITIONAL KNOWLEDGE Clients will demonstrate nutritional knowledge by identifying the correct food group for each food in a sample daily menu. They will recognize missing food groups and identify overrepresented groups. Clients will accurately assess the nutritional value of prepared foods, using label information. They will demonstrate the ability to select a nutritious, low-calorie, balanced daily menu for themselves.

NUTRITIONAL STATUS Clients will verbalize feelings that trigger overeating. They will verbalize feelings of increased self-control and greater self-esteem. Clients will progress steadily toward their personal weight-loss goals. They will demonstrate slower eating behaviors and avoid eating alone. They will describe how to order food in a restaurant yet adhere to their meal plans. They will participate in regular, structured exercise programs as well as self-help and/or support groups.

HOPEFULNESS Clients will voluntarily assume responsibility for hygiene and grooming. They will demonstrate commitment to a program of daily exercise. Clients will verbalize both positive and negative feelings and recognize life events over which they have no control. Clients will verbalize an intellectual understanding of the meaning of their compulsive overeating and techniques for its management.

SOCIAL INTERACTION Clients will demonstrate a willingness to socialize with others. They will voluntarily attend and participate in client group activities. Clients will approach other people appropriately for one-to-one interactions and will report minimal anxiety during social interactions.

Chapter Highlights

- Eating disorders can be considered maladaptive coping patterns characterized by obsession with food and compulsive overeating or undereating behaviors.
- Clients with anorexia nervosa and bulimia nervosa are predominantly young females from middle-class backgrounds.
- Obese clients are of both sexes; obesity is related to social class, being more common among the disadvantaged.
- Clients with anorexia nervosa experience fears of weight gain and markedly restrict their daily caloric intakes, denying hunger.
- Clients with bulimia nervosa are preoccupied with body size and shape. They experience hunger and respond to intense feelings with binge/purge behaviors.
- Clients who overeat compulsively may use food as a substitute for psychologic nurturance, which they desire.
- Nursing assessment of clients with eating disorders includes, but is not limited to, assessment of subjective emotional experiences, physiologic alterations, alterations in impulse control, impairment in family function, and impairment of social function.
- Nursing diagnoses for clients with eating disorders include Altered Nutrition, Ineffective Individual and Family Coping, Body Image Disturbances, Self-Esteem Disturbances, Anxiety, Fluid Volume Deficit, Knowledge Deficit, Hopelessness, and Social Isolation.
- Nursing interventions for clients with eating disorders and their families include a wide range of psychotherapeutic, behavioral, insight-oriented, cognitive, pharmacologic, environmental, family-oriented, and stress-reduction approaches.
- Nursing evaluation criteria for clients with eating disorders include reduction in physical and psychologic symptoms, increased cognitive understanding of the disorder, ability to use stress-reducing skills, accurate perception of body size, decreased preoccupation with food and eating, increased interest in others, and improved social skills.

References

American Psychiatric Association: *Diagnostic and Statistical Manual of Mental Disorders,* ed 4. American Psychiatric Association, 1994.

Bradshaw J: *Home-Coming: Reclaiming and Championing Your Inner Child.* Bantam, 1990.

Bruch H: *The Golden Cage: The Enigma of Anorexia Nervosa.* Harvard University Press, 1978.

Chitty KK: The primary prevention role of the nurse in eating disorders. *Nurs Clin North Am* 1991; 26(3):789–800.

Davis C, Durnin J, Dionne M, Gurevich M: The influence of body fat content and bone diameter measurements on body dissatisfaction in adult women. *Int J Ment Dis* 1994; 15(3):257–263.

Deering CG: Developing a therapeutic alliance with the anorexia nervosa client. *J Psychosoc Nurs* 1987; 25(3): 11–17.

Dippel NM, Becknal BK: Bulimia. *J Psychosoc Nurs* 1987; 25 (9):13–17.

Edmands MS: Overcoming eating disorders. *J Psychosoc Nurs* 1986; 24(8):19–25.

Halmi KA: Anorexia nervosa, in Kaplan HI, Freedman AM, Sadock BJ (eds): *Comprehensive Textbook of Psychiatry,* Vol. IV. Williams & Wilkins, 1985.

Herzog D: Eating disorders, in Nicholi AM (ed): *The New Harvard Guide to Psychiatry.* Belknap Press, 1988.

Holland AJ, Hall A, Murray R, Russell GFM, Crisp AH: Anorexia nervosa: A study of 34 twin pairs and one set of triplets. *Brit J Psychiatry* 1984; 145:414–419.

Kneisl CR: Healing the neglected, wounded inner child of the past. *Nurs Clin North Am* 1991; 26(3):745–756.

Kotler L, Katz L, Anyan W, Comite F: Case study of the effects of prolonged and severe anorexia nervosa on bone mineral density. *Int J Eating Dis* 1994; 15(4):395–399.

Krakoff DB: Eating disorders as a special problem for persons with insulin-dependent diabetes mellitus. *Nurs Clin North Am* 1991; 26(3):707–714.

Lam R, Goldner E, Solyom L, Remick R: A controlled study of light therapy for bulimia nervosa. *Am J Psychiatr* 1994; 151(5):744–750.

Leitenberg H, et al.: Comparison of cognitive-behavior therapy and desipramine in the treatment of bulimia nervosa. *Behav Res Ther* 1994; 32(1):37–45.

Love CC, Seaton H: Eating Disorders: Highlights of nursing assessment and therapeutics. *Nurs Clin North Am* 1991; 26 (3):677–697.

Miller KD: Body image therapy. *Nurs Clin North Am* 1991; 26 (3):727–736.

Miner CD: The physiology of eating and starvation. *Holistic Nurs Pract* 1988; 3(1):67–74.

Morley JE, Levine AS, Willenburg ML: Stress-induced feeding disorders, in Carruba MV, Blundell JE (eds): *Pharmacology of Eating Disorders: Theoretical and Clinical Developments.* Raven, 1986.

Orbach S: *Fat Is a Feminist Issue.* Medallion Books, 1978.

Orbach S: *Hunger Strike: The Anorectic's Struggle as a Metaphor for Our Age.* Norton, 1986.

Parent C, Whall A: Are physical activity, self-esteem, and depression related? *J Gerontol Nurs* 1984; 10(3):8.

Parks BR, Fischer RG: Misuse of syrup of ipecac. *Pediatr Nurs* 1987; 13(4):261.

Rock C, Curran-Celentano J: Nutritional disorder of anorexia nervosa: A review. *Int J Eating Dis* 1994; 15(2):187–203.

Ross CE: Overweight and depression. *J Health Soc Behav* 1994; 35(3):63–78.

Stunkard AJ (ed): *Obesity.* Saunders, 1980.

Taylor WB, White GL, Sargent R, Turan M: Anorexia nervosa and bulimia: Diagnosis and treatment update. *Clinician Rev* 1992; 2(8):65–89.

Telch CF, Agras WS: Obesity, binge eating and psychopathology: Are they related? *Int J Eating Dis* 1994; 15(1):53–61.

Welch SL, Fairburn DM: Sexual abuse and bulimia nervosa: Three integrated case control comparisons. *Am J Psychiatr* 1994; 151(3):402–407.

Wurtman RJ, Wurtman JJ (eds): *Human Obesity.* New York Academy of Sciences, 1987.

CHAPTER 19

CLIENTS WITH SLEEP DISORDERS

Marlene Reimer

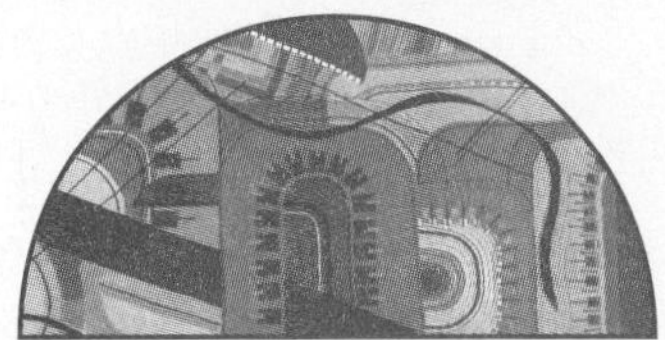

COMPETENCIES

- *List two examples from each of the three main* DSM-IV *categories of sleep disorders.*
- *Identify the sleep patterns most commonly associated with major depressive disorder, manic episodes in bipolar disorder, schizophrenia, and substance abuse.*
- *Define the four major symptoms that characterize the different types of sleep disorders.*
- *List three key assessments pertinent to each of the major symptoms.*
- *Compare and contrast the guidelines for good sleep hygiene with those for dealing with insomnia.*
- *Become aware of how your beliefs about what constitutes normal sleep have been influenced by your family and your cultural background.*

Cross-References

Other topics relevant to this content are: Psychobiology, Chapter 3; Substance-related disorders, Chapter 13; Mood disorders, Chapter 15; Medical conditions, Chapter 22; Psychopharmacology, Chapter 33.

Critical Thinking Challenge

Most people who say they have insomnia actually sleep more than they think they do, according to polysomnography studies. What are your interpretations of the difference between subjective reports about sleep and polysomnography as an objective measure of sleep? How might alternative explanations alter how you would apply the nursing process? Is any one view more correct than another?

Sleep is a basic human need that affects, and is affected by, mental health. It is so much a part of the normal rhythm of our lives that it tends to be taken for granted, until it is disrupted. Disrupted sleep is a particularly important consideration in mental health and illness because of its subtle but pervasive effects on mood, performance, and physical functioning (Bootzin et al. 1993; Totterdell et al. 1994). Lack of sleep tends to decrease our ability to cope, to deal with ambiguity, to make decisions, and to feel confident. Sleep pattern disturbance is often an early symptom of mental illness (Kaplan, Sadock, and Grebb 1994). For example, a change in sleep patterns is among the diagnostic criteria for major depressive disorder, manic episode, and dysthymic disorder in the *DSM-IV* (American Psychiatric Association 1994).

Sleep has been described as a neurobiologic window into the pathophysiology of psychiatric disorders (Gillin 1994). An association between depression and insomnia was observed as long ago as the time of Hippocrates. As a means of assessing the unconscious, Freud brought the study of dreams into the realm of science. The discovery of rapid eye movement (REM) sleep by Aserinsky and Kleitman in the early 1950s was a major breakthrough in the effort to understand the relationship between the mind and the body (Pivik 1994). Until that time, sleep had been seen as a quiet state, as is characteristic of non-

REM sleep. However, in REM sleep, the stage in which most dreaming occurs, brain waves show a level of cognitive activity comparable to the waking state, and physiological functions are also in a heightened state of activity. The major difference between REM sleep and the awake state is the almost total paralysis of skeletal muscle during REM sleep, a factor that essentially prevents the acting-out of dream states. More recent progress in the development of antidepressant medications, especially those that primarily target a particular neurotransmitter, has led to advances in our understanding of the physiologic aspects of mood disorders and sleep-wake states.

Characteristics of Normal Sleep

This chapter begins with a brief summary of the range of normal sleep patterns across the life span. The key points are as follows:

- There is a wide range of sleep patterns among "good sleepers."
- Changes in sleep patterns normally occur as individuals progress through the life span.
- Humans have considerable capacity to adapt to variations in sleep patterns.
- The functions of sleep are still poorly understood.

Optimal Sleep

A "good sleeper" can be identified in any of three ways: self-defined, behaviorally defined, or polysomnographically defined. Most people have a definite opinion about their sleep. Self-defined good sleepers generally describe themselves as getting enough sleep to feel refreshed in the morning, to have energy for the day, to fall asleep fairly quickly, and to wake up only briefly, if at all, during the night.

To hypothesize that a client is a good sleeper from a behavioral point of view, you would want to pay close attention to what he or she says about the quality of sleep, as well as observe alertness during sedentary, repetitive activity such as watching television or driving. You would note the ability to fall asleep in 10–30 minutes under usual circumstances, and final wakening at the habitual rising time, with or without an alarm clock.

Polysomnography is the simultaneous recording of several physical parameters during sleep, including brain wave activity, eye movements, muscle tone, and respiration. The technique is useful in determining the type and stages of sleep, as well as number of arousals and total sleep time. This electrophysiologic recording for a good sleeper would probably show recurrent sleep cycles about every 90 minutes, more slow-wave sleep (stages 3 and 4 of non-REM sleep) during the first part of the night combined with brief REM periods, changing to a greater percentage of REM sleep toward the end of the sleeping period (see Figure 19–1). Non-REM sleep consists of four stages, characterized by a progressive slowing of brain waves, decreasing muscle tone, and reduction in most physiologic functions. REM sleep is characterized by neurologic and physiologic activity that is similar to the waking state but with very low skeletal muscle tone.

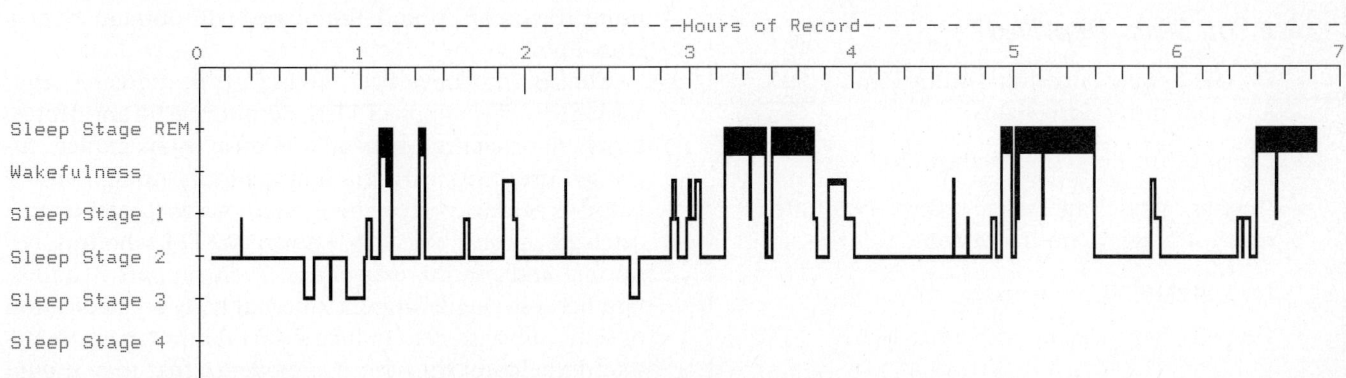

Figure 19–1 Sleep hypnogram summarizing pattern of sleep stages during an all-night polysomnograph recording on a young male. The hypnogram reading includes the following: REM sleep (note that the number and length of REM periods increased as the night progressed); Wakefulness (note that this client had a number of brief wakenings, or fragmented sleep); Sleep Stage 1; Sleep Stage 2; Sleep Stage 3 (note that stage 3 slow-wave sleep occurred during the earlier part of the night); and Sleep Stage 4 (note that this client did not have any stage 4 sleep on the night of the recording).

Sleep Pattern Variations

The average amount of sleep required to feel rested varies widely from person to person. Requiring an average of 7–8 hours sleep per night is most common for adults. However, a small percentage of the population are short sleepers, requiring an average of 6 hours or less. Another small percentage are long sleepers, requiring an average of 9 or more hours each night (ASDA 1990; Kaplan, Sadock, and Grebb 1994).

The distinction between average hours needed and average hours obtained is important. Short or long sleepers by definition are good sleepers; that is, they habitually feel rested and alert after *their* normal sleep time. However, they may experience social pressure and or even receive inappropriate pharmacologic intervention because they do not seem to conform to the norms of their family or peer group. More commonly, though, shortened sleep time is habitual, associated with the pressures of modern society. There is growing concern that whole populations in developed countries are becoming chronically sleep-deprived. As students, you are coping with pressures to study, to prepare for clinical experiences, and to complete assignments, as well as performing other roles that are important to you. Take the quiz in the accompanying Nursing Self-Awareness box below to see whether you are getting enough sleep.

You may also know of individuals who increase their habitual sleep time (or at least their total time in bed) as avoidance. In your psychiatric nursing practice, you may encounter clients who report the need for long periods of sleep and rest, often in association with depression. To distinguish normally long sleepers from clients who are trying to cope by spending more time in bed, it is useful to inquire about previous sleep patterns.

Sleep requirements also vary in relation to situational and developmental factors. With increased physical work, exercise, mental stress, or exposure to adverse weather conditions, total sleep requirements tend to increase. Specific needs for REM sleep increase in relation to periods of intense learning or other psychologic stimuli. Developmental changes in sleep patterns and requirements across the life span are not emphasized here because they are discussed in most fundamentals of nursing textbooks. The important point for the psychiatric nurse is to include a consideration of the client's developmental stage as part of sleep pattern assessment. For example, the tendency of adolescents to sleep late and of older adults to get up earlier appears to have some physiologic basis from age-related shifts in circadian rhythms. The number of arousals tends to increase as adults get older. This change is often greeted with concern that something is wrong. However, if clients are able to get back to sleep without much distress, and/or the wakenings are mainly associated with the need to void, you can help them see the change as normal and become amenable to minor adjustments such as reducing fluid intake after the evening meal.

We physiologically prioritize among types of sleep. Following periods of acute or chronic sleep deprivation, a rebound phenomenon occurs in which the recovery of REM sleep is given priority. You may have noticed how you seem to dream more after several nights of interrupted sleep. (Dreams can occur during non-REM as well as REM sleep, but dreams in non-REM sleep are usually more fragmentary and mundane, without much of a story line.)

Clients who have been taking medications or other substances that suppress REM sleep (tricyclic antidepressants, short-acting benzodiazepines) may notice increased dreaming with discontinuation. Through anticipatory teaching, you can help clients understand that this catching up on REM sleep, known as **REM rebound,** is a normal and passing experience. Such support is important because clients who have been relying on medication or other substances to induce sleep often interpret the reduced quality of their sleep as evidence that they should go back on the medication.

Recognition of the REM rebound phenomenon can be important with regard to physiologic function as well. Vital signs fluctuate during REM sleep, possibly putting added stress on weakened cardiovascular and respiratory systems. There is reduced stimulus to breathe, and ventilatory movement is limited to the diaphragm (because of very low skeletal muscle tone). Thus, clients who are al-

NURSING SELF-AWARENESS

Are You Sleep-Deprived?

- Do you usually fall asleep within 10 minutes after you turn off the lights?
- Do you struggle to stay awake in lectures?
- Do you "get by" all week and then try to catch up by sleeping in on the weekend?
- Do you do shift work?
- Do you often wake up with a headache?
- Do you have trouble getting going in the morning?
- Do you push yourself to keep going?

If you answered yes to more than two of these questions, you may not be getting as much sleep as you need.

ready compromised (as from drug overdose, sleep apnea, chronic obstructive lung disease, or major trauma) may become hypoxic during REM sleep in the first night or two after REM-suppressing drugs are withdrawn.

Functions of Sleep

Sleep is commonly believed to be restorative, but the evidence is actually quite conflicting (Hodgson 1991). Arguments for sleep as a time of body restitution are based on the common observation that rest seems to promote healing; that growth hormone, which is anabolic, has its peak release during slow-wave sleep, whereas catabolic hormones such as the corticosteroids are at their lowest point of release during the night; and that conditions seem optimum for protein synthesis. However, protein synthesis is stimulated by amino acid absorption, little of which occurs during the nighttime fast; there is no sleep-related change in insulin release, a requirement for cell growth; and the release of growth hormone changes immediately with a change in sleep time, whereas change in corticosteroid release requires up to 2 weeks after a change in the sleep period. Alternative theories about the function of sleep range from protective (there are fewer admissions to hospital emergency departments during the night) to adaptive (you cannot do much without light), from energy conservation to somewhat optional. Horne, the chief proponent of the latter view, suggests that there is a core amount of required sleep but that the excess sleep time is not really required. There is more agreement on the role REM sleep plays in memory storage, consolidation of experience, and learning.

The important point is although the functions of sleep are still poorly understood, client beliefs about the functions of sleep are important in psychiatric nursing practice. Through a recognition and an exploration of client beliefs about sleep, you may be able to reinforce healthy attitudes and offer alternative perspectives based on your knowledge of sleep and its disorders.

Sleep Disorders

There are two similar sets of diagnostic codes used to categorize sleep disorders. In psychiatric nursing, you may become more familiar with the *DSM-IV* coding scheme for sleep disorders. However, you should also be aware of the more comprehensive International Classification of Sleep Disorders (ICSD) (American Sleep Disorders Association 1990). You may notice that the comparable ICSD coding is described in the *DSM-IV* as the last point in each sleep disorder description. In this chapter, the commonalities rather than the differences will be emphasized. Table 19–1 provides a comparison of the main categories in each classification system.

Table 19–1 Selected DSM-IV and ICSD Sleep Disorder Categories Compared

DSM-IV Classification	***ICSD Classification***
Primary sleep disorders	***Dysomnias***
Primary insomnia	Psychophysiological insomnia
	Idiopathic insomnia
	Sleep state misperception
	Environmental sleep disorder
	Inadequate sleep hygiene
Primary hypersomnia	Idiopathic hypersomnia
Breathing-related sleep disorder	Obstructive sleep apnea syndrome
	Central sleep apnea syndrome
	Central alveolar hypoventilation
Narcolepsy	Narcolepsy
Circadian rhythm sleep disorder	
Jet lag type	Time zone change (jet lag) syndrome
Shift work type	Shift work sleep disorder
Delayed sleep phase type	Delayed sleep phase syndrome
Unspecified type	Advanced sleep phase syndrome
Parasomnias	***Parasomnias***
Sleepwalking disorder	Sleepwalking
Sleep terror disorder	Sleep terrors
Nightmare disorder	Nightmares
Parasomnia not otherwise specified	Sleep paralysis
	Sleep bruxism
	Sleep enuresis
Sleep disorders related to another mental disorder	***Sleep disorders associated with medical/psychiatric disorders***
Insomnia related to . . .	Psychoses
Hypersomnia related to . . .	Mood disorders
	Anxiety disorder
	Panic disorder
Substance-induced sleep disorder	Alcoholism
Sleep disorders related to another medical condition	Dementia

DSM-IV Diagnostic Criteria for Primary Insomnia

A. The predominant complaint is difficulty initiating or maintaining sleep, or nonrestorative sleep, for at least 1 month.

B. The sleep disturbance (or associated daytime fatigue) causes clinically significant distress or impairment in social, occupational, or other important areas of functioning.

C. The sleep disturbance does not occur exclusively during the course of Narcolepsy, Breathing-Related Sleep Disorder, Circadian Rhythm Sleep Disorder, or a Parasomnia.

D. The disturbance does not occur exclusively during the course of another mental disorder (e.g., Major Depressive Disorder, Generalized Anxiety Disorder, a delirium).

E. The disturbance is not due to the direct physiological effects of a substance (e.g., a drug of abuse, a medication) or a general medical condition.

Source: American Psychiatric Association 1994, p. 557.

Sleep disorders fall into three main categories: the dysomnias, the parasomnias, and those associated with medical/psychiatric disorders. **Dysomnias** are sleep disorders characterized by difficulty initiating or maintaining sleep, or excessive sleepiness. **Parasomnias** are abnormal sleep disorders that intrude into sleep, including disorders of arousal and sleep stage transition (such as sleepwalking).

Dysomnias

Dysomnias are further divided into those that arise within the body, intrinsic sleep disorders; those that primarily develop from external factors, extrinsic sleep disorders; and those that are related to the timing of sleep in the 24-hour day, circadian rhythm sleep disorders. The most common or most relevant of the disorders characteristic of each category will be discussed next. The first five disorders come from the intrinsic category, the next four are extrinsic, and the final four are circadian rhythm disorders.

INSOMNIA **Insomnia,** difficulty falling asleep or maintaining sleep, is a common complaint. Up to 15% of adults report severe or frequent insomnia, and another 15% report occasional episodes. It is important to try to distinguish between transitory insomnia, commonly associated with change in environmental or situational stressors, and insomnia as a sleep disorder.

Primary insomnia is the term used in the *DSM-IV* to describe difficulty initiating or maintaining sleep, or nonrestorative sleep that lasts for at least a month and does not occur exclusively in association with another sleep disorder or mental disorder (see the accompanying box). Subtypes of insomnia are identified in the ICSD classification: psychophysiological insomnia, sleep state misperception, and idiopathic insomnia. Idiopathic insomnia, a less common type, has no known cause but persists from childhood.

Psychophysiological Insomnia The most common type of insomnia is a pattern of delayed sleep onset and/or broken sleep that can be verified by polysomnography and that is perpetuated by an interaction between physically manifested tension (increased arousal) and learned associations that prevent sleep (negative conditioning). A careful history often identifies the onset of psychophysiological insomnia at the time of acute stress. The initial stressful event subsided, but the associations of frustration in trying to get to sleep persist.

Sleep State Misperception By ICSD criteria, sleep state misperception is perceived insomnia that cannot be verified by polysomnography. The idea of differing perceptions of sleep state is gaining support through recent research. For example, triazolam (Halcion) was shown to affect the subjective experience of sleeping in 15 chronic insomniacs tested at five time points per night after placebo or varying doses of triazolam (Mendelson 1993b). The strongest effect of triazolam on sleep perception when compared to placebo occurred at 5 minutes after lights-out and before polysomnograph-defined sleep onset. After receiving triazolam, subjects were less certain about whether they had been awake or asleep and the elapsed time since lights-out. Nurse researchers found that 14.6% of a volunteer sample of women in midlife reported habitual sleep disturbance but had relatively normal sleep as defined by polysomnography (Shaver, Giblin, and Paulsen 1991). Mendelson (1993a) has suggested that this subjective sense of poor sleep may occur prior to objective evidence, but there has not yet been sufficient follow-up of clients with this problem. He also notes that these clients may share a common personality type in that they have been found to score high on the hysteria scale of the Minnesota Multiphasic Personality Inventory (MMPI).

To determine your thoughts and feelings about sleep state misperception, see the accompanying Nursing Self-Awareness box on page 451.

NURSING SELF-AWARENESS

Is Sleep State Misperception a Type of Sleep Disorder?

- How would you feel about being told you have sleep state misperception?
- What thoughts and feelings does that arouse?
- Do you think it is useful to recognize individual differences in describing the state of being or not being asleep?
- If yes, is there an alternative term that could be used?
- If no, what would it take to convince you that your perception of whether or not you had been asleep is wrong?

SLEEP APNEA Apnea is the absence of breathing. The most common form of **sleep apnea** is the obstructive type, in which the upper airway partially or totally collapses in spite of repeated respiratory effort. Opening of the airway requires a partial arousal. With polysomnography, up to 200–300 arousals per night may be observed, even though the client may say he or she slept soundly. The outcome of the numerous arousals preceded by drops in oxygen saturation is **hypersomnia,** or excessive sleepiness. Clients with obstructive sleep apnea may report difficulty staying awake, even in social situations, at work, or driving in spite of a normal or longer nighttime sleep period, in addition to dozing off regularly when watching television.

People with obstructive sleep apnea are often obese middle-aged males with thick necks and a history of severe snoring. The loudness of the snoring, irregularity of nocturnal breathing, irritability, and constant sleepiness of the affected partner add strain to the interpersonal relationship. Bed partners often report that they, too, have a sleep pattern disturbance related to environmental noise and/or vigilance about breathing (Reimer and Remmers 1991). Women may also develop obstructive sleep apnea, with incidence increasing after menopause. Elderly clients with obstructive sleep apnea may present with insomnia rather than hypersomnia. The explanation may be that they have more difficulty getting back to sleep after their frequent arousals. Clients suspected of sleep apnea should be seen by a sleep specialist. Overnight sleep monitoring is important for diagnosis and treatment. These clients often experience significant REM rebound when first treated.

The principle underlying the treatment of obstructive sleep apnea is reduction or removal of the obstruction. Conservative measures include weight loss, avoidance of alcohol and other CNS depressants (which reduce muscle tone in the upper airway), and a change in habitual sleep positions (such as wearing something like a backpack to bed to prevent sleeping supine). Continuous positive airway pressure (CPAP) by nasal mask is the most common form of treatment. Surgical treatment includes removal of a portion of the soft palate, uvula, and residual tonsillar tissue. Dental splints are the newest form of treatment for reducing apnea and the associated snoring.

In central sleep apnea, the airway remains open but the stimulus to breathe is missing or abnormal. This type of breathing-related sleep disorder is less common, except after some neurologic insults (such as brain stem lesions). Clients may present with hypersomnia or insomnia, or be asymptomatic. It is not unusual to observe some central apneas mixed with obstructive episodes. Rather than actual apneas, there may be prolonged hypoventilation resulting in low oxygen saturation, a condition called central alveolar hypoventilation syndrome. For the DSM-IV diagnostic criteria for breathing-related sleep disorder, see the accompanying box below.

As a psychiatric nurse, you must be vigilant for sleep apnea for several reasons. Clients may be unaware of a breathing-related sleep disorder and yet be concerned about hypersomnia, disrupted interpersonal relationships, or poor work performance. Depression secondary to obstructive sleep apnea is not uncommon. Other symptoms of mood disturbances, irritability, memory loss, and impaired concentration are similar to the

DSM-IV Diagnostic Criteria for Breathing-Related Sleep Disorder

A. Sleep disruption, leading to excessive sleepiness or insomnia, that is judged to be due to a sleep-related breathing condition (e.g., obstructive or central sleep apnea syndrome or central alveolar hypoventilation syndrome).

B. The disturbance is not better accounted for by another mental disorder and is not due to the direct physiological effects of a substance (e.g., a drug of abuse, a medication) or another general medical condition (other than a breathing-related disorder).

Source: American Psychiatric Association 1994, p. 573.

presenting symptoms of various mental disorders. Furthermore, people with Alzheimer's disease have sleep apnea more frequently than healthy people of similar age, and the severity of apnea and severity of dementia are positively correlated (Hoch, Reynolds, and Houck 1988). Thus, it is important to assess nocturnal breathing patterns in clients with dementia (Jensen and Herr 1993). Do not assume that their sleep pattern disturbance is the phenomenon called **sundowning**—increased restlessness and agitation during the evening and night hours.

NARCOLEPSY **Narcolepsy** is brief episodes of deep sleep. But unlike sleep apnea, the sleep is followed by a sense of refreshment. The urge to sleep can be almost irresistible, and there is association with other symptoms such as cataplexy, sleep paralysis, and hypnagogic hallucinations. **Cataplexy**, which refers to the sudden collapse of muscle tone usually associated with intense emotion, occurs in about 70% of individuals with narcolepsy (APA 1994). **Sleep paralysis**, which is a sense of being totally unable to move for a brief period after wakening or at sleep onset, occurs in 30–50% of those with narcolepsy. It may also occur occasionally in people who do not have narcolepsy or any other sleep disorder. **Hypnagogic hallucinations** are vivid dreamlike images that appear just before sleep onset and are reported by 20–40% of individuals with narcolepsy. All these symptoms are thought to be related to the recurrent intrusion of REM-like mechanisms into waking or the waking-sleep transition.

Polysomnography in the form of a multiple sleep latency test (MSLT), preceded by an all-night sleep study, will confirm the diagnosis. The MSLT consists of five or six scheduled daytime naps at 2-hour intervals, during which the subject is monitored for 20 minutes in a quiet, darkened room with instructions to try to go to sleep. At the end of 20 min, subjects are wakened and not allowed to sleep until the next scheduled nap. One or more recordings of sleep latency less than 10 min, REM sleep latency (time from sleep onset to first REM period) less than 20 min, MSLT evidence of two or more sleep-onset REM periods, or a mean sleep latency of less than 5 min plus the associated symptoms are diagnostic of narcolepsy, according to ICSD diagnostic criteria (ASDA 1990). For the DSM-IV diagnostic criteria, see the accompanying box.

As a psychiatric nurse, be aware of narcolepsy because about 40% of people with this disorder also have a concurrent or prior-onset mental disorder. With onset typically occurring in adolescence, often exacerbated by an acute psychosocial stressor, these clients have experienced a life-changing and poorly accepted chronic illness during an important developmental stage. The frequency of daytime sleeping and cataplexy attacks is embarrassing and disruptive in relation to occupational and social activities (Fredrickson et al. 1990). Various theories have been offered about the association between narcolepsy and mental disorders, but no clear cause-and-effect explanation is anticipated. Stimulants such as amphetamines are the most common treatment for the hypersomnia. Tricyclic antidepressants (TCAs) are useful in controlling the associated symptoms of cataplexy, sleep paralysis, and hypnagogic hallucinations (Guilleminault 1994).

The accompanying Research Note reports on a nonpharmacologic intervention approach for narcolepsy.

DSM-IV Diagnostic Criteria for Narcolepsy

A. Irresistible attacks of refreshing sleep that occur daily over at least 3 months.

B. The presence of one or both of the following:
   1. cataplexy (i.e., brief episodes of sudden bilateral loss of muscle tone, most often in association with intense emotion).
   2. recurrent intrusions of elements of rapid eye movement (REM) sleep into the transition between sleep and wakefulness, as manifested by either hypnopompic or hypnagogic hallucinations or sleep paralysis at the beginning or end of sleep episodes.

C. The disturbance is not due to the direct physiological effects of a substance (e.g., a drug of abuse, a medication) or another general medical condition.

Source: American Psychiatric Association 1994, p. 567.

PERIODIC LIMB MOVEMENT DISORDER Periodic limb movement disorder usually involves the legs, which repeatedly move in a jerking, stereotypic manner during sleep, often causing partial arousals. This disorder can contribute to excessive sleepiness, unrefreshing sleep, and multiple awakenings. Prevalence tends to increase with age; it occurs in up to 34% of individuals over age 60 (ASDA 1990). It should be distinguished from restless legs syndrome (RLS) which may occur prior to sleep and is characterized by disagreeable sensations in the legs which are only relieved by movement. Persons with RLS usually have PLMD as well, but PLMD is not necessarily associated with RLS.

As a psychiatric nurse, it is important to know that TCAs and monamine oxidase inhibitors (MAOIs) can trigger or worsen periodic limb movement disorder (ASDA

RESEARCH NOTE

Citation

Rogers AE, Aldrich MS: The effect of regularly scheduled naps on sleep attacks and excessive daytime sleepiness associated with narcolepsy. *Nurs Res* 1993; 42(2):111–117.

Study Problem/Purpose

The effectiveness of nap therapy in improving alertness and reducing the number of sleep attacks was investigated in this pilot intervention study.

Methods

A convenience sample of 16 individuals, age 21–65, with narcolepsy was recruited through a university hospital sleep disorder center. The intervention consisted of three regularly scheduled 15-minute naps each day. Subjects maintained their usual medication and nocturnal sleep schedules. Sleep diaries were kept for 1 week prior to and throughout the 4-week period of intervention. The Maintenance of Wakefulness Test (MWT), a test similar to the MSLT but in which subjects are asked to try to stay awake, was administered at the beginning and end of the intervention period. The Narcolepsy Symptom Status Questionnaire was also used for measuring subjective symptoms.

Findings

The average sleep latency on the MWT increased significantly after 4 weeks of intervention, suggesting that subjects were better able to stay awake after 4 weeks of nap therapy. However, there was no change in the frequency of sleep attacks or other symptoms. Responders (subjects who had longer sleep latency on at least four of the five test periods in the second MWT) (n = 6) were compared to nonresponders (n = 10). The two groups were similar on most of the outcome measures, but before treatment, the responder group tended to report more troublesome symptoms and more napping. Only 7 of the subjects were able to maintain the nap schedule with an average of two or more naps per day, but even the 9 subjects who averaged less than two naps a day during the test period showed increased sleep latency on the second MWT.

Implications

On the basis of these findings, it would be premature to recommend nap therapy to all clients with narcolepsy. However, this nurse-led pilot study is an important step toward systematic investigation of a potential intervention within the scope of nursing practice. Although limited by small sample size and lack of a control group, it suggests a direction for further study. For example, improvement in alertness between naps and sleep attacks may be important to the quality of life of clients with narcolepsy, even if nap therapy is ineffective in reducing the number of sleep attacks or other symptoms. And, while you cannot yet tell clients nap therapy has been supported by research, it is an alternative with which they may want to experiment themselves.

1990). Withdrawal of anticonvulsants, benzodiazepines, and other hypnotic drugs can also exacerbate the condition of periodic limb movement disorder.

Idiopathic Hypersomnia Idiopathic hypersomnia is prolonged nocturnal sleep time, especially slow-wave sleep, and excessive sleepiness. Although the cause is unknown, it is thought to be related to the central nervous system (ASDA 1990). In the *DSM-IV,* the corresponding term is primary hypersomnia (see the box on page 454).

Inadequate Sleep Hygiene This first of the extrinsic sleep disorders, according to the ICSD classification, is seldom seen as a diagnosis but is commonly encountered in clients. Inadequate sleep hygiene is having behaviors that contribute to either insomnia or hypersomnia. These behaviors may not have been problematic for the person earlier in life, or for other individuals, but they are now contributing to sleep pattern disturbance. Examples are wide variations in sleep schedule; the regular use of stimulants such as caffeine and/or nicotine; using the bedroom as a work area; and doing intense mental or physical activity immediately before going to bed.

Environmental Sleep Disorder Like inadequate sleep hygiene, environmental sleep disorder is seldom written that way as a diagnosis, but nurses and other health care professionals frequently encounter clients for whom a specific environmental factor is the main contributor to either insomnia or excessive sleepiness. The environmental factor may be noise, temperature, or light; it may be interpersonal, such as the snoring of a bed partner or caretaking vigilance for an infant, sick child, or adult; or it may be vigilance related to a perceived personal threat, as

> ### DSM-IV Diagnostic Criteria for Primary Hypersomnia
>
> A. The predominant complaint is excessive sleepiness for at least 1 month (or less if recurrent) as evidenced by either prolonged sleep episodes or daytime sleep episodes that occur almost daily.
>
> B. The excessive sleepiness causes clinically significant distress or impairment in social, occupational, or other important areas of functioning.
>
> C. The excessive sleepiness is not better accounted for by insomnia and does not occur exclusively during the course of another Sleep Disorder (e.g., Narcolepsy, Breathing-Related Sleep Disorder, Circadian Rhythm Sleep Disorder, or a Parasomnia) and cannot be accounted for by an inadequate amount of sleep.
>
> D. The disturbance does not occur exclusively during the course of another mental disorder.
>
> E. The disturbance is not due to the direct physiological effects of a substance (e.g., a drug of abuse, a medication) or a general medical condition.
>
> *Source: American Psychiatric Association 1994, p. 562.*

during a critical illness. The environmental factor might also be fear of a violent attack. Sensitivity to environmental stimuli increases whenever the client is in stage 1 or 2 of slow-wave sleep and toward the end of the sleep period. Older adults are usually more sensitive to environmental disturbance than younger adults. However, there is great variation among and within individuals, including the ability to respond to certain meaningful sounds such as a baby's cry or a footstep and yet ignore other sounds such as routine traffic noise.

NOCTURNAL EATING (DRINKING) SYNDROME Nocturnal eating or drinking syndrome is characterized by repeated nighttime awakenings and the inability to get back to sleep without eating or drinking. Such a pattern is common among young children who have always been breast-fed or bottle-fed as a means of going to sleep. It is thought to be a learned behavior that can also occur in adults, and it can become obsessional (ASDA 1990).

STIMULANT OR ALCOHOL-DEPENDENT SLEEP DISORDER This type of sleep disorder does not have a clear counterpart in the *DSM-IV*. It is characterized by sustained use of stimulants for staying awake, or of alcohol to induce sleep. You will probably work with many clients who use stimulants or alcohol periodically for their effect on sleep. For example, the use of stimulants is not uncommon among long-distance truck drivers. Alcohol is and has been one of the most frequently used hypnotics. While a drink at bedtime reduces sleep latency, it usually induces wakening later in the night.

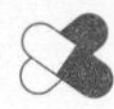

A wide range of biochemical substances can contribute to this sleep disorder by their presence in sufficient quantities (such as caffeine and prescription drugs like fluorazepine), their unaccustomed absence (alcohol), or their abuse (street drugs). Clients with psychiatric disorders, especially schizophrenia or mania, are particularly vulnerable to sleep disorders from these chemical imbalances, as are clients with a history of traumatic brain injury.

TIME ZONE CHANGE (JET LAG) SYNDROME As a result of jet travel, a client's manic phase may be further exacerbated by jet lag and associated sleep deprivation.

Mr J traveled from the United States to the Middle East on business. Upon his return to the United States, he made a series of irrational business decisions that he blamed on the stress of jet lag. However, it was subsequently determined that Mr J had bipolar disorder.

Recent research, based on a chart review, suggests that first episodes of mania may be rapidly reversed in clients who are able to sleep (with haloperidol) during the first night of hospitalization (Nowlin-Finch et al. 1994). The response was most evident in clients who also reported a known stressor, which may have precipitated the first manic episode. The stressor may have also contributed to sleep deprivation, like clients experiencing major sleep disruption through jet travel across seven time zones.

SHIFT WORK SLEEP DISORDER As you might expect, shift work is a major source of circadian rhythm disruption. If you choose hospital nursing, you may be concerned about this disorder for yourself as well as for clients.

Jane was working rotating shifts in an intensive care unit. She noted that she had worsening insomnia, and feared that her judgment would become affected by increasing sleep deprivation.

The science of chronobiology is rapidly expanding and has implications for coping with shift work. Inquiries about shift work should be a routine part of sleep assessment because the impact on sleep patterns and sleep disturbance often extends beyond the period of shift work.

Years after he had retired from his bakery business, Mr W continued to awaken very early in the morning. This pattern further complicated a sleep disorder related to his medical condition of Parkinson's disease.

Delayed Sleep Phase Syndrome An abnormality in sleep phase can contribute to what may appear to be socially inappropriate or uncooperative behavior. Clients with this circadian rhythm disorder seem programmed to stay up late and sleep in late. This syndrome should not be confused with normal tendencies to be either a "night owl" or "morning lark." Delayed sleep phase syndrome is a persistent problem that is resistant to standard attempts to get up earlier. It is not unusual to encounter people with this disorder who have adapted by seeking types of employment and entertainment that are conducive to late nights and late rising. The disorder can also contribute to social isolation.

Advanced Sleep Phase Syndrome Advanced sleep phase syndrome is the reverse of delayed sleep phase syndrome in that early evening sleepiness regularly accompanies early wakening. A mildly advanced sleep phase is common among older adults and should not be confused with the early wakening associated with depression. With depression, other symptoms and sleep changes are evident.

The main consequences of delayed or advanced sleep phase syndrome are the disruption of family, work, and/or social activities. If the circadian pattern is problematic, phase shifting can be modified through chronotherapy or light therapy. Chronotherapy consists of systematically delaying bedtime, usually in 3-hour increments, over a period of several weeks until the client reaches the desired bedtime hour, after which the new schedule must be carefully maintained (Roehrs and Roth 1994). Light therapy is timed to coincide with the time of day that sleepiness should be reduced. For people with advanced sleep phase syndrome, light therapy may be administered in the early evening.

For the DSM-IV diagnostic criteria for circadian rhythm sleep disorders, see the accompanying box.

DSM-IV Diagnostic Criteria for Circadian Rhythm Sleep Disorder

A. A persistent or recurrent pattern of sleep disruption leading to excessive sleepiness or insomnia that is due to a mismatch between the sleep-wake schedule required by a person's environment and his or her circadian sleep-wake pattern.

B. The sleep disturbance causes clinically significant distress or impairment in social, occupational, or other important areas of functioning.

C. The disturbance does not occur exclusively during the course of another Sleep Disorder or other mental disorder.

D. The disturbance is not due to the direct physiological effects of a substance (e.g., a drug of abuse, a medication) or a general medical condition.

Specify type:

Delayed Sleep Phase Type: a persistent pattern of late sleep onset and late awakening times, with an inability to fall asleep and awaken at a desired earlier time.

Jet Lag Type: sleepiness and alertness that occur at inappropriate time of day relative to local time, occurring after repeated travel across more than one time zone.

Shift Work Type: insomnia during the major sleep period or excessive sleepiness during the major awake period associated with night shift work or frequently changing shift work.

Unspecified Type:

Source: American Psychiatric Association 1994, p. 578.

Parasomnias

The parasomnias include **somnambulism** (sleepwalking), sleep talking, nightmares, sleep terrors, **sleep bruxism** (teeth-grinding), and **sleep enuresis** (bed-wetting). They are characterized by CNS activation, including autonomic nervous system changes and skeletal muscle activity (ASDA 1990). The parasomnias will be discussed in relation to the sleep stages during which they typically occur.

Parasomnias that emerge during slow-wave (non-REM) sleep include sleepwalking and night terrors. Certain medications used for psychiatric disorders, such as lithium, desipramine, and thioridazine, may exacerbate or induce sleepwalking, as can fever or sleep deprivation (ASDA 1990). Sleep terrors (also known as night terrors) are sudden arousals from slow-wave sleep, associated with intense autonomic and behavioral reactions characterized by fear. Unlike nightmares, which occur in REM sleep, there is little or no memory of the frightening episode. Both of these parasomnias are more common in children prior to puberty, but they may also occur in adults, particularly at times of intense stress (see the boxes for diagnostic criteria for these disorders, opposite).

DSM-IV Diagnostic Criteria for Sleepwalking Disorder

A. Repeated episodes of rising from bed during sleep and walking about, usually occurring during the first third of the major sleep episode.

B. While sleepwalking, the person has a blank, staring face, is relatively unresponsive to the efforts of others to communicate with him or her, and can be awakened only with great difficulty.

C. On awakening (either from the sleepwalking episode or the next morning), the person has amnesia for the episode.

D. Within several minutes after awakening from the sleepwalking episode, there is no impairment in mental activity or behavior (although there may initially be a short period of confusion or disorientation).

E. The sleepwalking causes clinically significant distress or impairment in social, occupational, or other important areas of functioning.

F. The disturbance is not due to the direct physiological effects of a substance (e.g., a drug of abuse, a medication) or a general medical condition.

Source: American Psychiatric Association 1994, p. 591.

DSM-IV Diagnostic Criteria for Sleep Terror Disorder

A. Recurrent episodes of abrupt wakening from sleep, usually occurring during the first third of the major sleep episode and beginning with a panicky scream.

B. Intense fear and signs of autonomic arousal, such as tachycardia, rapid breathing, and sweating, during each episode.

C. Relative unresponsiveness to efforts of others to comfort the person during the episode.

D. No detailed dream is recalled and there is amnesia for the episode.

E. The episodes cause clinically significant distress or impairment in social, occupational, or other important functioning.

F. The disturbance is not due to the direct physiological effects of a substance (e.g., a drug of abuse, a medication) or a general medical condition.

Source: American Psychiatric Association 1994, p. 587.

Parasomnias associated with REM sleep include nightmares, sleep paralysis, and REM sleep behavior disorder. REM sleep behavior disorder is a rare but potentially serious disorder in which motor activity occurs during REM sleep and may be associated with the apparent acting-out of dream sequences. Injuries to the individual or bed partner have been reported. It is thought to be more frequent during REM rebound following alcohol or sedative-hypnotic withdrawal. It has also been reported in association with the use of tricyclic antidepressants (ASDA 1990). See the box for nightmare disorder on page 457.

Sleep bruxism, or teeth-grinding, is strongly associated with stress and anxiety. Sleep enuresis (bed-wetting) can occur during any sleep stage. A normal behavior in infancy, sleep enuresis may persist for some children into the early teens.

Sleep Disorders Associated with Medical/Psychiatric Disorders

The sleep disorders discussed prior to this point are those that any individual, with or without a mental disorder, may have. Their importance to psychiatric nursing is that they are so common that you can expect some of your clients to be also coping with a sleep disorder. A psychiatric illness and/or its treatment may have an interactive effect on a preexisting or concurrent sleep pattern disturbance. The importance of this final category to psychiatric nursing is obvious. Sleep disturbances that are symptomatic of underlying psychiatric illness are troublesome to clients. These symptoms are an important part of the experience of mental illness for clients, even though they may not meet the DSM-IV criteria of being a predominant complaint (see the boxes on page 457 and 458 concerning insomnia and hypersomnia).

Sleep pattern disturbance may be related to psychoses, mood disorders, anxiety disorders, panic disorder, or alco-

DSM-IV Diagnostic Criteria for Nightmare Disorder

A. Repeated awakenings from the major sleep period or naps with detailed recall of extended and extremely frightening dreams, usually involving threats to survival, security, or self-esteem. The awakenings generally occur during the second half of the sleep period.

B. On awakening from the frightening dreams, the person rapidly becomes oriented and alert (in contrast to the confusion and disorientation seen in Sleep Terror Disorder and some forms of epilepsy).

C. The dream experience, or the sleep disturbance resulting from the awakening, causes clinically significant distress or impairment in social, occupational, or other important areas of functioning.

D. The nightmares do not occur exclusively during the course of another mental disorder (e.g., Delirium, Posttraumatic Stress Disorder) and are not due to the direct physiological effects of a substance (e.g., a drug of abuse, a medication) or a general medical condition.

Source: American Psychiatric Association 1994, p. 583.

DSM-IV Diagnostic Criteria for Insomnia Related to . . . (Axis I or Axis II Disorder)

A. The predominant complaint is difficulty initiating or maintaining sleep or nonrestorative sleep, for at least 1 month that is associated with daytime fatigue or impaired daytime functioning.

B. The sleep disturbance (or daytime sequelae) causes clinically significant distress or impairment in social, occupational, or other important areas of functioning.

C. The insomnia is judged to be related to another Axis I or Axis II disorder (e.g., Major Depressive Disorder, Generalized Anxiety Disorder, Adjustment Disorder with Anxiety), but is sufficiently severe to warrant independent clinical attention.

D. The disturbance is not better accounted for by another Sleep Disorder (e.g., Narcolepsy, Breathing-Related Sleep Disorder, a Parasomnia).

E. The disturbance is not due to the direct physiological effects of a substance (e.g., a drug of abuse, a medication) or a general medical condition.

Source: American Psychiatric Association 1994, p. 596.

hol use or abuse. Sleep disturbances associated with dementia and other cerebral degenerative disorders will also be considered.

Sleep Pattern Disturbance Associated with Psychoses Significant sleep disruption often occurs in conjunction with an exacerbation of schizophrenia (ASDA 1990; Kaplan, Sadock, and Grebb 1994). Great difficulty in getting to sleep may accompany extreme anxiety and concern about delusional and hallucinatory phenomena. The overall circadian cycle may also be disrupted. Clients with schizophrenia have reduced REM sleep and do not experience REM rebound. Deficit of slow-wave sleep, particularly stage 4, has been found in acute, chronic, and remitted schizophrenia (Benson, Faull, and Zarcone 1991). A link with serotonin, a neurotransmitter associated with non-REM sleep, has been hypothesized. Depressed, alcoholic, and elderly clients also have reduced stage 4 sleep.

Sleep Pattern Disturbance Associated with Mood Disorders As discussed previously, insomnia of the maintenance or early wakening type commonly occurs in major depressive episodes. The sleep pattern disturbance may actually precede other symptoms of depression and likewise may respond to antidepressant medication more rapidly than the depression (ASDA 1990). Partial sleep deprivation, particularly of REM sleep, has been associated with modest improvement in depression but the mechanism for this process is not well understood (Kaplan, Sadock, and Grebb 1994; Sutker and Adams 1993). Most antidepressants suppress REM sleep and lengthen latency to the first REM period.

Seasonal affective disorder (SAD) is related to fluctuations in melatonin levels by variation in the hours of sunlight. The positive response of SAD to light therapy lends strength to the argument that its development is related to weakened circadian rhythmicity (Sutker and Adams 1993).

In the manic phase of bipolar disorder, sleep time is significantly reduced but clients do not complain of

DSM-IV Diagnostic Criteria for Hypersomnia Related to . . . (Axis I or Axis II Disorder)

A. The predominant complaint is excessive sleepiness for at least 1 month as evidenced by either prolonged sleep episodes or daytime sleep episodes that occur almost daily.

B. The excessive sleepiness causes clinically significant distress or impairment in social, occupational, or other important areas of functioning.

C. The hyposomnia is judged to be related to another Axis I or Axis II disorder (e.g., Major Depressive Disorder, Dysthmic Disorder), but is sufficiently severe to warrant independent clinical attention.

D. The disturbance is not better accounted for by another Sleep Disorder (e.g., Narcolepsy, Breathing-Related Sleep Disorder, a Parasomnia) or by an inadequate amount of sleep.

E. The disturbance is not due to the direct physiological effects of a substance (e.g., a drug of abuse, a medication) or a general medical condition.

Source: American Psychiatric Association 1994, p. 597.

insomnia. They have reduced slow-wave sleep and reduced REM latency. During the depressive phase, these clients may experience excessive sleepiness, as may clients with SAD (ASDA 1990).

Sleep Pattern Disturbance Associated with Anxiety Disorders Sleep onset or maintenance insomnia is commonly associated with heightened anxiety. The proportion of stages 1 and 2 non-REM sleep tends to increase as part of the overall state of hyperarousal.

Sleep Pattern Disturbance Associated with Panic Disorder Panic episodes may be associated with sudden wakenings, after which clients may find it very difficult to return to sleep. Sleep-associated panic episodes are most likely to occur during non-REM sleep, particularly stage 2.

Sleep Pattern Disturbance Associated with Alcohol Use or Abuse With acute alcohol intoxication, there is increased sleepiness for 3–4 hours. Sleep may be deep (increased stages 3 and 4) with REM suppression. However, after that, sleep tends to be fragmented, restless, and often accompanied by bizarre dreaming. During alcohol withdrawal, sleep tends to be very fragmented, with REM rebound. The vivid dreaming may be associated with alcohol withdrawal delirium (APA 1994).

Sleep pattern disturbances persist even after a year or more of abstention. The pattern of prolonged sleep latency, increased number of arousals, higher proportion of stage 1 sleep at the expense of slow-wave sleep, and more interrupted REM sleep is thought to be due to a chronically high arousal (Monti et al. 1993). A range of other biochemical substances can also contribute to sleep disorder if they are present in sufficient quantities (caffeine, prescription drugs such as fluorazepine). Some substances contribute to sleep disorder by their unaccustomed absence (stimulants); and still others contribute to sleep disorder by their abuse (street drugs). Clients with psychiatric disorders, especially schizophrenia or mania, or clients with a history of traumatic brain injury are particularly vulnerable to sleep disorders due to chemical imbalances. The vulnerability may be twofold: direct effects of biochemical imbalance, plus the use of alcohol or drugs as an attempted means to cope with a psychiatric disorder.

Ms K and Ms W participate in a maintenance program for people with schizophrenia. They often meet for a drink together at the conclusion of a meeting. While they consume similar amounts of alcohol, Ms K, who also has a history of minor brain injury, experiences much more disordered sleep.

Other abused drugs follow a similar pattern of exacerbation of their usual effect (sedation or stimulation) after excessive intake, along with rebound effects upon withdrawal (see Chapter 13).

Sleep Pattern Disturbance Associated with Dementia and Other Cerebral Degenerative Conditions The tendency for individuals with dementia to become more agitated, more verbal, and more restless as nighttime falls is known as sundowning. Unfortunately, definitions of this phenomenon have been vague, limiting the usefulness of much of the related research (Bliwise 1994). However, it has been suggested that sundowning may be the most common trigger to the institutionalization of clients with dementia because of the additional demands on caregivers (Bliwise 1994). In an exploratory nursing study, activity patterns of clients with dementia were found to increase between 4:00 and 6:00 PM, whereas cognitively healthy clients had decreased activity at that time, corresponding to general population norms (Beel-Bates and Rogers 1990). The most common causal assumption has been a temporal relationship to conditions of decreased light and other environmental stimulation. Apparent deterioration of circadian patterns may be associated with deterioration of the suprachiasmatic nucleus in the brain (Bliwise 1994). Frequent arousals from sleep apnea, incontinence, or caregiver checks have also been implicated. This population is particularly difficult to study because with increasing dementia, there is less and less tolerance of polysomnography. Other cerebral degenerative diseases that involve neurotransmitter imbalance such as Parkinson's disease and Huntington's chorea are also characterized by increasingly fragmented sleep.

The Nursing Process and Clients with Sleep Disorders

The nursing process for sleep disorders will be discussed according to four major symptoms: insomnia, hypersomnia, parasomnia, and sleep-wake schedule disturbance.

Assessment of sleep patterns should become part of your regular assessment with all clients (see the accompanying box). The depth with which you pursue potential problems will vary according to the presenting problems and context of care.

ASSESSMENT

Sleep Patterns

Sleep-Wake Schedule

What time do you usually go to bed?

How long does it usually take you to fall asleep after you have turned off the light?

What time do you usually wake up?

What is different about your sleep-wake schedule on the weekend/days off?

How often do you take naps? (Be alert here for cultural influence, such as taking siestas, or occupational influence.) Under what circumstances?

Getting to Sleep

What helps you get to sleep?

What makes it difficult for you to get to sleep?

Staying Asleep

On average, how many times do you wake up during the night?

What seems to waken you?

How long does it usually take to get back to sleep?

What do you do if you are having trouble getting back to sleep?

Waking Up

How difficult is it for you to wake up?

How soon after waking up do you usually get up?

How do you feel when you first get up?

Daytime Functioning

At what time of day do you usually feel most energetic?

At what time of day do you feel most sleepy?

Would you call yourself a "morning person" or an "evening person"?

Satisfaction with Sleep; Potential Problems

How satisfied are you with the sleep you usually get?

Do you think you get enough sleep on average? How do you know?

How has your sleep been during the past two weeks in comparison to what is normal for you?

Are you concerned about any of the following things?

- Getting to sleep
- Waking up too many times during the night
- Waking up too early
- Having to fight sleepiness during the day
- Snoring, restlessness, talking or walking in your sleep
- Bad dreams
- Drinking too much coffee (or other caffeine/nicotine sources)

When do you enjoy sleep the most?

CLIENT/FAMILY TEACHING

Improving the Quality of Your Sleep

1. Think about the kind of sleep schedule that seems to fit you best.
2. Make a list of things that help you get to sleep (how dark you like it to be, what temperature, how you get ready for bed).
3. Jot down all the "rules" and "suggestions" you have heard about how to get better sleep. Cross out the ones that don't seem to fit. (Some people sleep better by not having a bedtime snack; other people sleep better after having a snack. Do what feels best for you. If you aren't sure, try an experiment doing it one way for a week and then the other way for the next week.) Put a question mark by the rules and suggestions you have never really tried, and underline the ones you think are important for you.
4. Consider what you could change to get an extra half-hour of sleep each night.
5. Keep a sleep diary for 2 weeks. For the first week, just keep track of your usual pattern (time you went to bed and got up, number of hours actual sleep, how you felt in the morning, etc.). At the end of the first week, review the diary and your responses to items 1–4 above. In the second week, experiment with one change you think would be helpful to you.
6. Carry on the process a bit longer if you like, but remember:
   - You can manage on very little sleep if you have to.
   - You know better than anyone else what works for you.
   - Your needs and preferences regarding sleep may change a bit as you get older or take on different roles and activities.

Through sleep assessment, you may also create opportunities for teaching or reinforcing healthy sleep behaviors, such as sleep hygiene (see the box above). There has been a tendency to be overprescriptive in terms of healthy behaviors. For example, a carefully designed English study provided evidence that people who usually have a snack before bedtime sleep better after a bedtime snack than without one; but people who usually do not have a snack before bedtime sleep better without a snack than with one (Adam 1980). Likewise, guidelines intended for people with insomnia are often generalized to the rest of the population. For example, napping is not recommended for people with insomnia. However, having a nap is common in some cultures, such as in countries where the siesta is part of the daily routine, in some farming communities, and among many retired and elderly people. 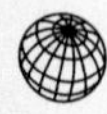 Broughton, a Canadian sleep researcher, proposes, on the basis of his research and that of others, that humans are biphasic, having a natural tendency for two sleep periods per 24-hour day, one major sleep period (commonly at night), and another shorter one (a nap) (Dinges and Broughton 1989).

Sleep Pattern Disturbance is the appropriate NANDA diagnosis for any disruption of sleep time that causes discomfort or interferes with desired lifestyle (Cox et al. 1993). It should be differentiated from the nursing diagnoses of Fatigue and Activity Intolerance. Fatigue is described by clients as a lack of energy that persists regardless of the amount or quality of sleep. Activity Intolerance is a state of insufficient physical or psychologic energy to complete daily activities without report of inadequate sleep.

The Nursing Process and Clients with Insomnia

Assessment

Building from the basic sleep pattern assessment, it is particularly useful to follow up on history of onset of insomnia, and possible contributing intrinsic and extrinsic factors. An ability to sleep better away from the usual bedroom suggests a conditioned response to that setting from many sleepless nights. Explore potential environmental factors, from condition of the mattress to sounds heard from outside the personal dwelling. Inquiry into thought processes while trying to go to sleep may help detect fears, anxiety, or work/family/financial pressures. Listen for evidence of a perceived need for increased vigilance, either currently or at the time the problem developed. Explore beliefs about sleep and its importance. Particularly among individuals with a history of mental

ASSESSMENT

A Client with Sleep Pattern Disturbance (Insomnia)

Nature of the Insomnia

What do you have the most difficulty with?

- Getting to sleep,
- Waking up and then taking a long time to get back to sleep, or
- Waking up earlier than you want to and not being able to get back to sleep.

Possible Contributing Factors

Does it help if you try to sleep somewhere else in your home?

Is your sleep better or worse when you are away from home?

Do you usually sleep with someone? If yes, does it make a difference if they are not with you? (Be alert here for possible disturbance by a partner, or poorer sleep when a habitual partner is not present. Note also that sharing the bed with infants and children varies across and within different cultures.)

How many cups of coffee a day do you have? (Follow up regarding caffeinated or decaffeinated, timing, other caffeine-containing substances such as tea, chocolate, colas.)

Do you smoke? How many packs a day?

What medications and drugs are you using? (Note that many of the psychotropic medications alter sleep patterns, as do most substances of abuse.)

What do you tend to think about while you are trying to get to sleep?

What do you associate with sleep?

What do you think is the single greatest factor affecting your ability to sleep?

or physical disorders, there may be associated fears about death, disturbing dreams, or vulnerability to external threat (see the Assessment box above).

Nursing Diagnosis

Specify that insomnia is the type of Sleep Pattern Disturbance, and further identify it as sleep-onset, maintenance, or early-wakening as appropriate. If the insomnia seems secondary to a mental disorder, that can be specified; but even for those clients, it is helpful to include other contributing factors. Even if environmental factors were not contributory initially, the client may begin to associate them with sleeplessness and/or they may become disturbing because of chronic hyperarousal.

Planning and Implementing Interventions

A few basic interventions for insomnia will be discussed in this section, but the overall treatment may be quite complex, requiring the skills of a specialist. If the insomnia is related primarily to a mental or physical disorder, management of that condition usually brings relief of associated symptoms. Antidepressants are often effective in reducing sleep pattern disturbance before the antidepressant effect can be noticed (see Table 19–2 on page 462).

The interventions that are discussed in this section may be appropriate with clients in a variety of settings. If the insomnia is relatively recent or mild, information on the basic principles of sleep hygiene may be adequate (see the Intervention box on page 462). If the insomnia is chronic and more severe, more rigorous intervention is warranted.

Encouraging Hope Insomnia is such a discouraging and worrisome problem to clients that creating a sense of realistic hope that they will eventually learn to manage the problem is an important part of therapy (Engle-Friedman et al. 1992). The goal is to change perception of the problem from something against which they are helpless to something over which they can gain control.

Providing Information Clients with severe insomnia are often well-acquainted with the self-help literature. However, it is important to review what they have come to understand about managing insomnia. They may have misconceptions or difficulty applying some of the information to themselves. For example, some people are not aware that chocolate is also a source of caffeine. Others may not be aware of normal developmental changes in sleep patterns. Normalizing the experience of occasional times of prolonged sleep latency (more than 30 min) or

Table 19–2 Medications Used in the Treatment of Insomnia

Type	*Examples*	*Comments*
Antihistamines	Chlorpheniramine (Chlor-Trimeton)	Available over the counter, may be used to facilitate sleep onset because of the drowsiness they induce
	Pseudoephedrine compounds (Benylin cold capsules)	
Hypnotics	Benzodiazepines such as	
	Temazepan (Restoril)	Useful for sleep onset
	Flurazepam (Dalmane)	Sleep onset and maintenance
	Zopiclone (Imovane)	Chemically different from benzodiazepines, useful for sleep onset and maintenance
Antidepressants	Tricyclic antidepressants (especially those with more sedative effects such as amitriptyline (Elavil) and Trimipramine (Surmontil))	Effect on insomnia evident earlier than antidepressant effect. Supress REM sleep

INTERVENTION

Basic Principles of Sleep Hygiene

1. Maintain regularity in the sleep-wake schedule.
   - Avoid staying up too late or sleeping in too long on days off.
   - Enjoy an occasional nap, but stop taking naps if you notice that it is harder to get to sleep at night.
   - Be consistent in the time you get up, even if you have had less than usual sleep.
2. Go to bed only when you are reasonably sleepy and relaxed.
   - For a half-hour or so before you go to bed, engage in activities that are relaxing to you, even if you feel some pressure of things needing to be done. There is even research to support the belief that a good night's sleep is associated with better mood and social interactions the next day (Totterdell et al. 1994).
   - If you are not drowsy when it is time to go to bed, engage in some activity that usually makes you drowsy, like reading something light.
   - Learn relaxation exercises (but practice them at other times of the day first).
   - Increase the physical exercise that you get during the day.
3. Maintain some sleep rituals as part of getting ready for bed.
   - Bring your day to a close with prayer or meditation if that is meaningful to you. Make this a time to focus on the good things that have happened, the accomplishments of the day, no matter how minor they may seem to be.
   - Get into a routine (brushing your teeth, winding the clock, opening the window, etc.).
4. Avoid the intake of stimulants or other substances that affect sleep patterns.
   - Instead of an alcoholic drink to induce sleep and relaxation, try a warm bath.
   - Experiment with decreasing the amount of coffee you drink, especially later in the day.
5. Enjoy what sleep you do get rather than thinking about what you think you need.
   - Move the clock so you cannot see what time it is every time you look in that direction.
   - Snuggle under the covers and think how nice it is that you can be resting in bed. If you are starting to feel restless or your mind is racing, get up and do some quiet activity such as reading until you feel drowsy again.

wakenings during the night may be helpful as an intervention, as well as facilitating the setting of realistic goals. Clients with insomnia may also need some help in differentiating between myth and research-based evidence, between beliefs and facts. Of particular importance is recognizing that insomnia can be managed and that clients can continue to function adequately even on minimal sleep.

SHORTENING THE OVERALL SLEEP PERIOD WITH CONSISTENT RISING TIME The time of rising is under voluntary control; the time of actually getting to sleep is not. With shorter total time in bed, sleep usually becomes more consolidated. These two principles are the basis for one of the most effective means of gaining control over insomnia:

1. Clients must not go to bed until they feel sleepy.
2. They must get up at the same time each morning.

Initially this prescription may seem threatening to clients who have usually gotten into a pattern of getting sleep whenever and wherever they can. They will need support during this initial phase, possibly through a contracting process in which they go one week at a time. Reinforce that they will be able to get by and that their body will eventually begin to respond to the regularity of schedule, and that you believe in their ability to accomplish this goal. Clients with insomnia should not be permitted to nap. (For the very old or very ill, naps should be restricted to a brief, set time period.)

REDUCING KNOWN STIMULANTS AND OTHER SOURCES OF AROUSAL Help clients with insomnia realize that they are susceptible to any stimulation, even though such stimulating factors may not have been contributory initially. Encourage them to avoid all sources of caffeine, nicotine, and other stimulants. However, in working with psychiatric clients, as with any client population, this intervention and all others must be considered in the context of the overall health problems, goals, and treatment plan as negotiated with the client, family, and other members of the health care team.

You may wish to collaborate with the client in making a list of possible contributing factors to the sleep pattern disturbance. For example, the client may identify interaction with a particular family member as generating a lot of emotion that is tough to deal with before going to bed. If fear or a perceived need for vigilance is a factor, it may be possible to modify the environment.

An elderly widow, initially referred to our Sleep Clinic with possible obstructive sleep apnea, had become increasingly depressed. On a recent visit she confided that she had been sexually abused a few years prior and was extremely afraid to venture out of her apartment building. She felt especially vulnerable because of living in a basement suite, which could be readily broken into. Through the efforts of one of the nurse clinicians, the social welfare agency that was involved agreed to pay the slight additional cost involved in moving her to a second-story apartment, where she felt much safer. Through ongoing counseling with the nurse clinician, she began a modest exercise program in her own small apartment, and medical treatment for her sleep disturbance and depression resulted in clinically significant improvement over the next few months.

As discussed earlier, the state of arousal may be conditioned by objects in the bedroom environment or certain activities. Ways to alter these associations can be explored with the client. An assessment of the bedroom environment and its uses may call for relocating certain activities, such as paying bills or studying, to another part of the home. Rearranging furniture or even changing the color of pillowcases may help reestablish associating the bedroom with sleep.

RELAXATION TRAINING Relaxation exercises are discussed in Chapter 29. The important point in using them as an aid to sleep is that developing the skills should occur apart from the sleep period, so that they, too, do not become associated with the inability to sleep.

Evaluation and Outcome Criteria

Early collaboration with the client in establishing realistic goals will help result in a satisfactory outcome. Regardless of behavioral or polysomnography-defined changes, it is important that the client can express some sense of mastery over his or her sleep problem. Whether that sense of control is achieved through reframing of essentially the same sleep patterns, a modest improvement in one or more parameters of sleep latency or number and length of awakenings, or an improved sense of energy for the day's activities, is not important clinically. However, a better understanding of which interventions are most effective through carefully designed research studies would be a definite asset in helping nurses and others to choose among intervention alternatives.

The Nursing Process and Clients with Hypersomnia

The focus in this section will be on clients who present with excessive sleepiness as part of their mental disorder. Basic assessments to identify clients who might benefit from referral to a sleep specialist are included. However,

CASE STUDY

A Depressed Client with Hypersomnia

Identifying Information

Maha is a 42-year-old woman presently living in a small apartment with her unmarried 22-year-old son.

Client's Description of Problem

Maha states she has been having trouble with periodic wakenings and daytime sleepiness since before her divorce two years ago. She has been steadily gaining weight, feels that she has no energy, and says that the only thing she feels like doing is "watching my soaps on TV."

Family History

Never an energetic person, Maha feels that her present problems started years ago when she had to spend long hours with the children while her husband traveled. His homecomings usually included verbal abuse about her "slovenly" housekeeping and lack of discipline with the children. Having immigrated as a young wife she has deeply missed her family and made few friends here. Food has always been a source of comfort to her, particularly the traditional dishes of her homeland.

Health History

Maha was heavy even as an adolescent and has snored for as long as she can remember. When she was still married, her husband usually slept in another bedroom because of her snoring. Maha's current depressive episode was diagnosed six months ago when her son insisted she see their family doctor. Treatment was initiated with fluoxetine (Prozac) 20 mg which has now been increased to 40 mg daily in the morning.

Current Mental Status

Maha appears somewhat drowsy with a paucity of movement. Her speech is slow but coherent. She acknowledges some problems with short-term memory and concentration.

Other Significant Subjective and Objective Clinical Data

Maha is 163 cm tall and weighs 160 kg. She has a thick neck and large abdomen. Her son describes her snoring as disruptive with periods of escalating noise cumulating in a half minute or longer silence which ends abruptly with a gasp and gradual resumption of quiet breathing until the next episode. She goes to bed about 9:00 PM and stays there until 11:00 AM or later the next morning, sleeping most of the time. She often wakens with a headache, feeling as tired as she did the night before.

Diagnostic Impression

Nursing Diagnosis

Sleep Pattern Disturbance: Hypersomnolence
Breathing-Related Sleep Disorder (i.e., obstructive sleep apnea)

DSM-IV Diagnosis

Axis I: 307.44 Hypersomnia related to Major Depressive disorder;
296.3x Major Depressive Disorder, recurrent
Axis II: None
Axis III: Obesity
Axis IV: Problems with progress in support group
Axis V: Current GAF = 55

principles of treatment for most of the primary sleep disorders characterized by hypersomnia (obstructive sleep apnea, narcolepsy) were briefly discussed earlier.

Assessment

Building from the basic sleep pattern assessment, explore potential contributing factors. With respect to the possibility of sleep apnea or periodic limb movement disorder:

- Try to interview the client's bed partner, or, if the client is institutionalized, to arrange for observation during sleep. If the bed partner describes recurrent periods of erratic breathing including pauses of 20 seconds or longer interspersed between snoring, gasping, or snorting sounds, the client may have sleep apnea.
- Determine whether the problem disappears when the client is in a side-lying position, is worse after ingesting alcohol (even one or two drinks), is accompanied by morning headaches or wakening with a feeling of still being tired.
- Ask the bed partner about the client's restlessness, repetitive jerking of one or more limbs, and/or gasping or choking noises.

NURSING CARE PLAN

A Depressed Client with Hypersomnia

Nursing Diagnosis

Sleep Pattern Disturbance: Excessive somnolence related to inactivity secondary to depression, obstructive sleep apnea, and obesity.

Expected Outcome

Client will spend less time in bed, and less time sleeping

Nursing Interventions

- Explore previously enjoyed activities, involvement in exercise or sporting activity and establish a contract with client for increasing activity based on what she thinks she can manage.
- Support continued therapy for depression.
- Report symptoms of hypersomnolence, snoring, and disordered nocturnal breathing to physician for possible referral to a sleep specialist.
- Encourage 30 min of outdoor activity to increase exposure to natural sunlight to restore circadian rhythm
- Establish a regular time for getting up that is 30 min earlier than current rising time. Each week set that time 30 min earlier than previous week until client reaches what was previously an adequate amount of sleep for her.

Outcome Met If

- Client increases activity level by 25%.
- Client reports decrease in level of depression.
- Client seeks assessment and treatment from sleep specialist.
- Client appears more alert.
- Client spends 10% less time sleeping.
- Client reports daily sunlight exposure.
- Client modifies rising time between the hours of 7 and 9 am and reports feeling refreshed upon awakening.
- Client gradually loses weight to upper end of normal weight for height and age.

An occasional apnea or myoclonic jerk about the time of sleep onset is not unusual. These are common occurrences as part of the normal wake-sleep transition. It is the recurrent episodes accompanied by some daytime somnolence that are of particular concern.

In the psychiatric context, you will encounter clients whose excessive sleepiness is associated with a coping mechanism, hopelessness, or an underlying mental disorder. Eliciting information about onset, patterns, and perceived causes may be difficult with these clients. Regular observation and recording of states of waking-sleeping in relation to clock time, activities, and environment may provide some clues about the pattern. For example, if the client is sleeping quite soundly whenever left undisturbed, chronic sleep deprivation or post-traumatic hypersomnia could be a factor (ASDA 1990). Clients with secondary depression following a physical illness may also sleep more. In contrast, the lethargy that may accompany a major depressive episode or schizophrenia may be associated with lying with the eyes closed but not actually sleeping. (Such assessment will not be elaborated here, as it is best considered as part of the overall assessment for these clients.)

Nursing Diagnosis

Specify that the type of Sleep Pattern Disturbance is hypersomnia, and describe contributing factors, if known. Frequently, contributing factors will be unknown or hypothetical at best. It is better to say unknown than to label a client in the absence of adequate evidence.

Planning and Implementing Interventions

The commonly observed interaction of aging, depression, and concurrent physical disease as contributors to excessive sleepiness (Reynolds and Kupfer 1987) illustrates the difficulty of planning and implementing specific interventions. Focus the interventions as follows:

1. Treat the underlying mental and physical disorders.
2. Ensure client safety, because of the frequently associated problems with loss of concentration and memory.
3. Regularize the client's schedule, alternating periods of activity and rest, to help gain a sense of control over the excessive sleepiness.
4. Expose the client to natural sunlight or light therapy in the morning; encourage walking outdoors.

5. Plan favorite events, such as a television program or visitor.
6. Maximize the use of environmental time cues, such as regular mealtimes and the visibility of a clock and windows.

Evaluation and Outcome Criteria

The setting of short-term, achievable, and meaningful goals is important for clients with this condition. For them, time otherwise seems to become a blur of sleeping and eating.

The Nursing Process and Clients with Parasomnia

Clients with parasomnias are often encountered in psychiatric settings because of the frequency of associated psychopathologic problems. The exception is young children, in whom parasomnias are considered a normal phenomenon or, at most, a transient sleep disorder (Fredrickson et al. 1990). In adults, parasomnias are often associated with major stressful events.

Assessment

Besides the basic sleep pattern assessment, focus on the circumstances at the time of onset of the current and previous episodes, and on family history.

- Clients with a single parasomnia may have a history of one or more other parasomnias, so ask about wakening with a sense of terror, vivid nightmares, etc.
- Clients may be only partially aware of their parasomnias (they are usually amnesic about sleepwalking episodes), so question family members.
- The occurrence of subjective experiences like sleep terrors or sleep paralysis may never have been disclosed out of embarrassment or lack of adequate descriptive language; therefore, use normalizing statements followed by a question. "Many people who have trouble with sleepwalking have also experienced times when they wake up feeling terribly frightened but aren't sure why. Has anything like that ever happened to you?"
- Inquiry about family history should not be limited to the same parasomnia, as there is some mixing of types among family members. The prevalence is higher among first-degree relatives than in the general population (Fredrickson et al. 1990).
- Help clients explore stressors that might be associated with initial or recurrent episodes. "What else was happening in your life about then?"
- Ask about current and prior medications. Medication changes may also be a precipitator, particularly of the REM-related parasomnias such as nightmares. Remember that what was prescribed and what the client has actually taken may be different, so be sure to ask.

Nursing Diagnosis

As with the other sleep pattern disturbances, specify the type(s), but the contributing factors may be unknown or just hypotheses.

Planning and Implementing Interventions

Promoting Client Safety Physical and emotional safety is the major goal in planning and implementing interventions for clients with Sleep Pattern Disturbance related to parasomnias. Physically active parasomnias, such as somnambulism and REM Sleep Behavior Disorder, pose the risk of injury to the client and/or others. At a children's camp, safety may be a matter of seeing that the affected child is assigned a lower bunk and that the cabin counselor is aware of the potential problem. Among older children or adults the behaviors may be elaborate. Clients have been known to remove barricades, silence alarms, open exterior doors, and cross streets while sleepwalking. Protective intervention must be highly individualized and must involve close collaboration with the family. Caution family members to avoid wakening or arguing with the client.

Subjective parasomnias, such as sleep terrors and nightmares, can be extremely frightening to clients, particularly those who are already compromised by a mental disorder. The dreams of clients with posttraumatic stress disorder may likewise be one of the most frightening factors for them. Clients who are aware that they have somnambulism or REM sleep behavior disorder also tend to carry some burden of fear as to what might happen during this phenomenon that seems beyond their control. Offer assistance by helping them explore these feelings and understand the physiologic basis. They can be guided in the decisions they make about taking their medication and other substances by understanding the possibility of REM rebound.

Administering Pharmacotherapy Clients with REM sleep behavior disorder respond to the regular administration of clonazepam (Mahowald and Schenck 1994). However, there have been reports of breakthrough behavior even a year after beginning drug therapy. Somnambulism usually responds to clonazepam (Clonopin), diazepam (Valium), or imipramine (Tofranil) (Fredrickson et al. 1990). As noted earlier, many of the antidepressants suppress REM sleep and therefore offer some protection against nightmares. Caution clients against abruptly discontinuing the medication; REM rebound is less of a problem with gradual reduction of dosage.

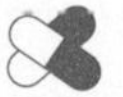

Managing Psychosocial Stressors and/or the Underlying Mental Disorder These interventions will be part of the overall therapeutic plan and are not specific to the sleep disorders.

Evaluation and Outcome Criteria

Reducing the risk factors is the most important outcome criterion. It is unrealistic to say you will prevent injury, because that is usually not within your realm of responsibility, nor is it realistic for any other care provider to guarantee injury prevention. In an environment of increasing litigation, the choice of words used in documentation is important.

The Nursing Process and Clients with Sleep-Wake Schedule Disturbance

The information in this last section is on the kind of disorganized sleep-wake patterns that are common among depressed and psychotic clients (Kaplan, Sadock, and Grebb 1994).

Assessment

Much of the information that you need will come from the basic sleep pattern assessment, if clients can participate and recall accurately. The next step is a combined assessment-intervention: a sleep diary. By keeping a diary, they may confront their own irregularities and be more amenable to developing a regular schedule. Other psychiatric clients may be unable or unwilling to maintain a diary and may require help. It is also useful to obtain information about previous patterns, tendencies toward being a morning or evening person, and the type of schedule to which they will most likely return as their condition improves. In that way, they will not have to cope with further schedule change upon discharge or resuming family and work roles.

Nursing Diagnosis

The nursing diagnosis is Sleep Pattern Disturbance, but for this problem it is usually easier to identify contributing factors, at least to the immediate situation. For example, a client may live alone and be on an indefinite leave from work because of a major depressive episode. The mental disorder is an underlying cause, but the immediate and more rectifiable contributing factor is that there are few markers of time in the client's daily life, other than therapy appointments. Some clients, such as those with dementia, may have lost their ability to estimate time or even interpret cues. Other clients may live in such a chaotic environment that it is very difficult to achieve any regularity of schedule.

Planning and Implementing Interventions

Establishing Regularity and Cues in Daily and Weekly Schedules Interventions will be highly individualized, as previously discussed. For the client who lives alone, external cues may be introduced through the help of family, friends, or social agencies. For example, a family member may agree to phone the client at the same time each day. A volunteer may agree to invite the client and two or three others to dinner every Wednesday evening. A service such as Meals on Wheels may be warrented, providing the combined benefit of better nutrition and another regular daily event. Scheduling morning appointments for these clients gives them a reason to get up early. As their condition gradually improves, they can take increasing responsibility for structuring their own schedule. Markers of the days of the week and even the season may further help them once again participate in life around them.

Clients who live in a chaotic environment and/or experience multiple role demands present a very different challenge. For example, a young single mother with a colicky baby and a toddler may find her days and nights have become a blur of child care. Overall sleep deprivation, particularly REM sleep because of caregiving responsibilities, may reduce her coping skills. Reliance on alcohol or drugs may further fragment sleep, as may memories of abuse or trauma. Crisis intervention may be necessary (see Chapter 30). However, a long-term plan of helping her reestablish control in her life will also be an important part of her overall therapy.

Evaluation and Outcome Criteria

A sleep diary, as suggested for assessment, is an excellent resource for evaluation. Reviewing the diary with the client suffering from sleep-wake disturbance can provide further opportunity for positive reinforcement on accomplishments and for revised goal setting.

The Nursing Process and Clients with Psychiatric Disorders Characterized by Associated Sleep Disturbance

Sleep disturbances that are secondary to psychiatric disorders generally fall into one of the four symptom categories already discussed. While recognizing that a cyclical relationship is usually involved, it is helpful to try to differentiate primary sleep disorders from those that are secondary to a psychiatric disorder. Such differentiation can be particularly important for clients with depression, anxiety, and/or dementia. Sleep deprivation can lead to restlessness, reduced concentration, and, if prolonged, hallucinations and delusions (Kaplan, Sadock, and Grebb 1994). Likewise, chronic sleep deprivation may exacerbate dementia behaviors.

Maria, an elderly client, was recently hospitalized for acute management of a chronic medical condition. She was known to have early dementia of the Alzheimer's type but had been managing alone in her apartment up to this point. Over a period of several days, she became increasingly agitated, demanding cigarettes from nursing staff, other clients, and visitors. Attempts at distraction or providing unsolicited attention were unsuccessful. A student nurse began questioning how much sleep this woman had been getting. At that point the nurse's only cues were the lack of Maria's success with other interventions and her knowledge that sundowning is common in clients with dementia. The brief chart notes made by the night staff offered little information. From a neighbor who came to visit, she found out that prior to the hospitalization, Maria had been phoning her a couple of times during the night in an agitated state. The night staff agreed to observe and record the amount of time the client spent sleeping. Day staff did the same. With this additional data it was soon apparent that Maria was averaging no more than 4 hours of sleep per 24-hour period. Meanwhile, her agitated behavior was increasing.

After a client conference in which the student nurse offered her hypothesis of Sleep Pattern Disturbance, the physician agreed to try a mild short-acting hypnotic for the next three nights. Nursing staff continued to monitor Maria's sleep patterns and behavior. By the end of the three nights during which she did appear to sleep for longer periods, the agitated behavior and demands for cigarettes subsided considerably.

The use of hypnotics was not a long-term solution for the client in the above example, but it broke the escalating cycle of increasing agitation and decreasing sleep. Recognition of the role of sleep deprivation in contributing to a daytime behavior problem can facilitate effective short-term intervention and create a context for more comprehensive assessment of possible contributing factors, such as fear, relocation stress, powerlessness, or sensory and/or perceptual alterations.

Differentiation of sleep disorder secondary to psychiatric disorder from primary sleep disorder is a complex process that requires collaboration among clients, families, and health professionals. The sequence of onset may provide a clue. Many persons with unipolar depressive disorder initially present to family physicians or sleep clinics with insomnia. As in the example above, it may take a trial of an intervention known to be effective for one or the other type of disorder to help clarify the primary diagnosis.

As a psychiatric nurse, you will often need to be vigilant for the potential effects of a mismatched primary diagnosis with intervention. A depressed client misdiagnosed as having a primary sleep disorder of insomnia may be at risk of suicide if given a usual supply of hypnotic medication; likewise, obstructive sleep apnea with modest ingestion of alcohol can be mislabeled as alcohol abuse. As in any area of nursing practice, all components of the nursing process must be carefully and critically used.

Chapter Highlights

- Sleep pattern disturbance frequently accompanies mental disorders. Certain sleep disorders are also common in the general population, such as sleep apnea, and they will also be seen in a portion of the psychiatric population.
- REM rebound occurs after the abrupt discontinuation of REM-suppressing substances such as alcohol or most antidepressant medications.
- Dysomnias are characterized by difficulty initiating or maintaining sleep, or excessive sleepiness. They may arise from internal factors, environmental factors, or as a result of disruption in circadian rhythms.
- Parsomnias are disorders of arousal or sleep stage transition. Abnormalities in the normal loss of muscle tone during REM sleep are thought to account for parasomnias such as sleepwalking and sleep paralysis.
- Sleep pattern disturbances accompany and sometimes precede mental disorders such as schizophrenia and unipolar and bipolar disorder.
- Four major symptoms characterize the different types of sleep disorders: insomnia, hypersomnia, parasomnia, and sleep-wake schedule disturbance.
- Establishing a consistent rising time regardless of the amount of sleep is one of the most important interventions for insomnia. Reducing the total time in bed helps consolidate sleep and improve its quality.
- Establishing a regular sleep-wake schedule and increasing environmental time cues can be helpful in managing insomnia, hypersomnia, and sleep-wake schedule disturbance.
- Management of underlying mental disorders and other major stressors usually has reciprocal benefits in reducing sleep pattern disturbances.

References

Adam K: Dietary habits and sleep after bedtime food drinks. *Sleep* 1980;3(1):47–58.

American Psychiatric Association: *Diagnostic and Statistical Manual of Mental Disorders,* ed 4. American Psychiatric Association, 1994.

American Sleep Disorders Association (ASDA): *The International Classification of Sleep Disorders: Diagnostic and Coding Manual.* ASDA, 1990.

Beel-Bates CA, Rogers AE: An exploratory study of sundown syndrome. *J Neurosci Nurs* 1990;22(1):51–52.

Benson KL, Faull KF, Zarcone Jr, VP: Evidence for the role of serotonin in the regulation of slow wave sleep in schizophrenia. *Sleep* 1991;14(2):133–139.

Bliwise DL: Dementia, in Kryger MH, Roth T, Dement WC (eds): *Principles and Practice of Sleep Medicine,* ed 2. Saunders, 1994.

Bootzin RR, Manber R, Perlis ML, Salvio MA, Wyatt JK: Sleep disorders, in Sutker PB, Adams HE (eds): *Comprehensive Handbook of Psychopathology,* ed 2. Plenum, 1993.

Cohen-Mansfield J, Marx MS: The relationship between sleep disturbances and agitation in a nursing home. *J Aging and Health* 1990;2(1):42–57.

Cox HC, Hinz MD, Lubno MA, Newfield SA, Ridenour NA, Slater MM, Sridaromont K: *Clinical Applications of Nursing Diagnosis: Adult, Child, Women's, Mental Health, Gerontic and Home Health Considerations,* ed 2. FA Davis, 1993.

Dinges DF, Broughton RJ: *Sleep and Alertness: Chronobiological, Behavioral, and Medical Aspects of Napping.* Raven Press, 1989.

Engle-Friedman M, Bootzin RR, Hazlewood L, Tsao C: An evaluation of behavioral treatments for insomnia in the older adult. *J Clin Psych* 1992;48(1):77–90.

Fredrickson PA, Richardson JW, Esther MS, Lin S: Sleep disorders in psychiatric practice. *Mayo Clinic Proc* 1990;65: 861–868.

Gillin JC: Sleep and psychoactive drugs of abuse and dependence. Kryger MH, Roth T, Dement WC (eds): *Principles and Practice of Sleep Medicine,* ed 2. Saunders, 1994.

Guilleminault C: Narcolepsy syndrome, in Kryger MH, Roth T, Dement WC (eds): *Principles and Practice of Sleep Medicine,* ed 2. Saunders, 1994.

Hoch C, Reynolds C, Houck P: Sleep patterns in Alzheimer's patients and healthy controls. *Scholarly Inquiry for Nurs Prac* 1988;1:221–235.

Hodgson LA: Why do we need sleep? Relating theory to nursing practice. *J Adv Nurs* 1991;16:1503–1510.

Horne JA: *Why We Sleep,* Oxford University Press, 1988.

Jensen DP, Herr KA: Sleeplessness. *Nurs Clin N Am* 1993; 28(2):385–405.

Kaplan HI, Sadock BJ, Grebb JA: *Kaplan and Sadock's Synopsis of Psychiatry,* ed 7. Williams & Wilkins, 1994.

Mahowald MW, Schenck CH: REM sleep behavior disorder, in Kryger MH, Roth T, Dement WC (eds): *Principles and Practice of Sleep Medicine,* ed 2. Saunders, 1994.

Mendelson WB: Insomnia and related sleep disorders. *Psychiatr Clin N Am* 1993a;16(4):841–851.

Mendelson WB: Pharmacologic alteration of the perception of being awake or asleep. *Sleep* 1993b;16(7):641–646.

Monti JM, Alterwain P, Estevez F, Alvarino F, Giusti M, Olivera S, Labraga P: The effects of Ritanserin on mood and sleep in abstinent alcoholic patients. *Sleep* 1993;16(7): 647–654.

Nowlin-Finch NL, Altshuler LL, Szuba MP, Mintz J: Rapid resolution of first episodes of mania: Sleep related? *J Clin Psychiatr* 1994;55(1):26–29.

Pivik RT: The psychobiology of dreams, in Kryger MH, Roth T, Dement WC (eds): *Principles and Practice of Sleep Medicine,* ed 2. Saunders, 1994.

Reimer M, Remmers J: Outcomes of CPAP treatment as perceived by OSA patients and their families. *1991 Annual Meeting Abstracts, Association of Professional Sleep Societies,* 5th Annual Meeting, Toronto, Canada, 1991.

Reynolds III, CF, Kupfer DJ: Sleep research in affective illness: State of the art circa 1987. *Sleep* 1987;10(3):199–215.

Roehrs T, Roth T: Chronic insomnias associated with circadian rhythm disorders, in Kryger MH, Roth T, Dement WC (eds): *Principles and Practice of Sleep Medicine,* ed 2. Saunders, 1994.

Rogers AE, Aldrich MS: The effect of regularly scheduled naps on sleep attacks and excessive daytime sleepiness associated with narcolepsy. *Nurs Res* 1993;42(2):111–117.

Shaver JL, Giblin E, Paulsen V: Sleep quality subtypes in midlife women. *Sleep* 1991;14:18–23.

Sutker PB, Adams HE: *Comprehensive Handbook of Psychopathology,* ed 2. Plenum, 1993.

Totterdell P, Reynolds S, Parkinson B, Briner RB: Associations of sleep with everyday mood, minor symptoms and social interaction experience. *Sleep* 1994;17(5):466–475.

CHAPTER 20

CLIENTS WITH PERSONALITY DISORDERS

Judy Banks Campbell
Noreen King Poole

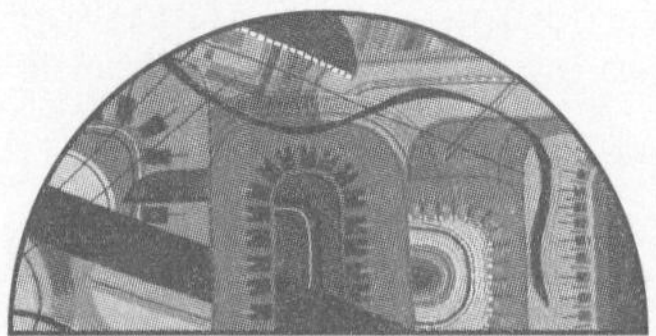

COMPETENCIES

- *Differentiate personality traits and styles from personality disorders.*
- *Compare and contrast biopsychosocial characteristics of various personality disorders.*
- *Correlate the* DSM-IV *with the nursing process in providing care for clients with personality disorders.*
- *Apply the nursing process in a variety of clinical and community settings with clients identified as having personality disorders.*
- *Distinguish the developmental and psychobiologic characteristics of selected personality disorders.*
- *Relate selected concepts, supported by research, to the nursing assessment, diagnosis, planning, implementation, and evaluation of clients who have personality disorders.*
- *Apply the nursing process in caring for clients who manifest angry and/or manipulative behavior.*
- *Discuss positive and negative effects of your emotional responses to clients who have personality disorders.*

Cross-References

Other topics relevant to this content are: Persistent mental illness, Chapter 21; Communication techniques, Chapter 7; Nursing process, Chapter 6; Psychiatric theories, Chapter 2; Clients with a dual diagnosis, Chapter 25.

Critical Thinking Challenge

As a newly employed nurse on a crisis stabilization unit, you get a request from one of your clients to bend the rules for her and extend her pass for two hours longer in order that she may meet her boyfriend for dinner before her return to the unit. When you question the legitimacy of this request and suggest that she get approval from the treatment team, the client becomes angry and accuses you of "not being the caring nurse" she thought you were. She states that she will remember this incident and warn her friends about the unfeeling nurses at this facility. What effect can clients with manipulative, perfectionistic, aggressive, impulsive, and resistive behavior have on the milieu of a therapeutic unit? How would you handle this situation with the client? What ethical dilemmas can you identify in this situation?

Working with an impatient, manipulative, self-centered, or overly suspicious person can be trying, at best. Many people demonstrate persistent behavioral patterns that do not significantly interfere with their lives but may charm, annoy, or frustrate others. Such behavioral patterns may be called **personality traits** or styles, and they often define the uniqueness of the individual.

Frank consistently compliments his female coworkers. They, in turn, prepare his lunches, lend him money, and make excuses for his sloppy work performance.

Alice interrupts a supervisory meeting to borrow a stapler. She is surprised when her behavior is criticized.

Whenever Keith is asked a personal question, he responds, "Why do you want to know?"

Jill contributes to daily team conferences only when her input is solicited. She prefaces her comments with, "You probably won't think this is important, but. . . ."

Lance offers detailed descriptions of his personal life to anyone who will listen. Quickly bored with his monologues, his listeners do not return for "seconds."

These lifelong patterns are exhibited in a variety of social and personal experiences, and generally anxiety is absent (Eaton, Peterson, and Davis 1976). These relatively stable patterns, however, may become rigid and maladaptive, cause significant personal distress, and impair social functioning. When this happens, these personality traits or styles are called **personality disorders.** Since people with personality disorders experience problems in living rather than clinical symptoms, they may not seek professional help unless there is extreme external stress and/or internal distress (APA 1994).

The psychiatric nurse encounters people with personality disorders in a variety of settings, including the workplace, counseling centers, general hospitals, and forensic facilities. Widiger and Frances (1985) point out that the essential features of personality disorders are chronicity, pervasiveness, and maladaptation. These authors state that all three features must be present to make a psychiatric diagnosis.

The *DSM-IV* delineates diagnostic criteria for personality disorders on the Axis II. Essential features of these disorders include significant distress or impairment in at least two of the following areas of functioning: cognition, affect, interpersonal relationships, or impulse control. The *DSM-IV* points out that these behavior patterns must be evident by early adulthood and not accounted for by other mental disorders or the effects of substance use (drugs, alcohol, medications, etc.) (APA 1994). It is important to distinguish the behaviors that define personality disorders from responses that may emerge from specific situational stressors or transient mental states. Therefore, it is often necessary and important to conduct more than one interview with the client, over a period of time. While personality-disordered people display enduring, inflexible, and pervasive maladaptive behaviors in a broad variety of personal, occupational, and social situations, they may or may not view their lifestyles as abnormal or intrusive. For the general diagnostic criteria for a personality disorder, see the accompanying box.

DSM-IV Diagnostic Criteria for a Personality Disorder

A. An enduring pattern of inner experience and behavior that deviates markedly from the expectations of the individual's culture. This pattern is manifested in two (or more) of the following areas:
   1. Cognition (i.e., ways of perceiving and interpreting self, other people, and events).
   2. Affectivity (i.e., the range, intensity, lability, and appropriateness of emotional response).
   3. Interpersonal functioning.
   4. Impulse control.

B. The enduring pattern is inflexible and pervasive across a broad range of personal and social situations.

C. The enduring pattern leads to clinically significant distress or impairment in social, occupational, or other important areas of functioning.

D. The pattern is stable and of long duration and its onset can be traced back at least to adolescence or early adulthood.

E. The enduring pattern is not better accounted for as a manifestation or consequence of another mental disorder.

F. The enduring pattern is not due to the direct physiological effects of a substance (e.g., a drug of abuse, a medication) or a general medical condition (e.g., head trauma).

Source: American Psychiatric Association 1994, p. 633.

If we assume a common developmental course for the emergence of a person's personality, different levels of adjustment may occur. Consequently, one individual may view peculiarities as "natural" or "eccentric"—**ego-syntonic**—and seek no change, while a second person may feel tension and conflict as the behaviors become increasingly rigid and lead to difficulties in a variety of social activities—**ego-dystonic.** The person may begin to view a characteristic once valued to be unique as a weakness. This changed perspective leads to dissatisfaction and disequilibrium, which may motivate the person to seek therapy. Our society contributes to such lack of insight by discouraging direct confrontation and feedback about self-defeating behaviors, thus delaying intervention.

Personality disorders may coexist with extreme psychopathology, considered under *DSM-IV* Axis I groupings. In addition, under stress, the individual with a

Table 20–1 Clusters of Personality Disorders

Odd-Eccentric	*Dramatic-Emotional*	*Anxious-Fearful*
Paranoid	Borderline	Avoidant
Schizoid	Histrionic	Dependent
Schizotypal	Narcissistic	Obsessive-compulsive
	Antisocial	

Source: Adapted from American Psychiatric Association 1994, pp. 629–630.

personality disorder may progressively deteriorate even to the point of psychosis.

Three major clusters of personality disorders guide psychiatric nurses in diagnostic, treatment, and research issues (see Table 20–1). These clusters are Cluster A, odd-eccentric, Cluster B, dramatic-emotional, and Cluster C, anxious-fearful. The **odd-eccentric** category includes paranoid, schizoid, and schizotypal personality disorders. The **dramatic-emotional** category includes borderline histrionic, narcissistic, and antisocial personality disorders. The **anxious-fearful** category includes avoidant, dependent, and obsessive-compulsive personality disorders.

These clusters establish criteria for distinct disorders according to the presence or absence of symptoms that do not characterize major thought, perceptual, or mood disorders. Because individuals often have personality characteristics that overlap DSM-IV categories and clusters, mental health care professionals are encouraged to use multiple Axis II diagnoses in order of importance. It should be noted that while these cluster groupings may be useful in some research and educational situations, they have not been consistently validated (APA 1994).

As the psychiatric nurse becomes familiar with the psychodynamics and behaviors of people with personality disorders, the following common features emerge:

- Restricted or exaggerated development of a particular pattern or trait.
- Restricted or exaggerated moral development.
- Restricted or exaggerated problem-solving skills.
- Seriously impaired ability to develop meaningful interpersonal relationships and communications.
- Difficulty in adjusting to social or occupational relationships.
- Defensive coping strategies against real or perceived threats to the sense of self.
- A lifelong pattern of responding that is consistent in most situations and that becomes accentuated in stressful situations.
- A self-stabilizing and self-perpetuating level of functioning despite distorted coping strategies.
- Exaggerated or restricted affective responses to the environment (overly sensitive, unemotional, "cold").
- Conflict with others, either in the immediate family or in society.
- Lack of awareness that others view the lifestyle as different or unusual.
- Impulsive behavior seeking immediate gratification.

Biopsychosocial Theories

Our styles of perceiving, thinking, and responding shape our ability to adapt and defend our sense of self (Shapiro 1965). As the individual experiences life, adaptive-defensive operations solidify, ultimately crystallizing into an automatic response style. When the response style is based on misperceived or distorted object relations, a personality disorder may emerge. Given these premises, the psychiatric nurse using a biopsychosocial model views clients with personality disorders as people whose communication and behavior are greatly influenced by past experiences, a need to maintain self-direction and control, and a unique style of interpreting their world.

Little systematic research has been conducted on the causes or treatment of personality disorders (Widiger and Frances 1985). Furthermore, debate continues about the developmental course of personality disorders. Some theorists argue that their course of development is different from that of anxiety-related and psychotic forms of maladaptation. Other theorists see personality disorders as belonging in a developmental continuum that includes personality disorders, anxiety-related disorders, and psychoses. The accompanying box presents characteristics of the personality disorders as described in the *DSM-IV.*

Biologic Factors

Recent literature points to genetic and biologic factors in the development of some personality disorders. Using studies from 15,000 pairs of monozygotic and dizygotic twins in the United States, Kaplan and Sadock (1991) identified significant familial correlations of schizotypal personality disorder (Cluster A) among people with family members who are schizophrenic. Cluster B illnesses (borderline, histrionic, narcissistic, and antisocial) are often correlated with histories of mood disorders, alcoholism, and somatization disorders among family members. Loranger and Tulis (1985) also report that borderline clients have a significantly higher family history of alcoholism compared to healthy clients.

McCormick (1993) notes that biologic factors may play a major role in the development of obsessive-compulsive

Characteristics of Personality Disorders

Odd-Eccentric Styles (Cluster A)

Paranoid

Is pervasively and unjustifiably suspicious and mistrustful, as evidenced by jealousy, accusations of infidelity, and guardedness. Is hypersensitive and usually feels mistreated and misjudged. Restricts feelings, as evidenced by lack of humor, absence of sentimental or tender feelings, and pride in being cold and unemotional. Bears grudges and is quick to counterattack.

Schizoid

Is emotionally cold and aloof. Shows indifference to the praise or criticism of others. Has little or no desire for social or sexual involvement. Does not desire or enjoy close relationships. Has few friends.

Schizotypal

Manifests various oddities of thought, perceptions, speech, affect, and behavior, such as ideas of reference, bizarre fantasies, and preoccupations. Is suspicious and hypersensitive to real or imagined criticism. Isolates self from society because of acute discomfort.

Dramatic-Emotional Styles (Cluster B)

Borderline

Is impulsive and unpredictable in areas of life that are self-damaging. Has unstable but intense interpersonal relationships involving manipulation of others. Displays temper inappropriately. Has unstable moods (including rage); is uncertain about identity, and may experience severe dissociative symptoms. May inflict physical damage on self. Has chronic feelings of boredom and emptiness. Fears abandonment.

Histrionic

Is overly dramatic and reactive, and responds intensely. Engages in attention seeking, self-dramatization, sexual provocation, and irrational outbursts of emotion. Is perceived by others as shallow, self-indulgent, and demanding. Uses appearance and style of speech to draw attention to self. Is suggestible and overrates the intimacy of relationships.

Narcissistic

Has grandiose sense of self-importance. Is preoccupied with fantasies of unlimited success, power, beauty, brilliance, etc. Needs attention and admiration. Shows an arrogant attitude based on feelings of entitlement and envy. In relationships with others, expects special favors. Takes advantage of others; shifts between overidealizing others to disregarding them. Lacks ability for empathy.

Antisocial

Engages in behavior that causes conflict with society, such as theft, vandalism, fighting, delinquency, truancy, lying. Is unable to sustain consistent work or to function as a responsible parent or spouse. Cannot maintain an enduring attachment to a sex partner. Lacks respect and loyalty; is irritable and aggressive. Manipulates others for personal gain, does not plan ahead, lacks guilt, does not learn from past experiences, blames others. Disregards the safety of self and others.

Anxious-Fearful Styles (Cluster C)

Avoidant

Is hypersensitive to rejection and interprets innocuous events as ridicule. Is unwilling to become involved with others unless given a guarantee of acceptance. Withdraws socially in interpersonal and work roles; avoids new situations. Desires affection and acceptance, yet shows restraint in intimate situations for fear of ridicule. Feels inept and infuriated.

Dependent

Passively allows others to assume responsibility for major areas of life. Subordinates own needs. Lacks self-confidence and initiative. Has difficulty disagreeing with others. Fears being alone so urgently seeks a close relationship.

Obsessive-Compulsive

Is overconscientious, overmeticulous, and perfectionistic. Is excessively concerned with conformity. Adheres rigidly to strict standards of morality and values. Is preoccupied with trivial details, rules, schedules, and lists. Keeps worthless objects. Is unable to delegate without control. Is miserly and stubborn.

Source: Adapted from American Psychiatric Association 1994, pp. 629-673.

personality disorder (Cluster C), with basal ganglia and frontal cortex dysfunctions being suspect. Because selective serotonin reuptake inhibitors (SSRIs) have proven so effective as both antidepressive and antiobsessive agents, Zetin and Kramer (1992) suggest that there may be biologic factors common to both these disorders. Dillon and Brooks (1992) discuss possible links between changes in progesterone levels in college-age women and obsessive-compulsive disorders. This study was based on a small sample, and subjective recordings and discussions were the primary methodologies used. It is also reported that people with obsessive-compulsive personality disorder have biologic indicators associated with clinical depression (shortened REM latency period and abnormal Dexamethasone Supression Test results). It is worth noting that among monozygotic twins, the concordance for personality disorders was much higher than that of dizygotic twins (Kaplan and Sadock 1991). This literature review also suggests that CNS dysfunctions in early childhood and children with minimal brain damage are at higher risk for the development of some types of Cluster B personality disorders. This speculation is supported by Andrulonis et al. (1980), who reports organic involvement, including episodes of minimal brain dysfunction and episodic dyscontrol syndromes among subjects in an intensive study of borderline personality disorder.

Additional biologic factors associated with personality-disordered individuals as reported by Kaplan and Sadock (1991) include alterations in hormone levels and platelet MAO levels, smooth-pursuit eye movements, levels of endorphin and 5-HIAA (a metabolite of serotonin), and EEG changes.

Psychosocial Theories

Psychologic fixations in the genital stage of development may account for many of the behaviors noted in the dramatic-emotional cluster of personality disorders (Cameron and Rychlak 1985). Research data lend support to the concept of **separation-individuation** as the psychodynamic basis of borderline personality disorder (Mahler, Pine, and Bergman 1975; Masterson 1981). Benner and Joscelyne (1984) also suggest that the borderline personality is the foundation for dissociative identity disorder.

As a result of research done with borderline personality clients, several theoretic concepts have been identified as applicable to this group. Erik Erikson (1964) coined the term **identity diffusion** to describe the failure to integrate various childhood identifications into a harmonious adult psychosocial identity. Kernberg (1975) suggests that when, as infants, borderline clients perceive their mothers as both nurturing and punishing, the child learns to reduce anxiety and resolve resulting conflicts by the use of primitive defensive strategies including splitting, projective identification, primitive idealization, omnipotence, devaluation, and denial. These will be discussed later in the chapter.

In summary, a person's style of functioning is shaped by the following:

- Biopsychosocial characteristics
- Object relations
- Reinforcement of behavioral responses

Table 20–2 describes the preceding developmental concepts and their interaction. It is only when we acknowledge the individual's response style and definition of a situation that we can identify the subjective meaning of a thought, feeling, or behavior for that person.

Martha, a 49-year-old secretary, is a perfectionist and shows exaggerated loyalty to her company. Most of her energies are directed toward work and being indispensable to her employer. She consistently takes work home at night and on weekends, even postponing her vacation to complete elaborate, detailed reports. Martha's relationships with coworkers focus on work only; she is unable to socialize with coworkers without experiencing extreme anxiety. Consequently, others view her as rigid, isolated, cold, and tense. They try to avoid relating to her. During a performance evaluation, when her employer pointed out her defensive peer relationships, Martha became irritable and pressured, stating, "I was not hired to socialize. Those people who complain should be doing their work and earning the paychecks they receive."

In the example above, Martha's definition of any situation is based on her narrow view of the world and her purpose in it. When confronted with her behavior, she does not attend to personal issues but rather focuses on the technical details of the situation. Martha justifies her position by falling back on the rules and regulations that reinforce her own moral convictions. Even with her distorted strategies, she is able to achieve stable functioning. As a result, people interacting with Martha generally choose not to confront the frustrating behaviors. Instead, they accept her "peculiarities" as a trade-off for her work performance. The likelihood that Martha will change her response style is minimal unless she experiences deep dissatisfaction and begins to examine her own personality traits.

Odd-Eccentric Personality Disorders

As mentioned earlier, the *DSM-IV* categorizes as odd-eccentric the **paranoid**, **schizoid**, and **schizotypal personality disorders.** The major features of these disorders are pervasive distrust, social detachment, and consequent impairment in social and occupational functioning.

Table 20–2 Factors Influencing Style of Functioning

Factor	*Definition*	*Example*
Biopsychosocial characteristics	Unique endowment of qualities, including genetic factors, biologic factors, mental ability, and social group	An 8-year-old Korean child is adopted by white American parents. The child experiences rejection from his classmates because of his physical characteristics. Consequently, he begins to avoid situations, and he scrutinizes the behavior of others for hidden motives.
Object relations	Interaction between the individual and objects in the environment (people, material things, symbols)	An upwardly mobile professional couple demand perfection and conformity from their 7-year-old daughter. They discourage fantasy and creativity. The daughter procrastinates and follows directions half-heartedly in coping with her parents' demands.
Reinforcement of behavioral responses	A reward or punishment that strengthens or weakens a person's responses	A highly anxious mother gives in to her child's demands when the child has a temper tantrum; she fails to respond positively to the child's "good" behaviors. The child rarely makes polite requests, but interrupts, screams, and shouts for attention.

Interaction of Factors

The medicine man of the Hopi Indians sometimes uses meditation to diagnose illnesses. He may even use a crystal ball as his focal point during meditation. At other times the Hopi medicine man chews roots of jimsonweed (datura) to go into a trance as he meditates. The Hopis believe that the ensuing hallucinations are visions of the evil that caused the sickness. After the meditation, he prescribes an appropriate herbal treatment; for example, a fever is "cured" by a plant that smells like lightning. Indeed, the Hopi phrase for fever is "lightning sickness" (Spector 1985).

These disorders have been observed in family members of people with schizophrenia (Kendler et al. 1984).

Familial patterns vary among disorders in the odd-eccentric cluster. Some studies show a 2:1 male-to-female ratio in clients with schizoid personality disorder (Kaplan and Sadock 1991). Schizotypal personality disorder is seen in approximately 3% of the population and is often apparent during childhood or adolescence. Of the disorders in this group, the one most commonly seen in inpatient psychiatric settings is paranoid personality disorder (APA 1994).

People with odd-eccentric personality disorders have been identified as having more cognitive style impairments than people with the disorders in the other *DSM-IV* clusters (Torgensen 1984; Widiger and Frances 1985). The odd-eccentric disorders are the most peculiar and reflect the most maladaptive defensive styles.

The Nursing Process and Clients with Paranoid Personality Disorder

Assessment

When conducting an interview with a client who has paranoid personality disorder, maintain an open, nonpressuring style of questioning. Do not argue with or interpret the client's responses. Because these clients may hold grudges and be quick to counterattack, consider safety provisions. For the diagnostic criteria for paranoid personality disorder, see the box on the next page.

SUBJECTIVE DATA Paranoid clients will report that others plot against them or attempt to use or deceive them. They will talk about disloyal friends and coworkers and the irreversible harm others' actions have caused. They may be surprised and mistrustful of loyalty shown to them. They may refuse to answer questions, saying, "This is no one's business." If you, the nurse, are unavoidably late, the client may interpret it as premeditated and may hold a grudge and be unwilling to forgive. Clients may report anger and disappointment at the actions of others. The self-fulfilling prophecy occurs when the client is rejected by those he or she mistrusts and accuses. A frequent theme in client interviews is one of pathologic suspicion of spousal or partner infidelity. During the interview, grandiose, unrealistic fantasies often emerge; clients may discuss activities with others who share their beliefs, such as special interest groups or cults. Client affect may be labile with hostile, stubborn sarcasm predominant.

OBJECTIVE DATA

Suspiciousness and Mistrust Suspiciousness and mistrust reflect an attitude of doubt toward the trustworthiness of objects or people. The suspicious person is usually preoccupied with being maneuvered, tricked, or framed. Suspiciousness is also a way of thinking and includes such manifestations as expectations of trickery or harm, guardedness, secretiveness, pathologic jealousy, and overconcern with hidden motives and special meanings. For example, the suspicious person may perceive a birthday gift as a trick to create an obligation. Legal disputes may arise from the client's response to perceived threats.

DSM-IV Diagnostic Criteria for Paranoid Personality Disorder

A. A pervasive distrust and suspiciousness of others such that their motives are interpreted as malevolent, beginning by early adulthood and present in a variety of contexts, as indicated by four (or more) of the following:
   1. Suspects, without sufficient basis, that others are exploiting, harming, or deceiving him or her.
   2. Is preoccupied with unjustified doubts about the loyalty or trustworthiness of friends or associates.
   3. Is reluctant to confide in others because of unwarranted fear that the information will be used maliciously against him or her.
   4. Reads hidden demeaning or threatening meanings into benign remarks or events.
   5. Persistently bears grudges, i.e., is unforgiving of insults, injuries, or slights.
   6. Perceives attacks on his or her character or reputation that are not apparent to others and is quick to react angrily or to counterattack.
   7. Has recurrent suspicions, without justification, regarding fidelity of spouse or sexual partner.

B. Does not occur exclusively during the course of Schizophrenia, a Mood Disorder With Psychotic Features, or another Psychotic Disorder and is not due to the direct physiological effects of a general medical condition.

Note: If criteria are met prior to the onset of Schizophrenia, add "Premorbid," e.g., "Paranoid Personality Disorder (Premorbid)."

Source: American Psychiatric Association 1994, p. 637.

Rigidity Paranoid people are inflexible in their perception of the world. They are preoccupied with their expectations of others and relentlessly try to confirm these expectations, often through argumentation. They closely examine rational arguments and contrary information, but with prejudice. The paranoid person justifies a position by excessive rationalization, rejecting any evidence refuting the original notion. It is not unusual for a paranoid person to suspect people with opposing ideas. Paranoid clients go to great lengths to prove a point, making mountains out of molehills. A need to be in control and have power is another characteristic, as is a preoccupation with the rank and status of oneself and others. The need to be self-sufficient may give rise to difficulty in working with others.

Hypervigilance Hypervigilance refers to a tendency to be a keen, penetrating observer, far more attentive and acute than the ordinary person (Shapiro 1965). Constant sensitivity to nuances in social relations, interpretation of both open and hidden attitudes of others, and scrutiny are modes of operation.

Following a bomb threat that occurred one year ago, a unit clerk opens and inspects every package brought into the ICU by staff and visitors, anticipating that someone will bring weapons into the unit.

Distortions of Reality Although paranoid people may perceive facts accurately, they invest them with a special significance. In this way, they create a private reality. They have a special interest in hidden motives, underlying purposes, special meanings, and the like. They do not necessarily disagree with the average observer about the existence of any given fact, only about its meaning and significance. Therefore, even severely paranoid people can recognize various essential facts well enough to achieve a limited adjustment to the normal social world. At the same time, however, they continue to interpret substantial portions of this world autistically. They often have difficulty distinguishing real from imagined offenses. The individual's distorted attitudes antagonize others and may lead to real discrimination.

Ellen is a paranoid woman who is quick to detect signs of anger, jealousy, and rejection in the actions of her coworkers. She magnifies these negative aspects and overlooks such positive behaviors as humor, support, and empathy. Eventually, Ellen's coworkers begin to snicker when she makes public statements, and they gossip about her.

Projection Paranoid people attribute to external figures their own intolerable motivations, drives, or feelings. Some psychiatric theorists believe that paranoid people use projection to attribute to others the evil intentions that they themselves feel. In this way, the idea that one may be harmed really reflects the individual's own wish to harm others.

Nancy's idea that her boyfriend is seeing another woman may reflect her wish to terminate their relationship.

Restricted Affect Labile emotional expressiveness and a lack of spontaneity characterize paranoid people. They often appear cold, humorless, and devoid of tender, sensitive feelings, although they may demonstrate temper outbursts. Usually, they pride themselves on remaining objective and reasonable and frequently use intellectualization and rationalization to avoid affective experiences. Some paranoid people may appear friendly, but in fact this friendliness is a "script" that helps them adapt to social situations or achieve their goals.

The Process of Exclusion Because of the paranoid person's antagonism, suspiciousness, and restricted object relations, tension develops between the person and significant others. The persistent strain on relationships causes others to define the paranoid person as more than simply "different." Instead, they see the individual as unreliable or untrustworthy, and others begin to interact according to their perceptions. These behaviors reinforce the suspicions and beliefs of the paranoid person. The effects of this process include the following:

- Blocked communication, which increases the process of exclusion.
- Emergence of a crisis, which formally excludes the paranoid person.
- Reinforcement of the paranoid person's beliefs, interpretations, or ideas of reference.

Because paranoid people are generally intelligent, persuasive, and creative in justifying their beliefs, these clients may adapt in one of two ways. They may join quasipolitical groups, esoteric religions, cults, or quasiscientific organizations that reinforce their interpretations of reality. Or they may join organizations that challenge societal norms and trends in an effort to direct and thus control hostile feelings. An example of a paranoid person's behavior is given below.

Jim, a 39-year-old engineer, suspects that his employer is withholding significant data from him pertaining to an important job assignment. Jim began to question others about the reliability and integrity of his boss. Jim went to the plant one Sunday morning without authorization. A security guard found him going through the filing cabinets of his employer, who confronted him the following day and sent him to the employee assistance program nurse. During the interview, Jim states, "I knew he [the employer] was dishonest from the start. He never could give me a straight answer. As soon as I was almost on him, he sets me up to lose face and maybe my job."

Nursing Diagnosis

When conducting interviews or engaging in staff conferences involving clients with paranoid personality disorder, it is very important to remember that behavior is culturally defined. Many individuals, particularly those from minority and/or immigrant groups, are erroneously labeled mentally ill because their behaviors are not congruent with the expected standards of the health care team. Indeed, the clinical evaluation may reinforce suspiciousness, hostility, and acting-out behavior because the client is unfamiliar with and frightened by the process. It is also important to remember that paranoid traits may be adaptive in threatening situations. The diagnosis of paranoid personality disorder should be made only when the behavior is long-standing, maladaptive, and causes significant distress (APA 1994).

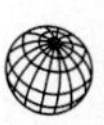

After gathering objective and subjective data about the paranoid client's behavior, you must categorize the information into problem areas designated as nursing diagnostic categories. It is critical to involve the client in all steps of the treatment planning process to enhance participation and promote planned changes. The general nursing diagnostic groupings that follow focus on psychosocial needs only. You will develop individualized care plans to address the unique needs of each client assessed.

DEFENSIVE COPING The client demonstrates impairment of adaptive behaviors in meeting life's demands. The paranoid personality may exhibit these forms of ineffective coping, among others:

- Suspiciousness
- Limited affect
- Reluctance to confide in others
- Carrying grudges
- Pessimistic regard for others

IMPAIRED THOUGHT PROCESSES The paranoid client experiences impaired cognitive functioning without loss of reality contact. Behaviors often observed include the following:

- Preoccupation with theories of conspiracies
- Hypervigilance and hypersensitivity
- Misinterpretation of benign remarks as threats
- Egocentricity and grandiosity
- Perseveration
- Impaired problem solving

IMPAIRED SOCIAL INTERACTION The predominant interactional dysfunctions of the paranoid personality are distortions and the overuse of defense mechanisms related to high levels of fear and anxiety. Interactional impairments include the following:

- Failure to interpret messages accurately
- Stereotyping others
- Judgmental attitudes toward others
- Failure to listen actively

INTERVENTION

The Paranoid Client

Nursing Diagnosis: Defensive Coping (Related factors: exclusion, restricted and controlled affect, guardedness, reclusiveness, and secretiveness)

Nursing Intervention	***Rationale***
• Respect client's privacy and preferences as much as is reasonable.	• Predictable environments (schedules, consistent caregivers, etc.) foster trust.
• Give feedback to client based on observed nonverbal cues of responsiveness, such as eye movement, posturing, voice tones.	
• Point out inconsistent behaviors such as affect and verbalization.	
• Provide a daily schedule of activities and inform client of changes as needed.	• Activity schedules will diminish anxiety about social interactions and may help ensure participation.
• Help client identify adaptive diversionary activities (leisure, recreation) in one-to-one sessions and groups.	• Participation in groups may increase client's support system.
• Use role playing to help client identify feelings, thoughts, and responses brought on by stressful situations.	• Rehearsing social behaviors in a safe environment provides immediate feedback and time for altering responses as necessary.
• Encourage an evaluation of how client behaviors led to the current crisis.	

Nursing Diagnosis: Impaired Thought Processes (Related factors: suspiciousness, rigidity, distortions of reality, projection, and hypersensitivity)

Nursing Intervention	***Rationale***
• Say firmly and kindly that you do not share client's interpretations of an event but do acknowledge client's feelings.	• Responding to client feelings will diminish anxiety even though the delusional thinking is not supported.
• Follow through on commitments made to client, including contracts.	• Direct, clear communication will diminish opportunities for misunderstanding, misinterpretation, and search for hidden meanings.
• Assign the same staff member to work with client to establish consistency and trust.	
• Give positive reinforcement for successes in a matter-of-fact manner.	
• Respond honestly to client at all times.	
• Refocus conversation to reality-based topics, and set limits on duration and frequency of suspicious concerns during one-to-one sessions and groups.	• It may not be possible for client to give up a delusional belief quickly or completely; spending a limited amount of time discussing the idea will decrease anxiety and help client slowly relinquish the delusion or suspicion.
• Do not argue with illogical assertions; simply point out that you do not share the same beliefs.	

→

INTERVENTION *(continued)*

Nursing Intervention	*Rationale*
• Remain calm, nonthreatening, and nonjudgmental at all interactions.	
• Give clear information regarding confidentiality and job-related consequences of counseling sessions.	
• Help client identify and verbalize feelings.	
• Respond to suspicious ideas by focusing on feelings: "It must be distressing . . ."; "You see him as vindictive. . . ."	
• Include client in formulating the treatment plan.	• Client-centered goals increase compliance.

Nursing Diagnosis: Impaired Social Interaction (Related factors: argumentativeness, critical comments about others, arrogance, aggressiveness, and defensiveness)

Nursing Intervention	*Rationale*
• Use an objective, matter-of-fact approach with client.	• Client will identify the nurse as a reliable person who will respect him or her without argument.
• Use concrete, specific words rather than global abstractions.	
• Give feedback concerning behavior.	• Giving reality-based feedback while acknowledging client's feelings will establish trust and facilitate problem solving.
• Identify feelings presented by client during interactions. For example, "I notice some reluctance on your part to tell me about that"; or "From the way you are looking at me, I wonder if you think I'll break my promise."	
• Direct client to clarify the person or object when pronouns are used.	
• Keep verbal and nonverbal messages clear and consistent.	
• Conduct brief one-to-one sessions daily (avoid prolonged sessions).	• Shortened one-to-one sessions decrease fear and anxiety.
• Encourage client to express feelings through creative modes (drawing, writing) and to discuss them.	• Nonverbal expression of feelings is often safer for client.
• Involve client in communication skills groups, such as assertiveness training, current events clubs.	• Identifying behaviors that impair social interactions may help client gain awareness of personal behaviors contributing to isolation.
• Gradually introduce client to group situations.	
• Inform client of the emotional cues he or she gives to others, such as suspiciousness, intimidation, or contempt. Encourage client to validate your perceptions.	• Self-awareness is enhanced with nonthreatening feedback (mirroring).

- Arrogance
- Aggressiveness
- Overuse of defense mechanisms of denial, rationalization, projection and intellectualization

Planning and Implementing Interventions

Nursing interventions with paranoid clients focus on mutual decision making. The goal of all interventions is to diminish the client's pervasive suspiciousness, distortions of thought, communication problems, and resulting impairment of role performance. See the Intervention box on page 478 for strategies for working with paranoid clients.

Because clients with paranoid personality disorder often appear arrogant as well as suspicious and antagonistic, staff members may feel intimidated in their presence. A paranoid client's persistent use of projection (targeted at both staff members and other clients) creates tension, frustration, and even a sense of powerlessness among staff members who may attempt to control the situation by becoming defensive and argumentative with the client. Clinical supervision, team meetings, and the consistent application of care plan intervention strategies will help the staff provide care while remaining objective in their responses to the client's maladaptive behavior patterns. Role playing is also useful in defusing staff anxiety.

DEFENSIVE COPING Clients with paranoid personality disorder have been using maladaptive and primitive defenses for a long time before experiencing sufficient distress to become involved in a psychotherapeutic program. Therefore, appropriate goal setting should include lessening of the client's suspicious behavior and establishing satisfying client interactions with the staff and significant others. Intervention strategies include:

- Give clear, simple directions, respecting client privacy as much as possible and maintaining confidentiality at all times.
- Because clients may not view their behavior as maladaptive or contributing to the difficulties being experienced, give feedback based on observed nonverbal and verbal cues; help clients see themselves as others see them.
- Point out inconsistencies between affect and verbalizations. While clients may become defensive and argumentative, your calm, objective, concerned approach will help diminish their anxiety.
- Provide clients with activity schedules, keep appointments, and inform clients of schedule changes as quickly as possible to increase participation in unit activities and acquaint them with a potential support system.
- As trust is established, encourage clients to examine their behavior to determine what changes would be desirable. Role playing also helps clients identify feelings, thoughts, and responses brought on by stressful situations.

IMPAIRED THOUGHT PROCESSES The patterns of suspiciousness, distrust, rigidity, hypervigilance, grandiosity, and aloofness that characterize clients with paranoid personality disorder lend themselves to setting goals that include developing a sense of reality, which is validated by others.

- Remain calm, nonthreatening, and nonjudgmental; an overly friendly approach may be threatening and may foster mistrust and misinterpretation.
- Answer the client's questions and requests honestly, and follow through with promises and commitments.
- Assign the same staff member to the client, to foster trust. Involve the client in treatment planning efforts.
- Give honest answers to questions concerning confidentiality and job-related consequences of treatment.
- When the client expresses beliefs that are not validated by reality, respond by saying, "I sense you are frightened by. . . ." Do not argue with the client's illogical assertions, but simply point out that you do not share the belief.
- Clients will experience heightened anxiety if not permitted to discuss their beliefs at all; therefore, set limits on the duration and frequency of such discussions during one-to-one sessions, and refocus the conversation to reality-based topics after an agreed-upon time.

All clients need positive reinforcement for appropriate behavior. With paranoid clients, offer such rewards in a matter-of-fact manner in order to avoid any misinterpretation of motives.

IMPAIRED SOCIAL INTERACTION Much of the basis for poor social relationships in clients with paranoid personality disorder is related to their lack of communication skills. These clients are argumentative, critical of others, arrogant, intrusive, aggressive, and often emotionally labile, which may lead to unpredictable outbursts. When others avoid them, they find their projections reinforced, and further alienation occurs. During the course of treatment, help clients express their thoughts and feelings verbally in a nonaggressive manner.

- Give direct, clear, matter-of-fact verbal messages.
- Use concrete terms rather than abstract generalities.
- Ask clients to clarify statements when they use pronouns.
- Conduct brief one-to-one sessions.
- Use communication and social skills groups to teach and reinforce verbal and nonverbal messages.

Evaluation and Outcome Criteria

Defensive Coping It is unlikely that paranoid clients will give up coping responses developed over a lifetime. Consistently used interventions, however, should reduce anxiety and allow clients to identify at least one significant person as trustworthy. At minimum, paranoid clients should be able to relax sufficiently in the presence of the nurse to explore how personal coping modes have created problems and to identify ways to avoid future conflicts with others.

Outcome criteria may include the following measurable behaviors:

- Expresses feelings without intellectualizing, threatening, or extreme sarcasm.
- Consensually validates perceptions of events with a staff member or significant others.
- Makes assertive, nonjudgmental statements to staff and other clients.
- Responds to feedback without rationalizing, projecting, or intellectualizing.
- Demonstrates decreased suspicion by interacting with the nurse at least once a day.

Impaired Thought Processes Consistency and structure help direct the client's thoughts to present reality. You can use role modeling to reach this goal—that is, the nurse tests reality appropriately to encourage the client to do the same. When clients begin to voice doubts about their interpretations or to identify alternative interpretations, you are in a position to reinforce their achievements. Many paranoid clients simply learn not to discuss their illogical or irrational beliefs with others.

Outcome criteria may include the following measurable behaviors:

- Focuses on ideas that are reality-based.
- Accepts positive feedback without questioning motives or hidden meanings.
- Accepts responsibiltiy for own feelings and thoughts without attributing them to others; makes "I" statements.
- Remains in a group activity for the duration of the activity.
- Realistically applies the problem-solving process, including making plans for after discharge.

Impaired Social Interaction The client should learn to make global statements concrete and to clarify verbal expressions. The client may learn to defuse anxiety-producing situations by making "I" statements rather than responding aggressively and judgmentally. Creative modes of expressing feelings are perceived as an acceptable, nonthreatening outlet. Behavior in groups should reflect the paranoid client's increasing ability to accept varying opinions without attaching personal significance to them.

Outcome criteria may include the following measurable behaviors:

- Attends and spontaneously participates in short one-to-one sessions and activity groups (less than 1 hour).
- Initiates one-to-one sessions with assigned staff member.
- Approaches other clients and staff without encouragement.
- Identifies personal behaviors that precipitated hospitalization.
- Demonstrates a variety of moods appropriate to the situation encountered.
- Attends to individual and group tasks without attaching unusual meanings to them.
- Identifies support systems outside the therapeutic relationship.
- Identifies feelings that minimize and maximize social interaction.

The Nursing Process and Clients with Schizoid and Schizotypal Personality Disorders

Assessment

When assessing both schizoid and schizotypal clients, it is imperative to consider the person's ethnicity, cultural milieu, and spiritual belief system. Within many cultures, speaking in tongues, rooting, voodoo, and psychic phenomena are natural experiences and should not be deemed pathologic. People who are making a transition from one environment to another—from a rural to an urban setting, for instance—may seem different because of their constricted affect and solitary activities. Immigrants must be assessed from a multicultural viewpoint in order to differentiate between lack of understanding and indifference. What may seem odd in Parker, Georgia, may be commonplace in New York City.

Individuals who are diagnosed with schizoid personality disorder are rarely seen in clinical settings, but schizotypal personality disorder is found in about 3% of the population, and these clients are frequently treated for symptoms associated with anxiety, depression, or dysphoric affect. Kaplan and Sadock (1991) have reported low platelet MAO in some schizotypal clients. Clients in both categories may experience transient psychotic

DSM-IV Diagnostic Criteria for Schizoid Personality Disorder

A. A pervasive pattern of detachment from social relationships and a restricted range of expression of emotions in interpersonal settings, beginning by early adulthood and present in a variety of contexts, as indicated by four (or more) of the following:
   1. Neither desires nor enjoys close relationships, including being part of a family.
   2. Almost always chooses solitary activities.
   3. Has little, if any, interest in having sexual experiences with another person.
   4. Takes pleasure in few, if any, activities.
   5. Lacks close friends or confidants other than first-degree relatives.
   6. Appears indifferent to the praise or criticism of others.
   7. Shows emotional coldness, detachment, or flattened affectivity.

B. Does not occur exclusively during the course of Schizophrenia, a Mood Disorder With Psychotic Features, another Psychotic Disorder, or a Pervasive Developmental Disorder and is not due to the direct physiological effects of a general medical condition.

Note: If criteria are met prior to the onset of Schizophrenia, add "Premorbid," e.g., "Schizoid Personality Disorder (Premorbid)."

Source: American Psychiatric Association 1994, p. 641.

episodes which may last a few minutes to several hours (APA 1994). For the diagnostic criteria for the two disorders, see the accompanying boxes.

SUBJECTIVE DATA When being interviewed, clients with schizoid personality disorder claim to enjoy being alone and to prefer occupations where there is minimal social interaction. They may decline job promotions because social demands (meetings, supervisory responsibilities, etc.) accompany the change. When asked if they think this loner-type behavior is unusual, a typical response is, "I never thought about it much . . . it doesn't much matter to me." Accompanying disclaimers about social needs, schizoid clients acknowledge that they rarely become excited, angry, upset, or joyful.

In contrast, clients with schizotypal personality disorder report a great deal of subjective anxiety in social situations. They report bizarre fantasies, especially of paranormal events. During an interview, they may remark,"I know what you're going to ask me before you say it," believing they are endowed with special powers or have the ability to control others' behavior by simply "willing it to happen." Often, these clients have speech patterns so loose, digressive, or vague that an interview is difficult to

DSM-IV Diagnostic Criteria for Schizotypal Personality Disorder

A. A pervasive pattern of social and interpersonal deficits marked by acute discomfort with, and reduced capacity for, close relationships as well as by cognitive or perceptual distortions and eccentricities of behavior, beginning by early adulthood and present in a variety of contexts, as indicated by five (or more) of the following:
   1. Ideas of reference (excluding delusions of reference).
   2. Odd beliefs or magical thinking that influences behavior and is inconsistent with subcultural norms (e.g., superstitiousness, belief in clairvoyance, telepathy, or "sixth sense"; in children and adolescents, bizarre fantasies or preoccupations).
   3. Unusual perceptual experiences, including bodily illusions.
   4. Odd thinking and speech (e.g., vague, circumstantial, metaphorical, overelaborate, or stereotyped).
   5. Suspiciousness or paranoid ideation.
   6. Inappropriate or constricted affect.
   7. Behavior or appearance that is odd, eccentric, or peculiar.
   8. Lack of close friends or confidants other than first-degree relatives.
   9. Excessive social anxiety that does not diminish with familiarity and tends to be associated with paranoid fears rather than negative judgments about self.

B. Does not occur exclusively during the course of Schizophrenia, a Mood Disorder With Psychotic Features, another Psychotic Disorder, or a Pervasive Developmental Disorder.

Note: If criteria are met prior to the onset of Schizophrenia, add "Premorbid," e.g., "Schizotypal Personality Disorder (Premorbid)."

Source: American Psychiatric Association 1994, p. 645.

conduct. The client may acknowledge this behavior by stating, "I was never talkable" (APA 1994).

While indifference is a hallmark of the schizoid personality, suspicion, including paranoid ideation, is noted in the schizotypal client. "Those people don't like me and have been trying to get rid of me since the day I was hired." Maintaining eye contact may be difficult during the interview, and interviewing strategies such as humor to defuse anxiety may be met with a stare and questions about the meaning of or purpose for the joking.

Onset of schizotypal personality disorder is believed to be in childhood or early adolescence, as clients report poor academic achievement and peer relationships as well as social anxiety, even as children. When questioned about sexual activity, clients in both groups usually deny interest in or involvement in intimate relationships.

People with schizoid and schizotypal personality disorders generally have a detached and aloof social style. The schizotypal personality, however, has more cognitive impairments than the schizoid personality does. There is a range of adjustment in clients with these personality disorders. Some are fairly well-adjusted individuals who are loners; others live out their lives in protective environments, such as group homes, mental hospitals, and prisons. When conducting assessments, rule out the possibility of a crisis response or chemical dependence.

Objective Data

Lifelong Patterns of Social Isolation These clients show a preference for solitary interests and occupations. They have a history of being loners and neither desire nor enjoy close relationships. Friends and confidants are not part of their lifestyle. They are indifferent to feedback and insensitive to others. These clients will choose solitary hobbies such as solitaire and computer games, and jobs such as night security guard or bridge worker. The detachment from social relationships is also noted in the schizoid or schizotypal personality's lack of interest in having intimate or sexual relationships.

Blunted Affective Response Clients may appear cool, aloof, humorless, "in a fog," bored, and perhaps even mentally retarded, although IQ would negate this perception (Cameron and Rychlak 1985). These individuals appear "joyless" and are slow to anger.

Detachment from the Environment These clients appear absent-minded: they daydream, are vague about goals, are indecisive, and lack social skills. They do not respond in a usual manner to social cues and may seem like social misfits.

The schizotypal personality demonstrates eccentricities in communication and behavior not seen in the schizoid personality. Examples include such oddities of thought as magical thinking and ideas of reference; altered perceptions, such as illusions, depersonalization, and derealization; speech alterations, including circumstantiality (giving detailed, factual but nonessential information), digression, metaphorical speech patterns, and overly concrete or abstract responses; and an odd or unkempt manner of dress, which includes ill-fitting, stained, and mismatched clothing.

Some researchers have found that schizoid and schizotypal personality disorders are significantly more common among first-degree relatives of schizophrenic clients. At this time, however, there is no substantial evidence that these personality disorders are early indicators of a future schizophrenic process (Kaplan and Sadock 1991; Kendler et al. 1984; Torgensen 1984).

Rhoda is a 40-year-old female seen in the emergency room of a large metropolitan hospital. She was brought in after experiencing a hypoglycemic episode at the factory where she has been employed for 15 years as a night maintenance worker. Rhoda's appearance is unkempt and eccentric. She is wearing three layers of clothing and mismatched shoes. Rhoda reports living in a one-room apartment 5 minutes' walk from her place of employment. During the nursing admission interview, Rhoda reports no family or significant others who are available to assist her. Rhoda makes frequent inappropriate grimaces and mutters to herself about getting "back home." She avoids eye contact and direct answers to the nurse's questions. She states, "I don't need any help. I have my own remedies that work just fine. Leave me alone." Following stabilization of her condition, Rhoda is released because she insists she must return to work.

Nursing Diagnosis

People with schizoid or schizotypal personality disorder are not a danger to themselves or others, a criterion used to authorize long-term hospitalization. However, 30–50% of those diagnosed with schizotypal personality disorder have a concurrent diagnosis of major depressive disorder when admitted to a mental health facility. It is also noted that other personality disorders in the odd-eccentric cluster occur concurrently in the schizotypal client (APA 1994).

These clients are found among homeless or marginal populations with limited resources, although some have the financial reserves to lead more adaptive lifestyles. They often come to the attention of health care professionals as a result of cluttered, negligent lifestyles that are considered ascocial, unaesthetic, and unhygienic. Assessment of these clients may be hampered by their preference for independence, in spite of the negative consequences such "freedom" may have. If you can sustain a relationship with these clients, the following NANDA nursing diagnoses are often the basis for guiding nursing care.

Impaired Social Interaction These clients have a narrow range of coping skills and tend to resist acquiring new skills if they must give up their independence as a result. The following problems signal impaired social relationships:

- Social isolation
- An absence of warm feelings for others
- Inadequate social skills
- Little or no desire for social encounters
- Lack of ongoing support systems
- Oddities of thinking

Impaired Verbal Communication Schizoid and schizotypal clients have minimal verbal and nonverbal interactions with others. Typical behaviors may include but are not restricted to the following:

- Aloofness
- Restricted affect
- Indifference or excessive social anxiety
- Peculiar word selection
- Loose, fragmented speech patterns

Bathing/Hygiene Self Care Deficit This deficit is characteristically seen, particularly in clients who are homeless. All aspects of activities of daily living may be involved, including the following:

- Inadequate hygiene
- Bizarre grooming
- The presence of vermin
- Failure to seek health care or adhere to prescribed regimens

Feeding Self Care Deficit This deficit may be the result of lack of knowledge, inadequate living arrangements, or lack of interest and motivation. This deficit often leads to physical problems that precipitate visits to emergency rooms and neighborhood clinics. Problems are:

- Obesity
- Anorexia
- Malnutrition
- Dehydration

Impaired Home Maintenance Management Impaired home maintenance is often detected when neighbors report that the person is living in an unhealthy or unsafe environment. This diagnosis includes all aspects of one's ability to make the environment healthful and safe. Problem areas include:

- Inadequate housing or lack of housing
- Inadequate sanitation facilities
- Rodent- or vermin-infested living quarters
- Inability to manage finances
- Insufficient income or lack of income

Planning and Implementing Interventions

The goal of nursing interventions is to provide an uncomplicated, supportive environment that is safe and nonthreatening to the client. It is hoped that this approach will prevent deterioration and will enhance the client's level of adaptation and functioning. Because schizoid and schizotypal clients have extreme difficulty with emotional commitments, you must be watchful of stressful conditions that could precipitate a psychotic episode.

Social isolation resulting from inadequate social skills and lack of a support system may improve with the use of community-based resources by these clients. While most of them disdain involvement with "busybodies," case management techniques are useful for identifying needy clients who might accept basic services, as well as for monitoring other associated health problems. Encourage clients to accept meals offered by community or private agencies, attend outings and activities in the community, and to avail themselves of the services of the case manager at the community mental health center.

Nursing interventions include the following:

- Focus on low-stress topics during one-to-ones to facilitate appropriate speech patterns.
- Teach basic hygiene measures, providing the client with necessary supplies (soap, towels, toothbrush, and toothpaste).
- For clients living in a group home or being monitored by community health nurses, offer intense nutritional counseling.
- Provide clients with a list of community facilities that offer meals and a place to sleep during inclement weather.
- Link clients with governmental and/or private agencies that may qualify them for financial and/or health care assistance, or that may act as a resource when a crisis occurs; for example, Crisis Hotline, Salvation Army, shelters for the homeless, etc.

Evaluation and Outcome Criteria

It is often difficult to persuade schizoid or schizotypal clients to cooperate with and adhere to structured treatment plans after discharge from inpatient settings, halfway houses, or crisis intervention programs. In structured settings, these clients perform on the fringe of the

CASE STUDY

A Client with Borderline Personality Disorder

Identifying Information

Wendy S is a 27-year-old divorced woman. She was brought into the hospital by the staff of a substance-abuse treatment facility after threatening to commit suicide if not released from the program. Wendy is a dental hygienist who has been employed for 6 months. Her employer confronted her 1 week ago about her rapid mood swings, irritability, and absenteeism related to her chemical dependence. At that time, she agreed to enter treatment. Wendy has an A.S. degree in dental hygiene. She was in treatment for 1 week prior to this admission. She cut both wrists, lacerating tendons, 6 months ago following her graduation from the hygiene program.

Client's Description of the Problem

Wendy states that she does not need to be on a psychiatric unit because she didn't really mean that she was going to kill herself. She was merely looking for attention. Wendy states that her employer is overly critical of her and was jealous that the male patients were very attracted to her. She thought it unfair that her employer asked her not to see patients socially after hours. She also stated that her employer was jealous of her figure and cute uniforms, and decided to have her admitted for an alcohol problem that Wendy didn't believe she really had. Wendy would like to get back to work immediately, as she needs the money and knows that her patients miss her. She feels she can handle her alcohol intake herself. She relates that she just uses alcohol to help her unwind. Jogging, racquetball, and aerobic dancing are her major coping strategies.

Wendy states that she has had problems getting along with female employers before. She prefers the company of men, even though she relates a history of physical and sexual abuse as a child. Her ex-husband abused her verbally and physically. She began drinking more heavily after she had her second abortion. Wendy's "bad temper" has gotten her into problems recently. She was given a citation for speeding and has a pending court date for failure to appear for an old violation.

Psychiatric History

Hospitalized for 3 days in a crisis stabilization unit for attempted suicide 6 months ago. History of counseling in high school for acting out and self-mutilating acts.

Family History

Wendy's parents are divorced and both alcoholic. They wish to have no contact with Wendy. Wendy's two younger brothers are addicted to opioids and crack cocaine. Wendy's older sister is living out of state and has limited contact with her. Wendy feels that she is alone and has no family support. Her two ex-husbands call her occasionally seeking money or sex.

→

group. They need encouragement and reinforcement to become involved in self-care, meal planning, and leisure activities, as might be found in a drop-in center that provides a variety of services the client may select.

IMPAIRED SOCIAL INTERACTION These clients may not achieve dramatic behavioral and personality changes. If, however, the client is able to maintain a therapeutic alliance with the psychiatric nurse as an outpatient in individual or group settings, the goal of increasing the client's level of attachment may be met.

Outcome criteria may include the following measurable behaviors:

- Participates in ongoing support systems offered by community mental health clinic.
- Initiates at least one interaction with a staff member or significant other daily.
- Writes a list of at least two people with whom to speak about a concern.
- Identifies the name(s) of the case manager and/or nurse.

IMPAIRED VERBAL COMMUNICATION If the client remains linked with the support system, increasing levels of interaction should occur. Any appropriate verbal or nonverbal response by the client may indicate motivation and progress toward meeting the goal of effective communication. To encourage the client to use more direct and meaningful speech patterns, focus on low-stress topics during interaction (like the weather, travel, current events, games, cards) and use clear, concise speech.

Outcome criteria may include the following measurable behaviors:

- Selects one activity for the group three times weekly.

CASE STUDY *(continued)*

Social History

Although a good student in college, Wendy was anxious about tests and being evaluated by her instructors. She states that she was usually able to talk her way out of problems while in school, when she would arrive late or be absent because of problems with her boyfriends who were jealous of each other. She has no girlfriends but feels close to several boyfriends. She has experimented with drugs offered by her brothers, but prefers alcohol. She expresses concerns about returning to her job and not losing her license.

Health History

Wendy has had no serious physical health problems other than occasional problems with vaginal herpes. She expresses concern about whether her past abortions will affect her ability to have children later in life. Her blood pressure is 110/80 with a pulse rate of 80. There is evidence of scars on her wrist and forearm from past self-inflicted lacerations and burns.

Current Mental Status

Wendy is hyperactive and frequently gets up to move around the room. She talks a great deal about how she is not crazy and feels like she is being treated unjustly. She is critical about the care she has received at the substance-abuse treatment facility and on this unit. She is oriented to time, place, and person. Her judgment is impaired. Her affect is labile, even though she attempts to be cheerful when meeting new people. She frequently lashes out at them later for a perceived infraction. Mood swings alternate between crying and excessive smiling. She is often angry when staff members do not meet her needs immediately. She is easily distracted, especially when she notices a male client or physician walk by. She denies delusions or hallucinations. Her speech is clear and coherent, though pressured at times. She uses projection, seeking to blame others for her present hospitalization.

Other Subjective or Objective Clinical Data

She is taking no prescribed medications at this time but is seeking medication for her "nerves." Suicidal/homicidal violence potential present.

Diagnostic Impression

Nursing Diagnoses

Ineffective Individual Coping
Personal Identity Disturbance
Risk for Violence

DSM-IV Multiaxial Diagnosis

Axis I:	305.00 Alcohol abuse
Axis II:	301.83 Borderline personality disorder
Axis III:	Vaginal herpes
Axis IV:	Occupational problems
Axis V:	GAF=50 (current); Serious impairment in social and occupational functioning; GAF=80 (highest level in past year)

- Remains out of the room at least 4 hours daily.
- Speaks for 5–10 minutes without introducing circumstantial material.

Bathing/Hygiene Self Care Deficit Some of these clients carry all their belongings with them and frequently bathe in bus terminal restrooms. For this reason, it may be difficult to teach and monitor adequate self-care activities. If the client is not homeless, help develop weekly schedules for self-care activities.

Outcome criteria may include the following measurable behaviors:

- Bathes and changes clothing three times weekly.
- Prepares dirty laundry for washing.
- Uses hygiene/grooming checklist daily.

Feeding Self Care Deficit Linking these clients with meals-on-wheels or congregate dining facilities following discharge from inpatient settings not only promotes adequate nutrition but also encourages increased social interactions. Because many of their physical problems are the result of poor nutrition, use a variety of resources to teach nutritional concepts, for example, pictures, activity groups, cooking classes, and outings to grocery stores.

Outcome criteria may include the following measurable behaviors:

- Eats two to three balanced meals a day.
- Participates in a complete physical exam within 48 hours of hospitalization.
- Gains 2–3 lb weekly while hospitalized.

text continues on page 489

NURSING CARE PLAN

A Client with Borderline Personality Disorder

Nursing Diagnosis

Ineffective Individual Coping related to destructive behavior toward self and others; use of defenses such as splitting, projecting, and regression; verbal manipulation; and employment crisis.

Expected Outcome

Client will demonstrate moderate and stable means of expressing feelings and relating to others.

Nursing Interventions

- Assign nonjudgmental staff to work with client; maintain consistency.
- Schedule frequent staff meetings; establish behavioral expectations.
- Schedule family meetings if possible.
- Inform client of acceptable behavior and unit rules.
- Enforce limits when client attempts to manipulate.
- Delegate to one staff member the final authority and responsibility for the treatment plan.
- Use problem-solving techniques to help client make changes.
- Point out when client is experiencing both positive and negative responses toward the same person.
- Challenge client's idealizations of staff.
- Point out discrepancies in client's behavior.
- Tell client you do not feel the way he or she imagines that you do.
- Draw a parallel between how you respond to client's behavior and how others are likely to respond.
- Remain neutral to client's comments, being neither flattered nor offended.
- Do not seek client's approval.
- Explore feelings and experiences rather than making interpretations.
- Use group techniques to teach responsibility for self.
- Discuss behaviors that were problematic at work.
- Use role playing to demonstrate adaptive communications.
- Teach client to recognize needs requiring immediate attention and those that may be delayed.
- Avoid rescuing or rejecting client; rather, deal with the manipulative behavior.
- Have client record daily experiences, feelings, and responses in a journal; use the journal to enhance the nurse-client relationship.
- Use a "transitional object" (an appointment card, a postcard) when out of town or out of touch with client.
- Discuss the effects of alcohol use on client's ability to cope and to succeed in personal and professional life.
- Share with client how the behavior affects you and others.

Outcome Met If

- Client develops a therapeutic relationship with at least one staff member.
- Client verbally acknowledges both positive and negative characteristics about self and others.
- Client explores responses to others' behavior and relates these responses to feelings about oneself.
- Client describes feelings rather than somatizing them.
- Client identifies situations in which manipulation is employed and verbalizes the consequences.
- Client identifies and uses modes of responding that are assertive and responsible.
- Client verbalizes consistent stories or reports to a variety of staff.
- Client adheres to unit rules and regulations.
- Client engages in constructive and satisfying activities during free time.
- Client sustains a meaningful relationship without using primitive defenses such as projection and splitting.
- Client explores the past use of chemicals as a means of coping and options available.
- Client takes time to process a problem, using problem-solving skills, rather than acting impulsively.
- Client sustains a long-term therapeutic relationship.
- Client lists behaviors at work indicative of acting-out and manipulation.
- Client verbalizes some responsibility for the present problems.

Nursing Diagnosis

Personal Identity Disturbance related to history of physical and verbal abuse.

Expected Outcome

Client will identify and resolve the immediate crisis and initiate the development of a secure sense of self.

Nursing Interventions

- Develop a consistent treatment plan involving all staff members.
- Encourage staff to discuss feelings directed toward client in staff meetings.
- Encourage client to discuss per-

NURSING CARE PLAN *(continued)*

sonal body image.

- Help client deal with loss of body image associated with history of abuse.
- Help client examine belief systems and identify how perceptions and beliefs influence responses.
- Encourage client to write an autobiographical essay or story, and give feedback.
- Encourage client to set daily objectives, and assist in meeting goals.
- Give positive reinforcement for the achievement of goals.
- Have client evaluate personal progress weekly.
- Point out to client when affective responses are inappropriate or incongruent to situations.
- Help client identify rewards of both appropriate and inappropriate responses.
- Encourage participation in a variety of group situations.
- Help client accept disappointments by altering thoughts with such statements as "It would be nice if . . ." rather than magnifying losses.
- Confront client with various ways he or she denies pleasure.
- Discuss with client ways to change feelings and behavior.
- Ask client to use "I" statements when sharing personal experiences and concerns.

Outcome Met If

- Client behaves and dresses appropriately in social situations.
- Client develops a realistic view of self by identifying strengths and weaknesses.
- Client explores how beliefs and perceptions of situations influence responses and roles played.
- Client establishes goals that can be reached in a specified time period.
- Client identifies consequences of behaviors.
- Client evaluates personal progress.
- Client sustains a situation-appropriate mood and avoids mood swings.
- Client discusses modes of sexual expression and ways of achieving satisfaction.
- Client refers to self using "I" or "me."

Nursing Diagnosis

Risk for violence: Self-Directed or Directed at Others, related to inability to verbalize frustration and anger, history of impulsive self-mutilating acts, and hostile verbalizations.

Expected Outcome

Client will eliminate destructive acting-out behavior such as suicidal/homicidal threats and gestures.

Nursing Interventions

- Assess history of previous self-mutilation.
- Observe behavior and document every shift.
- Use suicide precautions as necessary.
- Tell client that staff will not permit injury to self or others.
- Search client's belongings for contraband.
- Contract with client to notify staff members when suicidal or self-mutilating thoughts occur.
- Help client identify alternatives to self-destructive behavior.
- Explore self-destructive fantasies.
- Help client identify situations in which self-destructive ideas occur or are triggered.
- Explore hostile relationships in the past.
- When client verbalizes anger during one-to-one sessions, point out that anger is not caused by the current situation but by perceptions of things in the past.
- Modulate the amount of warmth shown to client.
- Help client explore ways to express anger constructively.
- Encourage verbal expression of anger, and give positive reinforcement for same.
- Explore with client how to direct the energy of anger toward positive ends, motivation for change, problem solving.
- Deal with client's transference phenomena, which are expressions of anger and hatred.
- Use treatment contracts, including expectations, between client and team with mutually agreed-upon goals.
- Give consistent feedback for goal achievement or lack thereof.

Outcome Met if

- Client verbalizes feelings of anger and frustration when they occur.
- Client requests time-out periods, physical activities, and PRN medications when anger cannot be defused by verbalizing.
- Client identifies precipitating factors, such as rejection, separation, loss, disappointment.
- Client seeks out staff member with whom to discuss anger or releases anger in constructive activity.
- Client identifies alternatives to self-mutilating behavior.
- Client uses "I" statements when dealing with anger and frustration.
- Client does not harm self or others.

- Takes vitamin supplements as ordered.
- Reports any problems of elimination to nursing staff.

Impaired Home Maintenance Management Because schizoid or schizotypal clients value independence highly, take into account their preferences and former lifestyle when planning interventions. If the client has a history of transience, provide a list of community resources and discuss other options to prevent life-management crises. Guardianship by government agencies may be necessary and desirable for clients who are not competent to care for themselves.

Outcome criteria may include the following measurable behaviors:

- Accepts social service plan to locate adequate housing, food, and medical care.
- Accepts referral to human services for evaluation and support.
- Demonstrates how to use all appliances in the boarding home setting.
- Discusses how to pay rent and other bills.
- States what to do in the event of fire or other emergency in the home setting.

For a summary of client/family teaching guidelines for clients with schizoid or schizotypal personality disorder, see the box on the next page.

Dramatic-Emotional Personality Disorders

The *DSM-IV* identifies the **borderline, histrionic, narcissistic**, and **antisocial personality disorders** as dramatic, emotional, erratic dysfunctions. Individuals with these disorders are often in conflict with society because of their impulsive behavior. Impulsive people view the world as a discontinuous, fragmented conglomerate of opportunities, frustrations, and affective experiences. They live only in the present and lack the ability to examine hunches and to formulate long-range plans. They act decisively without critical evaluation of consequences. The focus of their intellectual and emotional goals is to achieve immediate gain and satisfaction. This lack of impulse control and inability to delay gratification often result in both verbal and nonverbal outbursts of anger, which may be self-directed or other-directed. Indeed, clients with dramatic-emotional personality disorders may experience rapid escalation of anxiety when their own angry impulses are not controlled by others. The Assessment and Intervention boxes on pages 491 and 492 illustrate some common angry behaviors and provide guidelines for nursing interventions.

Most researchers agree that psychologic fixations in the genital stage of development account for many of the behaviors noted in this cluster of disorders (Cameron and Rychlak 1985). Specifically, parental deprivation; inadequate, excessive, or inconsistent discipline; and failure of the child to develop integrated cognitive, affective, and behavioral modes in early life may lead to these disorders. Clients have generalized feelings of low self-esteem, need to control people and situations, and are unable to delay gratification. In response, dramatic-emotional clients tend to interact by negatively manipulating others. Although manipulation is a standard response in the repertoire of people with these personality disorders, its occurrence escalates with increased stress. The Assessment and Intervention boxes on pages 494 and 495 illustrate some manipulative behaviors and provide guidelines for nursing interventions.

Common features of the dramatic-emotional cluster of personality disorders are summarized in the Assessment box on page 497. Because of its instability and the potential for transient psychotic symptoms, borderline personality disorder is discussed first.

The Nursing Process and Clients with Borderline Personality Disorder

Assessment

Although the person with a borderline personality disorder (BPD) is unstable in a variety of areas (relationships, mood, self-image) no single feature is invariably present. Of the nine DSM-IV diagnostic criteria, at least five must be observed to diagnose this disorder (see the box on page 497). Some theorists characterize BPD as occupying a place on a continuum between neurotic and psychotic disorders. Prevalence of this disorder is about 2% of the general population (APA 1994).

Recent literature addresses the role of biologic factors in the genesis of borderline personality disorder. Hormones are being implicated to the extent that increased levels of testosterone, 17-estradiol, and estrone have been observed in people with impulse control problems. Dexamethasone suppression test (DST) findings have also been abnormal in some people with depressive symptoms who are diagnosed with BPD. The serotonin metabolite 5-HIAA has been shown to be low in people who attempt suicide and in those with aggression and impulse control problems (Kaplan and Sadock 1991). Recent research suggests that core symptoms of BPD can be altered by pharmacologic manipulation of serotonergic function. For futher details, see the Research Note on page 498.

Surprisingly, little research has been conducted in the area of family interactional patterns that may predispose to BPD. Although the *DSM-IV* reports that this disorder is

CLIENT/FAMILY TEACHING

A Client with Schizoid or Schizotypal Personality Disorder

Strategies to Enhance Personal Hygiene

- Provide step-by-step, concrete self-care instructions when client is unable to make decisions.
- Establish schedules for personal care activities, and provide sufficient time for client to complete tasks.
- Instruct client in bathing, nail care, use of deodorants, mouth care, and changing/washing underwear.
- Teach female clients the appropriate use of cosmetics; encourage male clients to shave frequently or how to care for facial hair.
- Encourage client to make a list of daily grooming/hygiene tasks, including medications.

Strategies to Enhance Nutrition

- Help client prepare a list identifying foods he or she eats and has access to daily.
- Teach client minimum daily requirements for an adequate diet and how to provide these requirements from the foods currently used in the diet.
- Discuss with client ways to obtain food necessary for good nutrition, for example, food stamps, social service agencies, church organizations, social clubs, etc.
- Teach client how to chew small bite-sized pieces of food slowly.
- Help client understand the connection between dietary intake and physical state: bowel movements, level of hydration (skin, urinary patterns), feelings of energy and fatigue.
- Help client identify ways to get two or three balanced meals daily.

Strategies to Enhance Social Adjustment and Home Maintenance

- Determine the level of client's interest in and motivation for social activity.
- Help client understand that increased contact with people will maximize his or her choices and provide more, not less, freedom.
- Ask client to identify one family member or friend he or she would trust to help with personal needs.
- Ask client to make a list of people (including phone numbers) with whom he or she may need to interact; include case manager, physician, store clerk, landlord, etc.
- Encourage client to use a notepad to write requests to discuss with the nurse or carry out at a later time.
- Teach client how to use a telephone to make calls to professional offices or agencies.
- Role-play with client how to detect social cues given to him or her by others.
- Teach client social manners: eating with mouth closed, how to use eating utensils, use of tissue for blowing nose, how to sit at a table, etc.
- Ask client to make a list of hobbies/activities enjoyed as a child that can be engaged in now; have client identify activities/hobbies he or she might enjoy, in the present, that would involve limited "people" contact, such as computer games, crossword puzzles, checkers, backgammon, and double solitaire.
- Meet with client and family member, roommate, or significant other to discuss realistic expectations for the client.
- Teach client home management skills necessary for independent living: how to buy a money order or use a checking account, paying bills, purchasing necessary items for self-care and home care, accessing public transportation, how to use coupons and rebates for food and other purchases, how to make a shopping list, how to find a repair person, how to use the Yellow Pages.
- Ask client if he or she desires testing, placement services, job skill retraining, or employment.
- Refer client to agencies such as sheltered workshops, Goodwill Industries, State Employment offices, vocational/technical centers for employment assistance.
- Teach client to prepare a resume of vocational qualifications and how to fill out an application for employment or social services such as food stamps or housing.

ASSESSMENT

The Angry Client

Nonverbal

Glaring, piercing stares

Tight facial muscles

Facial flushing

Distended neck veins

Hyperalertness

Knitted brows

Tense body posture

Arms crossed over chest or placed on hips

Finger pointing

Fist clenching, waving, or pounding

Slamming, throwing, or punching inanimate objects

Irritability

Overreaction; temper outbursts

Intimidation

Physical assault/injury to animals or people

Homicide/suicide ideation, plan, or gesture

Verbal

Derogatory statements and sarcasm

Malicious gossiping

Angry voice tone

Pressured speech

Shouting, screaming, cursing

Overly critical, impatient

Threatening

Scapegoating

Negativity

Statements such as, "You make me mad. I could kill you."

Overuse of defense mechanisms of denial, rationalization, projection, and displacement

five times more prevalent among first-degree relatives (APA 1994), Feldman and Guttman's (1984) research in this area reported findings that indicated that **biparental failure**, rather than failures during the separation-individuation process with the primary caregiver, may lead to the development of symptoms. Biparental failure is evident in those homes where the male parent fails to offset the child's troubled relationship with the mother by providing positive experiences for the child. For example, the male parent fails to become involved in day-to-day parenting, generally lacks interest in the child, gives little approval, is passive, or affectively neglects the child.

The following subjective and objective nursing assessment criteria for clients with BPD have been adapted from the DSM-IV diagnostic criteria. Because most people with this disorder are encountered in the workplace or socially, it is important to recognize and intervene appropriately to prevent crises (Rimpey and Davidson 1994; Wester 1989). Else et al. (1993) concluded that men who commit spousal abuse may not only have poor problem-solving skills, but also appear to have borderline-antisocial personality traits, certain types of hostility, and a history of childhood abuse, which predispose them to violent behavior. Given the societal attention to problems of family violence today, researchers may well identify some biologic markers for violence; family interactional issues have been well documented in this area. The Nursing Self-Awareness box on page 499 will help you identify strategies for dealing with the feelings of anger and helplessness that are often triggered by the behavior of borderline personality clients.

Subjective Data

Instability or Unpredictability Impulsiveness may be observed in self-damaging ways, demonstrating a lack of responsibility and disregard for the consequences of the behavior. "I just told my boss to take this job and shove it" may be the response to a work situation that is perceived as intolerable. "I just got another credit card with a $5000

INTERVENTION

The Angry Client

Nursing Intervention	*Rationale*
• Use a calm, unhurried approach.	• Calmness promotes security.
• Do not touch indiscriminately.	• Touch may be misinterpreted as aggressive or sexual.
• Respect personal space.	• Space provides insulation/protection.
• Use active listening skills.	• Attention and direct eye contact promote trust.
• Remain aware of personal feelings.	• Avoids countertransference reactions.
• Use statements to provide feedback and to identify sources of anger: "I notice your fists are clenched . . . what's happening?"	• Feedback on feelings increases client awareness.
• Set verbal limits on behavior.	• Conveys external controls.
• Use adult-adult rather than parent-child communications.	• Promotes mature responses.
• Offer time-out periods/one-to-one sessions in a quiet area.	• Diminishes sensory stimuli.
• Assure client that the staff will not allow the client to hurt self or others.	• Conveys external controls.
• Observe for escalation of anger (increased activity, verbal and nonverbal acting-out).	• Prevents crisis.
• Institute precautions against suicide, homicide, assault, or escape, as indicated.	• Ensures safety of client and others.
• Document patterns of acting-out, including trigger situations.	• Identifies precursors to anger and violence.
• Discuss alternate means of releasing tension and physical energy.	• Increases self-esteem through adaptive outlets.
• Provide physical outlets to reduce tension, like exercise, punching bags, gardening, clay, music, art (avoid competitive or contact sports).	• Exercise releases anxiety/tension.

limit, so I don't have to worry about going over the limit on my other three cards." "I only drink wine when I'm driving, so I don't worry about DUIs." "I don't worry about AIDS; all my partners come from the high-rent districts, so they are clean and safe." Responses such as "I did it; I don't know why I did it, I just did" are common when clients are questioned about the reasons for particular actions.

Unstable Interpersonal Relationships When being interviewed, borderline client statements such as "He told me he'd love me forever and then he wanted to go bowling on a Friday night" are not uncommon. Clients relate stories of "one-night stands" in search of the perfect partner. Any real or perceived threat of abondonment results in the client's "switching" to another partner. "He's never there when I need him" may be used in conjunction with "I always see to it that his shirts are ironed and his dinner is ready when he gets home from work." These clients need a payback in return for any giving they do.

Intense Anger These clients are unable to tolerate their own "bad" image and project it onto others, often raging at the perceived attributes of the other. Anger tends to be greatest toward those people who remind

INTERVENTION *(continued)*

Nursing Intervention	*Rationale*
• Use humor to reduce tension and avoid a power struggle.	• Humor defuses anxiety/confrontation.
• Offer medication if appropriate.	• Chemical interventions may reduce anxiety.
• Be prepared to use seclusion and restraints.	• Diminishes stimuli to increase self-control.
• Recognize client's potential to act on threats.	• Impulsivity is a hallmark of angry people.
• Initially ignore derogatory statements.	• Avoids reinforcement of negative behavior.
• Protect other clients from verbal/physical abuse.	• Ensures safety of all clients.
• Clearly communicate and enforce unit regulations concerning acting-out behavior.	• People behave according to expectations.
• Postpone discussion of anger and consequences of acting-out until client is in control.	• Anger narrows perceptual field.
• Role-model appropriate assertions of angry feelings: "I dislike it when . . . ."	• New behaviors can be learned.
• State desire to help client maintain/regain control.	• Offering self establishes trust.
• Hold client responsible for behavior; remind client that he or she can make choices.	• Promotes internal control.
• Do not argue or criticize.	• Negative feedback may escalate violence.
• Give feedback regarding client's ability to maintain control in similar situations.	• Positive validation increases ability to control self.
• Do not threaten punitive action.	• Ultimatums increase confrontation.
• Involve in treatment planning.	• Client-centered goals increase compliance.
• Use contracts for behavioral control, including seeking out staff people when feelings emerge.	• Establishes responsibility.
• Teach assertiveness skills, relaxation, imagery, thought stopping, thought control, etc.	• Defuses anxiety and reinforces ability for self-control.

them of a nurturing/ frustrating parent. "I can't stand that fat slob of a nurse. She acts like God went on vacation and appointed her to substitute for Him." "So what if I yell when I get angry; I'm paying a lot of money to be here. If you don't like it, leave."

Identity Diffusion The borderline individual displays behaviors that show confusion about values and goals in life: "I can't make up my mind if I should stay in nursing or try interior design" (after completing 1 year in a 2-year nursing program). "I feel so totally empty inside. I burned my wrist with the cigarette just to see if I could still feel." "I'd really prefer to have you as my nurse counselor than the one they assigned me to because you are my age and *really* understand me."

Affective Instability "Of course I knew I wouldn't kill myself when I took those pills—do you think I'm stupid or something?" "I only told him [partner] I was HIV-positive to see if he really cared for me as much as he said."

Feelings of Emptiness and Aloneness "I get depressed and I think about taking some pills, but then my boyfriend calls and we'll go out and I won't be depressed anymore."

ASSESSMENT

The Manipulative Client

Nonverbal

Smiling to excess

Touching inappropriately

Crying, whining in public

Appearing confused and helpless

Drawing attention to self (falling, dramatic displays of somatic problems, etc.)

Gift giving

Tardiness

Selective forgetting

Refusal to participate in activities

Seductive dressing, eye movements, body language

Decreased frustration tolerance

Self/other destructive acting-out

Verbal

Compliments, flattery

Sarcasm

Threats

Demanding behavior

Induction of guilt: "I thought we had a relationship of trust."

Excessive criticism of others

Wheeling and dealing

Bargaining for special privileges

Being overly solicitous of others

Requesting exemption from rules: "Couldn't I have my medication just one hour earlier?"

Mimicking therapeutic responses used by staff: "I have a feeling you're angry with me."

Confronting staff in the presence of other clients

Lying

Reporting great "insights" early in the relationship

Telling the nurse what he or she "wants" to hear

Using information about others to exploit them

Excessive involvement in the problems of others

Aggressive questioning about personal matters

Rationalizing, projecting, and minimizing blame for behavior

Self-pity

Role reversal

Self-Damaging Acts "I don't see what's the big deal, so I tried to cut my wrists a couple of times—doesn't everybody?" "Yeah, I vomit after I eat; it keeps my weight down and I still get to have all the desserts I want."

Objective Data

Instability or Unpredictability The individual with BPD has fluctuating responses in situations that are subjectively interpreted and often distorted. Impulsiveness is manifested in spending habits, sexuality, substance use, eating habits, shoplifting, and frequent job changes.

Unstable Interpersonal Relationships The failure to resolve the separation-individuation process described by Mahler et al. (1975) is reflected in the person's attitudes toward self and others. Normal autism and symbiosis must occur before the separation-individuation process, referred to as "psychologic birth," can begin. The inability to unify the "good and bad" objects into one whole is demonstrated by the inability to integrate the self as both "good and bad" or to separate or individuate from the maternal object.

The sense of self originates with the earliest mother-child interactions. If the mother is not sensitive and attuned to the child's needs, she will fail to confirm the child's emerging sense of reality. Consequently, the child distorts reality and develops an unreal "as-if" personality that shifts to meet the demands of cues in the outer world

INTERVENTION

The Manipulative Client

Nursing Intervention	Rationale
• Assign one staff member as primary resource person.	• Consistency prevents opportunities for splitting staff.
• Provide for staff conferences on a regular basis.	• Communicates treatment goals and interventions.
• Allow sufficient time to develop a relationship.	• Time is essential to develop trust.
• Use group and peer supervision for staff.	• Promotes awareness of countertransference phenomena.
• Provide for consistency in limit setting.	• Promotes self-control.
• Make limits realistic with enforceable consequences.	• Unpleasant consequences may help decrease negative behavior.
• Give reasons for limits and consequences.	• Helps client make appropriate choices.
• Identify personal feelings (anger, frustration, discomfort, rescuer needs) in response to client's behavior.	• Promotes self-awareness.
• Model respect, honesty, openness, and assertiveness.	• Learning promotes behavioral change.
• Avoid power struggles and focus on need for self-control.	• Avoids client-focused issues.
• Seek times to interact with client when he or she is not acting out.	• Reinforces positive behavior.
• Confront client each time manipulation occurs.	• Consequences must follow behavior closely.
• Describe impact of client's manipulation in an unemotional way: "I feel angry when you scream at me in front of all the staff members."	• Honesty enhances client empathy.
• Explore the meaning and effects of the client's manipulations.	• All behavior has meaning.
• Discuss with the client alternative ways of dealing with people or situations.	• Promotes personal responsibility.
• Do not express nonverbal amusement (eye rolling, smiling) when client manipulates others.	• Reinforcement of negative behavior increases it.
• Avoid accepting gifts.	• Prevents unprofessional alliances.
• Explore meaning of gift giving with client.	• Client learns to recognize manipulative patterns.
• Enlist client's participation in treatment plan.	• Client-centered goals increase compliance.
• Encourage control over routine decisions about activities of daily living.	• Independence fosters feelings of control.
• Encourage participation in group activities in both member and leader roles.	• Provides opportunity for successes.

→

INTERVENTION *(continued)*

Nursing Intervention	*Rationale*
• Help client write a self-assessment identifying both assets and liabilities.	• Promotes self-esteem.
• Remove limits from treatment plan when client adheres to objectives consistently.	• Rewards appropriate behavior.
• Evaluate effectiveness of limit setting.	• Clarifies discharge planning goals.
• Jointly develop contracts for behavioral change.	• Establishes client responsibility.
• If client refuses to comply with contracts or treatment recommendations, avoid negotiating; enlist staff team to resolve issues.	• Group pressure enhances personal responsibility.
• Offer support to other clients who may be targets of manipulation.	• Ensures safety of all clients.
• Involve both client and significant others in identifying and managing manipulative behavior.	• Clear expectations foster behavioral change.
• Teach stress-reduction techniques (guided imagery, relaxation, thought stopping).	• Defuses anxiety and reinforces ability for self-control.
• Involve in assertiveness training and problem solving.	• Differentiates aggression from assertion.
• Practice role rehearsal skills.	• Decreases threats to self.

(Brainerd 1978; Mahler et al. 1975). The implications for the child's later relationships include such behaviors as:

- Manipulation of others.
- Pitting individuals against one another.
- Intense attachment.
- Explosive separations.
- Sudden shifts in attitude toward others perceived as good or bad.
- Clinging, demanding.
- Controlling, exploitive behavior.
- Sadism or masochism in close relationships.
- Relationships motivated by a need to avoid being alone rather than the need to be with others.
- Lack of empathy.
- Diminished capacity to evaluate others realistically.
- Transient, brief, close relationships.

Intense Anger Borderline clients tend to instigate problems as they become involved in therapeutic relationships. The anger may manifest itself in accusations, frequent displays of temper, inability to control anger (acting-out), irritability, sarcasm, argumentativeness, devaluing others, and overreaction to minor irritants.

Identity Diffusion Clients with BPD display behaviors that show confusion about values and goals in life. These clients cannot genuinely experience feelings and emotions; their core personality is hollow. They do not assume responsibility for their actions but project blame and credit onto others.

Problems of identity diffusion are also apparent in the areas of sexual intimacy and gender identity. Sexual intimacy is disturbed as a result of the person's fears of being engulfed and destroyed or abandoned by another. An approach-avoidance conflict emerges as a consequence of the mother having thwarted independence and rewarded dependent behavior. As a result, the borderline client develops two major fears: the fear of abandonment, which leads to clinging behavior, and fear of engulfment, which leads to distancing from others. The client desperately wants intimate relationships but is terrified of losing the self. These fears are reminiscent of the early choice between mother's love and autonomy, which is the core of

ASSESSMENT

Common Features of the Dramatic-Emotional Personality

- Labile affective responses
- Intense episodes of anger/rage
- Self-centeredness/egocentricity
- Unstable personal relationships
- Superficiality, exploitiveness, and manipulativeness
- Lack of empathy for others
- Inability to postpone gratification
- Boredom or need for constant attention
- Poor judgment
- Failure to learn by experience
- Failure to assume responsibility for behavior
- Poorly integrated sexual identity
- Ability to test reality and absence of major thought or affective disorders

the borderline conflict. This conflict is managed by using the primitive dissociation defense, also called splitting (discussed further below).

Gender identity disturbance may be manifested by the selection of rejecting or abusive partners, the preference for homosexual relationships while maintaining a heterosexual lifestyle, bizarre fantasies, and transsexualism (Akhtar 1984). False accusations of sexual involvement and sexual acting-out with one's therapist are additional examples of identity diffusion problems (Gutheil 1989).

Another area of identity diffusion is temporal discontinuity, which is manifested by a searching for one's origins or keeping detailed chronologic journals. Borderline individuals seem unable to integrate past, present, and future into a continuum. They may frantically plan for the future while reminiscing about past events. These behaviors often lead to difficulty in choosing long-term goals, making career choices, and reassessing personal values.

Affective Instability The failure to resolve object permanence issues is also related to the inability of the borderline person to maintain a consistent, satisfying, affective state. Characteristic of this individual are intense fluctuations of mood, normally of short duration (a few hours or a few days); intense, discrete episodes of depression with accompanying suicidal ideation and gestures; and hypomanic or elated episodes.

DSM-IV Diagnostic Criteria for Borderline Personality Disorder

A pervasive pattern of instability of interpersonal relationships, self-image, and affects, and marked impulsivity beginning by early adulthood and present in a variety of contexts, as indicated by five (or more) of the following:

1. Frantic efforts to avoid real or imagined abandonment. **Note:** Do not include suicidal or self-mutilating behavior covered in Criterion 5.
2. A pattern of unstable and intense interpersonal relationships characterized by alternating between extremes of idealization and devaluation.
3. Identity disturbance: markedly and persistently unstable self-image or sense of self.
4. Impulsivity in at least two areas that are potentially self-damaging (e.g., spending, sex, substance abuse, reckless driving, binge eating). **Note:** Do not include suicidal or self-mutilating behavior covered in Criterion 5.
5. Recurrent suicidal behavior, gestures, or threats, or self-mutilating behavior.
6. Affective instability due to a marked reactivity of mood (e.g., intense episodic dysphoria, irritability, or anxiety usually lasting a few hours and only rarely more than a few days).
7. Chronic feelings of emptiness.
8. Inappropriate, intense anger or difficulty controlling anger (e.g., frequent displays of temper, constant anger, recurrent physical fights).
9. Transient, stress-related paranoid ideation or severe dissociative symptoms.

Source: American Psychiatric Association 1994, p. 654.

RESEARCH NOTE

Citation

Hollander E, et al.: Serotonergic sensitivity in borderline personality disorder: Preliminary findings. *Am Psychiatr* 1994;151(2):277–280.

Study Problem/Purpose

This study examined the effects of single doses of oral m-chlorophenylpiperazine (m-CPP), a partial 5-HT agonist, and a placebo on 12 clients with borderline personality disorder and 15 healthy comparison subjects. The purposes of this study were to determine a role for 5-HT (central serotonin) in BPD and to determine whether the core symptoms of the disorder can be altered by pharmacologic manipulation of serotonergic function.

Methods

The structured clinical interview for *DSM-IV* personality disorders (SCID-II) was used to select 12 adult clients who met the criteria for borderline personality disorder. Fifteen healthy comparison subjects were selected from a recruiting unit for healthy subjects. The subjects received single doses of oral m-CPP (0.5 mg/kg) and placebo under double-blind, randomized conditions at least 48 hours apart. The subjects were assessed by the clinical rater on a 13-item affect analog scale, which included feelings of being high, calm, and mellow. Blood samples for determining prolactin, cortisol, and m-CPP levels were collected 45, 90, 180, and 210 minutes after insertion of the intravenous line. Comparisons within subject groups used analysis of variance (ANOVA).

Findings

Behavior measures among BPD clients suggested improvement in mood, with decreases in anger of all subjects and decreases in fear in the male subjects following administration of m-CPP, but not placebo. Ratings of rigidity, impulsivity, and destructiveness did not significantly change. The analog scale revealed that clients with BPD became more calm.

Implications

The results suggest that core symptoms of borderline personality disorder can be altered by pharmacologic manipulation of serotonergic function. A possible disinhibiting effect of m-CPP in BPD will require further study, but it presents hope for pharmacologic interventions.

Feelings of Emptiness and Aloneness Individuals with borderline personality disorder report hollow, empty feelings, lack of peaceful solitude, a sense of being disconnected, and anhedonia (absence of pleasure in performing ordinarily pleasurable acts). The person may attempt to combat these feelings by compulsive eating, drinking, drug abuse, sexual encounters, and self-mutilation. It is believed that excessive anxiety associated with unresolved separation-individuation issues underlies these behaviors (Perlmutter 1982).

Self-Damaging Acts Impulsiveness, together with identity disturbances, often leads to self-destructive behaviors. People with BPD are often depressed, but they may make self-destructive gestures to affirm their reality and relieve tension rather than to express a wish to die. Variations in the severity of suicide attempts may be related to age, history of self-directed violence, the presence of an eating disorder, and psychotic features (Shearer et al. 1988). Additional self-damaging behaviors include self-mutilation (cigarette burns, cutting, taking drug overdoses), recurrent accidents, and physical fights.

Overuse of Primitive Defenses According to Lego (1984), clients with BPD consistently use the following defenses:

- Primitive dissociation, also called **splitting.** The client keeps the opposing affective states of love and hate separate, fearing that the bad aspects (hate) will poison the good aspects (love).

Sharon, a graduate student, loves her instructor during laboratory instruction when she receives individual attention from him but detests the same instructor in the role of the distant lecturer.

- **Projective identification.** The client projects personal feelings onto another, thereby justifying expressions of anger and self-protection.

NURSING SELF-AWARENESS

Recognizing and Working with Borderline Personalities

Patty, a 25-year-old RN, has been working on your acute medical-surgical unit for 8 months. During this time she has had several run-ins with the nurse manager and other staff members. After 2 months of employment, it was obvious that Patty was intent on developing a "special" relationship with the nurse manager. Patty would stay after shift changes to talk with her and frequently asked the nurse manager to go out for drinks after work. When the nurse manager did not respond to these overtures or grant Patty's special requests (vacation, shift changes, time off for personal reasons), Patty became angry and spoke of her supervisor in a disparaging way to the other nurses on the unit. Patty told one coworker, "She [the nurse manager] made me so mad I almost got mugged after I got drunk the night she refused to go out with me." Patty confessed that she had anonymously phoned the nurse manager three times after midnight, hanging up each time, just to "harass her and let her know she isn't as great as she thinks she is."

At the time of her 6-month evaluation with the nurse manager, Patty denied that she had abused sick leave, even though she had called in sick 10 days and failed to report for duty twice. Patty steadfastly insisted that she did comply with hospital policy, even though she had failed to complete CPR and Infection Control inservices, failed to have her PPD test done, and had gone directly to the hospital administrator with a complaint about the nurse manager. Patty had also refused to care for a client diagnosed with AIDS. She tried to justify her behavior by saying that no one had ever explained these policies to her. After Patty was placed on probationary status, she became overtly hostile toward the nurse manager and attempted to turn her coworkers against this supervisor. Much of Patty's days were spent gossiping about the unfairness of her situation and blaming the nurse manager for her own escalating use of alcohol, which Patty said she needed to "calm myself." When Patty's maneuvers failed to elicit a sympathetic response from either her coworkers or the nurse manager, she threatened to sue the supervisor for "harassment and interference with employment stability."

Behavioral Characteristics

- High potential, but low achievement levels.
- Excessive interest in the personal lives of those in authority.
- Idealistic, oversolicitous responses to supervisory personnel.
- Demands for special considerations or privileges.
- Inconsistent work performance.
- Mood swings, argumentativeness, and manipulativeness with others.
- Hostile acting-out, including sick calls, dishonesty, noncompliance with policies, and broken promises.
- Impulsive behavior, temper tantrums, splitting of work staff and friends.
- Substance abuse.
- Chronic expressions of boredom.
- Malicious gossip; anonymous phone calls and letters of complaint.
- Sexual overtures toward physicians, administrators, supervisors, clients, and other nurses.
- Verbal attacks on superiors, threats of litigation, failure to follow chain of command.

Never underestimate the potential for crisis that borderline personalities may create. People in supervisory positions should use a consultant to maintain objectivity when identifying and developing strategies to deal with such employees.

Intervention Strategies

- Establish clear guidelines for workplace behavior; set firm, consistent limits on behavior.
- Give equal treatment in group situations.
- Avoid showing favoritism, emotional involvement, or permissiveness.
- Make work assignments appropriate to level of education, experience, and ability.
- Encourage adult-level communication.

→

NURSING SELF-AWARENESS (continued)

- Be alert for substance use and/or sexual acting-out on duty.
- Do not "diagnose"; document problem behavior.
- Avoid behavioral interpretations; document facts only.
- Maintain confidentiality of records.
- Maintain communication with hospital administrators or human resource personnel regarding "problem" employees.
- Carefully screen all applicants for employment to identify borderline characteristics that may result in disruptive activities in the workplace.

Source: Adapted from Wester 1989, pp. 49–51.

Paul, a borderline client, accuses a second client, whom he dislikes, of disliking him. Paul refuses to attend any activities at which the other client is present.

- **Primitive idealization.** Dependent on someone, the client assigns unrealistic powers to that individual.

Francisco tells his nurse, "You are the perfect nurse; I always know nothing bad can happen when you're around."

- **Omnipotence:** Omnipotence is signaled by fantasies of greatness or exaggerated importance.

In response to a question about a suicidal gesture, Brenda states, "Don't worry. I knew I wouldn't die."

- **Devaluation:** The client criticizes another to defend against a sense of inadequacy.

Phyllis repeatedly criticizes those nursing staff members who do not have master's degrees as being "nontherapeutic."

- **Denial:** Denial is keeping disturbing thoughts and feelings out of conscious awareness.

Sue, a medical student, was expelled from school for academic and clinical incompetence. When the new term began, she attempted to register for the next class. Sue acted dumbfounded when told she could not register.

Distortions of Reality When identity diffusion reaches panic proportions, the borderline individual may experience the following:

- *Depersonalization:* feeling of strangeness or unreality about one's self.
- *Derealization:* feeling of disconnectedness from the environment.

Steve has multiple cigarette burns but reports no pain or discomfort and smiles when the lesions are being cleaned and dressed.

Nursing Diagnosis

Because of the nature of the borderline personality, the aim of therapy is generally to resolve the immediate crisis and then develop a long-term therapeutic alliance. The long-standing history of affective instability, impulsiveness, and intense, immature relationships leads to persistent maladaptive behavior. The following NANDA nursing diagnoses are integral parts of any nursing care plan for these clients.

PERSONAL IDENTITY DISTURBANCE People diagnosed with BPD experience feelings of self-devaluation because of a failure to negotiate the separation-individuation. Personal Identity Disturbances may be identified from the following problems:

- Chameleonlike behavior
- Superficial interactions
- Intense but disruptive relationships
- Play-acting roles
- Mood swings

INEFFECTIVE INDIVIDUAL COPING These clients tend to overuse primitive defenses to the extent that learning adaptive coping skills is highly impaired. These behaviors are frequently observed:

- Splitting, projection, and regression
- Devaluation or idealization of others
- Potential for chemical dependence
- A persistent sense of boredom and loneliness
- Inadequate responses to life stresses and expectations

Risk for Violence: Self-Directed or Directed at Others Because of the borderline client's mood swings, limited problem-solving ability, and self-concept disturbances, the following problems may be observed:

- Intense and often contagious rage
- Impulsiveness
- Self-mutilation or suicidal gestures
- Hostile, threatening verbalizations
- Property destruction

Planning and Implementing Interventions

When providing care, be alert to the often intense feelings that the borderline client may precipitate. These feelings (anger, guilt, overgiving, rescuing, rigidity) may cloud judgment and lead to nursing decisions the client may interpret as abandonment, distancing, engulfment, or lack of empathy. Staff members who work with these clients should be skillful in nurturing the "adult" side of the client while simultaneously protecting and empathizing with the vulnerable "child" within (Johnson and Silver 1988).

Inez presents herself as a pathetic victim of involuntary hospitalization. As a result, the staff becomes guilt-ridden and prematurely grants an out-of-hospital pass. Inez, in turn, acts out her sense of abandonment by making a serious suicide attempt.

Responding to seductive, angry, or solicitous behavior in either a negative or rescuing manner may reinforce the inappropriate responses of the client. An ideal therapeutic relationship is one in which the nurse: maintains a matter-of-fact but caring approach; establishes and maintains consistent, firm limits; makes regular appointments; and mobilizes the healthy aspects of the client's personality.

As with all clients with personality disorders, use clinical supervision, staff counseling sessions, and team meetings to identify the client's underlying dynamic issues and to work toward decreasing distortions in communications between the client and others.

Evaluation and Outcome Criteria

Although borderline clients often appear relatively healthy, you may find it difficult to maintain a therapeutic alliance with them because of their intense and contagious affects, impulsiveness, and the intense feelings they trigger in others. The quality of object relationships, especially that between the therapist and the client, is crucial to the outcome of therapy.

Personal Identity Disturbance Successful integration of fragmented aspects of the borderline client's personality ("healing the split") depends on the client's ability to remain in a sustained therapeutic relationship (Platt-Koch 1983). Among clients who do remain in therapy, those who demonstrate likability, warmth, reliability, interest in people, talents, and social as well as occupational skills have the most favorable treatment prognosis (Woollcott 1985).

Ineffective Individual Coping The use of primitive defenses may be replaced by more adequate problem-solving skills over time. Encourage the client who has innate cognitive psychomotor talents to sublimate feelings of intense rage into a productive outlet, such as art, music, or dance. Receiving positive reinforcements for these achievements may enhance the development of effective coping strategies.

Risk for Violence: Self-Directed or Directed at Others According to Woollcott (1985), those clients who are most infantile and regressed (as opposed to those who have more narcissistic features) tend to achieve greater affective stability. Confront the client's anger during one-to-one sessions by comparing the client's responses to those of others. This strategy may cause the client to think before acting.

The borderline personality has established patterns of responding to others in any situation. This pattern may sabotage the client's objectives. Furthermore, these clients usually terminate therapy when the acute crisis has ended. The following are among the factors that influence the likelihood of successful change:

- The severity of the client's emotional deprivation.
- The rigidity of the client's personality structure.
- The client's ego strengths.
- The client's motivation to change.
- The nurse's skill and commitment.
- Social support systems in the client's family or milieu that favor the desired change.

The Nursing Process and Clients with Histrionic Personality Disorder

Assessment

People with histrionic personality disorder (HPD) show a lifelong tendency for dramatic, egocentric, attention-seeking response patterns. Their seeming lack of sincerity and emotional commitment contributes to disturbances in interpersonal relationships. These people appear to be continually "on stage" and acting a role. Their extensive use of coping patterns based on repression, denial, and dissociation leads them to deal with problems as though

DSM-IV Diagnostic Criteria for Histrionic Personality Disorder

A pervasive pattern of excessive emotionality and attention seeking, beginning by early adulthood and present in a variety of contexts, as indicated by five (or more) of the following:

1. Is uncomfortable in situations in which he or she is not the center of attention.
2. Interaction with others is often characterized by inappropriate sexually seductive or provocative behavior.
3. Displays rapidly shifting and shallow expression of emotions.
4. Consistently uses physical appearance to draw attention to self.
5. Has a style of speech that is excessively impressionistic and lacking in detail.
6. Shows self-dramatization, theatricality, and exaggerated expression of emotion.
7. Is suggestible, i.e., easily influenced by others or circumstances.
8. Considers relationships to be more intimate than they actually are.

Source: American Psychiatric Association 1994, p. 657.

they do not exist. Because more females than males are diagnosed with this condition, the diagnosis of histrionic personality disorder may reflect the bias of the clinician (Ford and Widiger 1989).

As with other personality disorders, it is important to consider cultural and ethnic background. Approximately 3% of the general population are diagnosed with this disorder (APA 1994). For the DSM-IV diagnostic criteria, see the accompanying box.

Linda, a 33-year-old woman who is twice divorced, was observed at the outpatient clinic responding flirtatiously to male staff members. She was neatly groomed but dressed in a low-cut peasant blouse, a tight miniskirt, and bright red knee-high boots. When called by the female therapist for her appointment, Linda screamed that she had waited too long, complaining loudly about patients' rights to rapid treatment. She quickly captured the attention of others in the waiting room. Then Linda feigned dizziness and "fell" as she arose from her chair. During the ensuing session, Linda complained that several men had made passes at her on the bus. When the therapist failed to share her outrage, Linda accused her of being jealous. Linda terminated the interview at that point and left the office, slamming the door behind her and stating, "My problems are physical, and no one cares whether I live or die. You'll be sorry for treating me this way!"

Subjective and Objective Data

Dramatic, Exhibitionistic, and Egocentric Responses Responses are characterized by exaggerated emotional expression; craving for attention, activity, and excitement; overreaction to minor stessors; irrational emotional outbursts; and temper tantrums. "I need someone to see me right now. . . . What kind of physicians staff this emergency room—sadists?"

Difficulty Sustaining Interpersonal Relationships Histrionic clients constantly need love, reassurance, and validation of their existence because of their feelings of dependence and helplessness. For this reason, they have problems with significant relationships. These individuals are likely to manipulate others to hold on to a love object while being highly inconsiderate and lacking empathy.

Calling her current boyfriend at 3:00 in the morning, Mary says,"Oh, Jim, I couldn't sleep and I knew you would want to be with me, at least in spirit."

Sexual Expression People with HPD are generally provocative and seductive and use sexual expression to manipulate and control others in relationships. Clients are often unaware of this flamboyance and how others perceive it. Individuals are often competitive with those of the same sex and seductive with the opposite sex. This personality disorder is more frequent in women than men, although men may express themselves in terms of their athletic prowess (APA 1994). A potential problem is promiscuous sexual activity and risk of HIV transmission.

Client to spouse: "I can't stand the way Julie rubs her body against you when she greets you."

Dysphoric Moods Dysphoria is a sense of disquiet or restlessness. Histrionic clients may experience depression when their demands for attention and affection are not met. They may act out in a suicidal fashion in order to manipulate or coerce others. Often, these individuals behave frivolously, acting silly and making nuisances of themselves.

Client to spouse who is threatening to leave him: "If you won't stay with me, there's no point in living. You'll be very sorry you are doing this."

Cognitive Dimensions Clients with histrionic personality disorder are much more interested in creative or imaginative pursuits than in analytic or academic achievements. They tend to be impressionable and highly suggestible and tend to look to authority figures for magical solutions to problems.

Health Patterns Regression and the development of somatic and/or dissociative disorders are frequent among histrionic people. These disabling symptoms may serve the purpose of calling attention to the person. They generally occur when an audience is present or when an unpleasant situation is anticipated. Substance use, depression, seizurelike activity, blackouts, falling, dizziness, or reactive psychoses may lead to hospitalization.

Nursing Diagnosis

Nurses' responses to clients who have Cluster B personality disorders may be similar to the behaviors displayed by the clients—anger, helplessness, increased anxiety, rescuer notions, defensiveness, and guilt from a sense of powerlessness. Although histrionic clients may look and act as though they have few problems, major dysfunctions are present. Nursing diagnoses may include those that follow.

Risk for Injury The dramatic, impulsive responses of HPD clients may lead to injuries or suicidal gestures. Problems often include the following:

- Increased potential for accidents, especially falls and automobile accidents.
- Self-inflicted injury or suicide attempt.
- Misdiagnosis of physical illness.
- Physical and verbal altercations.

Ineffective Individual Coping Ineffective coping is manifested by behavior resulting from high anxiety levels, limited judgment, and need for attention and reassurance. These behaviors are often observed:

- Seductiveness (in dress, makeup, mannerisms, conversational tone and content).
- Substance use.
- Manipulation of others; lack of consideration.
- Emotional lability.
- Low tolerance of frustration.
- Irresponsibility, vanity, silliness, frivolity.
- Lack of insight.
- Overuse of denial.
- Inability to deal with stress.
- Frequent physical complaints.
- Angry outbursts.

Planning and Implementing Interventions

Nursing care for histrionic clients closely resembles that for borderline clients. Because many health care professionals view these clients as feigning illness, it is imperative to carry out a thorough physical assessment. Do not permit a client to use physical complaints to avoid responsibilities. In addition, the potential for self-injury is a risk, and suicidal assessment should be a component of daily interviews when the client is in crisis.

Treatment plans should emphasize that staff members must avoid paying attention to the sexual provocations of these clients. Clients should be taught safer-sex practices to prevent the transmission of disease. Limit setting, as well as positive reinforcement for appropriate behavior, should be stressed. In inpatient settings, clients should be removed from an "audience" when attention-seeking behaviors occur. Routine teaching emphasis should be on assertiveness training and appropriate social behavior.

Evaluation and Outcome Criteria

Even when intervention strategies are implemented consistently, histrionic clients tend to manifest more denial than clients with other disorders in the dramatic-emotional cluster.

Risk for Injury When acting-out behavior is eliminated, the potential for self-destructive acts will be decreased. Hopefully, the client will also develop communication skills sufficient to avoid physical altercations with others.

Ineffective Individual Coping It is not unusual for histrionic clients to exaggerate all aspects of living and loving. If the client can learn to be less conspicuous and to express emotions appropriately, then many seductive, attention-seeking behaviors will diminish. But there is always the possibility that when the client's needs for affection and attention are thwarted, vulnerability to depression may increase.

The Nursing Process and Clients with Narcissistic Personality Disorder

Assessment

People with narcissistic personality disorder (NPD) have difficulty regulating self-esteem and self-expression (Masterson 1981). Jacobson (1979) advises that the term **narcissism** should apply to clients whose self-esteem is too low, as well as inappropriately high. Characteristics most frequently observed include a sense of entitlement,

DSM-IV Diagnostic Criteria for Narcissistic Personality Disorder

A pervasive pattern of grandiosity (in fantasy or behavior), need for admiration, and lack of empathy, beginning by early adulthood and present in a variety of contexts, as indicated by five (or more) of the following:

1. Has a grandiose sense of self-importance (e.g., exaggerates achievements and talents, expects to be recognized as superior without commensurate achievements).
2. Is preoccupied with fantasies of unlimited success, power, brilliance, beauty, or ideal love.
3. Believes that he or she is "special" and unique and can only be understood by, or should associate with, other special or high-status people (or institutions).
4. Requires excessive admiration.
5. Has a sense of entitlement, i.e., unreasonable expectations of especially favorable treatment or automatic compliance with his or her expectations.
6. Is interpersonally exploitative, i.e., takes advantage of others to achieve his or her own ends.
7. Lacks empathy: is unwilling to recognize or identify with the feelings and needs of others.
8. Is often envious of others or believes that others are envious of him or her.
9. Shows arrogant, haughty behaviors or attitudes.

Source: American Psychiatric Association 1994, p. 661.

interpersonal manipulations, lack of empathy, and indifference toward others.

About 1% of the general population has NPD, and it is increasing steadily. Of those diagnosed, 50–75% are male (APA 1994). There may be a higher than usual risk in children of narcissistic parents who impart to them an unrealistic sense of omnipotence, grandiosity, beauty, and talent (Kaplan and Sadock 1991). While narcissistic traits are quite common in adolescents, they do not necessarily go on to develop NPD (APA 1994). For the diagnostic criteria, see the accompanying box.

Subjective and Objective Data

Grandiosity Grandiosity is evidenced by expressions of exaggerated self-importance, self-absorption, and egocentricity. This inflated self-concept may be a compensation for feelings of diminished self-worth. Isolating a child from the feedback of others and the parents' failing to mirror the child's behavior may contribute to this disorder. **Mirroring** or "mirror images" reflect what the parents think of and how they treat the child. When coming in contact with people outside the home, the child may discover a discrepancy between the way others treat him or her and the mirror images developed at home. Excessive boasting may result from this inconsistency in self-concept. Humility is not a characteristic.

Preoccupations The narcissistic person is generally preoccupied and fantasizes about power, success, idealized love, morals, and intelligence. These behaviors may be the result of overidealization of the child by the parents. Concern over declining physical attractiveness and occupational limitations may lead them to seek cosmetic surgery.

Exhibitionism Exhibitionistic behavior is evidenced by the constant seeking of support and admiration from others. Because of their limited interests, these clients perseverate about themselves to the point of boring others.

Vacillation of Affective Response In spite of the narcissistic individual's extensive use of rationalization for failures, there is an underlying sense of rage, shame, and diminished self-esteem. The perceptive nurse may observe cool indifference, emptiness, humiliation, uncontrolled anger, or desire for revenge. They lack empathy for others, especially those who are perceived to be of lower status.

Dysfunctional Interpersonal Relationships Clients with NPD feel entitled to special favors and attention. Further, they refuse to assume mutual responsibilities in relationships. They tend to exploit others and disregard their rights. Kernberg (1975) emphasizes that chronic, intense envy and defenses against envy lead to idealization or devaluation of others. Responses to others may include lack of concern, mistrust, lack of intimacy, accusations of incompetence, and demand for unattainable perfection.

They see interpersonal relationships as a means of enhancing their own self-esteem. A narcissistic person often will select a spouse or a mate who will be dutiful and subservient in return for assurances of security and faithfulness.

Socialization In addition to having problems forming and sustaining interpersonal relationships, the narcissistic person may experience occupational divergences. Kohut (1971) describes work inhibitions as peculiar to this group. In contrast, Cameron and Rychlak (1985) note that these individuals often assume active leadership roles, putting their power needs to work and attacking the established working order. One may also consider the effect of the culture on the development of socialization skills. The post–World War II philosophy of "looking out for number one" may well have contributed to a rise in identification of narcissistic disorders and their inclusion as a diagnostic category in the *DSM-III* (Widiger and Frances 1985).

Sexual Expression Perverse sexual fantasies, promiscuity, or homosexuality may be associated with this disorder. There may be confusion regarding sex-role behavior as a result of learned defenses against libidinal and ego-need conflicts (Wilson and Prabucki 1983).

Alicia is a 40-year-old teacher who seeks professional counseling after dropping out of a graduate program. She presents as a slender, well-groomed individual. Alicia makes it clear upon initial contact that she has a wide circle of friends. Indeed, she devotes the first 30 minutes of the session to recounting sexual encounters and venting anger that concern about AIDS is limiting her sex partners. She states she had a live-in relationship with one partner for 15 years but that recently this partner became discontented with her need to "party." Consequently the two are not "communicating." Alicia defends her desire to seek out a variety of partners by focusing on her personal needs and the "lack of consideration" of her significant other.

When questioned about dropping out of graduate school, Alicia rationalizes her failure by blaming it on a "hostile major professor" and further proclaiming, "I know more than he does." She describes herself as the "leader" in her group of six graduate students and interprets this to mean that they have great respect for her.

She tells the therapist that she attempted to call two friends following her withdrawal from school. She dramatically and self-righteously expresses anger and disappointment that they were not available to her. (One was vacationing out of state and the other was hospitalized for major surgery.) When the therapist inquires how her friend was doing following surgery, Alicia responded, "How in the world should I know? That's not my problem. She never even bothered to call me back."

Alicia requests that the therapist set up Saturday morning appointments (no office hours were normally scheduled on this day) because she becomes very tired in the afternoons and always takes a nap. When the therapist refuses to meet this request, Alicia becomes angry and shouts, "You're just like all the rest of them. No one considers my needs! I'll see to it that your supervisor hears about this, and I'll let all my friends know how incompetent you are as a therapist."

Nursing Diagnosis

Like people with BPD and HPD, people with NPD have problems associated with disturbed self-concept and coping abilities. Nursing diagnoses will usually include those that follow.

Personal Identity Disturbance

- Self-centeredness.
- Exaggerated sense of importance and intelligence.
- Setting unrealistic goals.
- Indifference to the feelings of others.
- Interpersonal exploitiveness.
- Concern over aging and physical attractiveness.
- Entitlement.

Ineffective Individual Coping

- Excessive use of denial of shortcomings, rationalization of errors, and projection of blame.
- Inconsistent and intense emotional responses to interpersonal relationships.
- Occupational dysfunctions.
- Preoccupation with or fantasies of power.
- Exhibitionism.

Planning and Implementing Interventions

Objectives for the care of narcissistic clients are helping them accept feedback without defensiveness and rationalization, increasing their capacity to tolerate frustration and disappointment, and helping them appreciate the rights and needs of others. Interventions are geared toward using the therapeutic alliance to work through feelings of abandonment, rejection, shame, and self-doubt, thereby heightening self-esteem. Heterogeneous group therapies have been successful with some narcissistic clients (Wong 1980). However, the client often terminates both individual and group work prematurely.

You must be attuned to personal feelings and reactions when working with clients with NPD. Do not criticize their haughty, uncaring attitude, but demonstrate by actions that they are accepted regardless of wealth, position, or status.

Prevention of this disorder may be facilitated by teaching parents how to praise and reward their children in a realistic fashion that acknowledges them as people, not as the sum of their accomplishments.

Evaluation and Outcome Criteria

The goal is for the narcissistic individual to learn how to empathize with others by recognizing that it is not necessary to be right all the time, that imperfections in self and others exist. Although some clients develop positive roles through the use of creativity and humor, most substitute hypochondriacal behavior and a sense of emptiness and lowered self-esteem for previous behaviors and feelings.

The Nursing Process and Clients with Antisocial Personality Disorder

Assessment

The antisocial personality was one of the earliest to be identified. It has been labeled *psychopathy, sociopathy, dyssocial disorder,* and *moral insanity.* Without question, it is the most researched and validated of the personality disorders (Widiger and Frances 1985). Yet there have been no great strides in our understanding of the syndrome or the successful treatment of these individuals (Reid 1985). One reason is that most antisocial people do not seek medical help but often come to the attention of authorities because of criminal activity. Such criminal behavior creates anger toward the person committing it, which precludes medical research support. It is difficult to identify antisocial personality disorder as an illness when the behaviors are seemingly intentional, antagonistic, and self-serving.

Some clinicians are concerned about the term *antisocial* because it connotes criminality. In fact, the behaviors may be adaptive in people with certain lifestyles, such as transient pieceworkers, people holding high-risk jobs, and even the chronically mentally ill (Cameron and Rychlak 1985; Reid 1985; Travin and Protter 1982). Remember that manipulation, which is a hallmark of the antisocial client's behavior, may be a normal, nondestructive mode of meeting one's needs. However, when used to control others, manipulation interferes with interpersonal relationships. In antisocial clients, the drive to manipulate others is paramount, because these clients feel a need to be "number one" at all times.

The essential features of antisocial personality disorder (ASPD) are found in the accompanying box and are used as criteria for making the diagnosis. In clinical settings, 3–30% of the population may have this disorder. Higher prevalence rates are found in substance abuse treatment centers and forensic settings (APA 1994).

DSM-IV Diagnostic Criteria for Antisocial Personality Disorder

A. There is a pervasive pattern of disregard for and violation of the rights of others occurring since age 15 years, as indicated by three (or more) of the following:
   1. Failure to conform to social norms with respect to lawful behaviors as indicated by repeatedly performing acts that are grounds for arrest.
   2. Deceitfulness, as indicated by repeated lying, use of aliases, or conning others for personal profit or pleasure.
   3. Impulsivity or failure to plan ahead.
   4. Irritability and aggressiveness, as indicated by repeated physical fights or assaults.
   5. Reckless disregard for safety of self or others.
   6. Consistent irresponsibility, as indicated by repeated failure to sustain consistent work behavior or honor financial obligations.
   7. Lack of remorse, as indicated by being indifferent to or rationalizing having hurt, mistreated, or stolen from another.

B. The individual is at least age 18 years.

C. There is evidence of Conduct Disorder with onset before age 15 years.

D. The occurrence of antisocial behavior is not exclusively during the course of Schizophrenia or a Manic Episode.

Source: American Psychiatric Association 1994, p. 649.

The study of developmental considerations has been hampered by the fact that most investigators have used prisoners as research subjects. Although many criminals are sociopaths, not all sociopaths are found in prisons. While the course of this disorder tends to become chronic, it has been noted that by the fourth decade of life, there is a decrease in criminal behavior as well as other manifestations.

Research indicates strong familial tendencies toward this disorder. It is more common among first-degree relatives; having a female biologic relative with the disorder tends to increase the risk. While adoption studies show that more genetic and environmental factors contribute to the risk, adopted children are at a higher risk for development of this psychopathology (APA 1994).

In workplace, social, and clinical contacts with antisocial people, you may find them initially attractive. They are often intellectually "bright," conversationally "glib," and they will "tell you what you want to hear." Because they are so astute in identifying others' vulnerabilities, nurses are frequently amazed at the "empathy" they show for others. These behaviors are manipulative and are used to create a situation which the antisocial person can control. The arousal of feelings of anger, powerlessness, a sense of having been "conned," disappointment, and even guilt and shame is common among health care professionals.

Subjective Data During the initial interview, it is common for the person diagnosed with ASPD to refuse responsibility for admission to the mental health or forensic facility. In fact, this individual will probably claim that the victim of his or her actions is at fault; in addition no remorse will be shown. "Well, you know, the only reason I'm here is because those cops made a mistake and thought I was the one who was assaulting that woman. Actually I stopped to help her and she told them I was trying to rape her. You know if she hadn't parked her car in the mall garage, then she wouldn't have been at risk for an assault in the first place."

Manipulation, another hallmark of this disorder, often shows in the client's attempt to form alliances with the staff. Once alliances are formed, splitting occurs and the client is in control. "You know, you are the only nurse on this unit who knows anything about the meds that we get. I always feel so safe when you are at the med station. You know when I really need my tranquilizers. The other nurses look at me suspiciously like I'm some kind of criminal. Thank God you're on duty tonight." This same client may tell the nurse on the following shift, "That night nurse does nothing but pass pills all night long; she never spends time with the patients or even tries to talk to them before she drugs them up. I think something should be done about her."

Impulsiveness is manifested in the client's making quick decisions without any regard for the consequences. "I'm going on pass right now; it doesn't matter if you discharge me AMA." Aggression may be shown in picking fights with other clients, often when the antisocial person feels a need for excitement or has not received sufficient attention from the staff. "Hey, if you guys would get more sports going for us here, we wouldn't be getting on each other's nerves so much."

Disregard for the welfare and safety of others may be noted in sexual acting-out, including having intimate relationships with others on the unit. "I've been talking to the social worker about the need for conjugal visits; maybe now you'll understand how important it is to meet our biological as well as our psychological needs."

Objective Data Lack of anxiety is notable with these clients, unless there is extreme external stress, in which case they may act out in ways that put them at high risk for accidents, physical injury, or suicidal acts. History of violence toward others is very common, including sex offenses (rape, child pornography, child molestation) and murder. You will also notice a considerable lack of empathy, along with pathologic lying. These clients give histories of drug dealing and substance abuse, prostitution, homelessness, erratic job histories, and exploitive sexual relationships. While these individuals can identify correct and appropriate behavior, they do not believe that rules apply to them, only to others.

They need immediate gratification in most situations but can delay rewards to the extent that they need planning time to achieve what they want. Most antisocial people are extroverted and make good first impressions because they can be charming and persuasive. They are often admitted to mental health facilities for depressive symptoms, suicidal attempts, substance abuse, somatic disorders, and/or anxiety disorders.

Nursing Diagnosis

Despite the quantity of assessment data, the primary nursing diagnoses for the antisocial client are the two that follow, with the accompanying problems often observed.

Ineffective Individual Coping

- Altered participation in society.
- Verbal and nonverbal manipulation.
- Destructive behavior toward self and others.
- Overuse of defense mechanisms of denial, splitting, projection, rationalization, and intellectualization.
- Impaired problem-solving abilities.

Impaired Social Interaction

- Altered self-esteem evidenced by affective disturbances (grandiosity, depression).
- Lack of responsibility, accountability, or commitment.
- Lying.
- Distancing relationships.
- Nonparticipation in therapy.
- Impulsiveness.

Planning and Implementing Interventions

Because antisocial people manipulate others so successfully, it is unlikely that they will seek change unless faced with severe external stress. In clinical situations, your responses to these clients are critical to developing and maintaining a therapeutic alliance as well as preserving the hospital or prison milieu. The accompanying

INTERVENTION

The Antisocial Client

Nursing Intervention	Rationale
• Use a concerned but matter-of-fact approach.	• Appropriate distance must be given all clients.
• Set, communicate, and maintain consistent rules and regulations for all clients.	• Provides security.
• Do not argue, bargain, or rationalize.	• Decreases power struggles.
• Confront inappropriate behaviors without anger, punitiveness, or personalization.	• The behavior, not the person, should be addressed.
• Do not seek approval, or coax; use choices and consequences.	• A professional relationship increases client self-control.
• Set limits on all interactions and behaviors.	• Conveys external control.
• Be alert for flattery or verbal attacks.	• Decreases the chances of manipulation.
• Do not permit client to dictate the therapeutic regimen.	• The therapeutic structure decreases manipulative attempts.
• Using contracts and relaxation techniques, teach client how to delay immediate gratification and impulsiveness.	• Provides other outlets for anger and aggression.
• Teach client to redirect thrill-seeking impulses into socially acceptable outlets, such as race car driving versus speeding.	• Negative behaviors can be replaced with positive ones.
• Use peer pressure (groups, buddy systems) to modify manipulative behaviors.	• Peer feedback is a greater reinforcement than staff input.
• Use reinforcing techniques and consequences to achieve desired behaviors.	• Increases the frequency of positive outcomes.

Intervention box provides guidelines for developing a relationship. It is important to recognize, however, that these clients identify unit power structures and pit staff members against one another. Because these clients tend to be intelligent and charming, staff members may fail to recognize manipulations and may excuse such behavior. In addition, clients may actively resist directives while appearing to be compliant. Short-term therapy is usually ineffective, and long-term hospitalization or incarceration may be indicated.

In general, you must present the "brick wall" that antisocial clients must face (Dighton 1986) as they attempt to manipulate others to achieve personal ends. Because of their charm, air of superiority, and persuasiveness, antisocial people sometimes manipulate nurses to assume the roles of nurturers and rescuers. Never give out your telephone number, assign special privileges, or make yourself available to these clients outside the therapeutic relationship. These clients have lifelong patterns of victimizing others.

Incorporate clear, concise, and consistent limit setting and directions into all intervention strategies. Develop these strategies using a team approach, and contract with the client. When infractions of the rules or manipulations occur, apply consequences immediately. Do not include clients in any discussions about other clients or staff members.

The use of reinforcing techniques for behavior is important, but the approach should be direct and matter-of-fact. When clients become anxious or impulsive, or when acting-out occurs, relaxation techniques, journal writing, and/or physical activity may be useful. Point out for the

INTERVENTION (continued)

Nursing Intervention	Rationale
• Role-model self-discipline.	• New behaviors can be patterned after those of others.
• Participate in staff meetings and clinical supervision to work through transference and countertransference phenomena.	• Consistency and open communication decrease manipulation.
• Encourage the connection between client behavior and consequences.	• Increases a sense of responsibility.
• Positively reward appropriate behavior, such as honesty or empathy, in a gradually increasing manner.	• Positive reinforcement increases self-esteem and compliance.
• Do not discuss other staff or clients with the antisocial person.	• Keep client as the focal point in order to decrease manipulation.
• Ask client to keep a log of daily frustrations, along with perceived options.	• Understanding triggers, and alternatives increase, self-control.
• Assess for suicidal/homicidal intent.	• Safety of all clients is a priority.
• Place client in a room where he or she may be monitored easily.	• Elopement risk is minimized.
• Staffing should be sufficient to control aggressive behavior.	• Conveys external control and increases a sense of security.
• Help client identify true sources of anger.	• Angry outbursts are often displaced feelings.
• Point out and process rationalization when it occurs.	• Increases client awareness.

antisocial client when lying, intellectualizations, rationalizations, or projections occur so that he or she may become conscious of these behaviors.

Evaluation and Outcome Criteria

Extensive studies indicate that antisocial clients:

- Do not respond to drug therapy.
- Remain in psychodynamic therapies only long enough to decrease their anxiety and ingratiate therapists.
- Respond to cognitive-behavioral therapies only if someone is available to reinforce the desired behaviors.

Court-ordered hospitalization tends to be more successful than voluntary treatment because the antisocial individual is generally highly manipulative and may easily disrupt the milieu or leave the facility. Some therapeutic success has been observed with "back-to-nature" programs in which survival depends on developing skills and relationships with others (Reid 1985). The treatment outcome may improve if the antisocial client is able to form a working relationship with the therapist (Gerstley et al. 1989).

Some antisocial people "burn out" in later life (after age 40), giving up extreme forms of antisocial responses (APA 1994). These people do not become model citizens, but they tend to avoid the criminal and welfare systems.

When evaluating short-term inpatient objectives, the nurse looks for the following client behaviors as evidence that coping abilities and self-concept are within normal boundaries.

INEFFECTIVE INDIVIDUAL COPING

- Increased impulse control and ability to delay gratification.
- Decreased verbal and nonverbal manipulations.
- Adherence to unit rules and regulations.
- Acceptance of personal responsibility and accountability for actions.

IMPAIRED SOCIAL INTERACTION

- Realistic identification of assets and liabilities.
- Identification of personal problem areas.
- Absence of aggression directed to self or others.
- Assertive communications with others.

Anxious-Fearful Personality Disorders

According to the *DSM-IV*, individuals who present primarily as anxious or fearful may be diagnosed with **avoidant, dependent,** or **obsessive-compulsive personality disorder.** Anxious-fearful people generally experience both social and occupational impairments as a result of their restricted affect, nonassertiveness, problems expressing feelings, unrealistic expectations of others, and impaired decision making and problem solving. These individuals tend to have arrested development during the oral or anal stages of psychosexual development (Cameron and Rychlak 1985). Developmental precursors to these disorders include early anxiety associated with parental attitudes and fears of abandonment and rejection. Overly critical, demanding, and punitive parenting practices coupled with diminished opportunities to express feelings may be contributing factors. Reich's study (1989) indicates the significance of family history in the development of the anxious-fearful cluster of personality disorders (Cluster C). The lifestyle of the anxious-fearful person is characterized by intense emotional repression and behaviors that are socially isolating and self-defeating. The behaviors of anxious-fearful personalities tend to overlap, and common features are described in the accompanying Assessment box.

The Nursing Process and Clients with Avoidant Personality Disorder

Assessment

SUBJECTIVE AND OBJECTIVE DATA The essential feature of people with avoidant personality disorder (APD) is a pattern of social withdrawal along with a sense of inadequacy, and fear and hypersensitivity to potential rejection and shame. These people withdraw socially even though they avidly desire affection and acceptance. Their avoidant behavior results in visiting public places (movies, museums, and ballparks) simply to experience the presence of other people because they do not enjoy being alone. When in public places, however, they maintain a safe distance from others. For example, in a movie theater, one can be physically close to people without feeling that one's personal space is being invaded.

Avoidant people devalue their own achievements. They appear overly serious, humorless, and painfully shy. Speech is often slow, and they do not express feelings. Thought content is generally serious. For the DSM-IV diagnostic criteria for APD, see the box on page 512.

Mary Jane is a 27-year-old single female who sought counseling because of her feelings of loneliness and lack of friends. She describes herself as having grown up on a midwestern farm where she was "pretty much a homebody." In high school she made good grades but did not participate in any extracurricular activities. She studied library science in college and admits to receiving secondhand pleasure from reading about experiences of others. Historical novels are her favorites. She is currently employed as a reference librarian in a large computer software company where she has minimal contact with other people. She says she wants to establish both male and female friendships but feels afraid that "people will laugh" at her. Mary Jane joined the company bowling team at the suggestion of a coworker but quit after the first evening because she felt she would "hold them back." Mary Jane rationalized her decision by stating, "I think I would be more comfortable pursuing an intellectual hobby."

Although the schizoid and avoidant personalities have many similar characteristics, the avoidant person's motivation to form a therapeutic relationship differentiates the two. The avoidant person also tends to lead a fairly productive life, particularly regarding occupation and self-care maintenance.

Nursing Diagnosis

The primary nursing diagnoses for avoidant personality disorder are given below. The social isolation is self-induced, and the feelings that promote distancing are very painful.

SOCIAL ISOLATION

- Feelings of being "different."
- Lack of significant purpose.
- Insecurity in public.

ASSESSMENT

Common Features of the Anxious-Fearful Personality

Aloof, Ambivalent Social Style

The anxious-fearful person restricts social contact to those typified as safe and nonrejecting. Because they anticipate rejection and criticism from others, their relationships may be either clinging or detached. The dependent person seeks to replace an ended relationship with another one as soon as possible.

Restricted Affect

The affective responses of anxious-fearful people range from insensitivity to the feelings of others to overconcern and oversensitivity to evaluation by others. The inability to express underlying feelings is generally based on a fear that others will reject them unless they are perfect. Avoidant and dependent people tend to see themselves as inferior to others and subordinate their needs accordingly. In contrast, the compulsive person views authority as overly restrictive; consequently, he or she is insensitive to others' needs.

Fear of Success or Failure

Active or passive avoidance of responsibility characterizes all the anxious-fearful personalities. Resistant behavior may be deliberately avoidant, as seen in dependent and avoidant people. The behavior may be covert, as evidenced by the compulsive person's obsessive attention to details, leading to ineffective overall performance.

Fear of Loss of Control

When a person's quest for autonomy is thwarted at an early age, response patterns manifested by rigidity are often noted. Needs to control, to have guarantees of others' love, to avoid relaxation and fun, and to maintain structure and orderliness are seen in anxious-fearful people. These responses seem to provide some reassurance of predictability and control in their lives. The dependent person fears being left to care for himself or herself. The obsessive-compulsive person is unable to delegate duties to others. They assume errors will be made if their method is not used.

Fear of Embarrassment

People with any of the personality disorders in the anxious-fearful cluster manifest response patterns indicating low self-esteem and lack of self-confidence. An insignificant act by a waitress or salesperson may be construed as rejecting or overly solicitous. The avoidant person assumes that shame, ridicule, and rejection will accompany any intimate or significant relationship.

Difficulty with Decision Making

Related to low self-esteem and fear of criticism is a fear of making an incorrect choice or recommendation. Consequently, anxious-fearful people either tend to focus on details and procrastinate, or they may give responsibility for decision making to others, to avoid loss of approval. The obsessive-compulsive individual cannot discard worthless objects even when they have no sentimental value.

Negativity

Anxious-fearful people view the world as potentially disappointing. They exude an air of pessimism, irritability, sulkiness, discontent, and submissiveness that colors all their interactions. They tend to dampen everyone's spirits, thus confirming their perceptions and expectations.

- Verbalized fears of rejection.
- Shyness, inhibition.

CHRONIC LOW SELF-ESTEEM

- Inability to accept positive reinforcement.
- Inability to evaluate one's own worth realistically.
- Belittling oneself in daily activities; a pervading sense of inferiority.
- Condemning oneself for failing to develop adequate social skills.
- Fearful, tense demeanor.

Planning and Implementing Interventions

Intervention strategies are focused on developing a therapeutic alliance with the client. In this relationship, the nurse confronts clients' illogical beliefs about themselves

DSM-IV Diagnostic Criteria for Avoidant Personality Disorder

A pervasive pattern of social inhibition, feelings of inadequacy, and hypersensitivity to negative evaluation, beginning by early adulthood and present in a variety of contexts, as indicated by four (or more) of the following:

1. Avoids occupational activities that involve significant interpersonal contact, because of fears of criticism, disapproval, or rejection.
2. Is unwilling to get involved with people unless certain of being liked.
3. Shows restraint within intimate relationships because of the fear of being shamed or ridiculed.
4. Is preoccupied with being criticized or rejected in social situations.
5. Is inhibited in new interpersonal situations because of feelings of inadequacy.
6. Views self as socially inept, personally unappealing, or inferior to others.
7. Is unusually reluctant to take personal risks or to engage in any new activities because they may prove embarrassing.

Source: American Psychiatric Association 1994, p. 664.

and their perceptions of others and helps them test reality. Because these clients are so sensitive to teasing and ridicule, avoid these situations. Systematic desensitization techniques are useful in helping clients form social relationships. Behavioral techniques, such as contracting with the client to network with others in support groups and employment activities, may also be useful. Underlying any intervention strategies should be the knowledge that avoidant personalities, because of their intense fear, are prone to episodes of depression, phobias, and periods of intense inner-directed rage. Consequently, be prepared to prevent and deal with intermittent crises as psychodynamic issues are uncovered.

Evaluation and Outcome Criteria

Unless the cycle of timidity and fear in social situations is interrupted, avoidant clients continue to reinforce their apprehension by their own interpersonal restraint. In a clinical setting, expectations for the client would include:

- Establishing a positive relationship with the person.
- Describing himself or herself in a positive way.
- Demonstrating the ability to communicate socially.

Cognitive-behavioral therapies are often useful in helping these clients look at their own behaviors and at the erroneous meanings they may assign to the comments of others.

The Nursing Process and Clients with Dependent Personality Disorder

Assessment

Subjective and Objective Data The essential features of dependent personality disorder (DPD) include a pervasive, excessive, and unrealistic need to be cared for; fear of separation; lack of self-confidence; an inability to make decisions; and an inability to function independently. In sharp contrast to the avoidant person, dependent people cling to others and passively accept their dictates and leadership. Dependent people view themselves as "helpless" or "stupid" and seek out dominant others or objects to lean on for guidance, control, and support as well as for "permission" to behave. They have difficulty initiating projects and function adequately only when assured of approval and supervision.

The dominant other or object relationship stems from the normal life-sustaining bond between mother and infant. In dependent people, this normal symbiotic relationship has been excessively prolonged, impairing their capacity for thinking, feeling, and responding on their own. They believe they must be taken care of and consequently rely on others to mirror their feelings to them.

Dependent people subordinate their desires and needs to the wishes of others in order to maintain relationships. They often appear friendly, helpful, and indispensable. Indeed, they will volunteer for unpleasant tasks if they think it will be reciprocated with nurturing. When the dominant other or object is unavailable, or perceived as unavailable, dependent people experience intense anxiety. This may lead to feelings of unhappiness, anger, resentment, or depression. It is also noteworthy that significant others may eventually respond to dependent people with anger and resentment because of their continuous clinging and ingratiating behaviors.

The early childhood environment, which is characterized by premature separation from parents, neglect, overprotection, or lack of parental responsiveness, may predispose to DPD (Moyer and Snider 1984). Like people with other personality disorders, the dependent person may have multiple DSM-IV Axis II diagnoses. See the accompanying box for the diagnostic criteria. DPD is among the most frequently reported of the personality disorders (APA 1994).

The following example illustrates how a dependent client might behave.

Marie is a 40-year-old single parent of two teenage daughters. She has gained 70 lbs since her divorce 2 years ago. Currently, Marie is sporadically attending a group for displaced homemakers, where she has shared a great deal of information about herself. She states that she is essentially a "homebody" and feels most satisfied when baking, cooking, and sewing for her daughters. Marie describes her secondhand pleasure in their activities, including ballet, gymnastics, and modeling. In fact, Marie becomes visibly saddened when she discusses her daughters' eventual departure for college. When her daughters expressed concern about Marie's weight gain and general health, Marie giggled and said, "Better to be fat and jolly than skinny and mean."

Marie has made no attempt to develop new friendships or social outlets since her divorce. She is poorly groomed and haphazardly dressed, in contrast to her impeccably groomed daughters. When confronted by group members about setting priorities and the need to direct some energy toward herself, Marie responded, "My life is devoted to my daughters; their needs are more important than mine, and that's why I agreed to make the thirty costumes for their dance recital next week."

DSM-IV Diagnostic Criteria for Dependent Personality Disorder

A pervasive and excessive need to be taken care of that leads to submissive and clinging behavior and fears of separation, beginning by early adulthood and present in a variety of contexts, as indicated by five (or more) of the following:

1. Has difficulty making everyday decisions without an excessive amount of advice and reassurance from others.
2. Needs others to assume responsibility for most major areas of his or her life.
3. Has difficulty expressing disagreement with others because of fear of loss of support or approval. **Note:** Do not include realistic fears of retribution.
4. Has difficulty initiating projects or doing things on his or her own (because of a lack of self-confidence in judgment or abilities rather than a lack of motivation or energy).
5. Goes to excessive lengths to obtain nurturance and support from others, to the point of volunteering to do things that are unpleasant.
6. Feels uncomfortable or helpless when alone because of exaggerated fears of being unable to care for himself or herself.
7. Urgently seeks another relationship as a source of care and support when a close relationship ends.
8. Is unrealistically preoccupied with fears of being left to take care of himself or herself.

Source: American Psychiatric Association 1994, p. 668.

Nursing Diagnosis

Nurses frequently avoid or voice dislike for dependent clients because of their cloying, clinging, and demanding behaviors. This avoidance response tends to reinforce the clients' perceptions that other people are unwilling to help and that they are unable to help themselves. As a result, clients increase their clinging responses because they know no other way to behave. This increased clinging only leads to further avoidance by others. The primary nursing diagnoses and problem areas are those that follow.

Chronic Low Self-Esteem

- Is verbally and nonverbally compliant.
- Lacks initiative.
- Avoids decision making or changes mind frequently; has difficulty making decisions.
- Is unable to meet own needs independently.
- Is unwilling to make assertive requests of others for fear of rejection.
- Belittles personal assets and abilities.
- Feels uncomfortable when alone.

Bathing/Hygiene, Dressing/Grooming, and Feeding Self Care Deficits

- Altered activities of daily living (grooming, hygiene, and nutrition).
- Inattention to medical and dental needs unless supervised.

Planning and Implementing Interventions

The long-term goal of nursing interventions is to help the client achieve independent functioning. Short-term goals would help the client do the following:

INTERVENTION

The Dependent Client

Nursing Intervention	Rationale
• Evaluate client's ability to perform self-care activities; encourage grooming and personal hygiene.	• Fosters independent living skills.
• Schedule regular sessions as a way to anticipate client needs *before* he or she demands attention through inappropriate responses.	• Anticipatory guidance minimizes anxiety and acting-out.
• Help client identify assets and liabilities, including plans for change; emphasize strengths and potential.	• Self-assessment can enhance a positive self-concept.
• Encourage client to take responsibility for own opinions; point out when client negates own feelings or opinions.	• Fosters independence.
• Encourage client to verbalize feelings of anxiety related to independent functioning.	• Identification of feelings enhances ability to problem-solve.
• Encourage client to talk about how needs for affection, control, and responsibility are currently being met.	• Verbalization of feelings decreases fears and anxieties.
• Share with client your observations of his or her manipulative behavior. For example, client may offer to accompany a physically impaired client to a group activity in order to minimize the amount of time spent in productive therapy.	• Feedback from staff and peers fosters self-awareness.
• Set realistic limits about what can and cannot be done for the client.	• Minimizes client dependence on others.
• Using group therapy to provide support, emphasize that client is not alone in experiencing fear of failure or of success.	• Group support minimizes feelings of isolation.
• Work through feelings of disappointment with client when new behaviors are not immediately successful.	• By processing disappointment, learning can occur.
• Explore with client the consequences of behaviors; for example, clinging tends to result in avoidance by others.	• Clients may not be aware of how certain behaviors affect others.
• Discuss personal responsibilities and make client aware that he or she has choices.	• Choices optimize independent functioning.

- Ask for assistance only when realistically needed.
- Develop an awareness of dependent behaviors and make a decision to change.
- Increase social skills.
- Learn assertiveness skills such as the ability to say no and to meet his or her own needs first.

To these ends, nursing interventions include helping clients make realistic appraisals of their assets and liabilities; encouraging them to assume responsibility for self-care by providing schedules, supplies, and reminders as needed; giving clients feedback about how their behaviors influence responses from other people; setting realis-

INTERVENTION *(continued)*

Nursing Intervention	Rationale
• Teach client problem-solving techniques, including goal setting, making alternative responses, and evaluating consequences.	• A logical rather than emotional method of problem solving builds self-confidence.
• Provide opportunities for client to have successful experiences, and encourage participation in such activities.	• Positive affirmations enhance the repetition of behavior.
• Help client develop a realistic time frame in which to achieve independent living activities (getting a job or apartment).	• Time management enhances feelings of self-control.
• Do not do for client what he or she is capable of doing without help.	• Reduces dependence.
• Give positive reinforcement for successful achievements.	• Reinforces client's ability to succeed.
• Teach and role-model assertive behavior; teach client to develop strategies for confrontations by others.	• Clients often confuse assertive and aggressive communication.
• Prevent secondary gains from negative statements about self by refocusing interactions.	• Subject changes diminish reinforcement of negative self-talk.
• State goals for nursing care in terms client and staff can understand.	• Teaching must be appropriate to the learner's level of understanding.
• Involve staff members in conferences and clinical supervision to deal with transference and countertransference issues.	• Consistency and open communication decrease negative consequences.
• Introduce client to termination and discharge planning from admission and throughout stay.	• Termination can be a positive experience if client works through feelings.
• Help client identify present and future supports available in the community.	• A community support system dilutes dependence on the hospital/clinic.
• Gradually introduce different staff members to do one-to-ones with client.	• Fosters feelings of independence and decreases anxiety in new situations.
• Introduce client to social skills training groups (such as cooking and money management classes).	• Social interaction and successful experiences build self-confidence.

tic limits on what the staff will do for the client; establishing tasks that clients can initiate, complete, and get approval for independently; and teaching clients goal-setting, planning, and implementing techniques. Additional strategies are found in the accompanying Intervention box.

Evaluation and Outcome Criteria

Clients with DPD commonly experience crises when the dominant support system is altered. Often, they will frantically seek another caregiver upon the death of a significant other. Unrealistic fears of abandonment are not uncommon (APA 1994). During crisis episodes, these clients may be open to cognitive-behavioral strategies, but the outlook for major personality restructuring is dim. Instead, dependent people tend to transfer dependence needs to others.

The Nursing Process and Clients with Obsessive-Compulsive Personality Disorder

Assessment

People with obsessive-compulsive personality disorder (OCPD) demonstrate anxiety and fearfulness by behavior that shows fear of losing control over situations, objects, or people. The obsessive-compulsive personality strives at all times to keep the world predictable and organized. The major features of this disorder are an excessive dedication to work, productivity, and perfectionism to the exclusion of feelings and pleasure. A person with OCPD may be likened to a drill sergeant in the military who is rigid, serious, detail-oriented, and stingy with emotions.

A focus on trivial details often leads this person not only to "miss the forest for the trees, but also fail to see the tree while counting its leaves" (Eaton, Peterson, and Davis 1976). Although these people may be highly praised for their organizational skills and work ethic, eventually their rigidity causes them to fear making mistakes. Because they repeatedly check their work, they are not good time managers. Projects may not get completed. They are self-critical and adhere strictly and concretely to rules. Consequently, they postpone making decisions. They tend to resent authority but rarely express this resentment openly. Instead, they may engage in passive-aggressive behavior, such as procrastination and stubbornness.

The obsessive-compulsive personality, according to some theorists, evolves from the need to exert control and autonomy over one's bodily functions and the world during the second stage of psychosexual development. The struggle with parental figures over bowel control and the resultant anxiety and frustration may lead to characteristics of stinginess, pompous bookishness, and touchiness. Consequently, there is a lifelong struggle for independence, which is hampered by equally strong feelings of inadequacy, self-doubt, and ambivalence toward authority figures (Cameron and Rychlak 1985).

Interestingly, excessively conscientious, rigid people often exhibit a contradictory pattern of slovenliness, which is also compulsive. Thus, a compulsive housewife may scrub her kitchen floor daily but allow bags of garbage to accumulate and become infested.

Learning and behavioral theories about obsessive-compulsive behavior hold that society positively reinforces the ritualistic patterns people use to adapt to the world. It is also likely that the parents of an obsessive-compulsive individual disciplined the child excessively during the early years of development. Whether a compulsive response is adaptive or symptomatic depends on its effectiveness and the person's ability to modify the response when inappropriate. As noted earlier in the chapter, recent studies point to a biologic basis for OCPD. Clinical reports on the use of selective serotonin reuptake inhibitors (SSRIs) indicate that symptom relief is possible, especially with clomipramine (Anafranil Hce) (Zetin and Kramer 1992).

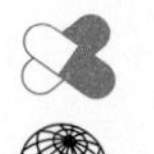

Because many cultures emphasize and positively reinforce adherence to a work ethic, it is important to consider cultural factors when assessing these clients. This disorder appears in males more often than females and in about 1% of the general population. Nurses often experience a range of responses to obsessive-compulsive clients, including pity, disgust, anger, frustration, anxiety, and intense discomfort. Because anxiety may be contagious, it is wise to limit the duration of one-to-one sessions and make contracts with clients to avoid spending an entire session on obsessional material. For the DSM-IV diagnostic criteria see the accompanying box.

Subjective and Objective Data When obsessive-compulsive clients describe their lifestyle, you will quickly become aware of their rigidity, concreteness, and need for order and perfection.

John, an OCPD client, explained, "I have all my clothes hanging in the closet according to the day of the week, including my socks and underwear, so I know if it's a Tuesday after a long weekend with a Monday holiday that I need to wear the clothing on the hanger marked Tuesday."

To manage their procrastination, obsessive-compulsive people often initiate work on a project far in advance of the due date.

Peter set himself a deadline in early fall for ordering his family's Christmas gifts. His family found this deadline something of an annoyance. Yet Peter persisted in his attempts to get commitments from everyone about what they wanted. Often, he would mislay his early purchases by the time Christmas arrived, and he would rush out to do last-minute shopping anyway.

In the above example, Peter appears to be concerned with his family and interpersonal relationships, but he is really more concerned with meeting the Christmas deadline and checking off his list than in his relatives' enjoyment of their gifts. Although Peter suffers under the pressure of his deadlines, he sets them for himself. He functions as his own overseer, issuing commands, direc-

DSM-IV Diagnostic Criteria for Obsessive-Compulsive Personality Disorder

A pervasive pattern of preoccupation with orderliness, perfectionism, and mental and interpersonal control, at the expense of flexibility, openness, and efficiency, beginning by early adulthood and present in a variety of contexts, as indicated by four (or more) of the following:

1. Is preoccupied with details, rules, lists, order, organization, or schedules to the extent that the major point of the activity is lost.
2. Shows perfectionism that interferes with task completion (e.g., is unable to complete a project because his or her own overly strict standards are not met).
3. Is excessively devoted to work and productivity to the exclusion of leisure activities and friendships (not accounted for by obvious economic necessity).
4. Is overconscientious, scrupulous, and inflexible about matters of morality, ethics, or values (not accounted for by cultural or religious identification).
5. Is unable to discard worn-out or worthless objects even when they have no sentimental value.
6. Is reluctant to delegate tasks or to work with others unless they submit to exactly his or her way of doing things.
7. Adopts a miserly spending style toward both self and others; money is viewed as something to be hoarded for future catastrophes.
8. Shows rigidity and stubbornness.

Source: American Psychiatric Association 1994, p. 672.

tives, reminders, warnings, and admonitions about what should be done. People like Peter are also keenly aware of society's and other people's expectations, of the threat of possible criticism, of the weight and direction of authority, of rules, regulations, and conventions, and of a great collection of moral or quasimoral principles. These people feel required to fulfill unending duties, responsibilities, and tasks that are, in their view, not chosen, but simply there.

Compulsive people do not view taking work home and working long hours as an imposition, since work organizes their lives and binds their anxiety. Indeed, the compulsive person will manage to make work out of pleasurable activities.

Jennifer planned her European vacation in meticulous detail. She scheduled exhausting daily tours and activities from 6:30 A.M. until 12:00 P.M. Jennifer planned to visit every attraction available as quickly as possible. So as not to waste time, she wrote her postcards to her family while she rode tour buses. The cards were crammed with information about weather, prices of goods and services, menus, and daily time tables. She wrote nothing about how she felt or what she was experiencing. Upon returning home, she spent two weeks cataloging all her photographs and typing short paragraphs to accompany each photo. She passed her album around at work during lunch hour expecting that her coworkers would read all the captions. She became insulted and irate when several coworkers flipped through the album quickly. Jennifer found it difficult to forgive them for "slighting" her in this way.

When a coworker was planning a trip, Jennifer suggested that he record details of the trip in a diary so that he could compile an album similar to her own. Jennifer was not aware of the resentment, hurt, and irritation her behavior generated in others.

Specific defining characteristics of the obsessive-compulsive personality are listed in the Assessment box on the next page. However, always consider how clients will react to the realization that years of denying themselves satisfaction, working hard, saving, and restricting the quality of life have not produced the expected rewards (career advancement, status, promotions). This realization often leads to the potential for depression, especially during middle life. As the following example shows, the obsessive-compulsive person may even postpone acting on major decisions to avoid the reality of life without work.

Millie, a 61-year-old college professor, seeks counseling one year prior to her planned retirement. She complains of insomnia, weight loss, and pervasive anxiety about "what life will be like without anything to do." Millie is retiring early because she feels that in spite of 25 years of loyal service to the university and diligent work, she has been passed over

ASSESSMENT

Common Features of the Obsessive-Compulsive Personality

- Shows excessive dedication to work.
- Is sensitive to criticism and rejection.
- Is preoccupied with organization, details, procedures, and rules.
- Is a perfectionist.
- Fails to complete tasks because of repeated checking and redoing.
- Is indecisive and ambivalent.
- Demands conformity to his or her standards.
- Resists authority or help of others.
- Excludes pleasure; makes work out of play; treats hobbies as serious tasks.
- Is moralistic and judgmental about self and others.
- Concentrates on minute details and trivia.
- Restricts emotional expression; has difficulty expressing feelings.
- Is stingy and miserly with both emotions and material objects; has lower standard of living than can be afforded.
- Harbors anger and resentment against others.
- Shows little empathy.
- Expresses anger indirectly.
- Is status-conscious.
- Fears making mistakes.
- Has potential for depression.
- Has difficulty discarding worn-out or worthless objects with no sentimental value.

repeatedly for promotion to the position of department chairperson. Millie is an unmarried, slender woman who is meticulously dressed in very conservative clothing.

During the interview, she says that she made most of her own clothing and purchased only items that were on sale. In describing her daily activities, Millie states that she is a "hard worker who always took things home to finish." She voices resentment that neither the department chairperson nor other faculty did likewise. Millie says that she spent more than 10 years caring for an elderly mother because "my sisters didn't have time for her." Millie devoted a great deal of time to church and university activities. The therapist's impression is that Millie performed these functions out of duty rather than for spontaneous enjoyment or satisfaction. Millie states that she volunteered to be secretary of the local humane society because she knew she could keep the detailed records better than any of the other members.

When questioned about her relationships with other faculty, Millie says that she communicated with them by memos to avoid being misquoted. She further states that she kept copies of all these memos because "They can't keep things straight most of the time." Millie becomes visibly angry when relating a recent experience: She overheard two colleagues ridiculing a memo requesting, 6 months in advance, that guest lecturers be permitted to use the colleagues' parking spaces. When challenged about the lack of immediacy of her request, Millie states that she has "stopped speaking to them [the faculty] entirely." When the therapist questions Millie about her interests for retirement, Millie says, "I don't really know; I've never had time for frivolous activities." By the end of the session, Millie has become indecisive about whether she should retire, after all.

Nursing Diagnosis

Ineffective Individual Coping and Social Isolation are the primary nursing diagnoses with obsessive-compulsive clients. These are evidenced by responses that show restricted cognitive, affective, and motor behavior, along with resentment, self-doubt, and the exclusion of pleasure.

Planning and Implementing Interventions

The goal is to help clients examine and evaluate their lifestyle and goals so they can modify troublesome compulsive traits and develop new behavior patterns that will enhance well-being and increase their capacity for intimacy. Help them express dissatisfaction with their lives and encourage realistic planning for future changes. Guidelines for nursing interventions are given in the accompanying Intervention box, right.

Interventions should help clients express their feelings in ways other than obsessing or compulsively acting out rituals. Exploring pleasurable activities, providing role modeling and social skills training, and helping clients evaluate their feelings about such activities will enhance their awareness of their level of anxiety and ineffective coping methods.

The administration of medication as ordered is an important nursing measure with these clients. It may not be possible for them to "give up" all their maladaptive behaviors, so goal setting must be realistic.

INTERVENTION

The Obsessive-Compulsive Client

Nursing Intervention	Rationale
• Confront nonconstructive, compulsive responses gently and be alert for anxiety when you confront the client.	• Increases self-awareness.
• Ask client to record feelings in a daily journal, highlighting situations where a mistake was made.	• Use of a journal increases client's connection between feelings and behavior.
• Show approval of recreation and enjoyment.	• Positive reinforcement encourages repetition of behavior.
• Do not demand that client engage in leisure or recreational activities (clients will "work" at them instead of enjoying them).	• Choices increase client's sense of control.
• Make a contract with client, stating how much time during one-to-one sessions will be used to discuss obsessive thoughts or rituals; gradually decrease the time allotted to these activities.	• Contractual agreements increase feelings of automony.
• Help client identify feelings of anxiety generated in stressful situations and the usual responses to this anxiety.	• Future behavior can be altered based on understanding the past.
• Help client identify alternative coping methods to deal with stressful situations.	• Reinforces that choices are available.
• Help client identify and differentiate between "shoulds" (behaviors expected by others) and "wants" (desirable activities).	• Differentiation of "should" from "wants" releases guilt and reduces anxiety.
• Explore activities that were or are pleasurable or satisfying.	• Client may not be aware of the feeling of pleasure.
• Plan activities and interventions around pleasurable memories and events.	• Learning to "play" occurs more easily in a relaxed setting.
• Encourage physical activity.	• Physical exertion reduces tension and fosters relaxation.
• Encourage verbalization of feelings, especially those of anger and resentment.	• Client must feel free to express negative as well as positive feelings.
• Provide examples of appropriate ways to handle emotion through role modeling, skills training, and group activities.	• Mirroring of appropriate behavior fosters positive changes.
• Discuss with client how to recognize behavior changes.	• Discussion of personal behaviors strengthens self-awareness.
• Monitor levels of compulsive behavior after initial baseline assessment.	• Documentation aids the evaluation of progress.

→

INTERVENTION (continued)

Nursing Intervention	Rationale
• Give gentle feedback, identifying weaknesses as well as strengths.	• Honest evaluation promotes growth.
• Provide progressive opportunities to make decisions.	• Encouragement should proceed from the simple to the complex.
• Encourage client to evaluate progress in meeting goals.	• Client involvement enhances compliance.
• Teach client how to use humor in situations of stress.	• Humor and laughter provide a release of tension and anxiety.
• Maintain routine schedules and appointments.	• Consistency enhances trust and reduces anxiety.
• Explore family responses to client's rigid behaviors.	• Family interactional patterns affect treatment outcome.

Evaluation and Outcome Criteria

As always, when evaluating any client with a personality disorder, consider the potential for major psychiatric conditions such as depression and anxiety-related disturbances. Even though people with obsessive-compulsive personalities often seek treatment for subjective distress, the course of treatment may be drawn out and ineffective as a result of the rigidity of their defensive operations. If the behavior is confronted directly, the client might develop acute psychiatric conditions because of intense anxiety.

Whenever possible, include family members or significant others in some aspects of therapy. Clients should be able to identify and verbalize their fears and some specific areas where change is indicated.

Personality Disorder Not Otherwise Specified

In addition to the *DSM-IV* categories discussed in this chapter, a category exists for disorders that do not meet criteria for any specific personality disorder: **personality disorder NOS.** An example would be when there is clinically significant distress or impairment in one or more important areas of functioning, such as work or socialization, with the presence of features from more than one specific personality disorder that do not meet the full criteria for any single disorder.

Chapter Highlights

- When personality traits (consistent, enduring response patterns) become inflexible, maladaptive, and cause social or occupational impairments, they may be diagnosed as personality disorders.
- Personality disorders are modes of functioning that include ways of thinking and perceiving, ways of experiencing emotion, and modes of subjective experience that are generally consistent patterns over broad areas of living.
- Personality disorders are best characterized by lifestyle responses that may create problems both for clients and, to some extent, for society.
- Personality disorders are best understood as defensive modes of living rather than as psychiatric illnesses.
- Examples of personality disorders include three major DSM-IV clusters: odd-eccentric (Cluster A), dramatic-emotional (Cluster B), and anxious-fearful (Cluster C).
- The odd-eccentric lifestyle is generally associated with people who are emotionally cold, aloof, guarded, and reclusive, and who exhibit various degrees of odd behavior.
- The dramatic-emotional lifestyle is generally associated with people who are impulsive, demonstrative, emotionally labile, needy, lacking in empathy, and unmindful of the consequences of behavior.

- The anxious-fearful lifestyle is generally associated with people who are hypersensitive, fearful of losing control, and lacking spontaneity.
- Nursing interventions for clients with personality disorders are based on the understanding that defensive operations such as anger and manipulation allow the client to avoid anxiety and maintain an ego-syntonic state.

References

Agras WS: *Behavior Modification Principles and Clinical Applications*. Little Brown, 1978.

Akhtar S: The syndrome of identity diffusion. *Am J Psychiatr* 1984;141:1381–1385.

American Psychiatric Association: *Diagnostic and Statistical Manual of Mental Disorders*, ed 4. APA, 1994.

Andrulonis PA, et al.: Organic brain dysfunction and the borderline syndrome. *Psychiatr Clin North Am* 1980;4:47–66.

Benner DG, Joscelyne B: Multiple personality as a borderline disorder. *J Nerv Ment Dis* 1984;172:98–104.

Brainerd CJ: *Piaget's Theory of Intelligence*. Prentice-Hall, 1978.

Braverman B, Shook J: Spotting the borderline personality. *Am J Nurs* 1987;2:200–203.

Cameron N, Rychlak JF: *Personality Development and Psychopathology: A Dynamic Approach*. Houghton Mifflin, 1985.

Chitty KK, Maynard CK: Managing manipulation. *J Psychosoc Nurs Ment Health Serv* 1986;24:8–13.

Cleckley H: *The Mask of Sanity*. Mosby, 1964.

Cloninger CR: The antisocial personality. *Hosp Pract* (Aug) 1978;97–106.

Cull A, Chick J, Wolff S: A consensual validation of schizoid personality in childhood and adult life. *Br J Psychiatr* 1984;144:646–648.

Dighton S: Tough-minded nursing. *Am J Nurs* 1986;86:48–51.

Dillon KM, Brooks D: *Psychological Reports* 1992;70(1):35–39.

Eaton Jr MT, Peterson MH, Davis JA: *Psychiatry*, ed 3. Medical Examination Publishing, 1976.

Ellis A: *Humanistic Psychology*. McGraw-Hill, 1973.

Else L, et al.: Personality characteristics of men who physically abuse women. *Hosp Commun Psychiatr* 1993;44: 54–58.

Erikson EH: *Childhood and Society*. Norton, 1964.

Feldman RB, Guttman HA: Families of borderline patients: Literal-minded parents, borderline parents, and parental protectiveness. *Am J Psychiatr* 1984;141:1392–1396.

Ford MR, Widiger TA: Sex bias in the diagnosis of histrionic and antisocial personality disorder. *J Consult Clin Psychol* 1989;57:301–305.

Frank H, Paris J: Recollections of family experience in borderline patients. *Arch Gen Psychiatr* 1981;38:1031–1034.

Freeman SK: Inpatient management of a patient with borderline personality disorder: A case study. *Arch Psychiatr Nurs* 1988;2:360–366.

Frosch J: The psychosocial treatment of personality disorders, in Frosch J (ed): *Current Perspectives on Personality Disorders*. American Psychiatric Press, 1983.

Gallop R: The patient is splitting: Everyone knows and nothing changes. *J Psychosoc Nurs Ment Health Serv* 1985;23: 6–10.

Gallop R, Lancee W, Garfinkel P: How nursing staff respond to the label "borderline personality disorder." *Hosp Commun Psychiatr* 1989;40:815–819.

Garfinkel T: A reconsideration of psychotherapy of narcissistic personality disorder. *Am J Psychoanal* 1982;42:207–220.

Genetic traits predispose some to criminality. *U.S. News and World Report* (Sept) 1985;54.

Gerstley L, McLellan AT, Alterman AI, Woody GE, Luborsky L, Prout M: Ability to form an alliance with the therapist: A possible marker of prognosis for patients with antisocial personality disorder. *Am J Psychiatr* 1989;146:508–512.

Gorenstein E: Frontal lobe functions in psychopaths. *J Abnorm Psychol* 1982;91:368–379.

Gutheil TG: Borderline personality disorder, boundary violations and patient-therapist sex: Medicolegal pitfalls. *Am J Psychiatr* 1989;146:597–602.

Haaken J: Sex differences and narcissistic disorders. *Am J Psychoanal* 1983;43:315–324.

Hickey BA: The borderline experience: Subjective impressions. *J Psychosoc Nurs Ment Health Serv* 1985;23:24–29.

Hollander E, et al.: Serotonergic sensitivity in borderline personality disorder: Preliminary findings. *Am J Psychiatr* 1994;151:277–280.

Jacobson G: Personality disorders, in Lazare A (ed): *Outpatient Psychiatry*. Williams & Wilkins, 1979.

Johnson AG: *Human Arrangements: An Introduction to Sociology*. Harcourt Brace, 1986.

Johnson M, Silver S: Conflicts in the inpatient treatment of the borderline patient. *Arch Psychiatr Nurs* 1988;2: 312–318.

Kaplan HI, Sadock BJ: *Synopsis of Psychiatry*, ed 6. Williams & Wilkins 1991.

Kendler KS, Gruenberg AM: Genetic relationship between paranoid personality disorder and the schizophrenic spectrum disorders. *Am J Psychiatr* 1982;139:1185–1186.

Kendler KS, et al.: A family history study of schizophrenia-related personality disorders. *Am J Psychiatr* 1984;141: 424–427.

Kernberg O: *Borderline Conditions and Pathological Narcissism*. Aronson, 1975.

Kohut H: *Analysis of the Self*. International Universities Press, 1971.

Kreisman J, Straus H: *I Hate You—Don't Leave Me*. Avon Books, 1989.

Kuhlman TL: Gallows humor for a scaffold setting: Managing aggressive patients on a maximum-security forensic unit. *Hosp Commun Psychiatr* 1988;39:1085–1090.

Lego S (ed): *The American Handbook of Psychiatric Nursing*. Lippincott, 1984.

Loomis ME, Horsley JA: *Interpersonal Change: A Behavioral Approach to Nursing Practice*. McGraw-Hill, 1974.

Loranger AW, Oldham JM, Tulis EH: Familial transmission of DSM-III borderline personality disorder. *Arch Gen Psychiatr* 1982;39:795–799.

Loranger AW, Tulis EH: Family history of alcoholism in borderline personality disorder. *Arch Gen Psychiatr* 1985;42: 153–157.

Mahler MS, Pine F, Bergman A: *The Psychological Birth of the Human Infant: Symbiosis and Individuation*. Basic Books, 1975.

Masterson JF: *The Narcissistic and Borderline Disorder*. Bruner/Mazel, 1981.

McCormick M: New hope for patients with obsessive-compulsive disorders. *J Am Acad Physician Assistants* 1993;6 (4):283–290.

McEnany GW, Tescher BE: Contracting for care: One nursing approach to the hospitalized borderline patient. *J Psychosoc Nurs Ment Health Serv* 1985;23:11–18.

Moyer RL, Snider MJ: Interpersonal problems of adults, in Howe J et al. (eds): *The Handbook of Nursing*. Wiley, 1984.

O'Brien P, Caldwell C, Transeau G: Destroyers: Written treatment contracts can help cure self-destructive behaviors of the borderline patient. *J Psychosoc Nurs Ment Health Serv* 1985;23:19–23.

Perlmutter R: The borderline patient in the emergency department: An approach for evaluation and management. *Psychiatr Q* 1982;54:190–197.

Perry JC, Flannery RB: Passive-aggressive personality disorder: Treatment implications of a clinical typology. *J Nerv Ment Dis* 1982;170:164–173.

Platt-Koch LM: Borderline personality disorder: A therapeutic approach. *Am J Nurs* 1983;83:1666–1671.

Poldrugo F, Forti B: Personality disorders and alcoholism treatment outcome. *Drug Alcohol Depend* 1988;21: 171–176.

Reich JH: Familiality of DSM-III dramatic and anxious personality clusters. *J Nerv Ment Dis* 1989;177:96–100.

Reid WH: The antisocial personality: A review. *Hosp Commun Psychiatr* 1985;36:831–837.

Rimpey M, Davidson S: Chaos, perfectionism, sabotage: Personality disorders in the workplace. *Iss Ment Health Nurs* 1994;15(1):27–36.

Rowe CJ: *An Outline of Psychiatry*. Brown, 1984.

Runyon N, Allen C, Ilnicki S: The borderline patient on the med-surg unit. *Am J Nurs* 1988:88:1644–1650.

Schaefer RT, Lamm RP: *Sociology*. McGraw-Hill, 1986.

Schlesinger LB: Distinctions between psychopathic, sociopathic, and anti-social personality disorders. *Psychol Rep* 1980;47:15–21.

Schwarz G, Halaris A: Identifying and managing borderline personality patients. *Am Family Physician* 1984;29: 203–208.

Shapiro D: *Neurotic Styles*. Basic Books, 1965.

Shearer SL, Peters CP, Quaytman MS, Wadman BE: Intent and lethality of suicide attempts among female borderline inpatients. *Am J Psychiatr* 1988;145:1424–1427.

Slavney PR, Teitelbaum ML, Chase GA: Referral for medically unexplained somatic complaints: The role of histrionic traits. *Psychosomatics* 1985;26:103–109.

Smoyak SA: Borderline personality disorder (editorial). *J Psychosoc Nurs Ment Health Serv* 1985;23:5.

Spector RE: *Cultural Diversity in Health and Illness*. Appleton & Lange, 1985.

Standage K, et al.: An investigation of role-taking in histrionic personalities. *Can J Psychiatr* 1984;29:407–411.

Torgensen S: Genetic and nosological aspects of the schizotypal and borderline personality disorders. *Arch Gen Psychiatr* 1984;41:546–554.

Travin S, Protter B: Mad or bad? Some clinical considerations in the misdiagnosis of schizophrenia as antisocial personality disorder. *Am J Psychiatr* 1982;139:1335–1338.

Waldinger R: Intensive psychodynamic therapy with borderline patients: An overview. *Am J Psychiatr* 1987;144(3): 267–274.

Wester CM: Managing the borderline personality. *Nurs Management* 1989;20:49–51.

Widiger TA, Frances A: Axis II personality disorders: Diagnostic and treatment issues. *Hosp Commun Psychiatr* 1985;36: 619–627.

Wilson JP, Prabucki K: Psychosocial antecedents of narcissistic personality syndrome. *Psychol Rep* 1983;53:1231–1239.

Wong N: Combined group and individual treatment of borderline and narcissistic patients: Heterogeneous versus homogeneous groups. *Int J Group Psychother* 1980;30: 389–494.

Woollcott Jr P: Prognostic indicators in the psychotherapy of borderline patients. *Am J Psychother* 1985;39:17–29.

Zetin M, Kramer MA: Obsessive-compulsive disorder. *Hosp Commun Psychiatr* 1992;43(7):689–699.

PART FOUR

CONTEMPORARY CLINICAL CONCERNS

CONTENTS

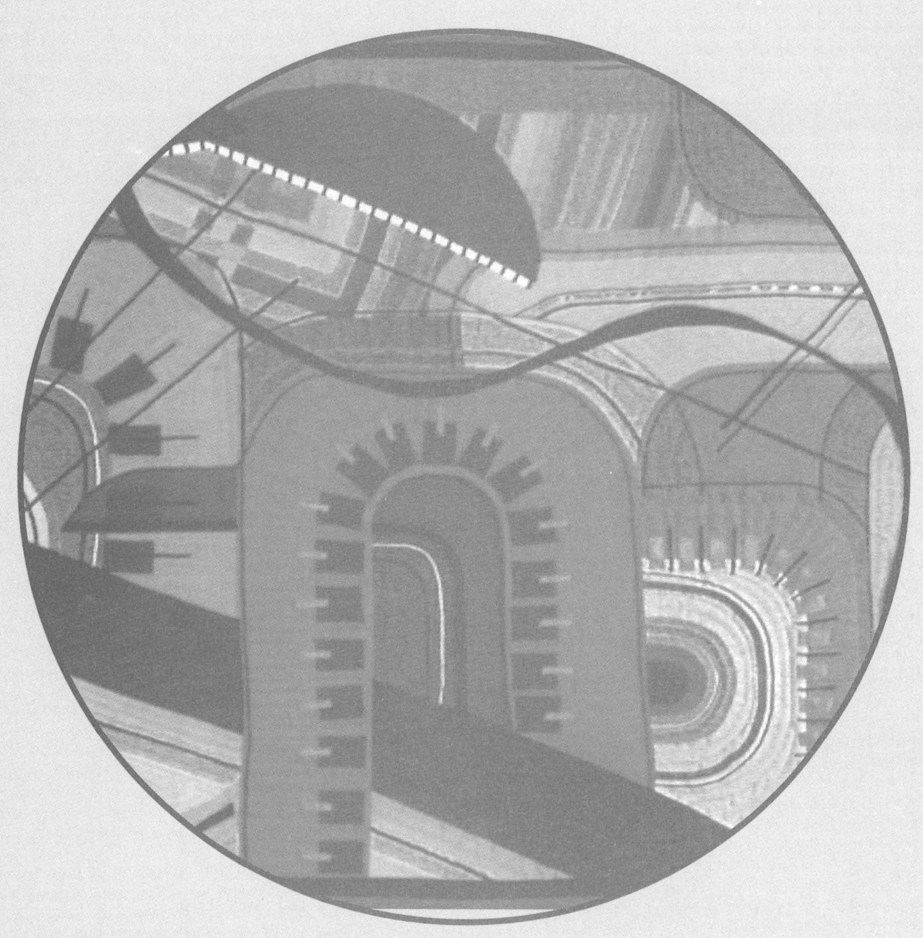

CHAPTER 21

THE SEVERELY AND PERSISTENTLY MENTALLY ILL IN THE COMMUNITY

Linda Chafetz

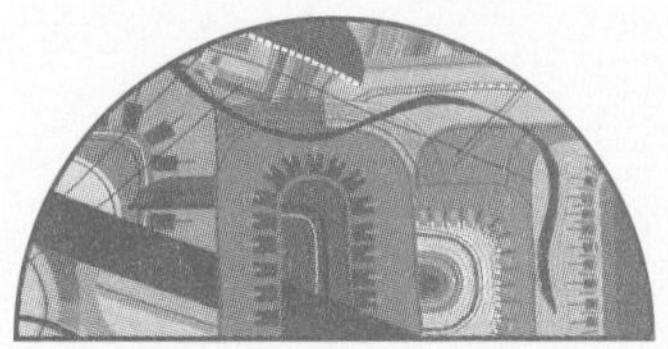

COMPETENCIES

- *Define the severely and persistently mentally ill.*
- *Distinguish between psychiatric disorders and psychiatric disabilities.*
- *List three or more areas of community living significantly influenced by severe and persistent mental disorders.*
- *Identify the components of community support programs.*
- *Identify the core concepts underlying psychiatric rehabilitation programs.*
- *Discuss the impact of severe disorders and psychiatric disability on families.*
- *Discuss the programs that address the needs of high-risk clients in the community.*
- *Identify roles for psychiatric nurses in community support systems.*

Cross-References

Other topics relevant to this content are: Prevention levels, Chapter 5; Substance-related disorders, Chapter 13; Schizophrenia and other psychotic disorders, Chapter 14; Mood disorders, Chapter 15; Personality disorders, Chapter 20; Dual diagnosis, Chapter 25; HIV/AIDS, Chapter 27.

Critical Thinking Challenge

Some psychiatric nurses believe that the goal of mental health care is to make the client as independent as possible. Others consider providing support to be a long-term commitment to the client and do not see a need to move the individual to a more autonomous level of functioning. Where do you stand on this issue? Why? Do you see this as a matter of psychiatric nursing practice or as a question of moral beliefs?

This chapter is concerned with psychiatric disorders that have two core features: severe impairment and long-term course. Some psychiatric problems discussed in other chapters of this book may involve intense symptoms that are more short-lived. Many crisis reactions fall into this category. Other disorders, such as phobias or low-grade affective problems, may follow a long-term course without impairing major role function. Severe and persistent psychiatric disorders are those that impinge on major role functioning and that do so over time. They involve some level of disability, or they would be disabling in the absence of appropriate services and treatment.

Who are the severely and persistently mentally ill in the community? What kinds of services support their overall quality of life, and how have these services evolved? Are there special subgroups who have special needs? This chapter addresses these questions with an emphasis on emerging service delivery models: community support programs, psychosocial rehabilitation services, intensive case management services for high-risk clients, consumer and family-guided programs. It also highlights psychiatric nursing interventions within these programs, including nursing case management, psychiatric home care nursing, family support interventions, and nursing services focusing on symptom management and psychoeducation.

Who Are the Severely and Persistently Mentally Ill?

Clinical Diversity

The term **severely and persistently mentally ill** came into general professional acceptance during the past decade because it avoids some of the more undesirable features of its predecessor term, the *chronically mentally ill,* including its connotation of inevitable and progressive deterioration (Goldman and Manderschied 1987). In fact, the severely and persistently mentally ill do not experience a common course of illness. They are clinically diverse, with different diagnoses and with varied patterns of illness. Schizophrenic disorders provide the prototype for severe and persistent illness; many decades of research affirm that they are typically disabling, on an intermittent or ongoing basis (Fenton and McGlashan 1991; Hegarty et al. 1994). However, even schizophrenic disorders vary considerably in terms of symptomatic profile, pattern of acute exacerbations, and quality of long-term functional outcomes (Carpenter and Strauss 1991). Bipolar disorder, recurrent depressions, and severe personality disorders can be as disabling as some forms of schizophrenia and also show great variation in outcomes (Winokur et al. 1993). Whether mild or severe, whether ongoing, recurring, or remitting, these disorders require services that go beyond the limits of an acute disease model. The core feature of a severe and persistent disorder is not diagnosis nor prognosis, but the experience of psychiatric disability.

Defining Psychiatric Disability

In 1980, the World Health Organization (WHO) developed and published a classification for the phases of a long-term illness. This classification may help identify common factors among the severely and persistently mentally ill that go beyond the treatment of discrete disorders. As Figure 21–1 shows, the etiology of the disorder, known or unknown, gives rise to changes in structure or functioning, manifest as signs and symptoms, collectively known as **impairment.** If the impairment alters functional performance or behavior, it produces **disability.** When the impairment or disability places the person at a disadvantage within the community, a **handicap** occurs.

Bachrach (1987) proposes a classification of levels of psychiatric disability that parallels the WHO formulation, but it is more specific to psychiatric illness. **Primary disability** refers to actual symptoms of illness, such as problems organizing thoughts or interpreting perception. **Secondary disability** refers to the person's reactions to the illness, such as low self-esteem and loneliness. **Tertiary disability** includes the social handicaps associated with severe mental illness, such as discrimination in housing and unemployment. Bachrach's terminology is compatible with the WHO schema. In both classifications, the core assumption is that the illness need not produce inevitable forms of social handicap. Rather, preventive approaches may be mobilized at any stage of illness.

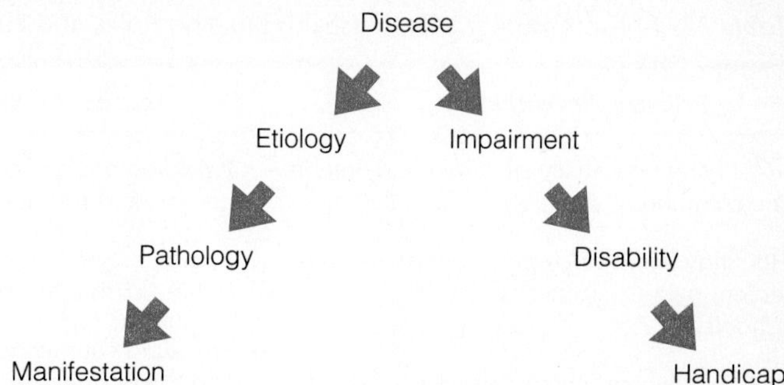

Figure 21–1 The WHO parallel sequence for long-term illness.

Levels of Prevention

In community mental health, prevention can occur at three levels (Table 21–1). **Primary prevention** activities focus on avoiding new cases of mental disorder by counteracting harmful stressors or other risk factors. **Secondary prevention** attempts to shorten the duration of a mental disorder through early case finding and treatment, and to reduce the prevalence of disorder in a given segment of the population. In **tertiary prevention,** treatment and rehabilitative services for clients with diagnosed illnesses prevent and reduce disabilities that are consequences of those disorders. At this level, preventive activities help the severely and persistently mentally ill to manage their symptoms and adjust their environments to permit optimal quality of life as defined by the individual.

Epidemiologic Considerations

Recent epidemiologic studies have increased our understanding of the extent of severe and persistent diagnosis among the general population and within treatment settings. According to a report by the National Advisory Mental Health Council (1993), about 5 million individuals, or 2.8% of the adult population in the United States, experience severe mental disorders annually. Excluding the mentally ill in nursing homes, the report estimates

Table 21–1 Community Mental Health Nursing Roles and Functions

Primary Prevention	*Secondary Prevention*	*Tertiary Prevention*
Identifying potentially stressful conditions in the community and high-risk populations.	Providing brief psychotherapy to individuals, groups, and families.	Helping plan for a client's discharge from the hospital.
Holding effective parenting classes for adolescent parents, at day care centers, in schools.	Suicide prevention hotline counseling and staffing crisis intervention programs.	Coordinating and monitoring follow-up care in home, halfway house, foster care home, or other transitional service.
Holding divorce therapy groups for couples, families, and individuals.	Providing counseling to victims of violence and their significant others.	Teaching clients self-care activities before discharge from the hospital using psychosocial rehabilitation.
Providing mental health consultation to health care providers.	Holding stress-reduction groups for health care providers.	Serving as a client advocate.
Providing mental health education to members of the community.	Case finding and referring clients in need of treatment.	Providing individual, group, and family psychotherapy.
Consulting with self-help groups.	Providing emergency mental health services.	Referring clients to self-help groups or after-care services.
Being politically active in relation to mental health issues.	Intake, screening, and assessment of clients.	Staffing partial hospitalization programs.

that treatment costs $20 billion yearly, or 4% of all national health expenditures, with a far larger cost in terms of social services, forensic services, and loss of individual productivity.

The National Institute of Mental Health **Epidemiological Catchment Area (ECA)** study shows us how these disorders are distributed. The ECA study employed sophisticated survey techniques in five sites across the United States and administered a standardized instrument, the Health Diagnostic Interview Schedule (Regier et al. 1993). The ECA data show that very prevalent problems, including anxiety disorders (with an annual prevalence rate of 12.6%), depression and dysthymia (8.3%), and substance abuse (9.5%), are frequently managed outside of formal treatment systems, if they are managed at all. Diagnoses associated with severe and persistent illness are far less common. For example the annual prevalence rate for schizophrenic and schizophreniform disorders is only 1.1%; the rate for bipolar disorder is 1.2%. In fact, only 2–3% of the adult population have severe problems that persist throughout a year. However, the relatively small proportion of adults with severe and persistent disorders are overrepresented in treatment settings. For example, while only 28.5% of people with psychiatric diagnoses sought formal treatment overall, more than 60% of the schizophrenic and bipolar subgroups received treatment.

The ECA study also indicated that people with serious problems might have more than one concurrent problem. For example, the existence of a psychiatric diagnosis greatly increased the risk of a substance-related disorder (Regier et al. 1990). More recently the **National Comorbidity Study (NCS)** is the first survey to use a structured psychiatric interview for a national probability sample of people age 15–54 (Kessler et al. 1994). NCS data indicate that more than 50% of all lifetime disorders occur among 14% of the population with multiple disorders. This very comorbid group included many of the severely mentally ill.

Recent epidemiologic studies confirm the enduring association between severe and persistent disorders and low socioeconomic status. In the ECA study, for example, the odds of having any NIMH Diagnostic Interview Schedule disorder were twice as high among the lowest socioeconomic group (Regier et al. 1993). To some extent this reflects the effects of disability on the ability to maintain social and economic assets. However, social factors can also act as stressors and contribute directly to disorder.

The profile that emerges is that of a highly vulnerable subgroup in our mental health care system, and one of the groups least likely to assess social resources to protect that vulnerability. While the severely mentally ill account for a relatively small proportion of our overall population, they account for the largest major subgroup in acute psychiatric services and in many community programs. They are at risk for developing secondary or concurrent psychiatric problems and for problems associated with socioeconomic status. These multiple, interacting problems require complex approaches to services. However, the development of systems that can reply to this complexity began relatively recently.

Service Models

The Community Mental Health Movement and Deinstitutionalization

From the early nineteenth century until the 1950s, state and county mental hospitals constituted the major treatment resource for the severely mentally ill, often serving as their long-term place of residence. **Deinstitutionalization** in the United States began in the post–World War II period, when large public mental hospitals were overcrowded and had fallen into disrepair, and when they were widely criticized for "warehousing" or "institutionalizing" their residents (Chafetz, Goldman, and Taube 1983; Deutsch 1948; Goffman 1961). New therapies such as crisis intervention showed much promise and raised hopes that effective treatments might be delivered in community settings. With the development of neurologic medication in 1955, and the enactment of statutes restricting involuntary detainment in psychiatric facilities, the resident population of state and county mental hospitals began to decline from 560,000 in 1955 to 140,000 by the late 1970s (Chafetz, Goldman, and Taube 1983).

This phase-down of large institutions occurred within the context of a much broader movement for community mental health that reached its apex in the 1960s (see the accompanying box). In 1961, the Joint Commission on Mental Illness and Health presented a report to Congress called *Action for Mental Health* that called for not only a shift from institutional to community care, but also a new emphasis on access to all levels of mental health prevention and treatment in the community. The Community Mental Health Centers Act of 1963 authorized federal matching funds for the construction of comprehensive community mental health centers and set a model for the essential service packages to be offered in communities, including acute care and ambulatory services. These services were not developed for the severely mentally ill per se, but it was widely assumed that they would integrate into community systems to meet their treatment needs.

By the mid 1970s, a number of disturbing trends cast this assumption into doubt. First of all, hospital care remained the main treatment modality for the severely mentally ill, with repeated readmissions replacing long-term institutional residence (Chafetz, Goldman, and Taube 1983). Although the outpatient sector expanded by more than 100%, it frequently served people with less severe disorders. Even where the severely mentally ill had access to outpatient treatment, they did not receive the full range of nontreatment support services formerly provided by hospitals, including housing, social support, and even a place of refuge. Communities were unwelcoming, often enacting restrictive zoning statutes and other mechanisms to exclude the mentally ill from the mainstream (Aviram and Segal 1973; Wahl 1993).

Landmarks in Community Mental Health

The 1950s

- The National Mental Health Study Act established the Joint Commission on Mental Illness and Health.
- Psychotropic drugs were introduced to control psychotic symptoms, facilitating a transition to community care.

The 1960s

- The Joint Commission presented its report, *Action for Mental Health,* to Congress, recommending a shift to community-based care.
- The Community Mental Health Centers Act authorized $150 million in federal matching funds to states to develop services.

The 1970s

- President Carter established a President's Commission on Mental Health.
- The National Institute of Mental Health began the Community Support Program.
- Congress passed the Omnibus Budget Reconciliation Act, placing services formerly directed by the NIMH in federal block grants to states.
- The National Institute of Mental Health established an Office of Programs for the Homeless Mentally Ill.

The 1990s

- The NIMH funded research demonstration programs authorized by the Stewart B. McKinney Homeless Assistance Act.
- The Federal Task Force on Homelessness and Severe Mental Illness made recommendations for the expansion of housing and service options to the homeless mentally ill.
- The Americans with Disabilities Act affirmed the rights of those with psychiatric disabilities.

Consequently, an alarming number of the severely mentally ill appeared to be living very marginal and isolated lives in the community. Some resided in group homes that reproduced the institutional atmosphere of the state hospital (Lamb and Goertzel 1971). Many resided in the single-room occupancy rentals that have traditionally served the single poor in central urban areas, providing few opportunities for social integration in any meaningful sense (Shapiro 1972). A disturbing number of these displaced people began to cycle through the criminal justice system (Whitmer 1980), often because of problems that were clearly illness-related. The severely mentally ill began to comprise a very prominent subgroup among the homeless (Baxter and Hopper 1981).

Some model programs developed in the 1960s and 1970s seemed to produce better outcomes for the severely mentally ill. Compared to hospital-based programs, they resulted in very modest gains, if any, in terms of symptomatology and function (Test and Stein 1978). However, compared to standard outpatient treatment, they reduced readmission rates, and by inference delayed or prevented relapse (Stein 1993). They provided alternatives to institutions and received generally positive evaluations from consumers. Examples are the Program for Training in Community Living in Dane County, Wisconsin (Thompson, Griffith, and Leaf 1990), and the Psychosocial Clubhouse model pioneered by Fountain House in New York (Beard, Malamud, and Rossman 1978).

Certain critical elements appeared to contribute to their success, including accessibility and flexibility. The Wisconsin model provided services in the client's environment, without the demands that treatment conform to a "therapy" hour, and with a range of support services that promote function in a broad sense. The Clubhouse model offered a place for the mentally ill to visit on their own terms; a range of services was accessible but not intrusive or coercive. In general, promising programs focused on functional adaptation through both skill development and environmental support. They deemphasized the idea of "cure" and accepted the long-term nature of psychiatric disability. These programmatic features were incorporated into many developing service systems to better address the needs of the severely mentally ill.

Community Support Programs

In 1977, the NIMH **Community Support Program (CSP)** was established to help states implement programs that provided a full range of support services, and to offer them through a single provider or provider team, thus assuring coordination and monitoring of services (Turner and TenHoor 1978). The CSP covers a limited number of actual service sites, but it established a widely accepted model for mental health services targeting the severely and persistently mentally ill. Systems adhering to this model offer a range of treatment and rehabilitation services, with a case management component to assess needs, coordinate care, and monitor outcomes.

CASE MANAGEMENT **Case management** is the linchpin for community support programs. The case manager works with the client to assess individual needs and to develop individualized treatment objectives. The case manager then works to link the client with the services available for meeting these needs and objectives. Because service needs can change over time, the goals and referrals for a given client may change as well. However, the case manager remains a consistent figure in the treatment plan. This avoids duplication and overlap of services. It also avoids shunting vulnerable clients between services because of fluctuations in their clinical status.

Case managers often find that they are fulfilling many roles for their clients that have not been satisfied by other clinical resources, including a sense of social support (Meeks and Murrell 1994). At first they must build relationships, assess their clients, and connect them with pertinent services. As time passes, these functions evolve into monitoring client needs by touching base with them and responding to periodic crises. High-risk groups such as the dually diagnosed, the homeless mentally ill, and frequently hospitalized patients may receive more intensive and clinically sophisticated forms of case management to address their unique service requirements.

The case management philosophy has generated enthusiasm in systems for the psychiatrically disabled, because it acknowledges the pervasive nature of their problems, their need for multiple services, and the oscillating or unpredictable course of illness. Case management in mental health care and elsewhere increasingly has a cost-containment function as well. This function will play a critical role in future managed-care environments for the delivery of mental health services.

SUPPORT FOR BASIC NEEDS, INCOME, AND MONEY MANAGEMENT Community mental health programs generally emphasize the importance of self-support and gainful employment whenever possible. However, surveys of the severely mentally ill indicate generally low rates of competitive employment. This situation reflects general economic conditions as well as work disability. In times of high unemployment, people with psychiatric disabilities may be pushed out of jobs that can be performed by competing groups in the labor force. Certainly many mentally ill individuals without "gainful" employment are meaningfully occupied in supported employment and/or volunteer work. However, low rates of competitive employment among members of this population underscore their dependence on income assistance programs such as Supplemental Security Income (SSI).

A community support system helps assure the severely mentally ill both access to and linkage with appropriate services to secure income and obtain other entitlements (such as health benefits) and basic resources such as food, clothing, and transportation. This may be a more complex task than it appears to be because accessing financial resources may mean helping the client through difficult applications procedures and even appeals. It may also involve providing money management services to help the severly mentally ill who cannot budget their monthly income independently.

RESIDENTIAL SERVICES Recent reports continue to document the lack of affordable and decent housing options for many of the severely mentally ill and their consequent concentration in what may be marginal or unsafe areas (Newman 1994). Many of the severely and persistently mentally ill live with families, but those who live alone frequently depend on residential hotels and boarding homes. It is difficult to generalize about the quality of these housing options because they vary a great deal. For example, some boarding arrangements encourage autonomy and provide a warm, stable environment for residents. Other arrangements, however, fall far below standards that should be applied to living environments for the chronically disabled.

The question of housing satisfaction can also be highly subjective. Some people prefer the privacy of a hotel, despite what may be other negative features, such as location or small living space. Programs with an active treatment component may be attractive to some people, but others appreciate a fairly calm and nondemanding environment despite its monotony. For this reason, a community support system focuses not only on assessing some form of acceptable housing but on evaluating the quality of that housing for the individual, working with the client to find "a good fit" (Baker and Douglas 1990).

MEDICATION MANAGEMENT Medication regimens are the mainstay of treatment programs for the severely and persistently mentally ill. Research on the efficacy of medication, particularly neuroleptic regimens for schizophrenia, demonstrates that these agents reduce rates of relapse and hospital readmission. However, they have not been problem-free. Drug regimens demand compliance, tolerance of temporary side effects, and acceptance of the risk of long-term problems such as tardive dyskinesia. Secondary effects of medications can be uncomfortable and embarrassingly visible.

Medication services for the severely and persistently mentally ill should address the impact of medications on quality of life and should promote collaboration with clients to develop a regimen that is tolerable and beneficial. **Depot medication therapy**, usually consisting of an injection every 2 to 4 weeks, does not require the client to take medications several times a day and is a valuable strategy for some people. Current advances in psychopharmacology have produced new classes of medications that may prove less uncomfortable and socially limiting than standard treatments, and that may help people who have been resistant to medication, or noncompliant, in the past. The introduction of newer therapies makes the medication component of community care all the more important, particularly for advanced practice nurses with prescriptive authority for the severely mentally ill (Talley and Caverly 1994).

Ms L is a 57-year-old widow who came into the medication clinic for her monthly injection, accompanied by her case manager. Ms L has carried a diagnosis of schizophrenia, paranoid type, for many years but she was maintained well with outpatient care and medications, requiring only brief crisis intervention and two short hospital stays by the time she was 50. Ms L was married but unable to maintain employment. Her husband participated in a support group at the local clinic.

After her husband died, Ms L had a severe decompensation, experiencing frightening hallucinations and delusions, and was threatening her neighbors. Police were called and she was hospitalized; during this time, all her belongings were stolen from her apartment. Ms L was stabilized on depot medications and was referred to a Community Support Program (CSP) for assistance with both housing and rehabilitation. A case manager helped Ms L apply for SSI, arranged for a shared apartment, facilitated medication and clinic appointments, visited her weekly, and encouraged regular participation in a social rehabilitation program. Ms L has not required hospitalization in the six years since being enrolled in the CSP. Although she still "hears voices," she is able to monitor her symptoms and advises her son or her case manager when her symptoms increase.

OUTPATIENT TREATMENT Traditional outpatient psychotherapies that address *problems in living* may not meet the needs of all the various types of people composing the severely and persistently mentally ill. This is because disabled people often require a broader range of support services to function well in the community. Many of the severely mentally ill also require rehabilitation interventions that address their specific functional deficits and treatment goals, rather than insight-oriented therapies.

Nevertheless, these clients need individual, family, and group treatments that are sensitive to their particular problems and needs. Much individual treatment emphasizes support to the individual coping with a severe disorder (Weiden and Havens 1994). Family treatment with the severely mentally ill frequently follows a psychoeducational model that has been applied very successfully by nurses (Gamble 1993). Group treatments often have a socialization or peer support function.

CRISIS STABILIZATION, EMERGENCY AND ACUTE INPATIENT CARE The severely and persistently mentally ill are at risk for acute exacerbations of an illness. This may be particularly true during times of stress or transition. But in some cases, acute exacerbations are entirely unpredictable and are probably less indicative of the effects of environmental stressors than of the fluctuations of a disease process. In any case, this population requires access to

RESEARCH NOTE

Citation

Newman, Sandra J. (1994). Housing and Neighborhood Conditions of Persons with Severe Mental Illness, *Hosp Commun Psychiatr*, 45(4), 338–344.

Study Problem/Purpose

Research over the past 15 years has considered housing as an essential component of community services for the mentally ill. However, little research has addressed attributes of the homes and neighborhoods offering that housing. What are the attributes of housing settings for the mentally ill, including their physical condition, size, cost, neighborhoods? And how do these attributes compare with those of the general population? This study reports on these questions, comparing a systematic sample of severely mentally ill adults with representative samples of the general population.

Methods

This study used two sets of data. Information on housing of the severely mentally ill was obtained from the baseline data collected in 1988 and 1989 for a national evaluation of the Robert Wood Johnson Foundation Program on Chronic Mental Illness. The sample included 307 cases being discharged from acute care in Cincinnati, Columbus, and Baltimore. Data included information on demographic and clinical factors as well as housing conditions prior to and after the index treatment episode. Information on housing of the general population was obtained through the American Housing Survey conducted by the U.S. Bureau of the Census for the Department of Housing and Urban Development. This comprehensive data set offered data on the metropolitan areas sampled in the Robert Wood Johnson Foundation survey. The National Housing Survey does not report on the types of housing that many of the mentally ill may occupy, such as group homes or short-term hotels. However, these data sets permitted a statistical comparison of the mentally ill in independent housing with their counterparts in the general population.

Findings

People with serious mental illness were more likely to report living in a dwelling other than a house or apartment (such as a shelter or group home) and less likely to own homes. The mentally ill showed lower median years of residence in current housing and disposed of less space. In terms of affordability, housing was more costly for the mentally ill than for the general population in these index cities. Crowding was not a discriminating factor between these groups, but physical adequacy of housing for the mentally ill was more problematic (heating, window, plumbing problems, problems with rats in one city), leading to lower subjective ratings of housing quality by mentally ill subjects. Neighborhood attributes for the mentally ill were mixed. In some cases, the mentally ill reported no more or fewer difficulties than the general population, for issues such as shopping availability and noise levels. However, the crime rates in neighborhoods of the mentally ill were elevated, contributing to lower subjective ratings.

Implications

This survey focuses on the living conditions of adults with severe mental illness who occupy independent community residences. By definition, it concerns the more "mainstream" segment of this population, and not the subgroups who reside in short-term or crisis housing. Nevertheless, by standard and objective criteria, and in comparisons with geographically appropriate controls, the mentally ill report housing conditions that appear inferior to the general population. They pay elevated rates for housing that they occupy on a more short-term basis, with higher incidence of environmental problems that decrease individual satisfaction and quality of life. Even in comparisons with low-income renters in the general population, these differences remain. A population at high risk for reaction to environmental and household stressors is thus subject to some of the more problematic housing settings in our cities. The author points out that while we lack information connecting housing attributes to specific outcomes, current studies suggest that affordable and acceptable housing may promote quality of life. As home care providers, case managers, and family care specialists, nurses deal with the issue of housing and neighborhoods in their daily work with the mentally ill. It is critical to attend to these attributes in the total plan of care. It is also essential to advocate for residential resources that can support the quality of life for this population.

acute asessment and treatment services as part of a package of community support.

Twenty-four-hour emergency and crisis units and outreach programs are mandated in community mental health statutes to provide for people with problems that exceed the resources of the outpatient sector, such as dangerous behavior, suicidal ideation, and/or grave disability. They provide a point of entry to hospital care as needed, but they also allow diversion from hospitals where crises can be managed in the community. Nursing expertise is extremely important in these emergency settings because of the need for skilled and comprehensive assessment of acute problems.

General Health Care The severely mentally ill are a medically underserved group in the community, with needs in the areas of primary health care, dental care, and vision care. Health needs are most pronounced in such subgroups as substance-abusing clients and the elderly mentally ill, who have concurrent physical disorders. However, many of the severely mentally ill are to some extent at risk from lifestyle factors (problematic housing or nutrition) or from the consequences of psychiatric treatment (problematic medication side effects or drug interactions). Any person with a serious psychiatric diagnosis risks underdiagnosis of medical illness by both primary care and psychiatric providers. In the general health care sector, physicians and nurses tend to have a poor understanding of psychiatric illness and have difficulty working with these clients effectively (Adler and Griffith 1991).

In psychiatric services, many clinicians focus on mental disorders with inadequate attention to the total person. A recent study by d'Ercole et al. (1991) indicated that evaluating psychiatrists identified only a small proportion of the medical problems that were later diagnosed in physical assessments. Those most likely to be underdiagnosed were substance abusers, elderly clients, and women. Community support and case management interventions can help the severely mentally ill obtain services despite these problems of "falling between the cracks" in systems that are poorly organized to meet the needs of clients with multiple diagnoses.

Vocational Programs When the severely mentally ill are surveyed about their preferences, they usually indicate a strong desire to work. Work not only provides income, it also helps create a sense of self-worth and social belonging. However, psychiatric disability limits access to employment by its impact on healthy functioning and because of the stigma attached to mental disorders (Solinski, Jackson, and Bell 1992). Vocational services address this problem by providing training and protected alternatives to the competitive workplace.

Vocational training may occur in specialized programs, or it may be integrated into other mental health modalities such as day treatment. It provides assessment of work capacities and preferences, technical preparation, and social skills training to prepare people for the workplace. However, not all people with psychiatric disabilities enter the competitive workplace. Many, by desire or by necessity, work within protected environments. Sheltered workshop programs have a long history of offering work in a low-stress, low-demand environment. Transitional vocational programs also provide a low-stress environment but emphasize the development of skills for movement to the competitive workplace.

Much recent attention has focused on **supported employment**, an approach that provides training and support in the place of employment. For example, a job coach might accompany a group of psychiatrically disabled workers to a place of employment where the coach learns the same job as the team, provides on-the-job training, and provides daily back-up and support. This approach is based on the principle that the mentally ill learn skills best in the environment where they will be practiced. Supported employment models may become increasingly prominent because the recent Americans with Disabilities Act guarantees people with psychiatric disabilities the right to reasonable accommodation in the workplace.

Day Programs A complete system of community-based services for the severely mentally ill offers some forms of day programs. Day treatment and partial hospitalization programs provide continuity of care between the hospital and the outpatient sector. They provide a less restrictive setting than the hospital for people who require structure and support but not actual treatment or nursing supervision (Kluiter et al. 1992). These programs can also provide an alternative to hospital care for individuals who need complex treatment monitoring.

Day treatment programs offer groups and activities that provide for recreation and socialization and that help people function in the community. They may be used on a short-term basis for specific goals or on a long-term basis for relapse prevention. Day programs are increasingly incorporating a rehabilitation philosophy that maximizes opportunities for meaningful activities in environments that are as "normal" as possible, focusing on strengths rather than on pathology.

Family and Network Support Family therapies for the severely and persistently mentally ill generally are based on a model of stress and vulnerability. Family support interventions are directed at reducing stress in the client's interpersonal environment and minimizing the burden of care for family members (Chafetz and Barnes 1989; Maurin and Boyd 1990). If clients have little contact with families, interventions may target the people in their networks that provide them with support: friends, landlords, service providers. For example, Barnes (1993) has conducted research on the special needs of residential care providers who occupy a position somewhere between family and professionals in the client's network.

With this emphasis on support to the supporters, interventions include psychoeducational activities that increase knowledge about the disorder and reduce family stress (Gamble 1993). Family or network support can also mean very practical assistance. Information about homemaking or legal services can be as welcome as information about treatment. Respite services (or short-term placements to relieve the family of the burden of care) give families the help they need to continue in a caregiving role. Such services have been widely recommended as a way to reduce the family's burden and enhance the quality of life of both the client and relatives for the long term.

Nurses working with families of the severely and persistently mentally ill need to become attuned to their concerns. Families may express ambivalence about caregiving. For example, they may want to promote the client's autonomy yet feel discomfort or guilt about the type of living situation the client is able to maintain independently. Clear information and nonjudgmental attitudes from nurses and other providers can do much to alleviate a family's distress and assure them that there may not be a single ideal solution to their problems.

COMMUNITY EDUCATION AND ADVOCACY Many of the difficulties the severely mentally ill experience in the community reflect a poor understanding of psychiatric illness among the general population and inadequate resources for their needs. For example, access to housing is a function of resources and community acceptance. Attention to housing is futile if no residential resources exist; vocational programs require access to employers. For this reason, one component of community support for the severely mentally ill is **advocacy**, or activities increasing access to resources. Advocacy can occur on an individual basis; for example, a case manager might intervene with a landlord to help a client obtain housing. Advocacy activities also occur at the level of the community, such as in programs for community education or outreach to employers.

Rehabilitation Approaches

Although the components of community support models provide the structure for services to the severely and persistently mentally ill, their effectiveness depends on the content of these component services. **Psychiatric rehabilitation** has emerged during the past decade as a guide for the content of practice at many levels of care, and it includes an overall treatment philosophy as well as specific interventions and programs.

REHABILITATION PHILOSOPHY Psychiatric rehabilitation has its roots in theory about physical disabilities (Anthony and Liberman 1986). Considering WHO's phases of a long-term illness, psychiatric rehabilitation separates the treatment of disease from the prevention or reduction of impairment and handicap. Treatment (medication) addresses the disease process and its consequent symptoms. Rehabilitation approaches emphasize specific interventions to address targeted areas of functioning. Rehabilitation approaches are also strongly grounded in beliefs about empowerment of the mentally ill, emphasizing client feelings of control and worth.

Rehabilitation-oriented services begin with functional assessment and identification of highly individualized goals. A plan is developed to meet objectives by behavioral interventions that target specific functional deficits, or by environmental interventions that enable functioning with an existing deficit. From a rehabilitation perspective, it is important to extend support as long as possible. Support is not necessarily withdrawn because a client improves. For example, clients doing well in supported employment programs would not be expected to necessarily "graduate" to independent employment and thereby forfeit the support.

Because rehabilitation services reduce social distance between clients and providers, they may run counter to the training of some mental health care clinicians. Nevertheless, as Anthony and Liberman (1986) note, they are entering the mainstream of community mental health programs as a viable, credible, intervention approach. Further, rehabilitation philosophy is entirely consistent with self-care and symptom management interventions for the mentally ill developed by psychiatric nurses. In fact rehabilitation theory and conceptual models in nursing share a common focus on functional adaptation in supportive environments.

THE CLUBHOUSE MODEL Although a rehabilitation philosophy can inform and enhance many treatment modalities, some specific rehabilitation programs make a unique contribution to service systems. One of the most important types of psychiatric rehabilitation programs are Psychosocial Rehabilitation Centers, modeled after Fountain House and other clubhouse programs (Beard, Malamud, and Rossman 1982). Under a community support system structure, these would fall at the level of day programming, but the content of Psychosocial Rehabilitation Centers or Clubhouse models may be very different than the program contents of "maintenance" day treatment centers, which do not apply a rehabilitation perspective.

As Anthony and Liberman (1986) explain, Psychosocial Rehabilitation Centers grew out of clubs formed by former psychiatric hospital patients in order to provide mutual support and assistance. These evolved into service centers providing multiple services such as group activities, assistance with employment, and housing. Psychosocial Centers emphasize a collaborative relationship between staff and members, and provide experiences in a supportive but realistic milieu, for the development of abilities for functioning in the real world.

VOCATIONAL REHABILITATION While all mental health programs have some emphasis on vocational rehabilitation, not all vocational programs conform to a psychiatric rehabilitation model. Supported employment models reflect a rehabilitation perspective because of their emphasis on adding support to the normal environment. Danley, Sciarappa, and MacDonald-Wilson (1992) point out that supported employment is the end-point in a vocational rehabilitation process based on personal choice, called "choose, get, keep" (Table 21–2). This model delineates three basic competencies that are necessary for employment and offers classes that prepare the client to set goals and choose a job focus. Once clients are placed, they are supported by job coaches, who act as role models, provide feedback, and act as liaisons to employers.

Table 21–2 Phases of Supported Employment

Choose	*Get*	*Keep*
Identifying interests	Identifying assets	Appropriate behavior
Assessing capabilities	Locating potential employment	Being on time
Matching traits to job	Writing a resume	Responding well to training
Evaluating options	Job applications	Interacting well with others

SOCIAL SKILLS TRAINING **Social skills training** methods are based on principles of social learning and use behavioral techniques such as role playing, practicing, and reinforcement to promote the learning of instrumental role behavior as well as problem-solving abilities and interpersonal skills. Social skills training modules have been developed to permit dissemination of these techniques in comprehensive programs (Wallace et al. 1992).

Social skills training techniques may be incorporated into individual, group, and family treatment modalities, where they may add measurable benefits. For example, social skills training to remedy specific functional deficits appears to be more effective than group psychotherapy, when the two conditions are studied experimentally (Wirshing et al. 1992).

Programs for High-Risk Clients

Subgroups of the severely and persistently mentally ill are at particularly high risk for poor outcomes and are also extraordinarily difficult to serve in conventional programs. These include those with substance-related problems, homelessness, frequent readmissions to acute care, and frequent criminal justice system involvement. Their interrelationships among these problems are complex, making it difficult to separate them, or to distinguish root problems from their consequences (Chafetz 1992). For example, substance use may exacerbate symptoms and lead to rehospitalization. This in turn may disrupt stability of residence, increasing the possibility of arrest and reducing the likelihood of medication compliance. In other words, if individuals belong to one subgroup at risk, it is possible that they belong to several, increasing their overall vulnerability.

Concurrent Substance-Related Disorders

Psychiatric illness greatly increases the odds of having a substance-related disorder. Alcohol has typically been the drug of choice with the severely mentally ill, perhaps because of its relative cheapness and accessibility (Barbee et al. 1989). During the recent past, psychostimulant use has increased among this population, a phenomenon partially attributed to the emergence of crack cocaine as a major drug of abuse (Bunt et al. 1990). Concurrent substance-related disorders are probably the most consistent predictor of readmission to psychiatric hospitals noted in the literature. In fact, Drake, Osher, and Wallach (1989), in their research on substance use in schizophrenia, note that even "mild" alcohol use (not considered problematic by clinicians) increased the likelihood of readmission.

Dual diagnoses of severe mental illness and psychoactive substance-related disorders are most common among younger males, although women are well represented. This corresponds to the distribution of these disorders in the general population. Substance use contributes to a host of undesirable outcomes (Bartels et al. 1993). It is highly correlated with homelessness and criminal justice system involvement. It is also a cause of concurrent medical morbidity, including exposure to HIV. Several hospital surveys indicate a high rate of seropositivity among severely mentally ill adults. Triple diagnosis patients—those with HIV disorders, substance-related disorders, and psychiatric disorders—require a complex and demanding range of services.

For a variety of reasons involving different funding streams and different treatment philosophies, substance abuse services and psychiatric care are often poorly integrated (see Chapter 25). In mental health care systems, the dually diagnosed client encounters little specific expertise related to drug or alcohol use. The severely mentally ill sometimes do poorly in substance abuse programs stressing confrontation or demanding sobriety as a precondition to treatment. Integrated programs for the dually diagnosed mentally ill include inpatient programs (Minkoff 1989) and some of the assertive treatment models discussed below. Adjusting the psychotropic medications for these clients may help them deal with problems such as dysphoria and anxiety that lead to self-medication with drugs and alcohol.

The Homeless Mentally Ill

Mr R is a 29-year-old man who was referred to an intensive case management team after his third hospital admission within one year. Mr R has a diagnosis of schizoaffective disorder but it is unclear whether his diagnosis accounts for his frequent acute episodes, or whether the episodes are precipitated by his use of stimulants and alcohol. Mr R has no stable place of residence and has used shelters over the past few years. He describes himself as too preoccupied with his survival needs to seek treatment between emergency episodes. He claims that alcohol helps him to manage his anxiety and his "voices" when he is on the streets. The case management team will first address Mr R's need for safe housing. The team will then work with Mr R to help him acknowledge that alcohol and drugs can increase his discomfort, and to support his use of psychotropic medication. When Mr R is stabilized, he will work with the team and consider other treatment goals.

Several government reports in the 1980s documented the prominence of the mentally ill among the urban homeless. They accounted for approximately 25–30% of the homeless in most major studies, including an Institute of Medicine Report published in 1988. The problem of homelessness has continued into the 1990s, and the goal of providing acceptable and long-term housing for the mentally ill remains elusive, particularly in urban centers (Bachrach 1992; Dennis et al. 1991). The proportion of the mentally ill in the community who are permanently homeless is relatively small. However, a large and heterogeneous group experiences spells of residential instability (Dixon, Friedman, and Lehman 1993; Goldfinger and Chafetz 1984; Mowbray, Bybee, and Cohen 1993).

Whether these periods of homelessness involve movement between transient accommodations or actual street dwelling, they impose very harsh living conditions on people who are highly vulnerable. Homelessness interferes with the ability to use services, including the use of psychotropic medications. It increases the risk of trauma, substance abuse, infectious disease exposure, and victimization. Homelessness also makes conventional services unworkable, since the undomiciled can rarely store medication and utilize regular outpatient services (Chafetz 1992; Goldfinger and Chafetz 1984).

A great deal of work has gone into developing models for services to the homeless population, including supported housing models with case management components (Morse et al. 1992; Wasylenki et al. 1993); shelter-based rehabilitation and substance abuse services (Canton et al. 1990; Canton et al. 1993); and mobile outreach teams to identify cases and to link them with services (Cohen and Tsemberis 1991). It is clear that while shelters and emergency programs serve a critical short-term need, they also contribute to instability. Recent initiatives by the federal government link the Department of Housing and Urban Development (HUD) with local public health departments to increase the development of permanent housing for people with psychiatric disabilities (Federal Task Force on Homelessness 1992).

Frequent Readmissions

Recidivism, or frequent readmission, in acute psychiatric settings is a problem for several reasons:

1. It represents a considerable expense.
2. It is a proxy (albeit a very approximate one) for relapse, indicating severe difficulties for the individual.
3. It suggests a failure of the community system to link the client between acute episodes and to institute the type of treatment and monitoring that might manage symptomatic shifts without hospitalization.

Since virtually all severe and persistent disorders will involve some kind of relapse at some time, high acute service utilization is considered to be readmission at a much more frequent rate than that suggested by the illness process. Generally more than one or two admissions in 12 months exceeds norms (Chafetz 1992).

Client-based factors that contribute to recidivism include substance abuse, which may be the best predictor of readmission (see Chapter 13). Younger adults are readmitted at higher rates than clients over 40 (Safer 1987). Cycling through emergency and acute care has been attributed to a "chronic crisis" style among some diagnostic groups, particularly those with severe *DSM-IV* Axis II disorders (Sullivan et al. 1993). However, many younger clients with schizophrenia and bipolar disorder use alcohol and drugs to combat boredom and medication side effects, and to treat symptoms in what they consider to be a "normal" way. Their frequent admissions may form the early phase of a process of coping with a long-term diagnosis (Test et al. 1989).

On a systems level, readmission may reflect a failure to link the client with services that he or she considers meaningful and accessible. The most successful programs for the severely and persistently mentally ill have served clients with superior treatment histories and intact social resources (Braun et al. 1981). The system as a whole may respond best to clients who "fit" into programs and benefit from treatment alone. Those with more social needs or less acceptance of their illness may not consider current ambulatory services relevant to their needs and may require more assertive outreach to link with outpatient providers.

The Severely Mentally Ill in Forensic Settings

Prevalence rates of major psychiatric disorders in the jails have increased gradually but continuously over the past 20 years, at least in part because of deinstitutionalization policies (Jamelka, Trupin, and Chiles 1989). Society has a low tolerance for disordered behavior, and the lack of services for the severely and persistently mentally ill in the mental health care system may lead to a funneling of these people into the criminal justice system.

Unemployment, homelessness, and substance abuse contribute to the profile of the severely mentally ill forensic client (Whitmer 1980). Nearly 25% of forensic inpatient services are filled to capacity (Way et al. 1990). Most mentally ill offenders end up in county jails rather than forensic mental hospitals; they rarely become connected with local mental health networks and are frequently counted among the homeless because they have no fixed address.

Intensive Treatment Models for High-Risk Populations

Assertive programs have shown much promise in terms of service delivery to high-risk groups. These are expensive, sophisticated programs that are believed to be cost-effective because they offset still more expensive hospital episodes (Bond et al. 1990; Hu and Jerrell 1991; McGurrin and Worley 1993). Many employ the **Continuous Treatment Team** model to deliver services in the client's own environment. Treatment teams not only provide a mobile outreach capacity, they also provide consumers with access to multidisciplinary providers and comprehensive services.

The team structure is believed to reduce stress and burnout of individual case managers by sharing the load of difficult clients. The client benefits from both reduced dependence on an individual clinician and the support of a multidisciplinary group for back-up during crisis. These teams have been widely implemented (Bush et al. 1990; Thompson, Griffith, and Leaf 1990) and show promising results with the homeless (Cohen and Tsemberis 1991) and with other high-risk groups (Arana, Hastings, and Herron 1991).

Other intensive services for high-risk clients use a single case manager to provide **clinical case management**, which combines service brokerage with the role of outpatient therapist (Kanter 1989). From this perspective, the case manager's visits to clients in the community not only provide instrumental assistance but also offer opportunities for psychoeducation, social skills training, and supportive psychotherapy. For example, Fariello and Scheidt (1989) integrate substance abuse counseling into clinical case management.

Case management programs may be defined in terms of conceptual framework or core philosophy. The rehabilitation model does not focus on preventing readmissions but emphasizes reducing impairment and handicap. This model has been studied extensively in Toronto, with generally positive outcomes (Goering et al. 1988). The strengths, or developmental acquisition model, builds on capacities rather than deficits and provides environmental opportunities to use and develop functional abilities (Sullivan 1992).

It is difficult to assess the specific benefits of intensive programs for high-risk clients because in general they have been compared to nonintensive and nonassertive services, not to each other (Chamberlain and Rapp 1991; Solomon 1992). However, there appears to be consensus on several points:

- The more difficult-to-treat subgroups appear to benefit from assertive, intensive services that can be delivered in the client's own environment, and that have a crisis-response capacity.
- Those services depend on maintaining a fairly low ratio of client to provider, with small caseloads for individual case managers (Dietzen and Bond 1993).
- In comparison to simple service brokerage models, staff members must be clinically sophisticated and capable of managing acute care in the community.

It is likely that advanced practice psychiatric nurses will work within these programs increasingly in the future, as the context of complex care shifts to the community (Goering 1993).

Home Care for the Severely Mentally Ill

While the U.S. population has tripled since 1900, the over 65 age group has grown eightfold. Currently there are approximately 2 million severely and persistently mentally ill elderly people in the United States. This number is growing continually, reflecting the aging of the baby-boom population, and resulting in a subgroup of the severely mentally ill with multiple concurrent health problems (Krach 1993; Sheline 1990).

The aging of the severely mentally ill in the community has created a marked need for specialized nursing case management (Knight and Carter 1990). It has also created a growing demand for psychiatric home care nursing (Duffy, Miller, and Parlocha 1993; Mellon 1994). In addition to the elderly with severe mental disorders, the triply diagnosed mentally ill with AIDS also require **psychiatric home care** services to manage issues related to the ongoing illness, the experience of a life-threatening illness, and neuropsychiatric problems that may occur as a result of HIV infection (Hurley and Ungvarski 1994).

Psychiatric home care nursing has a long history in community mental health. Some of the most successful programs for the severely mentally ill in the early years of community mental health employed visiting nurses to deliver home-based services with a family support component (Keener 1975; Pasamanick, Scarpitti, and Dinitz 1967). Today, advanced practice nurses working for home care agencies generally work as intensive case managers, coordinating a range of services that include direct psychiatric nursing care.

Consumer and Family-Guided Programs

The consumer movement in mental health care has diverse roots. It is based to some extent on the self-help movement in health care in general and peer support models for recovery. It is also based in the mutual aid "clubs" of former patients that gave rise to the Psychosocial Clubhouse model. Patient rights organizations and "antipsychiatric" protest groups of the 1960s and 1970s also contributed to today's consumer movement, which has moved from an adversary position to the role of collaborator in mental health care planning and evaluation of services.

Mental health care consumers have conducted several major surveys, including a study of housing preferences among the severely mentally ill (Campbell et al. 1989). It has become increasingly common for consumers to participate in program reviews and evaluations conducted by mental health authorities (Anagnos et al. 1993). Consumers have also entered mental health care systems in the role of peer counselors (Mowbray,Wellwoodm and Chamberlain 1988), consumer advocates (Moxley and Freddolino 1991), and case managers (Sherman and Porter 1991). Connelly et al. (1991) describe a consumer-run drop-in center where increases in consumer empowerment appeared to increase mutual support. In fact, a sense of mastery and control, or empowerment, has been identified as a powerful predictor of quality of life for the severely mentally ill, and therefore an important feature of any program (Rosenfield 1992).

Families of the severely and persistently mentally ill have also assumed a much greater advocacy role than in the past. Sommer (1990) points out that family advocacy arose in response to problems accompanying the deinstitutionalization process that placed an enormous burden of care on families. It also developed in reaction to the stigmatization of parents by people who attributed serious mental disorders to child-rearing practices. The major family organization for people with severe and persistent mental disorders is the **National Alliance for the Mentally Ill (NAMI).** The national and local chapters of NAMI have grown tremendously over the past decade and now comprise a recognized force in mental health policy development (Hatfield 1991).

Nursing Contributions to Community Support and Rehabilitation Programs

Nurses occupy a pivotal position in mental health care systems that serve the severely and persistently mentally ill. Because of nursing's traditional concern with such issues as self-care, environmental support, and family-oriented health services, psychiatric nurses can integrate their skills into community support and rehabilitation programs.

On the inpatient level, psychiatric nurses coordinate services and prepare clients for connection or reconnection to community support services (Goering 1993). Rehabilitation goals must begin with the nursing care plan. Inpatient care often involves psychoeducational interventions to teach the client about the illness, required medications, and symptom management techniques that contribute to self-care (Buccheri and Underwood 1993; Hamera et al. 1992; Murphy and Moller 1993; O'-Connor 1991). Acute care nurses also participate in psychoeducational interventions with families to help them learn to problem-solve effectively and to cope with the illness (Drysdale, Nelson, and Wineman 1993; Gamble 1993).

In the community, nurses practice at all levels of the community support systems (Mound et al. 1991; Connelly 1992). They are prominent in intensive case management programs, rehabilitation centers and home care programs. Advanced practice roles in these settings require the skills and knowledge of an expert clinician and the ability to work within complex organizations. In psychiatric rehabilitation programs, nurses have the opportunity to teach self-care and symptom management skills and to offer the general health services that maximize the quality of life. Psychiatric home care promises to expand over the coming decade and to offer nurse case managers a unique role with the severely mentally ill at home and with their families (Blazek 1993; Duffy and Miller 1993).

Nursing Research and Education

In 1989, Judith Krauss wrote: "Comprehensive care, continuity of care, community-based care—these words have a far better chance of being actualized through the practice and research of nursing than through the work of any of the other . . . core disciplines." If nursing is to meet this challenge, we must develop and test the nursing interventions that can benefit the severely and persistently mentally ill. The research base for psychiatric nursing has grown dramatically over the past decade. It has benefitted from research initiatives by the NIMH and the establishment of the National Institute for Nursing Research (McBride et al., 1992).

In the future, as we move into an era of health care reform, it will be critical to produce outcome studies that examine nursing contributions in emerging systems of service delivery for the severely mentally ill in the community. It is far from clear what role advanced practice nurses will play in these systems and how much nursing will contribute to their development. Should clinical specialists also be prepared for primary care of the severely and persistently mentally ill? What are the benefits and drawbacks of prescriptive authority for advanced practice psychiatric nurses? Will the expansion of a direct clinical role distract nurses from participating in policy making regarding the community services for the psychiatrically disabled? What educational preparation is necessary to meet the demands of the future? These are questions that can be answered through research, if we allow emerging knowledge to shape our educational programs and inform our practice.

Chapter Highlights

- Case management is central to the operation of community support programs, because it is the mechanism for coordination of a range of treatment and support services.
- Essential services address needs in the area of entitlements and money management, housing, medication, acute and outpatient mental health services, general health services, vocational and social activities, family education and support, and education and advocacy.
- Community programs with a rehabilitation philosophy emphasize support to function in a normalized environment and emphasize client self-care and determination.
- Intensive programs for high-risk clients generally involve flexible and assertive programming that takes services to the client. Continuous treatment teams provide one increasingly important way to deliver intensive services.
- Psychiatric nurses provide skilled assessment and management of the acute exacerbations of illness that characterize severe and persistent disorders.
- Psychiatric nurses provide educational and support interventions to families who are coping with serious illness of a relative.
- Psychiatric nurses in case management roles coordinate care across settings and attend to a complex range of health needs.
- Psychiatric nurses in home care settings provide comprehensive care to medically complex severely mentally ill adults, whose numbers are growing because of the aging population.

References

Adler LE, Griffith JM: Concurrent medical illness in the schizophrenic patient: Epidemiology, diagnosis, and management. *Schizophrenia Res* 1991;4(2):91–107.

Anagnos A, McConnell W, Chafetz L, Barto S: A consumer-oriented program review process for mental health care. *New Directions for Mental Health Services* 1993;58:77–83.

Anthony WA, Blanch A: Supported employment for persons who are psychiatrically disabled: an historical and conceptual perspective. *Psychosoc Rehab J* 1987;11(2):5–23.

Anthony WA, Liberman RP: The practice of psychiatric rehabilitation. Historical, conceptual, and research base. *Schizophrenia Bull* 1986;12(4):652–559.

Arana JD, Hastings B, Herron E: Continuous care teams in intensive outpatient treatment of chronic mentally ill patients. *Hosp Commun Psychiatr* 1991;42(5):503–507.

Aviram U, Segal SP: Exclusion of the mentally ill. *Arch Gen Psychiatr* 1973;29:126.

Bachrach LL: The context of care for the chronic mental patient with substance abuse problems. *Psychiatric Quarterly* 1987;58(1):3–14.

Bachrach LL: What we know about homelessness among mentally ill persons: An analytical review and commentary. *Hosp Commun Psychiatr* 1992;43(5):453–464.

Baker F, Douglas C: Housing environments and community adjustment of severely mentally ill persons. *Commun Ment Health J* 1990;26(6):497–505.

Barbee JG et al.: Alcohol and substance abuse among schizophrenic patients presenting to an emergency psychiatric service. *J Nervous and Mental Disease* 1989; 177(7):400–407.

Barnes LE: Residential care operators: perspectives on mental illness and caregiving roles. *New Directions for Mental Health Services* 1993; Summer (58):33–42.

Bartels SJ, Teaque GB, Drake RE, Clark RE, Bush PW, Noordsy DL: Substance abuse in schizophrenia: Service utilization and costs. *J Nervous and Mental Disease* 1993;81(4): 227–232.

Baxter E, Hopper K: *Private Lives/Public Spaces: Homeless Adults in the Streets of New York City.* Community Service Society, 1981.

Beard JH, Malamud TJ, Rossman E: Psychiatric rehabilitation and long-term rehospitalization rates: The findings of two research studies. *Schizophrenia Bull* 1978;4:622.

Beard JH, Propst RN, Malamud TJ: The Fountain House model of psychiatric rehabilitation. *Psychosoc Rehabilitation J* 1982;5(1):47–53.

Blazek LA: Development of a psychiatric home care program and the role of the CNS in the delivery of care. *Clinical Nurse Specialist* 1993;7(4):164–168.

Bond GR, Witheridge TF, Wasmer D, Webb J, DeGraaf-Kaser R: Assertive community treatment for frequent users of psychiatric hospitals in a large city. *Am J Commun Psych* 1990;18(6):865–891.

Braun P, Kochansky G, Shapiro R, Greenberg L, Gudeman JE, Johnson S, Shore MF: Overview: Deinstitutionalization of psychiatric patients, a critical review of outcome studies. *Am J Psychiatr* 1981;138:736.

Buccheri R, Underwood P: Symptom management: In-patient nursing care of persons with schizophrenia, in Chafetz L (ed): *A Psychiatric Nursing Perspective on Severe Mental Illness: New Directions in Mental Health Services,* no. 58. Jossey-Bass, 1993.

Bunt G, Galanter M, Lifshutz H, Castaneda R: Cocaine/crack dependence among psychiatric inpatients. *Am J Psychiatr* 1990;147(11):1542–1546.

Bush CT, Langford MW, Rosen P, Gott W: Operation outreach: Intensive case management for severely psychiatrically disabled adults. *Hosp Commun Psychiatr* 1990; 41:647–649.

Campbell J, Schraiber R, Tempin T, ten Tusscher T: The well-being project: Mental health clients speak for themselves. California Network of Mental Health Clients, 1989.

Canton CL, Wyatt RJ, Felix A, Grunberg J, Dominguez B: Follow-up of chronically homeless mentally ill men. *Am J Psychiatr* 1993;150(11):1539–1542.

Canton CL, Wyatt RJ, Grunberg J, Felix A: An evaluation of a mental health program for homeless men. *Am J Psychiatr* 1990;147(3):286–289.

Carpenter WT, Jr, Strauss JS: The prediction of outcome in schizophrenia. IV: Eleven-year follow-up of the Washington IPSS cohort. *J Nervous and Mental Disease* 1991; 179(9):517–525.

Chafetz L: Why clinicians distance themselves from the homeless mentally ill, in Lamb HR, Bachrach LL, Kass FI (eds): *Treating the Homeless Mentally Ill.* American Psychiatric Association, 1992.

Chafetz L, Barnes LE: Issues in psychiatric caregiving. *Arch Psychiatr Nurs* 1989;3(2):61–68.

Chafetz L, Goldman HH, Taube CA: (1983). Deinstitutionalization in the United States. *Int J Ment Health* 1984; 11(4):48–63.

Chamberlain R, Rapp CA: A decade of case management: a methodological review of outcome research. *Commun Ment Health J* 1991;27(3):171–188.

Cohen NL, Tsemberis S: Emergency psychiatric intervention on the street. *New Directions for Mental Health Services* 1991;52:3–16.

Connelly PM: Services for the underserved: a nurse-managed center for the chronically mentally ill. *J Psychosoc Nurs Ment Health Serv* 1991;29(1):15–20.

Connelly PM: What does a nurse need to know to maintain an effective level of case management? *J Psychosoc Ment Health Nurs* 1992;30:35–39.

Danley KS, Sciarappa K, MacDonald-Wilson K: Choose-get-keep: A psychiatric rehabilitation approach to supported employment. *New Directions for Mental Health Services* 1992;53:87–96.

Dennis DL, Buckner JC, Lipton FR, Levine IS: A decade of research and services for homeless mentally ill persons. Where do we stand? *Am Psychologist* 1991;46(11): 1129–1138.

D'Ercole A, Skodol AE, Struening E, Curtis J, Millman J: Diagnosis of physical illness in psychiatric patients using Axis III and a standardized medical history. *Hosp Commun Psychiatr* 1991;42(4):395–400.

Deutsch A: *The Shame of the States.* Harcourt Brace, 1948.

Dietzen LL, Bond GR: Relationship between case manager contact and outcome for frequently hospitalized psychiatric clients. *Hosp Commun Psychiatr* 1993;44(9):839–843.

Dixon L, Friedman N, Lehman A: Housing patterns of homeless mentally ill persons receiving assertive treatment services. *Hosp Commun Psychiatr* 1993;44(3):286–288.

Drake RE, Osher FC, Wallach MA: Alcohol use and abuse in schizophrenia: A prospective community study. *Schizophrenia* Bull 1989; 16(1):57–67.

Drysdale AE, Nelson CF, Wineman NM: Families need help too: group treatment for families of nursing home residents. *Clinical Nurse Specialist* 1993;7(3):130–134.

Duffy J, Miller MP, Parlocha P: Psychiatric homecare: A framework for assessment and intervention. *Home Healthcare Nurse* 1993;11:22–28.

Fariello D, Scheidt S: Clinical case management of the dually diagnosed patient. *Hosp Commun Psychiatr* 1989;40(10): 1065–1067.

Federal Task Force on Homelessness and Severe Mental Illness. *Outcasts on Main Street.* Dept Health and Human Services, 1992.

Fenton WS, McGlashan TH: Natural history of schizophrenia subtypes. II. Positive and negative symptoms and long-term course. *Arch Gen Psychiatr* 1991;48(11): 978–986.

Gamble C: Working with schizophrenic clients and their families. *Br J Nurs* 1993;2(17):856–859.

Goering P: Psychiatric nursing and the context of care, in Chafetz L (ed): *A Psychiatric Nursing Perspective on Severe Mental Illness: New Directions in Mental Health Services,* no. 58. Jossey-Bass, 1993.

Goering PN et al.: Improved functioning for case management clients. *Psychosoc Rehabilitation J* 1988;12(1):3–17.

Goffman E: *Asylums.* Doubleday, 1961.

Goldfinger SM, Chafetz L: Developing a better service delivery system for the homeless mentally ill, in Lamb HR (ed): *The Homeless Mentally Ill: A Task Force Report of the American Psychiatric Association.* American Psychiatric Association, 1984.

Goldman HM: Mental illness and family burden: A public health perspective. *Hosp Commun Psychiatr* 1984;33: 557–561.

Goldman HH, Manderscheid RW: Chronic mental disorder in the United States. Manderscheid RW, Barrett SA (eds): *Mental Health, United States.* Dept of Health and Human Services, 1987.

Hamera EK, Peterson KA, Young LM, Schaumloffel MM: Symptom monitoring in schizophrenia: Potential for enhancing self-care. *Arch Psychiatr Nurs* 1992;6:324–330.

Hatfield AB: The national alliance for the mentally ill: A decade later. *Commun Ment Health J* 1991;27:95–103.

Hegarty JD, Baldessarini RJ, Tohen M, Waternaux C, Oepen G: One hundred years of schizophrenia: A metamanalysis of the outcome literature. *A J Psychiatr* 1994;151(10): 1409–1416.

Hu TW, Jerrell J: Cost-effectiveness of alternative approaches in treating severely mentally ill in California. *Schizophrenia Bull* 1991;17(3):461–468.

Hurley PM, Ungvarski PJ: Mental health needs of adults with HIV/AIDS referred for home care. *Psychosoc Rehabilitation J* 1994;17:117–126.

Institute of Medicine Committee on Health Care for Homeless People. *Homelessness, Health, and Human Needs.* National Academy Press, 1988.

Jamelka R, Trupin E, Chiles J: The mentally ill in prisons: A review. *Hosp Commun Psychiatr* 1989;40(5):481–491.

Joint Commission on Mental Illness and Health. *Action for Mental Health.* Basic Books, 1961.

Kanter J: Clinical case management: Definition, principles, and components. *Hosp Commun Psychiatr* 1989;40: 361–368.

Kasten BP, Monteleone MP: Psychiatric nursing and the emergency setting. *New Directions for Mental Health Services* 1993;Summer (58):13–22.

Keener ML: The public health nurse in mental health follow-up. *Nurs Res* 1975;24:198–201.

Kessler RC, McGonagle KA, Zhao S, Nelson CB, Hughes M, Eshleman S, Wittchen HU, Kendler KS: Lifetime and 12-month prevalence of DSM-III-R psychiatric disorders in the United States: Results from the National Comorbidity Survey. *Arch Gen Psychiatr* 1994;51(1):8–19.

Kluiter H, Giel R, Nienhuis FJ, Ruphan M, Wiersma D: Predicting feasibility of day treatment for unselected patients referred for inpatient psychiatric treatment: Results of a randomized trial. *Am J Psychiatr* 1992;149(9):1199–1205.

Knight BG, Carter PM: Reduction of psychiatric inpatient stay for older adults by intensive case management. *The Gerontologist* 1990;30:510–515.

Krach P: Nursing implications: Functional status of older persons with schizophrenia. *J Gerontological Nurs* 1993;19(8): 21–27.

Krauss JB: New conceptions of care, community, and chronic mental illness. *Arch Psychiatr Nurs* 1989;3(5):281–287.

Lamb HR, Goertzel V: Discharged mental patients: Are they really in the community? *Arch Gen Psychiatr* 1971;24:29.

Maj M, Magliano L, Pirozzi R, Marasco C, Guarneri M: Validity of rapid cycling as a course specifier for bipolar disorder. *Am J Psychiatr* 1994;151(7):1015–1019.

Maurin JT, Boyd CB: Burden of mental illness on the family: A critical review. *Arch Psychiatr Nurs* 1990;4(2):99–107.

McBride AB, Friedenberg EC, Babich KS, Bush CT: Nursing research at NIMH: an update. *Arch Psychiatr Nurs* 1992; 6(2):138–141.

McGurrin MC, Worley N: Evaluation of intensive case management for seriously and persistently mentally ill persons. *J Case Management* 1993;2(2):59–65.

Meeks S, Murrell SA: Service providers in the social networks of clients with severe mental illness. *Schizophrenia Bull* 1994;20(2):399–406.

Mellon SK: Mental health clinical nurse specialists in home care for the 90's. *Issues Ment Health Nurs* 1994;15:237.

Minkoff K: An integrated treatment model for dual diagnosis of psychosis and addiction. *Hosp Commun Psychiatr* 1989;40(10):1031–1036.

Morse GA, Calsyn RJ, Allen G, Tempelhoff B, Smith, R: Experimental comparison of the effects of three treatment programs for homeless mentally ill people. *Hosp Commun Psychiatr* 1992;43(10):1005–1010.

Mound B, Gyulay R, Khan P, Goering P: The expanded role of nurse case managers. *J Psychosoc Ment Health Nurs* 1991;29:18–22.

Mowbray CT, Bybee D, Cohen E: Describing the homeless mentally ill: Cluster analysis results. *Am J Commun Psych* 1993;21(1):67–93.

Mowbray CT, Wellwood R, Chamberlain P: Project stay: a consumer-run support service. *Psychosoc Rehabilitation J* 1988;12(1):33–42.

Moxley DP, Freddolino PP: Needs of homeless people coping with psychiatric problems: findings from an innovative advocacy project. *Health and Social Work* 1991;16(1): 19–26.

Murphy MF, Moller MD: Relapse management in neurobiological disorders: The Moller-Murphy symptom management assessment tool. *Arch Psychiatr Nurs* 1993;7:226–235.

National Advisory Mental Health Council. Health care reform for Americans with severe mental illness: A report. *Am J Psychiatr* 1993;150(10):1447–1465.

Newman SJ: The housing and neighborhood conditions of persons with severe mental illness. *Hosp Commun Psychiatr* 1994;45(4):338–343.

O'Connor FW: Symptom monitoring for relapse prevention in schizophrenia. *Arch Psychiatr Nurs* 1991;5:193–201.

Pasamanick D, Scarpitti FR, Dinitz S: *Schizophrenics in the Community.* Appleton-Century-Crofts, 1967.

Regier DA, Farmer ME, Rae DS, Locke BZ, Keith SJ, Judd LL, Goodwin FK: Comorbidity of mental disorders with alcohol and other drug abuse: Results from the Epidemiologic Catchment Area (ECA) Study. *JAMA* 1990;264(19):2511–2518.

Regier DA, Narrow WE, Rae DS, Manderscheid RW, Locke BZ, Goodwin FK: The defacto US mental and addictive disorders service system: Epidemiological Catchment Area—prospective 1 year prevalence rate of disorders and services. *Arch Gen Psychiatr* 1993;50(2):85–94.

Rosenfield S: Factors contributing to the subjective quality of life of the chronic mentally ill. *J Health and Social Behavior* 1992;33(4):299–315.

Safer DJ: Substance abuse by young adult chronic patients. *Hosp Commun Psychiatr* 1987;38(5):511–514.

Shapiro J: *Communities of the Alone.* Associated Press, 1972.

Sheline YI: High prevalence of physical illness in a geriatric psychiatric in-patient population. *Gen Hosp Psychiatr* 1990;12(6):396–400.

Sherman PS, Porter R: Mental health consumers as case management aides. *Hosp Commun Psychiatr* 1991;42(5):494–498.

Solinski S, Jackson HJ, Bell RC: Prediction of employability in schizophrenic patients. *Schizophrenic Res* 1992;7(2):141–148.

Solomon P: The efficacy of case management services for severely mentally disabled clients. *Commun Ment Health J* 1992;28(3):163–180.

Sommer R: Family advocacy and the mental health system: The recent rise of the alliance for the mentally ill. *Psychiatric Quarterly* 1990;61(3):205–221.

Stein LI: A system approach to reducing relapse in schizophrenia. *J Clin Psychiatr* 1993;54:7–12.

Sullivan PF, Bulik CM, Forman SD, Mezzich JE: Characteristics of repeat users of a psychiatric emergency service. *Hosp Commun Psychiatr* 1993;44(4):376–380.

Sullivan WP: Reclaiming the community: The strengths perspective and deinstitutionalization. *Social Work* 1992; 37(3):204–209.

Talley S, Caverly S: Nursing update: Advanced-practice nursing and health care reform. *Hosp Commun Psychiatr* 1994;45:545–557.

Test LI, Stein MA: Community treatment of the chronic patient: Research overview. *Schizophrenic Bull* 1978;4(3):350–364.

Test MA, Wallisch LS, Allness DJ, Ripp K: Substance use in young adults with schizophrenic disorders. *Schizophrenia Bull* 1989;15(3):465–475.

Thompson KS, Griffith EE, Leaf PJ: A historical review of the Madison model of community care. *Hosp Commun Psychiatr* 1990;41(6):625–634.

Turner JC, TenHoor WJ: The NIMH Community Support Program: Pilot approach to a needed social reform. *Schizophrenia Bull* 1978;4:319.

Wahl OF: Community impact of group homes for mentally ill adults. *Commun Ment Health J* 1993;29(3):247–259.

Wallace CJ, Liberman RP, MacKain SJ, Blackwell G, Eckman TA: Effectiveness and replicability of modules for teaching social and instrumental skills to the severely mentally ill. *Am J Psychiatr* 1992;149(5):654–658.

Wasylenki DA, Goering PN, Lemire D, Lindsey S, Lancee W: The hostel outreach program: Assertive case management for homeless mentally ill people. *Hosp Commun Psychiatr* 1993;44(9):848–853.

Way BB et al.: Staffing of forensic inpatient services in the United States. *Hosp Commun Psychiatr* 1990;41(2):172–174.

Weiden P, Havens L: Psychotherapeutic management techniques in the treatment of outpatients with schizophrenia. *Hosp Commun Psychiatr* 1994;45(6):549–555.

Whitmer GE: From hospitals to jails: The fate of California's deinstitutionalized mentally ill. *Am J Orthopsychiatr* 1980;50(1):65–75.

Winokur G, Corvell W, Keller M, Endicott J, Akiskal H: A prospective follow-up of patients with bipolar and primary unipolar affective disorder. *Arch Gen Psychiatr* 1993;50(6):457–465.

Wirshing WC, Marder SR, Eckman T, Liberman RP, Mintz J: Acquisition and retention of skills training methods in chronic schizophrenic outpatients. *Psychopharmacology Bull* 1992;28(3):241–245.

World Health Organization: *International Classification of Impairments, Disabilities, and Handicaps*. World Health Organization, 1980.

CHAPTER 22

PSYCHOLOGIC FACTORS AFFECTING MEDICAL CONDITIONS

Jerry D. Durham

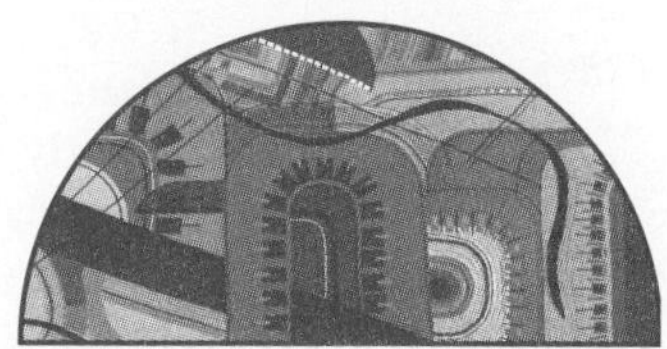

COMPETENCIES

- *Explain how psychology, emotions, personality, and health are related.*
- *Recognize illness as influenced by multiple biologic, psychologic, social, and environmental factors.*
- *Recognize the DSM-IV diagnostic features of psychologic factors affecting medical conditions.*
- *Identify psychologic factors that increase an individual's risk of physical illness.*
- *Define key terms associated with psychologic factors affecting medical conditions.*
- *Identify common medical conditions whose onset and course are influenced by psychologic and behavioral factors.*
- *Discuss how you can incorporate a holistic view of health and illness into your nursing practice.*

Cross-References

Other topics relevant to this content are: Stress, anxiety, and coping, Chapter 4; Techniques for managing stress, Chapter 29.

Critical Thinking Challenge

Some clinicians hold that certain medical conditions (such as peptic ulcer or asthma) result primarily from unresolved conflict and problematic emotions. Others believe that most medical conditions have a biologic or genetic basis and that once these causes are fully understood, a medical intervention will cure or ameliorate them. Nurses and certain other practitioners have traditionally viewed disease as being multifactorial in origin. What are your beliefs concerning the cause(s), progression, and treatment of disease? How do client views on disease affect treatment choices by clinicians?

This chapter discusses the ways in which the mind and body interact and how this interaction can potentially result in healthy or unhealthy states. Certain conditions and illnesses have an important emotional component in their onset, course, and outcome, which has been demonstrated by evidence from systematic research and case reports (Stoudemire 1993).

Health-Illness States: Interaction Between the Mind and Body

In the recent past, physical illnesses with a major emotional component were referred to as **psychophysiologic disorders.** This term has largely been abandoned because it is vague and has limited value for diagnosis, treatment, and research. Many (perhaps most) clinicians do not use this term today, although it still appears as a category in the *Cumulated Index Medicus.*

Prior to the publication of the *DSM-III*, **psychosomatic disorder** was the term for such conditions. However, the word *psychosomatic* suggests a restrictive and dualistic view of physical illness and psychologic factors that does not adequately account for the complex interaction of biologic, environmental, and psychosocial variables. Moreover, the very use of the word *psychosomatic* may suggest a special class of disease, thereby suggesting the absence of psychosomatic factors in other diseases—a duality inconsistent with the view that disease stems from multiple causes (Fava 1992). Nonetheless, "psychosomatic" is still in common usage as evidenced by the titles of several journals that focus on the relationship between physical illness and psychologic factors: *Psychosomatics, Journal of Psychosomatic Research, International Journal of Psychosomatics,* and *Psychosomatic Medicine.*

Much debate about the classification of and diagnostic criteria for conditions at the interface of physical illness and psychologic factors has appeared in the literature (Fava 1992; Sensky 1994; Stoudemire 1993; Stoudemire and Hales 1991). The *DSM-IV* lists **psychological factors affecting medical condition (PFAMC)**, a category that includes "factors that interfere with treatment and factors that constitute health risks to the individual" (APA 1994). The essential feature of this category is the presence of one or more specific psychologic or behavioral factors that adversely affect a medical condition. These factors may influence the course of a medical condition, interfere with the condition's treatment, or constitute an additional health risk. They may be any one or a combination of the following:

- A mental disorder affecting the course or treatment of a general medical condition, such as bipolar I disorder (manic episode) complicating hemodialysis.
- A psychologic symptom affecting the course or treatment of a general medical condition, such as anxiety complicating the ability to carry out self-care for diabetes mellitus.
- A personality trait or coping style affecting the course or treatment of a general medical condition, such as denial interfering with the timely treatment of cancer.
- A maladaptive health behavior affecting the course or treatment of a general medical condition, such as sedentary lifestyle and overeating affecting treatment for coronary artery disease.
- A stress-related physiologic response affecting the course or treatment of a general medical condition, such as stress-related dysrhythmias in a person recovering from myocardial infarction.

In using the *DSM-IV,* the clinician specifies the psychologic factors affecting the client's medical condition (Kaplan and Sadock 1994). Such factors may also precipitate or exacerbate a medical condition. According to the *DSM-IV* (APA 1994, p. 676), the PFAMC category should be reserved for situations in which:

1. the psychologic factors significantly affect the course or outcome of the medical condition, or
2. the psychologic factors place the individual at significantly higher risk for an untoward outcome.

In addition, there should be evidence of a relationship between the psychologic factors and the medical condition even though it may not be possible to specifically pinpoint the psychologic factors as a direct cause or to identify exactly how they operate.

The *DSM-IV* distinguishes PFAMC from several related disorders. In mental disorder due to a general medical condition, the presumed causality is in the opposite direction. For example, an individual may have catatonic disorder due to a neurologic condition such as a neoplasm, encephalitis, or cerebrovascular disease. Personality change may be due to HIV disease, head trauma, or lupus erythematosus. For situations in which delirium, dementia, amnestic disorder, mood disorder, psychotic disorder, anxiety disorder, sleep disorder, or sexual dysfunction are factors, see the appropriate chapters related to these diagnoses in this text. While somatoform disorders are characterized by both psychologic and physical symptoms, no medical condition completely accounts for the physical symptoms seen in people with this disorder. Other psychiatric disorders excluded from PFAMC include conversion disorder, hypochondriasis, physical complaints associated with a mental disorder, and substance-related physical complaints.

The psychiatric diagnostic criteria for PFAMC are discussed in the accompanying DSM-IV box.

Personality Type and Health-Illness Potential

Evidence from epidemiologic, clinical, and animal studies has begun to demonstrate that various psychologic factors (personality type, mood, emotions, behavior) influence the onset, exacerbation, and clinical course of physical illness, although the exact nature and the extent of this influence are not always easily measured (Stoudemire and Hales 1991). Moreover, epidemiologic, stress and coping-related, and laboratory animal studies strongly suggest that many people have "self-healing" or "disease-prone" personalities (Eysenck 1991; Friedman and VandenBos 1992).

People with self-healing personalities are described as enthusiastic, alert, responsive, energetic, calm, conscientious, content, curious, secure, and constructive. In terms of behavior, "self-healers" smile naturally, have unforced

DSM-IV Criteria for Psychologic Factors Affecting Medical Condition

A. A general medical condition (coded on Axis III) is present.

B. Psychological factors adversely affect the general medical condition in one of the following ways:
   1. the factors have influenced the course of the general medical condition as shown by a close temporal association between the psychological factors and the development or exacerbation of, or delayed recovery from, the general medical condition
   2. the factors interfere with the treatment of the general medical condition
   3. the factors constitute additional health risks for the individual
   4. stress-related physiological responses precipitate or exacerbate symptoms of the general medical condition

expressions and smooth gestures, and walk and talk smoothly. They are viewed as people others like to be around and as capable of forming close relationships. When confronted with stressful situations, the self-healing individual demonstrates resilience and emotional stability (Friedman and VandenBos 1992).

Several commonly cited chronic negative emotions appear to predispose an individual to chronic physical illnesses such as arthritis, pain (especially headache), ulcers, coronary artery disease, stroke, certain neurologic conditions, and asthma. These negative emotions include chronic hostility, anxiety, depression, and repressed feelings (Friedman 1992; Rogers et al. 1994). It is important to note, however, that there is no evidence for the conclusion that any one personality trait can account for the development of a physical illness (Stoudemire 1993). Those who are said to be disease-prone exhibit such characteristics as suspiciousness, cynicism, and despair. Negative emotions, mediated through complex neuroendocrinologic pathways, are believed to cause stress in vulnerable people, predisposing them to physical illness.

Friedman and VandenBos (1992) summarize how the environment and negative emotions may interact to cause physical illness:

> When vulnerable people encounter psychosocial environments that are a poor match for their needs, they often develop chronic negative emotional patterns. These reactions are accompanied by physiological disturbances such as high levels of activation of the sympathetic nervous system, of cortisol, and possibly other hormones; unhealthy behaviors, such as substance abuse, may also occur. Finally, these disturbances interact with disease-proneness caused by environment, such as high-fat diets, and by heredity, such as predisposition to cancer. Although the resulting risk of illness is not overwhelming, it is comparable to that of many other commonly noted health risks (p. 1177).

Although the relationship between negative emotions and chronic conditions has historically been a focus of research, scientists and clinicians have recently also turned their attention to how stress and negative emotions may suppress the immune system, increasing vulnerability to acute illnesses (such as infectious diseases) and the development of cancers (see the Research Note on page 544). The increasing interest in biologic regulatory mechanisms associated with behavioral and psychologic variables has greatly accelerated the development of such fields as psychoneurophysiology, psychoneuroendocrinology, and psychoneuroimmunology (Ader, Felton, and Cohen 1991; Schmoll, Tewes, and Plotnikoff 1992).

Because all illnesses may ultimately stem from multiple factors, a holistic theory of illness serves as a basis for understanding all human disorders. By appreciating the complex, interwoven pattern of emotional and physical elements, the nurse can more fully comprehend the essential unity of the body and the mind. For a partial list of physical conditions having psychologic components, see Table 22–1 on page 545.

Clients who come to the attention of health care professionals because of physical complaints frequently have their psychologic needs neglected. Those unmet needs may be contributing to the complaint, may be the primary cause of symptom development, or may be the reason for the client's decision to seek help. Even if the most technologically advanced diagnostic and treatment approaches are applied, ignoring the psychologic components of illness can be as disastrous as ignoring the biologic components. Such psychologic components can undermine medically appropriate treatment.

Therefore, in all illness, a holistic approach is necessary if each facet of the client's overall problem is to be addressed. For each of the disorders, we suggest nonmedical interventions that reduce stress while increasing the client's understanding and control over troublesome symptoms. Promoting healthy lifestyle and advocating lifestyle modifications are important nursing responsibilities regardless of the clinical area in which you practice.

RESEARCH NOTE

Citation

Malarkey W, Kiebolt-Glaser D, Glaser R: Hostile behavior during marital conflict alters pituitary and adrenal hormones. *Psychosom Med* 1994; 56(1):41–51.

Study Problem/Purpose

Many disease processes are induced or aggravated by stressful events. This study examined problem-solving behaviors among newlywed couples under controlled, stressful conditions. The purpose of the study was to describe the impact of stress on the release of the hormones norepinephrine, epinephrine, ACTH, cortisol, growth hormone, and prolactin.

Methods

Ninety newlywed couples, selected on the basis of stringent mental and physical health criteria, were admitted for 24 hours to a research unit. Admissions were scheduled around the follicular phase of the woman's menstrual cycle. Nurses drew blood samples at set intervals through a long polyethylene tube out of the subjects' visual field. Five blood samples were drawn before, during, and after a 30-minute structured problem-solving or conflict task. The conflict session was recorded on videotape and was scored with a standard system.

Findings

Marital conflict and hostile/negative behavior were closely linked to changes in five of the six hormones studied. This finding persisted in spite of the high marital satisfaction of the couples and the stringent study criteria. Hostile behavior was associated with decreased levels of prolactin and increases in all other hormones except cortisol. Blood pressure also increased in high-hostile subjects. The researchers believe that their findings reflect, and even underestimate, the physiologic impact of marital discord in the real world.

Implications

Hostile behavior activates adrenal and pituitary hormones during marital conflict. An unhappy marriage characterized by conflict may pose a risk for the development of stress-related illnesses, including hypertension and atherogenesis.

Biopsychosocial Theories

The relationship between the mind and the body has always been a subject for speculation. Early humans had a holistic approach to disease, making no distinction between physical and mental illness. From Socrates, we have, "As it is not proper to cure the eyes without the head, nor the head without the body, so neither is it proper to cure the body without the soul." And from Hippocrates, "In order to cure the body it is necessary to have a knowledge of the whole of things." Then, during the Middle Ages, medicine became dominated by mysticism and religion. Sin was thought to be the cause of disease. In reaction to this view, and in conjunction with the scientific discoveries of the Renaissance (autopsy and microscopy), the study of the psyche was completely divorced from the study of medicine. In the nineteenth century, the rift was deepened by further scientific advances. It was thought that all disease must be associated with structural cell changes. Hence, the disease and not the client was the focus. Now, in the twentieth century, we have come full circle, and the treatment of the mind and body are again united. How the mind and body affect each other is still not completely understood, although many theorists have attempted to explain the nature of the relationship. Kaplan and Sadock (1994) provide an excellent overview of psychosomatic medicine from 10,000 BC to the present.

The Specificity Model

One theory is the specificity model of Franz Alexander (1950). Alexander believed that prolonged psychologic stress could sometimes lead to a medical condition via activation of the autonomic nervous system. The development of the disorder is mediated by genetic predisposition and vulnerability. According to Alexander, specific types of emotional conflict cause anxiety in the individual. In defending against this anxiety, the individual regresses to an earlier psychologic and physiologic stage of development. For instance, a person may regress into the oral receptive stage, in which there is an unconscious wish to be fed by the mother. This results in gastric hypersecretion. If the person has a vulnerable duodenal mucosa, peptic ulcer may result. Alexander hypothesized seven psychosomatic disorders: essential hypertension, neurodermatitis, bronchial asthma, rheumatoid arthritis, hyperthyroidism, ulcerative colitis, and peptic ulcer. The following case example illustrates how the specificity model is applied:

Linda, a 20-year-old nursing student, has been diagnosed with a small peptic ulcer, treatable with diet and medication. Because she mentioned that she was having difficulties at school, she is also referred to the psychiatry service, where she meets with a psychoanalytically inclined therapist. He

Table 22-1 Examples of Physical Conditions Having Psychologic Components

System	Condition
Cardiovascular	Essential hypertension, angina pectoris, tachycardia, arrhythmia, cardiospasm, coronary artery disease, mitral valve prolapse, myocardial infarction, migraine headache.
Gastrointestinal	Irritable bowel syndrome, gastric ulcer, duodenal ulcer, pylorospasm, regional enteritis (Crohn's disease), ulcerative colitis, nausea and vomiting, gastritis, chronic diarrhea.
Hormonal	Hypoglycemia, diabetes mellitus, hyperthyroidism, hypothyroidism, hyperparathyroidism, hypoparathyroidism, premenstrual syndrome, obesity.
Immune	Allergic disorders, cancer, autoimmune disorders (systemic lupus erythematosus, rheumatoid arthritis, Hashimoto's thyroiditis, myasthenia gravis, psoriasis), AIDS.
Integumentary	Neurodermatitis (atopic dermatitis), pruritus, psoriasis, hyperhidrosis, urticaria, alopecia, acne, herpes, genital warts.
Neuromuscular/skeletal	Chronic pain, headache, sacroiliac pain, temporomandibular joint (TMJ) pain, rheumatoid arthritis, Raynaud's disease.
Respiratory	Asthma, hyperventilation syndrome, tuberculosis.

asks Linda about her childhood and discovers that she was cared for by her grandmother while both her parents were away at work during the day. Later, Linda had to take care of a younger sister and brother after school and on weekends. She says she never had a "real childhood" and doesn't ever remember her mother being there when she needed her. According to Alexander's model, the therapist would deduce that Linda has a dependence conflict deriving from her early childhood. Current academic stress causes her to wish for a time when she was protected and nurtured by her mother. These unconscious feelings produce gastric hypersecretion, and eventually a peptic ulcer.

Other investigators made further attempts to relate specific personality characteristics to certain diseases. People with ulcerative colitis were found to be passive, conforming, and dependent. Those with hypertension had counterdependence strivings. Diabetic people were passive, needed affection, and wished to be cared for. Women with dysmenorrhea were infantile and expressed hopelessness and self-denial. Cancer clients were found to be selfless and undemanding (Sachar 1975).

On closer scrutiny, the specificity theory is actually not very specific. Certain emotional states, such as dependence, appear to be common to all disorders. Furthermore, research does not indicate whether dependence is a cause or an effect of the disease process. Another criticism is that some of the relationships described above have been based on faulty physiologic premises. For instance, ulcerative colitis was thought to be caused by an inability to express anger openly. Instead, the client's rage "explodes" in uncontrollable bouts of diarrhea. It was believed that the frequent evacuations caused inflammation of the bowel lining. However, research has shown that *before* the persistent diarrhea appears, small ulcerations are already forming in the bowel (Sachar 1975). Many early studies linking specific conditions to personality traits or emotions have also been criticized as suffering from research bias and faulty design.

The Nonspecific Stress Model

A second theory is the nonspecific stress model of Gustav Mahl (1953). Unlike Alexander, who focused on specific types of emotional conflict, Mahl theorized that the psychosomatic process can be activated by any stressful event, such as an earthquake, or a more subtle intrapsychic event, such as a fear of elevators. Whatever the source of the stress, the physiologic responses are identical for everyone. Selye (1950, 1976) also studied these physiologic responses. Selye's general adaptation syndrome (GAS) has been widely featured in nursing literature and is the theoretic underpinning of much stress-related nursing research (see Chapter 4). These responses include gastric and cardiovascular hyperfunctioning and hormonal changes, such as increased adrenal steroid secretion. A person who experiences chronic stress may develop a biologic symptom, whose nature is determined by organ susceptibility and early learning experiences involving pathologic responses. According to this theory, physical illness can occur in individuals with a genetic predisposition, usually as a result of anxiety. Studies in animals support this nonspecific stress model (Kaplan and Sadock 1994).

This nonspecific model can be applied to the same case study used to illustrate Alexander's specificity model.

Linda, the nursing student, still has a small peptic ulcer, but with this model it is explained differently:

Linda experienced the usual school stresses along with the rest of her classmates. But Linda develops an ulcer because her stomach is particularly vulnerable to stress. She may naturally produce an excess of hydrochloric acid, or her stomach lining may have some congenital defect. Along with organ susceptibility, Linda may have a parent who had a peptic ulcer. She may have seen a parent react to stress with abdominal disturbances and learned to react in a similar manner.

This viewpoint is consistent with the clinical research data that have been gathered from studying people under stress. However, this theory fails to account for the influence that meaning has in an individual's interpretation of stressful events.

The Individual Response Specificity Model

A third theory is the individual response specificity model formulated by Lacey, Bateman, and Van Lehn (1953). According to this model, individuals tend to show highly characteristic and consistent physiologic responses to a wide range of stimuli. These responses were formed in childhood. This model contradicts the nonspecific model in which everyone is seen as responding in much the same way to stress. Instead, according to the individual response model, there are "cardiac reactors," "gastric reactors," and "hypertensive reactors."

To illustrate this model, we return to Linda and her peptic ulcer:

Linda always has indigestion when she becomes upset. However, Monica, her roommate, never has indigestion. Instead, she frequently has migraine headaches.

This theory is compatible with the previously mentioned theories of organ susceptibility and early learning experiences. Because it encompasses current research data, this theory has become increasingly popular.

The Multicausational Concept of Illness

It is readily apparent that the preceding models do not fully illuminate the relationships between emotions and physical functioning. By taking some other factors into account, researchers developed a more useful model. Some of these factors are presented in the research by Holmes and Rahe (1967), Mutter and Schleifer (1966), and Rahe and Arthur (1978). These studies show that physical illness is commonly preceded by stressful life changes. Their findings thus indicate that emotions play a role in all disease processes. The studies further suggest that physical disorders, like mental disorders, are related to socioeconomic status. Furthermore, individuals in similar social situations defined those situations differently and consequently had different reactions to the similar situations.

These findings underscore the following:

- The concept of the separation of mind and body is not useful in understanding the total disease process.
- Stress comes in many forms—psychologic, physiologic, and sociologic—and is a causative factor in all illness.
- Stress is perceived differently, depending on the individual and the specific context.

Figure 22–1 and the following clinical example illustrate these ideas.

Peter G, 5 years old, was admitted for the fourth time in 6 months because of an acute asthma attack. While Peter was being treated medically, his parents waited in the family room. Mrs G sat crying and wringing her hands while Mr G paced the floor with a strained expression on his face. A staff nurse was able to talk to them and trace the sequence of events leading up to Peter's admission to the hospital.

It was a Saturday afternoon, and Mr and Mrs G had been arguing about whether to send Peter to kindergarten in the fall. Two points of view had emerged. Mr G was all for it. He wanted Peter to grow up quickly and leave his "babyish ways" behind. Mrs G was against it. Peter was the baby of the family, and Mrs G felt that her husband was always pushing him to do things too advanced for a 5-year-old. Peter had awakened from his nap to hear his parents shouting at each other. The quarrel ended abruptly when Peter started to wheeze, and both parents rushed to his bedside, united in their concern for him.

What factors brought on Peter's asthma attack at that particular time? The biologic factors include Peter's physiologic makeup. His mother had been asthmatic as a child. She and Peter are both allergic to chocolate, eggs, feathers, and dust. Peter inherited certain genetic features that make him susceptible to certain environmental stressors—in this case, the specific allergens. Sociologic components of Peter's illness revolve around his family's functioning. Mr and Mrs G have different viewpoints on what Peter's role in the family should be. Their conflicts create a second source of stress for Peter. A third component is Peter's psychologic state. A 5-year-old boy views the integrity of his family as extremely important, and parental conflicts may threaten his sense of security. Peter had discovered that his parents rallied together when he was ill.

In view of these contributing factors, the treatment plan for Peter should not end when Peter stops wheezing. To reduce the number of such emergencies, caregivers need to devise a long-range treatment plan. This plan

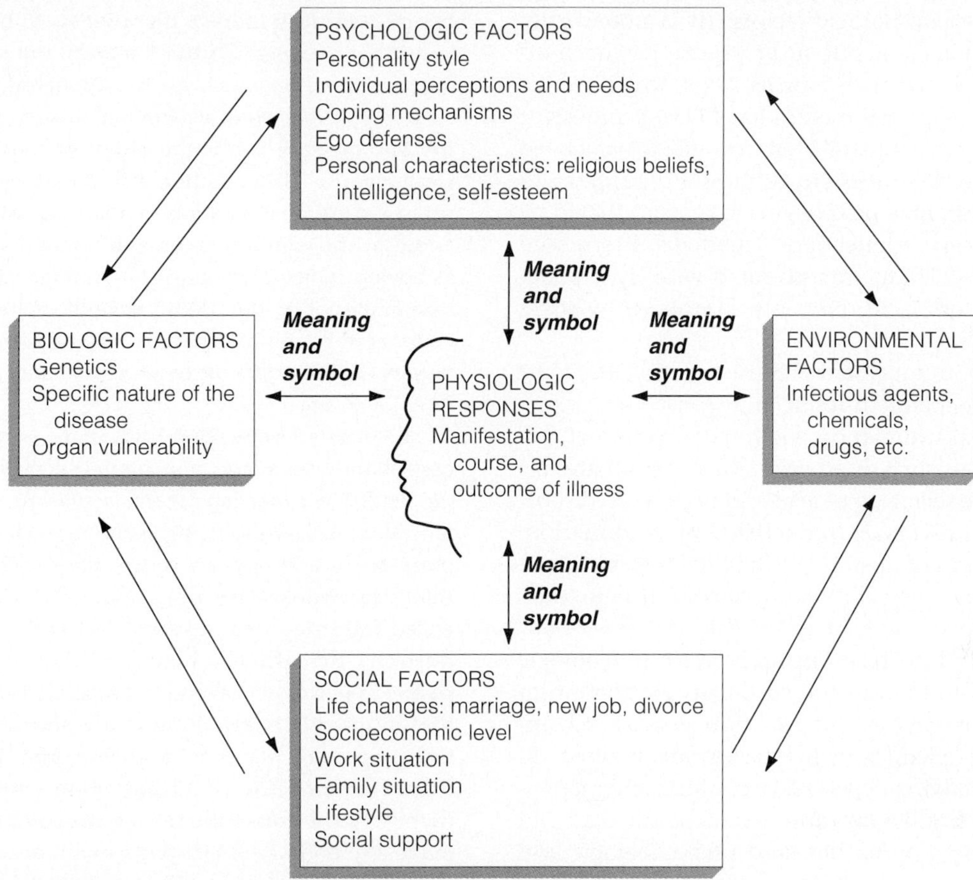

Figure 22–1 The multicausational concept of the illness process. The phrase "meaning and symbol" refers to the fact that clients interpret all experiences in a highly individual manner according to their specific meaning and the broader meaning in the client's culture.

should encompass the physiologic, psychologic, and sociologic components of Peter's asthma attacks. Peter's condition further illustrates the importance of examining cultural, environmental, developmental, genetic, constitutional, and historical factors in all disease processes.

Selected Conditions Affected by Psychologic Factors

The following sections review the characteristics of several conditions often considered to be affected by psychologic factors. For most of these conditions, an exact etiology is unknown. Current research focuses on the complicated interrelationships among such factors as stress, personality, environment, hormones, and genetic susceptibility.

Gastrointestinal Disorders

Gastrointestinal (GI) functional disorders may be defined as "variable combination(s) of chronic or recurrent gastrointestinal symptoms not explained by structural or biochemical abnormalities. They include symptoms attributed to the pharynx, esophagus, stomach, biliary tree, small or large intestine, or anorectum" (Drossman et al. 1993, p. 1970). GI symptoms are widespread throughout the population and vary according to such factors as gender and socioeconomic status. Women, for example, tend to more frequently report irritable bowel syndrome or functional constipation, while men more frequently report bloating symptoms (Drossman et al. 1993). Social, economic, and lifestyle factors all appear to affect susceptibility to GI disorders to varying degrees, although whether such increased susceptibility results from differences in social stress, dietary factors, or other socioeconomic factors is unclear. The medical literature is replete with studies demonstrating a relationship between psychologic factors and the GI system, particularly such conditions as irritable bowel syndrome, regional enteritis, ulcerative colitis, dyspepsia, and peptic ulcer (Folks and Kinney 1992b).

Peptic Ulcer Disease Peptic ulcer disease (PUD) has been one of the most thoroughly studied illnesses thought to be influenced by psychologic factors. (It is noteworthy that some individuals' peptic ulcer disease has been attributed to the bacterium *Heliobacter pylori,* which can be treated with antimicrobial medication.) PUD is prevalent among people with stressful lifestyles and is associated with "getting ahead" in Western cultures. PUD appears to run in families and may be brought on or exacerbated by diet, stress, and certain infections. Duodenal ulcers, seen more frequently in men, are associated with hypersecretion of hydrochloric acid, probably stimulated by stress and anxiety.

Alexander (1950) suggested that frustrated wishes to be loved and to be dependent result in unconscious conflict that leads to vagal stimulation and hypersecretion of gastric acid. Emotions such as anxiety and anger are also associated with the secretion of acid and pepsin, predisposing susceptible individuals to duodenal ulcer formation. Personality features of hostility, irritability, hypersensitivity, and impaired coping ability may also contribute to ulcer formation (Folks and Kinney 1992b).

While studies of the relationship between psychologic factors and ulcer formation and chronicity are somewhat controversial, psychologic intervention is often recommended for PUD clients. Such intervention is often directed toward resolving dependence conflicts and may include biofeedback and relaxation therapy, individual and group educational approaches, and pharmacologic and dietary management. The following clinical example illustrates the emotional and psychologic factors involved in ulcer formation and in illness progression:

Cynthia, a 42-year-old trial lawyer, married and the mother of two children, is referred for consultation by her gastroenterologist following her third hospitalization for duodenal ulcer disease. Her ulcer disease was first diagnosed 4 years ago, but an upper GI series at that time showed evidence of both an active ulcer and scarring secondary to previously healed ulcers. The gastroenterologist requested the consultation for help in considering the possibility of surgery, prompted by the seriousness of the bleeding episode that precipitated Cynthia's last admission and by the fact that she seems to "ignore pain." His referral note indicates that he sees no clear connection between the bleeding episodes and her highly stressful occupation.

Cynthia arrives exactly on time for her appointment; she is neatly and conservatively dressed. She presents an organized, coherent account of her medical problem and denies any past or immediate family history of significant mental disorder. Appearing genuinely worried by her recent hospitalization and frightened by the prospect of surgery, Cynthia is doubtful that speaking to a psychiatrist will produce any meaningful help. As she points out, "Ulcers are supposed to be related to stress, and that just isn't true with me." She then produces a detailed, written outline of her professional life over the past 5 years, accompanied by a chronology of her ulcer attacks. Indeed, there seems to be no temporal relationship between Cynthia's attacks and several highly taxing court cases in which she has appeared.

During the second evaluation session, Cynthia discusses her background. She is the oldest of four children and the clear favorite of her father, also an attorney. He communicated a strong expectation that she would become a lawyer and that she would succeed in his field. Cynthia sees herself as having fulfilled this expectation admirably and displays a rare smile while describing several of her more dramatic courtroom triumphs. There is no evidence that Cynthia experiences these difficult cases as stressful; in fact, she seems to enjoy them.

She married a law school classmate, who is also quite successful and who works noncompetitively in an unrelated legal field. Their marriage seems sound. As Cynthia begins to talk about her two sons, age 8 and 4, she becomes noticeably more tense and appears much more concerned and upset than usual while describing minor crises they have experienced with friends or in school. With great surprise, Cynthia discovers that the chronology of these crises corresponds clearly to five of her seven ulcer attacks, including all of those that resulted in hospitalization. Cynthia admits that despite being upset by her sons' problems, she finds it difficult to share her concerns about parenting with her husband or friends. At the end of the session she comments, "You'd have made a good lawyer. I'm glad I'm not arguing against you." Cynthia herself suggests that some further sessions may be in order.*

Gastric functioning becomes intimately tied to dependence needs through the feeding process from earliest infancy. The baby's mouth and digestive system are its early means of relating to the external world and its principal sources of gratification and frustration. Through complex learning processes, humans associate feeding and being taken care of and nurtured in a general sense. The mouth, through biting and chewing, also becomes the first mechanism through which the human infant can express anger and disappointment at being frustrated. It is well known that gastric secretion increases when infants and children are emotionally involved in either a positive or a negative sense.

INFLAMMATORY BOWEL DISORDERS Ulcerative colitis and Crohn's disease are chronic inflammatory disorders of unknown etiology. They are characterized by diarrhea, abdominal pain, anorexia, fever, weight loss, vomiting, urgency to defecate, and incontinence. In severe cases, an ileostomy or colostomy may be necessary.

The role of psychologic factors in inflammatory bowel disorders is unclear (Folks and Kinney 1992b). Autoim-

**Adapted from Spitzer et al. 1981, pp. 23–24.*

mune factors and infections, coupled with psychologic factors, may contribute to these disorders. Clients with ulcerative colitis tend to have a compulsive personality style with the following features: neatness, orderliness, punctuality, indecisiveness, emotional guardedness, humorlessness, conscientiousness, obstinacy, conformity, moral rigidity, and worry. Recent research, however, raises many questions about the validity of these personality features (Folks and Kinney 1992b). Contemporary researchers say that the psychologic traits these clients display are similar to those of clients with other chronic illnesses, with dependence being the most common trait. In many cases, onset and flare-ups seem linked to stressful life events, such as separations, failures, and disappointments.

Regardless of the source of the client's illness, treatment should focus on present troublesome areas, particularly concerns about the uncertain nature of the disease. Because of inherent differences between Crohn's disease and ulcerative colitis, the clinician must consider different approaches in planning treatment. The plan may include individual psychotherapy, family therapy, and environmental manipulation along with the medical regimen. These clients do best when they are involved in solid and long-term supportive relationships with their nurses and physicians who help them develop coping and self-care skills.

Cardiovascular Disorders

The cardiovascular system is a sensitive indicator of emotional arousal, whether it be fear, anger, or pleasurable excitement. High levels of stress are suspected to have harmful effects on the heart and vascular system, especially if stress is chronic or repeated. Experience, learning, and symbolic meaning, along with their emotional content, can influence heart rate, heart rhythm, and blood pressure. These cardiovascular changes can in turn create emotions, mostly unpleasant, that affect perception and ideation.

A number of indicators have been identified as high-risk factors for heart disease. They include genetic, physiologic, social, and psychologic influences:

- Family history of heart disease.
- A diet high in saturated fats and cholesterol.
- High level of blood cholesterol, triglycerides, sugar, uric acid.
- Hypertension, diabetes, hypothyroidism, renal disease, gout.
- Low level of physical activity.
- Heavy smoking and eating.
- High-pressured lifestyle (type A personality).
- Suppressed anger and hostility.

A variety of psychosocial factors are believed to contribute to coronary artery disease (CAD). Many of these have been studied extensively, including affective states, personality or coping style, psychologic reaction to environmental stimuli, sociocultural factors, and interpersonal factors (Goldstein & Niaura 1992). Psychologic factors that have been linked to CAD, sudden death, and ventricular arrhythmias include anxiety and depression, a behavior pattern involving feelings of hostility and anger, work overload, life stress, and a lack of social support.

The highly competitive, driving **type A personality** displays the classic constellation of personality characteristics associated with CAD, angina pectoris, and myocardial infarction. Adverse conditions in the client's environment, either social or economic, can also create the stress that leads to cardiac dysfunction.

Essential hypertension, cardiac dysrhythmias, and so-called cardiac neurosis are three syndromes of cardiovascular functioning with major psychologic inputs. The classical hypothesis in hypertension has been that people have conflict between their dependent and aggressive inclinations. This causes chronic repression of all displays of anger or resentment. The repressed emotions are eventually transformed into disorders of blood pressure regulation. Although this specific hypothesis has been difficult to prove, experiments have shown that fear, anger, frustration, and guilt all cause rises in diastolic blood pressure in vulnerable individuals. Likewise, anxiety, hostility, depression, interpersonal conflict, and disruptive life events have all been shown to potentially precipitate dysrhythmias, such as sinus tachycardia, paroxysmal atrial tachycardia, and both atrial and ventricular ectopic beats.

Cardiac neurosis is a syndrome consisting of cardiac distress, exercise intolerance, easy fatigability, respiratory discomfort, and dizziness. These features are similar to those found in panic disorder and mitral valve prolapse.

The treatment of cardiac disease must be multifaceted. In addition to medical or surgical treatment, other approaches involve stress management, relaxation training, biofeedback, weight control through diet and exercise, and behavioral interventions to help people give up smoking. More efforts are being geared toward prevention, including programs by industry and corporations to promote healthy lifestyles among employees.

Asthma

Asthma is among the most widely studied psychophysiologic illnesses of the respiratory system. Because breathing is essential to life, there has been much speculation about the emotional and symbolic significance that can become attached to the processes of air exchange. Asthma is characterized by labored breathing and wheezing resulting from spasm, secretions, and swelling in the bronchial tree.

There are allergic, immunologic, and emotional inputs to asthmatic attacks. The emotional components may lead directly to alterations in bronchus size. They may also affect the allergic and immunologic systems through hypothalamic nuclei in the central nervous system. According to Moran (1991), the "psychosomatic" basis of asthma is postulated as follows: "Childhood trauma leads to unconscious conflict, which leads to somatic manifestations of conflict (asthma). . . . Psychoanalysts came to see the wheeze as the suppressed cry of the child for its mother" (p. 15). More contemporary researchers examine the interplay of both psychologic and physiologic aspects of asthma, particularly the neurologic and humoral bases of asthma pathogenesis. However, certain personality types are linked by some researchers and clinicians to asthma susceptibility: those with extreme inhibition, covert aggression, marked dependence needs, a high need for affection, and those prone to depression, anxiety, and disturbances of self-esteem (Moran 1991).

Asthmatic people may be extremely frightened by asthmatic attacks, particularly in childhood. This fear may make them feel helpless and vulnerable. In response, they often adopt a clinging style of relating. The emotional and physical aspects of the illness seem to interrelate in a complex system of feedback loops. See the clinical profile of Peter G (p. 546) for an example.

Each person with asthma must be assessed individually to determine what factors are contributing to the disease process. A treatment plan may include, along with medication, family therapy, relaxation training, behavior modification, and hypnosis.

Arthritis

Rheumatoid arthritis (RA) has long been identified as an illness that is strongly influenced by emotional life. Its etiology remains uncertain (Moran 1991). RA is a progressive inflammatory disease, primarily of the joints, believed to be immunologically based. Family prevalence studies indicate a genetic predisposition to the disease. RA is three times more common in women than men.

Psychologic stresses are thought to precipitate attacks and flare-ups. The mechanism of transformation from idea or affect into tissue alteration appears to be via hormonal and autonomic nervous system pathways. Specifically, levels of growth hormone, sex hormones, thyroid hormone, and adrenal corticosteroids all change in stages of emotional arousal, and all are involved in the production of connective tissue, especially collagen. The hypothalamus and the limbic system also mediate.

Early psychologic studies of individuals with RA attempted to define the "rheumatic personality" (Moran 1991). These people were described as self-sacrificing, masochistic, inhibited, perfectionistic, and retiring. While a high percentage of people with RA are depressed, they do not differ from others with chronic illness in this respect; that is, chronic illness increases the risk of depression. Thus, in RA, depression may stem from actual and perceived functional and other losses (such as mobility). The diagnosis cannot be based on personality type, however, because there are many exceptions to the rule. Physical findings, deformities, subcutaneous nodules, and blood studies remain the criteria for identification.

A treatment plan for clients with arthritis may include pain control, surgery, drugs, vocational counseling, occupational therapy, and interventions to alleviate or prevent depression and to deal with depression and anger more directly.

Headache

The experience of headache resulting from emotional tension is common. Headaches account for many physician visits and for job absenteeism. Headaches are also highly associated with depressive and anxiety disorders. Headaches may be divided into the five following types:

1. Vascular headache of migraine type.
2. Muscle contraction headache (tension headache).
3. Combined vascular–muscle contraction headache.
4. Delusional, depressive, conversion, or hypochondriacal headache.
5. Structural or disease-related headache.

The mechanism of vascular headache seems to involve the release of various vasoactive substances in the brain, such as serotonin, catecholamines, histamine, bradykinin, and prostaglandins. This release frequently occurs with stress. In genetically susceptible individuals, the substances cause vasodilation and inflammation of the arterial walls. There are generally early warning symptoms of migraine attacks. These range from mood changes and GI upset to gross neurologic findings in the visual and contralateral sensorimotor systems. A number of upsets in physiologic functioning can actually be migraine equivalents. These include nausea and vomiting, diarrhea, tachycardia, cyclical edema, vertigo, periodic fever, pain, depression, confusion, and insomnia.

A tension headache results from muscular contraction in the neck, shoulders, face, or scalp. These are steady, persistent headaches with no warning signs that commonly feel like a "band wrapped around the head." Some theorists support the notion that headache sufferers are likely to maintain rigid control over emotions, feel hostility toward others, use introjection as a defense, and be perfectionists.

Structural or disease-related headache arises from systemic infections, primary or metastatic tumors, hematomas, abscesses, cranial infections, cranial nerve inflammations, and eye, ear, nose, sinus, or tooth diseases. Interventions are based on the diagnosis and the contributing factors that have been identified. Possible treatments and approaches include measures that increase circulation, such as massage or heat application; use of medications; alterations in diet, rest, and exercise patterns; psychotherapy; and biofeedback, meditation, hypnosis, relaxation, and other stress-management approaches (Kaplan and Sadock 1994).

Endocrine Disorders

A large number of disorders of endocrine functioning are associated with psychologic factors (Beardsley and Goldstein 1993). The endocrine system has particular significance for psychiatry, because there is a close relationship between the emotions and a variety of active chemical substances released in tissues by nerve impulses (Hellhammer and Wade 1993). In physical medicine, the feedback loop has long been accepted as the model for the functioning of the endocrine organs.

Extensive research on the endocrine feedback system has led to a sophisticated model that includes several kinds of feedback loops. The levels of circulating hormones released by endocrine glands, such as the thyroid and gonads (the sex glands), are controlled by long feedback loops that send information to the cerebral cortex and limbic system. Short feedback loops of pituitary hormones affect the hypothalamus. Very short loops of releasing hormones from the hypothalamus determine their own production and control. Studies on the relationship between emotions and endocrine function have shown that:

- Various neurotransmitters affect hormone-releasing factors.
- Psychoactive drugs whose action is mediated by neurotransmitters also affect the release of releasing factors.
- Stress stimulates the autonomic nervous system, which can stimulate the adrenal medulla to produce epinephrine or the pancreas to secrete insulin.
- Corticosteroid production of the adrenal cortex increases greatly during some psychotic episodes of schizophrenic clients.
- Steroid levels also increase in agitated or anxious depressive people.

It seems fair to conclude that the emotional centers of the brain—the cerebral cortex and limbic system—are intimately tied to the endocrine organs, through the axis of the hypothalamus and the anterior pituitary. Their secretions act as communication messengers. It is not surprising, then, to find expressions of emotional arousal through endocrine changes and major effects on emotional states from endocrine diseases. These are both, in fact, common. Endocrine disorders and their physical and mental symptoms are listed in the Assessment box on the following page.

Adrenal dysfunction characteristically produces prominent mental as well as distinctive physical symptoms. Thyroid disorders are commonly accompanied by cognitive or emotional changes. Stress has been implicated, though inconclusively, in the precipitation of thyrotoxic crises. Stress may influence the course of diabetes, either directly by promoting a flare-up or indirectly by causing the client to neglect a usually rigid medical regimen (Beardsley and Goldstein 1993). So many mental symptoms are associated with hypoglycemia that many clients are classified and treated as "classic neurotics."

It is evident that numerous problems can be caused by endocrine dysfunction. The treatment approach must be individualized to meet the client's physical and psychologic needs.

An important role for the nurse is primary prevention. Adequately preparing a person for developmental changes by offering accurate information about likely physical and emotional alterations can help prevent severe psychiatric disturbances during these periods. Reliable support and open channels of communication are necessary. New coping strategies can be successful if their design, timing, and presentation are appropriate.

Skin Disorders

Allergic illnesses, particularly those involving the skin, have been shown to have psychologic elements in etiology or course (Folks and Kinney 1992a). The skin, with its critical sensory functions, mediates between the outside world and internal states. Itching (pruritus), excessive sweating (hidrosis), urticaria, and atopic dermatitis are all commonly classified as psychophysiologic conditions.

A variety of stressful or emotional states are associated with flare-ups of allergic skin disorders. Attempts have been made to correlate the following specific emotional states or stresses with individual disorders:

- Generalized pruritus: aggression.
- Genital and anal pruritus: sexuality (heterosexual and homosexual).
- Hyperhidrosis: anxiety.
- Urticaria: anger.
- Atopic dermatitis: longing for love.

In truth, these feelings and conflicts are seen in normal, disordered, and other psychophysiologic states. Nurses should therefore be cautious about accepting pathogenic mechanisms and explanations.

ASSESSMENT

Common Features of Endocrine Disorders

Disease	Physical Symptoms	Mental Symptoms
Cushing's syndrome (adrenal cortex hyperfunction)	Truncal obesity, moon facies, abdominal striae, hirsutism, amenorrhea, hypertension, osteoporosis, weakness.	Impotence, decreased libido, anxiety, increased emotional lability, apathy, insomnia, memory deficits, confusion, disorientation.
Addison's disease (adrenal insufficiency)	Weakness, fatigue, anorexia, weight loss, nausea and vomiting, pigmentation of skin, hypotension.	Depression, irritability, psychomotor retardation, apathy, memory defect, hallucinations.
Hyperthyroidism	Staring, exophthalmos, goiter, moist warm skin, weight loss, increased appetite, weakness, tremor, tachycardia, heat intolerance.	Anxiety, tension, irritability, hyperexcitability, emotional lability, depression, psychosis, or delirium.
Hypothyroidism	Dull expression, puffy eyelids, swollen tongue, hoarse voice, rough dry skin, cold intolerance.	Psychomotor retardation, decreased initiative, slow comprehension, drowsiness, decreased recent memory, delirium, stupor, depression or psychosis.
Diabetes mellitus	Polydipsia, polyuria, polyphagia, weight loss, blurred vision, fatigue, impotence, fainting, paresthesia.	Stupor, coma, fatigue, impotence.
Hypoglycemia	Tremor, light-headedness, sweating, hunger, nausea, pallor, tachycardia, hypertension.	Anxiety, fugue, unusual behavior, confusion, apathy, psychomotor agitation or retardation, depression, delusions, hallucinations, convulsions, coma.
Premenstrual syndrome	Headache, breast engorgement, lower abdominal bloating, GI complaints, increased sweating, craving for sweets, other appetite changes.	Irritability, depression, anxiety, emotional lability, fatigue, crying spells.

The location of the lesions has, historically, had symbolic significance. Thus, conflict over an extramarital affair has been associated with dermatitis in the wedding ring area. Head and face locations have been classically associated with conflict over affective display. Affliction of the hands is associated with practical or professional conflicts. A genital distribution may be associated with sexual concerns.

Chronic Fatigue Syndrome

Fatigue—an ancient complaint—is a common presenting symptom seen by clinicians, estimated to lead to 10 million visits to primary care physicians each year in the United States (Manu, Lane, and Matthews 1992). During the past decade, much interest has focused on chronic fatigue syndrome (CFS). Because the symptom of fatigue is not easily measured or categorized, studies of fatigue have suffered. While so-called epidemics of fatigue have been reported (Dawson and Sabin 1993), the search for an infectious cause of chronic fatigue has not been successful. For research purposes, CFS has been defined as lasting at least 6 months and not attributable to a known cause, including a psychiatric condition. In addition, those with CFS must have other symptoms or physical criteria. People with CFS often have signs and symptoms that are suggestive of a mild infection (elevated temperature, sore throat, muscle and joint pain, headaches, neuropsychologic symptoms, sleep disturbance, and lymph node pain).

While controversy continues about the existence of CFS, and its possible causes, one major clinical study involving 327 clients with CFS found that 81% of these had a standard medical or psychiatric disorder (76% had a psychiatric disorder) (Manu, Lane, and Matthews 1992). The most common cause of chronic fatigue in this study was major depression (56.5%—five times greater than in the general population), followed by panic disorder (13.5%), and somatization disorder (11.9%). The researchers reported that a high percentage of clients in the study thought they had CFS. Although many reported that their depression resulted from chronic fatigue, the researchers' findings did not support this contention. The prevalence of depression in CFS clients is also supported by other studies.

Treatment of CFS is usually comprehensive and aimed at reducing symptoms and helping the client gain control. Thus psychiatric, pharmacologic, social, occupational, and spiritual dimensions of care are considered and tailored to individual client needs. It is important to acknowledge the client's beliefs about the cause(s) of fatigue while at the same time suggesting that several approaches may be needed to reduce or alleviate the fatigue. Group and individual psychotherapy, in combination with antidepressants, are common treatments. Cognitive-behavioral therapy has also shown promise. Those with somatization disorder are the most challenging to treat because their symptoms have been of long duration. The following clinical example illustrates the presentation and treatment of a client with chronic fatigue:

Louise M, 43, was referred to the community mental health center by her physician, who had been treating her for more than 2 years for symptoms of fatigue. She had had a variety of tests over that period of time and had taken several antibiotics. Louise had been hospitalized twice for severe fatigue. Her fatigue was now so draining that she needed a nap in the late morning and frequently in the afternoon in order to complete minor household chores. She had been unable to work as a teacher for more than 2 years since her fatigue had worsened. Louise and her husband had withdrawn from most social activities because of her fatigue. She had not been sexually active for more than a year. Physical symptoms included occasional low-grade fever, intermittent diarrhea, headache, and loss of appetite. Louise had never entertained the possibility that her fatigue might stem from a psychiatric condition and had been insulted when her physician suggested that she visit the mental health center for an evaluation.

Following an evaluation of Louise's mental health status, the nurse therapist began weekly psychotherapy sessions that helped her gain insight into the possible causes of her condition. Louise also entered into a contract with the therapist to take only one nap daily, and eventually her naps were discontinued altogether. After one month of therapy, the nurse therapist prescribed a tricyclic agent that helped Louise gain enough energy to engage in former social activities. After 1 year of therapy and continued medication, Louise was able to return to a part-time teaching position.

Resistance to Psychosocial Intervention

Behavioral therapy, cognitive therapy, biofeedback, hypnotherapy, and psychotherapy have all been used successfully with appropriate clients (Cottraux 1993; Sharpe, Peveler, and Mayou 1992). However, despite the wealth of psychosocial interventions available to people with psychophysiologic disorders, many are resistant to approaches that are not strictly medical. Some reasons for this are the following:

- These clients are believed to lack insight because they express conflict through somatic complaints rather than verbalization.
- Conflicts over unresolved dependence and aggressive wishes may make it difficult to relate to these clients interpersonally.
- These clients focus steadfastly on their somatic complaints, apparently indicating that alternative defense mechanisms are unavailable or inadequate.
- They are rarely highly motivated to heighten their self-awareness, which is the goal of many forms of psychotherapy.
- Even when they are somewhat motivated, they may be unable or unwilling to delay gratification and thus are impatient with the slow process of growth usually required in psychotherapeutic work.

For these reasons, traditional psychotherapy is not the most useful intervention. Approaches that enhance medical and surgical intervention and allow the client's primary bond to remain with nonpsychiatric health care providers are more successful. Programs geared toward stress management (such as those discussed in Chapter 29) are very useful because they present stress as part of the human condition and the participants do not feel labeled as having psychiatric problems. Behavioral and cognitive approaches have also gained favor because they may alleviate symptoms over a short period of time and thus prove effective in terms of outcome and cost.

Chapter Highlights

- The multicausational concept of illness acknowledges the biologic, psychologic, social, and environmental components of the illness/disease process.

- Psychologic factors should always be considered among those factors that lead up to, worsen, or perpetuate any physical illness.
- Ignoring the psychologic components of illness can undermine appropriate treatment.
- Psychophysiologic disorders are those that have an important emotional component in their onset and future course.
- The psychophysiologic disorders in particular illustrate the complicated interactions of mind, body, and environment because they present physical symptoms with a strong psychologic component.
- Syndromes in which physical and psychologic factors interact by means of feedback loops include peptic ulcer; asthma; arthritis; headache; and certain bowel, cardiovascular, endocrine, and skin disorders.
- Promoting a healthy lifestyle and advocating lifestyle modifications are important nursing responsibilities.
- Regardless of the clinical area in which they practice, nurses must have a knowledge of stress management approaches to offer clients a useful plan of care.
- Many clients resist the idea that emotions may play a part in their disorders. Therefore, the plan of care should be thoughtfully managed by a health care professional whom the client trusts.

References

Ader R, Felton D, Cohen N (eds): *Psychoneuroimmunology II.* Academic Press, 1991.

Alexander F: *Psychosomatic Medicine: Its Principles and Application.* Norton, 1950.

American Psychiatric Association: *Diagnostic and Statistical Manual of Mental Disorders,* ed 4. American Psychiatric Association, 1994.

Beardsley G, Goldstein M: Endocrine disease literature review. *Psychosomatics* 1993; 34(1):12–19.

Cottraux J: Behavioral psychotherapy applications in the medically ill. *Psychother Psychosom* 1993;60:116–128.

Dawson D, Sabin T: *Chronic Fatigue Syndrome.* Little, Brown, 1993.

Drossman D, Zhiming L, Andruzzi E, Temple R, Talley N, Thompson G, Whitehead W, Janssens J, Funch-Jensen P, Corazziari E, Richter J, Koch G: U.S. householder survey of functional gastrointestinal disorders. *Digestive Diseases and Sciences* 1993;38(9):1569–1580.

Eysenck H: Personality, stress, and disease. *Psychological Inquiry* 1991;2:221–232.

Fava G: The concept of psychosomatic disorder. *Psychother Psychosom* 1992;58:1–12

Folks D, Kinney F: The role of psychological factors in dermatologic conditions. *Psychosomatics* 1992a;33(1):47–60.

Folks D, Kinney F: The role of psychological factors in gastrointestinal conditions. *Psychosomatics* 1992b;33(3): 257–270.

Friedman H (ed): *Hostility, Coping, and Health.* American Psychological Association, 1992.

Friedman H, VandenBos G: Disease-prone and self-healing personalities. *Hosp Commun Psychiatr* 1992;43(12):1177–1179.

Goldstein M, Niaura R: Cardiovascular disease literature review, Part I. *Psychosomatics* 1992;33(2):134–145.

Hellhammer D, Wade S: Endocrine correlates of stress vulnerability. *Psychother Psychosom* 1993;60:8–17.

Holmes TH, Rahe RH: The social readjustment rating scale. *J Psychosom Res* 1967;11:213–218.

Kaplan H, Sadock B: *Synopsis of Psychiatry,* ed 7. Williams & Wilkins, 1994.

Lacey JI, Bateman DE, Van Lehn R: Autonomic response specificity. *Psychosom Med* 1953;15:8.

Mahl GF: Physiological changes during chronic fear. *Ann N Y Acad Sci* 1953;56:240.

Malarkey W, Kiebolt-Glaser PD, Glaser R: Hostile behavior during marital conflict alters pituitary and adrenal hormones. *Psychosom Med* 1994;56(1)41–51.

Manu P, Lane T, Matthews D: Chronic fatigue syndromes in clinical practice. *Psychother Psychosom* 1992;58:60–68.

Moran M: Psychological factors affecting pulmonary and rheumatologic diseases: A review. *Psychosomatics* 1991; 31(1):14–23.

Mutter AZ, Schleifer M: The role of psychological and social factors in the onset of somatic illness in children. *Psychosom Med* 1966;28:333–343.

Rahe R, Arthur R: Life change and illness studies: Past history and future directions. *J Hum Stress* 1978;4:3–15.

Rogers M, White K, Warshaw M, Yonkers K, Rodriguez-Villa F, Chang G, Keller M: Prevalence of medical disorders in patients with anxiety disorders. *Int J Psychiatr Med* 1994; 24(1):83–96.

Sachar EJ: Current status of psychosomatic medicine, in Strain J, Grossman S (eds): *Psychologic Care of the Medically Ill,* Appleton-Century-Crofts, 1975.

Schmoll H, Tewes U, Plotnikoff N (eds): *Psychoneuroimmunology.* Hogrefe & Huber, 1992.

Selye H: *The Physiology and Pathology of Exposure to Stress.* Acta, 1950.

Selye H: *The Stress of Life,* McGraw-Hill, 1976.

Sensky T: Somatization: Syndromes or processes. *Psychother Psychosom* 1994;6(1):1–3.

Sharpe M, Peveler R, Mayou R: The psychological treatment of patients with functional somatic symptoms: A practical guide. *J Psychosom Res* 1992;36(6):515–529.

Spitzer RL, et al.: *DSM-III Casebook.* American Psychiatric Association, 1981.

Stoudemire A: Psychological factors affecting physical condition and the DSM-IV. *Psychosomatics* 1993;34(1):8–11.

Stoudemire A, Hales R: Psychological and behavioral factors affecting medical conditions and DSM-IV: An overview. *Psychosomatics* 1991;32(1):5–13.

CHAPTER 23

RAPE AND INTRAFAMILY ABUSE

Karen Lee Fontaine

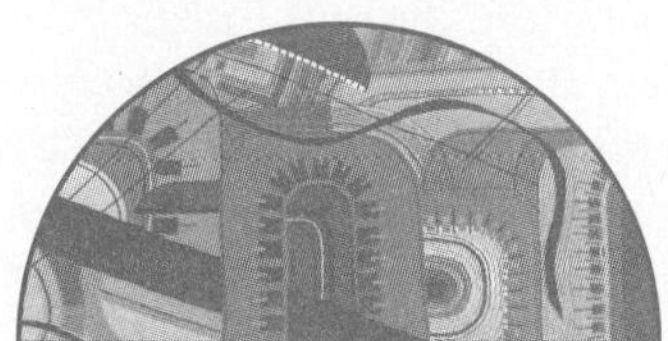

COMPETENCIES

- *Describe the biopsychosocial causes of rape and intrafamily violence.*
- *Identify principles common to most treatment plans for victims of violence.*
- *Assess your personal values regarding perpetrators of physical and sexual abuse.*
- *Demonstrate sensitivity to the long-term effects on victims of rape and intrafamily violence.*

Cross-References

Other topics relevant to this content are: Family dynamics and family therapy, Chapter 32; Recovered memory (see the Mind-Body-Spirit box), Chapter 4; Stress management techniques, Chapter 29.

Critical Thinking Challenge

Much of the current sociocultural climate encourages beliefs and practices about abuse that can subtly or overtly support abuse. Do you believe that men would not be abusive if women did not make them angry? Do you believe that a wife should be below her husband in status as evidenced by giving up her birth name and adopting his last name, by never making more money than he does, and by making sure his needs are met such as meals and laundry? Do you believe that a man has a right to hit a woman if she nags or yells at him incessantly? Do you believe that violence against children, women, and the elderly flourishes due to tolerance for violence within American institutions such as the courts and police? What do you think about the studies that show that the men who rape or commit incest are within the range of what is considered "normal" for men in our society?

Violence that is demonstrated as rape or that occurs as physical or sexual abuse within the family is a national health problem that confronts not only psychiatric nurses but also nurses in many different clinical settings. Victims are seen in the community, in pediatric units, in intensive care units, in medical-surgical units, in maternal care settings, in ambulatory care facilities, in geriatric units, and in psychiatric settings.

Nurses must assess and provide appropriate intervention for the emotional consequences, as well as the

Portions of this chapter appeared in another form in Fontaine KL, Fletcher JS: Essentials of Mental Health Nursing, *ed 3. Addison-Wesley, 1995.*

physical trauma, of rape. Nurses may be called on to give legal evidence in the prosecution of a rapist. Within the community, nurses can establish, or refer victims to, support groups. They can also become active in increasing public awareness of rape through formal and informal teaching activities. Because of their unique position, nurses can be active in the prevention of rape and the treatment of rape survivors.

Nurses also need to be involved in the prevention, detection, and treatment of intrafamily violence. Developing a knowledge base and being able to identify factors that contribute to domestic violence help nurses assume a preventive role. Part of this role is providing public education and becoming active in changes in public policy. This knowledge, along with increased awareness of the extent of the problem, helps nurses arrive at earlier, more accurate detection of intrafamily violence. Nurses must comply with state laws on the reporting of violence and referral for treatment. Some nurses with advanced education in family therapy are part of the therapy teams that intervene with violent families.

Rape

Rape is a crime of violence. It is second only to homicide in its violation of a person. The motivation is not one of sex but one of force, domination, and humiliation. If you think rape is about sex, you have confused the weapon with the motivation. **Rape** refers to any forced sexual activity; the key factor is the absence of consent.

There is no typical rape victim. Of reported rapes, however, 93% of the victims are female and 90% of the perpetrators are male. One can be a victim of rape at any age, from childhood through old age. Police records indicate that a women is raped every 6 minutes in the United States. And experts believe that 70% of rapes are unreported. It is believed that 1 out of every 3 women will be raped or sexually assaulted at least once in her lifetime; 40–60% of victims are raped by a spouse, partner, relative, or friend (Vachss 1993).

Of all women raped on college campuses, 50% are date rapes. In surveys of college men, 10–15% admitted that they had committed date rape on at least one occasion, and another 22% admitted they had used verbal coercion and deception to pressure a date into having sex. Women very rarely report rapes when they know their attackers, especially if they were in a dating relationship. The victim is often blamed, by herself and others, for being naive or provocative. A cultural value, slow to die, is: If a woman accepts a date and allows the man to pay all the expenses, she somehow "owes" him sexual access and has no right to refuse. One researcher found that 25% of acquaintance rapists called their victims to ask them for a date after the initial rape (Stacy, Prisbell, and Tollefsrud 1992).

Traditionally, husbands have not been charged when they raped their wives. It was not until 1974 in the United States and 1991 in Great Britain that the first cases of marital rape were prosecuted. Marital rape is often accompanied by extreme violence and is the most underreported type of rape.

The myth of male rape has been that it occurs only where heterosexual contact is not possible, such as in prisons or in isolated living conditions. As more male rape victims report the crime, however, this myth is being exploded. Male rape is not a homosexual attack. Just as in female rape, the issue is one of violence and domination rather than one of sex.

Rape Trauma Syndrome

Rape is a violent act against an innocent person. It changes lives forever because once people become victims, they never again feel completely safe. The victim's response to this act of violence is referred to as **rape trauma syndrome.** Members of each gender's response to and recovery from rape is influenced by cultural and gender values and beliefs. Some rape survivors do not develop major symptoms in response to the trauma, while as many as 25% continue to have signs of impairment a year after the assault. A variety of factors contribute to the response, including age or developmental state, a history of prior victimization, the relationship to the offender, precrisis coping abilities, and the ability to use support resources. Response factors related to the rape itself include the severity of the rape, the duration, the frequency, the number of offenders, and the degree of violence. Environmental factors contributing to a rape victim's response are the quality and continuity of social supports and community attitudes and values (Koss and Harvey 1991; Mezey and King 1992).

During the actual rape, some victims use the defense mechanism of depersonalization or dissociation to cope with the attack. By perceiving the attack as "not really happening to me," a victim protects her sense of integrity. Other victims rely on denial to block out the traumatic experience.

Some rape victims respond immediately with agitated and nonpurposeful behavior. They appear in the emergency department emotionally distraught and unable to respond to questions about what has occurred. Their level of anxiety may be so high that they may not be able to follow simple directions. After a period of shock and disbelief, many experience episodes of fear.

Doreen, a graduate student at the local university, was brought to the hospital by the police who found her running down the street half-clothed. In the hospital she was able to tell the staff that she had been raped by her date, Mike, another graduate student. She exhibited outward calmness but

kept repeating "This cannot have happened to me. My friends introduced us and he seemed so nice." She was unable to decide who to call to take her back to the dorm or what to tell her friends about what happened.

Fears may arise in response to any stimulus that brings back the rape memories. There are also fears of rape consequences such as pregnancy; sexually transmitted infections, especially HIV; talking to the police; and testifying in court. In addition, there are fears related to potential future attack, which underlie fears of getting close to men, of being alone, and of being in a strange place.

Rape often results in a number of physical injuries. The victim may be beaten, stabbed, or shot. Profuse bleeding and trauma to vital organs may be critical problems. Most likely, the vagina or rectum will be sore or swollen. There may be tearing of the vaginal or rectal wall from forceful insertion of the penis or a foreign object. The throat may be traumatized from forced oral sex.

Rape trauma syndrome may have long-term consequences. Depression frequently develops within a few weeks of the assault. This posttrauma depression usually lasts about 3 months, and it is not unusual for the survivor to experience suicidal ideation. For some, the depression will develop into a major depressive disorder requiring medical intervention (Koss and Harvey 1991). Some survivors develop obsessional thoughts about the rape, which may be severe enough to interfere with daily functioning. Some experience flashbacks, some have violent dreams, and others may be preoccupied with thoughts of future danger.

Rape profoundly affects a person's beliefs about the environment. If the assault occurred in the home, the normal feeling of safety within the home will most likely be destroyed. A woman who is a survivor of marital rape suffers additional problems. Often, she must continue to interact with her rapist because she is dependent on him. She may be forced to pretend, to herself and to family members and friends, that the rape never occurred. Until it becomes more socially acceptable and legally feasible to report marital rape, many of these survivors will suffer in silence.

Sexual dysfunction is one of the longest-lasting effects of rape. Nearly all adult rape survivors feel the need to withdraw from sexual activity for a period of time. For some, a period of celibacy is necessary to reestablish control and autonomy. Others may choose abstinence because they feel unclean or contaminated. Both the survivor and the sex partner must understand that the need for closeness and nondemanding physical contact continues. Expressing caring and affection through nonsexual touching minimizes the partner's feelings of rejection and reduces the rape survivor's feelings of self-blame and uncleanliness. The accompanying box describes the phases of response to rape.

Phases of Response to Rape

Anticipatory Phase

Begins when the victim realizes the situation is potentially dangerous.

The victim may think about how to get away, may reason or argue with the offender, and recall advice people have given about rape.

Use of dissociation, suppression, or rationalization to preserve the illusion of invulnerability.

Possible physical action.

Impact Phase

The period of actual assault and immediate aftermath.

Intense fear of death or serious injury.

Expressive styles:

- Open expression of feelings—crying, sobbing, pacing.
- Controlled style—numbness, shock, disbelief.
- Compound reaction—reactivated symptoms of previous conditions, such as psychotic behavior, depression, suicidal behavior, substance abuse.

Somatic reactions—tension headache, fatigue, increased startle reaction, nausea, gagging.

Reconstitution Phase

Outward appearance of adjustment with an attempt to restore equilibrium.

Life activities are renewed, but superficially and mechanically.

Periods of anxiety, fear, nightmares, depression, guilt, shame, vulnerability, helplessness, isolation, sexual dysfunctions.

Resolution Phase

Anger at the assailant, at society, and at the judicial system.

The need to talk to resolve feelings.

The survivor seeks family and professional support.

Biopsychosocial Theories

Theorists in many disciplines have studied the crime of rape in an effort to understand the causes and develop preventive measures. Most agree that rape is a crime of violence generated by issues of power and anger rather than by sex drive.

Intrapersonal Theory

The intrapersonal perspective views rapists as emotionally immature individuals who feel powerless and unsure of themselves. They are incapable of managing the normal stresses of everyday life. The causes of rape are many, but the dynamics of the act are that perpetrators abuse their own and others' sexuality as a method of discharging anger and frustration. From this perspective, there are five types of rape: anger rape, power rape, sadistic rape, gang rape, and date or acquaintance rape.

An **anger rape** is distinguished by physical violence and cruelty to the victim. Believing that he is the victim of an unjust society, the rapist takes revenge on others by raping. He uses extreme force and viciousness to demean and humiliate the victim. The ability to injure, traumatize, and shame the victim provides an outlet for his rage and temporary relief from his turmoil.

In a **power rape**, the intent of the rapist is not to injure someone but to command and master another person sexually. The rapist has an insecure self-image, with feelings of incompetence and inadequacy. The rape becomes the vehicle for expressing power and strength. Seeing his victim as a conquest, the rapist temporarily has the feeling of omnipotence.

A **sadistic rape** involves brutality, bondage, and torture as stimulants for the rapist's own sexual excitement. For the rapist, the assault is an erotic experience. He plans very carefully, and the process of rape may be ritualized. Victims are often murdered after being raped.

A **gang rape** involves a number of perpetrators and may be part of a group ritual that confirms masculinity, power, and authority. The perpetrators may range in age from 10 to 30, but they are most typically adolescents. Victims are usually the same age as the gang members (Holmes 1991).

A **date rape**, or **acquaintance rape**, is forced sexual activity by a perpetrator who is known to the victim. Typically, there is less physical violence and more coercion and deception involved. Even during the high school years, it is estimated that 30% of female students are sexually or physically abused in their dating relationships (Ellis 1994).

Not all rapists are alike. Their motives and expectations vary. Most convicted sex offenders do not suffer from major mental disorders. Many meet the criteria for sociopathic, schizoid, paranoid, and narcissistic personality disorders. Rapists are typically young; 80% are under the age of 30, and 75% are under age 25. The majority report having been sexually and physically abused as children or adolescents (Holmes 1991).

Interpersonal Theory

Most rapists do not have normal interpersonal involvements. Preoccupied with their own fantasies, they want to control and dominate others rather than engage in mutually satisfying relationships. With this model in mind, a rapist sees no need for consent to sexual activity, particularly from his wife. The husband may view the rape as merely a disagreement over sexual behavior. If the wife has said she does not want to engage in sex and the husband uses force, her control and autonomy have been violated. When sex occurs without consent, it is, in fact, rape (Holmes 1991).

Social Learning Theory

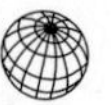

The acceptance of interpersonal violence in a culture contributes to a higher incidence of rape. Society's approval of the use of intimidation, coercion, and force to achieve a goal promotes an excessive level of violence. Violent behavior is an expression of power and strength, and individual rights are disregarded.

Aggression is learned through three primary sources: family and peers, culture/subculture, and the mass media. The modeling effect occurs when potential offenders see rape scenes and other acts of violence against women in real life or in the media, in slasher and horror films and in violent pornography. The media contribute to the process of desensitization; with repeated exposure, viewers become numb to the pain, fear, and humiliation of sexual aggression (Ellis 1989).

Feminist Theory

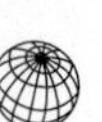

From the feminist perspective, rape is the result of long and deeply rooted socioeconomic traditions. Men dominate most political and economic activities, and women are viewed as subservient and relatively powerless. At the farthest extreme, women are viewed as property. Sexual gratification is not the prime motive in rape; rather, it is used to establish or maintain control of one person by another. When women are considered inferior to men, tacit approval is given for coercion and force. These stereotypes support the false beliefs that at times women deserve to be raped, that they may want or need to be raped, and that rape does not cause them much physical or emotional damage.

Sexist values affect people of all ages, both female and male. When 1700 middle school children were asked questions about rape, 65% of the boys and 57% of the girls replied that it was acceptable for a man to force a woman to have sex if they have been dating more than 6 months. College students responded in the following ways to the question of when forced sex is acceptable: It is acceptable if the woman agrees and then changes her mind, 13%; while dating exclusively, 24%; if the woman allows him to touch her genitals, 24%; if she touches his genitals, 29%; and if both partners willingly have their clothes off, 35% (Koss and Harvey 1991).

The Nursing Process and Victims of Rape

Before the assessment process, clients must be informed of their rights, which include the following:

- A rape crisis advocate present in the emergency department.
- Their personal physician notified.
- Privacy during the assessment and treatment process.
- Family, friends, or an advocate present during the questioning and examination.
- Confidentiality maintained by all members of the staff.
- Gentle and sensitive treatment.
- Detailed explanations of, and giving consent for, all tests and procedures, including photographs.
- Referrals for follow-up treatment and counseling.

As a nurse, you must respect the victim's autonomy and give the victim as much control as possible through every step of the assessment and treatment process. If this is not done, clients are susceptible to revictimization by members of the health care team.

Assessment

Rape victims must be assessed physiologically from head to toe for any serious or critical injuries that may have resulted from the assault. With the victim's permission, a vaginal or rectal examination is performed to determine necessary treatment and to provide evidence for legal action. With permission, photographs of the injuries may be taken for legal documentation. The physiologic assessment process must be carefully documented in writing to assist with possible prosecution of the perpetrator. Guidelines for physical assessment are given in the Assessment box on page 560.

Victims who respond to rape in a controlled manner may be able to answer assessment questions, but those in a state of emotional shock and disbelief may find it difficult to engage actively in the assessment process. The method by which you complete the assessment depends on the person's response to the trauma. Documentation of assessment should be in subjective terms and objective quotes. Clear and concise depicting of the client is necessary for possible court proceedings. Guidelines for assessing the victim's mental status are given in the Assessment box on page 561.

Nursing Diagnosis

Physical and mental status priorities must be quickly established by the health care team. Attention must then be given to long-range physical, emotional, social, and legal concerns of the survivor.

The nursing diagnosis for clients who have been raped is Rape Trauma Syndrome. If clients suffer from reactivated symptoms of a previous physical illness or mental disorder, or if they rely on alcohol or drugs to manage their trauma, they are given the more specific nursing diagnosis of Rape Trauma Syndrome: Compound Reaction. The nursing diagnosis of Rape Trauma Syndrome: Silent Reaction is applied when the client experiences high levels of anxiety, an inability to discuss the trauma, abrupt changes in relationships with men and/or changes in sexual behavior, and the onset of phobic reactions.

There is no corresponding DSM-IV diagnosis. Rape is, however, mentioned specifically as the type of trauma that may result in posttraumatic stress disorder. Rape victims may also experience one of the anxiety disorders, mood disorders, or sexual dysfunctions discussed in the *DSM-IV.*

Planning and Implementing Interventions

It is important to *support defense mechanisms* until clients are able to cope with the reality of the assault. Give them ample time to respond to simple questions; anxiety will decrease their ability to perceive input, thereby slowing down their response time. If clients are unable to express feelings, acknowledge the difficulty by saying, "I understand that it's difficult for you to describe your feelings right now. That's okay. You may be able to talk about them later." Communicate your knowledge and understanding of the usual emotional responses to rape. Statements such as "People usually experience a number of feelings, like anxiety, fear, embarrassment, guilt, and anger" will reassure clients that their feelings are a normal reaction to rape. Use the Nursing Self-Awareness box on page 562 to help you in understanding your own feelings and attitudes.

Encourage the client to *talk about the rape.* Many clients will have a compulsive need to recount the assault. The emotional arousal of the trauma contributes to this intense pressure to talk. Listen patiently and supportively, understanding that compulsive retelling is a natural way by which the victim is gradually desensitized to the trauma.

ASSESSMENT

Physical Assessment of the Rape Victim

Complete a head-to-toe physical assessment with particular attention to the following:

Head

Evidence of trauma

Facial bruises

Facial fractures

Eyes: swollen, bruised, hemorrhages

Skin

Bruises

Genital trauma

Rectal trauma

Musculoskeletal

Fractures of the ribs

Fractures of arms/legs

Dislocated joints

Impaired mobility

Abdomen

Bruises or wounds

Evidence of internal injuries

Other

Have physical injuries such as scratches, bruises, and cuts been recorded and photographed?

Have fingernail scrapings been taken and preserved?

Has blood typing been done?

Have smears for sexually transmitted infections been taken of the mouth, throat, vagina, and rectum?

Have combings of the pubic hair been made and preserved?

Has genital trauma been recorded and photographed?

Has rectal trauma been recorded and photographed?

Have semen specimens been preserved?

When was the client's last menstrual period?

Has the clothing been inspected for rips, blood, and stains?

Has the clothing been preserved?

Identify specific *coping behaviors* clients used during the rape such as screaming, fighting, talking, blacking out, and/or remaining passive. Initially, clients may experience distortions related to self-blame or guilt. Recognizing that their behavior was an adaptive mechanism for survival will raise their self-esteem and decrease their feelings of guilt. Repeatedly tell clients it was not their fault. Emphasize that *survival is the most important outcome.* Reassure them that their responses were all that was possible under the degree of fear that rape induces. A helpful statement might be, "I know you handled the situation right because you are alive."

Help clients *identify immediate concerns* and prioritize them. Focusing on immediate problems lessens the client's confusion and the feeling of being overwhelmed. Next, help the client use the *problem-solving process.* Clients need to be empowered to make their own decisions and act on their own behalf. Restoring personal choice is a primary antidote to rape trauma. Informed choices help clients regain control and autonomy, both of which were violated during the rape.

Help clients *identify who to tell* about the rape. Rape is both a personal and a family crisis. Victims often fear how family and friends will respond to the situation. Anticipatory guidance on your part will help them take advantage of available support systems. When significant others are involved, prepare them before they join the victim because they may not know how to best support their loved one. Use the Client/Family Teaching box on page 563 as a guide to family education.

Discuss beliefs about postcoital contraception and abortion if appropriate. Pregnancy may result from the rape, and clients must have information about available options. The most common medical intervention is a course of hormonal treatment. Elevated doses of oral contraceptive or DES (diethylstilbestrol) may be administered if the woman chooses to prevent conception (Krueger 1988). Mifepristone (RU-486), a pill that is currently being tested

ASSESSMENT

Nursing History Tool for Assessment of the Rape Victim

Behavioral Assessment

Is the client able to respond verbally to questions?

Is the client able to follow simple directions?

Has the client bathed, douched, changed clothes, or done any self-treatment before coming to the hospital?

Affective Assessment

Which of the following emotions is the client experiencing? Describe with objective and subjective data.

Disbelief	Anxiety
Shame	Fear
Embarrassment	Guilt
Humiliation	Anger
Hopelessness	Depression
Vulnerability	Alienation from others

Cognitive Assessment

Evidence of defense mechanisms:

Is the client confused?

Has the client been informed of her rights?

Describe the client's attention span.

Is the client able to describe what occurred?

Is the client able to make decisions?

Who has the client informed about the rape? Family? Friends? Police?

Does the client need assistance in telling others?

Is the client blaming self for the attack?

Is the client experiencing flashbacks to the attack?

What does this event represent to the client?

Sociocultural Assessment

Who and where are the available support systems for the client? Family? Friends? Advocate? Clergy?

Is the client in need of temporary shelter?

Does the client know about available counseling?

by the FDA in various parts of the country, is a chemical that greatly diminishes the chances that a fertilized ovum will be implanted or that a placenta will develop (Nevid et al. 1995). Inform clients about the need for follow-up medical evaluation and treatment for sexually transmitted infections, including a test for HIV.

Provide a *written list of referrals* of community resources before clients are discharged from the emergency department. Crisis intervention counseling can help minimize the long-term emotional impact of rape. Every effort should be made to connect clients with aftercare services while they are still in the emergency department.

Group therapy provides an opportunity for victims to meet with other survivors of rape in a safe, supportive, and egalitarian setting. In this therapeutic environment, clients have their feelings validated as normal reactions to the assault and receive confirmation of their survival behaviors. The long-term goal of group therapy is to help survivors understand their distress and take charge of their own recovery. Recovery is accomplished by counteracting self-blame, sharing grief, and by affirming the self and life.

Evaluation and Outcome Criteria

The long-term goal of intervention is to help survivors of rape return to their precrisis level, or achieve a higher level of functioning. The following outcome behaviors demonstrate that the crisis has been resolved in an adaptive fashion (Koss and H3arvey 1991):

- Control over remembering—can elect to recall or not recall the rape; decreased flashbacks and nightmares.
- Affect tolerance—feelings can be felt, named, and endured without overwhelming arousal or numbing.
- Symptom mastery—anxiety, fear, depression, and sexual problems have decreased and are more tolerable.
- Reconnection—increased ability to trust and attach to others.
- Meaning—has discovered some tolerable meaning to the trauma and to self as a trauma survivor; feels empowered.

As a nurse, you must challenge cultural values and beliefs that promote and condone sexual violence. Myths

NURSING SELF-AWARENESS

Working with Rape Victims

Take some time to think about and consider your reactions to the following questions:

- Are people being conditioned by their families, movies, and television into accepting rape as something allowable?
- Have you ever been in a situation in which genital or oral sex occurred without your complete consent or your partner's complete consent? How did you feel after it was over?
- Is acquaintance rape more emotionally destructive than stranger rape?
- Is it rape if the victim is under the influence of alcohol or drugs?
- Can a person who is mentally retarded, or suffering from a mental disorder, give consent to sexual activity?
- Is our society too tolerant of rapists?

that support rape in any way must be confronted, and a new understanding of rape and rape victims must be developed. It is only through this process that long-term changes will occur.

Intrafamily Violence: Physical Abuse

Domestic violence—violence within the family—occurs at all levels of society. The myth is that violence occurs only among the poor and undereducated, but the reality is that violence occurs also among the middle and upper classes and professional elite. In the past, these problems among wealthy or prominent people were kept hidden from the general public. With an increase in national concern, however, more publicity is being given to cases of domestic violence at all socioeconomic levels.

In this text, the word "family" refers to any one of these three categories: those who are related by birth, adoption, or marriage; those in an intimate relationship; and those who are in a domestic relationship, that is, sharing the same household. Although the image of the American family is one of happiness and harmony, this ideal is often in conflict with the underlying reality of domestic violence. **Battering**, a pattern of repeated physical assault, can be considered an epidemic in the United States.

The incidence of domestic violence can only be estimated. Studies often include only those people who are willing to respond to surveys. Typically underrepresented in such studies are those who do not speak English, the very poor, the homeless, and those who are hospitalized or incarcerated at the time of the survey. The actual rates of domestic violence are probably much higher than reported.

In all 50 states, nurses are *required by law* to report suspected incidents of child abuse, and in every state, there is a penalty—civil, criminal, or both—for failure to report child abuse. State laws vary for reporting the abuse of adults and the elderly. Domestic violence is now considered to be a violent crime against which the victim has the right to be protected and for which the perpetrator can be arrested and prosecuted.

Sibling Abuse

The most common and unrecognized form of domestic violence occurs between siblings. Many people assume it is natural and even appropriate for children to use physical force with one another. Parents say things like "It's a good chance for him to learn how to defend himself," "She had a right to hit him; he was teasing her," and "Kids will be kids." With these attitudes, children learn that physical force is an appropriate method of resolving conflict among themselves. Parents should not be complacent about sibling aggression; 3% of all child homicides in the U.S. are caused by siblings. Even though violence decreases with age, studies indicate that 63–68% of adolescent siblings use physical violence to resolve conflict (Gelles and Cornell 1990).

Child Abuse

Each year, approximately 2.5 million American children experience at least one act of physical violence. Younger children are spanked, punched, grabbed, slapped, kicked, bitten, and hit with fists or objects. Adolescents are more likely to be beaten up and have a knife or gun used against them. Both men and women are equally likely to abuse young children. During adolescence, however, the abuser is more likely to be male (Browne 1993).

In the U.S., homicide is one of the five leading causes of death before the age of 18. Some 72% of children killed between the ages of 1 week and 1 year are killed by a parent. Between ages 1 and 17, 23% of homicides are caused by parents, 3% by stepparents, and 6% by other family members (Brown 1991; Gelles and Cornell 1990).

Acts of violence against children range from a light slap to a severe beating to homicide. Hitting or spanking

CLIENT/FAMILY TEACHING

Rape Myths Versus Rape Facts

Myth: Sexual assault is caused by uncontrollable sex drives.

Fact

Sexual assault is an act of physical and emotional violence, not of sexual gratification. Men assault to dominate, humiliate, control, degrade, terrify, and violate. Studies show that power and anger are the primary motivating factors.

Myth: Women provoke sexual assault, and sex appeal is of prime importance in selecting targets.

Fact

Women who have been sexually assaulted range in age from infants to the elderly. Appearance and attractiveness are not relevant. A man assaults someone who is accessible and appears vulnerable.

Myth: Women are usually sexually assaulted by strangers.

Fact

Studies show that the majority of those sexually assaulted are acquainted with their assailants.

Myth: Most sexual assaults are interracial.

Fact

As a national average, more that 90% of all sexual assaults occur between people of the same race, although attacks by men of color against white women are given more publicity. There is evidence of racial bias in our legal system: Although men of color are estimated to constitute a small proportion of sexual assailants, they are 48% of those convicted and 80% of those jailed for assault.

Myth: Sexual assault is unplanned and spontaneous.

Fact

Studies show that a majority of sexual assaults are planned in advance.

Myth: Women make false reports of sexual assault.

Fact

Statistics show that 2% of reports of alleged rape are unfounded; this is the same proportion as for all other crimes.

Myth: Men do not have to be concerned about sexual assault because it affects women.

Fact

Men, both straight and gay, are sexually assaulted. In addition, men have wives, friends, mothers, and daughters who may someday need help coping with the aftereffects of sexual assault. Rape will not cease until men stop raping.

Source: Adapted from Resources Against Sexual Assault, *1987, pp. 5–6.*

children is condoned and even approved of as being necessary and good for the child. Many parents, however, do not realize the underlying messages they are giving the child by hitting (Straus, Gelles, and Steinmetz 1980):

- If you are small and weak, you deserve to be hit.
- People who love you, hit you.
- It is appropriate to hit people you love.
- Violence is appropriate if the end result is good.
- Violence is an appropriate method of resolving conflict.

Parental violence often becomes chronic in that it occurs periodically or regularly. In extreme cases, it ends in the death of the infant or child. In the United States, three children are killed every day. Of these, 84% are younger than 5 years old, and 43% are less than 1 year old. Child victims are helpless captives because they are dependent on the adults in the family. Abused children often try to please the abusing parent and may become overly compliant to all adults. They may avoid peers and withdraw from outside contacts. It is not unusual for child victims to act out with aggressive behavior later, during adolescence (Baldacci 1993).

Countless other children are scarred by neglect. **Child neglect** refers to a child's health or welfare being compromised by negligence from the person or persons who are responsible for the care. Neglect consistently accounts for the majority of child abuse reports and actual incidents. Neglect is not only the most frequent form of abuse but can be just as fatal as physical abuse. It is believed that neglect leads to at least one-third of all child fatalities (McCurdy and Daro 1994).

Partner Abuse

The number of women who are abused by their spouse, live-in partner, or lover is unknown. In heterosexual partner abuse, it is estimated that 95% of the perpetrators are men. It is thought that 1 woman in 3 will be assaulted by her domestic partner in her lifetime, and that 4 million women are severely assaulted every year. If verbal and emotional assaults were included, the numbers would be much higher. Violence is the single largest cause of injury to women in the United States, with 20% of emergency department visits resulting from physical abuse. As many as 50% of female homicide victims are killed by their husbands or lovers. At least two-thirds of these women have been abused by their murderer prior to their deaths. Fifty-three percent of the men who are violent toward their partners are also violent toward their children. Women sometimes kill their husbands or lovers, almost invariably in response to years of abuse. They most often murder their partners in self-defense, fearing for their lives and the lives of their children (Bean 1992; Campbell 1992; Smolowe 1994; Urbancic, Campbell, and Humphreys 1993).

Overwhelmingly, the first acts of partner violence occur in dating relationships. Physical abuse occurs among as many as 30–40% of adolescent and college students who are dating. Sadly, more than 25% of victims and 30% of offenders interpret violence as a sign of love (Bean 1992; Gelles and Cornell 1990).

Half the women who are abused suffer beatings several times a year. The other half may be beaten as often as once a week. The intensity and frequency of attacks tend to escalate over time. Compared to nonabused women, abused women are 5 times more likely to attempt suicide, 15 times more likely to abuse alcohol, and 9 times more likely to abuse drugs (Bean 1992).

Among adult family members, women commit fewer violent acts than men. Women do more hitting, kicking, and throwing of objects, while men are more likely to push, shove, slap, beat up, and even use knives or guns against their partner. The acts that men commit against women are more dangerous and result in more severe injuries. While the victim is being beaten, she is also being verbally abused, often by being called a slut, an incompetent housekeeper, or an inadequate mother. The abuser attacks aspects of life that women use to measure their success: homemaking, child care, attractiveness, sex appeal, and sexual fidelity.

Elder Abuse

Elder abuse takes many forms. Some older adults may have their basic physical needs neglected and suffer from dehydration, malnutrition, and oversedation. Families may deprive them of necessary articles such as glasses, hearing aids, and walkers. Some older people are psychologically abused by verbal assaults, threats, humiliation, and/or harassment. Families may violate an older person's rights by refusing appropriate medical treatment, forcing isolation or unreasonable confinement, denying privacy, providing an unsafe environment, or demanding involuntary servitude. Some are financially exploited by their relatives through theft or misuse of property or funds. Others are beaten and even raped by family members.

A number of factors contribute to the abuse of older adults. Perpetrators may have personal problems such as lack of support in caring for the older family member, alcohol or drug addiction, and a family history of violence. Family factors include unresolved previous conflicts and power struggles. When the culture devalues older people, abuse is more likely to occur. There are similarities with child abuse in that in both situations, the perpetrator is usually a family member and the victim is dependent on the perpetrator (Brown 1991).

Homosexual Abuse

Until very recently, there has been a public minimization or denial of physical abuse in lesbian and gay relationships. This denial has been supported by the myths that women are not violent people and that men can defend themselves. In reality, violence does occur in some gay and lesbian families, for the same reasons as in heterosexual families: to demonstrate, achieve, and maintain power and control over one's partner. In addition to physical or emotional abuse, the violent partner may use homophobic control—the threat of telling family, friends, neighbors, or employers about the victim's sexual orientation.

In the United States, domestic violence is the third largest health problem for gay men, following substance abuse and AIDS. It is estimated that 11% of coupled gay men are victims. Men rarely talk about being victims for fear of being considered feminine if they admit that their partners are hurting them. Homophobia and hatred of homosexuals in the U.S. contributes to the difficulties of battered lesbians and gays. They are cut off from the usual support systems available to heterosexual victims such as specialized counseling services and shelters. Fear of bad press and hostile response adds to the silence about the violence. Members of lesbian and gay communities are currently making an attempt to intervene with and support victims (Island and Letellier 1991; Rothblum and Cole 1989).

Abuse of Pregnant Women

Pregnancy is a time of increased risk for abuse. There are more incidents of violence during pregnancy than of either gestational diabetes or placenta previa, both of which are screened for regularly. Recent studies indicate that 4–20% of pregnant women are physically abused (O'Campo et al. 1994).

A past history of abuse is one of the strongest predictors of abuse during pregnancy. Nonpregnent women are usually beaten in the face and chest. But pregnant women tend to be beaten in the abdomen, which can lead to miscarriage, placenta abruptio, fetal loss, premature labor, fetal fractures, pelvic fractures, rupture of the uterus, and hemorrhage. Physical abuse during pregnancy may be related to ambivalent feelings about the pregnancy, increased vulnerability of the woman, increased economic pressures, and decreased sexual availability. Parents, not male partners, are the main perpetrators of violence against pregnant adolescents.

Unfortunately, the abuse of pregnant women is often overlooked by health care professionals even when the victim appears in the emergency department with bruises, cuts, broken bones, and abdominal injuries (O'Campo 1994; Stewart and Cecutti 1993).

Emotional Abuse

Although the focus of violence in this chapter is on physical abuse, it must be remembered that emotional abuse is often equally as damaging. Words can hit as hard as a fist, and the damage to self-esteem can last a lifetime. Emotional abuse involves one person shaming, embarrassing, ridiculing, or insulting another either in private or in public. It may include destruction of personal property or the killing of pets in an effort to frighten or control the victim. Such statements as "You can't do anything right," "You're ugly and stupid—no one else would want you," and "I wish you had never been born" are devastating to self-esteem.

The Cycle of Violence

The first incident of domestic violence may be precipitated by frustration or stress. If the victim immediately refuses to accept the violence and seeks outside help, there are often no further episodes. If the victim submits to the violence, then physical force, without the stimulus of frustration or stress, becomes a way of relating, and the pattern becomes resistant to change. A typical cycle occurs when conflict escalates into a violent episode, after which the perpetrator begs for the victim's forgiveness. The victim stays in the system because of promises to reform. With the next episode of conflict, the cycle of violence begins again and becomes part of the family dynamics (O'Leary and Vivian 1990).

Violent people are often extremely jealous and possessive. They view other family members in terms of property and ownership. Abusers use violence in an attempt to prove to themselves and others that they are superior and in control. Their use of physical force temporarily obliterates their sense of inadequacy and compensates for a lack of internal resources.

The abuser is the most powerful person in the life of the abused. The abuser's purpose is to enslave the victim, while simultaneously demanding respect, gratitude, and love. Control over the victim is established by repetitive emotional abuse that instills terror and helplessness. Threats of serious harm or threats against other family members keep the victim in a constant state of fear. In order to have complete domination, the abuser isolates the victim. She often is forced to give up work, friends, and family. He may stalk her, eavesdrop, and intercept letters and phone calls. Control and scrutiny of the victim's body and bodily functions further destroy her sense of autonomy. She is shamed and demoralized when told what to eat, when to sleep, what to wear, when to go to the bathroom, and so on. For a victim who has been deprived long enough, the hope of a meal, a bath, or a kind word can be a powerful reward. All this abusive behavior alternates with unpredictable outbursts of physical violence. Such domestic captivity of women, along with traumatic bonding to the abuser, often goes unrecognized.

Victims can be further immobilized by feelings of anxiety and depression. Feelings of self-blame may be expressed in such statements as "If I hadn't talked back to my mother, she wouldn't have hit me," and "If I were a better wife, he wouldn't beat me." Guilt can contribute to depression, which further immobilizes victims and keeps them from leaving or seeking help for the family system.

Fear contributes to women's inability to leave abusive relationships. Often threatened with death at the idea of leaving, they live in fear of physical reprisal. Fearing loneliness, some women may believe being in a bad relationship is better than being alone. And leaving the relationship would not necessarily ensure the end of the abuse. The abuser is often most dangerous when threatened or faced with separation (Smolowe 1994).

Maria, age 20, met Brad at work. In the beginning of their dating relationship, Brad bought her small gifts and said sweet things to her. He told Maria he'd never loved anyone else as much. Maria believed him, quickly fell in love, and moved in with Brad. Several months later she called her parents from work and begged them to come and get her. Maria told them that she didn't like the relationship with Brad but she didn't know how to get out of it. Brad had taken over Maria's life, even controlling the use of the car her parents had helped her buy. He followed her everywhere and rarely let her out of his sight. Maria insisted on returning to the apartment that night to get her car, telling her parents that Brad was not a violent person. However, Brad brutally beat her for having called her parents. Maria moved back home and began trying to put her life back together. Even so, Brad continued to make harassing phone calls to Maria. Because she had moved out so quickly, there were still financial matters she and Brad needed to clear up, so Maria

Why Do They Stay? Why Do They Go Back?

Fear Of physical reprisal if they resist, of being found and beaten again, of their children being hurt; those who attempt to leave risk suffering worse violence and even death.

Learned Helplessness They believe they have no choices and no control; have come to believe that violence is an accepted way of life.

Traumatic Bonding Results from alternating good and bad treatment; they have no sense of autonomy.

Emotional Dependence They are convinced that they are weak, inferior, and do not deserve better treatment; insecure over potential autonomy.

Financial Dependence They may not have a source of income; if the abuser is arrested, he may lose his job and the family will have no income; have been taught that they have to be submissive in exchange for financial support.

Guilt and/or Shame They have been convinced that they provoked the abuse; guilt over failure of the relationship; family/religious/cultural values against divorce or separation; shamed about remaining in the abuse relationship.

Isolation They have few, if any, friends; little support from family; no phone, no mail, no car.

Children They may believe two parents are better than one; they may be threatened with loss of custody; the abuser may threaten to harm or kidnap the children.

Hope They hope that if they change in the way the abuser wants them to, the abuse will stop; hope that the abuser will keep promises and stop the assaults.

agreed to meet with him one evening. But instead of allowing her to end their 16-month relationship, Brad pulled out a gun and shot Maria once in the back of the head.

For a partial list of reasons people remain in abusive relationships, see the accompanying box.

Fear also contributes to the inability to leave a partner in an abusive gay or lesbian relationship. Because many couples share close friends within the same community, victims may fear shaming their partners. They may also fear that friends will either deny the problem or take the abuser's side. Homophobia contributes to the victim's reluctance to seek help. Calling the police may result in ridicule or hostile responses from the officers. Victims may not seek help from family members to avoid reinforcing negative stereotypes about homosexuality, which might exacerbate the family's homophobia (Island and Letellier 1991).

Biopsychosocial Theories

Domestic violence is easy to describe but difficult to explain. There is no single cause of this type of violence. It results from an interaction of neurobiologic, personality, situational, and societal factors that have an impact on families.

Neurobiologic Theory

Neurobiologic theorists propose that genes and neurotransmitters may contribute to causing violent behavior. Although a genetic predisposition may make certain behaviors more likely, it does not make them inevitable. Two genetic mutations have been added to a growing body of evidence that supports a genetic-environmental link to violence. One defect appears to decrease serotonin (5-HT) levels and the other raises norepinephrine (NE) levels in susceptible people exposed to certain environmental stresses such as violence and substance abuse. Low levels of 5-HT and high levels of NE are implicated in a lack of control, loss of temper, and explosive rage. These two neurotransmitters may work separately or together in different abnormal combinations to produce a strong tendency toward a variety of violent behaviors (Kotulak 1993).

Intrapersonal Theory

Intrapersonal theory suggests that the cause of violence lies in the personality of the abuser. It is thought that people who are violent are unable to control their impulsive expressions of anger and hostility. As many as 80% of male abusers grew up in homes in which they were abused or observed their mothers being abused. With these family dynamics, the child sees the father as frightening and intimidating and sees the mother as helpless and nonprotective. This early emotional deprivation contributes to an adult who is very needy of nurturance and support. He comes to adult relationships with unrealistic demands for time and attention. As the relationship develops, he discourages his partner's relationships with other people because of his low self-esteem and fear of abandonment (Gelles and Cornell 1990).

Social Learning Theory

Social learning theory proposes that violence is a learned behavior. Children learn about violence from having observed it, from being a victim, and/or from behaving violently themselves. If the use of violence is rewarded by a gain in power, the behavior is reinforced. If there is immediate negative reinforcement within the family, a decrease in violent behavior will result.

In addition to family models, the media provide many models of violence to which children are exposed. Some movies and television shows demonstrate that "good" people use force to achieve "good" ends. Many of the stories make no attempt to justify the use of force for "good" ends; they simply present endless, senseless acts of cruelty by one human being upon another—violence without consequences. With these types of family and media examples, children develop values that tolerate, and even accept as normal, everyday violence between people.

Feminist Theory

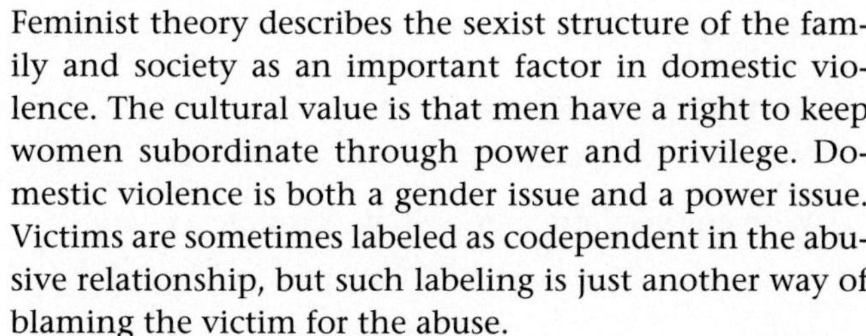

Feminist theory describes the sexist structure of the family and society as an important factor in domestic violence. The cultural value is that men have a right to keep women subordinate through power and privilege. Domestic violence is both a gender issue and a power issue. Victims are sometimes labeled as codependent in the abusive relationship, but such labeling is just another way of blaming the victim for the abuse.

The sexist economic system helps entrap women, who are often forced to choose between poverty and abuse. It is often difficult for women to find advocates and solutions within the male-dominated legal, religious, mental health, and medical systems. Society sanctions male violence by neglecting female victims. This neglect includes a lack of resources, a minimal response to domestic violence, and inadequate laws. Financial resources have been reduced during recent years; an example is the 1992 abolishment of the toll-free national domestic violence hotline, due to lack of funding (Birns, Cascardi, and Meyer 1994).

The Nursing Process and Intrafamily Physical Abuse

Assessment

Nurses in all clinical settings must routinely assess clients for evidence of intrafamily violence. Considering the extensiveness of the problem, ask one or two introductory questions of every client. In assessing a child, say, for example, "Moms and dads try to help their children learn how to behave well. What happens to you when you do something wrong?" Or ask, "What is the worst punishment you ever received?" In assessing adults, you may begin with this approach: "One of the sources of stress in our lives is family disagreement. Could you describe how disagreements affect you? What happens when you disagree?" If the responses to these questions are indicative of violence, conduct a more in-depth nursing assessment. Guidelines for assessment are given in the Assessment box on the following page.

Nursing Diagnosis

The most important outcome of nursing assessment is identifying the existence of domestic violence. Priority must be given to critical and serious physical injuries. The severity and potential fatality of the situation must be considered, as well as the needs of dependent children and legal issues surrounding the case. Consider the following nursing diagnoses when analyzing your assessment data:

- Ineffective Family Coping, Disabling, related to an inability to manage conflict without violence.
- Ineffective Individual Coping related to being a victim of violence.
- Altered Parenting related to the physical abuse of children.
- Powerlessness related to feelings of being dependent on the abuser.
- Self Esteem Disturbance related to feeling guilty and responsible for being a victim.
- Social Isolation related to shame about family violence.
- Risk for Violence, Directed at Others, related to a history of the use of physical force within the family.

Planning and Implementing Interventions

Most victims of domestic violence would like it to end, but they may not know how to seek the help they need. It is extremely important that you be nonjudgmental in your interactions with all family members. Initially, clients may be unwilling to trust you because of family shame and fears of being accused for remaining in the violent situation. It is vital that you not impose your own values by offering quick and easy solutions to the very complicated problem of domestic violence. The Client/Family Teaching box on page 569 will help you to debunk myths about family violence. Use the Nursing Self-Awareness box on page 570 to help you in understanding your own feelings and attitudes.

The treatment of families experiencing violence requires a multidisciplinary approach, with a broad range of interventions. Nurses, social workers, physicians, family

ASSESSMENT

Nursing History Tool for Assessing Victims of Family Violence

Behavioral Assessment

Tell me about how people communicate within your family.

What types of things cause conflict within your family?

How is conflict managed or resolved?

Who in your family loses control of themselves when angry?

Have you received verbal threats of harm?

Have you ever been threatened with a knife or gun?

In which ways have you been at the receiving end of a family member's violent outbursts? Slapped? Hit? Punched? Thrown? Shoved? Kicked? Burned? Beaten up?

Is there a history of the need for emergency medical treatment?

In what ways have you attempted to stop the violence?

Have you attempted to leave the situation in the past?

What occurred when you attempted to leave?

Describe the use of alcohol in the family.

Describe the use of drugs in the family.

Affective Assessment

Who do you think is responsible for the use of physical force within the family?

In what way is this person(s) responsible?

How much guilt are you experiencing at this time?

Tell me about your fears. Lack of security? Financial problems? Child care problems? Living apart from spouse? Further physical injury?

What kinds of factors contribute to your feeling of helplessness to leave or stop the abuse?

How hopeless do you feel about your situation?

How would you describe your level of depression?

Cognitive Assessment

Describe your strengths and abilities as a person.

If you were describing yourself to a stranger, what would you say?

What are your beliefs about keeping your family together?

Tell me about your reasons for remaining in this situation. Promises of reform? Material rewards?

Do you believe/hope the violence will not recur?

What are your expectations of how children should behave?

What rights do parents have with their children?

What rights do spouses have with each other?

What are the rules about physical force within your family?

Sociocultural Assessment

How did your parents relate to each other?

Who enforced discipline when you were a child?

What type of discipline was used when you were a child?

What was/is your relationship like with your mother?

What was/is your relationship like with your father?

How did you get along with your siblings?

In your present family, who is the head of the household?

How are decisions made in your family?

How are household jobs assigned in the family?

Describe the recent and current stresses on the family. Unemployment? Financial problems? Illness? New family members? Deaths or separations? Child-rearing problems? Change in job status? Increase in conflict? Change in residence?

Who can you turn to for support in times of stress?

Describe your social life.

What types of contact have you had with the legal system? Phoned police? Peace bonds? Obtained a lawyer? Court cases? Protective services?

CLIENT/FAMILY TEACHING

Myths and Facts About Domestic Violence

Myth: Family violence is rare.

Fact

Every year, 10 million Americans are abused by a family member.

Myth: Family violence is confined to mentally disturbed or sick people.

Fact

Fewer than 10% of all cases involved an abuser who is mentally ill. The vast majority seem totally normal and are often charming, persuasive, and rational.

Myth: Violence is trivial—a joking matter.

Fact

A woman is beaten every 15 seconds in the United States, and 2000–4000 women are murdered by their husbands or boyfriends every year. Every year, 2.5 million children are abused, and 1200 die from the abuse. There are 1 million cases of elderly abuse annually.

Myth: Family violence is confined to the lower classes.

Fact

Social factors are not relevant. There are doctors, ministers, psychologists, and nurses who beat their family members. Violence occurs at least once in two-thirds of all marriages.

Myth: All members of the family participate in the family dynamics, therefore, all must change in order for the violence to stop.

Fact

Only the perpetrator has the ability to stop the violence. A change in the victim's behavior will not cause the abuser to become nonviolent.

Myth: Family violence is usually a one-time event, an isolated incident.

Fact

Violence is a pattern, a reign of force and terror. It becomes more frequent and severe over time.

Myth: Abused women like being hit; otherwise, they would leave.

Fact

Abused women are forced to stay in the relationship for many reasons. The perpetrator dramatically escalates the violence when a woman tries to leave.

therapists, vocational trainers, police, protective services personnel, and lawyers must coordinate to intervene effectively in a situation of intrafamily violence.

In the initial contact with family members, *assure their physical safety* as much as possible. It is critical to assess the level of danger for the victim; homicide may be a real possibility if previous threats have been made. Also assess the level of danger for the abuser. The severity and duration of the violence are the factors that contribute most directly to victims killing their abusers in self-defense. If the level of danger is high, contact protective services or the police for emergency custody placement or removal to a shelter.

Provide interventions to *improve communication.* Families experiencing violence often have poor communication skills. Teach active listening with feedback, clear and direct communication, and communication that does not attack the personhood of others.

Identify the normality of conflict within all families by discussing how disagreements are inevitable. From there, discuss the use of the democratic process in conflict resolution and decision making. It is best to practice with minor, unemotional family problems at first.

Help family members identify *methods to manage anger appropriately.* All family members must assume responsibility for their own behavior. They can learn and practice talking out anger as it occurs. Make suggestions for appropriate expression, such as relaxation, physical exercise, and striking safe, inanimate objects (a pillow, a couch, or a punching bag). Guide the family in establishing limits and defining consequences if violence recurs. Emphasize that violence within the family will not be tolerated.

NURSING SELF-AWARENESS

Working with Victims of Domestic Violence

Take some time to think about and consider your reactions to the following questions:

- Is American culture violent compared to other cultures?
- The United States was founded by violence. How has this influenced the values and behavior of present-day Americans?
- What is the difference between spanking a child and beating up on a child?
- Do you think the stalking laws are decreasing the level of violence in the United States?
- Are you for or against gun control?
- Would it be more difficult for a person to stab a family member than to shoot that person?

Help parents who are physically abusive *develop and improve their parenting skills.* Begin by recognizing their current positive parenting skills, to increase their self-worth and help them engage in the learning process. Share your understanding that the use of violence is a desperate attempt to cope with their children. Confirming that they care about their children will increase the likelihood of their active participation in the treatment process. Because domestic violence is often transgenerational, discuss with the parents how they were punished as children. Teach them about the normal growth and development of children. Unrealistic demands for children to comply beyond their developmental ability often result in violence. The first step in the problem-solving process is helping parents identify specific problems they experience with raising children. They can then go on to identify solutions, other than physical force, that are age-appropriate for their children. They need support in implementing, practicing, and evaluating these new skills.

Practice *feminist-sensitive therapy.* This might also be called a survivor-centered approach—not specific techniques, but rather a perspective or way of seeing and understanding the context in which women and children live, recognizing the cultural values that underlie domestic violence. Using this approach, speak up and say that violence is wrong and will not be tolerated.

One of the primary goals of feminist-sensitive therapy is the *empowerment of victims.* The process of violence removes all power and control from a person resulting in low self-esteem, anxiety, depression, and somatic problems. The following principles are basic to the empowerment of victims:

- A commitment to the belief that women and men are inherently equal.
- An egalitarian approach to the nurse-client relationship. The client is viewed as an equal partner rather than a helpless recipient of nursing interventions.
- Interventions that focus on the enhancement of the victim's power.
- An emphasis on the victim's strengths and abilities.
- Respect for the victim's ability to understand his or her own experiences.
- Family interventions that change destructive roles and expectations within the family system.
- A willingness to state clear value positions about domestic violence.

Through this approach, clients can become aware that they have choices in, and control over, their lives.

Avoid trying to convince adult victims to leave their abuser. As difficult as it may be, you must be willing to support clients in their pain, rather than telling them what to do about their problems. For the most positive adaptive outcome, adult victims must be their own rescuers and take charge of their own safety and protection plan. If they need help with this process, teach them to ask for that help directly. This is not meant to imply in any way that you would abandon clients; rather, you stand by, support, and affirm the positive choices and decisions they make.

Help adult clients begin identifying ways in which they are dependent on their abusers. High levels of dependence make it difficult for victims to leave abusers without intense support. You can help them identify intrapersonal and interpersonal strengths to decrease their feelings of powerlessness. From there, clients can move on to identifying aspects of life that are under their control. Offer assertiveness training to help them develop new skills for relating to others in the future. But caution them, if they are still in the abusive relationship, because assertive behavior may escalate the violence.

Most abusers do not seek treatment unless it is court-ordered or there are custody issues involved. It is frustrating to intervene with abusers who deny the reality of or the responsibility for the violence. *Group therapy* for abusers is sometimes helpful. The group setting is more effective than individual therapy because interactions with a number of people more successfully address the anger and control problems. The responsibility for aggression is always placed on the aggressor. Issues regarding the patriarchal and power views of relationships are discussed in great depth. Abusers learn that anger *can* be controlled and that violence is always a *choice.*

Evaluation and Outcome Criteria

Nurses in acute care settings may not have the opportunity for long-term evaluation of the family system. Sengstock and Barrett (1984) state that short-term evaluation focuses on:

1. The identification of domestic violence.
2. The family's ability to recognize that a problem exists.
3. The willingness of the family to accept assistance by following through with referrals.
4. The removal of the victim from a volatile situation.

Nurses in long-term settings or within the community have an opportunity to evaluate the effectiveness of the multidisciplinary treatment plan over an extended period of time. When violence no longer exists within the family system, the plan has succeeded. Sharing in the process of family growth and adaptation can be a tremendous source of professional satisfaction.

Achievement of the following outcome criteria is evidence that the plan of intervention was successful. The victims have:

- Recognized that they are not to blame for the violence of others.
- Ended the denial and minimization of domestic violence.
- Demonstrated an awareness of strengths, skills, and competence.
- Reestablished a sense of power over their own lives.
- Verbalized their right to express their own needs and to satisfy them.
- Established social networks to decrease isolation and secrecy.

All nurses should evaluate their professional obligations and practice in counteracting those aspects of society that foster domestic violence. Domestic violence is a mental health problem of national and international importance, and nurses should be leaders in helping prevent it in future generations. Primary prevention includes the nursing interventions of parent education, family life education in schools, referral for appropriate child or elder care, establishment of support groups, and education of fellow nurses about the problem of domestic violence. It also includes community education about the pervasive effects of media violence upon individuals and society. Secondary prevention includes working with children who are victims or who have seen their mothers beaten, and making referrals for multidisciplinary intervention. Nurses must be community advocates in supporting hotlines, crisis centers, and shelters for victims of domestic violence. On the political level, nurses must make their voices heard in regard to policies and laws affecting children, women, and older people. Questions to guide the evaluation of nursing practice include the following:

- Have I, as a nurse, assessed each client for possible abuse?
- What action have I taken to decrease violence in the media?
- Have I been an advocate for gun control?
- Have I confronted the use of physical punishment within families?
- Have I volunteered to teach parenting classes at grade schools and high schools?
- Have I written to legislators to protest funding cuts in programs designed to help children, women, and older people?
- Have I spoken out on the need to increase the number of bilingual/bicultural counselors, lawyers, nurses, and physicians to attend to the needs of ethnic families?

Intrafamily Violence: Sexual Abuse

Childhood sexual abuse is a major health problem in the United States. The majority of cases are probably unreported. Health care professionals, as well as families, have used denial to cope with ambiguous evidence of the cultural taboos of incest and sex with children. Use the Nursing Self-Awareness box on the next page to help you in understanding your own feelings and attitudes. In order to respond appropriately to cues that signal sexual abuse, you must understand the characteristics and dynamics of families involved. A note of caution must be added, however. With the recent increased publicity, there is a real danger of a witch-hunt developing; any hint or accusation of sexual abuse may be interpreted as absolute proof of guilt. Individuals and families have been destroyed by rumors and false accusations. You must assess carefully and maintain a balance between the extremes of denial and automatic belief of guilt. Concerns about overreporting of suspected child abuse (especially sexual abuse) have generated studies such as the one discussed in the Research Note on page 573.

Sexually abused children and adult survivors of childhood sexual abuse (hereafter referred to as adult survivors) are crying out for help. A few cry out loudly in protest, but most cry inwardly in silence. It is thought that as many as 1 in 3 girls and 1 in 10 boys are abused sexually before the age of 18. Boys are more frequently molested outside the family system than are girls. The period of abuse tends to begin and end at a younger age in boys (Elliott and Briere 1992).

NURSING SELF-AWARENESS

Working with Victims of Child Sexual Abuse

Take some time to think about and consider your reactions to the following questions:

- Do you think the rate of child sexual abuse is increasing, or is there just better reporting?
- Do you think sex education can decrease the rate of sexual abuse?
- Which situation do you think is more devastating—when force is used or when no force is used?
- Does the fact that most perpetrators were sexually abused as children excuse their behavior? What if the perpetrator is only 11 years old?
- Many fewer women than men are accused of sexually abusing their children. How do you explain this?
- What needs to be done to decrease the incidence of child sexual abuse?

Sexual abuse occurs in all ethnic, religious, economic, and cultural subgroups. Affinity systems—immediate family, relatives, friends, neighbors, clergy, scout leaders—account for 75–80% of the abusers. Male perpetrators account for 92–98% of the reported cases; however, reports are now acknowledging more female perpetrators (Vanderbilt 1992).

Sexual abuse is defined as inappropriate sexual behavior, whose purpose is to sexually arouse the perpetrator or the child. The perpetrator may be an older child, adolescent, or adult. Behavior ranges from exhibitionism, peeping, explicit sexual talk, touching, caressing, masturbation, oral sex, vaginal sex, and anal sex, to forcing children to engage in sex with one another or with animals.

Types of Offenders

Some offenders prefer girls, others prefer boys, and some abuse both, as long as the victim is a child. Some are interested in adolescents or preteens, some in toddlers, and some in infants. Some offenders do not abuse until they are adults, but more than half start in their teens (Vanderbilt 1992).

JUVENILE OFFENDERS Many, if not most, of the cases that involve juvenile offenders are unreported. Family members often want to protect and shield the young offender. At other times, the behavior is rationalized as adolescent male experimentation. Most juvenile offenders were sexually abused as children; they gradually develop offending behaviors as they reach adolescence. Juvenile offenders may seek victims within or outside the family system. The type of sexual offense often parallels their own experiences of abuse. The most frequent offense is sexual touching, which often escalates to rape and other sex crimes.

MALE OFFENDERS One study of fathers who abused their daughters established five types of incestuous fathers (Vanderbilt 1992). *Sexually preoccupied abusers* (26% of the fathers) have a conscious and often obsessive sexual interest in their daughters. Many of them regard their daughters as sex objects, in some cases as early as birth. *Adolescent regressors* (33% of the fathers) become sexually interested in their daughters when they begin puberty. These men sound and act like adolescents around their daughters. *Self-gratifiers* (20% of the fathers) are not sexually attracted to their daughters per se, and during the abuse, they fantasize about someone else. In effect, they are simply using their daughters' bodies. *Emotional dependents* (10% of the fathers) see themselves as failures and feel very lonely and depressed. They see their daughters as romantic figures in their lives. *Angry retaliators* (10% of the fathers) abuse out of anger, either at the daughter or at the mother. This type of offender is most likely to have a criminal history of assault and rape.

FEMALE OFFENDERS Another study found that female sex offenders fall into four major types (Higgs, Canavan, and Meyer 1992). *Teacher-lovers* are older women who teach children about lovemaking. *Experimenter-exploiters* are often girls who have had no sex education growing up. Baby-sitting is often an opportunity to explore younger children. Many of the girls in this group do not even realize what they are doing or that it is inappropriate. *Predisposers* usually come from a family with a long history of physical and sexual abuse. These families have been dysfunctional over many generations. *Women coerced by males* are those who abuse children because men have forced them to abuse. Usually they have been victims as children and are easily manipulated and intimidated.

Ritual Abuse

Ritual abuse is emotional, physical, and sexual abuse that occurs in the context of bizarre and unusual rituals, torture "games," and cult or satanic worship activities. Children are frequently victimized and forced to participate in the abuse of other children. Types of abuse include drug-

RESEARCH NOTE

Citation

O'Toole AW, O'Toole R, Webster S, Lucal B: Nurses' responses to child abuse. *J Interpersonal Violence* 1994;9(2):194–205.

Study Problem/Purpose

In the past, there have been concerted efforts to increase the reporting of suspected child abuse. More recently, there has been some concern that health care professionals overreport suspected child abuse. According to interactionist theory, the recognition and reporting of child abuse varies because of a number of factors. These factors include the type of abuse (sexual, physical, emotional); the level of seriousness of the abuse; the relationship of the perpetrator to the victim (father, mother, sibling); victim age; victim sex; the psychologic characteristics of the perpetrator; and the justification or excuse offered by the perpetrator. Characteristics of the nurse and the clinical setting were also measured to use as controls in the analysis. The purpose of this study was to determine whether these factors influenced the identification and reporting of suspected child abuse.

Methods

Over 1000 nurses in Ohio were surveyed using a random sample of computer-generated vignettes containing a combination of the seven factors of a potential child abuse occurrance. Recognition and reporting were measured on a ten-point continuum from "not child abuse" to "child abuse," and "unlikely to report" to "likely to report." Each participant rated 28 randomized vignettes.

Findings

There was a strong correlation between the two steps of recognition and reporting of suspected cases of child abuse. The factors most closely associated with recognition and reporting were sexual abuse, the seriousness of the abuse, parental relationship, and the psychologic characteristics of the perpetrator. There were very small changes in variance when nurse and clinical setting factors were added.

Implications

This study demonstrates that sexual abuse is most likely to be recognized and reported, followed by physical abuse, and finally by emotional abuse. Sibling abuse is less often identified as abuse when compared to vignettes in which either parent was the perpetrator. Even though emotional abuse may have long-term harmful effects on a child, emotional abuse is not commonly identified, much less reported.

ging; brainwashing; leaving victims in total darkness for extended periods of time; temporary burial in graves or coffins; rape; bestiality; force-feeding of urine, feces, and/or blood; animal mutilating and/or sacrifice; and human torture and/or sacrifice. Victims are programmed to remain silent, and the thought of breaking the silence is terrifying. They are often programmed to commit suicide if they ever speak about what was done to them (Brown 1991; Ryder 1992; Uherek 1991). Cues to ritual abuse are listed in the box on page 574.

Abusive Behavior Patterns

Typically, adult perpetrators believe in extreme restrictiveness and domination. There is a characteristic enforcement of petty rules with intermittent rewards. Often the adult coerces the child and misrepresents the abuse as a game or "fun" activity. The behavior usually follows a progression of sexual activity, from exposure and fondling to oral, vaginal, and/or anal sex. Secrecy is imposed on the child by persuasion or threat. The abuser may say such things as "If you tell, you'll be sent away," "If you tell, I won't love you anymore," "If you tell, I will kill you," "If you tell, I'll do the same thing to your baby brother."

Secrecy and silence are used by abusers to escape accountability. When secrecy fails and the child victims or adult survivors begin to talk to others about the abuse, perpetrators usually attack the credibility of the victims and try to make sure no one will listen. Perpetrators make such statements as "It never happened, she's lying," "He's exaggerating some innocent touching," and "Even if it did happen, it's time to forget the past and move on." Other perpetrators acknowledge the abuse but minimize the impact with such statements as "Better for her to learn about sex from her father than from some horny teenager" and "She didn't really mind; in fact, we have a very close relationship." Others use the defense mechanism of projection and blame the child for the abuse, as evidenced by such statements as "She's a very provocative

Cues to Ritual Abuse

Children

- Preoccupation with or fear of urine, feces, and/or blood.
- Aggressive play that has mutilative themes.
- Preoccupation with animals being hurt, mutilated, or killed.
- Preoccupation with death and questions of a bizarre nature such as "Do we eat people after they die?"
- Fear of being tied up or caged.
- References to people at day care who dress in scary costumes, such as ghosts or devils.
- References to sexual activity with other children at day care.

Adults

- Vague memories of childhood.
- Inordinate fear of physical violence, knives, or guns.
- Hypersensitivity to unexpected touching and loud noise.
- Phobia about snakes.
- Dreams with recurring images of blood, robed figures, candles, demons, Satan.
- Self-mutilation.
- Fear of being photographed or videotaped.

child, and she seduced me," and "If he hadn't enjoyed it so much, I wouldn't have continued."

Child Victims

Children know adults have absolute power over them, so they obey. When they have been threatened with abandonment or harm, they frequently choose to protect others. When asked, "Why didn't you tell sooner?" the answers are, "I didn't know who to tell," "I was scared," and/or "I did tell and no one believed me."

Children often feel responsible for the adult's behavior and ashamed that they have not been able to stop the abuse. Secrecy and guilt keep these children isolated, causing them to feel alienated from their peers. They may act out sexually by initiating oral or genital sex with other children or adults. The feeling of powerlessness is extremely potent because what the victim says and does makes no difference. When the repressed rage comes to the surface, it may be directed against the self in self-defeating and self-destructive ways, such as self-mutilation and suicide (Glod 1993).

Adolescent victims may run away from home to escape an intolerable situation. Because they have learned, at home, that sexual behavior is rewarded by affection, love, and attention, some turn to prostitution. Others are forced into prostitution as a way to support themselves while living on the streets.

Some child victims use denial to cope with the trauma. Acknowledging the abuse would mean acknowledging that the world is dangerous and that those who are supposed to protect and nurture, failed and caused harm. Other victims minimize the impact, saying things like "It's not so bad; it only happens once a month" and "It's all right because it stopped when I was 11 years old."

Frequently, dissociation is the victim's major defense. The mind is "separated" from the body so the victim is not emotionally present during the sexual attack. Dissociation is evidenced by such statements as "I put myself in the wall, where he couldn't reach all of me" and "When he would come into my room, I would close my eyes and go to my favorite place. Only my body stayed on the bed; the rest of me wasn't there." When sexual abuse is severe and sadistic, the victim may develop dissociative identity disorder (DID).

Adult Survivors

Many adult survivors continue to believe that they were to blame for the abuse and should have been able to resist the adult. This self-blame often contributes to depression, anxiety, panic attacks, and low self-esteem. They feel worthless and different from other people. For some, anger is the only emotion experienced and expressed, all other feelings being repressed. Many adult survivors continue to hate their perpetrators, as well as nonabusing significant adults, for not protecting them (Hall 1993).

Sonja describes her current sexual life as one of promiscuity and relates this to being sexually molested by her grandfather when she was between the ages of 4 and 7. This is her description of the abuse: "Whenever I was alone with him in the car, he would fondle me and expose his penis to me. He would tell me I could touch it, it would be all right. So much of the time I tried to block everything out—it's hard for me to recall exactly what happened. Some of the things I remember clearly. I remember Grandpa's easy chair. When we were alone he would make me sit on his lap in that chair, he would stick his fingers in me. This happened many times.

One time he parked in an isolated area and played with me and made me touch him and kiss his penis. He tried to coax me to have intercourse. He told me it wouldn't hurt. But I cried and he masturbated into his handkerchief instead. Like most abuse victims, I was sworn to secrecy. He always bought me things or gave me money. I remember the day he died. I came home from school and when my mom told me, I cried. But deep down I was glad. I was really safe from him now. And I hated him for hurting me and making me lie all the time."

Adult survivors may believe they are only sex objects, to be used and abused by others. Some have a very strong aversion to sex and are filled with terror in sexual situations. Some are sexually inhibited and experience discomfort with sexual thoughts, feelings, and behaviors. Some engage in compulsive sexual behavior, perhaps as an unconscious way to validate their shame and guilt, or as a way to feel powerful. Many adult survivors go through a period of celibacy as they try to manage fear, anger, and distrust.

Confusion about sexuality is very common among male survivors. Sexual victimization of a male, by a male, carries a hidden implication that the victim is less than a man. Heterosexual survivors fear that the abuse has made, or will make, them homosexual. Intense homophobia and/or hypermasculine behavior may be an effort to disprove their fears. Gay survivors worry that their sexual preference may have caused the abuse. It must be remembered that childhood sexual abuse is not related to adult sexual orientation.

Some adult survivors engage in **self-mutilation**, as in cutting, slashing, or burning themselves. It is important to understand the meaning of such behavior. For some, the pain of self-mutilation proves their existence and reassures them that they are alive and real. Self-mutilation may be a plea for nurturance, as they come to the emergency department seeking care. Others nurture themselves by cleaning up the wounds after self-mutilation. For those who dissociate, self-mutilation may be a way to stop the dissociation with physical pain. Others self-mutilate as a form of self-punishment and a way to decrease guilt feelings. And finally, some self-mutilate as a way to reduce emotional pain through the feeling of physical pain. It is important to understand the function of the behavior in order to replace it with healthier behaviors that satisfy the same need.

False Memory Syndrome

The recently formed False Memory Syndrome Foundation (FMSF) is made up of adults who say that they have been falsely accused of sexually abusing their children; they believe that their children's memories are the product of suggestive therapy. If a person who is in therapy has no memories of abuse, but through the process of therapy comes to believe that abuse caused the present symptoms, it is very easy for that person to imagine memories. Some professionals who work with accused perpetrators of childhood sexual abuse believe that most repressed and now "recovered" memories are false memories implanted by overeager, undertrained therapists. Lief (1994) lists the following reasons a person may believe his or her memories of sexual abuse:

- To punish someone else.
- To punish oneself.
- To have a single explanation for current problems.
- To avoid blame.
- To attract attention.
- To explain self-injurious behavior.
- Suggestibility from self-help groups.

In the past several years, the FMSF has grown rapidly through advertising and media coverage. It now claims to represent 13,000 families that have been destroyed by false accusations of sexual abuse. However, the fine print reveals that the 13,000 families are not documented cases of false memories but in fact represent all the people who have ever contacted the foundation for more information. Even if all 13,000 adults were falsely accused, that number would only account for less than 1% of parents accused of sexual abuse (Perry 1994). For a more thorough discussion, see the Mind-Body-Spirit box in Chapter 4.

Biopsychosocial Theories

There is no single cause of childhood sexual abuse. Rather, the abuse results from a combination of personality and family factors.

Intrapersonal Theory

There are many types of perpetrators of sexual abuse of children. Some traits are contradictory, and there is no agreement on a composite personality. Certain characteristics apply to many people, not just abusers. The descriptions are guidelines for assessment, not proof that the person actually committed sexual abuse.

Abusers usually have low self-esteem and feel more secure in interactions with children than with adults. Some were emotionally deprived as children and thus have a great need for constant, unconditional love, which is more easily obtained from children than from adults. Some perpetrators are described as lacking impulse control and the ability to experience feelings of guilt. Others are described as rigid and overcontrolled, while others are dominant and aggressive.

If perpetrators were sexually abused themselves as children, they may have learned to associate all feelings of love with sexual behavior. Most people who were sexually abused as children do *not* go on to sexually abuse others. However, some victimized children develop offending behavior in late childhood, adolescence, or adulthood. Most likely, there are a number of factors involved in why some abuse and others do not. The world of abuse is comprised only of victims (powerless) and perpetrators (powerful). Victims become perpetrators in an unconscious attempt to master the trauma of their own experiences and take over the power. The move from victim to offender may also result when anger and hostility concerning the past are externalized and projected onto new victims (Higgs, Canavan, and Meyer 1992).

Family Systems Theory

Intrafamily sexual abuse most typically occurs in families who have difficulty with cohesion and adaptability. Families who are enmeshed, that is, the members are immersed in and absorbed by other another, may be at risk for sexual abuse. In addition, incestuous families tend to be either rigid or chaotic in their adaptability. Rigid family systems have strict rules and stereotyped gender-role expectations, with minimal emotional interaction. Children have no power and authority, even over their own bodies. They are not allowed to question or protest inappropriate sexual behavior. In contrast, chaotic family systems have either no rules or constantly changing rules. Within the chaotic system, there may be no assigned roles or no rules regarding appropriate sexual behavior, which may contribute to the incidence of sexual abuse (Gilbert 1993).

Communication patterns within the family system may contribute to the occurrence of sexual abuse. Incest depends on keeping the secret within the family. In family systems that avoid conflict, accusations of sexual abuse are not tolerated. Peace, and therefore silence, must be kept at all costs. (See Chapter 32 for a complete discussion of family dynamics.)

The Nursing Process and Intrafamily Sexual Abuse

A case study and nursing care plan for an adult survivor of childhood sexual abuse accompanies this section.

Assessment

It is vitally important that you acknowledge the reality of childhood sexual abuse. Nurses who deny the existence of the problem will miss the cues and fail to complete a detailed assessment. If you are knowledgeable about the incidence and the characteristics of the problem, you will be alert for cues that demand nursing assessment. Guidelines for assessment are given in the two Assessment boxes on pages 577 and 578.

When assessing children, remember that some will exhibit most of the characteristics presented in this chapter, others will exhibit only some, and still others will exhibit none of the characteristics. Also remember that these same behavioral, affective, and cognitive characteristics may be symptoms of other emotional problems. Once it has been discovered that one child in a family is a victim of sexual abuse, suspect the abuse of siblings, both boys and girls, as well. Sometimes entire families are sexually abused before someone "tells."

You must appreciate the power of secrecy and how difficult it is for adult survivors to disclose such information, especially for men, who, in our society, are expected to be anything other than victimized. Routine questions on nursing histories may provide an opportunity for survivors to share their pain and obtain treatments as adults.

As a nurse, you are responsible for initiating the topic. Shame and confusion may keep the adult survivor from doing so. If you avoid the topic, you will be contributing to pathology by supporting the client's denial of reality. Failure to initiate a discussion of sexual abuse sends a message to clients that such abuse does not occur or does not matter. Now that childhood sexual abuse has been identified as a major health problem, nurses in every clinical setting must be alert for cues from both individuals and families.

When working with adult survivors, you must continuously assess the client's comfort level with the physical setting. Closed doors will increase anxiety in some clients, while others will request that doors never remain open. Some will be uncomfortable in a room witha couch or a bed rather than chairs. How close you sit can be an issue for some clients. Even normally appropriate physical contact, such as a handshake, may increase anxiety. Always ask permission before touching a client.

Nursing Diagnosis

Based on assessment data, nursing diagnoses are formulated for the individual child victim, the family members, and/or the adult survivor. Possible diagnoses for the child victim include:

- Ineffective Individual Coping related to being a victim of sexual abuse.
- Powerlessness related to being a victim of sexual abuse.
- Post-Trauma Response related to being a victim of sexual abuse.
- Social Isolation related to keeping the family secret of sexual abuse.

For families that are experiencing sexual abuse, some possible diagnoses are:

- Ineffective Family Coping, Disabling, related to a child being sexually abused.
- Ineffective Family Coping, Disabling, related to an enmeshed family system that is either rigid or chaotic.
- Altered Parenting related to being a perpetrator of sexual abuse.
- Altered Family Process related to disruption of the family unit when abuse is discovered.

For adult survivors of childhood sexual abuse, some possible diagnoses are:

- Post-Trauma Response related to being an adult survivor.
- Spiritual Distress related to asking questions about fairness and justice in life or not being protected by a supreme being.
- Chronic Low Self Esteem related to self-blame for the abuse.
- Ineffective Denial related to amnesia for childhood events.
- Social Isolation related to difficulty in forming intimate relationships, mistrust of others.
- Sexual Dysfunction related to the trauma of abuse.
- Risk for Injury related to being revictimized as an adult.

ASSESSMENT

Physical Assessment of the Sexual Abuse Victim

Complete a head-to-toe physical assessment with emphasis on the following:

Weight and nutritional status

Throat irritation

Gag reflex

Episodes of vomiting

Abdominal pain near diaphragm

Smears of the mouth, throat, vagina, and rectum for sexually transmitted infections

Genital irritation or trauma

Rectal irritation or trauma

Chronic vaginal infections

Chronic urinary tract infections

Pregnancy

Planning and Implementing Interventions

The first priority of care with child victims is to *ensure the safety of the child.* Nurses are mandated by law to report any suspected child sexual abuse. Protective services will implement one of four plans if the abuse is occurring within the family system:

1. The most frequent option is when the abuser is removed from the family. The nonabusing parent must protect the child from any contact with the abuser.
2. When the nonabusing parent is unable to protect the child, both the child and the abuser are removed from the home. This option maximizes the child's safety and decreases the child's feelings of responsibility.
3. In a few cases where families have not used physical violence, where there is no substance abuse, and there is someone who can ensure the child's safety, the family may be allowed to remain intact while participating in intensive therapy.
4. In a few instances, the child may be removed from the family when that is the safest option. Unfortunately, this decision may place additional guilt on the child.

When families are enmeshed and either rigid or chaotic, help family members move to a *moderate position between the extremes.* With a rigid family, problem-solve ways in which the members can increase their flexibility of roles and rules. With a chaotic family, problem-solve ways to organize appropriate roles and formulate consistent rules. Throughout this approach, teach the family the problem-solving process.

Facilitate the child's ability to talk and to think about the abuse with decreasing anxiety. Create a safe and predictable environment in which the child feels supported. Make it clear to the child that you understand that talking about the abuse is difficult.

Plan interventions that will encourage affective release in a supportive environment. Child victims must be able to experience a range of emotions. *Play therapy* helps these children play out traumatic themes, fears, and distorted beliefs. It is a nonthreatening way to process thoughts and feelings associated with the abuse, both symbolically and directly. *Art therapy* provides an opportunity to express feelings for which there are no words. *Therapeutic stories* present the traumatic issues of abuse, link victims' feelings and behavior, and describe new coping methods. *Journal writing* can help children over age 10 cope with intrusive thoughts and feelings. They often choose to bring their journal into the one-to-one sessions with their therapist.

ASSESSMENT

Nursing History Tool for Assessment of Individuals and Families for Intrafamily Sexual Abuse

Behavioral Assessment

Individual Child

Have there been any signs of regressive behavior in the child?

Is the child having sleeping problems?

Is the child exhibiting clinging behavior to the parents or others?

Does the child have friendships with other children?

Has there been any sexual acting-out on the part of the child?

Has the child ever run away or threatened to run away?

Has the child ever attempted suicide?

Perpetrator

Describe how discipline is handled in the family.

Do you see yourself as the dominant person in the family?

At what age do you believe parents should give up control of their children?

How many adult friends do you have?

Describe your relationships with these friends.

Describe your relationship with your spouse.

What kinds of sexual difficulties are you and your spouse experiencing?

When you were young, who was the closest family member with whom you had any sexual activity?

Family System

Describe who has responsibility (mother, father, both parents, or children) in the following areas of home management:

- Caring for the younger children
- Cooking
- Cleaning
- Paying bills
- Shopping
- Outside home maintenance
- Budget planning
- Decisions about leisure time
- Supervising children's homework
- Taking children to activities
- Putting children to bed

Who are the best communicators in the family?

Who talks to whom the most?

Who is unable to talk to whom very much?

How are secrets kept from one another within the family?

How are secrets prevented from leaking outside the family?

Affective Assessment

Individual Child

How helpless does the child feel about changing any of the family's problems?

In what way is the child responsible for family problems?family?

Does the child get enough love within the family?

Practice feminist-sensitive therapy. Because the process of sexual abuse is disempowering, it is important to empower survivors. The focus on *traumatic stress therapy* treats the trauma while acknowledging the process and result of victimization. *Developmental therapy* focuses on the "gaps" in the personality that occurred during the abusive process such as trust issues, identity issues, and relationship issues. *Loss therapy* focuses on helping the survivors identify and grieve over the things that they have lost during their childhood sexual abuse such as innocence, trust, nurturing, and memories.

In working with adult survivors, remember that they

ASSESSMENT *(continued)*

Is the child more loved than the other children in the family?

Ask about the fears the child may have if any family secrets are told:

- Fears of not being believed
- Fears of being blamed for the problems
- Fears that your parents will not love you
- Fears that you will be moved to a foster home
- Fears that your parents will be taken away
- Fears of physical abuse

Perpetrator

Who loves you most within the family?

Who is able to give you unconditional support and affection?

How do you see yourself responsible for family problems?

How does fear of failure affect your life?

Family System

Describe the emotional relationships among family members.

Does everybody know each family member's business?

How is privacy protected within the family?

Do you have any fears of the family unit disintegrating?

What will happen if the family is separated?

Cognitive Assessment

Individual Child

Tell me about your nightmares.

How would you describe the family's problems?

What effect do these problems have on you?

What effect do these problems have on the rest of the family?

Who do you believe is responsible for these problems?

Perpetrator

Describe what kind of a person you are.

What are your personal strengths?

What are your personal limitations?

Describe how you handle new situations.

Do you enjoy changing situations?

Family System

Who sets the family rules?

Tell me about the most important family rules.

How do rules get changed within the family?

What are the expectations of the males in the family?

What are the expectations of the females in the family?

Sociocultural Assessment

What significant events have occurred for your family in the past year?

What support systems do you have outside the family?

How often do you visit with friends?

Who are the problem drinkers in the family?

How is the issue of drugs managed within the family?

have been robbed of a sense of power and feel detached from others. Recovery includes *restoring power and control.* Be sure to avoid becoming a "rescuer," as that might send the message that clients are not capable of acting for themselves. Also be careful not to set yourself up as a powerful authority because that might recreate the type of relationship in which the abuse occurred. The most helpful approach is being ally, collaborator, and supporter as clients struggle through the healing process. Point out ways they have taken control of their lives, and help them identify situations in which they are able to make self-respecting choices..

CASE STUDY

An Adult Survivor of Childhood Sexual Abuse

Identifying Information

Jill is a 35-year-old woman who is a full-time homemaker. Her husband, John, is president of an advertising firm. Jill and John have been married for 15 years and have three children, ages 14, 12, and 7.

Client's Description of the Problem

Jill was sexually abused by her grandfather from a very young age until about 11 or 12 years of age. At times, the grandfather would involve Jill's brother, who is three years older, by forcing Jill and her brother to have sex for the grandfather's enjoyment. She states that she told her mother about the abuse when she was 9 or 10 but that her mother just ignored it. Her mother now denies that Jill told her about the abuse when it was occurring. Jill has tried to ignore her abuse history until several months ago when she saw a television program about incest. She alternates between being immobilized with depression and filled with rage at her parents and grandfather.

Psychiatric History

No prior psychiatric history.

Family History

Jill was born and raised in Ohio and is the third child of five in an intact family. Jill describes her mother as "strict . . . she would threaten by saying 'wait until your dad comes home.'" When asked about her father, Jill states "He wasn't around . . . he was working . . . he was always distant." She describes the family communication as "dysfunctional; only certain people talk to certain other people. For example, none of us kids could talk directly to our father. We always had to go through our mother."

Social History

Jill describes herself as a "homebody." In the past, she attended social functions with her husband as necessitated by his employment position. These functions were not a great source of pleasure for her, however. Lately, she has had no desire to participate in any activities outside the home. She states that she has never had close friends. Her only friend is her husband, and she feels somewhat intimidated by him. She has a very close relationship with her children.

Health History

Jill has no current or past medical problems. She states she is in good health except for feeling "terribly depressed right now."

→

Support the client's *spiritual recovery.* Betrayal by abusing adults is a spiritual issue. As nurses, we sometimes ignore a client's need for spiritual healing. Victims and survivors are consumed with spiritual questions like "Why did it happen to me?" "What's wrong with me?" and "Am I some evil person?" When people are sexually abused, they must struggle with questions of a God who either overlooked their pain and did not respond or did not even see their pain at all. Questions arise, such as "What's wrong with God?" and "Why didn't God stop it?" It is not unusual for survivors to be angry with God and hold God responsible for the abuse. This anger may in turn trigger fear and guilt for hating someone so powerful.

To recover from sexual abuse, survivors must place responsibility for the abuse where it belongs—100% with the offender. If they fail to do this, they will continue to be paralyzed by self-blame and guilt. The adult self needs to reach out and care for the hurt inner child by breaking down the walls that have isolated that child. Fully experiencing the rage and grief enables the survivor to move on to self-forgiveness and more complete healing. Spirituality includes a sense of connectedness to others. Survivors must begin the long journey of developing trusting relationships. They need to experience human contact and the warmth of the nurse-client relationship. When requested, refer clients to religious counselors who understand the emotional issues surrounding sexual abuse and who are sensitive to the need of survivors to work slowly through their spiritual struggles.

Design interventions to *increase self-esteem.* Adult survivors have a continuous internal monologue of negative statements like "You're weak, stupid, incompetent, unlovable, and unattractive." Negative statements become self-administered abuse and keep the survivor weak and powerless. Help clients become aware of the frequency and intensity of these negative thoughts. Teach them to con-

CASE STUDY (continued)

Current Mental Status

Jill is oriented to person, place, and time. Her affect appears dysphoric, irritable, and constricted in range. At times she is filled with rage, saying "I am mad . . . mad at the world in general and at having to deal with all of this." She states that during her entire life she has spent much of her energy in "not thinking," "not imagining," and "not remembering" the abuse. She has attempted to keep a sense of distance and alienation from her inner emotional life. After viewing a televised program on incest, she now experiences "painful, bitter, brooding thoughts about the abuse." Jill is a depressed, anxious, and angry woman with extremely low self-esteem and intense feelings of inadequacy. On one hand she views herself as unable to function in an autonomous, self-directed, and self-reliant fashion. Yet she sees the world as untrustworthy, betraying, and often cruel. Unable to rely on her own resources or depend on the support of others, Jill feels a sense of bitter futility and resignation. She identifies herself as a victim who is inevitably betrayed and disappointed. Many of her dynamics are consistent with adult survivors of sexual abuse. There is an intense rage at her parents for being unsupportive, unprotective, and unable to provide Jill with an inner sense of safety and security in herself and the world around her. This contributes to Jill's fear of autonomy and her conflict between her need to depend on others and her intense mistrust of the sincerity and commitment that others can offer. There is no evidence of psychotic illness or of a manifest thought disturbance.

Other Subjective or Objective Clinical Data

Jill states that she needs more emotional support from her husband. Her husband states that he cannot give it to her lately because he is often irritated because the house is messy and dirty. She thinks he is being perfectionistic. He has offered to hire someone to help, but Jill sees that as another failure on her part.

Diagnostic Impression

Nursing Diagnoses

Post-Trauma Response
Social Isolation
Altered Role Performance

DSM-IV Multiaxial Diagnosis

Axis I:	300.4 Dysthymic disorder
Axis II:	301.6 Dependent personality disorder
Axis III:	No medical problems
Axis IV:	Victim of childhood sexual abuse
Axis V:	GAF=60 (current)

sciously replace negative thoughts with positive ones. Often difficult at first, it becomes easier with practice.

Because adult survivors are often anxious, interventions to *reduce anxiety* are also necessary. Clients who learn progressive relaxation and controlled breathing are often able to avoid full-blown panic attacks. Teach the process, and talk clients through the stages of relaxation until they are able to reduce anxiety by themselves. When they are relaxed, instruct them to imagine a scene in which they feel safe and comfortable. Any time they need to, they can return to this safe scene where they are in total control. Daily practice facilitates the usefulness of these techniques.

Art therapy helps adults in the healing process. Making group murals to express both individual progress and a sense of unity among clients can be very effective. *Music therapy*, combined with movement or dance, may be a way for clients to experience very early memories. *Journal writing* is used more than any other expressive therapy and can be expanded to include poetry, songs, and plays.

Group therapy allows survivors to share their feelings and experiences with others who believe their stories. The group setting fosters mutual understanding and decreases the sense of isolation. Many adult survivors find *self-help groups* to be very supportive in the process of healing.

Evaluation and Outcome Criteria

Nurses in acute care settings may not have the opportunity for long-term evaluation. Short-term evaluation focuses mainly on identifying child victims and adult survivors and referrals to appropriate community resources.

Nurses in long-term or community settings can evaluate the effectiveness of the treatment plan over an extended period. Questions to guide the evaluation of the child victim and family include the following:

NURSING CARE PLAN

An Adult Survivor of Childhood Sexual Abuse

Nursing Diagnosis

Post-Trauma Response related to being an adult survivor of incest.

Expected Outcome

Client will resolve associated anger and anxiety.

Nursing Interventions

- Discuss feelings of guilt. Repeat often that children are never responsible for the incest but rather the grandfather is totally responsible.
- Discuss feelings of anger toward the grandfather and anger toward the parents for not protecting the client.
- Explore childhood abuse issues that led to feelings of inadequacy.
- Connect feelings of low self-esteem to feelings of guilt and anger.
- Assign client to keep a journal about her thoughts, feelings, and memories.
- Help her identify and grieve over things lost in childhood, such as innocence and trust.
- Teach anxiety-reducing techniques such as muscle relaxation, deep breathing, and physical exercise.

Outcome Met If

- Client verbalizes decreased rumination about the abuse.
- Client verbalizes decreased anger.
- Client discharges the energy of anger appropriately.
- Client uses relaxation techniques.
- Client verbalizes increased trust in others.

Nursing Diagnosis

Social Isolation related to withdrawal and decreased desire to interact with others.

Expected Outcome

Client will increase interactions with people outside the family.

Nursing Interventions

- Help client identify the benefits of social interaction.
- Help client identify a variety of available supportive people.
- Give positive feedback when client expresses an interest in or engages in interactions with others.
- Provide assertiveness training.
- Provide information on self-help groups for adult survivors where she can share with others and establish trusting relationships.
- Refer for group therapy where members are able to identify with others' feelings of anger, anxiety, and isolation.

Outcome Met If

- Client contacts support persons.
- Client joins a self-help group.
- Client participates in group therapy.
- Client initiates relationships outside of family.

Nursing Diagnosis

Altered Role Performance related to apathetic and dysphoric mood.

Expected Outcome

Client will be able to fulfill her role responsibilities as homemaker.

Nursing Interventions

- Help client identify her own and her husband's expectations about role performance.
- Discuss impact on self and other family members when she is unable to fulfill role responsibilities.
- Help client assess self realistically and set appropriate goals.
- Help client identify new functions and purposes in life.
- Provide feedback for changes she makes.

Outcome Met If

- Client sets realistic goals for self.
- Client maintains positive changes.
- Client expresses satisfaction over chosen role performances.

- Has the child remained safe from further harm?
- Has the child returned to functioning at an appropriate developmental level?
- Is the child able to express feelings either verbally or through play or art therapy?
- Is the child verbalizing decreasing feelings of guilt and/or responsibility?
- Is the child developing peer friendships?
- Has the family structure become more flexible?
- Is communication more open within the family?

As a nurse, you have the opportunity to influence the care of adult survivors of childhood sexual abuse. Explain to others that the survivors' behavior is a posttrauma response that makes sense as an adaptation to trauma and perhaps a dysfunctional family. Intervene if staff members recreate the dynamics of the abusive relationship by assuming a position of power and control. It is very rewarding to share the growth of clients toward making self-respecting choices in their lives. Questions to guide the evaluation of adult survivors include the following:

- Has the person remained safe from further harm in adult relationships?
- Is the client able to talk about the childhood trauma? If not, is art therapy, music therapy, movement therapy, or journal writing effective in facilitating expression?
- Is the client able to identify situations in which he or she has been able, or hopes to be able, to make self-respecting choices?
- Is the client verbalizing increased spiritual comfort regarding the trauma?
- Is the client verbalizing less self-blame?
- Is the client verbalizing improved self-image?
- Is there evidence that the client is able to develop trusting and respectful relationships with adults?

Although, as a culture, we say that we protect our children, we do not in reality live out this value. We do not invest many of our energies—time, caring , and money—in the prevention of childhood sexual abuse. Our present approaches to treatment and to the social control of sexual abuse are not yet effective enough that we can be assured of the long-term safety of children. As nurses, we must all become active in the battle to stop childhood sexual abuse.

Chapter Highlights

- Rape is a crime of violence perpetrated against innocent victims of all ages and both sexes.
- Rape victims may use the defense mechanisms of depersonalization or dissociation to cope with the attack. Often victims respond with agitation, shock, disbelief, and fear.
- Physiologic consequences include trauma and injuries, pregnancy, STIs, and difficulties with sexual functioning.
- Most theorists agree that rape is a crime of violence generated by issues of power and anger. Theories relating to rape include revenge, dominance, eroticized assault, gang rituals, inadequate relationships, acceptance of violence within a culture, and sexist cultural values.
- Although the image of the ideal American family is one of happiness and harmony, in reality there is a great deal of domestic abuse and violence.
- Nurses are required by law to report suspected incidents of child abuse.
- Victims may be immobilized by anxiety, helplessness, depression, self-blame, and guilt. Multiple fears contribute to the victim's inability to leave the relationship.
- Theories relating to intrafamily physical abuse include genetic-environmental, personality, transgenerational, learned behavior, and sexism links.
- Sexual abuse occurs in all ethnic, religious, economic, and cultural subgroups in the United States.
- Adult perpetrators believe in extreme restrictiveness and domination. They often feel weak, afraid, and inadequate. They use secrecy and silence to escape accountability. If confronted by others, they will often deny the abuse.
- Child victims are at the mercy of adult perpetrators. Some become extremely affectionate, while others have problems with impulse control and aggression toward others. They may act out sexually with other children or adults.
- There is no single cause of childhood sexual abuse. Perpetrators may lack impulse control, or they may be rigid and overcontrolled or dominant and aggressive.

References

Baldacci L: State ranks near worst, but deaths drop in '92. *Chicago Sun-Times*, April 17, 1993.

Bean CA: *Women Murdered by the Men They Loved.* Haworth Press, 1992.

Birns B, Cascardi M, Meyer SL: Sex-role socialization: Developmental influences on wife abuse. *Am J Orthopsychiatr* 1994;64(1):50–59.

Brown SL: *Counseling Victims of Violence.* American Association of Counseling Development, 1991.

Browne A: Family violence and homelessness. *Am J Orthopsychiatr* 1993;63(3):370–384.

Campbell JCP: Violence against women. *Nurs & Health Care* 1992;13(9):464–470.

Elliott DM, Briere J: The sexually abused boy: Problems in manhood. *Med Aspects Human Sex* 1992;26(2):68–71.

Ellis GM: Acquaintance rape. *Perspect Psychiatr Care* 1994; 30(1):11–16.

Ellis L: *Theories of Rape.* Hemisphere, 1989.

Gelles RT, Cornell CP: *Intimate Violence in Families*, ed 2. Sage, 1990.

Gilbert CM: Intrafamily child sexual abuse, in Fawcett CS (ed): *Family Psychiatric Nursing.* Mosby, 1993.

Glod CA: Long-term consequences of childhood physical and sexual abuse. *Arch Psychiatr Nurs* 1993;7(3):163–173.

Hall LA, et al.: Childhood physical and sexual abuse: Their relationship with depressive symptoms in adulthood. *Image* 1993;25(4):317–323.

Higgs DC, Canavan MM, Meyer WJ: Moving from defense to offense: The development of an adolescent female sex offender. *J Sex Res* 1992;29(1):131–139.

Holmes RM: *Sex Crimes*. Sage, 1991.

Island D, Letellier P: *Men Who Beat the Men Who Love Them: Battered Gay Men and Domestic Violence*. Haworth Press, 1991.

Koss MP, Harvey MR: *The Rape Victim*, ed 2. Sage, 1991.

Kotulak R: Tracking down the monster within: Genes of aggression found. *Chicago Tribune*, December 12, 1993.

Krueger MM: Pregnancy as a result of rape. *J Sex Ed Theory* 1988;14(1):23–27.

Lief HI: Recovered memories and therapy abuse. *Contemporary Sexuality* 1994;28(6):4–7.

McCurdy K, Daro D: Child maltreatment. *J Interpersonal Violence* 1994;9(1):75–94.

Mezey GC, King MB: *Male Victims of Sexual Assault*. Oxford University Press, 1992.

Nevid JS, et al.: *Human Sexuality in a World of Diversity*, ed 2. Allyn and Bacon, 1995.

O'Campo P, et al.: Verbal abuse and physical violence among a cohort of low-income pregnant women. *Women's Health Issues* 1994;4(1):29–37.

O'Leary KD, Vivian D: Physical aggression in marriage, in Fincham FD, Bradbury TN (eds): *The Psychology of Marriage*. Guilford Press, 1990.

O'Toole AW, O'Toole R, Webster S, Lucal B: Nurses' responses to child abuse. *J Interpersonal Violence* 1994;9(2):194–205.

Perry JD: On repressed memories. *Contemporary Sexuality* 1994;28(6):5–9.

Rothblum ED, Cole E: *Lesbianism: Affirming Nontraditional Roles*. Haworth Press, 1989.

Russell DE: *Rape in Marriage*, ed 2. Indiana University Press, 1990.

Ryder D: *Breaking the Circle of Satanic Ritual Abuse*. CompCare, 1992.

Sengstock MC, Barrett S: Domestic abuse of the elderly, in Campbell J, Humphreys J (eds): *Nursing Care of Victims of Family Violence*. Reston, 1984.

Smolowe J: When violence hits home. *Time*, July 4, 1994:144(1):19–25.

Stacy RD, Prisbell M, Tollefsrud K: A comparison of attitudes among college students toward sexual violence committed by strangers and by acquaintances. *J Sex Ed & Therapy* 1992;18(4):257–263.

Stewart DE, Cecutti A: Physical abuse in pregnancy. *Can Med Assoc J* 1993;149(9):1257–1263.

Stopping Sexual Assault in Marriage. Center for Constitutional Rights, 1986.

Straus MA, Gelles RJ, Steinmetz SK: *Behind Closed Doors: Violence in the American Family*. Anchor Press/Doubleday, 1980.

Uherek AM: Treatment of a ritually abused preschooler, in Friedrich WN (ed): *Casebook of Sexual Abuse Treatment*. Norton, 1991.

Urbancic J, Campbell J, Humphreys J: Student clinical experiences in shelters for battered women. *J Nurs Ed* 1993;32(8):341–346.

Vachss A: *Sex Crimes*. Random House, 1993.

Vanderbilt H: *Incest: A Chilling Report*. Lear's, 1992.

CHAPTER 24

SUICIDE AND SELF-DESTRUCTIVE BEHAVIOR

Elizabeth A. Riley
Carol Ren Kneisl

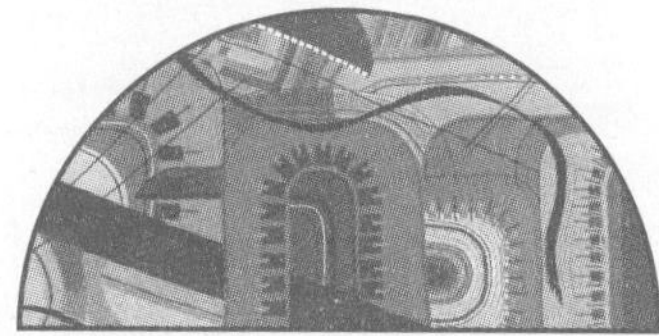

COMPETENCIES

- *Identify social, demographic, and clinical variables that influence suicidal or self-destructive behavior.*
- *Develop a plan for nursing interventions with a suicidal client.*
- *Explain the process of a lethality assessment.*
- *Suggest strategies for intervention with survivors of suicide.*
- *Differentiate among suicidal behavior, indirect self-destructive behavior, and self-destructive behavior.*
- *Discuss why you might feel anxious working with suicidal clients.*

Cross-References

Other topics relevant to this chapter are Stress, anxiety, and coping, Chapter 4; Therapeutic communication, Chapter 7; Advocacy, client rights, and legal issues, Chapter 11; Crisis intervention, Chapter 30; Rape and intrafamily abuse, Chapter 23; Mood disorders, Chapter 15; Ethical reasoning, Chapter 10; Substance abuse, Chapter 13; Stress management, Chapter 29.

Critical Thinking Challenge

It is a common practice on some inpatient units to take away articles of clothing (shoes, jackets, etc.) from clients believed to be a suicide or elopement risk. The rationale commonly cited is that the practice will stop clients who plan to run away or to harm themselves because they won't have the required clothing. Do you agree with this practice? In what way might this treatment philosophy have an impact on clients?

Suicide, the willful act of ending one's life, is a major public health problem in many countries. In the United States, suicide is the eighth leading cause of death across all age groups, the third leading cause of death among adolescents and young adults, and the leading cause of preventable death among older adults (age 60 and over). The rate of suicide for those of all age groups and both sexes in the U.S. is 11.5 per 100,000, and this rate has remained fairly constant since the 1960s (U.S. Bureau of the Census 1993).

Suicide as a response to overwhelming life crises cuts across all cultures, ages, religions, and socioeconomic classes, and it can affect every kind of person. It is conservatively estimated that 300,000 people will attempt suicide each year. However, these statistics are at best estimates of suicide and suicide attempts. No one knows for sure how many deaths that are labeled as accidents are truly suicides. Officials may be pressured not to cite a death as suicide, perhaps because of religious or insurance reasons. Some coroners will not rule a death to be a suicide unless a suicide note is present. Many doctors, families, and hospitals remain reluctant to label a youth or adolescent accident as a suicide.

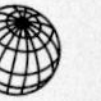

Nurses frequently find themselves face-to-face with suicidal or self-destructive people, and yet few clients elicit such intense feelings of anxiety and helplessness in nurses. The clients below have all considered suicide in the preceding 2 hours.

Sarah, age 17, is a petite brunette cheerleader. She comes to the school nurse stating that she just found out she has been rejected from the college of her choice.

Frank is 68 years old. His wife died last year and his children live two states away. He comes to the family nurse practitioner stating he just "feels sick."

Natalie is a 36-year-old divorced mother of two. She comes into the outpatient clinic stating she has taken thirty-two Valium, 10-mg tablets.

Tom is 24 years old. He is in the emergency room of the hospital and is comatose. He was found that way in his apartment by the landlord. There were bottles and pills all around him.

Purposeful self-destruction has been a part of the human experience since time began. Nurses need to be aware of that fact, because any client in a health care, occupational, or community setting may, under certain circumstances, contemplate suicide. All nurses must be competent to assess and intervene effectively with a suicidal client. It is critically important for nurses to be aware of and examine their own beliefs, values, and attitudes, because those attitudes can either impede or facilitate the methods by which a nurse intervenes with a suicidal client. The idea of suicide arouses intense and complicated emotions in others.

Biopsychosocial Theories

Suicide and self-destructive behavior are not well understood by the public or by the scientific community. (See the accompanying Client/Family Teaching box for a list of suicide myths and facts.) Suicide is a complex phenomenon, and there is no single explanation for its complicated process. There are as many reasons for suicide attempts as there is variation in the profiles of people who do commit suicide.

Theories about suicide are limited in that they do not give a comprehensive overview of all the factors, influences, or conditions that may have an impact on an individual who is considering suicide. Suicidologists (those who study suicide and suicide prevention) have focused on studying all the biopsychosocial factors associated with suicide. They tell us that although there are many reasons why people commit suicide, there are also some commonalities among those who do. The following several factors have been identified as having great significance to those individuals who are suicidal and are useful for the psychiatric mental health nurse to consider when working with suicidal people (Aguilera and Messick 1994; Mann and Arango 1992; Schneidman 1985):

- The meaning and motivation of suicide.
- The cognitive style of the suicidal person.
- Ambivalence and its relationship to suicide prevention.
- Communication and its relationship to self-destructive behavior.
- The importance of the significant other.
- Genetic predisposition.
- Neurochemical factors.

Psychodynamic Theories

Psychodynamic theories focus on the role of aggression and the inner world of the suicidal person. Freud (1964) conceptualized the act of suicide as a conflict between the instinct for life and the wish for death. Suicide occurs when the death wish predominates. Menninger (1938) postulated that the individual turns aggression intended for others inward against the self. This may be not only a reason for suicide but also a way of understanding self-destructive behaviors such as self-mutilation, smoking, eating disorders, and indirect self-destructive behaviors like self-neglect, excessive gambling, and compulsive overeating.

Sociologic Theories

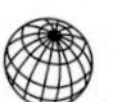

Sociologic theories about suicide propose that the social and cultural contexts in which the individual lives influence the expression of suicidality. Many of the sociologic concepts of suicide follow the initial work of Durkheim (1951), who described four types of suicide:

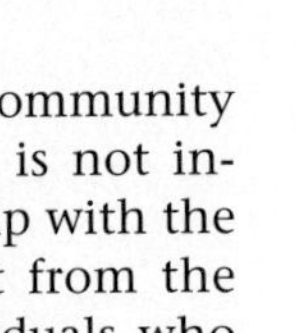

1. *Egoistic suicide.* An individual's ties to the community are too loose or tenuous, and the person is not invested in maintaining his or her relationship with the community. This person does not benefit from the usual social constraint on behavior. Individuals who have no close relationships are more likely to kill themselves.

Gerald had decided that life was not worth living after retiring from his job with the federal government. He realized that no one would even know or care if he succeeded in killing himself. Without family or friends, Gerald had not had a significant relationship since the death of his mother about 20 years ago.

2. *Anomic suicide.* An individual experiences the aloneness or estrangement that occurs when there is a precipitous deterioration in one's relationship with society (such as the loss of a job or a close friend).

CLIENT/FAMILY TEACHING

Suicide Myths Versus Suicide Facts

Myth: A suicide threat is just a bid for attention and should not be taken seriously.

Fact

All suicidal behavior should be taken seriously; a bid for attention may be a cry for help.

Myth: It is harmful for a person to talk about suicidal thoughts. The person's attention should be diverted when this occurs.

Fact

Of prime importance in planning nursing care is an accurate assessment of the lethality of the person's suicide plan.

Myth: Only psychotic people commit suicide.

Fact

The majority of successful suicides are committed by people who are not psychotic.

Myth: People who talk about suicide won't do it.

Fact

Most people do talk about their suicide intention before making a suicide attempt.

Myth: A nice home, good job, or an intact family prevents suicide.

Fact

People of all emotional, social, and economic backgrounds may commit suicide.

Myth: A failed suicide attempt should be treated as manipulative behavior.

Fact

Failed attempts are more likely to be evidence of a person's ambivalence toward suicide.

Myth: People who commit suicide are always depressed.

Fact

People who commit suicide are not always depressed, although depression is common. Also, people can be psychotic, agitated, organically impaired, or have personality disorders.

Myth: Once suicidal, always suicidal.

Fact

Often a suicide attempt is made during a particularly stressful time in one's life. If it is managed properly, people can go on with their lives without recurrent thoughts of suicide.

Myth: There is no connection between alcohol or drug use and suicide.

Fact

Alcohol, drugs, and suicide are often closely connected; a person who commits suicide may have become depressed, impulsive, and suicidal after using alcohol or other drugs.

Myth: Suicidal people rarely seek medical help.

Fact

According to studies, 50–60% of suicidal people sought help within 6 months preceding the suicide.

Danielle thought that suicide was the best way to solve her problems after she lost her job at a local factory, and her boyfriend of 10 years precipitously broke off their engagement, left the area, and remarried.

3. *Fatalistic suicide.* An individual is excessively regulated, or there are no personal freedoms and no hope of getting them.

Jamie, who is a battered woman, decides that at this point it doesn't make any sense to go on living. She has no close friends or relatives. Her husband will not allow her to drive, go shopping, go to work, etc. She is unable to see an alternative and decides that a life regulated to this extent is not worth living.

4. *Altruistic suicide.* Rules or customs demand suicide under certain situations, or self-inflicted death is considered honorable.

In November 1994, in the Gaza Strip, a suicide bomber on a revenge mission detonated explosives strapped to his body

as he rode his bicycle into an Israeli checkpoint, killing himself and three soldiers and wounding several other people. Those who claimed responsibility for the attack indicated that it was in protest of the Israeli presence in Gaza. Shortly afterward, a memorial service held by Islamic militants celebrated his honorable death.

Perhaps the most significant contribution sociologists have made is the understanding that suicide is not only an expression of intrapsychic conflict. Sociologists have been instrumental in reviewing the additional interpersonal, societal, and community components that we now know are critical to the understanding of suicide. Throughout history, the meaning of suicide to a culture has generally reflected the religious beliefs and traditions of that time.

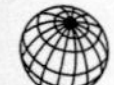

Some early societies forced members to commit suicide during rituals. During some eras, suicide was viewed as an appropriate alternative to military defeat, rape, or being taken hostage. Although suicide was mentioned in the Old Testament, it was not until the sixth century that suicide was viewed as "sinful," and the church refused certain religious rites or privileges, such as burial in sanctified ground or a religious cemetery, to people who committed suicide (Schneidman 1985).

In the fifteenth century, the bodies of people who committed suicide were often dragged through the streets, and their personal property was seized by the church or state. In countries such as India and Japan, suicide was expected of the widows and slaves of husbands or masters who died. In those cases, suicide was an expression of duty and fidelity.

According to Judeo-Christian tradition, life is a gift of God, and the taking of that life is forbidden. This belief is widely held and may account for the decreased rates of suicide in traditionally Jewish or Catholic countries (Israel, Ireland, and Italy). Modern culture and laws reflect society's ambivalence that surrounds this issue. We abhor youth or adolescent suicide and may believe that the person who opts for death over life is weak. At the same time, increasing respect for the individual's rights has led to movements that support suicide as a right of terminally ill clients. For those treating individuals with mental disorders, the question arises: Can suicide be a rational act? Can a person who is mentally ill opt for suicide as a reasonable course? (The overwhelming majority of suicides are individuals who are psychiatrically ill at the time of the suicide.) Although U.S. laws are lenient regarding suicide, suicide is considered a felony in some states.

Biologic Theories

Some promising results of research into the physiologic factors of suicidal behavior are becoming available. Studies of completed suicides suggest a much higher concordance rate for monozygotic twins and dizygotic twins. Later studies examining the biologic relatives of adoptees who committed suicide found a significantly higher incidence of suicide in biologic relatives than in adopted subjects. These results may indicate the possible evidence of a genetic predisposition toward suicidal behavior, although there is no conclusive evidence at this point. During the last decade, numerous studies have evaluated the neurochemical functioning of suicidal clients. Although several neurochemical factors have been investigated, the most promising studies have examined alterations in serotonergic neurotransmission in the central nervous system. These findings may one day yield a biologic work-up for clients who might be at risk for suicide. Future research needs to focus on the identification and prediction of suicidal behavior in individuals who possess a clustering of demographic, clinical, and biologic high-risk variables.

Direct and Indirect Self-Destructive Behavior

Self-destructive behavior is action by which people emotionally, socially, and physically damage or end their lives (Hoff 1989). Typical self-destructive behaviors include, but are not limited to, biting one's nails, pulling one's hair, scratching or cutting one's wrist, smoking cigarettes, driving recklessly, drinking alcohol, and using drugs. In general, these behaviors range from relatively innocuous acts at one end of the continuum, such as overeating and gambling, to more lethal ones at the other, such as driving recklessly in a blinding snowstorm.

A completed suicide is the most violent self-destructive behavior. In addition to completed suicide, there are three varying levels of self-destructive behavior:

- **Chronic self-destructive behavior:** behavior that harms the self; may be chronic or habitual and generally poses a low level of lethality to the individual. Behaviors may include smoking, gambling, substance abuse, and self-mutilation.
- **Suicide threat:** a threat that is more serious than a casual statement of suicidal intent and that is accompanied by other behavior changes. These may include mood swings, temper outbursts, a decline in school or work performance, personality changes, sudden or gradual withdrawal from friends, and other significant changes in attitude.
- **Suicide attempt:** a desperate call for help involving different levels of risk. It may be an attempt planned to avoid serious injury, or it may be an attempt in which the outcome depends on the circumstances and is not under the person's control. For example, someone who takes a heavy overdose of sleeping pills may or may not be discovered in time.

People who are self-destructive may manifest several of the behaviors listed above. For example, people who are chronically self-destructive may also make suicide attempts or complete suicides. This section focuses on chronic self-destructive behavior that is not highly lethal or imminently suicidal. Completed suicides, suicide attempts, and suicide threats are discussed in greater detail later in the chapter.

According to Van der Kolk (1988), people who are chronically self-destructive share these common family characteristics:

- Prior family history or tendency.
- Early trauma.
- Rigid, disorganized, or dysfunctional family system.
- Disturbed parent-child relationship.
- Unresolved loss.
- History of abuse.

Van der Kolk (1988) posits the possibility that the self-destructive behavior of self-mutilation is related to early childhood abuse or neglect and trauma. It may have a physiologic component. Elevations of endorphin levels have been reported following stress, surgery, gambling, and marathon running. Another study indicates the possibility that metenkephalins are elevated in some who habitually mutilate themselves (Coid, Allolio, and Rees 1983). No single theory or scientific study explains why some people are self-destructive.

Self-destructive people under stress perceive themselves as having very limited options. They tend to select self-destructive behaviors because these behaviors make the most sense to them, and these behaviors relieve them, at least temporarily, of their acute discomfort.

It is important to understand that not all self-destructive individuals intend to kill themselves. In fact, self-destructive behaviors are often maladaptive measures a person uses to restore inner equilibrium when overwhelmed or extremely stressed. People who have experienced early childhood neglect, abuse, or trauma frequently have difficulty understanding how to process feelings verbally and how to intervene in situations in a productive fashion—that is, to avoid problems. They often find themselves overwhelmed and unable to cope with stressful life events. Many of these individuals have learned to use self-destructive behaviors—such as cutting, burning with cigarettes, burning on a stove, pulling out one's hair, biting one's fingernails into the cuticles, or repeatedly purging—to deal with anxiety and distress. Self-destructive individuals do not see the behaviors as particularly problematic until it gets out of control. These clients feel that the experience of the painful behavior helps change or improve their mood and their level of awareness, thereby enabling them to reconnect with themselves. Clients who are self-destructive perceive their painful behavior as being adaptive and helpful to them in dealing with their anxiety and distress.

However, this does not mean that people who attempt to hurt themselves in these ways are never at risk for suicide. Approximately 10% of those who injure themselves will go on to kill themselves. Below are clinical examples of individuals involved in self-destructive behavior that should not be considered lethal.

Katy, 29 years old, has had trouble adjusting and being a part of things since "as far back as she remembers." She has no idea how to effectively manage her life problems and her feelings of increasing stress. She often cuts her abdomen or her arms to release stress. Katy is quick to point out that this is in no way a plan to kill herself. Rather, it helps relieve tension and changes her perspective.

Josie, age 33, is a compulsive overeater and manages anxiety by literally eating nonstop. Since she has been trying to lose weight, she now pulls out her hair (a different type of self-destructive behavior) to manage internal feelings of increasing stress and discomfort. Her hair is starting to fall out more readily, and she has required several haircuts to keep her hair looking appropriate while she continues to go to work.

Indirect self-destructive behavior may injure one's health and hasten one's own sometimes premature death. The goal of the behavior distinguishes direct from indirect self-destruction. When the primary conscious goal of the behavior is self-injury, the term *direct self-destructive behavior* is accurate. Suicide is its most extreme form. In *indirect self-destructive behavior,* self-injury is an undesired effect rather than the primary conscious goal.

The exact reason for indirect self-destructive behavior is unknown, although there is much speculation about it. Several interpretations are possible. For example, indirect self-destructive behavior may help people deny mental pain or cope with it, thus avoiding helpless depression. Indirect self-destructive behavior may also result from impulsivity in people who are unable or unwilling to consider the long-term effects of their behavior. Another possibility is that indirect self-destructive behavior is a coping mechanism that raises low self-esteem by denying helplessness. A self-punishing act tends to relieve unconscious guilt. Taking risks and overcoming them increase self-esteem.

People in crisis often resort to indirect self-destructive behavior in attempts to cope. They may get into fights, drink heavily, overeat, overwork, become preoccupied, and neglect their own health. When asked why they do what they do, clients often report that they have been experiencing or trying to avoid mounting anxiety, racing thoughts, depersonalization, inner rage, or a high level of distress. To work effectively with this group, the nurse must:

- Find out what the self-destructive behavior means at this time to this client.
- Perform a lethality assessment (discussed later in the chapter).
- Consider the possibility of a neurophysiologic component that may respond to medication, and evaluate the client accordingly.
- Help the client cope with dysphoria and loneliness.
- Help the self-destructive client by enlarging his or her repertoire of adaptive coping behaviors.
- Focus on interventions that diminish self-hatred, instill hope, build support, and stabilize the client's lifestyle (Farazza et al. 1989).

The Meaning of and Motivation for Suicide

Suicide is never a random act. Whether committed impulsively or after painstaking consideration, the act has both a message and a purpose. In general, the purpose or reason for suicide is to escape; to end an intolerable situation, crisis, or relationship, such as:

- Escaping a terminal (especially painful) illness.

Helen's lung cancer has metastasized to her bones; any exertion causes spontaneous fractures, and she is in constant pain. She has asked friends, family, and health care workers to help her escape her illness by ending her life.

- Avoiding being a burden to others.

Joan, a widow, fell three times last year and is now in a nursing home. She decided on suicide so that she would no longer be a burden to her family. Joan has not eaten in 7 days.

- Resolving an untenable family situation.

Matt, age 7, attempted to run into the path of a car. He had heard his mother say many times, "If it weren't for you, your Daddy and I would never have broken up." Matt believed that if he were dead, his parents would reunite, thus solving what he believes to be an untenable family situation.

- Resolving an untenable individual situation.

Kathy, age 33, had been admitted for the third time to a psychiatric unit because of suicidal ideation (thoughts of suicide). Michael, her husband, has broken the last two family therapy appointments and went on vacation when she came into the hospital this time. Kathy recognizes that Michael will not be available to her, and can't tolerate the idea of having to look for somebody else. She believes that she is unlovable and will attempt to leave the hospital tonight to finally stop the pain.

- Avoiding punishment or exposure of socially or personally unacceptable behavior.

John, 34, was a successful businessman. Last night, he was charged with drunken driving and vehicular homicide. Horrified that his unacceptable behavior would be exposed, he committed suicide after learning that his picture and the story would be in the morning newspaper.

Cognitive Style

Suicidologists have speculated about the cognitive style (method of thought processing) of clients who commit or attempt suicide. Although there is no single suicidal logic, some cognitive styles predispose to suicidal behavior.

Dichotomous thinking (the belief that there is only an either/or choice) is commonly seen in the suicidal person. The person falls into an imminently suicidal state when death seems the only escape. The thought processing of suicidal clients is generally constricted; that is, people who are suicidal have great difficulty (if they can do it at all) in considering alternatives to their current dilemma. This may be why clients agree to a request even if they have no intention of following through. *Constriction in thought* generally results in the belief that there are only two choices: a magical solution or death. The first nursing task is to maintain the client's safety and provide time and opportunity for discussion of alternatives. The second is to help the client explore other options. See the suggestions in the Research Note.

Ambivalence

People who are considering suicide are divided within themselves. They have two conflicting desires at the same time: to live and to die. To understand the thinking of someone who is acutely suicidal, nurses must understand the concept of **ambivalence.**

Ambivalence accounts for the fact that a suicidal person often takes lethal or near-lethal action but leaves open the possibility for rescue, allowing for the possibility of intervention (Aguilera and Messick 1994). A nurse may avert suicide by recognizing a cry for help (discussed later in the chapter) and intervening appropriately. Failing to intervene and provide life choices increases the person's desperation, and death becomes the more focused choice.

Communication

Many people who are self-destructive have lifelong difficulties communicating their needs to others (Hoff 1989).

RESEARCH NOTE

Citation

Botsis AJ, et al.: Suicide and violence risk: I. Relationship to coping styles. *ACTA Psychiatr Scand* 1994;89: 92–96.

Study Problem/Purpose

Suicidologists point out that individuals who ultimately commit suicide generally have trouble considering alternatives and thinking flexibly, and tend to persist in ineffective ways of solving problems. The overall coping style of the suicidal person is constricted. To date, there is limited empirical work describing particular coping styles commonly used by suicidal individuals. The purpose of this study was to study and identify the specific coping style of suicidal clients and the relationship of suicide and violence risk to these styles.

Methods

Thirty suicidal psychiatric inpatients (13 men and 17 women) were compared with a matched sample of 30 nonsuicidal psychiatric inpatients. A battery of self-report tests measuring suicide risk, violence risk, and coping styles were administered. No client in the control group had reported any history of suicidal and/or violent behavior. All were evaluated within 10 days of their admission; all were willing to participate. Candidates were adults over 18 and under 64, and those without acute severe cognitive impairment. No attempt was made to select subjects belonging to any particular diagnostic category. Each client was interviewed by a psychiatrist regarding the events leading to any suicidal behavior and the reasons for his or her admission. Other variables such as impulsivity and lifetime history of aggression and dimensions of psychopathology (such as depression and anxiety) were also measured.

Findings

Suicidal clients scored higher than subjects in the control group on both the suicide and violence-risk scales and showed a high correlation between the two scales. The control group did not show a correlation between the scales. Suicidal clients scored significantly lower on coping styles of minimization, seeking help, replacement, blame, sublimation, and reversal. Suicidal clients showed significant negative correlations between suicide risk and the coping styles of minimization, replacement, and blame. Coping styles were often predictive of suicide risk and violence in the suicidal group but not in the control group.

Implications

Coping styles can be used to predict the risk of suicide and violence in suicidal, but not nonsuicidal, individuals. This finding adds to the evidence that a person's reactions to stressors and perceptions of stressful events are far more important than the stressful event itself. An important implication for nurses who work with suicidal clients is to focus on an assessment of their coping skills. This study also serves to strengthen the belief that focusing on coping styles may not only be strategic and useful, but may also be critical. A nurse may need to demonstrate to a client how to use these skills. Helping an individual understand, develop, and practice additional coping skills may not only reduce the person's present suicide risk, but may also reduce his or her vulnerability to stressors and suicide in the future.

Some people cannot express their needs or feelings; or, when they do, they do not obtain the results they hope for. For them, suicide becomes a clear and direct, if violent, form of communication.

Suicidal thoughts and plans can almost always be traced back to feelings of hopelessness and helplessness, often as the result of separation from or loss of a significant person, place, or thing. People usually resort to suicide only when they believe there is no other way to express the depth of their despair. Clients feel driven to suicide because they believe they have exhausted all their coping abilities or that they cannot influence the behavior of others.

The message inherent in suicide is often aimed at a specific person, usually the significant other. The significant other's ability to recognize this message is the key to understanding and resolving the suicidal person's unmet need. Interrupting a suicide plan or suicidal thoughts requires hearing, understanding, and responding appropriately to messages of pain, loneliness, and hopelessness.

Intended Effect on Significant Others

Suicide is often thought to be an act, thought, or behavior that exists solely within one person. However, suicidologists believe that suicide is more accurately described as a dyadic event between two unhappy people, motivated by real or perceived rejection, abandonment, guilt, revenge, or pity (Schneidman 1985). Suicide can be better understood if viewed in the context of the relationship between two people: the suicidal person and the significant other. Broadly defined, the significant other can be a spouse, child, boss, landlord, friend, nurse, or other health care worker.

Suicidal people almost always communicate their intent to the significant others before the fact or attempt, although the meaning of the message may not be clear until after the attempt or death. Schneidman (1985) found a clear communication of intent in 80% of cases studied. Suicidologists have learned from such studies that another way to understand suicidal behavior is to look at the intended effect on significant others. A suicide threat or suicide attempt can arouse feelings of sympathy, anger, hostility, anxiety, or desire for connectedness on the part of a significant other, thus altering the current relationship to meet the need of the suicidal person.

The Nursing Process and Self-Destructive Behavior

This section discusses the nursing process for suicidal and self-destructive behavior in general. Specific guidelines for assessing and intervening with special populations—children, adolescents, the elderly, clients with HIV disease, psychiatric clients, and substance abusers—are discussed in the next section.

Assessment

When assessing a suicidal client, be aware of and monitor your own reactions to this potentially life-threatening situation, because your reactions may interfere with your ability to accurately assess the situation. The suicidal client presents a unique challenge and will call on all your resources. You must be able to ask the right questions, as well as manage your own fears and anxieties. Helping a person who not only may not want your assistance, but who wants to deliberately harm or kill himself, is a very complicated process. Most nurses want to help others and preserve life. Suicidal individuals will cause you to question your abilities to do so. Thus, it is critically important to be prepared for all of the emotional reactions—fear, anxiety, anger, and so on—that a suicidal client may evoke in you. Unless you understand them, these reactions may interfere with your ability to establish rapport.

The client will bring many feelings into the interaction. Whether the feeling is anger, fear, anxiety, irritability, or hostility, remember that all emotions need to be tolerated, worked through, and evaluated for a full understanding (Doyle 1990). To assess the suicidal client, you must be compassionate enough to be able to form an effective link. The goal is to encourage the client to see you as an ally. Yet you also need to maintain enough detachment to avoid being overwhelmed by the client's pain.

Effective assessment of a suicidal or self-destructive client requires having an understanding of the social, demographic, and clinical variables that place a person at high risk. Also consider the client's personal and family history, assess current medical and psychiatric status, determine what the individual's assets and liabilities are, and take into account the client's prior response to treatment. The most common variables are listed below.

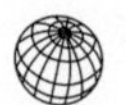

Social Variables Low suicide rates are noted among the following:

- Developing communities and groups in which hope and optimism are high.
- Cultures that are warm and nurturing, such as the Irish, Italian, and Norwegian cultures.
- Communities in which there is strong disapproval of suicide as an act, such as Italy, Spain, and Ireland, where the Catholic Church is highly influential.

High suicide rates are associated with the following:

- Societies in which social unrest, internal governmental problems, or a pessimistic outlook for the future predominate.
- Subcultures that are uncaring and cold and lack concern for people in trouble, such as skid rows and disorganized inner-city areas.
- Societies, such as the United States, Japan, Russia, and Germany, that value independence and individual performance.
- Social roles, occupations, and professions in which people exhibit a high degree of concern and nurturance toward others, such as physicians and police.
- Both ends of the socioeconomic scale.

Demographic Variables Suicide rates are higher among the following:

- Single people (twice the rate of married people).
- Divorced, separated, or widowed people (four to five times the risk of married people).
- People confused about their sexual orientation.
- People who have experienced a recent loss (divorce, loss of a job, loss of prestige, or loss of social status) or who are facing the threat of criminal exposure.
- Caucasians, Eskimos, and Native Americans.
- Protestants or those with no religious affiliation.

CLINICAL VARIABLES Suicide rates are higher among the following:

- People who have attempted suicide before.
- People who have experienced the loss of an important person at some time in the past or the loss of both parents early in life; or the loss of or threat of loss of their spouse, job, money, or social position.
- People who are depressed or recovering from depression or a psychotic episode.
- People with physical illness, particularly when the illness involves an alteration of the person's body image or lifestyle.
- People who abuse alcohol or drugs, especially among people who use two or more substances.
- People who are recovering from a thought disorder combined with depressed mood and/or suicidal ideation (especially those individuals who are experiencing any command hallucinations that tell them to kill or harm themselves or to join someone in the afterlife).

CLUES OR CRIES FOR HELP People intent on suicide almost always give either verbal or nonverbal clues of their plans or ideas. Suicidologists and crisis workers who work with suicidal people believe that people intending self-destruction can make a powerful attempt to communicate to others their hurt and desperation.

Some 75% of those individuals who commit suicide may signal their need for help by making contact with the health care system 3–6 months before the suicide because of various physical complaints (Roberts and McFarland 1986). Unfortunately, this message is not always clear until after the event. Because people do want help, it is important that questions about depression and suicide be asked. Always be alert to patterns that may at first seem coincidental.

A 21-year-old man was referred to a therapist by his physician. Although he described chronic "aches and pains" and "not feeling well," a physical exam revealed no physical problems. He did talk about how life was just not worth living, and he had a recent history of driving recklessly. After further discussion, he said that he had recently broken up with his girlfriend and admitted that his reckless driving had a suicidal intent.

The cry for help may be indirect or subtle. Examples of what a person might say are: "I just can't take it anymore," "There's no reason to go on," "Sometimes I think I'd be better off dead," "I won't be seeing you anymore," "Take care of my dog and cat," "Too bad I won't get to see my little brother grow up," and "Will you be sorry when I'm gone?" Sometimes the behavior of people intent on suicide provides the clue. They may:

- Give away prized possessions.
- Make out or change a will.
- Take out or add to an insurance policy.
- Cancel all social engagements.
- Be despondent or behave in unusual ways.
- Be unable to sleep.
- Feel hopeless.
- Have trouble concentrating at school or on the job.
- Suddenly lose interest in friends, organizations, and activities.
- Have a sudden, unexplained recovery from a depression.
- Plan their funeral.
- Cry for no apparent reason.

An assessment for suicide should *always* be done whenever you suspect suicidal thought or intent.

Because a Korean nursing student had failed the same major clinical course twice, she was asked to leave the BSN program. She desperately fought to be allowed to continue, even though the faculty had deemed her unsafe in the clinical area. The faculty could not understand her refusal to accept failure until they considered her cultural and family background, which sees failure as dishonorable. They decided to have the student speak with the psychiatric nursing instructor, who assessed the student's emotional state and found that she had no intentions of self-harm.

Nurses and others who may have contact with potentially suicidal people must be alert to both clear and veiled communications about suicide. Once clues have been identified, the next step is to perform an accurate lethality assessment.

LETHALITY ASSESSMENT A **lethality assessment** is an attempt to predict the likelihood of suicide. Certain signs help predict suicide risk (see the Assessment box on page 594). An accurate lethality assessment is essential in formulating a plan for helping a suicidal person. It also gives you cues about the client's possible need for hospitalization. Carrying out a lethality assessment requires direct communication between client and nurse concerning the client's intent. Part of assessment is a consideration of the lethality of the proposed suicide method. Table 24–1 on page 596 compares the lethality of various suicide methods.

Assessment of suicide risk is not easily accomplished. One barrier is the nurse's fear of asking the appropriate questions. *It is not possible to "cause" a person's suicide by assessing feelings and thoughts.* Suicide is not a spontaneous behavior, and inquiring about suicidal thoughts may alleviate a person's anxiety about considering

ASSESSMENT

Signs That Help Predict Suicide Risk: Comparing People Who Complete or Attempt Suicide with the General Population

Signs	*Suicide*	*Suicide Attempt*	*General Population*
Suicide plan*	Specific, with available, highly lethal method; does not include rescue.	Less lethal method, including plan for rescue; risk increases if lethality of method increases.	None, or vague ideas only.
History of suicide attempts*	65% have history of highly lethal attempts; if rescued, it was probably accidental.	Previous attempts are usually less lethal; rescue plan included; risk increases if there is a change from less lethal attempts to a highly lethal one.	None or less lethal with definite rescue plan.
Resources* Psychologic Social	Very limited or nonexistent; or person *perceives* self with no resources.	Moderate, or in psychologic and/or social turmoil.	Either intact or able to restore them through nonsuicidal means.
Communication*	Feels cut off from resources and unable to communicate effectively.	Ambiguously attached to resources; may use self-injury as a method of communicating with significant others when other methods fail.	Able to communicate directly and nondestructively concerning needs.
Recent loss	Increases risk.	May increase risk.	Is widespread but is resolved nonsuicidally through grief work, etc.
Physical illness	Increases risk.	May increase risk.	Is common but managed by effective crisis management (natural and/or formal).

→

suicide, not "give them the idea." Begin with "How bad are things for you?" "How down do you get?" "Are you worried about yourself?" "Do you ever think of harming yourself when you're down?" Then proceed with questioning the client gently, but directly.

It is critical that you evaluate the client's ability to and intent to act on an idea or plan. Beyond inquiring into the existence of a plan of suicidal action, ask questions and pay particular attention to whether or not steps have already been taken to implement such a plan. For example, has the person already stockpiled medication; written a suicide note; obtained (or have access to) knives or guns; spoken to others about purchasing a gun, writing a will, or giving away valued objects; recently purchased insurance? Also obtain information about prior suicide attempts as well as the client's history of violence and impulsiveness. Assess the availability of alcohol and its ongoing use, as alcohol abuse is closely associated with an increased risk of suicide. Family histories of suicide or violence might also be significant factors.

Do not use euphemisms. Some sample phrases are: "Do you have any thoughts of harming yourself?" "Have you ever thought of taking your own life?" "Have you ever been so sad that you have wanted to end it all, maybe by dying?"

The client who asks the nurse to promise not to tell anyone about a suicide plan poses a serious assessment problem. Never promise to keep clinical information a se-

ASSESSMENT (continued)

Signs	*Suicide*	*Suicide Attempt*	*General Population*
Drinking and other drug abuse	Increases risk.	May increase risk.	Is widespread but does not lead to suicide by itself.
Isolation	Increases risk.	May increase risk.	Many well-adjusted people live alone and manage isolation through social contacts.
Unexplained change in behavior	A possible clue to suicidal intent, especially in teenagers.	A cry for help and possible clue to suicidal ideas.	Does not apply in absence of other predictive signs.
Depression	65% have a history of depression.	A large percentage are depressed.	A large percentage are depressed.
Social factors or problems	May be present.	Often are present.	Widespread but do not by themselves lead to suicide.
Mental illness	May be present.	May be present.	May be present.
Age, sex, race, marital status	Statistical predictors useful for identifying if individual belongs to a high-risk group; not for clinical assessment of individuals.		

**If all four of these signs exist in a client, suicide risk is very high regardless of other factors. If other signs also apply, risk is further increased.*
Source: Adapted from Hoff 1989, pp. 207–208.

cret, and explain to the client that information is shared with the treatment team. You will probably need to discuss the issue of confidentiality further and explore the dynamics of the nurse-client relationship.

Many institutions and crisis centers use protocols for assessing suicide risk and have published these forms. However, research efforts to *predict* suicide by testing, using scales, or making clinical judgments have not been successful.

A comprehensive assessment, including a lethality assessment, will help you decide which interventions are indicated for the client. A complete assessment of level of lethality can prevent unnecessary hospitalizations. Hospitalizations in and of themselves can create a crisis. However, do not hesitate to admit a client when the suicide plan is lethal and there are inadequate supports to maintain the client in the community. This assessment tool helps clinicians develop and review the clinical rationale for the resulting treatment plan. The Assessment box on page 597 presents a lethality assessment scale.

Nursing Diagnosis

Core nursing diagnoses apply to most suicidal clients:

- Risk for Violence: Self-Directed
- Hopelessness

Table 24–1 The Lethality of Suicide Methods

Less Lethal Methods	*Highly Lethal Methods*
Wrist cutting	Gun
House gas	Jumping
Nonprescription drugs (excluding aspirin and acetaminophen [Tylenol])	Hanging
Tranquilizers, such as diazepam (Valium), flurazepam (Dalmane)	Drowning
	Carbon monoxide poisoning
	Barbiturates and prescribed sleeping pills
	High doses of aspirin and acetaminophen (Tylenol)
	Car crash
	Exposure to extreme cold
	Antidepressants, such as amitriptyline (Elavil)

- Ineffective Individual Coping
- Low Self Esteem

Several other nursing diagnoses (Anxiety, Impaired Verbal Communication, and Spiritual Distress) may be appropriate, depending on the situation.

Planning and Implementing Interventions

Do people have the right to commit suicide, and can or should nurses intervene when people try to kill themselves? Nurses should know that, ethical concerns aside, they may be prosecuted under state laws, making it a crime to aid or abet a suicide, under any circumstance, even when a terminally ill person decides to end his or her life. Questions about a client's right to suicide and society's right to control suicide have not been answered. The nursing interventions discussed below are based on the traditional belief that mental health care professionals should do everything possible to prevent suicide. Engaging in the process of ethical reasoning presented in Chapter 10 will help you in your search for a personal position.

General Guidelines for Any Setting The essential task is to work with the client to stop the constricted processing of suicidal thinking, long enough to enable the client and family members to consider alternatives to suicide. The nature of the nursing interventions are in large part determined by the setting in which you encounter the suicidal client. The following list of interventions and suggestions offers general guidelines that are applicable in most settings:

- Take any threat seriously. Evaluate the threat before dismissing it.
- Talk about suicide openly and directly. Asking about it will not put the notion in the client's head.
- Implement suicidal precaution status that includes checking on the client at least every 15 minutes or requiring the client to remain in public spaces.
- Search the client's room, especially if suicidal thoughts or a suicide attempt occurs after admission.
- Decide (usually along with other members of a team) if a **no self-harm/no-suicide contract** will be used (see the Intervention box on page 598).
- House the client in areas that are accessible for easy observation.
- Select a room that is near the nurses' station. A two-person room is best.
- Be careful not to encourage staff behaviors that give clients or staff members a false sense of security.

Staff members took Bob's shoes and reduced safety checks on him, thinking that, without shoes, he would not run away from the unit. He ran from the unit barefoot and suffered lacerations on both feet.

- Organize a plan of care with the client. Discuss all important problems, prioritize them, and list several approaches to each problem. Write down this plan, noting who is responsible for which actions.
- Do not make unrealistic promises such as, "Don't worry, I won't let you kill yourself." Remain honest, but hopeful. Making unrealistic promises diminishes your credibility with the client.

ASSESSMENT

Lethality Assessment Scale

Key to Scale	*Danger to Self*	*Typical Indicators*
1	No predictable risk of immediate suicide.	Has no notion of suicide or history of attempts; has satisfactory social support network; is in close contact with significant others.
2	Low risk of immediate suicide.	Has considered suicide with less lethal method; no history of attempts or recent serious loss; has satisfactory support network; no alcohol problems; basically wants to live.
3	Moderate risk of immediate suicide.	Has considered suicide with highly lethal method but no specific plan or threats; or, has plan with less lethal method, history of less lethal attempts, with tumultuous family history and reliance on Valium or other drugs for stress relief; is weighing the odds between life and death.
4	High risk of immediate suicide.	Has current highly lethal plan, obtainable means; history of previous attempts; has a close friend but is unable to communicate with him or her; has a drinking problem; is depressed and wants to die.
5	Very high risk of immediate suicide.	Has current highly lethal plan with available means; history of highly lethal attempts; is cut off from resources; is depressed and uses alcohol to excess; is threatened with a serious loss, such as unemployment, divorce, or failure in school.

Source: Adapted from Hoff 1989, p. 209.

- Encourage the client to continue daily activities and self-care as much as possible. Assign tasks for the client that are distracting, but not taxing.
- Decide with the client which family members and friends are to be contacted and by whom.
- Expect that the client will be experiencing shame, and work to help the client toward self-acceptance.
- Remove the client from immediate danger by confiscating pills or other harmful objects in the client's possession, or by moving the client to a physically safe environment.
- Relieve the client's obvious immediate distress. Does the client need a bath, clean clothing, food, sleep?
- Find out what, in the client's view, the most pressing need is. This may be to see a friend or family member, or to arrange for someone to pick up the children after school.
- Assume a nonjudgmental, caring attitude that does not engender self-pity in the client.
- Ask why the client chose to attempt suicide at this particular moment. The client's answer will shed light on the meaning suicide has for the client and may provide information that can lead to other helpful interventions.
- Provide for the client's safety through close observation and careful monitoring (see the section below on client safety).
- Review the safety of the environment (see the section below on safety in the therapeutic environment).
- Be prepared to deal with family members who may be confused, angry, or uninterested. Strive to remain neutral, and do not make assumptions about the family's behavior.
- Evaluate the client's need for medication.

INTERVENTION

Do's and Don'ts of No Self-Harm/No-Suicide Contracts

No self-harm/no-suicide contracts are effective in many situations, and they work well with certain clients. They can be used in hospital or outpatient settings as a means of providing additional support to people who are likely to harm themselves. It is imperative to establish a trusting relationship with the person prior to making a contract.

Do's

- Do fully assess a client to decide if a contract will be a helpful aid to treatment.
- Do establish a relationship with the client prior to initiating the contract.
- Do use the contract as a way of connecting with and staying connected with the client.
- Do specify in the contract the intervals for reevaluation. In outpatient work, the interval may be 1 week; the inpatient interval may range from every shift to every 1–3 days.
- Do have both nurse and client sign the contract and date it.
- Do have the client write out the contract if at all possible. Be creative if a client is unable or unwilling to write it out; the contract could be audiotaped, or client and nurse might each write half.
- Do include possible alternatives in the contract, such as "If I'm feeling like hurting myself I'll call ______, or I'll ask for ______."

Don'ts

- Don't use a no-suicide contract before performing a full nursing assessment.
- Don't place more trust in a contract or emphasis on it than in clinical judgment. The contract is a helpful therapeutic tool but does not replace good clinical judgment. Clients who are acutely suicidal may agree to the contract even though they have no intention of adhering to it.

Sample No Self-Harm/No-Suicide Contract

I, Cathy Smith, will not harm myself in any way. If I feel I am going to lose control, I will tell the staff (call the crisis unit, call my therapist, etc.).

I will not bring nor will I ask others to bring harmful articles or substances on the unit.

This contract lasts until 1/10/96 and is renewable at that time.

Signed

Cathy Smith 1/3/96

Nancy Jones, RN 1/3/96

- Evaluate the plan developed in collaboration with the client, and arrange for appropriate follow-up.
- Monitor your personal feelings about the client, and decide how they may be influencing your clinical work.
- Work with other team members to evaluate the issues fully. The nurse doesn't always have all the pieces of the puzzle.
- Perform a physical examination. One woman had cut herself severely prior to coming to the hospital, but this injury was not discovered until the physical examination was performed.
- Recognize that people can and have hung or strangled themselves with shoelaces, brassiere straps, pantyhose, robe belts, craft materials, and so on. Remain alert: Razor blades may be found in pages of books; matches are relatively easy to hide; pills may be hidden in plastic wrap in a cake box and stuffed animals; light bulbs can be broken and used to cut oneself, as can wire from spiral notebooks. Clients are also able to drown in a bathtub, throw themselves through a plate-glass window, set themselves on fire, or drink bleach from the cleaning person's cart.

In the emergency department, the main goal of treatment is to save the person's life. Although the emergency staff may be excellent at technical interventions, they may voice or feel contempt for the client who is a "repeater," especially if the attempt is not a serious one. The client needs a professional, nonpunitive approach and a smooth transition to other caregivers or agencies. Leaving the person alone or with access to harmful objects is obviously a hazard to be avoided in a busy emergency department.

INTERVENTION

Basic Suicide Precautions: Sample Protocol

The following is a protocol for basic suicide precautions. The plan may be started without a physician's order, but a psychiatric consultation must be arranged as soon as possible.

- The client is to remain in the room with the door open unless accompanied by a staff or family member. The client may use the bathroom alone.
- Check the client's whereabouts and safety every 15 minutes. Have a check-off sheet on client's door to document safety checks.
- Stay with the client while all medications are taken.
- Search the client's belongings for potentially harmful objects. Make the search in the client's presence, and ask for the client's assistance while doing so.
- Check articles brought in by visitors.
- Allow the client to have a regular food tray, but check whether the glass or any utensils are missing when collecting the tray.
- Allow visitors and telephone calls unless the client wishes otherwise.
- Check that visitors do not leave potentially dangerous objects in the client's room.
- Maintain the protocol until it is canceled by a psychiatrist.
- Inform the client of reasons for and details of precautionary measures. This explanation must be made by the nurse and physician and documented in the chart.

INTERVENTION

Maximum Suicide Precautions: Sample Protocol

The following is a protocol for maximum suicide precautions. These measures can be instituted without a physician's order under emergency conditions. However, a psychiatric consultation must be obtained as soon as possible.

- Provide one-to-one nursing supervision. The nurse must be in the room with the client at *all* times. When the client uses the bathroom, the bathroom door must remain open. Stay within arm's reach of the client at all times. A staff member should sit next to the client's bed at night.
- Do not use restraints for suicidal clients on general hospital floors.
- Do not allow the client to leave the unit for tests or procedures.
- Allow visitors and telephone calls unless the client wishes otherwise. Maintain one-to-one supervision during visits.
- Look through the client's belongings in the client's presence, and remove any potentially harmful objects, such as pills, matches, belts, shoelaces, pantyhose, brassieres, razors, tweezers, mirrors or other glass objects (such as light bulbs), wire, and craft materials.
- If suicide precautions are initiated after the client has been on the unit for any length of time, make a complete search of the room.
- Check that visitors do not leave potentially harmful objects in the client's room.
- Serve the client's meals in an isolation meal tray that contains no glass or metal silverware.
- Prior to instituting these measures, explain to the client what you will be doing and why. A physician must also explain this to the client. Document this explanation in the chart.
- Do not discontinue these measures without an order from a psychiatrist.

Observing and Monitoring Client Safety; Suicide Precautions Maintain the client's safety in the least restrictive manner possible. The length of time on restrictive status is of concern to both the client and the staff. Remember that restrictions meet the safety needs of the client, but they do not constitute treatment. On an inpatient unit, times of highest risk for suicide are evenings, nights, and weekends. Two factors account for this. During these periods, clients' time is less structured, and fewer staff members are available.

Most psychiatric inpatient units have developed a set of protocols or guidelines for observing and monitoring client behavior, often referred to as **suicide precautions.** Systems of observation may have 3–6 levels. Restrictions may require a physician's order but can and should be implemented on an emergency basis by nurses or other clinical staff. These protocols are often labeled to reflect the rationale for their use. In addition to suicide precautions, they may be known by such names as *special awareness, observation, constant observation,* and *constant awareness.* For sample protocols, see the two Intervention boxes on the preceding page.

It is of critical importance that all staff members be familiar with the system being used and understand the rationale for its use. The responsibility for maintaining and observing clients on these protocols remains with the registered nurse.

Restrictive status should be reserved for the safety management of suicidal clients. Restrictions can confound therapeutic management, and their use simply to restrict the free movement of clients diminishes their effectiveness. In general, privileges and other components of unit restriction are better dealt with by other measures such as privilege systems. If staff members are in doubt as to the appropriate safety status, the client should remain on a more restrictive status until the team decides what measures are appropriate. If there is doubt or concern about moving a client to a different status, it is best to retain the more restrictive status until the clinical direction of treatment is clarified.

As the team begins to move the client off special status, it is important for all team members to keep communicating openly about the client. As the client begins to improve, the risk of suicide increases temporarily (especially if the client has increased energy and ability finally to act on the suicidal ideation). The following times are critical and call for careful evaluation:

- *When the decision is made to move the client off suicide precaution status.* Clients, especially those who have come to depend on the around-the-clock safety, comfort, and nurturance provided by a staff member, may experience the discontinuing of suicide precaution status as a loss. Gradual removal from suicide precaution status and careful monitoring of its impact on clients is indicated in these cases.
- *When the decision is made to increase access to "sharps"* (dangerous objects). This increased access may make it possible for a client to act on a suicidal impulse. Assess the client carefully before granting this access.
- *During the second or third week of antidepressive drug therapy.* At this time, clients have increased energy but their depression has not been resolved. 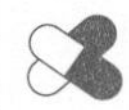
- *When the decision is made to grant a pass.* Decisions to grant pass privileges should be evaluated carefully. Where is the client going, and with whom? What time frame is being considered, and why? Perform a careful assessment both before and after the client goes on a pass. Additional searches may be needed at these times.
- *Prior to discharge and while formulating the discharge plan.* It is crucial to evaluate the "holding environment" in the community. Refer the client to resources in the community, and schedule a follow-up appointment at the time of discharge. Family and significant others should participate in discharge planning. It is generally not a good idea to discharge a client (especially one who lacks immediate family support and must rely on agencies or clinics) on a Friday, over a long weekend, or when the mental health care provider will be on vacation or otherwise unavailable.

Once a client has been recognized as a suicide risk and a safety plan has been implemented, the therapeutic work of addressing the depression, psychosis, and precipitating factors must begin. The treatment focus shifts as the client begins to show signs of clinical improvement.

The following signs usually indicate clinical improvement. They often signal the need to review or change treatment plans, grant privileges, or plan discharges:

- Verbalizing a range of options other than suicide.
- Making long-term plans or discussing future events.
- Verbalizing hope.
- Responding to antidepressant and/or antipsychotic medications.
- Wanting to reconnect or moving toward reconnecting with family or significant others.
- Showing more energy.
- Sleeping better.
- Feeling less hopeless.
- Demonstrating a wider range of affective responses to situations that occur on the unit.

Restrictions should be changed gradually, rather than all at once. A realistic plan is to change one or, at the most, two variables at a time while observing, monitoring, and documenting client responses.

CASE STUDY

A Suicidal Client

Identifying Information

Kevin is a 48-year-old lawyer who is married with two children and resides in the area. He is employed by a local law firm, he has been unable to work for the 3 weeks since his arrest for driving while intoxicated. The account of his arrest was published in the local paper 5 days ago. Four days ago, Kevin took an overdose of antidepressants, neuroleptics, and benzodiazepines and drank several liters of alcohol. He was found in a comatose state by his wife and transported to a general medical facility in which his acute symptoms were treated. He is transferred to a psychiatric inpatient unit after his 4-day stay in the ICU at the local hospital. At the time of transfer, Kevin states he has "no psychiatric problems and I don't know why I'm here." Kevin is admitted as an involuntary patient because he has been unwilling to come of his own accord. The treating physicians at the medical facility felt that he was a danger to himself and possibly others and needed to be in a psychiatric inpatient unit.

Client's Description of the Problem

Kevin relates his problems in a fairly matter-of-fact manner. He reports that up to approximately 6–8 months ago, things had been going fine for him. He felt like he was an up-and-coming attorney and that he was going to "make a spot for myself in this world." Approximately 6–8 months ago, the IRS placed a lien against his house because of tax problems. He began drinking heavily daily. As his financial problems increased, he became more depressed, especially when he was unable to find a way to manage his current situation. The relationship between Kevin and his wife deteriorated into frequent arguments and bickering. In addition, Kevin lost several large client accounts at his law office. He struggled with trying to understand what he was doing wrong and why these things were happening to him. His wife reports that as he became progressively depressed, she would frequently hear him talking loudly to himself. When she recognized that he was hallucinating, she became frightened of him and moved her belongings into the spare bedroom. Kevin and his wife have been very distant from each other. They describe the DWI arrest and publication of it in the paper as the "final straw."

Psychiatric History

Kevin has never been hospitalized for any psychiatric condition. He and his wife have attempted family counseling in the past to resolve problems, but Kevin was uncooperative because he "doesn't believe in that psychological stuff."

Family History

Kevin was raised in an affluent but emotionally cold family. Although his parents both died about 10 years ago, Kevin still talks of the anxiety and fears he knew as a young boy. He relates incidents from the past and remembers that he "excessively worried if I didn't know the right answer" to his parents' questions. He also relates that he was always the "dumbest of the kids," and his parents told him so frequently. He was sent away to boarding school from third grade through ninth grade. He relates that his brother was a better student, more attractive, and more athletic than he. This brother did not have to go away to boarding school like Kevin did. At age 21, he married his first and only girlfriend. He and his wife have two children, age 2 and 4.

Social History

Kevin has always been an insecure person who had to overcome his shyness to present himself in public. He is sensitive about a speech impediment that "the kids always made fun of." He now feels that he has been "exposed for the fake I really am." He had been able to be fairly successful in the past and feels that he and his wife have had good times together. He describes his marriage to his wife Sally as "a good one." He says he depends heavily on her to maintain the family and to be a constant source of support to him. When discussing his wife and their family, he becomes teary and quickly changes the subject. You find out later that Sally has been talking to him about filing for divorce. He has no leisure activities and uses alcohol to fill up his time. He has a few acquaintances, but no real friends and has not maintained a relationship with his brother.

Health History

Kevin had a repeat EKG on admission, which showed that there was no serious damage to his cardiac status as a result of the overdose. He completed intensive detox during the time that he was in the ICU. At this time, while he did not experience any negative physiologic effects of the detox from alcohol, he is irritable and complains of being shaky. He denies any additional medical problems. A physical exam yields no additional concerns.

CASE STUDY *(continued)*

Current Mental Status

Kevin presents as a casually groomed male who looks older than his stated age. He participates in the interview in an intermittently reluctant and irritated fashion. Kevin is oriented to person, place, and time. He exhibits an above-average fund of knowledge and at times uses multisyllabic words to either gain distance from or impress the interviewer. He appears hyperalert to any change in the environment. Judgment is seen as impaired because he denies having any problems.

Kevin says he has no feelings about his current life situation. His affect is limited to sarcasm or laughter when questioned about the past. He denies anger at himself or other people, although he seems quite irritable when you ask questions about his wife. His mood appears to be superficially within normal limits, but there is evidence of guardedness, depression, irritability, and a questionable paranoia. One gets glimpses of sadness from him, but he cannot tolerate these feelings for more than a few seconds.

Speech is normal in flow and volume. When asked personal questions by the interviewer, he becomes irritable. Posture during the interview is agitated and restless. There were no atypical movements noted, and Kevin denies the past use of medications that might result in abnormal and involuntary movements. Kevin's thoughts are coherent and logical, but they do tend to drift. He appears preoccupied and responded to internal stimuli on three occasions. He denies that he is hearing voices and is angry that he is asked this question. Later he says, "I've been covering it up so nobody will know that I'm really crazy."

Kevin denies having suicidal ideas or plans, but cannot relate why things have changed from a week ago. His plan prior to admission should be considered highly lethal because he had a highly lethal means to accomplish it, and he was discovered by accident, not by design. It is unclear at this point whether Kevin has any delusions, illusions, or hallucinations. At times he does seem to be speaking to himself, but when he recognizes that you have noted it, he becomes quite irritated and defensive.

At this time, Kevin appears to be using intellectualization, denial, rationalization, and avoidance as methods of coping. Although he has used these defenses for most of his life, they have been inadequate in helping him protect himself. There is no evidence that Kevin has any insight into his current situation. He denies current intent for suicide despite his recent elaborate plan to end his life.

Other Subjective or Objective Clinical Data

Kevin appears to be recovering uneventfully from his recent overdose. Vital signs are within normal limits. Prior to his transfer here, he was treated for alcohol withdrawal and initially showed signs of irritability and anxiety. No other overt signs are noted. It should also be noted that Kevin still continues to deny his use of alcohol as a problem. Kevin has also gained 20 lb in the last several weeks, and his wife says he has been eating literally night and day. He has also been unable to sleep and does not sleep for more than 2–3 hours at a time.

Diagnostic Impression

Nursing Diagnoses

Risk for Self-Directed Violence
Ineffective Individual Coping
Altered Nutrition: More than Body Requirements
Self Esteem Disturbance related to perceived feelings of loss of control
Altered Thought Process
Ineffective family coping

DSM-IV Multiaxial Diagnosis

Axis I: 296.24 Major depressive disorder, single episode, severe with psychotic features
Axis II: Deferred
Axis III: Status postoverdose, no current findings that affect treatment
Axis IV: Marital conflict and potential divorce, lack of friends, possible occupational problems related to the DWI, economic problems, financial conflicts with wife, recent DWI
Axis V: GAF = 30 (current); GAF = 80 (highest level in past year)

MONITORING SAFETY IN THE THERAPEUTIC MILIEU The safety of the therapeutic environment should be evaluated periodically. Does it meet the needs of the current client population, and is the level of restrictions consistent with the milieu philosophy? Here are specific questions to ask:

- Are areas free of glass or sharps?
- Are hazardous objects and areas kept locked?
- Are closet or shower rods of the breakaway type?
- Are craft items safe?

NURSING CARE PLAN

A Suicidal Client

Nursing Diagnosis

Risk for Self-Directed Violence related to ongoing suicidal ideation and suicide plan.

Expected Outcome

Client will not harm self during inpatient stay and will verbalize alternatives to suicidal behavior.

Nursing Interventions

- Assess client's level of suicidal ideation and evaluate his potential for self-harm.
- Evaluate for feelings, ideation, plans, and future orientation.
- Evaluate potential for self-harm at least every shift or more often if indicated.
- Implement basic suicide precautions.
- Explain suicide precautions to client.
- Explore with client how he came to decide on suicide as the method to solve the problem.
- Encourage client to verbalize ambivalence about suicidal ideation and plan.
- Ask the client if he has a future plan for suicide.
- Review how detailed and how feasible or lethal the plan is.
- Evaluate the possibility of using a no self-harm/no-suicide contract with client if indicated.
- Maintain close supervision of client in keeping with facility's policies and regulations.
- Know the whereabouts of client at all times.
- Designate a specific staff member to be responsible for client at all times during day and night to ascertain client's safety and whereabouts.
- Check on client at irregular intervals.
- Maintain especially close supervision of client at any time there is a decrease in number of staff or a decrease in the amount of structure or level of stimulation on the unit.
- Be especially aware of client during periods or turmoil or distraction, or when client is going to or from activities.

Outcome Met If

- Client can identify awareness of why he became suicidal.
- Client verbalizes suicidal ideation when it occurs.
- Client verbalizes decreased desire for self-harm.
- Client discusses two alternatives to suicide.
- Client participates in forming a no self-harm/no-suicide contract with his primary nurse.
- Client complies with suicide precautions.

Nursing Diagnosis

Ineffective Individual Coping related to extreme anxiety and distress.

Expected Outcome

Client will develop two additional coping strategies.

Nursing Interventions

- Encourage client to discuss current and past methods of coping.
- Encourage client to investigate alternative methods of effectively coping, such as communicating with others, asking for help when needed, developing leisure and recreational interests, developing increased ability to use defense mechanisms.

Outcome Met If

Client verbalizes connections between significant losses and low self-esteem resulting in depression.

Nursing Diagnosis

Self Esteem Disturbance related to perceived feelings of loss of control.

Expected Outcome

Client will verbalize connection between significant losses and problems in his life and his situational low self-esteem.

Nursing Interventions

- Use individual contacts every shift to encourage client to recognize and verbalize his losses. Encourage client to review a realistic evaluation of his part in these losses.
- Encourage client to explore areas that can be changed and which areas need acceptance.

→

- How many clients are there? What is the client population like now? Do they have character disorders? Serious depression?
- If the therapeutic environment is temporarily deemed to be unsafe—that is, if there are objects (such as liquor, razors, drugs) on the unit that can harm others—is there also a need to conduct a thorough "health-and-welfare search," in order to completely examine all areas of the unit for further contraband or other potential hazards?

NURSING CARE PLAN (continued)

- Discuss possible other methods to manage potential loss of wife and impact of DWI on his life.
- Engage client in milieu activities as much as possible, such as participation in client government, participation in groups.
- Encourage client as much as feasible to assume responsibility for his own treatment: discussing discharge dates, deciding what groups to attend, selecting outpatient therapists.

Outcome Met If

Client verbalizes connections between significant losses and his low self-esteem.

Nursing Diagnosis

Ineffective Family Coping related to impaired communication.

Expected Outcome

Husband and wife will be able to have full knowledge of what is happening and collaborate on alternatives to intervene effectively.

Nursing Interventions

- Assess both client's and wife's knowledge about current circumstances and suicidal ideation.
- Encourage the couple, and provide opportunities for them to talk through the problems to reevaluate possible alternatives.
- Give information about stress and crisis intervention, coping skills, alternatives, and the role of alcohol, and relate it to client's current situation.

Outcome Met If

Client and wife together come to agreement about how to take the next steps to resolve the problem.

Nursing Diagnosis

Altered Thought Processes related to auditory hallucinations of a self-deprecatory nature.

Expected Outcome

Client will demonstrate no signs of attending to internal stimuli and will identify stressors that have precipitated hallucinations.

Nursing Interventions

- Monitor client for signs of attending to internal stimuli and observe for precipitating stressors.
- Discuss observations with client and assess his awareness of hallucinations.
- Help client monitor events or interactions that increase hallucinations.
- Teach client and wife that hallucinations may be part of the current process.
- Support coping strategies that client has identified as personally effective in reducing hallucinations.
- Protect client who might be harmed by acting on hallucinated commands if these present themselves.

Outcome Met If

- Client expresses understanding and identifies episodes of hallucinations.
- Client verbalizes a decrease in hallucinations.
- Client and wife verbalize an understanding of the effect of stress on the symptom.
- Client takes medications that will decrease the hallucinations.

Nursing Diagnosis

Altered Nutrition: More Than Body Requirements related to binge eating to control anxiety.

Expected Outcome

Client will be able to discuss alteration in nutritional status as a consequence of current depressive mood and crisis situation.

Nursing Interventions

- Discuss with client the connection between altered nutritional status and current mental state.
- Discuss with client how current increase in weight affects his self-esteem.
- Allow client to make decision about whether he would like to pursue a nutritional consult and have meal trays during his inpatient stay.

Outcome Met If

- Client is able to identify how he uses food as a coping mechanism.
- Client verbalizes plan to resume pre-crisis nutritional habits.

It is also very important that the nurse educate the client's family and visitors about safety measures and their rationale. Taking this step helps ensure that family members and other visitors do not bring unsafe objects on the unit. Visitors must understand visit limits and unit policies in relation to passes. It is also necessary to explain the need for searches. Families and friends who repeatedly violate safety measures of the unit may require additional attention, and their visiting privileges may have to be restricted.

Documenting Client Behavior and Treatment Documentation is an essential duty for nurses working with suicidal clients on an inpatient unit. Documentation helps all staff members understand the rationale for changes and comply with ethical and legal requirements. In general, follow agency rules about documentation. Also be sure to document the following:

- All team reviews of client status and the names of the team members involved.
- Any decision to remove the client from a more restrictive status to a less restrictive one.
- The rationale for any changes in the treatment approach, especially changes in the level of restriction.
- Statements from clients about self-harm or denial.
- Client responses to changes, passes, family, visitors.
- All telephone calls or interactions with family members.
- All searches done and the reason for them.

Evaluation and Outcome Criteria

Suicide, like all crisis situations, calls for ongoing evaluation of the plan made by the nurse and client. Because events often occur rapidly, initial care plans may need to be changed almost daily. In addition to evaluating individual care plans, staff members who work with suicidal clients need to evaluate their overall approach and philosophy periodically.

Suicide in Special Populations

Children

Not long ago, most people believed that it was impossible for children to be depressed or suicidal. However, suicide by children has increased threefold over the last two decades. In 1990, for example, there were 300 suicides among children age 1–14 (U.S. Bureau of the Census 1993), and the numbers continue to rise despite increasing awareness by parents and professionals. These statistics probably underestimate the scope of the problem, because professionals and families still tend to label suicidal acts as accidents. Depending on age, children may not see death as irreversible, and to that degree, suicide may be accidental (Hurley 1991).

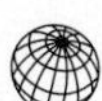

Some people cannot believe children would want to end their lives. Suicide attempts by children belie the myth of the "happy child" in our culture. One study revealed that, among children or adolescents who come to a general hospital emergency room with indications of suicidal intent or behavior, at least half are diagnosed as victims of accidents rather than suicide attempts, and no follow-up is planned (Hawton 1986). The following example illustrates denial and lack of information on the part of parents of a suicidal child:

A 10-year old boy set up a rope over a door to hang himself. His attempt was stopped by his parents. The door, a second entrance to the room, was painted shut, and the subject of suicide was not discussed. His parents failed to recognize the same symptoms in the child 2 years later. However, at this time, severe behavior problems in school and pressure by school personnel forced the parents to bring in the child for a psychiatric evaluation.

Children commit suicide by simple but lethal methods such as poisoning, shooting themselves with firearms, hanging, or darting into the path of moving cars. It is unclear what drives a child to commit suicide. Several authors have described characteristic presuicidal symptoms and life circumstances of the suicidal child. The symptoms are known as depressive equivalents; that is, the symptoms may indicate a masked depression. The symptoms of masked depression are:

- Boredom or restlessness.
- Irritability or lethargy.
- Difficulty concentrating.
- Apparently purposeful misbehavior.
- Somatic preoccupation.
- Excessive dependence on or isolation from others, notably adults.

Orbach (1984) and others reviewed many life and family factors that place a child at risk for suicide. These include depression, psychosis, impulsive traits, substance abuse, failure to complete developmental tasks, lack of family cohesion, overemphasis on achievement, frequent exposure to aggression, lack of religious identification, losses (peers, relationships), poor school performance, and family factors such as frequent moves, deprivation of love and attention, marital conflict, parental unemployment, parental loss, suicidal behavior in other family members, and poor management of divorce.

Although suicide in children under 12 occurs infrequently, Price (1991) indicates that suicidal ideation or suicide threats by a child always deserve attention and merit very careful study. Although suicide rates for children remain low, an explanation for the lower rate of completed suicide among children is that the association between mood disorders and suicide is less in children than in adults. Another possible theory is that children are basically less isolated than adults and therefore receive greater emotional support, thus reducing their chances of completing a suicide. A third hypothesis is that because children are not psychologically mature enough to experience hopelessness and despair, they are less likely to kill themselves. Children who attempt or have completed suicide do so sometimes in response to a frightening situation. A child's suicide threat is often perceived as a desperate attempt to change a scary circumstance.

A careful assessment of suicide risk should be done whenever a child expresses ideas about suicide or makes an attempt. The assessment interview should consider the degree of risk while exploring the family situation and the external events that preceded the thoughts or the attempt. The meaning behind the attempt must be explored. Young children are less able to verbalize and thus require more structure and planned activities to get at the heart of some of the information that may be needed to make an appropriate assessment. It is essential to obtain a promise from the child in the form of a contract not to cause himself or herself any harm for a specific period of time. It is equally important to secure the support of the family in creating a safe environment for their child. It is a good idea to ensure that all potentially lethal objects and medications are secured and out of sight. If the family appears to be unable or unwilling to agree to the contract or create a safe home environment, it may become necessary to hospitalize the child.

Adolescents

Adolescent suicide is a serious concern. In the past decade, there has been a dramatic rise in the rate of adolescent suicide. Among 15 to 24-year-olds, the rate of completed suicides over the past 20 years has doubled (U.S. Bureau of the Census 1993). Suicide is now the third leading cause of death among 15 to 24-year-olds in the United States. Only homicides and accidents account for more deaths in this population.

The rate of attempted suicide is also a major public health issue. Information on attempts is elusive, and some researchers speculate that many "accidents" of adolescents are actually suicide attempts. The ratio of adolescent suicide attempts to completed suicides is now estimated at 200 to 1; approximately 1 million young people annually engage in self-harmful behavior. As with suicide statistics for all age groups, it is likely that suicide rates for this group have been underestimated.

There are no clear rationales for the 173% increase in adolescent suicide since 1950. An important factor that may have contributed to this increase is the rise in depressive disorders among youths. Severe depression is the most prevalent characteristic of the suicidal adolescent. An increase in the divorce rate with the resulting dissolution of nuclear families, along with the availability of the means to commit suicide, all play a part in this phenomenon. Males are generally at greater risk than females, and whites are at greater risk than nonwhites for a completed suicide. Some speculate that our complex and dangerous world (nuclear threat, terrorism, war) contributes to a sense of depression or futility.

Some maintain that the very nature of adolescence contributes to the problem: that adolescent grandiosity and narcissism make the potentially suicidal adolescent believe, for instance, "I cannot die. Someone will find me before this overdose kills me." Others blame the increase in adolescent suicides on the nature of the media's reporting of suicides. They insist that the sensational and romantic quality of the reporting actually precipitates suicides, particularly cluster suicides. Critics allege that cluster suicides would never occur in the absence of publicity. (Cluster suicide is discussed later in this section.)

Although there are no studies that enable us to predict with certainty which adolescents will commit suicide, the

Table 24–2 Stressors Having Special Significance for Adolescents

Stressor	*Possible Meaning*
Anniversary date of death of loved one (particularly if death was suicide).	Can rekindle feelings of loss and mourning; may evoke feelings of guilt or anger, if unresolved; may prompt ideas of "rejoining" the loved one.
Developmental milestone (menarche, leaving grammar school and entering high school).	Can represent loss of childhood and decreasing dependence on parental figures; can evoke performance anxiety and fear of failure or embarrassment.
Holidays.	Can represent unfulfillment and disappointment; can trigger or intensify needs and longings; can be a source of increased family tension and fighting.
Loss, real or imagined.	Can intensify feelings of low self-esteem and unworthiness; can cause feelings of acute loss and loneliness, resulting in depression and despair.
Performance failure (failed exam, embarrassing school situation).	Can be devastating, particularly to overachieving adolescents with uncompromising parents; at the other extreme, can be the "last straw" for those with many failures.

ASSESSMENT

Factors Increasing the Risk for Suicide Among Adolescents

- Depression, usually related to the loss of someone or something of great value to the adolescent. Depression is usually marked by the following group of symptoms: feelings of helplessness, hopelessness, worthlessness, loss or deprivation, and guilt or rejection.
- Low self-esteem and lack of basic trust in self and others.
- Family system problems such as:

  Psychiatric illness in the family, particularly in one or both parents.

  Chronic depression in the family, particularly in one or both parents.

  Chronic or extensive history of family problems; conflicts in family, especially about discipline.

  Marital discord and unhealthy interactions between parents or among parents and the adolescent. Parents may scapegoat the adolescent, displacing their feelings of dissatisfaction and disappointment and leading the adolescent to accept the blame.

  Situations characterized by long-term neglect, abuse, or unstable home and family life.
- A handicap that makes the adolescent "different" and unworthy (such as a learning problem, a chronic illness, or a physical deformity). It is not the handicap that leads to the feelings of unworthiness but the negative messages the adolescent may receive if family and significant others do not provide frequent and consistent positive and accepting emotional experiences.
- Intrapersonal/interpersonal problems such as:

  School problems

  Pregnancy

  Drug use/abuse

  Worries about sexuality, sexual feelings, or sexual orientation

  Worries about breaking the law

  Feelings of anxiety

  Problems with a romantic relationship
- The presence of a "suicide model": having a close friend or relative who had either attempted or completed suicide, or having a parent who attempted suicide.

presence of certain stressors and risk factors can help you identify a potentially suicidal adolescent. Most suicides or suicide attempts are preceded by verbal or action threats, or a statement of intent. However, this is less true of adolescents, unless they have a history of long-standing problems and behavior changes. Adolescent suicides often occur without warning. They are frequently triggered by a seemingly trivial incident, such as a fight with a boyfriend or girlfriend, or a quarrel with parents. The suicide is a sudden, impulsive reaction to a stressful situation or a perceived loss, such as a separation, a divorce, a death, a loss in self-esteem (as in being cut from a high school team), or a transition or move that symbolizes loss (such as going away to college). The loss can also be an imagined one: "No one likes me," or "I'll never be pretty enough (or good enough)." The need to work through loss is a necessary developmental task of adolescence.

Adolescence is a time of increased internal and external stressors, and teenagers experiencing an abnormal number of life changes appear to be at even higher risk for suicide. What may be extremely stressful to one adolescent, however, may be a minor matter to another. The nature and severity of the precipitating stress can reveal a great deal about the person's coping abilities. Events and situations that have special significance as potential stressors and the possible meanings they may have for adolescents are listed in Table 24–2. Rather than assume a meaning, however, the nurse should, before developing a plan of care, explore a stressor with the client to identify the significance of the event.

Which adolescents are most likely to commit suicide? Certain risk factors can help the professional identify potentially suicidal adolescents (see the accompanying Assessment box). For example, it is possible to recognize individuals who are suffering from depression before it interferes with their ability to function in daily life and before the depression becomes so oppressive that the person considers suicide.

When assessing the youth for suicide or evaluating suicide attempts, consider some additional factors to determine the lethality of the behavior:

- Has the adolescent been exposed to suicide? Experiencing another person's suicide may make the adolescent more vulnerable to completing a suicide. Because someone else has done it, there is less conflict associated with it. This phenomenon may play a part in the incidence of the cluster suicides that are known to occur with teenagers.
- Are depression or psychological disturbance present? These high-risk factors for suicide in adults are also high-risk factors for suicide in adolescents.
- Is the adolescent's behavior hostile, aggressive, or assaultive?
- What is the motivation for the act—wanting to die, to get help, to get relief?
- How lethal is the suicide intent? More importantly, how lethal does the client consider the act to be? (If the client took ten aspirin tablets thinking this constituted an overdose, the attempt has high lethality.)
- What is the nature of the precipitating stress?
- What resources are available to the adolescent?
- What is the history of prior problems, and how good are the client's coping skills?

How can you effectively assess depression in individuals who characteristically act out their feelings rather than express them verbally? In fact, largely because of this acting-out behavior, in a setting with many adolescents, you have numerous opportunities to make such assessments. You will not only observe depressed adolescents for certain behavioral cues but also compare their behavior with that of peers who are not depressed. Assessments and interventions by the school or community nurse can be critical in this respect. The accompanying Assessment box lists possible behavioral cues indicative of adolescent depression.

The most common precursor of adolescent suicide is certainly depression. Adolescence is a volatile time characterized by rapid mood swings and great intensity of feelings. For this reason, adults may have trouble recognizing depression in teenagers. Moreover, adults tend to idealize adolescence and may refuse to accept the idea of adolescent depression. Adults, including mental health care professionals, are likely to view suicide attempts by adolescents as manipulative and hostile acts designed to punish or control significant others. A survey by Curran (1987) concluded that adults may view suicide attempts by adolescents as insincere acts because they are often of low lethality. However, the rising numbers of adolescents who complete suicide indicate the need to view all attempts as serious requests for help. It is imperative to assess and answer all such cries for help.

It is important to remember that in working with adolescents or children, involving the parent(s) is especially helpful in uncovering important events in the client's life and to accurately assess their problems and needs. Parents should be kept informed of the treatment progress and the interventions planned for their teenager. Parent education on childhood and adolescent development, behavior management, understanding illness, and suicidal ideation, can be an effective means of helping parents be a part of the treatment process. During these high-stress periods, parents may also appreciate the opportunity to meet with others whose children or teenagers have had similar problems.

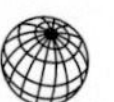

CLUSTER SUICIDES **Cluster suicide**—any excessive number of suicides occurring in close temporal or geographic proximity to each other—is a phenomenon of great concern to those who work with adolescents (Davies and Wilkes 1993). The terms contagion suicide, imitation suicide, copy-cat suicide, and mass suicide are sometimes used as if they were synonymous with cluster suicide. *Contagion suicide* is a process by which one person's suicide might encourage another's suicide, while *imitation suicide* is one way in which a suicide might become contagious to others. *Copy-cat suicide* is another term for imitation suicide, usually applied in the context of the depiction of suicide in the media. *Mass suicide* is the concurrent suicide of a large group of people such as that in Guyana in 1978. Mass suicide is best considered as a special and unusual form of clustering (O'Carroll, Mercy, and Steward 1992). From the viewpoint of prevention, a highly charged, dramatic environment heightens the potential contagious effect of a suicide. It is important to determine what segments of the community may be most vulnerable to cluster suicide. Gould (1990) found that clustering is most prevalent in the age group of 14–24, where it is two to four times more frequent than in older age groups. Because of the influence of and close connections with their peer group, adolescents are at risk for cluster suicide. At highest risk are hospitalized or institutionalized adolescents. Clustering has been estimated to account for about 5% of teenage suicides in the United States. While that might seem to be a small number, the rising suicide rate among the young is a particular public health concern.

The Elderly

Older adults are also at high risk for suicide. Suicide is the ninth leading cause of death and the leading cause of preventable death in this age group. It has long been recognized that the risk for this population is inordinately high (roughly two to three times that of all age groups). For example, in the United States in 1989, there were 6300 reported suicides among people 65 and older (U.S. Bureau of the Census 1993).

ASSESSMENT

Behavioral Cues Indicating Adolescent Depression

Changed mood	Reflects a persistent and pervasive unhappy mood rather than the transient and situation-specific mood typical of adolescence; may project a global anger that interferes with interpersonal relationships.
Low self-esteem	Results in feelings of unworthiness, guilt, and rejection; leads to behaviors that "set up" failure and rejection.
Decreased energy	Marked by extreme fatigue that is incapacitating at times; the person may "wake up tired"; leads to concern about possible underlying illness.
Problems with school involvement	Includes both academic performance and social activity; low grades or decline in academic performance can be a marker of emotional difficulty; changes in interpersonal relationships, particularly social withdrawal and isolation, are cues.
Somatic complaints	Will most likely be the reason to see the nurse in the school or community clinic; symptoms usually fall into three major categories: physical complaints with fatigue, alterations in sleep patterns, and changes in appetite and body weight.

The statistics on older adult suicides are probably not accurate because most studies on suicide in the elderly do not take into account two groups that likely have suicidal ideas or a plan:

1. Those who are terminally ill and request that no additional care be given.
2. Those who are in a precarious health state and "accidentally" take too much medication and die.

These facts are especially disconcerting when you consider that older adults may respond best to treatment for depression. Medications and supportive verbal therapy can make dramatic changes in the quality of their lives. Suicidologists speculate that the true suicide rate is at least double the reported rate (Boxwell 1988). Carney et al. (1994) point out that it becomes more difficult to detect suicidal ideations or plans with increasing age. Older adults tend to be much more covert about the nature of their suicidal ideations. It may be that some older adults avoid talking about their mental health concerns, thinking, "If I talk about this, everyone will think I'm crazy" or "If you have a problem, don't talk about it—do something." Suicide assessment and prevention should be a significant concern for the nurse working with the elderly in any health care setting.

The lethality index (ratio of suicide attempts to completed suicides) is also high among older adults. For all age groups, this ratio is between 10:1 and 20:1 (the ratio for adolescents is as high as 200:1). Among the elderly, the ratio of attempts to completed suicides is 4:1. Here are two significant concerns for this age group:

1. High lethality of intent. There is a notable lack of ambivalence about the decision to commit suicide.
2. High lethality of the methods utilized. In one study, older males most commonly shot themselves with guns (Boxwell 1988).

The elderly are also less likely to have the physiologic strength to recuperate after a suicide attempt.

Older adults tend to underutilize mental health services for several reasons. An elderly client may avoid seeking help from mental health care professionals because of the ethical, moral, and social stigma associated with suicide and suicide ideation and psychiatric illness. It is estimated that only 1–3% of calls to suicide prevention centers are from clients over the age of 65. Elderly people who have suicidal ideation or plans may have attempted to get help from primary health care providers (usually medical sources) and may complain of depression or somatic symptoms. Thus, nurses are in an ideal position to identify people at risk and provide services or make appropriate referrals.

Cynthia, a widow, is 84 years old and can no longer afford her apartment. Her Social Security payments are inadequate to cover the bills for heat, food, and rent. Cynthia's major source of support, her daughter Lauren, moved to England last year, and Cynthia refused to go with her, saying, "She needs her own life, not having me dragging her down." Last August, Cynthia realized she couldn't afford the rent and since then has become progressively more depressed. Cynthia worries all day about being "on the streets." She is too proud to let her daughter know she needs help. Cynthia has

been secretly saving up her pills and has decided that she cannot live if she is without a home. She has decided to take the pills tonight after she makes her weekly call to Lauren.

The following factors place older adults at an increased risk for suicide:

- Serious illness (terminal illness, debilitating illness, or chronic pain).
- Bereavement and loss (loss of spouse, significant friends, family).
- Use of alcohol and mood-altering drugs to cope with stress.
- Neurologic disorders (dementia).
- Changes in socioeconomic status, work status, prestige.
- History of prior suicidal behavior or prior requests for help.
- Use of medication that may precipitate depression (antidepressants, steroids, phenothiazines, rauwolfia derivatives).

To assess suicide potential in elderly clients, the nurse must be perceptive, listen actively, and pose direct questions. The suicidal elderly individual may give the following cues:

- Verbal cues ("I'm going to end it all," "Life is not worth living," "I won't be around much longer").
- Behavioral cues (completing a will, making funeral plans, acting out, withdrawing, somatic complaints).
- Situational cues (recent move, loss of a loved one, diagnosis of a terminal illness).
- Atypical cues (cognitive changes similar to dementia, excessive preoccupation with physical symptoms, a resigned attitude—"I'm supposed to feel this way because I'm old").

Clients with HIV Disease

The actual risk of suicide in people with AIDS is greater than that in the general population. In one recent study, the suicide rate for men with AIDS was 680 per 100,000 persons per year, whereas for a comparison group of men age 20–59 without a diagnosis of AIDS, the suicide rate was 18 per 100,000 per year (Marzuk et al. 1988). The suicide risk of AIDS patients is estimated to be 36 times that of those without AIDS.

One part of the problem with individuals who have HIV disease is that they may also, as a consequence of the progression of the illness, develop cognitive difficulties that are related to encephalopathy or other CNS impairment. (See Chapter 27 for a thorough discussion.) The risk of suicide for clients with HIV disease is also enhanced by the fact that in this group there are fewer cultural barriers and less stigma that are associated with suicide if a person does have AIDS.

Psychiatric Clients

There is a serious risk of suicide among those persons diagnosed with a psychiatric illness. Black and Winokur (1990) suggest that the risk of suicide among this group is three to twelve times greater than in the general population.

Among psychiatric clients in general, these factors are associated with increased suicidal risk:

- Being female.
- Young age.
- Diagnosis of depression or schizophrenia.
- History of a past attempt, living alone, unemployment, and/or being unmarried and recently admitted to psychiatric care.
- Being treated as either an inpatient or an outpatient with a diagnosis of depression, chemical dependence, schizophrenia, PTSD, or panic disorder.

The suicide rate for people with schizophrenia may be increasing because of stress from community living and frequent brief hospitalizations. The schizophrenic client most at suicide risk is a young white male who is in remission. He is well educated (several years of college) and has high expectations of himself. He feels hopeless, depressed, inadequate, and unable to cope with the chronicity of his illness. Other factors are previous suicide attempts and current threats or ideas. Suicide occurs most often early during hospitalization or soon after discharge.

The incidence of self-destructive behavior and suicide is also high among people with personality disorders. Suicidal behavior is an integral part of the clinical presentation especially of clients with a diagnosis of borderline personality disorder or histrionic personality disorder. In their study of suicidal behavior, Raczek et al. (1989) found the following:

- Suicidal behavior appears to be related to character pathology; the higher the number of pathologic personality traits, the higher the suicide risk.
- Borderline personality traits are the most common personality traits among clients with suicidal behavior.
- The combination of borderline and avoidant personality traits seems to be the most lethal.

Substance Abusers

It is estimated that 35–40% of completed suicides are alcohol related, as many as 50–60% of all suicide attempts are alcohol related, and the risk of suicide in alcoholics is

32 times the risk for suicide in the general population (Bukstein, Brent, and Perper 1993). Substance abuse is also related to many fatal automobile and boating accidents. It is often difficult to distinguish between suicides and accidental overdoses and accidents. When more than one substance is used (alcohol and sedatives, alcohol and cocaine), the impact on a person's mood and psychologic stability is even greater, increasing the risk for suicide or self-destructive behavior.

It is important to remember that drugs react chemically with the brain to produce altered moods, altered thought processes, and increased impulsivity. In general, the abuse of substances tends to:

- Diminish control and inhibition.
- Uncover or release impulses or thoughts.
- Diminish memory and concentration.
- Promote relaxation and feelings of stability. People believe they are seeing and understanding the situation exactly as it is. In these circumstances, suicide may seem to be the rational course, adopted without the anxiety or ambivalence that might normally accompany suicidal thoughts.
- Increase depression, especially after the initial response of relaxation.

The abrupt cessation or withdrawal from alcohol or other drugs is likely to precipitate suicidal thoughts or impulses. Habitual cocaine use can lead to life-threatening depression. This depression can last months and may require inpatient treatment.

Nurses' Attitudes About Self-Destructive People

Nurses' attitudes toward suicidal clients have many sources. In addition to direct experience with suicidal clients, societal and ethical issues as well as historical antecedents influence nurses' attitudes toward suicide and self-destructive behavior. These controversial issues include rational suicide, euthanasia, abortion rights, the right to commit suicide, and the responsibility to prevent suicide. Nurses often get caught up in the dilemma of how much responsibility to take for the self-destructive person and for how long.

Hoff (1989) points out that self-destructive people run counter to the socialized sick role that most clients assume in health care settings. They seemingly defeat our best efforts by choosing death over life, or by being self-destructive. Although it is the responsibility of the nurse to promote and maintain life, the nurse cannot battle the client to do so. Rather, the nurse joins clients in examining and understanding how it is that they have gotten to this point.

Nurses working with self-destructive or suicidal clients may feel frustrated and angry. Aggressive responses by nurses (such as choosing the largest nasogastric tube for gastric lavage in the emergency room, complaining that self-destructive clients are taking up the time they should be spending on their "real clients") are not unknown. Before working with someone who is suicidal or self-destructive, nurses must assess personal feelings, experiences, conflicts, and memories that might render them ineffective in performing this task. The inventory in the Nursing Self-Awareness box on the next page will help you explore your own attitudes.

Survivors of Suicide

A 27-year-old woman called her former boyfriend and told him to look out of his window so that he could watch her die. He hung up on her. Only minutes later, he heard a crash. She had driven her car into a tree in front of his apartment building. The impact killed her instantly.

A 17-year-old high school student killed himself in his home after holding his mother hostage for 3 hours, tying her to a chair and forcing her to type his four suicide notes. When she finished, he shot himself in the head.

The act of suicide has long-lasting ramifications for the survivors. Nurses who are working with the families or staff who have worked with the deceased must be alert to the potential aftereffects of the death. (Staff reactions are described later in the chapter.)

Farberow (1992) summarizes the emotional experiences of survivors of suicide:

- Strong feelings of loss accompanied by sorrow and mourning.
- Anger at being made to feel responsible for the behavior of the suicidal person.
- Feelings of separation because their help was refused.
- Anxiety, guilt, shame, or embarrassment because the person committed suicide.
- Relief that nagging, insistent demands from that suicidal person have ceased.
- Feelings of having been deserted.
- The arousal of impulses toward suicide.
- Anger caused by the belief that the suicide represents a rejection of social and moral responsibilities.

There are many people who should be considered as survivors of a suicide. Families and other survivors of suicide may not receive the support that other bereaved people generally receive. People in the support network (often including other family members) are uncomfortable

NURSING SELF-AWARENESS

Working with Suicidal Clients

To increase self-awareness about managing your own anxiety in working with clients who are suicidal, ask yourself the following questions:

- What kinds of things frighten me?
- How do I feel about asking for someone else's help with a client if I'm unsure of myself or uncomfortable?
- Is the client asking me to take responsibility for his or her behavior?
- Is the client able to assume responsibility for his or her own behavior?

To increase self-awareness of your own feelings about people who are self-destructive, ask yourself the following questions:

- How do I feel about people who deliberately harm themselves?
- How do I understand self-destructive behavior?
- Do I believe that clients are capable of change?
- Do I believe that everyone ultimately has the responsibility for his or her own life?
- How do I express and handle my own frustration?

To increase self-awareness about your own feeling of anger, ask yourself the following questions:

- What kinds of things make me angry?
- How do I deal with my own anger? Do I tend to ignore it or hide it?
- How do I react to others when they are angry?
- How do I feel about people who don't change immediately?
- How do I deal with people who appear to do illogical things?
- How do I feel when people don't change their behavior when I've asked them to or when I talk to them about it?

To increase self-awareness about your own feelings of control, ask yourself the following questions:

- In what areas of my life and my work do I feel the need to take control?
- How do I feel when treatment does not go the way I would like it to?
- How do I handle control issues with clients?
- How do I feel about control issues with clients?
- How do I feel about my lack of control over others?

and embarrassed and are more likely to stay away than to help. Family members are often blamed for not preventing the suicide. Very often, suicide is denied or concealed. This secrecy further impedes grief work, because survivors cannot resolve the loss unless they discuss it openly. Suicide exacerbates dysfunctional family dynamics, such as scapegoating or blaming other family members. Besides making the usual preparations after death, families need to deal with police investigations, the media, and insurance companies. This can precipitate extreme stress, especially if only limited support is available.

Survivors rarely seek assistance from mental health care professionals. They are much more likely to be furious with the group that "should have prevented this" and need to project their impotent rage on the professionals. A nurse working with survivors must be prepared for this reaction. Families and all significant others who survive a suicide need nursing intervention, but it is especially warranted for the following:

- Families who lack support from usual sources.
- Dysfunctional families who react by blaming, scapegoating, or covering up the death as an accident.
- Children whose parent has committed suicide.
- Adolescents exposed to the suicide of a friend.

Therefore, nurses should plan outreach services for these groups. A typical plan might include telephoning the family immediately after the suicide and periodically until the first anniversary of the death, and providing for staff or a staff representative to attend services, if appropriate. The family sometimes welcomes the assistance, but sometimes the family is angry and unable to relate to mental health professionals. The health care team must work together to formulate the most appropriate plan.

Children who experience a loss as the result of a parental suicide require urgent interventions to deal with the trauma. Children who have lost a parent to suicide require the nurse to be particularly sensitive because these children will not be able to grieve in the usual ways. A child who loses a parent is also at greater risk for suicide and depression (Price 1991).

Adolescents who are exposed to the suicide of a friend are at high risk for development of major depression and should be carefully screened, observed, and treated for depressive symptoms. A close relationship to the victim, visual exposure to the victim at the scene of death, having a conversation with the victim the day of the suicide, and both a personal and a family history of depression are all predictive of the development of depression subsequent to the suicide.

Staff Responses to a Client's Suicide

Staff members are also survivors of a client's suicide. Schneidman (1981) puts it especially well:

> The person who commits suicide puts his psychological skeleton in the survivor's emotional closet—he sentences the survivor to deal with the many negative feelings and, more, to become obsessed with thoughts regarding his actual or possible role in having precipitated or failed to abort the suicide (p. 30).

Client suicide during a course of treatment has sometimes been referred to as an "occupational hazard" (Brown 1987), and yet there seems to have been a general reluctance to examine and define the kinds of support needed for staff members after a suicide. Valente (1994) postulates that this may be related to a cultural influence that denies death and/or the hope or belief that if you are "a good enough nurse or therapist," you will be able to effectively prevent all suicides. An important point adapted from Valente is that there are two kinds of psychiatric nurses: those who have had a client die by suicide, and those who will in the future.

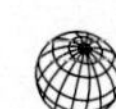

The reactions of staff members can be as varied as the roles they perform with clients. For example, the exact memories and reactions will vary with a nurse who finds a client hanging and administers first aid, a therapist who saw a client for his or her last session, and a psychiatrist who was the last person to evaluate the client. All are likely to experience the suicide as a traumatic event.

Support for staff members is critical after client suicide. Typical reactions to the suicide of a client may include sadness, anger, denial, and shame. Staff members may lack confidence and be unable to function. At this time, nurses may review their reasons for becoming nurses in the first place. Thoughts of reconsidering what they do or where they work are common. The range of other common reactions among nurses, therapists, and physicians range from refusing to admit suicidal clients to their caseloads or their units, to recognizing what the particular problems were and how they might manage them better in the future. Kottler and Blau (1989) developed a conceptual multistage model as a useful outline of how staff members may resolve the loss of a client by suicide. The stages are neither sequential nor time-limited. Staff members work through the process at their own speed.

- *Denial:* seeking to blame someone other than oneself.
- *Self-confrontation:* assuming total responsibility for what went wrong and painfully confronting the situation head-on. This usually results in self-doubt and self-deprecating thoughts.
- *The search:* seeking to find out what really happened by discovering some significant dimension of the experience and putting the situation in a more realistic light.
- *Resolution:* gaining new information and insight about the event by virtue of having opened up oneself to discovery; recognizing and accepting one's part in the entire process.
- *Application:* transferring new learning to future clinical work, being open to learning, and having a strong desire to work more effectively.

Staff members with little medical training or experience suffer more than those who have previously encountered illness and death. These workers need extra attention.

Chapter Highlights

- Suicide is a maladaptive response to a crisis.
- Nurses are in key positions to help clients resolve crises that lead to suicidal behavior.
- Suicidal behavior is affected by a number of social, demographic, and clinical variables.
- All suicidal ideation, threats, and attempts must be taken seriously and evaluated.
- A lethality assessment is the first step in helping self-destructive clients. The nurse uses this assessment to formulate a plan of care.
- The no self-harm/no-suicide contract is a useful tool for certain clients.
- Adolescents attempt suicide approximately 200 times as often as they complete a suicide.
- Older adults are the age group that is at the highest risk for suicide.

- To work effectively with self-destructive people, nurses must examine their own experiences and feelings.
- Suicide survivors are in need of special grief counseling but are unlikely to receive it.

References

Aguilera DC, Messick D: *Crisis Intervention: Theory and Methodology,* ed 7. Mosby, 1994.

American Psychiatric Association: *Diagnostic and Statistical Manual of Mental Disorders,* ed 4. American Psychiatric Association, 1994.

Black DW, Winokur G: Suicide and psychiatric diagnoses, in Blumenthal SJ, Kupfer DG (eds.): *Suicide Over the Life Cycle: Risk Factors, Assessment and Treatment of Suicidal Patients.* American Psychiatric Press, 1990.

Botsis AJ, et al.: Suicide and violence risk: I. Relationship to coping styles. *ACTA Psychiatr Scand* 1994;89:92–96.

Boxwell AO: Geriatric suicide: The preventable death. *Nurse Pract* 1988;13(6):10–19.

Brent DA, et al.: Bereavement or depression? The impact of the loss of a friend to suicide. *J Am Acad Child Adol Psychiatr* 1993;32:1189–1197.

Brent DA, et al.: Familial risk factors for adolescent suicide: A case-control study. *ACTA Psychiatr Scand* 1994;89: 52–58.

Brent DA, et al.: Firearms and adolescent suicide: A community case control study. *AJDC.* 1993;147:1066–1071.

Brown HN: The impact of suicide on therapists in training. *Comprehensive Psychiatr* 1987;28:101–112.

Bukstein OG, Brent DA, Perper JA: Risk factors for completed suicide among adolescents with a lifetime history of substance abuse: A case control study. *ACTA Psychiatr Scand* 1993;88:403–408.

Callias C, Carpenter MD: Self-injurious behavior in a state psychiatric hospital. *Hosp Commun Psychiatr* 1994;45: 170–172.

Carney SS, et al.: Suicide over 60. *The San Diego Study* 1994;42:174–180.

Coid J, Allolio B, Rees LH: Raised plasma metenkephalin in patients who habitually mutilate themselves. *Lancet* 1983;2:545–546.

Curran DK: *Adolescent Suicidal Behavior.* Hemisphere Publishing, 1987.

Davies P, Wilkes CR: Cluster suicide in rural western Canada. *Can J Psychiatr* 1993;38:515–519.

Doyle BB: Crisis management of the suicidal patient, in Blumenthal SJ, Kupfer DG (eds): *Suicide Over the Life Cycle: Risk Factors, Assessment and Treatment of Suicidal Patients.* American Psychiatric Press, 1990.

Dunn J: Psychiatric intervention in the community hospital emergency room. *J Nurs Admin* 1989;19(10):36–40.

Dunne-Maxim K: Survivors of suicide. *J Psychosoc Nurs* 1986;24(12):31–35.

Durkheim E: *Suicide.* Free Press, 1951.

Earle KA, et al.: Characteristics of outpatient suicides. *Hosp Commun Psychiatr* 1994;45:123–126.

Engberg M: Mortality and suicide rates of involuntarily committed patients. *ACTA Psychiatr Scand* 1994;89:35–40.

Farazza AR, et al.: Self-mutilation and eating disorders. *Suicide Life Threat Behav* 1989;19(4):352–361.

Farberow NL: The Los Angeles survivors—after suicide program: An evaluation. *Crisis* 1992;13:23–24.

Finch I: The effect of religion on clinical attitudes towards suicide. *Dissertation Abstracts International* 1993;53(9-A): 3146. French 1992.

Freud S: *New Introductory Lectures on Psycho Analysis: Lecture XXXII: Anxiety and Instinctual Life.* Hogarth, 1964 (originally published 1933).

Friedman S, et al: Suicidal ideation and suicide attempts among patients with panic disorder: A survey of two outpatient clinics. *Am J Psychiatr* 1992;149:680–685.

Gould MS: Suicide clusters and media exposure, in Blumenthal SJ, Kupfer DG (eds): *Suicide Over the Life Cycle: Risk Factors, Assessment and Treatment of Suicidal Patients.* American Psychiatric Press, 1990.

Hawton K: *Suicide and Attempted Suicide Among Children and Adolescents.* Sage, 1986.

Hazell P: Adolescent suicide clusters: Evidence, mechanisms and prevention. *Austral New Zeal J Psychiatr* 1993;27:653–665.

Hoff LA: *People in Crisis: Understanding and Helping,* ed 3. Addison-Wesley, 1989.

Hurley DJ: The crisis of paternal suicide: Case of Cathy, age 4½, in Webb NB (ed): *Play Therapy with Children in Crisis: A Casebook for Practitioners.* Guilford Press, 1991.

Kehoe NC, Gutheil TG: Neglect of religious issues in scale-based assessment of suicidal patients. *Hosp Commun Psychiatr* 1994;45:366–369.

Kottler JA, Blau DS: *The Imperfect Therapist: Learning from Failure in Therapeutic Practice.* Jossey-Bass, 1989.

Kovacs M, Goldston D, Gatsonis C: Suicidal behaviors and childhood onset depressive disorders: A longitudinal investigation. *J Am Acad Child Adoles Psychiatr* 1993;32: 8–20.

Kovansky RS: Loneliness and disturbed grief: A comparison of parents who lost a child to suicide or accidental death. *Arch Psychiatr Nurs* 1989;3(2):86–96.

Mann JJ, Arango V: Integration of neurobiology and psychopathology in a unified model of suicidal behavior. *J Clin Psychopharm* 1992;12(2, Suppl):2S–7S.

Marzuk PM, et al.: Increased risk of suicide in persons with AIDS. *JAMA* 1988;259:1333–1337.

Menninger A: *Man Against Himself.* Harcourt, Brace, 1938.

Nkongho NO: Suicide in the elderly: A beginning investigation. *J Nurs Admin* 1988;2(2):47–57.

O'Carroll PW, Mercy JA, Steward JA: CDC recommendations for a community for the prevention and containment of suicide cluster. *MMWR* 1992;Suppl. #6:1–12.

Orbach I: Personality characteristics, life circumstances, and dynamics of suicidal children. *Death Ed* 1984;8:37–52.

Pallikkathayil L, Morgan SA: Emergency department nurses' encounters with suicide attempters: A qualitative investigation. *Schol Inquiry Nurs Pract Int* 1988;2(3):237–253.

Pearce CM, Martin G: Locus of control as an indicator of risk for suicidal behavior among adolescents. *ACTA Psychiatr Scand* 1993;88:409–414.

Price JE: The effects of divorce precipitates a suicide threat: The case of Phillip, age 8, in Webb NB (ed): *Play Therapy with Children in Crisis: A Casebook for Practitioners.* Guilford Press, 1991.

Raczek SW, et al.: Suicidal behavior and personality traits. *J Pers Disord* 1989;3(4)345–351.

Read DA, Thomas CS, Mellsop GW: Suicide among psychiatric inpatients in the Wellington region. *Austral New Zeal J Psychiatr* 1993;27:392–398.

Reed PG, Leonard VE: An analysis of the concept of self-neglect. *Adv Nurs Sci* 1989;12(1):39–53.

Rissmiller DJ, et al.: Factors complicating cost containment in the treatment of suicidal patients. *Hosp Commun Psychiatr* 1994;8:782–788.

Roberts J, McFarland L: Assessment of suicide risk in the elderly. *Caring* 1986;5(7):20–23.

Savin-Williams RC: Verbal and physical abuse as stressors in the lives of lesbian, gay male, and bisexual youths: Associations with school problems, running away, substance abuse, prostitution, and suicide. *J Consult Clin Psych* 1994;62:261–269.

Schneider SG, Farberow NL, Kruks GN: Suicidal behavior in adolescent and young adult gay men. *Suicide Life Threat Behav* 1989;19(4):381–395.

Schneidman ES: *Definition of Suicide,* Wiley, 1985.

Schneidman ES: Postvention: The care of the bereaved. *Suicide Life Threat Behav* 1981;11:349–359.

Spirito A, et al.: Emergency department assessment of adolescent suicide attempters: Factors related to short-term follow-up outcome. *Ped Emer Care* 1994;10:6–12.

Stanford EJ, Goetz RR, Bloom JD: The no-harm contract in the emergency assessment of suicidal risk. *J Clin Psychiatr* 1994;55:344–348.

Stein E, et al.: Adrenal gland weight and suicide. *Can J Psychiatr* 1993;38:563–566.

Thompson J, Brooks S: When a colleague commits suicide: How the staff reacts. *J Psychosoc Nurs* 1990;28(10):6–11.

Traskman L, Asberg M, Bertilsson L: Monoamine metabolites in CSF and suicidal behavior. *Arch Gen Psychiatr* 1981;38:631–636.

U.S. Bureau of the Census: *Statistical Abstract of the United States,* ed 109, 1993.

Valente SM: Psychotherapist reactions to the suicide of a patient. *Am Orthopsychiatr Assoc* 1994;64:614–621.

Van der Kolk BA: The trauma spectrum: The interaction of biological and social events in the genesis of the trauma response. *J Traumatic Stress* 1988;1(3):273–290.

Wagner AW, Lineham MM: Relationship between childhood sexual abuse and topography of parasuicide among women with borderline personality disorder. *J Personality Disorders* 1994;8:1–9.

Walsh BW, Rosen PM: *Self-Mutilation: Theory, Research and Treatment.* Guilford Press, 1988.

CHAPTER 25

THE CLIENT WITH A DUAL DIAGNOSIS

Beth Phoenix Kasten

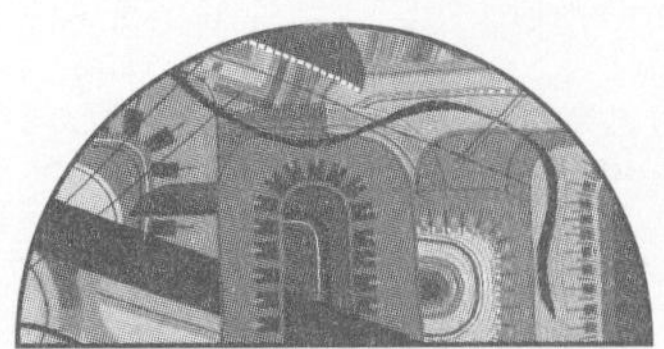

COMPETENCIES

- *Discuss at least two ways in which the use of nonprescription psychoactive substances can complicate the course of a mental disorder.*
- *Identify three ways in which mental health care and substance abuse treatment systems may fail to meet the needs of dual diagnosis clients.*
- *Be familiar with two theories about why people with mental illnesses have such a high rate of substance-related disorders.*
- *Identify two ways to ascertain the contribution of psychoactive substance use to a psychiatric emergency presentation, and two signs that would indicate a need for more extensive medical evaluation.*
- *Describe two ways in which an intoxicated client may be hazardous to self or others, and identify nursing interventions to prevent harm.*
- *Name three characteristics of an effective substance use assessment for a dual diagnosis client.*
- *Explain why you may find it difficult or unrewarding to work with dual diagnosis clients.*

Cross-References

Other topics relevant to this content are: Epidemiology, Chapter 5; Assessment, Chapter 8; Substance-related disorders, Chapter 13; The severely mentally ill in the community, Chapter 21; Codependence, Chapter 26.

Critical Thinking Challenge

Some mental health care settings have a policy of refusing to provide outpatient therapy for clients who are actively abusing drugs, reasoning that they cannot benefit from therapy until they "sober up," and that providing therapy to substance abusers condones their substance use. Do you agree with this policy? Is complete abstinence a precondition for therapy, or should it be a goal of therapy? What staff concerns might be reflected in such a policy? Is refusal to provide mental health services to those who are abusing drugs or alcohol an effective inducement to cease substance use?

Dual diagnosis is a term commonly used by providers in the mental health care and substance abuse treatment fields to refer to clients who experience both psychiatric and substance-related disorders. Most often, dual diagnosis connotes a complex of problems caused by the interaction of a disabling mental illness with substance abuse, although the term can be applied to any person who manifests both psychiatric and substance-related disorders.

Dual Diagnosis as a Mental Health Problem

The category of **substance-related disorders** in the *DSM-IV* includes both acute syndromes, such as **intoxication, delirium**, and **withdrawal**, and problems of longer duration (American Psychiatric Association 1994). Two DSM-IV categories, abuse and dependence, involve maladaptive patterns of substance use over time. **Substance abuse** involves continued use of the substance despite adverse consequences. **Substance dependence** may also include physical **tolerance**, withdrawal symptoms when substance use is stopped, and an eventual focus of most of the individual's energy on maintaining the habit. In this chapter, the terms *substance abuse* and *substance-related disorders* will be used interchangeably for the terms *abuse* and *dependence*.

Characteristics of Dual Diagnosis Clients

Ramon is a 25-year-old man who was diagnosed with schizophrenia 6 years ago, when he was a student at a local junior college. During the first few years of his illness, Ramon's relapses followed a familiar pattern: His family would bring him to the psychiatric emergency service (PES) after he had spent several weeks alone in his room, eating and sleeping little, talking to himself, and writing dozens of rambling, incoherent letters to a local talk show host. Ramon's mother believed he was smoking marijuana daily, but he denied this.

Ramon lost most of his high school and college friends because of his isolative and bizarre behavior, and also because he was preoccupied with his delusional relationship with the talk-show host. He dropped out of college because his periods of mental disorganization and his psychiatric hospitalizations interfered with his ability to attend classes.

Before Ramon's last hospitalization, he was convinced that his family was plotting to kill him and became threatening toward his sister. After Ramon's family refused to allow him to return home, he moved into a psychiatric halfway house for 6 months. After receiving weekly shots of a long-acting neuroleptic medication, he became much less delusional and developed some friendships with other residents of the halfway house. Several months ago, Ramon and two of his male friends from the halfway house moved into an apartment in a neighborhood known for its high incidence of crack cocaine use.

Ramon's case manager has become increasingly concerned that he may be using crack. Ramon's roommates have mentioned that he is spending a lot of time with another client of the mental health center who has a history of heavy crack use. He has lost weight, become more aggressive and paranoid, and has been threatened with eviction for failing to pay his rent. Ramon was brought into PES by the police after becoming loud, agitated, and incoherent in a convenience store, and threatening the owner of the store with a broken bottle when asked to leave. In PES, Ramon's urine toxicology screening was positive for cocaine.

Research on psychiatric/substance abuse **comorbidity**, as well as reports of clients receiving dual diagnosis treatment, indicate certain common clinical and demographic characteristics. As in people without mental illness, being young, male, unmarried, and poor are correlated with higher rates of substance abuse. However, as in the general population, no demographic segment is immune from substance-related disorders.

Results from several studies indicate that people with dual diagnoses are more socially competent than mentally ill abstainers. Some experts conclude that those whose mental illness is most severe lack the interpersonal skills and social contacts necessary to maintain drug or alcohol habits (Dixon et al. 1990; Kovaszny et al. 1993).

Dual diagnosis clients often suffer from the most disabling psychiatric conditions, such as schizophrenia, bipolar mood disorder, and antisocial personality disorder. Recent research on the prevalence of mental health problems indicates that those with severe disorders are highly likely to experience three or more comorbid disorders (Kessler et al. 1994), suggesting that "dual diagnosis" may be inaccurate to describe clients with multiple, interacting disorders.

Racial/Ethnic Differences in Substance Use

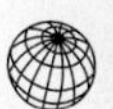

Information on racial differences in substance use by persons with mental illness is limited. Some studies comparing black and white clients with dual diagnoses indicate that while the overall rate of substance abuse was similar between the two groups, race was likely to influence the type of drug used. White clients were more likely to abuse alcohol, hallucinogens, or prescription sedatives; black clients had a higher rate of marijuana and cocaine use. Although these findings may be applicable primarily to the site of these studies (Philadelphia) and the time periods during which they were conducted, the authors emphasize that mentally ill persons are likely to demonstrate drug preferences similar to those of others in their ethnic or peer group.

Problems Resulting from Dual Diagnosis

Substance abuse compounds the already significant problems of daily living experienced by people who have multiple disorders. Difficulties with family and friends, lack of money, legal problems, accidents, and worsened physical problems have been cited by mentally ill clients as negative consequences of their substance abuse (Test et al. 1989).

Substance use can acutely aggravate symptoms of mental illness. For example, cocaine can increase psychotic symptoms and agitation in people with schizophrenia (Bunt et al. 1990), and alcohol can prolong depressive episodes (Mueller et al. 1994). Problematic behaviors more commonly seen in dual diagnosis clients, such as assaultiveness, incoherent speech, and disorganized behavior, may be a direct effect of intoxication, or may occur because substance use exacerbates the underlying mental illness (Drake and Wallach 1989).

The use of mental health services by clients with dual diagnoses reflects the tendency for substance use to cause acute exacerbations of illness. Mentally ill people who abuse substances make greater use of expensive emergency and acute care services, and make less use of community and rehabilitative services, than nonusers (Bartels et al. 1993).

Substance abuse appears likely to affect both the regular use and the effectiveness of psychotropic medication, which many people require to manage their mental disorders. Substance users are less likely to take psychotropic medication as prescribed (Drake and Wallach 1989), receive less effect from antipsychotic medication (Bowers et al. 1990), and are at greater risk for tardive dyskinesia, a nonreversible long-term side effect of antipsychotic therapy (Olivera, Kiefer, and Manley 1990).

Problems Resulting from Separate Treatment Systems

Some of the problems mentioned above are inevitable consequences of having combined psychiatric and substance-related disorders, each of which may complicate the course and management of the other. But other difficulties result from the failure of health care services to provide effective and coordinated treatment for clients with dual disorders. Historically, mental health care and substance abuse treatment systems developed separately, with different treatment philosophies and different types of staff training and expertise (Carey 1989).

- Because dual diagnosis clients do not fit neatly into the programmatic boundaries of either mental health care or substance abuse treatment, they may be considered "unsuitable" for treatment by both systems. Mental health care providers commonly fail to diagnose substance use problems, or may minimize their contribution to a client's difficulties. If substance abuse is recognized, mental health clinicians are apt to consider it a waste of time to treat psychiatric problems until the client has received substance abuse treatment and achieved sobriety (Fariello and Scheidt 1989).
- Substance abuse settings are also likely to exclude dual diagnosis clients. Their bizarre or disorganized behavior can disrupt the therapeutic environment, and the goal of being chemical-free may be unrealistic for clients who require psychotropic medication in order to maintain clear thinking and/or stable moods (Fariello and Scheidt 1989). Thus, dual diagnosis clients may be excluded from any medical treatment altogether.
- Clients who are able to receive both psychiatric and substance abuse treatment may find the advice they receive in the two settings difficult to reconcile. Compliance with psychotropic medication is often considered an essential component of treatment for a mental disorder but may be seen as "just another addiction" by staff members and peers in substance abuse treatment. Similarly, the confrontational approach used in addiction treatment to break down denial may be seen by mental health care professionals as precipitating psychiatric decompensation.

As the problem of psychiatric/substance abuse comorbidity began to receive wider attention in the mid-1980s, some areas began to establish special "dual diagnosis" treatment programs. However, the need to foster collaboration between mental health care and substance abuse treatment agencies, train staff capable of treating both problems simultaneously, and provide necessary funding for such programs has limited the availability of dual diagnosis treatment.

In the areas where dual diagnosis treatment programs have been offered, they have often demonstrated benefits, such as reducing hospitalization rates (Hellerstein and Meehan 1987; Kofoed et al. 1986) and promoting abstinence (Drake, McHugo, and Noordsy 1993). However, even state-of-the-art dual diagnosis treatment may be insufficient to adequately treat all the difficult and interlocking problems experienced by people whose severe mental illness is compounded by substance abuse.

A recent clinical trial involving a sophisticated dual diagnosis treatment program involving group education and case management failed to demonstrate improved client outcomes (Lehman, Herron, Schwartz, and Myers 1993). As well as noting problems with engaging clients in the experimental treatment, the authors suggested that, for those with multiple and deeply entrenched life difficulties, the one-year follow-up period may have been too short to demonstrate significant benefit from the treatment.

The Prevalence of Dual Diagnosis

Research in substance abuse treatment settings and psychiatric treatment settings has demonstrated high rates of psychiatric/substance abuse comorbidity (Caragonne, Emery, and Isser 1987; Hasin, Endicott, and Lewis 1989). In addition, large-scale epidemiologic studies indicate that people with mental illnesses are more likely than others to have substance-related disorders. The Epidemiologic Catchment Area (ECA) study, conducted in the early 1980s, surveyed over 20,000 people to determine the prevalence of mental health problems. Analysis indicated:

- Those with mental illnesses were much more likely than others to have a substance-related disorder.
- Those with schizophrenia were over four times as likely to be substance abusers.
- Those with mood disorders were over twice as likely to be substance abusers.
- Those with antisocial personality disorder were almost thirty times as likely as others to abuse substances (Regier et al. 1990). See Figures 25–1 and 25–2.

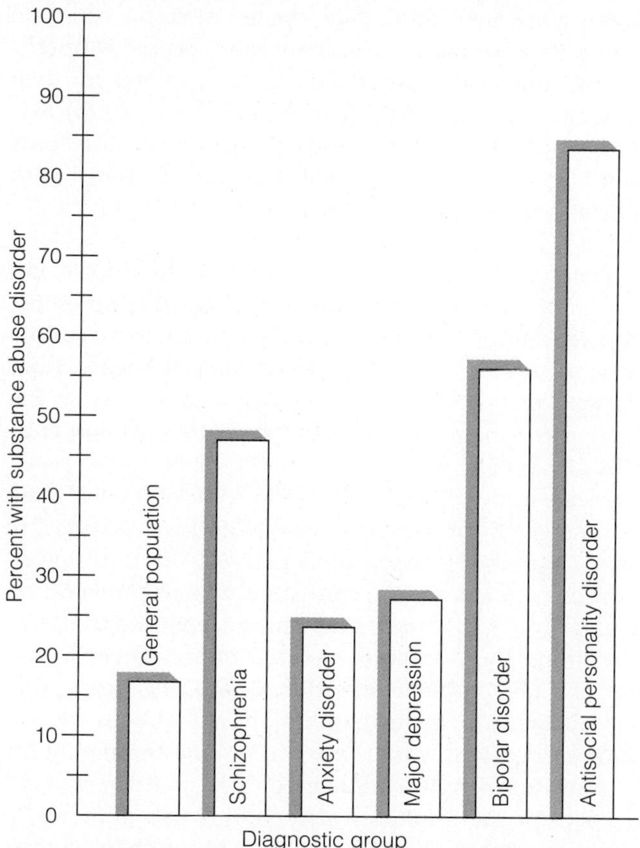

Figure 25–1 Lifetime prevalence rates for substance abuse disorder. *Based on data from Epidemiologic Catchment Area Study, Regier et al. 1990.*

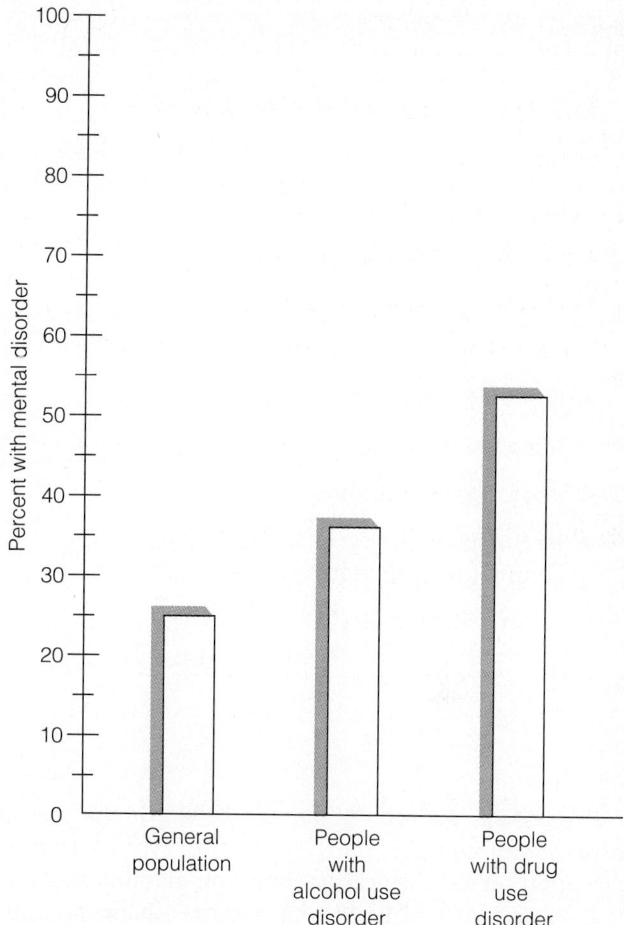

Figure 25–2 Lifetime prevalence rates for non–substance abuse mental disorder. *Based on data from Epidemiologic Catchment Area Study, Regier et al. 1990.*

As might be expected, people with substance abuse problems also have an elevated risk of mental illness. Each mental illness surveyed in the ECA study was more common in alcoholics than nonalcoholics (Helzer and Pryzbek 1988). Large studies of addiction treatment facilities have also shown high rates of mental illness in people with other types of chemical dependence (Ross, Glaser, and Germanson 1988; Rounsaville et al. 1987).

Biopsychosocial Theories About the Causes of Dual Diagnosis

A number of different factors—genetic predisposition, family and social background, the effects of psychoactive drugs on brain chemistry, among others—have been suggested as contributing to the high rate of psychiatric/substance abuse comorbidity. Lehman, Myers, and Corty (1989) suggest that any given dual diagnosis may be the outcome of different combinations of these factors and suggest a classification scheme that highlights the salient factors in each case. They propose four clinical explanations for how dual diagnosis conditions develop:

1. Primary mental illness with substance abuse sequelae.
2. Primary substance abuse with psychiatric sequelae.
3. Dual primary diagnosis.
4. Common etiology.

Primary Mental Illness with Substance Abuse Sequelae

This explanation assumes that having a mental illness predisposes individuals to substance abuse. As Lehman, Myers, and Corty (1989) point out, most of the risk factors for addictive behavior are also risk factors for mental illness. Risk factors for addictive behavior include the characteristics listed in the box on page 620.

SELF-MEDICATION One theory is that mentally ill clients self-medicate with nonprescribed psychoactive substances. **Self-medication** with substance-related disorders has been discussed from both psychologic and biologic perspectives.

Risk Factors for Addictive Behavior

- Negative affect states
- Impaired cognition
- Misinterpretation of internal cues
- Low self-esteem
- Lack of a sense of self-control and self-efficacy
- Poor role performance
- Impaired social skills
- Restricted coping abilities
- Disturbances of vegetative (eating, sleeping, eliminating) functions
- Lack of social supports

Psychologic Aspects Khantzian (1985) is the person most commonly associated with the psychodynamic viewpoint on self-medication. Based on his clinical observations and interventions with addicts, Khantzian concluded that deficits in ego functioning lead to an inability to modulate painful affects. The addict's "drug of choice" is chosen specifically for its ability to pharmacologically compensate for these difficulties the client experiences in regulating feeling states.

Compton (1989) reformulated Khantzian's ego/self theory of substance dependence to fit Orem's nursing model for self-care. Compton proposed that Orem's conceptualization of self-care, which includes all the actions that people take to maintain health and well-being, encompasses Khantzian's definition of self-care as a complex ego function that serves to alert and protect individuals from dangers in the environment. Using Orem's self-care deficit theory, Compton defines lack of self-protective behavior and difficulty in handling painful feelings as self-care deficits that require nursing intervention.

Khantzian's theory has helped clarify the adaptive function of substance use, making the behavior more comprehensible to health care providers, who are likely to see substance use as inherently self-destructive. However, this psychodynamic theory has some significant limitations when applied to clients with severe mental illness. Khantzian's focus on drug use to regulate unpleasant affects does not encompass other symptoms that mentally ill people may self-medicate, such as abnormal perceptions (hallucinations) and the physical discomforts associated with medication side effects. Also, his assertion that, after a period of experimentation, people will settle on one drug that most effectively compensates for their difficulties in managing their predominant painful feelings, is contradicted by research demonstrating long-standing patterns of multiple drug use in clients with schizophrenia (Test et al. 1989).

Biologic Aspects Biologic, as well as psychologic, factors are thought to contribute to the use of nonprescription substances to self-medicate symptoms of mental illness. In several studies that asked subjects their reasons for substance use, relief from anxiety and depression was cited as the main reason (Brady et al. 1990; Dixon et al. 1991; Test et al. 1989).

In the study by Test et al. (1989), three of the five main reasons given for substance use (to feel less anxious, to make it easier to sleep, and to make medication side effects more tolerable) are consistent with self-medication as a motive. When asked how substance use affected their symptoms, more subjects reported improvement in five out of eight problems mentioned (anxiety, sleep problems, depression, hallucinations, and side effects) than reported symptoms worsening. Further questioning by the investigators revealed that subjects were well aware of differences in the responses of their various symptoms to different substances and "attempted to self-manage their substance selection and amount in order to gain the most advantageous benefit-to-cost ratio of consequences."

Schneier and Siris (1987) consider different perspectives on the self-medication theory in their review of studies of drug choice by people with schizophrenia. They found that schizophrenic subjects used amphetamines, cocaine, cannabis, hallucinogens, inhalants, caffeine, and tobacco more often than controls. The researchers suggest that schizophrenics may prefer stimulants or hallucinogens for relief of depression or the negative symptoms of schizophrenia, such as apathy and lack of enjoyment. Increased use of tobacco and caffeine may be effective to combat extrapyramidal, sedative, or hypotensive effects of antipsychotic medications.

Schneier and Siris (1987) also suggest that some substances of abuse may stimulate neurotransmitter systems in the brain that have been altered both by the disease and by some of the agents used to treat schizophrenia. Animal studies indicate that addictive agents increase activity in brain systems dependent on dopamine (DA), a neurotransmitter whose functioning is known to be altered in schizophrenia. The use of stimulants by people with schizophrenia may be seen as an attempt to "normalize" certain brain functions that have been impaired by the disease.

As well as suggesting an adaptive function for substance abuse by mentally ill people, the self-medication theory has implications for treatment. Since studies of drug choice indicate that schizophrenics commonly use substances to relieve dysphoria and anxiety, Siris (1990) suggests careful consideration of using prescribed antidepressant and antianxiety medications for such clients.

Effects of Social Disadvantage Related to Mental Illness People with severe mental illness often experience social disabilities that may increase the risk of substance abuse. Estroff's well-known ethnographic 1981 study of chronic mentally ill clients paints a vivid picture of the employment difficulties, poverty, and social isolation too often experienced by people with long-term mental illness. Stressful conditions such as these are regarded by many experts as increasing the risk of substance-related problems.

Joblessness is likely to be a significant risk factor, because it leads to poverty and because unemployed people have lots of time on their hands. Large amounts of unstructured time and few affordable recreational outlets may make substance use an attractive way to kill time; "to relieve boredom" was cited as one of the most common reasons for substance use in a recent study (Test et al. 1989).

Poverty caused by living on disability income often limits mentally ill people to poor neighborhoods in which the widespread availability of such drugs as crack cocaine has become common (Bunt et al. 1990). Exposure to social norms condoning heavy substance use is likely to be particularly influential on those who are socially isolated because of stigma and impaired social skills. Studies of people with psychiatric disabilities have repeatedly found that being part of a group and having "something to do with friends" are the major reasons given for substance use (Bergman and Harris 1985; Dixon et al. 1991; Test et al. 1989).

Primary Substance Abuse with Psychiatric Sequelae

This explanation for the causes of dual diagnosis holds that the psychiatric difficulties experienced by substance abusers are direct effects of the abused substances. Acute effects of intoxication and withdrawal from drugs, such as psychoses produced by amphetamines and hallucinogens and rebound depression following a cocaine binge, resemble psychiatric disorders. However, if these symptoms resolve as the client detoxifies, such drug effects would not represent a true dual diagnosis.

The question of whether substance use can actually cause permanent alterations in brain physiology, leading to mental illness in the absence of continued substance abuse, remains unanswered. Although the long-term abuse of stimulants can produce chronic psychotic states, and the abuse of CNS depressants has been noted to produce persistent mood alterations, it has not been proven that these are direct results of the abused substances and not the result of a preexisting vulnerability to mental illness (Lehman, Myers, and Corty 1989).

Similarly, research to determine whether hallucinogenic drugs produce psychotic illness failed to demonstrate that drug use could produce long-term psychosis in the absence of underlying vulnerability to mental illness. 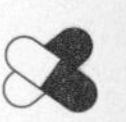 However, evidence that hallucinogenic drug use was associated with earlier and more frequent psychiatric hospitalizations led Bowers (1987) to conclude that such drugs may at least exacerbate psychotic disorders:

> Assuming that genetic liability to most psychotic disorders in the schizophrenia-mania spectrum is a continuous and not a dichotomous distribution, drugs may be playing a variety of roles. In some individuals, they may simply be causing a psychosis to become manifest at an earlier age. In others, they may be producing a psychotic disorder that would have remained dormant if drugs had not been used. Certain psychotogenic drug use becomes a significant risk factor for relapse in an individual who has previously suffered a psychotic disorder (p. 822).

Dual Primary Diagnosis

In this explanation, the individual suffers from two disorders that, although initially unrelated, interact to exacerbate each other. The fact that rates of psychiatric/substance abuse comorbidity are substantially higher than those predicted by chance indicates that the two types of disorder are in some way causally related, but certainly some mentally ill individuals have independent risk factors for both disorders.

In a recent study of clients in a dual diagnosis treatment group, most of the group members had family histories of substance abuse and had begun their own substance use in their teens or earlier, well before the onset of their psychiatric symptoms (Kasten 1993). These same individuals were likely to also have family histories of mental illness.

In such clients, diagnosis and treatment are likely to prove difficult because there is no history of psychiatric symptoms in the absence of substance abuse. Continued substance abuse, especially of multiple substances, is likely to mask the symptoms of mental illness.

Common Etiology

This explanation posits that a common underlying factor predisposes to both substance abuse and mental illness. Familial links between alcoholism and mood disorders raise the possibility of a genetic factor common to both (Lehman, Myers, and Corty 1989).

Psychosocial and historical factors may also predispose to dual disorders. The PTSD and substance abuse commonly seen in Vietnam veterans is an example of such a predisposing factor.

The Nursing Process with the Dual Diagnosis Client in an Emergency Setting

Clients with dual diagnoses are likely to constitute a significant part of the population served by nurses working in a psychiatric emergency setting. Intoxication is likely to lead to acute decompensations, and because dual diagnosis clients may be difficult to link with after-care services that do not address their special needs, a "revolving door" pattern of repeated emergency visits, with little psychiatric care between them, may emerge.

Substance use may be implicated in a variety of emergency presentations:

- Alcohol intoxication may lead to impulsive suicide attempts.
- Chronic cocaine use may produce intense paranoia.
- Stimulant or hallucinogenic drugs may produce or exacerbate psychotic symptoms, such as hallucinations and delusions.
- The "crash" that follows a cocaine or speed binge may cause severe depression and acute suicidality.

Given the high rate of substance abuse in individuals with mental illness, psychiatric nurses should always include a comprehensive evaluation for substance use in any emergency assessment. Substance-related diagnoses are often missed for several reasons:

- Drug effects may mimic symptoms of mental illness.
- The client may be too disorganized to provide accurate information about substance use.
- Psychiatric clinicians often receive inadequate training in assessing and treating substance-related disorders (Ananth et al. 1989; Szuster et al. 1990). See the Research Note.

Assessment

Subjective Data Gathering useful subjective data from clients who are intoxicated may be difficult because of their mental disorganization. If possible, ask clients if they have used any drugs or alcohol, and if so, how recently. As well as including alcohol and street drugs such as marijuana, speed, PCP, and cocaine, ask about over-the-counter drugs and inhalants, such as glue.

Even if clients are coherent enough to answer questions, the accuracy of their answers may be suspect. Clients may fear legal consequences if they admit to using illegal substances, may fear being stigmatized as a "junkie" or a "drunk," or may simply be unaware of what was in the street drugs they consumed (Drake, Osher, and Wallach 1989). Also ask anyone who accompanies the client about what substances were consumed, and the time and amount.

Other subjective data that may indicate substance use are the client's reported symptoms. Although auditory hallucinations are common in people with psychotic disorders, visual or tactile hallucinations are uncommon and may indicate substance use (Chafetz 1989).

Also ask about use of prescribed medications. Clients may overuse anticholinergic medications to get a "buzz," and narcotics and antianxiety agents may be taken in greater than the prescribed amounts for their euphoric effects. In addition to taking prescribed medicines for their pleasurable effects, clients may have misunderstood how the medications should be taken, or be too disorganized to take them correctly. Information about psychoactive medications is very important when clients have consumed drugs or alcohol, because both types of drugs can interact and cause serious complications, such as overdose or seizures (Chafetz 1989).

Objective Data Observe the client's appearance for signs of substance use. The smell of alcohol on the breath and the sight of "tracks" (needle marks) on the skin are immediate evidence of use. Slurred speech and ataxia may also indicate intoxication.

Vital signs are important indicators of substance-related problems. Elevated heart rate and blood pressure may indicate stimulant overdose or alcohol withdrawal. Hyperthermia may be a life-threatening complication of cocaine overdose (Kosten and Kleber 1988). Depressed vital signs may indicate sedative overdose. Although the cause of altered vital signs may not be immediately apparent and may be due to physical problems other than substance abuse, any abnormality in vital signs indicates a need for closer monitoring and more extensive physical examination.

Similarly, abnormal neurologic findings indicate a need for more extensive medical evaluation. Changes in levels of consciousness, such as delirium or stuporousness, are not caused by psychiatric illness and indicate an organic cause. Also observe the client's pupils: Pinpoint pupils can be caused by opiate use, marijuana or amphetamines dilate the pupils, and PCP use can cause nystagmus. Abnormal motor behavior, such as ataxia, should also be reported and further evaluated.

Abnormal mental status findings are seen in substance-induced disorders but are not specific to them. Confusion, disorientation, and agitation, while often seen in intoxicated individuals, may also indicate other problems, such as dementia, head injury, or metabolic abnormalities. Paranoia is common in stimulant abuse but may also indicate paranoid schizophrenia. Hallucinations can be caused by alcohol overuse, hallucinogenic drugs, or functional psychoses, such as schizophrenia or mania. However, signs of impaired thinking, such as loose associa-

RESEARCH NOTE

Citation

Dixon L, Dibietz E, Myers P, Conley R, Medoff D, Lehman AF: Comparison of DSM-III-R diagnoses and a brief interview for substance use among state hospital patients. *Hosp Commun Psychiatr* 1993;44(8): 748–752.

Study Problem/Purpose

Reported prevalence rates of psychiatric/substance abuse comorbidity have varied widely, partly because studies of this phenomenon have used different methods of identifying substance abuse in people with mental illnesses. This study used six different methods to identify substance abuse in a population of psychiatric inpatients and compared the prevalence rates obtained by these six strategies. Two substance abuse identification strategies were compared to see which better correlated with clinical determinations of the need for substance abuse treatment.

Methods

Chart reviews and brief interviews were conducted with a randomly selected sample of 474 state hospital inpatients. With this information, subjects were classified as having or not having a substance-use disorder based on six different criteria: DSM-III-R substance-use disorder; history of previous substance abuse treatment; any use of alcohol or drugs during the 30 days before admission; any past period of daily use of alcohol or drugs; any past period of daily or weekly use; and any past period of daily or weekly use plus any substance use in the 30 days before admission (referred to as "recent regular users"). Subjects were also rated as to their need for substance abuse treatment.

Multiple regression analysis was used to determine which demographic and clinical characteristics were most highly correlated with the presence of a substance abuse disorder. An additional analysis was done to compare subjects identified as "recent regular users" to those having DSM-III-R diagnosis of substance-use disorder to see which method was the better predictor of the need for substance abuse treatment services.

Findings

The survey found no indication of drug or alcohol use for 43% of the subjects. Those identified as having substance-use disorders were more likely to be male and to be younger, and less likely to have a diagnosis of schizophrenia. Prevalence rates for substance abuse found using the six methods ranged from 23% using DSM-III-R criteria to 55% based on having a past period of daily or weekly use. Thirty-seven percent of the subjects were classified as recent regular users. The different strategies did not always identify the same people as having substance-use disorders—for example, less than half of the recent regular users met DSM-III-R criteria for substance abuse, and almost one-quarter of those with DSM-III-R diagnoses had not engaged in recent regular use.

When the group identified as substance abusers by DSM-III-R criteria were compared to the recent regular users, the two groups were found to be similar in their rated need for substance abuse treatment. In contrast, those who were not in either group were generally considered unlikely to require, or to benefit from, substance abuse treatment.

Implications

These findings suggest that a brief screening for recent regular substance use is more useful than DSM-III-R substance abuse diagnosis in identifying psychiatric inpatients who need substance abuse treatment services. Since DSM-III-R criteria for substance-use disorder require evidence that life problems are caused by substance use, such diagnoses can be difficult to make in the presence of severe psychiatric impairment. Thus, reliance on such diagnoses may cause clinicians and service planners to underestimate the need for substance abuse treatment services by people with severe mental illness. A brief interview to establish a pattern of recent regular substance use is likely to be equally effective in identifying the need for substance abuse treatment.

tions, are unlikely to be caused by substance use and are more likely to be due to schizophrenia.

Toxicologic screening of the blood or urine may be extremely helpful in clarifying the contribution of substance use to the client's presentation. Studies have found that clients who denied drug use nevertheless showed evidence of drugs in their urine (Brady and Casto 1989; Elangovan et al. 1993). Toxicology specimens should be obtained as early as possible when the role of substance use is in question.

However, toxicology may also fail to detect covert drug use. Most toxicologic screenings do not identify inhalants, and other drugs may be missed unless the screening is done at the earliest possible time (Ananth et al. 1989). Because urine tests are inadequate to detect alcohol use, blood tests should be performed (Elangovan et al. 1993). Clients in withdrawal will test negative for substance use.

The client's history may offer some insight into his or her current presentation. If the client has been previously diagnosed with a mental illness, this is likely to be a contributing factor to the present difficulties. However, do not make the mistake of concluding that any symptoms of psychosis or mood alteration are due exclusively to the psychiatric illness, because these abnormalities may well be compounded by substance abuse.

Similarly, clients with documented histories of substance abuse cannot be assumed to be free of concurrent psychiatric illness. Although a conclusive psychiatric diagnosis cannot be made while the client is intoxicated or in withdrawal, any symptoms of mental illness should be noted and evaluated when the client is more stable.

Although dealing with the combination of mental illness and substance abuse is itself a significant challenge to the assessment skills of psychiatric nurses, dual diagnosis clients are at increased risk for other medical and psychosocial problems that can make the diagnostic picture even more complicated. For instance, HIV infection caused by intravenous drug use can cause many psychiatric syndromes, including mood disorder, dementia, and psychosis (Kasten and Monteleone 1993). Malnutrition in a homeless, alcoholic client can contribute to Wernicke's encephalopathy. Although the effects of all these interlocking disorders may be too complicated to sort out during an emergency visit, you should perform as thorough an assessment as possible of physical, psychologic, and social factors that led to the crisis admission. See the accompanying Assessment box.

ASSESSMENT

Substance Abuse by Persons with Mental Illness

Nursing History

- Comprehensive substance use history, including prescribed medication, over the counter (OTC) medications, alcohol, street drugs, and other potential substances of abuse, such as inhalants.
- Subjective perception of responses to use of each substance, prescribed or non-prescribed.

Physical Examination

- Visible or olfactory evidence of recent drug use such as alcohol on breath, "tracks" from injecting drugs.
- Altered vital signs.
- Signs of withdrawal such as agitation, tremulousness, and profuse sweating in alcohol withdrawal.

Mental Status Examination

- Delirium.
- Perceptual disturbances. Visual, tactile, or olfactory hallucinations are particularly likely to be caused by substance use or withdrawal.

Diagnostic Studies

- Blood or urine toxicologic studies.

Planning and Implementing Interventions

Stabilizing the client's physical and mental condition and preventing harm to the client and others are nursing care priorities for dual diagnosis clients in an emergency setting. Vital signs and neurologic status should be closely monitored to detect impending medical emergencies, such as seizures or delirium tremens. Serious complications such as these may require the client to be transferred to a medical emergency setting.

Intoxicated individuals are likely to be emotionally labile and impulsive, and to require close observation and vigilance. PCP users, in particular, may behave unpredictably, changing rapidly from being calm to being highly agitated. Clients who are highly agitated, threatening, or unpredictable may require seclusion and/or restraints to prevent them from becoming assaultive. Benzodiazepines, such as lorazepam, may be helpful in controlling agitation. To avoid harmful drug interactions, administer medications with caution if in doubt about what substances the client has consumed.

Suicidal intent is a concern with clients who are intoxicated, or who are acutely depressed from crashing after a cocaine or amphetamine binge. Suicide precautions should be instituted for clients whose admission was precipitated by a suicide attempt, who acknowledge suicidal ideation, or who appear acutely depressed.

Clients may require care for physical problems resulting from intoxication. Trauma may result from falls, fights, or self-inflicted injury. Encourage clients who are dehydrated or are withdrawing from alcohol to drink ample amounts of fluid.

In some emergency settings, client education is a component of crisis intervention. Wolfe and Sorenson (1989) describe the use of interactive computer programs and films to educate emergency clients about HIV disease and other consequences of substance abuse. Peer counselors, former clients who have been trained in counseling, are also available to share their experiences dealing with dual disabilities.

Patty, a 26-year-old woman with diagnoses of borderline personality disorder (BPD) and asymptomatic HIV infection and a history of alcohol and amphetamine abuse, was brought to the PES by the police. She had been found partially unclothed and wandering in traffic, mumbling incoherently to herself.

PES staff were quite concerned over Patty's condition, since this behavior was quite different from her usual presentation. When Patty was abusing drugs, she was often admitted to PES after a suicide attempt, having become severely depressed after a "speed run." However, 9 months ago, Patty had moved in with a boyfriend who did not use drugs, began attending twelve-step self-help groups, and remained "clean and sober."

Patty remained disorganized, incoherent, and intrusive, repeatedly disrobing and attempting to enter the nurses' station. She was secluded to protect herself and others. Patty's pulse and blood pressure were elevated, and her toxicology screen was positive for amphetamines. However, she showed no signs of head injury, metabolic abnormalities, or anything else that would explain her highly disorganized behavior. When this continued for over 24 hours, she was admitted to an inpatient unit.

Information subsequently obtained from Patty's boyfriend revealed that she had been behaving erratically. She was forgetful, irritable, and became easily confused. When Patty had bumped into a drug-using friend, she went off with her for a week and had apparently injected amphetamines.

Further psychologic testing revealed that Patty was suffering from AIDS dementia. Amphetamine use had dramatically increased her organic deficits, producing mental disorganization that required more than a week to clear.

The Nursing Process with the Dual Diagnosis Client in a Nonemergency Setting

Inpatient Psychiatric Wards: Guidelines for Care

Inpatient hospitalization presents an excellent opportunity for a more comprehensive nursing assessment of the dual diagnosis client. A study conducted by Ananth et al. (1989) found that substance abuse diagnosed in psychiatric inpatients was missed during the emergency admission in almost all of the cases. The research team attributed their success in identifying substance abuse to the fact that they conducted physical examinations and detailed histories, with probes for each type of drug, when the subjects' mental states had cleared enough for them to fully cooperate. The authors concluded that acutely psychotic emergency clients are often too disorganized to provide adequate information about their substance use.

ASSESSING SUBSTANCE USE Nurses performing assessments on dual diagnosis clients may find it helpful to use a standardized substance use questionnaire to guide their interviews and record data. Ask specifically about every drug, giving several examples of drugs in each category, using street names if possible. The use of alcohol, marijuana, stimulants, hallucinogens, narcotics, sedative/hypnotics, and inhalants should be covered in the interview, as well as caffeine and tobacco. Also inquire about over-the-counter (OTC) drugs, and whether prescription drugs are being used as prescribed. A matter-of-fact, nonjudgmental approach is most likely to elicit useful information.

SUPPORTING ABSTINENCE Given the likelihood that substance abuse contributed to the problems that led to the client's admission, substance use should be avoided while in the hospital. Clients in Veterans Administration facilities are particularly likely to continue substance use during psychiatric hospitalization (Galanter, Casteneda, and Ferman 1988), requiring particular clinical vigilance by nurses in these settings. Clients who are unable to abstain may require transfer to a more secure unit. Withdrawal must be treated and detoxification carefully monitored.

ASSESSING BASELINE FUNCTIONING Inpatient stays, during which the client is abstinent, are a good time to assess baseline functioning without the complicating factor of substance use, and to determine how substance abuse may be contributing to the client's psychiatric problems. Although the most prominent symptoms of withdrawal resolve in a few days, some substance-related symptoms require several weeks or more to completely clear (Brown, Irwin, and Schuckit 1991). Abbott (1992) found that a number of subjects had a "turning point" in their functioning and use of psychiatric services after a long hospitalization for a mental disorder. Abbott speculates that the opportunity to completely detoxify from all drugs, and to reflect on the consequences of drug use, contributed to the subjects' decreased use of street drugs and decline in number of hospitalizations.

CLIENT EDUCATION As well as providing general education about the effects of substance abuse on people with mental illness, encourage clients to reflect on the consequences of their own substance use. Rather than zealously preaching **abstinence**, a more useful nursing role is to help clients identify cause-and-effect relationships between the use of specific substances and the attendant consequences, and to help them make decisions about their use of drugs and alcohol (McKelvy, Kane, and Kellison 1987). In addition, eliciting information about the motivations for substance use may reveal symptoms, such as anxiety, that could be more effectively treated with prescribed medication.

Tom, an unemployed 28-year-old man with bipolar mood disorder, was admitted to an inpatient psychiatric unit after attempting suicide by overdosing on antianxiety medication. After recovering from the effects of the overdose, he described a period of depression that began a month before admission and became increasingly severe. His appetite was poor, he had little energy, he had difficulty getting to sleep, and was unable to sleep more than a few hours a night. In addition, he became preoccupied with fears of being unable to find a job and of being evicted from his apartment.

About 10 days before admission, he began to be bothered by auditory hallucinations telling him that nothing was going to get any better, and that he should kill himself. Although Tom had been taking the lithium and carbamazepine he had been prescribed until a few days before admission, he claimed, "They just weren't working for me any more."

Tom's discussions with his primary nurse revealed several substance-related problems that may have contributed to his psychiatric decompensation. As Tom's energy level had declined, he had begun drinking numerous cups of coffee each day, "just to keep me going." In addition to increasing his anxiety about his situation, Tom's high caffeine intake almost undoubtedly contributed to his sleep problems, and by so doing, exacerbated his depression.

Tom also revealed that he had begun drinking beer in increasing quantities during the few weeks before admission. At first, he drank only at bedtime "to help me get to sleep," but began drinking at other times during the day because he claimed "it fuzzed the voices out so I could ignore them."

Tom was surprised to learn that alcohol's diuretic effect could lead to an increased excretion of lithium in the urine, which may have caused his blood lithium level to drop below the therapeutic level. Although some individuals report that, in their experience, alcohol suppresses auditory hallucinations, it is also known to *increase* hallucinations after days or weeks of heavy alcohol intake. In addition, since alcohol is a physiologic depressant, it can prolong depressive episodes.

In discussing relapse prevention, Tom's nurse encouraged him to avoid consuming more than one or two alcoholic beverages per day, because it could affect his blood lithium level and because people with bipolar disorder are at unusually high risk for developing alcohol dependence. He was also encouraged to limit his caffeine intake to one or two cups a day, since caffeine's diuretic effect can increase lithium excretion, and because excessive caffeine consumption can disrupt sleep patterns.

As an alternative to self-medicating his depression and hallucinations with nonprescription substances, the nurse encouraged Tom to promptly report any worsening in his depressive symptoms, or the onset of new symptoms like auditory hallucinations, to his psychiatrist or the nurse at the outpatient clinic. In addition to allowing these professionals to intervene before Tom became suicidal, his medication regime might be altered to include such drugs as antipsychotic medication to decrease hallucinations, sleep medications, and an antidepressant.

Community Settings

Psychiatric nurses who work in community settings, such as day treatment, community mental health centers, case management agencies, and home care, are in a good position to help dual diagnosis clients lessen the negative consequences of their substance use. The frequency of contact and long-term nature of these nurse-client relationships allows for trust to develop, so clients feel able to talk about their drug use.

In addition, community mental health nurses can learn about the context of substance abuse in their clients' lives. Knowledge about the home situation, social milieu, and daily activities provides valuable information about which substances may be available, and under what circumstances they are used.

As you develop an awareness of how substance abuse is affecting a client's course of illness and daily functioning, you can help the client see cause-and-effect relationships between substance misuse and adverse consequences. Dual diagnosis clients may have a hard time making these connections, not only because of the denial commonly thought to be a feature of addictive disorders but also because thought disorder caused by their illness, or cognitive deficit produced by the toxic effects of the abused substances, inhibits logical thinking.

Watching clients repeatedly experience the often disastrous consequences of their substance use, despite your best efforts to encourage them to abstain, may be a frustrating experience. However, persistent outreach to dual diagnosis clients in the community has shown impressive results in decreasing both substance use and the necessity for psychiatric hospitalization (Durell et al. 1993).

Acceptance of the dual diagnosis client as a person, and a commitment to continue working with clients who are still abusing substances, does not mean tolerating threatening or disruptive behavior from people who are intoxicated. Similarly, those who are obviously intoxicated may appropriately be excluded from group sessions. Failure to allow clients to experience appropriate consequences of their substance-abusing behavior may be seen as condoning the abuse. However, it should be made clear to the clients that it is their disruptive behavior, and not their substance use habit per se that is objectionable, and that they are welcome back when they can maintain appropriate behavior.

In addition to focusing on the adverse effects of substance abuse, you may gain insight into the adaptive effects of the substance. Alternative coping strategies can then be taught. For instance, clients who use alcohol to relieve anxiety can be taught relaxation exercises or cognitive strategies to reduce anxiety. The use of prescribed antianxiety medications may relieve anxiety as effectively as alcohol, but with fewer deleterious side effects.

Substance Abuse Treatment Settings

Nurses in substance abuse treatment settings are also likely to work with dual diagnosis clients and face difficulties determining whether psychiatric symptoms result exclusively from substance abuse, or whether an underlying psychiatric disorder is present. Accurate history about the onset of symptoms and their relationship to substance use is usually difficult to obtain. If it can be adequately determined that such symptoms as depression, paranoia, or hallucinations were present before the substance use began, or during past periods of prolonged abstinence, you can assume the client has a mental disorder. Further consultation about managing the mental illness while in substance abuse treatment should be sought. Similarly, if symptoms present during periods of substance use or withdrawal persist after more than a few weeks of abstinence, refer the client for a more complete psychiatric assessment.

When abstinence is well established, previous psychiatric diagnoses may need to be reviewed. For instance, clients thought to be schizophrenic may have been diagnosed without knowledge of the role played by substance abuse in producing their psychotic symptoms. Clients with personality disorders may no longer meet the criteria for these disorders when substance abuse is no longer a factor. In a study by Dulit et al. (1990), almost 25% of their sample of subjects with BPD no longer met the diagnostic criteria for BPD when substance abuse was excluded.

In contrast, substance abuse may mask the presence of other psychiatric disorders, as in the example that follows.

Laura, a 28-year-old secretary, had been on methadone maintenance therapy for the past 4 years. Her nurse at the methadone clinic was encouraging when Laura asked to be detoxified from the methadone. She completed the detox program without incident, and did well for several months.

The nurse became concerned when she was informed by the leader of a Clean and Sober group Laura attended that Laura was becoming increasingly withdrawn, suspicious, and preoccupied. Another client asked the nurse to talk to Laura after she delivered a long, rambling diatribe against her ex-husband, who Laura believed was using his computer to broadcast "thought messages" that Laura was "a no-good whore" into her head.

Although the nurse had previously noticed that Laura was suspicious and that she seemed to be overly concerned she might be "poisoned by toxic rays" from her computer at work, the nurse had considered these merely to be Laura's eccentricities. However, when she talked to Laura, it became clear that she was now psychotic. Laura was talking to herself and believed that her ex-husband and his girlfriend were trying to control her and "substitute their own evil thoughts into my mind" by practicing "computer witchcraft."

The nurse suspected that Laura's paranoid symptoms might be the result of using street drugs, which Laura denied. A urine toxicology screen was negative. Laura was referred to the clinic's psychiatrist, who transferred her to PES on a psychiatric hold after she confided a plan to go to her ex-husband's workplace with an axe and "destroy that demon computer."

Information from Laura's family revealed that she had an uncle and a brother who had both been diagnosed with schizophrenia, and that Laura herself had always been suspicious and had "strange ideas." Laura acknowledged having heard voices since her late teens, before she began using drugs. She said that one of her motivations for using heroin, and then methadone, was that "it made the voices go away."

The PES nurse gave Laura a provisional diagnosis of schizophrenia, paranoid type. Since methadone is known to have antipsychotic properties, he suspected that Laura's psychotic symptoms had been suppressed by her use of methadone, and had become problematic after she stopped methadone maintenance.

Available Treatments for Dual Diagnosis Clients

Because nurses in many different settings may have occasion to refer dual diagnosis clients for treatment, they need to know what resources are available. The ideal referral is to a special dual diagnosis treatment program, which would concurrently address both treatment issues. Options range from inpatient programs to special case management teams, outpatient groups, and Double Trouble self-help groups.

The most psychiatrically disabled dual diagnosis clients usually require treatment in the mental health care system. As mentioned previously, their ability to get needed psychiatric treatment is often hampered by providers' attitude that it is a waste of time, or worse, "enabling" clients to continue substance abuse by treating those who are actively abusing substances (Osher and Kofoed 1989).

Mental health care systems also vary greatly in their degree of sophistication in dealing with dual disorders.

Diagnosis and treatment of substance-related disorders remains a neglected area of professional education (Peyser 1989), so mental health care providers may fail to recognize, or may underestimate, the role of substance abuse in aggravating their clients' difficulties.

Different types of substance abuse treatment services also vary in their ability to recognize and accommodate the special needs of dual diagnosis clients. Services run by professionals, such as psychiatrists and nurses, are more likely to recognize the need for psychotropic medications when treating mentally ill people than are settings run by laypeople recovering from addiction. The therapeutic community approach is likely to regard the need for psychotropic medications as another form of chemical dependence. Even professionally run services are apt to forbid the use of drugs with abuse potential, such as antianxiety agents like lorazepam. And other clients may express suspicion that dual diagnosis clients are using agents like antidepressants to "get high."

In addition, the use of group treatment techniques that are highly confrontational may aggravate symptoms in clients who are highly anxious or paranoid. Clients whose ability to perform activities of daily living is severely compromised by such symptoms as impaired concentration and anergia may be unable to fulfill their responsibilities in residential settings that require each resident to take responsibility for household maintenance.

A self-help group, such as Alcoholics Anonymous or Narcotics Anonymous, can be an important part of the treatment program for dual diagnosis clients, particularly if the group is oriented toward people with mental illnesses. In many areas, groups using the twelve steps of AA are available at least once a day, so individuals can attend as many groups as they desire. Groups are free and often provide refreshments—important considerations for people on fixed incomes.

Attending groups and finding a sponsor also provide alternative social supports that are not based on substance use. Peers in self-help groups are available to be called and to offer their support whenever the dually disordered individual is tempted to lapse. Few mental health services can provide this kind of network of support. People with dual diagnoses may also find that they are better able to accept feedback about the consequences of their behavior when it comes from those whose struggles are similar to their own.

Despite the progress made by groups like AA in recognizing that mentally ill people require medications, dually diagnosed individuals are still likely to receive well-meaning advice to stop taking their medications from twelve-step peers. The behavior of mentally ill people may also be too bizarre, paranoid, or disruptive to fit readily into such a group.

General Principles of Treatment

Although the magnitude and complexity of problems facing dual diagnosis clients may lead to feelings of frustration and inadequacy for nurses working with them, treatment gains can certainly be made if you are realistic and persistent. If nothing else, time is on your side—longitudinal studies show that substance use is likely to decline with age (Fillmore et al. 1989), and, in such long-term illnesses as schizophrenia, functioning is likely to improve with age (Harding et al. 1987).

The nurse working with a dual diagnosis client may feel confused by the different philosophical approaches to substance abuse treatment. In the United States, the predominant ideology of substance abuse treatment is heavily influenced by the disease concept of alcoholism, one of whose tenets is that alcoholics are incapable of controlling their drinking once they begin (Peele 1983). Based on this belief, abstinence is the only effective means of recovery from alcohol addiction.

However, the disease concept of alcoholism is not universally accepted as a model for understanding substance-related disorders. Studies in both the U.S. and Europe support the efficacy of controlled drinking as a treatment for alcoholism (Peele 1983), and some professionals working with drug users to decrease HIV infection have adopted a model that sees preventing the harmful consequences of drug use, rather than cessation of drug use, as its goal (Springer 1991).

This **harm-reduction model** conceptualizes abstinence as the top goal in a hierarchy of harm-reduction objectives. If the client is currently unwilling or unable to adopt abstinence as an objective, the goal is to help the client reduce the harmful consequences of his or her drug-using behavior (Springer 1991).

A pragmatic approach that measures progress in small steps toward an ultimate goal is probably better suited to working with dual diagnosis clients than an all-or-nothing expectation of sobriety. Clinicians working with dual diagnosis clients emphasize that improvement is likely to be slow, with lapses occurring as a predictable part of recovery (Fariello and Scheidt 1989; Osher and Kofoed 1989).

Osher and Kofoed (1989) identify the following four phases of treatment:

1. Engagement, in which the client is attracted to the treatment program.
2. Persuasion, the process of convincing engaged clients to accept long-term abstinence-oriented treatment.
3. Active treatment, in which clients learn the attitudes and skills necessary to remain sober.
4. Relapse prevention.

Relapses are anticipated and are used as learning experiences; they are not seen as failures. Analyzing "slips" can be a valuable way to help clients learn how to prevent future relapse.

Although it may be considered desirable for clients to avoid any use of nonprescription substances, the focus of treatment should be on controlling the types of substance use that are most problematic for that individual. Some individuals, for instance, are able to maintain moderate drinking without any problems, but decompensate when they use street drugs (Abbott 1992). As mentioned previously, discussion with the client about the effects of different substances may suggest ways to alter the medication regime to give better symptom relief.

As well as addressing biologic and psychologic factors involved with substance abuse, attention to relevant social and economic factors is an important part of the treatment plan. For example, helping a client living in a drug-saturated neighborhood find new housing may be an important aid to maintaining sobriety. Similarly, unemployed clients with large amounts of unstructured time may need help establishing a daily routine of inexpensive recreational, social, and self-help activities in order to avoid the temptation of substance use.

Chapter Highlights

- Nurses are likely to see clients with dual diagnoses of mental illness and substance abuse in both mental health care and substance abuse treatment settings. Because these disorders are commonly concurrent, clients identified as having either type of disorder are at high risk for the other.
- Substance abuse can complicate the course of a mental disorder by aggravating symptoms of mental illness, decreasing the effectiveness of treatment, and precipitating psychosocial stressors, such as arrest and financial problems.
- Although dual diagnosis clients require coordinated treatment for both disorders, mental health care and substance abuse treatment systems are usually designed to treat these problems in isolation. They often fail to give effective and comprehensive treatment, if they treat the client at all.
- Psychiatric/substance abuse comorbidity may develop in one of four ways: mental illness predisposes to substance abuse; substance abuse predisposes to mental illness; both disorders evolve from a common factor; or each disorder occurs because of risk factors independent of those for the other disorder.
- Although it may be difficult to sort out whether drugs or functional disorders are responsible for mental status abnormalities in an emergency psychiatric admission, abnormal physical findings such as elevated or depressed vital signs, pupillary changes, neurologic abnormalities, and altered motor behavior indicate a need for more extensive medical evaluation. Toxicology screening may help confirm the presence of drugs.
- Intoxicated clients, because of impulsivity and impaired judgment, are at risk of harming themselves or others. Seclusion, restraint, or suicide precautions may be necessary to prevent harm.
- Nursing substance use assessments can best be done in a nonemergency setting after the client's mental status has cleared. These assessments should include all classes of nonprescription psychoactive substances, as well as the misuse of prescription and OTC drugs, and should be done in a matter-of-fact and nonjudgmental manner.
- Since substance abuse may mask or alter the presentation of other psychiatric disorders, and since accurate information about the onset of symptoms may be difficult to obtain, dual diagnosis clients may require psychiatric reevaluation after several weeks of sobriety.
- Dual diagnosis clients may be challenging to work with because their problems are so numerous and so intertwined. But if the nurse is persistent, accepts the client as a person, and regards lapses in the course of recovery as learning experiences rather than failures, she can help the client reduce substance use and improve functioning.

References

Abbott FK: Daily lives of persons with schizophrenia living in the community. Unpublished doctoral dissertation, University of California, San Francisco, 1992.

American Psychiatric Association. *Diagnostic and Statistical Manual of Mental Disorders,* ed. 4. American Psychiatric Association, 1994.

Ananth J, Vandewater S, Kamal M, Brodsky A, Gamal R, Miller M: Missed diagnosis of substance abuse in psychiatric patients. *Hosp Commun Psychiatr* 1989;40(3):297–299.

Bartels SJ, Teague GB, Drake RE, Clark RE, Bush PW, Noordsy DL: Substance abuse in schizophrenia: Service utilization and costs. *J Nervous Ment Dis* 1993;181(4):227–232.

Bergman H, Harris M: Substance abuse among young adult chronic patients. *J Psychosoc Rehab* 1985;9:49–54.

Bowers MB: The role of drugs in the production of schizophreniform psychoses and related disorders, in Meltzer HY (ed): *Psychopharmacology: The Third Generation of Progress.* Raven Press, 1987.

Bowers MB, Mazure CM, Nelson JC, Jatlow PI: Psychotogenic drug use and neuroleptic response. *Schizophrenia Bull* 1990;16(1):81–85.

Brady K, Anton R, Ballenger JC, Lydiard RB, Adinoff B, Selander J: Cocaine abuse among schizophrenic patients. *Am J Psychiatr* 1990;147(9):1164–1167.

Brady K, Casto S: Illicit substance use by acutely psychotic patients (letter). *Am J Psychiatr* 1989;146(10):1349–1350.

Brown SA, Irwin M, Schuckit MA: Changes in anxiety among abstinent male alcoholics. *J Stud Alcohol* 1991;52(1):55–61.

Bunt G, Galanter M, Lifshutz H, Casteneda R: Cocaine/"crack" dependence among psychiatric inpatients. *Am J Psychiatr* 1990;147(11):1542–1546.

Caragonne P, Emery B, Isser S: *Mental Illness and Substance Abuse: The Dually Diagnosed Client*. National Council of Community Mental Health Centers, 1987.

Carey K: Emerging treatment guidelines for mentally ill chemical abusers. *Hosp Commun Psychiatr* 1989;40(4):341–349.

Chafetz L: Substance abuse and schizophrenia. Presentation to the American Psychiatric Nurses' Association Annual Meeting, Denver, 1989.

Compton P: Drug abuse: A self-care deficit. *J Psychosoc Nurs* 1989;27(3):22–26.

Dixon L, Dibietz E, Myers P, Conley R, Medoff D, Lehman AF: Comparison of DSM-III-R diagnoses and a brief interview for substance use among state hospital patients. *Hosp Commun Psychiatr* 1993;44(8):748–752.

Dixon L, Haas G, Weiden P, Sweeney J, Frances A: Acute effects of drug abuse in schizophrenic patients: Clinical observations and patients' self-reports. *Schizophrenia Bull* 1990;16(1):69–79.

Dixon L, Haas G, Weiden PJ, Sweeney J, Frances AJ: Drug abuse in schizophrenic patients: Clinical correlates and reasons for use. *Am J Psychiatr* 1991;148(2):224–230.

Drake RE, McHugo GJ, Noordsy DL: Treatment of alcoholism among schizophrenic outpatients: Four-year outcomes. *Am J Psychiatr* 1993;150(2):328–329.

Drake RE, Osher FC, Wallach MA: Alcohol use and abuse in schizophrenia: A prospective community study. *J Nervous Ment Dis* 1989;177(7):408–414.

Drake RE, Wallach MA: Substance abuse among the chronically mentally ill. *Hosp Commun Psychiatr* 1989;40(10):1041–1045.

Dulit RA, Fyer MR, Haas GL, Sullivan T, Frances AJ: Substance use in borderline personality disorder. *Am J Psychiatr* 1990;147(8):1003–1007.

Durell J, Lechtenberg B, Corse S, Frances RJ: Intensive case management of persons with chronic mental illness who abuse substances. *Hosp Commun Psychiatr* 1993;44(5):415–428.

Elangovan N, Berman S, Meinzer A, Gianelli P, Miller H, Longmore W: Substance abuse among patients presenting at an inner-city psychiatric emergency room. *Hosp Commun Psychiatr* 1993;44(8):782–784.

Estroff SE: *Making It Crazy*. University of California Press, 1981.

Fariello D, Scheidt S: Clinical case management of the dually diagnosed patient. *Hosp Commun Psychiatr* 1989;40(10):1065–1067.

Fillmore KM, Hartka E, Johnstone BM, Leino V, Moyotoshi M, Temple MT: Life course variation in drinking: A meta-analysis of multiple longitudinal studies from the Collaborative Alcohol-related Longitudinal Project. Paper presented at the Fifteenth Annual Alcohol Epidemiology Symposium, Maastricht, The Netherlands, 1989.

Galanter M, Casteneda R, Ferman J: Substance abuse among general psychiatric patients: Place of presentation, diagnosis, and treatment. *Am J Drug Alcohol Abuse* 1988;14(2):211–235.

Harding CM, Brooks GW, Ashikaga T, Strauss JS, Breier A: The Vermont Longitudinal Study of Persons with Severe Mental Illness, I: Methodology, study sample, and overall status 32 years later. *Am J Psychiatr* 1987;144(6):718–726.

Hasin D, Endicott J, Lewis C: Alcohol and drug abuse in patients with affective syndromes. *Comprehensive Psychiatr* 1989;26(3):283–295.

Hellerstein DJ, Meehan B: Outpatient group therapy for schizophrenic substance abusers. *Am J Psychiatr* 1987;144(10): 1337–1339.

Helzer JE, Pryzbek TR: The co-occurrence of alcoholism with other psychiatric disorders in the general population and its impact on treatment. *J Studies Alcohol* 1988;49(3):219–224.

Kasten BP: Perception of non-prescribed substance use by persons with long-term mental illness. Unpublished data, Department of Mental Health, Community, and Administrative Nursing, University of California, San Francisco, 1993.

Kasten BP, Monteleone MP: Psychiatric nursing and the emergency setting. *New Directions Ment Health Serv* 1993;58:13–22.

Kessler RC, McGonagle KA, Zhao S, Nelson CB, Hughes M, Eshleman S, Wittchen H, Kendler KS: Lifetime and 12-month prevalence of DSM-III-R psychiatric disorders in the United States: Results from the National Comorbidity Survey. *Arch Gen Psychiatr* 1994;51:8–19.

Khantzian EJ: The self-medication hypothesis of addictive disorders: Focus on heroin and cocaine dependence. *Am J Psychiatr* 1985;142(11):1259–1264.

Kofoed L, Kania J, Walsh T, Atkinson RM: Outpatient treatment of patients with substance abuse and coexisting psychiatric disorders. *Am J Psychiatr* 1986; 143(7): 867–872.

Kosten TR, Kleber HD: Differential diagnosis of psychiatric comorbidity in substance abusers. *J Substance Abuse Treatment* 1988;5:201–206.

Kovaszny B, Bromet E, Schwartz JE, Ram R, Lavelle J, Brandon L: Substance abuse and onset of psychotic illness. *Hosp Commun Psychiatr* 1993;44(6):567–571.

Lehman AF, Herron JD, Schwartz RP, Myers CP: Rehabilitation for adults with severe mental illness and substance use disorders: A clinical trial. *J Nervous Ment Dis* 1993;181(2):86–90.

Lehman AF, Myers CP, Corty E: Assessment and classification of patients with psychiatric and substance abuse syndromes. *Hosp Commun Psychiatr* 1989;40(10):1019–1024.

McKelvy MJ, Kane JS, Kellison K: Substance abuse and mental illness: Double trouble. *J Psychosoc Nurs* 1987;25(1):20–25.

Mueller TI, Lavori PW, Keller MB, Swartz A, Warshaw M, Hasin D, Coryell W, Endicott J, Rice J, Akiskal H: Prognostic effect of the variable course of alcoholism on the 10-year course of depression. *Am J Psychiatr* 1994;151(5):701–706.

Olivera AA, Kiefer MW, Manley NK: Tardive dyskinesia in psychiatric patients with substance use disorders. *Am J Drug Alcohol Abuse* 1990;16(1):57–66.

Osher FC, Kofoed LL: Treatment of patients with psychiatric and psychoactive substance abuse disorders. *Hosp Commun Psychiatr* 1989;40(10):1025–1030.

Peele S: Through a glass darkly. *Psych Today* 1983;17(8):38–42.

Peyser HS: Alcohol and drug abuse: Underrecognized and untreated. *Hosp Commun Psychiatr* 1989;40(3):221.

Regier DA, Farmer ME, Rae DS, Locke BZ, Keith SJ, Judd LL, Goodwin FK: Comorbidity of mental disorders with alcohol and other drug abuse: Results from the Epidemiologic Catchment Area (ECA) Study. *JAMA* 1990;264(19):2511–2518.

Ross HE, Glaser FB, Germanson T: The prevalence of psychiatric disorders in patients with alcohol and other drug problems. *Arch Gen Psychiatr* 1988;45:1023–1031.

Rounsaville BJ, Dolinsky ZS, Babor TF, Meyer RE: Psychopathology as a predictor of treatment outcome in alcoholics. *Arch Gen Psychiatr* 1987;44:505–513.

Schneier FR, Siris SG: Review of psychoactive substance use and abuse in schizophrenia: Patterns of drug choice. *J Nervous Ment Dis* 1987;175(11):641–652.

Siris SG: Pharmacological treatment of substance-abusing schizophrenic patients. *Schizophrenia Bull* 1990;16(1): 111–122.

Springer E: Effective AIDS prevention with active drug users: The harm reduction model. *J Chem Dependency Treatment* 1991;4(2):141–157.

Szuster RR, Schanbacher BL, McCann SC, McConnell A: Underdiagnosis of psychoactive-substance-induced organic mental disorders in emergency psychiatry. *Am J Drug Alcohol Abuse* 1990;16(3):319–327.

Test MA, Wallisch LS, Allness DJ, Ripp K: Substance use in young adults with schizophrenic disorders. *Schizophrenia Bull* 1989;15(3):465–475.

Wolfe HL, Sorenson JL: Dual diagnosis patients in the urban psychiatric emergency room. *J Psychoactive Drugs* 1989; 21(2):169–175.

CHAPTER 26

THE CODEPENDENT CLIENT

Eileen Trigoboff
Maryruth Morris

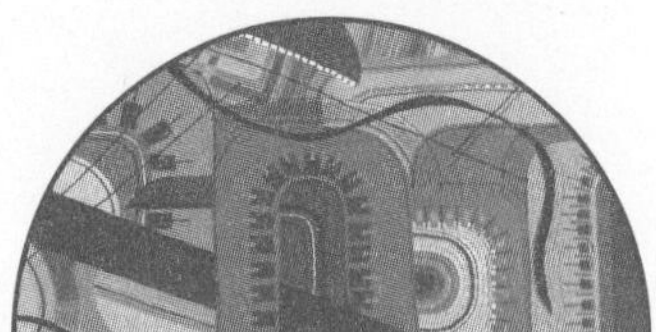

COMPETENCIES

- *Identify the characteristics of codependence.*
- *Relate codependence to a biopsychosocial theoretic model.*
- *Apply a codependence theoretic framework to a practical situation.*
- *Apply the nursing process with a codependent client.*
- *Formulate a healing-focused response to a client behaving within a codependent mind-set.*

Cross-References

Other topics relevant to this content are: Family therapy, Chapter 32; Personal integration, Chapter 1; Psychoactive substance use disorders, Chapter 13.

Critical Thinking Challenge

You are very close to a colleague at your new job. Even though you've only been there a short time, this nurse has stepped in for you and taken care of a number of problem situations. She tells you a lot about how often she does this and how well run the unit is because of her. She describes it as very hard work that people don't understand, but she will always be there to do the work no matter how little recognition she gets. You begin to see how the other staff members resent this colleague and how they don't know how to handle problems that arise when your colleague is not there. Her comments upon seeing the imperfect resolution of the problem are harsh and critical of the other staff members. What do you think is happening here, and how would you go about making changes?

The term *codependence* developed out of the alcohol addiction treatment movement. This term, coined in the 1970s, arises from the older idea of **co-alcoholic**, a term used in Al-Anon for the spouses and families of an alcoholic. Another phrase used during the formative years of alcoholism treatment was *co-ism,* a concept that implies that everybody in an alcoholic's family is emotionally impaired. Various authors estimate that the incidence of codependence in our culture ranges from about 33% to about 100% of the population. The latter estimate reflects a liberal and encompassing interpretation of codependent behavior.

Another rapidly growing part of the codependence movement is the focus on **adult children of alcoholics (ACoA).** Therapeutic endeavors in this area have been extensive, and many peer-support groups or therapist-led groups are available in most communities. The linking of the ACoA and the codependent styles of interacting is based on similar formative stages. Having prolonged exposure to a set of oppressive rules that prevent the open expression of feelings, such as an alcoholic home or a relationship that does not allow talking about problems, is believed to produce coping styles very much like codependence. An interesting (and controversial, for professionals) aspect of this movement is the commercial success of codependence-focused products and treatment groups. There are rehabilitation centers, books, manuals, videos, calendars, notepads, and wall plaques with inspiring messages on how to recover from codependence.

The most important aspect of codependence for nurses is that this notion is relatively new, and the professional literature has only recently begun to address the topic. It is our responsibility to be open to new information and ideas about the intrapersonal and interpersonal issues of codependence, process that information, and incorporate it into our view of this behavior pattern.

Mrs R is a new client with numerous physical problems for which she has been recently treated. When a nurse approaches her for treatment, Mrs R is on the telephone, emphatically discussing her 33-year-old daughter's finances. She insists that her daughter stop purchasing "those things" and learn to budget. Mrs R hangs up and quickly dials another number, ignoring the nurse, and agitatedly describes to another person her intent to pay her daughter's debt. It appears as if Mrs R, caught up in the behavior of her daughter and changing her own life to respond to her daughter, is left with little energy for attending to her own important physical care. Even as the nurse presses Mrs R for information, it is clear that Mrs R remains focused on her daughter's finances.

A set of behaviors like the one described above has been clinically observed for years, but the idea of codependence was not articulated. There were a lot of people involved in relationships that were problematic in a particular manner. The interactions were characteristic, and a way to describe them was needed. As attention to this interactive style of behaving came into sharper focus, a better understanding of what was behind the relationships became clear. It is commonly thought that a codependent person is someone who has a set of problematic interactions with another person or other people. These problems follow a particular path and vary in intensity.

Characteristics of Codependence

What does codependence mean? The definition is still being formulated and differs slightly from source to source. The most useful definition is based on the behavioral characteristics of the codependent client.

A codependent is a person who cannot detach from a bond even though there is a great deal of pain in the attachment (Levin 1991). Codependent individuals actually believe they can control the feelings and actions of others by willpower. They keep pushing others to do what needs to be done. At some point the codependent person will feel hopeless and inadequate if results are not forthcoming (Morgan 1991). Sensations of powerlessness and worthlessness from those experiences are coped with maladaptively.

People with codependent traits will not recognize or even know what their own feelings are. When asked how they feel, the response may be a thought, not a feeling. And even the thoughts are often really someone else's interpretation of events. Palpable **denial** is evident. Codependent clients actively believe that if they try hard enough, they will be able to change another person, even in the face of enormous amounts of evidence to the contrary. That can only be accomplished with a denial system that is well entrenched.

The codependent individual can be a highly organized achiever who works continuously at controlling events and people and attempting to maintain stability in the present situation. This behavior pattern emerges after routine exposure to a set of rules that prevents the open expression of feelings and direct discussion of problems. It is an effective, although maladaptive, coping pattern derived from routine contact with adverse circumstances.

Although codependence is effective in controlling the crisis situation, it is an unhealthy lifestyle because the exclusive focus on others promotes the neglect of the self. One of the "rules" of this lifestyle is to deny the existence of a problem, to deny one's feelings, and to adhere to a code of silence about the situation. There is an expectation that negative feelings are not to be voiced. The origin of these codependent styles is believed to be prolonged exposure to dysfunctional relationships. In other words, if you are predisposed to staying in a relationship where feelings are not and cannot be discussed and events crowd your identity, that is codependence.

Codependence, as defined in this chapter, is a group of learned behaviors that prevents individuals from taking care of themselves and has at its core a preoccupation with the thoughts and feelings of others. Codependent people gear their behavior toward helping others or taking charge of situations that appear to be out of control. Because codependents assume responsibility for others' lives, codependent relationships require the participation of at least one other dysfunctional person.

Codependent behavior can be learned at any point in life. Early learning is based on what the person learned as a child (meeting everyone else's needs) and what the family failed to model (the give-and-take of a healthy

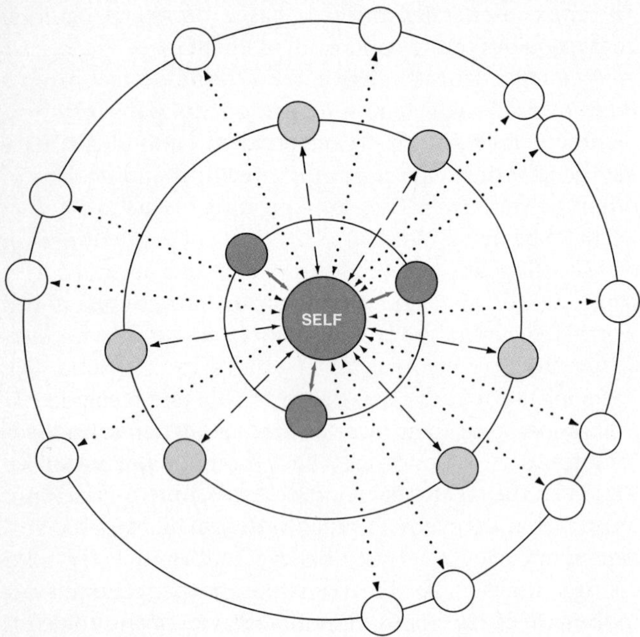

Figure 26–1 A normal pattern of interaction. The first level of intimates have the strongest lines of connection and are closest to the self, such as life partners and intimate friends. There are few people who can be this close, in contrast to the second and third level, which include acquaintances and work associates. These relationships are farther from the self and have a weaker claim. Each line of connectedness is reciprocal to indicate give and take in the relationships.

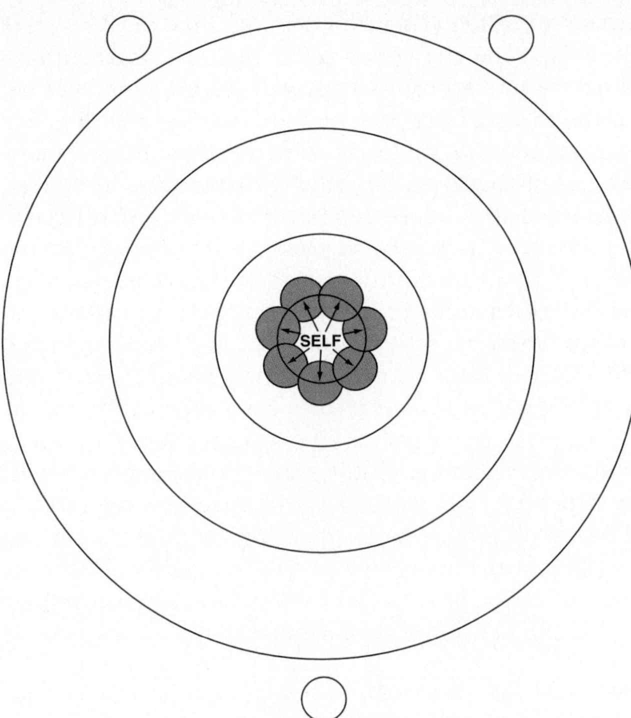

Figure 26–2 A codependent interaction pattern. The self is almost obscured by demanding individuals and intruded relationships. Every interaction that takes place is a relationship-focused interaction and there is no reciprocity in the relationships. The outer levels are empty because everyone is let in close to the self. Those outside the rings indicate individuals the codependent hasn't met yet, or those who have refused the dysfunctional relationship and left the unhealthy self system.

relationship). In a dysfunctional family, the child, to maintain some level of stability in the family, tries to sense what the adults need and want. Both the adults and the child see the child's needs, wants, feelings, and desires as unacceptable. Therefore, the child learns to ignore his or her own life.

These codependent behaviors can be learned as an adult, as well. Adult learning of codependence involves a relationship or a system that exploits the individual's overresponsibility, denial, control issues, and boundary problems. The relationship becomes more important than the individual, and enormous effort is expended to maintain it. The amount of energy that goes into relationship salvaging tends to equal the amount of evidence available that it cannot be salvaged. This activity thus crowds away who the codependent really is; it ignores his or her own life. Figures 26–1 and 26–2 represent the differences between normal and codependent relationships.

Biopsychosocial Theories

Several theoretic bases for codependence are summarized in the following sections.

The ACoA Perspective

Claudia Black (1987, 1990), well known for her work with children of alcoholics, has identified the characteristics of people who grew up in dysfunctional families. Although Black does not focus entirely on the codependent individual, her identification of the background common to codependent people and therapeutic recommendations for intervention are frequently cited in codependence literature. In Black's perspective, children of alcoholics learn that having feelings only makes things more of a problem—speaking about feelings usually makes situations worse rather than better. The child's solution is to stifle the feeling and say nothing. The child becomes unable to recognize what feelings are, to articulate them, or to address them in a caring manner. Personal conduct centers on the rules "don't feel; don't talk; don't trust." These individuals have not learned how to take care of themselves in an adult relationship.

The strong needs of codependent adults and ACoAs to control others originates, according to Black, in the child's need to have things done well and on time, before a parent or the neighbors see that things are not OK at home. The child hopes that being very good at everything will prevent negative consequences. Input from others is a nuisance and irrelevant when one knows how to do things the right way. As an adult, the person is not interested in hearing others' points of view. One manifestation of this attitude is cutting people off before they finish sentences. In addition, there are isolating repercussions from a childhood spent with an addict. Feeling cut off from people and perceiving oneself as alone in a crowd are telltale signs of the aftermath of growing up in an addiction-focused home.

According to Black's theoretic framework, healing involves verbalizing feelings and learning to trust oneself and others. Having the ACoA experience validated via therapy or peer-support groups breaks open the lock on talking about feelings.

Shame and Codependence

Shame as a major feature of codependence is the focus of John Bradshaw's (1988, 1990) work. In his view, the codependent is someone with a toxic form of shame. **Toxic shame** is a tremendous amount of shame that interferes with the ability to search outside of oneself for purpose and happiness.

Dysfunction in the family system is its basis. If a family does not meet each individual's needs and respond to the world in a healthy manner, unhealthy and dysfunctional patterns of response become ingrained. In Bradshaw's view, living a life that is **other-aided** is codependent because the person's concentration is always on someone else. Denial of one's own needs is one of the features of codependence. The goal of treatment is to return the focus to the self and work on breaking dysfunctional patterns of relating, by identifying one's needs and feelings and then making these needs and feelings a priority in one's life.

Proactive Approaches

John and Linda Friel, in *An Adult Child's Guide to What's "Normal"* (1990), define codependence, humorously but pointedly, as the "chase-your-spouse-around-the-room-with-the-self-help-book syndrome." The nurse can assess codependence by examining the amount of work each partner puts into a relationship. In a codependent relationship, one person routinely invests great energy keeping the relationship afloat, while the second person expends little or no effort. The Friels reinforce the idea that taking responsibility for another adult's life is not healthy caring. The move to health begins when codependents question whether they should continue, modify, or leave the relationship. Caring about others without being codependent involves paying attention to one's feelings and body, keeping one's identity, and undertaking a personal search that includes questioning the childhood styles of interacting that one learned along the way.

The Child Within Perspective

Charles Whitfield (1987, 1988) describes codependence as the result of growing up without nurturing or freedom of expression. He uses the term "our most common addiction" and describes it as a "disease of a lost selfhood." The **child within**, or the child who is in all of us, is an unnurtured child within the codependent adult. The codependent adult's child within maintains that unnurtured child's sense of the world. Adults who follow rules they made up when they were unnurtured children create a false self, one that is not true to the genuine and spirited part of a human being. In other words, the false self does not represent how a healthy adult interacts in the world.

To consider this further, speculate about what that child within the adult is feeling. It is frightening to see the world as a cold and critical place. Now imagine that grown-up person in situations that do not nurture or encourage freedom of expression. Old patterns start to play out. The person pretends to be strong—always—while in reality feeling vulnerable. Critical, perfectionistic, controlling self-righteousness becomes routine and prevents accepting oneself and others. The process of healing for the codependent person hinges on the healing of the child within. This healing addresses the needs of the child within, nurtures the child, and teaches the child healthy ways of relating to others.

The Undifferentiated Self Theory

Concepts from Bowen's family systems theory can be used in the interpretation of codependence (Fagan-Pryor and Haber 1992). Bowen (1985) observed specific patterns in family relationships and then classified the individuals according to a continuum of emotional maturity that ranged from undifferentiated to highly differentiated. The basic concept is that the more others influence an individual's thoughts, feelings, and behavior, the more undifferentiated that individual is. Poorly differentiated people have little sense of who they are. Approval or criticism from others decides how the individual feels about himself or herself. The sense of self comes from the outside. The concomitant anxiety that naturally arises from repeatedly being exposed to these experiences can lead to substance abuse. Further up the continuum is the more differentiated individual. The more someone is differentiated, the more he or she can actually participate in a relationship with emotions and not fear fusing with others.

The continuum aspect of Bowen's theory allows for gradations of codependence that are frequently seen in clients. Assessing a client within this framework would clarify some of the relationship difficulties clients experience. As this is a family-focused theory, it lends itself well to interpretation for intervention with the system within which the client lives—the family—instead of formulating care for the individual in isolation.

Feminist Theory

Codependence from a perspective of **feminism** requires confronting the social and political aspects of the definitions that may predispose a woman to a sense of powerlessness. Codependence is most frequently associated with women. Calling a woman "sick," when in reality she may be coping with and surviving in an abusive relationship, is just a version of blaming the victim (Babcock 1990). What hope is there if doing your best in a bad situation is also bad?

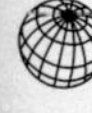

Feminist writers criticize the idea of codependence as an illness from which one recovers, because most of the characteristics ascribed to codependence are aspects of the traditional female gender role (Babcock 1991). So much is written about healing intrapsychic wounds that the external environment, which is likely oppressive and disconnected, is not taken to task for the problems. People can become involved with trying to clean up their own personal behavior, but meanwhile the possessive, demanding, and immature relationship going on around the codependent continues.

The feminist model of *growth in connection* (Jordon et al. 1991) is an interesting perspective from which to view codependence. The center of the model holds that in healthy relationships, mutual empathy and emotional connectedness between a mother and child form the basis for self-esteem and empowerment. Mutual empathy encourages the expression of feelings and needs so that both individuals become increasingly authentic in their interactions (Malloy and Berkery 1993). There is an interconnectedness of the growth of the individuals and the growth of the relationship that defines the health of the relationship. While 100% mutuality is not likely in relationships, there should be enough mutuality for both members of the interaction to feel that their needs in important areas are being met.

In codependence, a woman's attempt at healthy and mutual connectedness in an interaction is met with pain, rejection, and alienation. Despite this, the woman yearns to maintain the relationship and loses sight of her own needs and desires. Kaplan (1991) refers to this as the *futile connection syndrome,* where one is so disconnected from her own needs that she tries in vain to respond to the needs of others in order to maintain the relationship. Malloy and Berkery (1993) encourage women to examine the impact of the disconnections that occur in nonmutual, abusive, violent, and/or shaming relationships and put effort into not taking responsibility for the problems of other people or those relationships.

The Nursing Process with the Codependent Client

Assessment

Nurses and clients must recognize codependent behaviors in order to develop alternate patterns of interacting. The hallmark characteristic behaviors of codependence are as follows:

- Self-esteem is based on the ability to control others.
- There is an assumption that others' needs are more important than one's own needs.
- Situations of intimacy and separation result in excessive anxiety.
- Most relationships are based in enmeshment with another dysfunctional person (personality-disordered, substance-dependent, or another codependent).
- Certain other conditions will also exist, such as excessive denial, substance abuse, constriction of emotions (with or without outbursts), stress-related medical illness, depression, hypervigilance, compulsions, anxiety, having been (or being) the victim of recurrent abuse, remaining in an important relationship with a dysfunctional person or system without seeking outside help.

Characteristics of codependence, visible not only in the client population but also in everyday life, vary from mild to extreme. Mild traits can contribute to discomfort. Extreme codependence interferes with functioning, forcing individuals into awkward and untenable situations, totally ignoring their own needs. Intermediate levels of these traits and symptoms can also occur. Ask yourself this question: Do codependence symptoms to a large degree conflict with a healthy lifestyle? If so, then the client's behaviors are extreme.

Nursing Diagnosis

A number of nursing diagnoses apply to the codependent individual. As one client's level of codependence and dysfunction varies widely from that of others, focus the diagnosis on your client's current problems. Incorporate the client's other health problems into your conceptualization of this client as well.

Applicable nursing diagnoses include the entire range of individual and family coping diagnoses. Given that codependent individuals are not as likely to attend to their own needs, health maintenance skills also need to

CASE STUDY

A Codependent Client

Identifying Information

Terry is a 34-year-old single female who works full-time at a small restaurant as a chef. She comes to the clinic after a number of problems at work and home.

Client's Description of the Problem

Terry describes herself as being very busy and mentioned her schedule, which included a number of errands for other people but did not include anything that she did for herself. Terry lists several relatives and friends as supports but doesn't want them bothered with her problems. She has never been in a therapeutic relationship.

Terry states that she routinely keeps an eye out at work for "those crazy times when it gets so busy nobody can handle it." When she spots such a time, she goes out to the front of the restaurant and "makes everything OK." A new hostess had been working with Terry, and when Terry stepped in to "fix it," the new hostess told Terry she appreciated the intent but that Terry's help was not necessary. Terry was hurt and confused when this happened and was told she was "interfering." Terry's "helping out" this fellow worker had become such a problem that the difficulty prompted Terry to get help. In the clinic waiting room, Terry was talking with another client and began filling out the other client's insurance forms for her.

Psychiatric History

No prior psychiatric history.

Family History

Terry's parents are retired and living in a nearby community. Her father is an alcoholic "but has calmed down a lot in the past 15 years," although Terry denies that it was ever a problem. Her mother was always busy working and volunteering for extended family projects. She has three sisters; the youngest, 25 years old, lives with her parents. Although Terry is intimidated by her father as he still yells at her when she visits, she states she is very close to her family.

Social History

Terry has accomplished a great deal in her life. She lists raising her sister's three children for 2 years and paying for her parents' car insurance as her "pride and joy." She is a graduate of an associate degree program in cooking. Terry has been working 50–60 hours a week at the restaurant, always keeping involved, always willing to help. She is "very close" to a large number of people and has a male significant other. They have a 10-year relationship, but Terry does not list him to be contacted in case of an emergency "because he likes his privacy." Terry drinks "socially," denies any difficulty with alcohol, denies recreational drug use, and does not smoke.

Health History

Terry has some moderate health concerns. She is significantly underweight and has regular problems with constipation and occasional severe diarrhea. She has several headaches every week and has pain in her arms that she has not had examined.

Current Mental Status

Terry is attractive and appears younger than her stated age. She is neatly but plainly dressed. She is oriented to person, place, and time; but her judgment is impaired. She has no insight into her behaviors, and uses denial routinely. Her overall mood is anxious and has been for over 2 years; her affect is appropriate to topic (less anxious and more animated when talking about how helpful she is; appears sad regarding problem with coworker). Thought content includes concern about several other people (boyfriend, sister, father) and no recognition of her own difficulties. No delusions or hallucinations evident.

Other Subjective or Objective Clinical Data

Terry is not on any medications; suicide/violence potential minimal.

Diagnostic Impression

Nursing Diagnoses

Anxiety
Ineffective Individual Coping
Altered Health Maintenance
Altered Nutrition: Less than Body Requirements

DSM-IV Multiaxial Diagnosis

Axis I: 300.00 Anxiety disorder
Axis II: V71.09 (no diagnosis; frequent use of denial)
Axis III: Headache and arm pain, etiology unknown; rule out distal neuropathy vs. carpal tunnel syndrome
Axis IV: Occupational problems, interactions with coworker
Axis V: GAF = 51 (current); GAF = 56 (highest level in past year)

NURSING CARE PLAN

A Codependent Client

Nursing Diagnosis

Anxiety related to interpersonal difficulties.

Expected Outcome

Client will have less overall anxiety as she learns ways to recognize and intervene on her behalf and as she explores her own rights and limits her responsibilities.

Nursing Interventions

- Use simple statements and descriptions during communication with anxious client.
- Discuss options for client to choose from in responding to anxiety-provoking circumstances.
- Examine the source of some anxiety in taking on too much of other people's work and feeling responsible for others.
- Incorporate a sense of worth into client's self-speak, especially when she cares for herself.

Outcome Met If

Overall anxiety level is decreased.

Nursing Diagnosis

Ineffective Individual Coping related to excessive use of denial and attempts at controlling others.

Expected Outcome

Client will recognize use of denial and urge to control others as an ineffective coping mechanism, and be able to substitute more appropriate coping skills in time.

Nursing Interventions

- Discuss various defense mechanisms so that client recognizes pattern of denial and control.
- Explore alternative healthy coping styles.
- Design practice and role-play experiences so client can substitute preferable coping more easily.

Outcome Met If

Client recognizes use of denial and control and has, and uses, other coping skills.

Nursing Diagnosis

Altered Health Maintenance related to lack of caretaking, especially regarding unexplored physical pain.

Expected Outcome

Client will develop a personal desire to discover own physical and emotional needs and take steps to address them.

Nursing Interventions

- Initiate discussion regarding eventual consequences of client ignoring her health.
- Promote self-statements of worth.
- Encourage client to treat self with the same attention and caring as she now treats others.
- Reinforce client's movements toward self-care.
- Do not schedule medical tests for client so as not to model codependence.

Outcome Met If

Client prioritizes emotional and physical health needs by getting a physical and reducing energy expenditures on others.

Nursing Diagnosis

Altered Nutrition: Less than Body Requirements related to decreased food intake because of focus on others.

Expected Outcome

Client will have a realistic lifestyle pattern and get adequate nutrition.

Nursing Interventions

- Use client's superb organizational skills to arrange a schedule that prioritizes her nutrition.
- Discuss various routes client can take to keep her promise to herself regarding nutrition.

Outcome Met If

Client gains and maintains optimal weight.

be examined and addressed. Examples of nursing diagnoses with a codependent client are:

- Alteration in Coping related to a lack of sense of self-identity, as evidenced by codependent relationships.
- Self-esteem Disturbance related to feelings of shame and guilt, as evidenced by an inability to express needs and feelings.

Planning and Implementing Interventions

One of the goals of psychiatric–mental health nursing practice is to create a unique therapeutic approach based on a theory-centered nurse-client relationship. The ability to accomplish this goal requires the integration of theory, the effort of self-examination, and the reinforcement of a healthy self.

The Client's Decision to Change In psychiatric nursing with the codependent client, an important consideration is the client's readiness to change. Although many lifestyle patterns are unhealthy, individuals will only be able to change their behavior when they feel uncomfortable enough to want to learn something new. The hypothetical example below illustrates the point at which most people seek help with their codependent behavior.

Think of two people in two boats equipped with oars. They are in a calm river. Their mission is to row upstream. Mary is in one boat, and John is in the other. Mary lovingly gazes over to see how John is doing. John is standing up in his boat, only one of his oars is in the water, and he is going nowhere. Mary, trying to be helpful, calls over to John, instructing him to sit down and row correctly. After observing for a period of time Mary sees that, although John has followed some of her directions, he continues to have only one oar in the water and has not gone anywhere. As time goes on, Mary feels she should be more helpful in her efforts to get John on his way upstream. She decides that the best way to help is to get into John's boat, to be closer and more available to him. While in his boat, she continues to tell him how to row and what to do. Finally, in frustration, Mary takes over the oars of John's boat, leaving her own boat adrift and going nowhere. Mary does not concern herself with her boat—she spends all her energy rowing John's boat. She notices that the load is quite heavy with two in the boat and that she is working very hard. As the boat progresses upstream, Mary begins to feel resentful watching John sit and ride. However, she still feels it is better for her to row. She thinks to herself, "If John would appreciate all my work, I wouldn't mind rowing for two." But as they progress upstream, John becomes critical, not complimentary, of Mary. Eventually he asks her to get out of his boat. At this point Mary is devastated as well as astonished by John's request. She argues with him, pointing out all that she has done for him, to no avail, and he again asks her to leave his boat. Mary now realizes that she does not know where her boat is and that she is completely confused about how to find it.

Codependents like Mary often reach out for help at times like these.

Changing the Old to the New Changing codependent behavior is a long process and often includes several stages. Following each step listed below are illustrative statements.

1. An awareness of a problem.
   - "I find I can't live like this anymore."
   - "I have problems with almost all of my relationships."
2. Developing a desire to change how one looks at interpersonal relationships.
   - "It's possible that there is another way for me to handle these issues."
   - "I see how I end up doing different things in my relationships than she does, and she seems happier."
3. Developing an ability to learn functional rules of relationships.
   - "I like it, and it works better for me to be encouraged to talk about my hobbies."
   - "I see that there is nothing wrong with making mistakes, and the big deal that was made about them was not healthy."
4. Increasing an awareness of one's own thoughts, feelings, and desires.
   - "I like certain interactions, and I don't like others."
   - "I want to be able to talk about my fears with the person I am friends with."
5. Learning to accept one's own thoughts, feelings, and desires.
   - "It's OK for me to be scared."
   - "It's a good thing I know what I like and don't like."
6. Learning adaptive strategies to cope with the anxiety related to changing one's behavior.
   - "I will ask for a minute to think about the situation before I give you an answer."
   - "I will compliment myself privately when I am able to confront someone directly."
7. Learning and using assertive interpersonal skills.
   - "When you called and told me I had to cook for all those people, I felt my anxiety level go up. Let's figure out a way for this to be a potluck dinner instead."
   - "That was a nice experience for me; let's plan more of those together."

The Therapeutic Use of Self The role of the nurse in the change process is twofold: an appropriate role model of effective interpersonal relationships, and an effective teacher of functional relationship skills. Remember that codependent clients will most likely seek help at a time when they are feeling most vulnerable, confused, and angry that what they have learned to do in relationships does not work. Keeping this in mind will help you maintain a therapeutic role when the codependent person requests or demands to be rescued from this dilemma. As in the hypothetical example with Mary and John, you may see your client struggling, confused, and somewhat helpless, and you may wonder how you can be helpful. Such clients may also repeatedly request more than support from the nurse. Out of their confusion, clients often ask, "What should I do?" or "What would you do if you were in my situation?"

As a nurse, you must model an independent position and convey confidence in the client's own ability to work out a problem-solving strategy. Possible encouraging responses might be, "What alternatives have you already considered and how have they been working for you?" or "You seem unclear about what you want to do; I can appreciate how uncomfortable it is not knowing what to do." In these responses, you have redirected the codependent plea and reinforced the integrity of the client's self-concept while demonstrating concern and support during the client's struggle to learn new skills.

Establishing Personal Boundaries In teaching appropriate functional relationship skills, be aware that at the core of codependence is the lack of functional personal **boundaries** for the client. In simple terms, functional personal boundaries are the limits individuals have to indicate their personal rights and preferences. As a child, the codependent client learned to ignore and mistrust personal limits, feelings, needs, and wants. Therefore, when you introduce the ideas that the client has the right to limits, to have and express feelings, and to acknowledge needs and express desires, the client will find this information to be new and unfamiliar and perhaps anxiety-provoking.

The difficult aspect of maintaining a therapeutic demeanor with codependent clients is their desire to have you "help." The concept of "helping" may take many forms. In psychiatric nursing there are guidelines to maintaining the therapeutic relationship.

First, view your interactions with clients objectively and try to assess *whose* needs are being met by the interaction. If the client's needs for therapeutic contact with a professional are foremost in the interaction, then the prime directive for maintaining healthy associations has been met. It is important to avoid meeting your needs instead of the client's.

A client knows you have an interest in porcelain figurines and has briefly mentioned her relationship with someone who deals in rare figurines. At your next meeting, this client devotes several minutes to arranging your access to the dealer of rare figurines. The client feels like she has given something special to you, but you have spent this client's valuable time meeting your need and not getting to the business of helping the client move through treatment. Instead, you have "helped" this client perfect her method of meeting other people's needs.

Another guideline for maintaining your therapeutic barometer with codependent clients is to prevent the relationship from slipping into a social context. Pilette, Berck, and Achber (1995) discuss the boundary violation of relating to a client as one would relate to a friend. This article lists the items in the Nursing Boundary Index (Epstein and Simon 1990) to be used as an early warning system for boundary violations in psychiatric situations. The result of a boundary violation, such as insertion of the nurse's fears, concerns, and personal doubts into a conversation with a client, burdens the client and changes the focus of care from the client. This is especially true with a codependent client who is more at risk for seeking, engendering, and responding to others' needs and relegating personal needs to the status of being inconsequential.

As discussed in the following section, dealing with a codependent client is difficult. You may have issues that need to be explored and worked through. This can be accomplished through supervision or consultation (both routes are commonly taken by competent psychotherapists). Evaluate yourself in these situations to see if you are (a) focusing on the client's needs at all times, and (b) keeping your boundaries intact.

Relationship Work In working with the codependent client, remember that the client has established relationships with other dysfunctional people. The interpersonal systems in which the client functions often do not support the changes the client is struggling to make. A possible referral to a support group may help the client feel encouraged throughout the change process. An alternative may be an ACoA group. These groups and information about them are available through local AA organizations.

It is important to remember that the nurse-client relationship can be difficult. The codependent person has had years of practice with dysfunctional patterns that work, in a maladaptive way, in their relationships. The client will initially be confused and frustrated that the patterns that worked elsewhere do not work in healthy adult relationships. Establishing new interactional patterns will cost the client some acceptance within the dysfunctional relationships, but will give the client a stronger, healthier sense of self.

In the example of Mary and John, Mary is given an opportunity when she leaves John's boat to learn about herself and to learn how to stay in her own boat and row alongside another person. Mary can learn a new way of being helpful—by encouraging John to struggle and work out his own problems.

For suggestions about helping codependent clients change their behavior patterns, see the accompanying Client/Family Teaching box.

Evaluation and Outcome Criteria

Once a client is aware of dysfunctional approaches in his or her relationships and expresses a desire to change them, recovery has begun. Evaluating the recovery process of a codependent client involves acknowledging that it will not be a straight course but an up-and-down pattern winding through the various relationships and situations the client is involved in.

Becoming aware of one's feelings and validating that it is OK to have those feelings are remarkable events. How-

CLIENT/FAMILY TEACHING

Changing Codependent Behavior Patterns

Everybody has ways of coping with relationships, and sometimes that coping style is unhealthy. If responses to interactions focus on taking care of someone else, or prevent another adult from having to cope, or rescue a situation, then you need to take a fresh approach. Move toward healthier relationships. Replace what you would normally say with these new directions for your energies—you!

Old Thoughts, Behaviors, or Statements	***New Thoughts, Behaviors, or Statements***
(He's at it again, yelling and calling me names.) "Whatever you say."	"I'll talk to you later when we can be nicer."
(We've only been here an hour and he wants to go.) "OK, let's go. I have a lot of laundry to do."	"I am going to stay a while longer. You go ahead, and I'll be home later."
"I'd be happy to do that for you. That way you'd have more time."	"You certainly are busy lately. Could we make some time to be together when things aren't so hectic?"
"I never tell my father he's unreasonable. He'd only attack my mother."	"My father and I have an adult relationship. I will discuss rules and problems between the two of us. My mother has her own relationship with him, and she can design it or not as she wants."
Codependent interaction: You listen to a friend explain why another friend didn't keep an appointment with you.	*Resisting a codependent interaction:* "I will talk with her directly; that's between her and me. When can you and I go see that movie together?"
"I can't believe I did that wrong. It just doesn't make sense. I always do it the right way."	"I see that there's nothing wrong with making mistakes."

ever, there will be that one friendship, or work situation, or boyfriend, that pulls the client back into the maladaptive behavior pattern. Whenever someone is stressed, pushed too far, tired, or physically ill, the maladaptive coping mechanisms return because that is the path of least resistance. Prepare your clients for this event. It is not forbidden to "visit" the old maladaptive ways. Once there, the recovering client will feel the difference and will strive to regain the newly learned skills. It is important to emphasize this eventuality with clients who are struggling with new skills.

There is a difference between someone who is working on codependence issues and someone who is cured of codependence. The cure may never occur. These are lifelong issues, and the client will need to guard against them always. Discuss this timeline with clients so their expectations are realistic.

Be careful in evaluating interventions with codependent clients. Do not expect perfection from yourself or your clients. Make sure that you give clients and yourself the room to make mistakes and have it be OK. The effort of recovery from codependence is best directed toward decreasing the number of dysfunctional relationships and increasing involvement with a healthy and caring self.

Codependence and the Workplace

Codependence is not restricted to relationships and situations in one's personal life; the behavior pattern occurs in the workplace as well. A job may include helping others, focusing on details, minimizing mistakes, and rigidly adhering to technical policies and procedures. These are work-related characteristics that reinforce codependence.

Being in an occupation or profession that enhances codependence is an unhealthy and debilitating lifestyle when one is codependent. Because job choice is under the control of the individual—unlike the family of origin, where the behavior probably originated—there are options and alternatives. In choosing careers, it is essential that people with codependent traits carefully examine an attraction to an occupation or profession in which codependence is promoted or encouraged. If codependent

NURSING SELF-AWARENESS

Recognizing Codependent Behaviors in Yourself

Check your behaviors and see if you are exhibiting codependent traits. One of these does not make you codependent. Sets or clusters of these behaviors could be making your career or relationships much more work for you than they need to be. If you have all of these behaviors or just a couple, and they interfere with your life, it's a problem that needs care and attention soon. Do you:

- Spend time trying to control someone else?
- Bail others out of trouble?
- Feel responsible for what other people do?
- Feel guilty about what someone else has done?
- Avoid conflict?
- Threaten to quit, leave, report someone, or announce the problem to an authority and then not do it?
- Take over someone else's work?
- Not know how valuable you are when you're not working?

behaviors are being manifested on the job, or if one observes tendencies toward codependence, a reshaping of the interactions is a priority so that healthier behaviors can develop. First and foremost is the need to be aware of the problem. The next step is to obtain training to help stop bearing responsibility for others and "fixing" their problems. Placing priority on oneself and choosing to have the freedom to meet one's own needs in the work environment are powerful tools for career advancement.

Nursing and Codependence

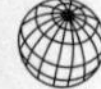

Nursing is a predominantly female field. Being involved in a woman-dominated profession involves careful examination of any theory or psychiatric label that defines women negatively. Lerner (1989) describes as normal the urge to want to help someone in trouble. The problem of codependence arises only when a woman becomes overinvolved with that trouble and becomes underfocused on herself. Keeping this distinction clear in our minds is paramount. Caring about others, which includes nursing as well as competence in many areas, does not justify labeling a person codependent. Doing so would encourage viewing involvement in the emotional health and growth of others, an activity that defines nursing, as a psychiatric problem. The innovative nurse who helps a team move through trying times is someone to be admired, supported, and promoted as an ideal. Codependence occurs when caring about others overshadows the individual's own needs and desires.

There are nursing situations where codependence exists. Professional codependence can be spotted in any act or behavior that shames and does not support the value, vulnerability, interdependence, level of maturity, and accountability or spirituality of a nurse, colleague, or client (Snow and Willard 1989). Burnout, staff turnover, absenteeism, unsatisfactory performance, flight from nursing—all may reflect ineffective adaptation or the progressive nature of a codependence problem (Chappelle and Sorrentino 1993).

Have you ever seen a nursing manager or supervisor solve *every* problem for the employees? This tends to stunt the professional growth of the staff. The result can be unmotivated and confused employees who resent their supervisor and may not understand why (Allen and Sevier 1992). Colleagues working together on a unit may have a member of the team that "barges in" and "takes over" at every opportunity. This nurse may be perfectionistic and feel underappreciated. Even when a nurse becomes overinvolved with a client, there are ways to restore emotional balance to the situation and assure support and understanding for the nurse (Heinrich 1992).

Nurses know that caring for each other and caring for our relationships can be mutually empowering. Even so, we must ensure that nursing care, or being a nurse and caring, is not reinterpreted as a license to martyr oneself (Malloy and Berkery 1993). We can be pivotal in helping ourselves, and our clients, cultivate mutual and accurate empathy in relationships that are empowering and self-affirming. But first we have to recognize codependent behaviors in ourselves. See the accompanying Nursing Self-Awareness box for an appreciation of the components of codependence. See also the Research Note on codependence in the nursing environment.

In addition to the interventions discussed earlier, a method for codependence intervention suggested by Farnsworth and Thomas (1993) can be used with groups of codependent nurses. It can also be adapted for use in group settings in which relationship difficulties involve codependence. This technique is called the Climb. It is a simulation/game teaching method using the metaphor of a mountain climbing expedition up Mt. Growmore. Each team of climbers is given Life Event cards to direct their movement up Mt. Growmore, including experiences such

RESEARCH NOTE

Citation

Chappelle LS, Sorrentino EA: Assessing co-dependency issues within a nursing environment. *Nurs Management* 1993;24(5):40–44.

Study Problem/Purpose

Nurses have been charged with being codependent in large numbers. The purpose of this study was to determine the level of codependence within one nursing environment.

Methods

A self-report survey/questionnaire format (Friel Co-Dependency Assessment Inventory, or CAI) was distributed to nursing staff in a southeastern U.S. government hospital. The nurses completed a demographic profile and the CAI during work hours and returned them in sealed envelopes; 383 questionnaires were distributed, and 160 were returned.

To determine the contribution of dysfunctional family histories, subjects were asked about immediate family members or significant others living with them. Involvement with alcohol dependence, other drug dependencies, compulsive gambling, anorexia, bulimia, sexual abuse, child abuse, and physical or mental health problems were specifically mentioned.

Each of the questions was classified based on Roy's definitions of effective adaptive modes, physiologic, self-concept, role function, and interdependence. T-test and frequency rates were the methodological approaches used.

Findings

The majority of the respondents reported few codependence concerns, and 27.5% reported mild to moderate codependence concerns. Moderate to severe levels of codependence were reported in 13.1% of the group.

The results for the ambulatory care and medical-surgical units showed positive differences for the interdependence adaptive mode as well as subjects who work in special care units. Role function mode focuses on the expected behaviors for maintaining a certain title. Special care units showed a negative difference. Self-concept mode is partly formed by perceptions of others' reactions. Subjects working on the medical-surgical units showed a negative significance.

Implications

Several aspects of this study require careful thought. One is the dysfunctional family self-assessment. Over half the subjects included in this study (57%, or 91 individuals) did not respond to this query. The possibility exists that these participants could be unaware of these problems in their families because of denial, a classic symptom of codependent behavior. It is also possible that these respondents did not answer the question because of privacy concerns. Yet another explanation is that they were ashamed of these problems. But even with this interesting gap in information, 25% of the subjects did report positive family history for codependence symptoms.

Adaptive modes were found in significant amounts in ambulatory care, medical-surgical, and special care units. Cultural and role definitions may have influenced these results.

The actual level, or intensity, of codependent behaviors derived from this self-assessment of nurses was surprising. Contrary to initial expectations that nurses are prone to high levels of codependence, most levels were mild to moderate in intensity. Given these results, the impression that nursing is rife with codependent behaviors at a fairly high level of intensity needs revision. However, the fact remains that codependence behaviors, when present, are uncomfortable at any level. Nurses, as well as everyone else, would benefit from having an awareness of codependence and available resources to address these interpersonal issues.

One of the cautions in the discussion of these results is not to dismiss that codependence exists in nursing at high levels because of the results of this single study. Could it be that nurses are considered codependent until proven otherwise? There seems to be an unfortunate bias that codependence is an illness as opposed to being seen as a continuum of behavior. Future research should clarify a continuous scoring of codependence rather than a categorical scoring. Self-esteem assessment instruments and specific objective criteria for determining the presence and level of codependence would strengthen research in this area.

as, "Nancy, an RN on your staff, tells you she can't work with another staff member. You encourage Nancy to talk directly to the other person. Offer to be available if they need your help. This is setting limits and not taking responsibility for others. Gain 25 feet." Climbers pass through areas reflecting the sequence of discovery and recovery aspects of codependence. This technique teaches about the course of codependence while indicating corrections to that course.

Research in Codependence

Research has been conducted on various aspects of codependence, such as its occurrence in specific populations, the combination of level of codependence with depressive features, and an examination of codependents' close relationships (Chappelle and Sorrentino 1993; Scher 1991; Wright and Wright 1990, respectively). Teaching views of codependence to nurses has been suggested for further study (Farnsworth and Thomas 1993). There are many opportunities to examine questions, issues, and hypotheses relating to the concept of codependence as well as opportunities to formulate nursing interventions to address codependent behaviors.

Treatment issues regarding codependence need to be thoroughly researched. It is important to study which combination of treatment interventions is most effective in remediating codependent symptoms. The best type of study would involve comparisons with randomly selected or noncodependent controls. However, as literature addressing intervention strategies based on empirical research is sparse, the field remains open for nurses to enact sound research to develop effective treatments.

Chapter Highlights

- Codependence is a fairly new concept in problematic interactions.
- Codependence is a learned behavior that affects one's ability to meet his or her own needs due to the overinvolvement of helping another adult.
- Biopsychosocial theories of codependence examine the variety of perspectives this topic is viewed through.
- Awareness of the definitions and implications of codependence require a sensitivity to issues affecting women.
- Nursing interventions include role modeling of effective interpersonal relationships and teaching relationship skills.
- Codependence may be treated once it has been recognized and when the desire to change is apparent in the client.
- Nurses may be at risk for being in job situations that encourage codependent traits.
- Graphic representations of healthy and codependent interaction styles show the dramatic differences between them.
- Adequate research in relation to codependence is beginning.

References

Allen BM, Sevier AJ: A key to empowerment. *Caring* (Sept) 1992:50–52.

Babcock M: Addicted women and women with addicts. Training session presented to Access—York, York, PA, 1990.

Babcock M: Who are the real codependents? *Focus: Education Professionals in Family Recovery* 1991;14:28–45.

Black C: *Double Duty.* Ballantine, 1990.

Black C: *It Will Never Happen to Me.* Hazelden, 1987.

Bowen M: *Family Therapy in Clinical Practice.* Jason Aronson, 1985.

Bradshaw J: *Healing the Shame That Binds You.* Health Communications, 1988.

Bradshaw J: *Homecoming: Reclaiming and Championing Your Inner Child.* Bantam, 1990.

Cermak TL: Diagnostic criteria for codependency. *J Psychoactive Drugs* 1986;28(1):80.

Chappelle LS, Sorrentino EA: Assessing co-dependency issues within a nursing environment. *Nurs Management* 1993;24(5):40–44.

Chesler P: *Women and Madness,* ed 2. Harcourt Brace Jovanovich, 1989.

Epstein R, Simon R: The exploitation index: An early warning indicator of boundary violations in psychotherapy. *Bul Menninger Clin* 1990;54(4):450–464.

Fagan-Pryor EC, Haber LC: Codependency: Another name for Bowen's undifferentiated self. *Perspec Psychiatric Care* 1992;28(4):24–28.

Farnsworth BJ, Thomas KJ: Codependency in nursing: Using a simulation/gaming teaching method. *J Continuing Ed Nurs* 1993;24(4):180–183.

Friel JC: Codependency assessment inventory: A preliminary research tool. *Focus Fam Chem Dep* 1985;8:20–21.

Friel J, Friel L: *An Adult Child's Guide to What's "Normal."* Health Communications, 1990.

Heinrich KT: What to do when a patient becomes too special. *Nursing92* 1992 (Nov):63–64.

Jordon JV, Kaplan AG, Miller JB, Stiver IP, Surrey JL: *Women's Growth in Connection.* Guilford Press, 1991.

Kaplan AG: Codependency: A reexamination. Paper presented at Women Teaching Women, conference at Harvard Medical School, Department of Continuing Education, Cambridge, MA, 1991.

Lerner H: *The Dance of Intimacy.* Harper & Row, 1989.

Levin JD: *Recovery from Alcoholism: Beyond Your Wildest Dreams.* Jason Aronson, 1991.

Malloy GB, Berkery AC: Codependency: A feminist perspective. *J Psychosoc Nurs* 1993;31(4):15–19.

Morgan JP: What is codependency? *J Clin Psych* 1991;47(5): 720–29.

Pilette PC, Berck CB, Achber LC: Therapeutic management of helping boundaries. *J Psychosoc Nurs* 1995;33(1):40–47.

Schaef AW: *Co-Dependence: Misunderstood, Mistreated.* Harper & Row, 1986.

Schaef AW, Fassel D: *The Addictive Organization.* Harper & Row, 1988.

Scher M: Codependency: Researchers investigate tools with which to validate codependence diagnosis. *Focus,* 1991 (April–May):35–39.

Snow C, Willard D: *I'm Dying to Take Care of You.* Professional Counselor Books, 1989.

Subby, R: *Codependency: An Emerging Issue.* Health Communications, 1984.

Tweed SH, Ryff CD: Adult children of alcoholics: Profiles of wellness amidst distress. *J Studies Alcohol* 1991;52(2):133–141.

Webster D: Women and Depression (Alias Codependency). *Family Commun Health* 1990;13(3):58.

Whitfield C: Co-dependence: Our most common addiction. *Wellness Associates J* 1988(Spring):1.

Whitfield C: *Healing the Child Within.* Health Communications, 1987.

Woititz JG: *Struggle for Intimacy.* Health Communications, 1985.

Wright PH, Wright KD: Measuring codependents' close relationships: A preliminary study. *J Substance Abuse* 1990;2: 335–344.

CHAPTER 27

HIV/AIDS IN VULNERABLE PSYCHIATRIC POPULATIONS

Carol Ren Kneisl

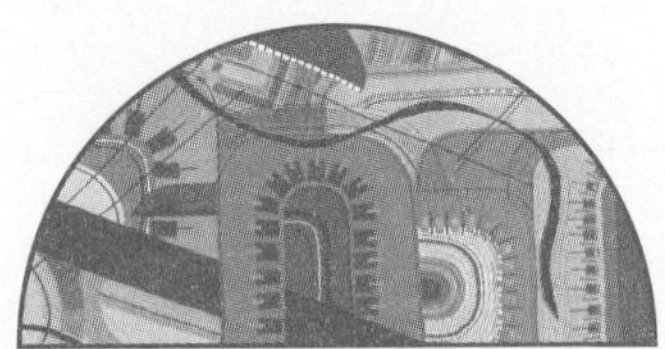

COMPETENCIES

- *Explain why certain psychiatric populations are at risk for acquired immune deficiency syndrome (AIDS).*
- *Describe the neuropsychiatric, developmental, sociocultural, economic, legal, political, and ethical impact of HIV infection.*
- *Provide direct nursing care to people with HIV disease in psychiatric settings.*
- *Incorporate HIV risk-reduction education and counseling regarding sexual behavior and substance abuse in work with clients and people in the community.*
- *Identify the means by which psychiatric nurses can support caregivers of people with HIV and AIDS and individuals experiencing AIDS-related bereavements.*

Cross-References

Other topics relevant to this content are: Caring for clients with dementia, Chapter 12; Caring for depressed clients, Chapter 15; Caring for substance-abusing clients, Chapter 13; Visualization and stress-management techniques for self-healing and pain and symptom control, Chapter 29.

Critical Thinking Challenge

The community in which you live is considering establishing a syringe and needle exchange program for injection drug users (IDUs) as an HIV/AIDS prevention strategy. At the town meeting, several people voice their concern that a needle and syringe exchange program would not only facilitate, but also stimulate, illicit drug injection. Because you are a psychiatric nurse, you are asked to comment. What would you say?

The contagious and potentially fatal condition of immune system depression known as **acquired immune deficiency syndrome (AIDS)** has no known cure and responds to limited treatments. A chronic, potentially life-threatening illness, AIDS is of clinical concern to all nurses, but especially to psychiatric–mental health nurses, who, by nature of their commitment and responsibility, become involved in human experiences. Clients with the **human immunodeficiency virus (HIV)**, the virus that causes AIDS, require care that promotes quality existence and personal growth in the face of serious illness.

Promoting quality existence and personal growth can be achieved only when psychiatric–mental health nurses are knowledgeable about the disease itself and are sensitive to the norms, customs, and lifestyle issues common to the communities hardest hit by the epidemic—gay/bisexual men, their partners, friends, children, and families of origin; and male and female injection drug users (IDUs), their partners, friends, children, and families of origin, disproportionately represented in the African-American and Latino communities. 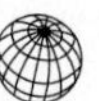

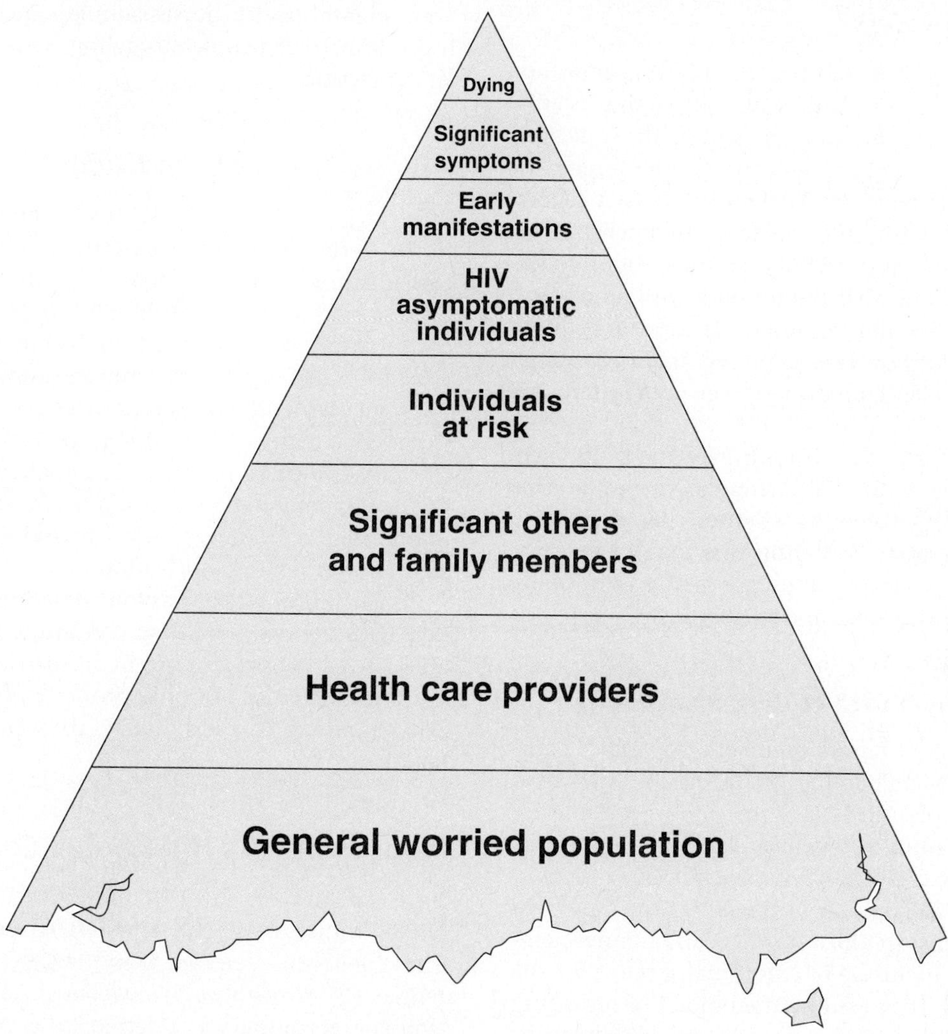

Figure 27–1 The HIV mental health spectrum. This model shows populations requiring mental health care services related to HIV. Cross-sectional size represents population size and diversity. Distance from the base represents increasingly direct emotional effects of HIV infection and the increasing need for mental health intervention. *Source: Adapted from Knox, Davis, and Friedrich, p. 77.*

This chapter has been written with the assumption that you have basic knowledge of HIV disease, its cause, incidence and distribution, and modes of transmission, and that you understand the basics of instituting universal precautions and providing physical care to people with HIV disease. The focus of this chapter is the understanding and skills essential to the mental health–psychiatric nurse's repertoire.

The HIV Mental Health Spectrum

According to Knox, Davis, and Friedrich (1994), there is a broad spectrum of people in the population with growing mental health care needs that are related to HIV. A model of the HIV mental health spectrum is illustrated above in Figure 27–1.

The General Worried Population

The general worried population makes up the majority of people in this country. Uninfected and personally unaffected by the AIDS epidemic, this group generally does not practice behaviors that put them at high risk of infection. Social naiveté in this group will lead to a speedier spread of the disease. Reducing fears, promoting knowledge, and encouraging behavioral change are crucial roles of mental health care providers with this population.

Health Care Providers

Irrational fears, prejudice, and stress can lead to burnout and reduce the quality of health care. Although it is crucial that mental health care workers help set the tone and example for others in the community for appropriate attitudes and practices regarding HIV infection, they report reluctance to work with HIV-infected individuals. They cite fear of contagion as a primary concern, followed by discomfort in working with the terminally ill, and then discomfort with IDUs and homosexuals (Dow and Knox 1991). Worries about how best to protect themselves and their families are also common concerns (Reutter and Northcott 1994).

Because nurses have the most intimate and prolonged contact with people with HIV infections, nurses are the primary determining factor in whether clients get empathic, supportive care. Providing this type of care requires confronting your own and your family's fear of infection and your own values and prejudices.

Significant Others and Family Members

Significant others and family members face many emotional challenges. Many families are facing the emotional challenge of multiple AIDS diagnoses and injection drug use within the family. Previously held family secrets about sexual or drug use behavior are publicly disclosed along with an AIDS diagnosis. At the same time they cope with these problems, significant others and family members are often the mainstay of emotional support for the person with AIDS. They assume the burden of providing emotional support while coping with their own fears, providing physical care, and anticipating, then grieving, their loss. The issue of bereavement associated with HIV and AIDS is addressed later in the chapter.

Individuals at Risk

Individuals at risk are those who are most likely to have or to contract HIV, due to past or current participation in high-risk activities (discussed later in the chapter). This specific group includes people who have not been tested for HIV and those who have received negative HIV antibody test results but are still considered at risk.

Individuals at risk often experience anxiety, ineffective coping, and decisional conflicts related to HIV infection. These human responses may be manifested in many ways, including fear of sexual expression related to the risk of transmission, denial of risk as a primary defense, and conflict over whether to take the HIV antibody test. Maladaptive human responses in individuals at risk could result in self-destructive behaviors such as suicide attempts, or irresponsible behaviors such as unsafe sexual practices. As the epidemic continues unabated, psychiatric–mental health nurses should expect to see increasing numbers of people struggling with issues related to HIV infection.

HIV Asymptomatic Individuals

This category of individuals affected by HIV is referred to in the Centers for Disease Control and Prevention (CDC) classification system as *HIV-seropositive (asymptomatic)*. This group has received validation of HIV status through confirmatory diagnostic test results but as yet exhibits no symptoms associated with immune system suppression.

People who are HIV-seropositive (asymptomatic) may experience many of the same responses as individuals at risk, in addition to problems of impaired adjustment and the development of a sense of powerlessness. This may be manifested in a variety of ways, including chronic depression and decreasing motivation.

As HIV-seropositive (asymptomatic) people begin to deal with the reality of their condition, the nurse may be able to help them engage in health-seeking behaviors. Wellness activities not only promote physical health but also empower the individual, thus promoting mental health.

Individuals with HIV-Related Conditions

This category on the HIV mental health spectrum includes individuals with HIV-related conditions (HRC). These people are referred to in the CDC classification system as *HIV-seropositive (symptomatic)*. In the past, this diagnostic grouping was referred to as AIDS-related complex (ARC). The specific physiologic symptoms associated with HRC are discussed later in the chapter.

Individuals with HIV-related conditions have begun to experience the physical effects of immune system deterioration. In addition to having physical manifestations, they may experience complicating psychosocial responses as well as the human responses previously discussed. These may include altered role performance and self-concept disturbance related to losses, and changes in their perceptions and abilities secondary to the development of physical symptoms and limitations.

People with AIDS

People with significant symptoms are those with a formal diagnosis of AIDS, as defined by CDC guidelines. These are characterized by the development of potentially life-threatening complications because of extensive immune system suppression.

People with AIDS (PWAs) may experience all of the human responses of individuals throughout the HIV mental health spectrum. In addition, PWAs may experience a sense of hopelessness, social isolation, impaired social interactions, or spiritual distress associated with the effects of a chronic life-threatening illness.

Long-Term Survivors

Although not listed in the HIV mental health spectrum, there is one other group of people of clinical concern to psychiatric–mental health nurses. People who have outlived the generally expected life span for people with HIV and AIDS are called long-term survivors. As more individuals with HIV infection are identified and treatments are discovered to slow or halt HIV progression in a predictable fashion, the number of long-term survivors will continue to increase. This has obvious implications for mental health care professionals working with people affected by HIV infection.

HIV Transmission Risks

The presence of HIV has been documented in blood, blood plasma, bone marrow, semen, cervical secretions, vaginal secretions, saliva, breast milk, lymph nodes, brain tissue, skin, tears, and cerebrospinal fluid. The presence of the virus in so many body fluids and tissues is one reason why the general public fears that HIV can be transmitted by casual contact. However, the research overwhelmingly indicates that the major modes of transmission of the virus are:

- Intimate unprotected sexual contact with an HIV-seropositive person.
- Parenteral injection of blood or blood products infected with HIV.
- Transfer of the virus from an HIV-infected mother to a fetus or newborn infant in utero, during labor or delivery, or in the early newborn period.

Because of the nature of these major modes of transmission and the epidemiology of the epidemic in the United States, two psychiatric–mental health populations have been identified as being at *high risk* for contracting HIV:

- Intravenous drug users (and their sex partners).
- The severely and persistently mentally ill.

Note that family members and friends in close contact with people with HIV are not listed among the high-risk categories. Research continues to confirm that there is little or no risk to those having long-standing household exposure to people with HIV.

Health care providers are also not in the high-risk category. In addition to having close contact with people with HIV, health care workers may be concerned about contracting HIV as the result of an accidental needlestick or being cut with a sharp instrument. Studies of health care workers that documented parenteral or mucous membrane exposure to the blood or body fluids of HIV-infected people indicated that the incidence is extremely low.

Injection Drug Users

The second largest transmission category for HIV in the U.S. and Europe is IDUs. The virus is believed to be transmitted among IDUs through the transfer of small amounts of blood in shared needles or syringes. IDUs also constitute a bridge to others—their fetuses, newborns, and sex partners—putting them at increased risk. It is believed that the category known as "heterosexual cases" is largely composed of the heterosexual partners of IDUs.

The incidence of AIDS among IDUs is highest in the New York/New Jersey metropolitan area (where the incidence of AIDS among IDUs has now surpassed the rate in homosexual men) and in neighboring Connecticut. Of heterosexuals whose only known exposure was through sex with a person at risk, approximately two-thirds are female partners of male IDUs.

The Severely and Persistently Mentally Ill

The prevailing stereotype that persons with serious mental illness are asexual or not interested in sex has been cited as the reason HIV infection has not been perceived as a serious risk for the mentally ill. However, we now know that people with serious mental illness do engage in sexual behaviors that put them at high risk for HIV infection (Cates, Bond, and Graham 1994). Just like any other psychiatric–mental health population or any general population, the severely and persistently mentally ill are at risk for HIV transmission if they have experienced any of the major modes of transmission mentioned earlier. However, this group is thought to be especially vulnerable for several reasons.

Unsafe heterosexual activity (rather than the risk factors of homosexual activity and drug injection) was by far the most common current risk behavior among the severely and persistently mentally ill in one study (see the Research Note). In a study of individuals diagnosed with schizophrenia, nearly half had been sexually active in the 6 months preceding the study, and sexual activity was almost always accompanied by HIV risk behavior (Cournos et al. 1994). Another study found that many subjects' sex partners had been met in bars or mental health clinics, and the sexual relations often involved the exchange of money or drugs (Kalichman et al. 1994). In all three studies, there were several consistent findings:

- Multiple sex partners.
- IDU sex partners.

RESEARCH NOTE

Citation

Cournos F, McKinnon K, Meyer-Bahlberg H, Guido JR, Meyer I: HIV risk activity among persons with severe mental illness: Preliminary findings. *Hosp Commun Psychiatr* 1993; 44(11): 1104–1106.

Study Problem/Purpose

The purpose of this study was to assess risk behaviors associated with HIV infection among severely mentally ill persons.

Methods

A structured set of face-to-face interviews using the Structured Clinical Interview for DSM-III-R, an adaptation of the Parenteral Drug Use High-Risk Questionnaire, and the Sexual Risk Behavior Assessment Schedule was carried out. Subjects had an average of five previous psychiatric hospitalizations.

Findings

Findings were for the first 95 subjects interviewed. Fifty-eight percent reported engaging in sexual activity in the past 6 months. Two-thirds under 40 years of age had multiple sex partners. Over half had never used condoms, and less than 10% consistently used them. Heterosexual anal intercourse was reported by 23% of men and 22% of women. Few subjects acknowledged homosexual activity or drug injection use within the past 6 months. However, 18.5% had engaged in homosexual behavior in the past, and 20% had injected drugs at some time (despite the exclusion from this study of those with a primary diagnosis of substance-related disorder).

Implications

Unprotected heterosexual intercourse was the most common HIV risk activity in this population of the severely and persistently mentally ill. Prevention education should focus on providing information on HIV infection and transmission, risk-producing characteristics of relationships, and proper condom use. Risk-reduction education is an important need in psychiatric settings and is an appropriate and necessary component of the psychiatric nurse's educator role.

- Absence of, or inconsistency in, condom use.
- Frequent use of alcohol and drugs in conjunction with sex.
- A history of sexually transmitted infections.

In addition, they are ambivalent about abstinence and reducing the risk of infection with a sex partner, and see themselves as more helpless to reduce risk than the general population (Cates, Bond, and Graham 1994).

The homeless mentally ill who live in urban areas, particularly those who live in municipal shelters, are at particular risk for both HIV and tuberculosis (TB) (Colson, Susser, and Valencia 1994). The upsurge in tuberculosis rates in the U.S. is thought to be directly related to the HIV epidemic.

The homeless mentally ill are likely to experience several barriers to beginning, maintaining, and completing treatment. Several practical matters—establishing a medication routine, having access to health care providers, and being supported by friends and family—are the usual barriers faced by homeless people. The specific cognitive barriers that result from mental illness and HIV infection add to the difficulty of obtaining prophylactic or early treatment.

The Biopsychosocial Impact of HIV/AIDS

HIV does not discriminate in its effects on the individual or society. It affects the biologic, psychologic, neurologic, developmental, sociocultural, economic, legal, political, and ethical spheres.

Neuropsychiatric (NPM) Manifestations

Neuropsychiatric manifestations represent one of the more complex aspects of people with HIV disease. Because the virus is able to invade central nervous system (CNS) tissue and because several of the opportunistic infections and neoplasms associated with AIDS also affect the CNS, significant numbers of people with HIV experience neuropsychiatric manifestations (Maj et al. 1994a, 1994b; Perkins et al. 1994).

Neuropsychiatric manifestations of HIV refer to a variety of disorders associated with psychologic and neurologic responses to HIV infection and/or HIV-related opportunistic processes. These can range from anxiety and depressive symptoms to delirium, dementia, and coma.

Psychologic HIV disease threatens psychologic integrity as well as physiologic integrity. The concept of loss is central to an understanding of the psychologic impact of HIV and the depression, anxiety, and suicidal ideation that often accompany it. HIV disease is frequently linked with several different loss experiences. These include loss of the following:

- Energy, appetite, strength, and physical stamina.
- Control of body functions such as elimination, mobility, speech, sight, hearing, and tactile sensations.
- Control of body appearance due to dramatic weight loss, oozing wounds, skin breakdown, hair loss, skin lesions, etc.
- Self-worth.
- Mental clarity and cognitive ability.
- Privacy.
- Self-sufficiency and self-determination.
- Employment, health insurance, salary.
- Personal competence.
- Physical intimacy, including sexual expression.
- Friends and lovers to earlier deaths from AIDS.
- Social support.
- Hope.
- Peace of mind and spirit.
- Life itself.

People with HIV and their families, friends, and caregivers experience these losses or fears.

Psychologic syndromes associated with HIV infection are generally related to the initial diagnosis of HIV, crisis points along the HIV mental health spectrum, or adjustment to the experience of chronic illness. Increased suicide risk can result from depression related to stress from the HIV diagnosis, treatment, and side effects of medications (Valente and Saunders 1994). The inherent lack of predictability and control, the fear of rejection and abandonment, and problems such as memory deficit and confusion play a role. Common psychiatric disorders frequently seen in people with HIV and AIDS are anxiety disorders, panic attacks, adjustment disorders with depressed mood, and major depression (Perkins et al. 1994; Sewell et al. 1994). Psychiatric disorders in people with HIV disease are probably grossly underdiagnosed. The reason may be that many health care providers assign higher priority to overwhelming physical needs.

NEUROLOGIC Studies suggest that physiologically based clinical neuropsychiatric manifestations or disorders are common among PWAs (Beason-Hazen, Nasrallah, and Bornstein 1994; Bedos et al. 1995; Maj et al. 1994b). It has been estimated that approximately 10% of people with AIDS develop neurologic syndromes as the first clinical manifestation of HIV disease (Navia and Price 1987; So, Choucair, and Davis 1987).

Focal Brain Processes The most common focal brain processes are toxoplasmosis (a parasitic opportunistic infection), cryptococcal meningitis (a fungal opportunistic infection), cytomegalovirus (CMV) encephalitis (a viral opportunistic infection), and CNS lymphoma (a neoplastic process). Signs and symptoms associated with these processes include focal deficits, altered level of consciousness, confusion, memory disturbances, headaches, and seizures.

HIV-Related Dementia An increasingly common neuropsychiatric disorder is HIV-related dementia. **HIV-related dementia,** a syndrome caused by direct HIV infection of the CNS, is characterized as a progressive dementia. It involves a progressive slowing and loss of precision in both cognitive and motor functions, with accompanying behavioral disturbances. The signs and symptoms of HIV-related dementia include the following:

- Cognitive indications: forgetfulness, loss of concentration, confusion, and slowness of thought.
- Motor deficiencies: loss of balance, muscle weakness, and deterioration in fine motor skills such as handwriting.
- Behavioral indications: apathy, withdrawal, dysphoric mood, organic psychosis, and regressed behavior.

In addition, people with HIV-related dementia may experience other symptoms such as headaches or seizures.

HIV-related dementia is often initially confused with psychiatric depression but generally progresses in a period of months to the point at which the affected individual is bedridden. Individuals with HIV-related dementia may quickly succumb to opportunistic infections because they are unable to take care of themselves.

Caregiver Concerns People with neuropsychiatric manifestations of HIV represent a tremendous challenge to both professional and nonprofessional caregivers. Working with this population requires participation as a client advocate, effective multidisciplinary collaboration, and the ability to make appropriate referrals. To address the needs of this group adequately, one needs the ability to empathize with the individual with HIV and with primary caregivers (PCGs) and to act on the basis of that empathy. A PCG is a person who is generally responsible for providing or coordinating daily care for a PWA who cannot perform self-care activities. Usually, a PCG is a nonprofessional who is a significant other (life partner, spouse, family member, or close friend) of the person with AIDS.

PSYCHONEUROIMMUNOLOGY There has been increasing emphasis in the scientific literature on the study of psychoneuroimmunology (PNI), introduced in Chapter 3. A growing body of evidence has demonstrated the interrelatedness of the body-mind-spirit connection and the immune system. Nurses need to be more aware of the psychologic and neurologic effects on immune system disorders. There is widespread support for the use of holistic nursing practices and treatment approaches to boost the immune system, in accordance with the findings in the growing field of psychoneuroimmunology (see the accompanying Mind-Body-Spirit Connection box).

Developmental Effects

Most people with HIV disease are young adults or adults in their middle years. The period known as young adulthood is normally the healthiest and is characterized by peaks in muscular strength. Cognitive development should be completed and cognitive abilities should be refined at this stage. Recall that the psychosocial task of identity consolidation is the major developmental task of young adulthood. HIV disease may disrupt the person's ability to negotiate this challenge successfully.

Typically, the middle years are very productive in the arenas of work and family. During this period, adults consolidate relationships and occupational status and goals. HIV disease may interfere with the individual's ability to accept the responsibilities inherent in such roles as parent, worker, mate or partner, and so on. Questions of dependence and independence, thought to have been resolved previously, are reawakened as illness forces a return to earlier developmental phases.

Children and adolescents with HIV infection face delays or changes in skills on all developmental fronts—physical, cognitive, and psychosocial—as they confront acute life-threatening illness and chronic disability. Failure to thrive is a striking feature of this illness in children; some are diagnosed with AIDS as early as 4 months of age.

Sociocultural and Economic Effects

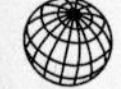

SOCIOCULTURAL HOSTILITY The sociocultural environment of most people affected by HIV is generally hostile to them. Several factors seem to account for this hostility. Most people with HIV are in one of two risk categories—homosexual/bisexual men and injection drug users—that engender fear, anger, and prejudice. **Homophobia** is the term used to describe an unrealistic fear of homosexuality and homosexuals based on myths and stereotypes. According to Hughes, Martin, and Franks (1987), homophobia may exist on both overt and covert levels and may be internalized, externalized, or institutional:

- Internalized homophobia is the self-rejection (feelings of shame, fear, guilt, and wrongdoing) that gay people may experience.
- Externalized homophobia is the rejection gay people experience from others.
- Institutional homophobia is evident in the rules and regulations of hospitals, churches, employers, and other institutions that, for example, restrict hospital visitors in intensive care units to blood relatives only or deny gay people the right to worship.

Moral indignation is a frequent response to both gay people and to injection drug users. Many people consider homosexuality, bisexuality, and substance use evidence of lack of character, criminal behavior, or a sinful lifestyle. The two risk groups share other common characteristics (Hughes, Martin, and Franks 1987):

- Friends and partners (or lovers) are nontraditional support systems. Families of origin may be unaware of, or may reject, the individual's behavior or lifestyle and thus may be unable or unwilling to provide support.
- People in both risk categories may be estranged from institutions, such as organized religion, that view their behavior or lifestyle as sinful or immoral.
- Both groups may be set apart from the mainstream because of differences in norms, values, and language.
- The caregivers and support systems of people in either of these groups may be members of the same high-risk groups, with which the nurse may not have had much previous contact.

On one hand, children with HIV disease or individuals who have contracted HIV from the transfusion of blood or a blood product are usually perceived as "innocents" rather than sinners. However, they may be as feared and subject to discrimination as gays and drug users.

In her book *Illness as Metaphor* (1977), Susan Sontag suggests that people with illnesses that evoke feelings of apprehension and vulnerability in others become objects of that dread. This is especially true of HIV and AIDS. Healthy people fear contamination by the sick with an illness for which there is no known cure.

ECONOMIC FACTORS For the individual, HIV disease can mean an unstable financial situation because of loss of employment, loss of private health insurance, and loss of income (Kass et al. 1994). Days lost from work because of illness may cost people with HIV infection or AIDS their jobs and insurance benefits. Some insurers are avoiding or reducing claims by isolating high-risk applicants with HIV antibody tests, denying new policies to those at risk, and aggressively fighting existing policyholders' claims in court. Family and friends may be unable or unwilling to assist financially. Young adults find themselves having to seek public assistance such as Medicaid for help in meeting the costs associated with HIV disease.

MIND-BODY-SPIRIT CONNECTION

Psychoneuroimmunology: Communication Between Mind and Cell in HIV Disease

Wars wage within our bodies every minute of every day. Most of the time we are unaware of the battles that go on within us. We have evolved legions of defenders—specialized cells that silently rout the unseen enemy. Their victories go unheralded. When our defenses are penetrated, our defenders are caught unprepared, or our defenders are routed and we've lost the battle, then we develop a cold, the flu, or something worse. Why did I catch a cold from the sick toddler on the plane when the woman next to me did not? Why didn't you come down with the flu when your roommate was sick? Why do only some of the people exposed to HIV develop the disease? Why do some people with HIV disease die within a year or two while others have survived, or even thrived, for five, ten, or more years? We don't, as yet, have all the answers to these questions.

One particularly exciting field of research that has contributed toward answering these questions is *psychoneuroimmunology (PNI),* the study of the communication between the mind, the brain, the endocrine system, and the immune system. How does this communication occur? Certain messenger chemicals—neuroendocrines, neurotransmitters, and immunotransmitters—are released by the immune and neurologic systems. In this multiple-process communication system, the brain serves as the central post for these messengers that carry instructions to body organs along heavily trafficked electrochemical pathways. The messages are actually picked up at the cellular level by cell receptors.

Belief in the interconnectedness of mind, body, and spirit has long been a tradition of nursing. Recent scientific advances in PNI are important to nurses because they support the mind-body-spirit connection. They demonstrate the way in which emotions register on the body and the way the mind is influenced by the body, and suggest the role of attitudes and emotions in combating serious illness such as AIDS.

Perhaps the most important common characteristics of people with AIDS who live long past the time predicted for them is their refusal to accept the diagnosis of HIV disease as a death sentence. They do not deny the diagnosis, but *they do defy the fatal outcome* that is supposed to be connected to it. Long-term survivors are extremely goal-oriented and social. They treat their symptoms as if they were minor impediments in their lives; they are determined to prevail. Their immune systems seem to function better. They have higher T-cell counts and, in many cases, other immune system cells compensate for the ravaged T-cells. Emotional distress, on the other hand, has been found to accompany negative immune function factors in HIV-infected individuals.

The highest incidence of illness and death occurs in people who experience stress after infection with HIV. This suggests that HIV-seropositive people should reduce their exposure to stressful events. Assertive coping, less stress, more self-nurturing, and regular exercise have been associated with a better immune status, suggesting that stress-reduction behaviors may be effective in slowing the progression of HIV disease.

The research describing the relationship between PNI and HIV disease is investigational and has not been controlled for factors such as mutational changes in the HIV, the amount of virus in the body, or the number and frequency of opportunistic diseases the person has experienced. This means that we cannot promote the idea that clients are in total control of the disease process and the state of their health, or that the mind can cure AIDS. However, nurses can and should teach clients the self-care behaviors that long-term survivors are using to maintain their health. Nurses should also assess the level of stress, quality of social support, and mood, factors that influence the quality and quantity of life of people with HIV disease. Standard and experimental drug therapies (especially psychotropic drugs) may bring about unexpected immunologic and neuroendocrine toxicities because of HIV-related defects in the person's cellular PNI communication system. For this reason, nurses must monitor these systems very carefully and teach their clients to do the same. Nursing interventions to help clients enhance neurologic, immunologic, and cognitive functioning should focus on improved nutrition, adequate sleep-wake patterns, hygiene, stress reduction, and social support. Case management of clients in stressful family, financial, or emotional situations should be directed toward supportive problem solving.

It was Norman Cousins (1989) who suggested that *positive attitudes are not merely "moods," but biochemical realities.* We need to learn more about the effects of mental events on the immune system. Lovejoy

→

MIND-BODY-SPIRIT CONNECTION *(continued)*

and Sisson (1989) propose the following nursing research questions related to PNI:

- Do state personality characteristics (those that are transitory) or trait personality characteristics (those that are stable individual differences) influence the incidence, severity, or course of immunologically resisted and autoimmune diseases, including HIV disease?
- Do early life experiences modulate the PNI systems of adults with HIV disease?
- Is longevity among people with HIV disease associated with superior psychologic defenses, interpersonal skills, and coping mechanisms?
- Are individuals who are out of touch with, unaware of, or unable to express emotions (particularly negative ones) most at risk for increased HIV progression rates?
- Are happiness, security, a sense of control, relaxation, and other positive emotions accompanied by immune enhancement?
- Is the onset of AIDS preceded by emotional distress or failure of coping mechanisms or psychologic defenses?
- What is the effect of chronic versus short-term stress on the HIV mental health spectrum?

Answers to these questions will help clients learn how to minimize the challenge of living with HIV disease and maximize the quality of their lives.

Carol Ren Kneisl, MS, RN, CS

Experts predict that during the 1990s, AIDS care will cost the nation more than the cost of kidney dialysis or the health care cost of people with cancer of the lung, breast, or colon. Only care for cardiac clients and auto accident casualties is expected to cost more. Federal authorities estimate that about 40% of all PWAs will eventually be without means of insurance and will need to rely on Medicaid.

Volunteer community programs provide a lifeline for people with AIDS. They provide emotional support counselors to the dying and their families; send out workers to clean, cook, shop, and provide transportation; run low-cost residences; and shuttle PWAs back and forth to hospital and clinic appointments. Programs such as these have helped lessen the financial impact. Unquestionably, HIV/AIDS presents an economic problem of severe proportions.

Homelessness An increasingly critical problem is the lack of decent, appropriate housing for the growing number of people with HIV disease. HIV disease is disproportionately prevalent among individuals already at the economic edge and those who are targets of discrimination in housing and medical care: people of color, homosexuals, injection drug users, and homeless and runaway youths. In many communities around the country, available housing and services fall short of the need for appropriate residential care for thousands of people who have been made homeless by HIV-related illnesses, or whose struggle to survive on the streets has been worsened by the disease (National Coalition for the Homeless 1990). Fatigue, repeated hospitalization, and recurring illnesses all require time off from work, resulting first in the loss of employment, then in the loss of housing. The lack of effective risk-reduction education programs among the homeless has led to predictable and dramatic increases in HIV-seropositivity among them.

Although most people with an impaired immune system can live independently, they require a safe environment that helps them avoid exposure to infectious disease, get adequate rest, meet their special nutritional needs, and have access to support services and home help when necessary. Many shelters for the homeless refuse to accept people with HIV or those at risk for HIV infection. Consequently, many homeless people are kept in hospital beds longer than necessary because they have no place to go. Others are discharged from hospitals without appropriate arrangements for residential care and find themselves on the street, where they are at high risk for infection and violence.

Legal Issues

Laws concerning HIV and AIDS are still in the formative stages. Several legal questions have not yet been answered. Some recommend legislation to ban discrimination against people infected with HIV, while others urge legislation to require mandatory testing and quarantine as two measures to protect the general public. Testing will probably not become common until people do not have to worry that they will lose their jobs or insurance if they test positive for HIV. The dilemma has to do with the violation of individual rights (by such activities as mandatory premarital or antepartal testing, or mandatory testing of those at high risk), as opposed to violation of the concept of societal good.

Bompey (1986) has reached the following conclusions on the direction of the law related to employment rights and HIV disease based on recent court decisions:

- HIV disease is a "protected handicap."
- An employer cannot deny employment to an applicant with HIV unless the disease is far advanced and renders the applicant incapable of performing the duties of the job.
- Segregation of people with HIV in the workplace is without medical justification and would probably violate prohibitions against discrimination on the basis of disability.
- Other employees generally cannot refuse to work with people who have HIV unless a claim can be substantiated that a dangerous work condition exists; such employees, after educational interventions, may be subject to discipline or dismissal if they still refuse to work with affected individuals.
- Employers may not discharge an employee with HIV merely because they believe that individual will soon become incapacitated.
- Employers may not generally ask job applicants if they have HIV or have been exposed to the virus.
- Employers can probably require blood tests as part of the preemployment physical examination, but the employer would be limited in using the test results. Disclosure of such information to others would be highly inadvisable.
- Employers cannot force employees with HIV disease to take a medical leave unless they are unable to perform their jobs.

There are several cases in the courts over denied HIV-related medical insurance claims and life insurance policy claims. Insurance companies have been accused of using legal tactics to delay the resolution of litigation on the theory that the life of a person with AIDS is shorter than the life of a lawsuit. The wills of people who have died from AIDS and bequeathed their estates to gay partners are also being contested by estranged blood relatives.

Because cognitive impairment is common in PWAs, decision making regarding treatment, investments, and other financial matters is often transferred to another person with power of attorney.

Political Issues

HIV activists have been concerned about the slow pace of the Food and Drug Administration (FDA) in approving new drugs for the treatment of HIV infection and argue that the FDA should be far more liberal in allowing the use of untested drugs by those who have no hope of a cure. The lack of easy access to drugs has encouraged the development of guerrilla AIDS clinics. These informal clinics, in living rooms and kitchens throughout the United States, provide a variety of medicines. Some are readily available prescription drugs. Others are more exotic mixtures of nutritional additives or items such as Brazilian tree bark and Chinese mushrooms. Still others are chemicals such as DNCB (a photographic solvent readily available at chemical supply houses, and traditionally used to treat warts), which is painted on Kaposi's sarcoma lesions with cotton-tipped applicators. Those who are desperate travel to Mexico and Europe to obtain drugs not yet approved for sale in this country.

The political climate also affects potential legislation to ensure confidentiality and to ban discrimination. For example, it may not be politically feasible for a legislator seeking reelection by a conservative, frightened, or unknowledgeable constituency to advocate measures the electorate would see as contrary to their best interests. Some politicians point to the HIV epidemic as graphically illustrating huge gaps in the health care system and the need for a comprehensive federal medical care program.

Ethical Concerns

According to Durham (1991), the mysterious nature of AIDS, the lack of a cure, and its highly lethal outcome combine to stigmatize people with HIV. Durham also suggests that they are doubly stigmatized because most of them are already members of other stigmatized groups—homosexuals, bisexuals, drug abusers, African Americans, and Latinos. The CDC reports that 45% of the reported adult and adolescent cases of AIDS are among African Americans (29%) and Latinos (16%), and 78% of the infant and child cases are also among African Americans and Latinos (CDC 1995).

The ethical issues surrounding HIV/AIDS probably prompt many emotional responses. Some of the ethical questions that have arisen are:

- Should HIV antibody testing be made mandatory? If so, who should be tested: gay men, IDUs, pregnant women, people admitted to hospitals, prisoners, couples applying for marriage licenses, food handlers, health care workers, child care workers, people applying for health and life insurance—everyone?
- Is it in the public interest to identify, report, and make public the names of HIV-infected individuals or those at risk for HIV?
- To what extent would the undertaking of preventive measures be a matter of public health responsibility?
- Should people infected with HIV be tattooed to protect potential sex partners from infection?
- Should people with HIV/AIDS be placed in quarantine for the public good?

- Can or should employers suspend, terminate, or refuse to hire people with HIV/AIDS? If they are teachers? Food handlers? Health care workers?
- Should people who have had sexual contact with people with HIV or received infected blood products be traced and informed by public health authorities?
- Do health care workers have a duty to inform those at risk when a person with HIV does not modify high-risk behavior?
- Is it appropriate to make experimental drugs and treatments that are not yet proven safe and effective available to people with HIV disease?
- Should research protocols that call for administering placebos to some (who thus remain untreated) and experimental drugs to others be allowed?
- Can nurses or other health care professionals refuse to provide care to people with HIV disease?

Engaging in the process of ethical reflection discussed in Chapter 10 can be used to analyze these and other issues so as not to further stigmatize people with HIV.

In 1985, the American Nurses' Association (ANA) reaffirmed its specific commitment to nursing care for people with AIDS. In addition, the first two statements in the ANA's code of ethics (ANA 1985) provide guidance to nurses with respect to these nursing care dilemmas:

1. The nurse provides services with respect for human dignity and the uniqueness of the client unrestricted by considerations of social or economic status, personal attributes, or the nature of health problems.
2. The nurse safeguards the client's right to privacy by judiciously protecting information of a confidential nature.

Several state nurses' associations have published statements relative to nursing practice that clarify the professional nurse's responsibility in relation to the care of HIV-infected people. These statements address the need to provide appropriate care (both direct and indirect), health teaching, and advocacy.

Roles for Psychiatric–Mental Health Nurses

Psychiatric–mental health nurses will work with clients all along the continuum of HIV infection and disability. You may be involved in working with people with HIV disease in inpatient settings in psychiatric hospitals, psychiatric units in general hospitals, mental health clinics, community health agencies, hospices or homes, private practice, industry, or schools, and as a citizen and neighbor. In addition, you will have an active role with healthy people, the family and friends of people with HIV, and bereaved survivors.

Providing a Therapeutic Milieu

Proactive Preparation Education of staff and clients is best begun before the first client with HIV disease is admitted to a unit. After-the-fact education about HIV is complicated by the surprise of the experience. Community-based AIDS service organizations (ASOs) provide education at the appropriate level for staff and clients. They give up-to-date information in a setting where people may feel most comfortable revealing feelings and biases.

Evans et al. (1990) emphasize the importance of proactive preparation and programming in allaying the anxiety of both staff members and clients when incorporating people with HIV disease into a psychiatric–mental health milieu. Both staff members and clients may have concerns about disease transmission, inadequate knowledge regarding HIV and AIDS, and lack of understanding of the unique needs and behavior of people with HIV disease.

Modifying Milieu Policies and Procedures Special arrangements may need to be made about the scheduling of activities, visiting policies, and the provision of physical treatments, depending on the physical and neuropsychiatric manifestations of the disease and the extent of HIV disease progression. Staff will need to make individual decisions case by case. Clear communication with staff members and other clients is necessary for promoting consistency and preventing disruption of the milieu as a result of perceived inequities.

Clients with neuropsychiatric manifestations of HIV may present a special challenge to the staff and to the therapeutic environment. Their behavior may be erratic, frightening, and unlike that of the usual psychiatric client. This may require modification of generally accepted milieu standards. For example, a client who is frequently incontinent may disrupt meal times and other community activities. It may become necessary to exclude some clients, such as those with HIV dementia, from certain activities. To prevent other clients from perceiving that the client with HIV disease is receiving special treatment, nurses should openly discuss these issues with the community while continuing to ensure individual client confidentiality, as appropriate.

In their experience with AIDS clients on an inpatient psychiatric unit, Baer et al. (1987) noted that not all clients react favorably to the presence of PWAs. They found that clients with paranoid disorders had the greatest difficulty accepting other clients who had AIDS. Among the behaviors they observed were hostility, incorporating AIDS into paranoid delusions, insisting on being transferred to another unit, and insisting that PWAs be transferred to another unit.

Ways to help other clients include providing education, offering support, allowing the other clients to vent their fears and express their concerns, and emphasizing that the care of HIV clients is an important and normal part of the unit routine. The clients most vocal in their protests use the AIDS issue to avoid dealing with some of their own problems (Baer et al. 1987). Keep this in mind when developing individual nursing care plans or dealing with milieu issues.

INFECTION CONTROL The use of universal infection control precautions in a psychiatric–mental health setting can also help minimize staff and client anxiety (Evans et al. 1990). Not all people with HIV (both staff and clients) are aware of their status or feel comfortable disclosing the information even if they are aware. Universal precautions, as prescribed by the CDC, will protect *all* staff members and clients against the transmission of HIV. This approach promotes confidentiality, because appropriate precautions are taken in the care of all clients. Therefore, it is unnecessary to identify HIV-infected individuals to the general community.

Giving Direct Care to Clients with HIV Disease

Psychiatric hospitalization may be needed because the client is depressed, suicidal, or psychotic or has an AIDS-related behavior disturbance, probably because of a focal brain disorder or HIV-related dementia. Psychiatric nurses caring for clients with HIV or AIDS on inpatient units encounter a number of issues that are uncommon in psychiatric settings:

- The client may have a multitude of physical problems.
- The client has a condition that calls for infection control precautions.
- The quality of the nurse-client relationship is intensified through the additional contact required in giving physical care.
- Psychiatric–mental health nurses, who very seldom work with dying clients, find it necessary to confront the issue of caring for clients with life-threatening illnesses.

A necessary modification has to do with the use of touch. The physical care needs of AIDS clients require modifying the usual psychiatric injunction of limiting physical contact with clients. Because AIDS is such an isolating and stigmatizing condition, giving a massage or holding the client's hand has therapeutic value.

The psychiatric nurse caring for clients with a dual diagnosis that includes HIV disease faces a challenge that requires creative modification. Nursing care for clients with depression, suicidal ideation, psychosis, or dementia has been discussed in earlier chapters in this text. With PWAs, it is important not to mistake delirium for depression (see Table 12–1 on page 220).

It may be beneficial to set up a separate support group for people with HIV disease, where they can discuss issues specific to HIV/AIDS in a supportive setting. If there aren't enough HIV clients for a group, then an ASO might provide support group services. An ASO can also be an important resource for HIV clients after discharge. The range of services available depends on the structure of the ASO but frequently includes support groups, buddy programs, educational programs, financial assistance, housing referral, legal aid, and client advocacy.

Clients with neuropsychiatric manifestations of HIV, such as HIV dementia, may offer the greatest challenge to the inpatient unit staff. Nursing diagnoses common to people with NPM are listed in the box on page 658. Three important but frequently ignored nursing diagnoses that apply to clients with NPM are:

- Impaired Communication
- Spiritual Distress
- Impaired Home Maintenance Management

Clients with neuropsychiatric manifestations of HIV disease often have special discharge planning needs or experience placement problems. Intervention strategies appropriate to these three selected nursing diagnoses are discussed in the following sections.

INTERVENING IN IMPAIRED COMMUNICATION Because a client's symptoms are generally progressive, interventions do not reverse the dementia but may enhance the quality of life for both the client and the primary caregiver. Here are several strategies:

- Convey unconditional positive regard, maintain a relationship, and maintain a sense of normality in interactions.
- Make verbal communication clear, concise, and unhurried; be sure to have the person's attention before starting; encourage the person to communicate; be comfortable with periods of silence; be aware of tone and volume of voice (this may prevent misperceptions).
- Use brief, direct statements: "Mike, eat this pudding" rather than "Why don't you and I have some pudding for dessert?"
- Ask questions that require only simple yes or no answers, and make only one request at a time.
- Be sensitive to the need to restate statements or questions at intervals.
- The client may have memory loss; therefore, reintroduce yourself as often as necessary.
- Remember that nonverbal communication and touch are important; nonverbal communication may eventually become the primary communication mode between the client and the nurse or the client and the primary caregiver.

Neuropsychiatric Manifestations (NPM) of HIV Infection

General Nursing Diagnoses

- Activity Intolerance (related to physical and psychologic impact of chronic HIV infection).
- Altered Health Maintenance (related to chronic HIV infection and NPM of HIV infection).
- Fatigue (related to chronic HIV infection and NPM of HIV infection).
- Risk for Infection (related to compromised immune system and NPM of HIV infection).
- Impaired Home Maintenance Management (related to NPM of HIV infection).
- Impaired Tissue Integrity (related to chronic HIV infection and NPM of HIV infection).
- Noncompliance (related to NPM of HIV infection).
- Self-Care Deficit (related to NPM of HIV infection).
- Sleep Pattern Disturbance (related to NPM of HIV infection).

Psychosocial Nursing Diagnoses

- Altered Sexuality Patterns (related to NPM of HIV infection).
- Altered Thought Processes (related to NPM of HIV infection).
- Anticipatory Grieving (related to issues associated with HIV infection and NPM of HIV infection).
- Anxiety (related to actual or perceived threats, losses, and/or changes associated with HIV diagnosis).
- Decisional Conflict (related to ethical dilemmas—qualify of life, life-support measures—and NPM of HIV infection).
- Fear (related to actual or perceived threats, losses, and/or changes associated with HIV diagnosis).
- Risk for Violence: Self-Directed (related to NPM of HIV infection).
- Hopelessness (related to chronic HIV infection and NPM of HIV infection).
- Ineffective Individual Coping (related to physiologic, situational, and/or maturational factors associated with HIV infection).
- Powerlessness (related to chronic HIV infection and NPM of HIV infection).
- Self-Esteem Disturbance (related to actual or perceived threats, losses, and/or changes associated with HIV diagnosis and/or NPM of HIV infection).
- Social Isolation (related to NPM of HIV infection).
- Spiritual Distress (related to NPM of HIV infection, diagnosis of HIV infection, unresolved identity crisis, confrontation of mortality).

Neurologic Nursing Diagnoses

- Acute Pain or Chronic Pain (related to chronic HIV infection, immobility, neuropathy).
- Altered Body Temperature (related to CNS infection and/or increased intracranial pressure, chronic HIV infection, and opportunistic infections).
- Altered Nutrition: Less than Body Requirements (related to altered level of consciousness or NPM of HIV infection).
- Altered Urinary Elimination (related to NPM of HIV infection).
- Bowel Incontinence, or Colonic Constipation, or Diarrhea (related to chronic HIV infection, opportunistic infections, immobility, and/or NPM of HIV infection).
- Risk for Injury (related to sensory or motor deficits such as neuropathy, gait disturbance, and dyskinesia associated with HIV infection).
- Impaired Physical Mobility (related to NPM of HIV infection).
- Impaired Verbal Communication (related to memory loss and/or decreased ability to process information, or related to CNS changes in function and motor control such as aphasia, echolalia, and dysphagia).
- Sensory/Perceptual Alterations (related to NPM of HIV infection).

- Remember who the person was in the past, because reminiscence and validation are important; provide familiar stimuli.
- Be sure not to equate aphasia or flat affect with the absence of feelings; use empathy and interpretation of behaviors/statements to understand what is happening (for example, when a person who is at home says, "I want to go home"); support the person's feelings.
- Provide an environment of sheltered freedom, that is, the least restrictive level that is safe (unhurried, consistent, structured, with decreased external stimulation).
- Avoid mechanical or chemical restraints as much as possible.
- Avoid infantilizing the person, but remember that you may need to set firm limits.
- Be flexible, try different approaches, and share information.

Intervening in Spiritual Distress Spiritual distress is usually evidenced by guilt, recriminations and self-blame, hyperreligiosity, rejection of significant others, and expressions of despair. The following list provides some guidelines for working with clients experiencing spiritual distress:

- Give the person permission to experience personal feelings, no matter what they are, and encourage appropriate expression of these feelings.
- Accept the fact that primary caregivers may not be able to listen to the client's feelings. If the PCG delegates this job, recognize the distress it may cause.
- Recognize the stages of grieving, and allow people to progress at their own rate; don't push the client into a stage that you think is necessary.
- Share spiritual resources as appropriate; encourage the person to find comforting spiritual outlets (poetry or other literature may be used to encourage reflection).

Enhancing Home Maintenance Management If clients return to their homes to be cared for by a nonprofessional, special preparations may be necessary. Impairment of home maintenance management is evidenced in several ways. The PCG may verbalize difficulty with maintaining the home environment or caring for the person with HIV. Other situations to look for are evidence of poor hygiene in the home, an impaired caregiver, or an unavailable support system. The following list gives guidelines for discharge planning and placement:

- Begin planning for discharge when the client is admitted to the hospital.
- Assess the client's abilities to function in the home, the family's or primary caregiver's abilities to function in the home, and the housing or home environment itself.
- Make referrals to home care professionals and other community agencies.
- Help the PCG determine the appropriate level of care and realistically assess his or her own ability to provide home care; explore all role responsibilities and related factors; assist in redefining and prioritizing roles and functions.
- Determine the PCG's learning needs, and facilitate the development of skills by identifying specific symptoms (such as memory loss) and developing strategies to address those symptoms.
- Provide respite care for PCGs.
- Provide emotional support to clients and PCGs, and refer them to additional support systems.

Risk-Reduction Education and Counseling

Taking a leading role in risk-reduction education and counseling is a crucial responsibility of all nurses. Risk-reduction education is directed toward three broad goals:

1. Educating clients, the public, other professionals, colleagues, friends, and neighbors in strategies to reduce the risk of contracting or spreading HIV.
2. Counteracting the myths, stereotypes, and hysteria that surround HIV and AIDS.
3. Correcting misinformation.

Because more is being learned about HIV and appropriate and effective risk reduction and prevention, *consult current CDC guidelines before implementing programs for people at risk for contracting HIV.*

Teaching risk reduction can best be accomplished by listening, informing, and supporting clients in making choices that reduce their risk. Bjorklund (1987) suggests that, to motivate clients to reduce their risks, nurses need to understand the following principles:

- Risk-reduction education is important for members of high-risk groups and their sexual contacts because a large percentage of high-risk group members have already been exposed to HIV.
- An HIV-positive person is at risk for developing AIDS and transmitting the virus even if healthy.
- The role of reexposure to HIV or other infectious organisms is not completely understood; reexposure may be implicated in the progression from either an asymptomatic state or HRC to AIDS.

- The change to low-risk behaviors for high-risk individuals may necessitate lifelong change. Lifelong change can be more effectively maintained if sexual activities that incorporate risk-reduction techniques are also satisfying.
- Clients need support in maintaining low-risk behavior in an environment that reinforces high-risk behavior.

SEXUAL BEHAVIOR Many experts fear that educating people about **safer sex practices** generates a false sense of security. In this AIDS era, these experts say, the only safe sex is no sex. Realistically, however, abstinence is not a lifelong change that will be maintained by many. Counseling about high-risk sexual behaviors, low-risk sexual behaviors, and risk-free sexual behaviors makes more sense, especially in terms of the principles outlined in the list above. High-risk sexual behaviors are those in which there is an exchange of blood or body fluids. Receptive anal intercourse is thought to be of highest risk because of the trauma caused to the mucous membranes of the rectum. Guidelines for counseling about risk reduction and safer sex are given in the accompanying Client/Family Teaching box.

The use of **condoms** (a barrier protection placed on the penis to prevent the transmission of body fluids during sexual activity) is important in minimizing risk, but they must be used correctly in order to be effective. Remember to include the following information about condoms in any risk-reduction program:

- Latex condoms are safer to use than natural or lambskin condoms. (HIV may be small enough to pass through the pores in natural condoms.)
- Condoms with reservoir tips are safer than those without. (A reservoir tip provides space for the semen and helps prevent breakage.)
- Condom packages should not be opened until use. Packages should be opened carefully (to help prevent damage that might result from rough handling or jagged fingernails).
- Condoms should be stored in a dark, cool, dry place. (Excessive heat or cold, sunlight, and moisture can damage the latex.)
- The condom should be applied before any genital contact. (Semen and seminal fluid may be discharged in advance of ejaculation.)
- The condom should be placed at the tip of the erect penis, and the air should be gently pressed out of the condom tip. (Air bubbles can cause condoms to break.)
- The condom should be held at the tip and rolled down and smoothed over the entire erect penis. Uncircumcised men should pull back the foreskin before applying the condom. (This provides a more effective seal.)
- A water-based product such as lubricating jelly or spermicidal jelly should be added before penetration. (Insufficient lubrication can cause condoms to tear or pull off. Oil-based lubricants such as petroleum jelly, baby oil, vegetable oil, mineral oil, cold cream, or hand lotion may cause the latex to disintegrate.)
- Spermicidal foams, creams, or jellies containing nonoxynol-9 can be used in conjunction with condoms. (Nonoxynol-9 may inactivate the virus if the condom should break.)
- After ejaculating, but before losing the erection, the man should hold the base of the condom firmly while gently withdrawing the penis. (This prevents the escape of semen from the condom.) The used condom should be safely discarded and never reused.

Since HIV is most commonly transmitted through sex, being sexually active without taking proper precautions is definitely high-risk behavior. In this AIDS era, it is crucial to understand that a person does not simply go to bed with one other person. When one calculates the possible length of the HIV latency period, a person goes to bed with the other person's entire sex history for approximately the past 10 years.

SUBSTANCE USE The transmission of HIV and injection drug use are linked in the following ways:

- Direct transmission of the virus through the sharing of IV drugs and equipment for injecting drugs (the most obvious link).
- Sexual transmission by infected IDUs to their sex partners.
- Neonatal transmission by infected women who are themselves IDUs or the sex partners of IDUs.

While these modes of transmission address injection drug users, there are other less well-known links to noninjection substance use and HIV. The use of poppers (volatile amyl and butyl nitrates in breakable glass capsules inhaled to enhance sexual pleasure) may be a cofactor in the susceptibility to HIV and in the development of AIDS because they are thought to lead to a generalized suppression of the immune system. Alcohol, as well as drugs such as amphetamines, cocaine, and marijuana, are also thought to damage the immune system. Another factor is lessened inhibition; that is, with loss of inhibition, a person under the influence of alcohol or drugs is more likely to engage in high-risk activities.

Realistic approaches to HIV risk-reduction education for IDUs consist of more than information about, and encouragement to obtain treatment for, substance abuse. Those who are not ready for treatment must be counseled on how to reduce the risk to themselves and to others.

CLIENT/FAMILY TEACHING

HIV Risk-Reduction Guidelines

Sexual Behavior

Risk-Free Behaviors *Most of these behaviors involve skin-to-skin contact only. The virus is unlikely to be transmitted from one person to another unless there are breaks in the skin.*

- Mutual masturbation (male or female).
- Body massage, hugging.
- Frottage (body-to-body rubbing without penetration).
- Dry (social) kissing.
- Using one's own sex toys (dildos or vibrators) that are not shared.
- Light S/M (sadism and masochism) activities (without bruising or bleeding).

Low-Risk Behaviors (Possibly Safe) *Small amounts of some body fluids may be exchanged during these activities. The risk of transmitting the virus is thought to be increased in proportion to the number of contacts.*

- Anal intercourse with condom (used properly).
- Vaginal intercourse with condom (used properly).
- Fellatio (oral-penile contact) without ingestion of seminal fluid or semen.
- Wet kissing (also called French kissing).
- Cunnilingus (oral-vaginal contact); risk is probably enhanced during menstruation.
- Using shared sex toys that are cleaned between uses and covered with a condom.
- Urine contact (also called watersports) when skin is unbroken and urine is not taken by mouth or by rectum.

High-Risk Behaviors (Unsafe) *These activities involve tissue trauma or exchange of blood or body fluids that may transmit HIV or other microbes.*

- Anal intercourse without condom (both receptive and insertive).
- Vaginal intercourse without condom.
- Fisting (manual-anal contact).
- Fellatio with ingestion of semen.
- Rimming (oral-anal contact).
- Using unclean, unprotected sex toys.
- Piercing or drawing blood.

Substance Abuse

- Remember that people who look healthy can carry the AIDS virus.
- Never share injectable drugs or works (equipment).
- If a new needle and syringe are not available or equipment must be shared, remember to clean the works. (See Figure 27–2.)
- Prevent sexual transmission.
- Avoid alcohol, marijuana, amphetamines, cocaine, and poppers.
- If you want to have children but have shared needles or may have been exposed to AIDS through sexual contact with someone who has, get medical advice.

Risk-reduction guidelines for IDUs are included in the Client/Family Teaching box. A counseling plan for clients with a dual diagnosis of HIV disease and substance use is given in the Intervention box on page 662.

Clients' risks to themselves derive from the practice of sharing drug use equipment with others. Teach clients to *never share injectable drugs, needles, syringes, or other drug paraphernalia with others.* As an HIV prevention strategy, increasing numbers of communities are providing needle and syringe exchange programs (Watters et al. 1994). The best way of preventing transmission through injection drug use is for clients to use new, sterile needles and syringes, from a reliable source, each time they inject drugs (Jones 1995).

Studies report that syringe exchange programs have played a significant role in lowering the rates of needle

INTERVENTION

Counseling Plan for Clients with a Dual Diagnosis of HIV and Substance Use

- Check the level of understanding of basic HIV information, and develop an education plan based on client needs.
- Confront denial or lack of commitment to minimize risk behavior.
- Offer hope for the stabilization of health through positive health care measures.
- Check the need for and depth of motivation for referral to chemical dependence or alcohol-treatment programs.
- Encourage joining or continuing commitment to the recovery process in treatment for chemical or alcohol dependence.
- Check the need for and refer to medical follow-up, emotional or sexual counseling, support groups, and other self-help programs.
- Help the client verbalize feelings of anger, grief, and loss generated by the diagnosis; the need for change in sexual and drug use behavior; or possible delay in childbearing.
- Reinforce the fact that taking action now may help stabilize the client's health and slow further deterioration.
- Discuss "contagion" issues with the client and family members to allay fears of spread by casual contact.
- Encourage and support client verbalization of such feelings as:

  Fear of dying of AIDS.

  Fear of having exposed others to HIV or doing so through continued risk behavior.

  Feelings of guilt over risk behavior in the past.

  Feelings of loss over necessary behavior changes and possible postponement of childbearing.

  Fear of what others will think or do, or fear of being isolated and rejected.
- Compile and distribute a list of community resources to serve people with HIV concerns or HIV/AIDS diagnosis.
- Stress the use of tools learned in recovering from chemical dependence and alcoholism in coping with this life crisis.
- Continue to confront the drug abuse as you would with other clients not diagnosed with HIV.
- Emphasize positive things the client can do to maximize health.
- Extend the hope that, with continued attention to health matters, the client may live longer, possibly extending life until more effective treatments become available.

Source: Adapted from O'Neil 1987, p. 137. By permission of the Visiting Nurses Association of San Francisco.

sharing in the Netherlands, Australia, the United Kingdom, and the United States. Studies also report that needle and syringe exchange programs have served as sources of referrals into drug treatment programs. Additionally, needle and syringe exchange programs recapture used and potentially infectious syringes for safe disposal (Watters et al. 1994).

If a new needle and syringe are not available, and the client will inject drugs anyway, the next best thing is for clients to clean their "works" (syringe and needle) as recommended in Figure 27–2.

Risks to sex partners are the same as those discussed earlier in this chapter. Prevention of risk to sex partners is important because IDUs serve as a bridge for transmitting HIV to their sex partners or to fetuses and newborns. Women who are IDUs or the sex partners of IDUs are urged to postpone pregnancy until more is known about the significance of a positive antibody test for a pregnant woman, the relationship between pregnancy and the onset of symptoms associated with HIV infection, and the risk of transmission to fetuses and infants.

Support for Caregivers

Psychiatric–mental health nurses can be a vital support link for the wide spectrum of people who are caregivers of

1. Before beginning, wash syringe thoroughly with soap and water. *Do this 3 times.*

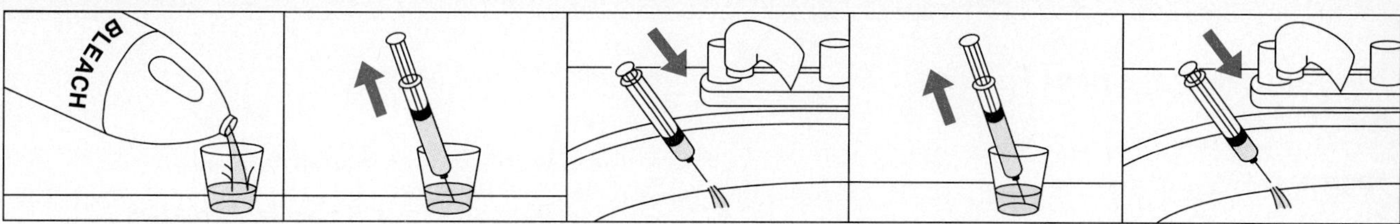

2. *Flush with bleach.* Pour bleach into glass. Fill syringe with bleach. Empty bleach from syringe. *Do this 3 times.*

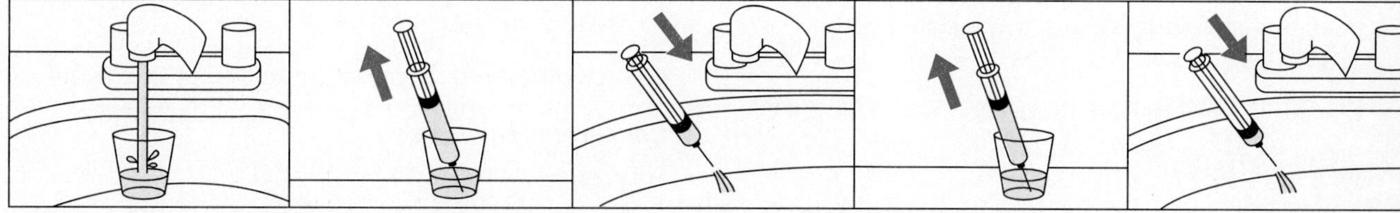

3. *Flush with water.* Fill a glass with clean water. Fill syringe with water. Empty water from syringe. *Do this 3 times.* (Caution: Be sure the client knows not to omit this important step.)

Figure 27–2 Cleaning the works.

persons with HIV disease. This spectrum includes nurses and other health care professionals; the family members, friends, and partners (those to whom gay people are committed in a long-term relationship) of people with HIV; firefighters, police officers, and correction officers; and community volunteers. Nurses are now and will continue to be the health care professionals who are the front-line workers in providing health care to increasing numbers of people with HIV/AIDS.

Special emotional stamina is needed to care for PWAs. Not only must nurses and other caregivers care for and comfort those who face great suffering and death, they also care for and comfort those infected with the virus who fear they will develop the disease. At the same time they provide help, nurses must cope with their fears for their own and their family's health (especially if the nurses themselves are members of a risk group) and their own pain in caring for people who do not get well or whose future is uncertain.

Specifically, the skills and knowledge of psychiatric–mental health nurses make them able to:

- Facilitate caregivers' expression of fears and concerns.
- Help caregivers acknowledge their susceptibility to increased stress and burnout in AIDS work.
- Instruct caregivers in stress-management strategies and relaxation techniques (see Chapter 29).
- Identify what needs to be reorganized and renegotiated in the work environment to maintain the health of caregivers and clients such as: staff support groups, networking with AIDS providers in other agencies and communities, respite time for staff, time off to attend funerals or memorial services, rearranging staff assignments to avoid overloading or overburdening particular staff members, creating getaway space for staff in the work setting.
- Provide help to caregivers unused to dealing with delirium and dementia, who may have unrealistic expectations about the client's ability to adhere to procedures and treatment as mental capacities diminish (see Chapter 12).
- Encourage administration to arrange time off and fund attendance at conferences and meetings that provide support and facilitate networking among people engaged in AIDS work.

Successful stress management is particularly important because neither a cure nor a vaccine is in sight. This means that increased numbers of people (those who are infected with the virus and have yet to develop HIV disease) will need nursing care in the coming years.

Bereavement Support

By the year 2000, millions of people will have experienced AIDS-related bereavements. There are several groups of people to whom the psychiatric–mental health nurse can provide bereavement support. The most obvious is the person with AIDS who grieves over a potentially fatal diagnosis, the loss of other friends or family to the disease, or any of the several other losses discussed in the section on the biopsychosocial impact of HIV/AIDS.

ASSESSMENT

High-Risk Bereavement Factors for SOPWAs

Stigma

Sources

- Discomfort with illness, death, and grief.
- Sexuality and drug use often associated with HIV/AIDS.
- Confusion and hysteria associated with HIV/AIDS.

Results for SOPWAs

- May perceive the need to mask the cause of death.
- May experience failure of the community to recognize the significance of relationship to the deceased.
- May perceive an absence of support to facilitate mourning the loss or expressing feelings associated with this bereavement.

Ambivalence

Sources

- Relationships strained due to lifestyle choices.

Results for SOPWAs

- Guilt related to bereavement may arise.
- Progress in the grief process may be blocked.

Untimely Nature of Death

Sources

- Faced with issues of mortality.
- Generally young age of people with AIDS.

Results for SOPWAs

- Anxiety, despair.
- Lack of time for preparation to accept the death.

Concurrent Life Crises

Sources

- Fear of the possibility of having been exposed to a fatal illness.
- Guilt if the survivor feels he or she may have transmitted HIV.

Results for SOPWAs

- Anger and helplessness associated with being a SOPWA.

Other Complicating Factors

- Lack of knowledge about HIV/AIDS.
- Lack of effective treatments; absence of a cure.
- Paucity of health care and social services resources.

Bereavement support to family, friends, and caregivers should continue after death has occurred. Home visits to friends, lovers, and family members demonstrate the nurse's continuing interest and concern for the survivor's well-being. Bereavement support groups and individual and family counseling can all be helpful, depending on individual situations and the availability of volunteers and professionals.

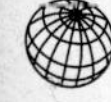

To provide adequate bereavement support to the survivors of people with AIDS (SOPWAs), the nurse must consider a number of factors. SOPWAs represent a diverse segment of society: gay and bisexual men, IV drug users, people who have received transfusions of blood or blood products, sex partners of PWAs, children of PWAs, parents and siblings of PWAs. Some SOPWAs may be in high-risk groups or may have HIV disease themselves, while some may have been unaware of the significant other's sexuality or lifestyle until diagnosis or death. Some survivors may have been responsible for the transmission of HIV, and many are members of minority groups and have few resources.

SOPWAs are often characterized by several factors that place them at high risk for complicated grief reactions (Geis, Fuller, and Rush 1986). These include:

- Perceived inability to share the loss with others.
- Lack of social recognition for the loss.
- Ambivalent relationships prior to the death.
- Traumatic circumstances of the death.
- Concurrent life crises at the time of the loss.

It is important to assess survivors for the presence of these factors, which can interfere with adaptive grieving. High-risk bereavement factors are discussed in the accompanying Assessment box.

Worden's Principles of Bereavement Intervention have been described as appropriate to guide psychiatric–mental health nurses in providing support to SOPWAs (Pheifer and Houseman 1988). These principles include:

- *Helping survivors actualize the loss by accepting its reality and finality* by encouraging them to talk about the death and the grieving rituals they participated in, and helping them develop meaningful grieving rituals in the absence of socially sanctioned opportunities.
- *Helping survivors identify and express feelings* by acknowledging their loss, validating their feelings and their right to express these feelings, and encouraging them to express their feelings in an atmosphere of understanding, relatedness, and acceptance.
- *Helping survivors continue living without the deceased* by identifying areas of their own lives that have been affected, and encouraging problem solving to promote independent functioning.
- *Facilitating survivors in the process of emotional withdrawal* by encouraging them, in time, to form new relationships (a particular issue for survivors who have been in spousal or lover relationships with a PWA); accepting the feelings of the survivor; being informed about HIV, AIDS, safer sex practices, and other topics that the SOPWA may need to discuss; referring to support groups that offer a forum for those with common concerns; and helping them recognize the benefits of relating to other people in their lives.
- *Providing survivors with time to grieve* by providing support for taking the time to grieve, allowing them to grieve at their own pace, and referring them to counseling or support groups.
- *Identifying and interpreting normal behavior for survivors* by recognizing and identifying for them the normal behaviors associated with grief (distractibility, forgetfulness, ruminations about the deceased, preoccupation with their own health, mood swings) and validating these as manifestations of grief.
- *Considering the individuality of survivors* by recognizing the broad spectrum of human responses to loss, supporting individual expressions of mourning, and helping support systems that recognize the individual's right to mourn in his or her own way.
- *Providing ongoing support for survivors* by allowing for support during critical periods, and by encouraging SOPWAs to use bereavement groups.
- *Analyzing survivors' defenses and coping mechanisms* by recognizing that each survivor has his or her own defenses and coping mechanisms, exploring the effectiveness and adaptability of these coping mechanisms, pointing out the maladaptive nature of any negative or self-destructive strategies, and helping them explore more adaptive means of coping.
- *Assessing survivors for pathologic grief responses* by assessing for depression, manic episodes, bizarre or acting-out behaviors, or suicidal ideation; and referring them to appropriate resources when the problems are beyond one's scope of practice.

The potential for dysfunctional grieving exists because multiple high-risk bereavement factors are characteristic of SOPWAs. Individual or group bereavement interventions can help survivors engage in the grief process in an adaptive fashion.

Self-Help Support

Self-help is one way in which persons with HIV disease can move to reestablish a sense of self-control and reduce feelings of helplessness and powerlessness. Self-help can occur on several levels, depending on the client's physical and mental abilities and motivation. Clients should participate as much as possible in their own care and in decision making that affects them. Nurses can encourage clients to join peer support groups and engage in AIDS advocacy activities in their communities.

Clients may benefit from such activities as nutritional counseling and psychologic counseling. Boosting the immune system also helps keep people healthy. Stress-management techniques and visualization and imagery for self-healing and pain and symptom control (such as those discussed in Chapter 29) are believed to boost the immune system by reducing stress.

Research

Not enough is known about HIV disease as an illness; the common nursing diagnoses in AIDS, HRC, and HIV-seropositivity; or the strategies that help people cope when HIV affects them or their loved ones. Psychiatric–mental health nurses have a direct role in research and an indirect role in supporting ongoing research and encouraging the undertaking and funding of new research. Being knowledgeable about the current research and incorporating it into clinical practice enables the psychiatric nurse to act on the basis of what is currently known or supposed. For example, there is a growing body of knowledge about quality of life and how it affects the physical, psychologic, and social well-being of people affected by HIV (Holzemer and Wilson 1995).

Advocacy and Political Activism

Persons with HIV disease and their loved ones need advocates. Psychiatric–mental health nurses can be effective advocates by speaking out against dehumanizing measures that threaten the well-being of these people.

A proposition was introduced in California that could have forced public health officials to establish camps to quarantine people with AIDS, as well as anyone infected by HIV, whether healthy or unhealthy. This measure would also have flatly banned HIV-seropositive people from attending or teaching in public schools or holding jobs that involve food handling. The California Nurses Association was among the groups that actively spoke against the proposition and contributed to its failure.

As citizens and as advocates, nurses should be politically aware of pending legislation and move to influence it in a positive direction.

Earlier in this chapter, brief mention was made of nurses' associations with published statements about the care of people with AIDS and nursing's role. Other national specialty groups such as the Association for Nurses in AIDS Care (ANAC) are also active in mobilizing the professional and political resources of the nursing community. It is every nurse's responsibility to find out what nursing groups are accomplishing or not accomplishing on local, state, and national levels. Beginning at the local level by becoming involved in community AIDS councils, self-help groups, and nursing organizations is a good way to start. Local involvement is a bridge to state and national involvement. Nurses can and should be part of a nationwide effort to lobby for adequate public and private funding for research, education, prevention, treatment, and a cure for HIV/AIDS.

Chapter Highlights

- HIV infection, a contagious and potentially fatal condition of immune system depression, is a clinical issue of concern to all nurses, including psychiatric–mental health nurses.
- HIV threatens the biopsychosocial integrity of individuals and of society.
- People with HIV/AIDS experience several different losses, may have neurologic or neuropsychiatric involvement because the virus invades the central and peripheral nervous systems, and find that their ability to successfully negotiate age-appropriate developmental tasks is disrupted.
- People with HIV/AIDS may experience social and familial rejection; discrimination in employment, housing, and health insurance; estrangement from institutions such as organized religion; and financial losses.
- Several ethical issues surround HIV and AIDS. Many of them revolve around questions of individual rights versus the public good.
- Psychiatric hospitalization may be needed if the client is depressed, suicidal, psychotic, or has an AIDS-related behavior disturbance, probably because of CNS involvement. The psychiatric–mental health nurse will have to creatively combine and modify the nursing care for clients with a dual diagnosis that includes HIV disease.
- Taking a leading role in risk-reduction education and counseling is a crucial role for all nurses during the HIV epidemic.
- Psychiatric–mental health nurses can be a vital support link for the wide spectrum of people who are caregivers of people with HIV disease.
- Psychiatric–mental health nurses have direct roles in HIV/AIDS research and indirect roles in supporting ongoing research and encouraging the undertaking and funding of new research.
- Psychiatric–mental health nurses can be effective advocates by speaking out against dehumanizing measures that threaten the well-being of people with HIV; influencing legislation in a positive direction; and becoming part of a nationwide effort by lobbying for adequate private and public funding for research, education, prevention, treatment, and cure.

References

American Nurses Association. *Code for Nurses*. ANA, 1985.

American Nurses Association. *Compendium of HIV/AIDS Positions, Policies and Documents*. ANA, 1994.

American Nurses Association. *Nursing and the Human Immunodeficiency Virus*. ANA, 1988.

Baer J, Hall J, Holm K, Lewitter-Koehler S: Challenges in developing an inpatient psychiatric program for patients with AIDS and ARC. *Hosp Commun Psychiatr* 1987;38(12):1299–1303.

Beason-Hazen S, Nasrallah HA, Bornstein RA: Self-report of symptoms and neuropsychological performance in asymptomatic HIV-positive individuals. *J Neuropsychiatr* 1994;6(1):43–49.

Bedos J-P, et al.: Early predictors of outcome for HIV patients with neurological failure. *JAMA* 1995;273(1):35–40.

Bjorklund E: Prevention: Reducing the risk of AIDS, in Durham JD, Cohen FL: *The Person with AIDS: Nursing Perspectives*. Springer, 1987.

Bompey S: AIDS—An employment issue for the eighties. *Digest Publication of International Foundation of Employee Benefit Plan* 1986;23(2):6–10.

Burack JH, et al.: Depressive symptoms and CD4 lymphocyte decline among HIV-infected men. *JAMA* 1993;270(21):2568–2573.

Cameron ME, Crisham P: The content of ethical problems experienced by persons living with AIDS. *JANAC* 1994;5(5):32–42.

Cates JA, Bond GR, Graham LL: AIDS knowledge, attitudes, and risk behavior among people with serious mental illness. *Psychosoc Rehab J* 1994;17(4):19–29.

CDC National AIDS Clearinghouse: *HIV/AIDS Surveillance Report.* 1995:6(1).

Colson P, Susser E, Valencia E: HIV and TB among people who are homeless and mentally ill. *Psychosoc Rehab J* 1994; 17(4):157–160.

Cournos F, et al.: Sexual activity and risk of HIV infection among patients with schizophrenia. *Am J Psychiatr* 1994; 151(2):228–232.

Cournos F, McKinnon K, Meyer-Bahlberg H, Guido JR, Meyer I: HIV risk activity among persons with severe mental illness: Preliminary findings. *Hosp Commun Psychiatr* 1993; 44(11):1104–1106.

Dow M, Knox M: Mental health and substance abuse staff: HIV/AIDS knowledge and attitudes. *AIDS Care* 1991;3: 75–87.

Durham JD: The ethical dimensions of AIDS, in Durham JD, Cohen FL: *The Person with AIDS: Nursing Perspectives* ed 2. Springer, 1991.

Evans C, Kasoff M, Beckman E, Handel-Kindred J: Reducing AIDS anxiety on the unit with preventive infection control. *J Psychosoc Nurs* 1990;28(1):36–39.

Feingold A, Slammon WR: A model integrating mental health and primary care services for families with HIV. *Gen Hosp Psychiatr* 1993;15:290–299.

Fetter MS, Larson E: Preventing and treating human immunodeficiency virus infection in the homeless. *Arch Psychiatr Nurs* 1990;4(6):379–383.

Foley ME, Fahs MC: Hospital care grievances and psychosocial needs expressed by PWAs: An analysis of qualitative data. *JANAC* 1994;5(5):21–29.

Geis SB, Fuller RL, Rush J: Lovers of AIDS victims: Psychosocial stresses and counseling needs. *Death Studies* 1986; 10:43–53.

Grimes DE, Grimes RM: *AIDS and HIV Infection.* Mosby, 1994.

Hestad K, et al.: Neuropsychological deficits in HIV-1 seropositive and seronegative intravenous drug users. *J Clin Exper Neuropsych* 1993;15(5):732–742.

Holzemer WL, Wilson HS: Quality of life and the spectrum of HIV infection. *Ann Rev Nurs Res* (in press, 1995).

Hughes A, Martin JP, Franks P: *AIDS Home Care and Hospice Manual.* AIDS Home Care and Hospice Program, VNA of San Francisco, 1987.

Jones TS: Personal Communication, CDC, June 5, 1995.

Kalichman SC, Kelly JA, Johnson JR, Multo M: Factors associated with risk for HIV infection among chronic mentally ill adults. *Am J Psychiatr* 1994;151(2):221–227.

Kaplan EH, Heimer R: HIV incidence among needle exchange participants: Estimates from syringe tracking and testing data. *J Acq Immune Def Synd* 1994;7:182–189.

Kass NE, et al.: Changes in employment, insurance, and income in relation to HIV status and disease progression. *J Acq Immune Def Synd* 1994;7(1):86–91.

Katz RC, Watts C, Santman J: AIDS knowledge and high-risk behaviors in the chronic mentally ill. *Commun Mental Health J* 1994;30(4):395–402.

Kelly JA, et al.: Outcome of cognitive-behavioral and support group brief therapies for depressed, HIV-infected persons. *Am J Psychiatr* 1993;150(11):1679–1686.

Kneisl CR: Psychosocial and economic concerns of women affected by HIV infection, in Cohen F, Durham J: *Women, Children, and HIV/AIDS.* Springer, 1993.

Knox MD, Davis M, Friedrich MA: The HIV mental health spectrum. *Commun Ment Health J* 1994;30(1):75–89.

Knox MD, Friedrich MA, Gaies JS, Achenbach K: Training HIV specialists for community mental health. *Commun Mental Health J* 1994;30(4):405–413.

Lovejoy N, Sisson R: Psychoneuroimmunology and AIDS. *Holistic Nurs Pract* 1989;3(4):1–15.

Maj M, et al.: WHO neuropsychiatric AIDS study, cross-sectional phase I: Study design and psychiatric findings. *Arch Gen Psychiatr* 1994a;51:39–50.

Maj M, et al.: WHO neuropsychiatric AIDS study, cross-sectional phase II: Neuropsychological and neurological findings. *Arch Gen Psychiatr* 1994b;51:51–61.

National Coalition for the Homeless. *Fighting to Live: Homeless People with AIDS.* The Coalition, March 1990.

Navia B, Price R: The acquired immunodeficiency syndrome dementia complex as the presenting or sole manifestation of human immunodeficiency virus infection. *Arch Neurol* 1987;44:65–69.

O'Neil M: AIDS and bereavement: Partners, families, friends, in Hughes AM, Martin JP, Franks P: *AIDS Home Care and Hospice Manual.* VNA of San Francisco, 1987.

Perkins DO, et al.: Mood disorders in HIV infection: Prevalence and risk factors in a nonepicenter of the AIDS epidemic. *Am J Psychiatr* 1994;151(2):233–236.

Pheifer W, Houseman C: Bereavement and AIDS: A framework for intervention. *J Psychosoc Nurs* 1988;26(10): 21–26.

Reutter LI, Northcott HC: Achieving a sense of control in a context of uncertainty: Nurses and AIDS. *Qual Health Res* 1994;4(1):51–71.

Sacks M, Dermatis H, Looser-Ott S, Burton W, Perry S: Undetected HIV infection among acutely ill psychiatric inpatients. *Am J Psychiatr* 1992;149:544–545.

Scherer P: How AIDS attacks the brain. *Am J Nurs* 1990;90(1):44–52.

Schmitz D: When IV drug abuse complicates AIDS. *RN* January 1990;53(1):60–66.

Sewell DD, et al.: HIV-associated psychosis: A study of 20 cases. *Am J Psychiatr* 1994;151(2):237–242.

Silberstein CH, et al.: A prospective four-year follow-up of neuropsychological function in HIV seropositive and seronegative methadone-maintained patients. *Gen Hosp Psychiatr* 1993;15:351–359.

So Y, Choucair A, Davis R: Neoplasms of the central nervous system in the acquired immunodeficiency syndrome, in Rosenblum J, Levy R, Bredesen D (eds): *AIDS and the Nervous System.* Raven, 1987.

Sontag S: *AIDS and Its Metaphors.* Farrar, Straus & Giroux, 1988.

Sontag S: *Illness as Metaphor.* Vintage Books, 1977.

Swanson B, Cronin-Stubbs D, Colletti MA: Dementia and depression in persons with AIDS: Causes and care. *J Psychosoc Nurs* 1990;28(10): 33–39.

Torres RA, Mani S, Altholtz J, Bricker PW: Human immunodeficiency virus infection among homeless men in a New York City shelter. *Arch Intern Med* 1990;150:2030–2036.

Valente SM, Saunders JM: Management of suicidal patients with HIV disease. *JANAC* 1994;5(6):19–29.

Watters JK, Estilo MJ, Clark GL, Lorvick J: Syringe and needle exchange as HIV/AIDS prevention for injection drug users. *JAMA* 1994;271(2):115–120.

References for Mind-Body-Spirit Connection Box

Burack JH, et al.: Depressive symptoms and CD4 lymphocyte decline among HIV-infected men. *JAMA* 1993;270(21): 2568–2573.

Coward DD, Lewis FM: The lived experience of self-transcendence in gay men with AIDS. *Oncol Nurs Forum* 1993; 20(9):1363–1368.

Cousins N: *Head First: The Biology of Hope*. Dutton, 1989.

Kertzner RM, et al.: Cortisol levels, immune status, and mood in homosexual men with and without HIV infection. *Am J Psychiatr* 1993;150(11):1674–1678.

Lovejoy NC, Sisson R: Psychoneuroimmunology and AIDS. *Holistic Nurs Pract* 1989;3(4):1–15.

Lyketsos CG, et al.: Depressive symptoms as predictors of medical outcomes in HIV infections. *JAMA* 1993;270(21): 2563–2567.

Saah AJ, et al.: Factors influencing survival after AIDS: Report from the multicenter AIDS cohort study (MACS). *J Acq Immune Def Synd* 1994;7(3):287–295.

PART FIVE

INTERVENTION MODES

CONTENTS

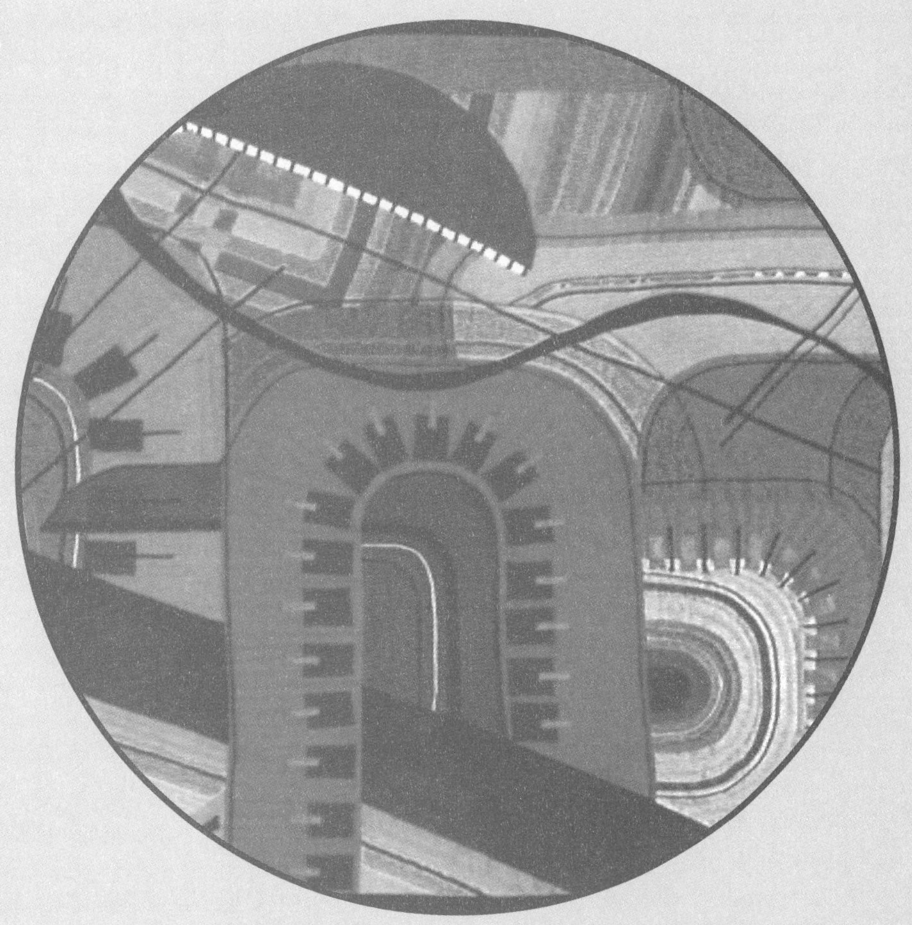

CHAPTER 28

THE NURSE-CLIENT RELATIONSHIP AND INDIVIDUAL THERAPY

Beth Moscato

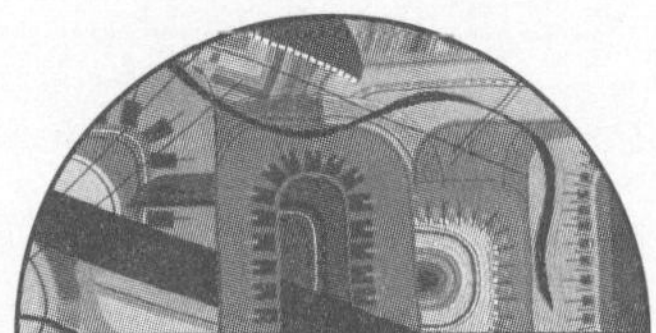

COMPETENCIES

- *Identify the common characteristics of one-to-one relationships.*
- *Recognize types of individual therapies.*
- *Delineate the client abilities and behaviors most often associated with growth-producing outcomes.*
- *Analyze the following special concerns as they relate to psychiatric nurses: critical distance, self-disclosure, gift giving, the use of touch, and values.*
- *Explain the three phases of therapeutic relationships and the main objectives and therapeutic tasks of each phase.*
- *Apply the nursing process in establishing and maintaining one-to-one relationships within the context of the client's cultural background.*

Cross-References

Other topics relevant to this content are: Assessment, Chapter 8; Communication skills, Chapter 7; Cultural considerations, Chapter 5 and Appendix C; Facilitative personal characteristics of the nurse, Chapter 1.

Critical Thinking Challenge

You have just met with your first psychiatric client to develop a therapeutic one-to-one relationship. Despite your best efforts to learn and apply the nursing process within the session, your client "gave you a hard time." There were long periods of silence broken by explosive statements directed toward you as a nursing student. You are uncertain whether the client will meet with you again. How do you feel about the client, these client behaviors, and your performance as a nursing student? What steps can you take to deal with this first contact and the uncertainty of subsequent contacts with this client?

The psychiatric–mental health nurse entering into a one-to-one relationship with a client will find it to be intriguing, challenging, and anxiety provoking. The one-to-one relationship between nurse and client has evolved as the cornerstone of psychiatric nursing theory and practice. In this century, nurses have moved from being primarily responsible for observing, reporting, and maintaining order on the unit to being functioning members of an interdisciplinary treatment team. Although psychiatric nursing has expanded to include group, family, milieu, and a host of other therapies, one-to-one relationships remain the cornerstone.

A one-to-one relationship may evolve in any nursing situation: between a nurse who makes home visits and an ailing client, between a hospital nurse and a child intermittently hospitalized with leukemia, or between a nurse-counselor and a high-risk pregnant woman. Of particular relevance is the one-to-one relationship that evolves between the psychiatric nurse and the client. This may occur in medical facilities, psychiatric institutions, community mental health centers, and private practice settings.

How is it possible to define, initiate, and effectively use a one-to-one relationship? This chapter demystifies the characteristics, processes, phases, and problems of one-to-one relationships so that beginning psychiatric nurses can approach them with increased awareness of their own interpersonal effectiveness. Practical guidelines on how to facilitate interpersonal effectiveness with clients are included. The principles, processes, and phases discussed in this chapter also apply to family, group, and community interventions or therapies.

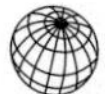

Because cultural context influences nursing care, a sensitive and systematic consideration of the client's cultural and ethnic background is an essential part of the psychiatric nursing process in one-to-one relationship work. The nurse consistently evaluates the influence of culture within the one-to-one relationship as well as the effects of the therapeutic relationship on the client's cultural and ethnic background. General considerations of cultural diversity are interwoven within this chapter and are further described in Chapter 6.

Common Characteristics of One-to-One Relationships

The **one-to-one relationship** between psychiatric nurse and client is a mutually defined, collaborative, and goal-oriented professional relationship. A one-to-one relationship has three distinct phases:

1. The **orientation** (beginning) **phase**, characterized by the establishment of contact with the client.
2. The **working** (middle) **phase,** characterized by the maintenance and analysis of contact.
3. The **termination** (end) **phase,** characterized by the termination of contact with the client.

Each phase of a one-to-one relationship is distinguished by important goals and therapeutic tasks, discussed in detail in the nursing process sections of the chapter.

The major task and overriding characteristic of the one-to-one relationship is the creation of a therapeutic alliance between nurse and client. The **therapeutic alliance** is a conscious relationship between a facilitative person and a client. In this process, the nurse forms a mature alliance with the growth-facilitating aspects of the client. Each implicitly agrees to work together to help the client address personal problems and concerns. More specifically, the nurse identifies and provides feedback regarding the client's patterns of reaction, abilities, and potentials. The client can use these assets to handle unresolved problems constructively. The establishment of the therapeutic alliance enhances informal one-to-one relationships and is essential in formal one-to-one relationships. Such a binding alliance between nurse and client allows the one-to-one relationship to continue, especially when the client experiences increased anxiety and resistance to change.

Professional

One-to-one relationships reflect a professional, rather than social, relationship. Psychiatric nurses use their personalities, interpersonal skills and techniques, and theoretic knowledge of psychiatric nursing practice in a purposeful, goal-directed manner to facilitate a useful change in their client's lives. This professional relationship differs from a social relationship in several significant ways. Table 28–1 summarizes the major differences between professional and social relationships.

The one-to-one relationship may also be differentiated from the nurse-client interaction. An interaction is some segment of actual behavior that takes place between the psychiatric nurse and the client. The one-to-one relationship may be viewed as a series of sequential nurse-client interactions with the following additional elements:

- The interactions occur over a designated period of time (daily, weekly, monthly).
- The interactions take place in a unique nurse-client structure, characterized by specific phases, processes, and problems.
- The interactions occur in a designated setting that tends to remain stable over time (home, private practice office, mental health clinic, inpatient psychiatric unit, medical unit).

A professional one-to-one relationship can be either informal or formal. Spontaneous, informal nurse-client relationships are at one end of the continuum, and formal individual counseling or psychotherapy is at the other end.

Clinical supervision is an essential aspect of professional one-to-one relationships. Supervision provides novice, as well as experienced, nurses with the opportunity to learn therapeutic techniques and attitudes and receive support during the difficult times that may accompany therapeutic relationships, and enables them to analyze how they affect the one-to-one relationship and its outcome. In addition, clinical supervision helps one to examine the experience, expression, reporting, and evaluation of psychiatric disorders as influenced by cultural diversity. Supervision is further discussed later in this chapter.

INFORMAL Informal nurse-client relationships may be prearranged and planned, but more often they occur spontaneously. They consist of a set of interactions limited in time. There is minimum structure and a sense of

Table 28–1 Differences Between Professional and Social Relationships

Characteristic	*Professional Relationship*	*Social Relationship*
Purpose	Systematic working-through of troublesome thoughts, feelings, and behaviors. Planned evaluation (through stages).	Companionship, pleasure, sharing of interests. Evolves spontaneously.
Role delineation	Roles for nurse and client with explicit use of psychiatric nursing skills and interventions.	Generally not present, except for broad social norms governing the particular type of relationship (friend versus lover).
Satisfaction of needs	Client is encouraged to identify, develop, and assess ways to meet own needs more effectively. Does not address personal needs of the nurse.	Mutual sharing and satisfaction of personal and interpersonal needs.
Time frame	Usually time-limited interactions with an expected termination.	Usually not time-limited, in either duration or frequency of contact. No planned termination.

immediacy. These relationships occur in numerous medical and nonmedical settings and are particularly common in psychiatric institutions and community mental health settings.

FORMAL The more formal one-to-one relationship is used in crisis intervention, counseling, or individual psychotherapy. It requires more planning, structure, consistency, nursing expertise, and time. The formal one-to-one relationship occurs in various psychiatric settings, including psychiatric institutions, community mental health centers, and private practice.

The choice and effectiveness of informal or formal relationships depend upon:

- The client's level of functioning.
- The psychiatric nurse's current abilities and skills.
- To some degree, the time that is available to both participants.

Table 28–2 highlights the similarities and differences of informal and formal relationship work. The differences are discussed throughout this chapter.

Mutually Defined

A one-to-one relationship is mutually defined by the two participants. Both psychiatric nurse and client voluntarily enter the relationship and specify the conditions under which it is to evolve. For example, the client may seek immediate alleviation of symptoms rather than long-term individual psychotherapy. Nurse and client identify together where and when they will meet and other conditions of their participation. This contractual aspect of the one-to-one relationship is explored further in the discussion of the beginning (orientation) phase of therapy later in the chapter. Once the one-to-one relationship is established, its maintenance depends on the commitment of both participants.

Collaborative

Both participants enter a relationship in which goals, strategies, and outcomes evolve within the context of the therapeutic work together. Mutual collaboration implies that each participant brings personal abilities, capabilities, and power to the relationship. Thus, the psychiatric nurse does not assume responsibility for client behaviors but actively works with the client to assess the self-defeating and growth-promoting aspects of specific behaviors. Mutual collaboration also means that nurses assess and are accountable for their own behavior with clients. Ongoing supervision often helps the nurse meet these particular goals. The psychiatric nurse can increase the chances of success by knowing the client's abilities. Schuable and Pierce (1974) have demonstrated that the following client characteristics are conducive to effective relationship work:

- The nurse-client relationship is more effective if clients are aware of and show a willingness to assume responsibility for their feelings and actions. In contrast, some clients act as if their problems are entirely external and beyond their control.
- Clients must admit their feelings and show an awareness that the feelings are tied to specific behaviors. By contrast, clients who avoid accepting their personal

Table 28–2 Similarities and Differences of Informal and Formal One-to-One Relationships

Characteristic	*Informal Relationship*	*Formal Relationship*
Setting	Varied.	Generally psychiatric settings.
Frequency and duration of contact	Flexible, depending on client need or tolerance. Example: short, frequent intervals daily.	Structured. Example: once weekly, with possible crisis sessions. Duration usually set at 30 minutes or 1 hour.
Duration of relationship	May or may not involve time commitment. Generally a few days to a few weeks.	Involves time commitment: weeks to months, for short-term work; months to years, for long-term work.
Type of dysfunction	In general, more effective with severe dysfunction.	In severe dysfunction, may be useful after client is stabilized on medication.
Use of therapeutic contract	May involve simple therapeutic contract.	Utilizes therapeutic contract; the more specific, the better.
Fees	Usually not relevant.	May be relevant. May be part of therapeutic contract.
Degree of skill required	Nursing student or psychiatric nurse.	Advanced degree beneficial but not essential.
Degree of supervision	Some degree and type of supervision always necessary.	Consistent supervision or consultation usually necessary.
Degree of effectiveness	For both, depends on client's level of functioning, skills of the psychiatric nurse, and time allotment.	

feelings and view them as belonging to others or as situational and outside themselves are not likely to benefit from relationship work.

- Clients must express a desire to change and cooperate with the nurse, as opposed to resisting involvement.
- Clients must show a willingness to learn how to differentiate feelings, concerns, and problems and must recognize their unique reactions and individuality.

Only an ideal client has all these abilities. Such a client is not typically found in long-term care situations. Nurses who work with chronic, resistant, long-term clients may learn that clients can make improvements if both the client and nurse work with one client ability over time. An awareness of client abilities conducive to one-to-one relationships is essential regardless of the setting.

Goal-Directed

A one-to-one relationship is always goal-directed. The client is expected to identify and achieve specific physical, emotional, and social goals within the context of the relationship. Client goals vary widely in type and depth. For example, in informal relationship work, a client's goal may be to initiate one peer relationship within an inpatient psychiatric unit. Other examples include resolution of a divorce involving children and shared personal possessions, or coming to terms with the client's impending death. Often the client's initial goal is to solve an immediate problem, and this serves as a basis for establishing more extensive psychosocial goals. The psychiatric nurse also formulates personal therapeutic goals to enhance the growth-producing elements of the relationship.

Open

The one-to-one relationship between nurse and client may be viewed as an experience in *shared dignity*. The psychiatric nurse adapts to allow clients to reveal their humanness freely and openly. Each aspect of the nurse's verbal and nonverbal behavior either encourages or inhibits clients from further revealing their humanness.

Negotiated

In the one-to-one relationship, the client is an active decision maker, determines the type and length of involvement, and is personally accountable for the work. The atmosphere of give and take within the relationship emphasizes mutuality, reciprocity, and interpersonal fairness. Establishing a clearly defined, mutually agreed-on therapeutic contract represents a prime example of negotiation in one-to-one work. (The therapeutic contract is covered later in the chapter.)

RESEARCH NOTE

Citation

Heifner C: Positive connectedness in the psychiatric nurse-patient relationship. *Arch Psychiatr Nurs* 1993;7(1):11–15.

Study Problem/Purpose

Positive connectedness within the psychiatric nurse-client relationship is believed to enhance the effectiveness of the therapeutic relationship. The purpose of this study was to explore how psychiatric nurses experience a positive connectedness in the nurse-client relationship, including an identification of factors that contributed to establishing connectedness.

Methods

This exploratory, descriptive study consisted of a convenience sample of 8 nurses who worked in acute psychiatric–mental health settings with clients who had a variety of psychiatric diagnoses. Nurse subjects were asked to focus on one client with whom they felt connectedness. Data were collected by tape-recorded structured interviews, which were later transcribed, coded, and analyzed.

Findings

Several themes in a particular order of occurrence were identified through analysis of the interview transcripts. Connectedness developed progressively, beginning when the client expressed vulnerability. The nurse encouraged further disclosure in the vulnerable area. The nurse recognized commonalities (the nurse was able to relate to the patient's life situation or to similar values and beliefs) that the nurse did or did not disclose. The client's ability to respond resulted in a mutual investment, with mutual trust and risk taking.

Implications

This exploratory study emphasizes a sequential interactional process and key themes associated with the development of positive connectedness in the psychiatric nurse-client relationship. Emphasis on the dynamics of this process is noteworthy, because the nurse and client were able to confront sensitive issues sooner, more frequently, and with less difficulty when connectedness had developed within the context of the therapeutic relationship.

Committed

Commitment is based on the therapeutic contract between nurse and client. The contract establishes the limits of the relationship as well as the time and energy allotted to it. At some point in the relationship, the nurse is confronted by the reality of the client's dysfunction. The beginning psychiatric nurse may respond by actively colluding with the client to deny or ignore the dysfunction and remain on a superficial, social level of communication. This collusion protects the nurse from having to address the client's helplessness, desperation, hostility, or raw grief. The nurse who does not let the client express these feelings is not sufficiently committed to the client. The opposite is also nontherapeutic. The overcommitted psychiatric nurse may assume an omnipotent or rescuer role to "cure" the client. This role robs the client of active decision-making power and accountability. The client will test the nurse's commitment in some phase of the relationship. Both nurse and client need to deal with this test explicitly on verbal and nonverbal levels. A sense of positive connectedness with the client strengthens the sense of commitment. See the Research Note.

Responsible

Personal responsibility for the one-to-one relationship is also based on the therapeutic contract between nurse and client, and it, too, will be tested by the client in some phase of the relationship. Beginning psychiatric nurses usually encounter responsibility problems as they begin to perceive unattractive, dysfunctional, or blatantly offending interpersonal behavioral patterns or habits in their clients. Both nurse and client must deal explicitly with "who is responsible for what." In addition, the nurse should avoid making any agreements with a client that the nurse may be unable to fulfill.

Authentic

Spontaneity and authenticity are important in one-to-one relationships. Psychiatric nurses need to create an atmosphere that conveys permission to express pain and pleasure. Expressions of joy and assessments of client abilities, talents, and capabilities are an often neglected, yet essential, aspect of relationship work.

Meaningful

Psychiatric nurses work with clients in a search for meaning in their lives. It is essential that nurses establish their own personal meaning and integration of self, for these are key resources in treatment. For psychiatric nurses to be effective, they must already possess the personal skills to deal with the client's symptoms. They must have personally worked through any problems that resemble those of the client. For example, nurses who cannot cope with their own feelings of depression cannot be effective with severely depressed clients.

Types of Individual Therapies

Psychotherapeutic treatment in recent years has moved from intensive psychoanalysis to diversified techniques and systems of psychotherapy. **Psychotherapy** is a process in which a client enters into an implicit or explicit contract to interact in a prescribed way with a psychotherapist. Goals of psychotherapy may include personal growth, resolving problems in living, and relieving symptoms.

Numerous systems of psychotherapy include reality therapy, rational-emotive therapy, gestalt therapy, primal therapy, transactional analysis, and logotherapy. A critical discussion of these approaches is beyond the scope of this chapter, but selected current therapies are highlighted. Concerns regarding a decrease in the availability of long-term psychotherapy are discussed. Other systems of psychotherapy are addressed elsewhere in this text (Chapters 29–32).

Supportive Therapy

The goal of this type of psychotherapy (often called relationship therapy) is to restore or strengthen an individual's defenses and capacities that have been impaired by illness or turmoil. The nurse-therapist avoids probing and may help the individual suppress emotional conflicts to reinforce existing coping mechanisms. Techniques include reassurance, suggestion, persuasion, counseling, and reeducation. The expression of strong feelings within the context of a safe, caring relationship may bring considerable relief and a reduction of inner tension and anxiety. The client's participation in this corrective emotional experience may be brief (such as during a situational crisis) or may extend over a period of years (such as when associated with a chronic and severe mental disorder).

Cognitive Therapy

This short-term structured therapy attempts to identify and modify an individual's dysfunctional cognitions (faulty thinking and self-defeating basic assumptions) that are assumed to underlie various mental disorders. An important therapeutic goal is to increase awareness of the relationship between dysfunctional cognitions, painful emotions, and maladaptive behaviors. The nurse-therapist actively collaborates with the client to pinpoint, challenge, and eventually correct these dysfunctional cognitions. Therapeutic activity is oriented toward current problems and their resolution. Cognitive therapy is one of the most useful interventions currently available for depression and shows promise in the treatment of other disorders.

Behavior Therapy

This form of treatment is based on principles of learning theory, using classical and operant conditioning techniques within a structured format. Behavior therapy is most effective when specific current problems and desired therapeutic goals are clearly defined.

Behavior modification is one type of behavior therapy used in inpatient settings. It operates on the following general principle: A behavior tends to be strengthened and occurs more frequently if it is followed by a rewarding event (such as food, praise, or avoidance of pain). Clients may be rewarded for performing a desired behavior with tokens that may be used to buy luxury items or special privileges. Such a process is referred to as a *token economy.* Although behavior therapy requires less time and expense than other therapies, it is most effective in targeting specified symptoms rather than global areas of dysfunction.

Short-Term Dynamic Psychotherapy

Short-term dynamic psychotherapy (STDP) is the synthesis of several approaches. STDP has evolved to treat a maximum number of clients with numerous issues in a minimum amount of time. This has gained increasing importance because clients are now seen for briefer periods of time. Characteristics of STDP include brief duration (usually 16–20 hour-long sessions), a very active therapist role, identification of a central issue or "core conflict," limited goals that address the specific problems for which the client seeks treatment, and a wide range of therapeutic techniques.

Prospective clients are carefully assessed for their potential to benefit from STDP. Best results are obtained with fairly well-functioning clients with circumscribed personality difficulties. A high degree of motivation for change and not just symptom relief on the part of the client is critical for selection. Other selection criteria include psychologic sophistication, the ability to respond to interpretation, flexibility, problem-solving ability, and a history of good interpersonal relationships in childhood (Sifneos 1989).

Long-Term Therapy

The recent emphasis on efficiency in client selection and therapeutic outcome has decreased the emphasis on long-term psychotherapy. The extensive selection criteria for STDP may leave the severely dysfunctional client with minimal programs in today's mental health care delivery system. As discussed in Chapter 21, the staggering increase in the number of homeless people across America is a symptom of our nation's inefficiency in providing comprehensive programs to meet the needs of people with chronic and complex problems.

In addition to formal long-term psychotherapy, specific skill training can address the chronic problems of long-term psychiatric clients. Such training may include communication skills, skills needed in the activities of daily life, community living skills, stress-management skills, problem-solving skills, and medication education.

Phenomena Occurring in One-to-One Relationships

Sometimes you may initially sense confusion about what is happening in the nurse-client therapeutic relationship. This uneasiness may be difficult to identify, describe, and explore. Remember to keep the following phenomena in mind when you are attempting to "make sense" of a one-to-one relationship.

Resistance

Resistance refers to all the phenomena that interfere with and disrupt the smooth flow of feelings, memories, and thoughts. It inevitably surfaces in the course of one-to-one work and most often occurs as the client begins to address self-defeating thoughts, feelings, and behaviors. Resistance in the traditional psychoanalytic sense means anything that inhibits the client from producing material from the unconscious. Conscious phenomena (feelings, memories, thoughts) may be forceful or weak, significant or unimportant. The same is true of unconscious material. However, in the psychoanalytic view, some unconscious productions may be intense forces under pressure to be discharged (archaic sexual and aggressive impulses), regardless of whether they are unrealistic, inappropriately timed, or illogical. These intense forces can be controlled only by another force equal in strength, which is labeled resistance.

Resistance is often mistakenly seen as the client's struggle against the nurse. Instead, the client is struggling against change, against self-awareness, and against responsibility for actions. Although the client's behavior patterns may have self-defeating aspects, they have also provided some satisfaction or prevented some discomfort. The client may also resist giving up a defense that offered protection from the anxiety associated with unbearable thoughts and impulses. Thus, resistance in therapeutic one-to-one relationships is best understood as the client's struggle against change.

Resistance occurs in varied situations and settings. It may surface as a primary concern in the following examples: during therapeutic work of any kind (one-to-one, group, family) in community liaison services, home visitation programs, or consultative activities.

MANIFESTATIONS In general, you may suspect resistance when the client's behavior appears to block the progress of the relationship. Resistance can be expressed by:

- Forgetting events.
- Focusing on the past to avoid talking about the present (or vice versa).
- Consistently avoiding certain topics or inquiries.
- Expressing antagonism toward the nurse.
- Falling in love with the nurse.
- Acting-out.

Some manifestations of resistance are more subtle. For example, a client may introduce an abrupt crisis, an alarming childhood memory, or an intense new relationship whenever a certain topic is approached. Likewise, a client may use flirtatious or seductive behaviors that embarrass you to avoid working on a particular problem. Silence may indicate resistance, and so may an invigorating clinical discussion that is intended as a filibuster or "smoke screen" to avoid expressing emotions or resolving problems.

You must exercise caution in evaluating a client's behavior as resistive. The client's silence may indicate pensiveness, a pause before emotive expression, or a sense of completion. The client who is habitually late may have real difficulties adjusting a full personal schedule to accommodate the sessions. Resistance to specific topics or concerns may indicate that the client is not ready for investigative work. Likewise, the client may resist giving up a defense that is desperately needed to keep anxiety about a present situation at manageable levels.

Remember that the client has a right to resist one aspect of or the entire therapeutic process, as a matter of choice. The client's resistive behavior should be openly discussed, rather than ignored. The humanistic nurse views the client as exercising free will—as an active participant in decisions that shape the client's well-being, including the one-to-one relationship.

ACTING-OUT **Acting-out** is a particularly destructive form of resistance in which the client puts into action (that is, "acts out") a memory that has been forgotten or repressed. It is important to recognize that the client is externalizing an inner conflict to people in the immediate environment. Rather than verbalizing conflicts or feelings, the client displays inappropriate behaviors. Examples of acting-out include forcefully slamming a door, dressing provocatively, or slapping someone. In acting-out, the client acts toward a mate, friend, relative, or other person those feelings and attitudes that the client does not express toward the nurse. An example of acting-out is developing third-person relationships to absorb the emotions and fantasies that belong in the therapeutic relationship. Exaggerated feelings of intense hostility toward the nurse may lead to violence or physical harm to the client, nurse, or the third person. Intense feelings of love for the nurse or therapist may precipitate an affair or marriage with the third person.

Acting-out is difficult to deal with because the client does not talk about the feelings that precipitate the behavior and later tends to conceal or rationalize the behavior. Acting-out can abruptly break up treatment, unless it is identified and dealt with explicitly. Specific nursing interventions regarding acting-out include the following:

- Bring acting-out to the attention of the client.
- Encourage the client to *talk about* impulses rather than to act them out.
- Encourage identification of feelings *before* putting them into action.
- Increase frequency of contact.
- Look for evidence of transference phenomena toward the nurse.
- With repeated dangerous acting-out, consider withdrawing from the relationship unless the client sets limits on these behaviors.

The following example illustrates acting-out in a clinical setting:

Sharon is a 15-year-old with a history of self-abusive behavior. She had been the victim of repeated incestuous experiences with her stepfather over several years, despite her mother's knowledge of such activity. On an inpatient adolescent evaluation unit, she met daily in an informal one-to-one relationship with a nursing student, of whom she seemed fond. One day Sharon received a message from the team leader stating that the student had the flu and was unable to meet with Sharon that day but planned to meet again the following day. When the team leaders asked about Sharon's reactions to this, Sharon refused to speak. She rushed out of the dayroom area, ran to her room, and pounded her fist into the cement wall numerous times, fracturing her right hand in two places.

The next day, the nursing student approached Sharon. Sharon offered no comment. The student's inquiry regarding the previous day's message also met with no comment. The student stated her concern for Sharon's welfare and her confusion regarding Sharon's injury. Sharon remained silent. The student stated her wish to sort things out together as they had done in the past and then sat quietly with Sharon. After a couple of minutes, Sharon began crying, and talked about feeling alone.

The nonverbal behaviors of nurses affect clients. Acting-out can be demonstrated by the nurse who manifests parental, erotic, sexual, or hostile behaviors, such as:

- Placing hands on hips or pointing a finger while setting limits on a client's behavior (parental).
- Patting a client on the shoulder and offering reassurance (parental).
- Blushing and giggling when a client makes a sexual remark (sexual).

These behaviors by the nurse encourage gross acting-out by the client.

Parental or caretaker behaviors are the most common among beginning psychiatric nurses. They express the nurse's need to nurture the client. These behaviors may indicate a countertransference problem for the nurse and discount the client's ability to ensure his or her own well-being. Recognition of acting-out by the psychiatric nurse is essential and reinforces the need for formal supervision.

General Intervention Strategies Several consecutive approaches are used as general nursing intervention strategies for resistance. They begin with the nurse's awareness of the resistance. Helpful intervention strategies include the following:

- Labeling the resistant behavior with the client. The nurse may allow the resistance to occur several times to demonstrate its presence to the client. It is as if the nurse were holding up a mirror for the client, reflecting and clarifying the specific resistant behavior.
- Exploring the accompanying emotion and history of its development.
- Exploring what function the resistance may serve, especially any self-defeating aspects.
- Facilitating working through the resistance by fully understanding and appreciating its implications in the client's life.

This sequence may occur repeatedly before a resistant behavior is resolved. Many examples of specific interventions are presented later in the chapter.

Transference

Transference is a normal phenomenon that may surface and inhibit effectiveness in any phase of one-to-one relationship work. The term *transference* originated in psychoanalytic theory. Transference is the result of unresolved childhood experiences with significant others.

Instead of remembering the past, the client "transfers" unresolved feelings, attitudes, and wishes into present significant relationships in an attempt to resolve them in a more satisfying manner. Thus, the client misunderstands the present according to the unresolved problems of the past. The client is unaware of the nature of this action.

It is important to understand that transference is a form of resistance. The client unknowingly resists any recollection of childhood conflicts. Instead, the client transfers these conflicts to present relationships, including the nurse-client relationship.

You may suspect that a client is in transference when the client repeatedly assigns meanings to the nurse-client relationship that belong to one or more of the client's past relationships. It is as if the client's ability to assess the nurse-client interactions becomes confused and thwarted by the unfinished conflicts belonging to past interactions with significant others. Thus, you may be viewed as parent, sibling, lover, or friend.

The psychiatric nurse explores the meaning of individual words, gestures, events, and situations in the current one-to-one relationship to determine how these reflect or replay distortions in past relationships. The therapeutic task is to separate feelings, thoughts, and behaviors that belong to the current one-to-one relationship from those that represent unresolved conflicts in past relationships.

Increasing awareness of the transference process often frees the client to work through past conflicts and explore the more creative, self-actualizing aspects of personal identity as they evolve in the current relationship. You must not behave like the client's parent or any other transference figure has behaved. Rather, help the client bring an unconscious event into consciousness, to examine its cause and meaning. The following example illustrates how transference may surface in a clinical setting:

Conrad Wilson is a 40-year-old married man hospitalized with moderate depression, which is manifested by restless agitation, an inability to complete tasks, and subjective feelings of hopelessness. Conrad was assigned to a primary counselor, a male psychiatric nurse. Over the course of several meetings with his counselor, Conrad assumed a cowering, ingratiating manner. He seemed to resemble a little boy awaiting punishment from an intimidating, punitive father. This interpersonal orientation was observed by other male staff members who informally initiated interaction with Conrad on the unit. In this instance, the transference figure appeared to be a father figure.

The counselor chose not to explore Conrad's past relationships. The aim of short-term work was to focus on concrete ways to decrease depressed feelings in Conrad's present life situation. The counselor addressed ingratiating behaviors in the nurse-client relationship only when they had an adverse effect on their short-term work together.

In this example, the primary counselor chose to focus on present rather than past relationships in an effort to stabilize the hospitalized client. Transference may be dealt with in many ways, depending on the client's functioning, the counselor's theoretic orientation, and the type of therapy.

Transference may be positive or negative. **Positive transference**—that is, positive feelings for the therapist—occurs when the client generally has had satisfying past relationships with significant others during childhood. The therapeutic relationship is usually able to progress in this instance. (Negative transference is discussed shortly.)

Countertransference

While transference involves the client's reactions to the psychiatric nurse, **countertransference** involves the nurse's reactions to the client. The psychiatric nurse may develop powerful counterproductive fantasies, feelings, and attitudes in response to the client's transference or personality.

Countertransference is suspected when the nurse repeatedly assigns meaning to the nurse-client relationship that belongs to the nurse's other past relationships. In countertransference, the psychiatric nurse's ability to assess the nurse-client interactions becomes confused or thwarted by unresolved past conflicts. Thus, the nurse may unconsciously use behaviors (as parent, sibling, lover, or friend) that attempt to replay in the current situation some past identity with significant others. Countertransference indicates unresolved conflict in the nurse. This conflict may be expressed in acts of omission or commission and in irrational friendliness or annoyance. These expressions may be covert or overt.

Countertransference is a normal occurrence, requiring supervision or consultation to prevent degeneration of the one-to-one relationship. Supervision may enable the nurse to separate feelings, thoughts, and behaviors that belong to the current relationship from those that represent unfinished conflicts in past relationships. Awareness of the existence of countertransference is crucial. The nurse may act out unrecognized countertransference, confusing the client. Unrecognized countertransference can undermine the entire psychotherapeutic process.

Intervening in Problems with Transference and Countertransference

NEGATIVE TRANSFERENCE In **negative transference**, the client shows a number of reactions based on forms of hate (hostility, loathing, bitterness, contempt, annoyance). Although there are both positive and negative aspects to every transference, a predominantly negative transference is uncomfortable for client and nurse alike. The client does not like to be aware of and express this hate, and the nurse does not like to be the target of it. When negative transference appears unresolvable, it may be advisable to terminate relationship work rather than run the risk of further client dysfunction.

It is important to note that negative transference responses that seem related to deep-seated depression or paranoia are usually not dealt with in relationship work. The reason is that exploration may stir up issues and intense emotions that cannot be dealt with in a limited time span (Arieti 1974–1981).

PSYCHOTIC TRANSFERENCE In psychotic transference, or transference psychosis, the relationship with the psychiatric nurse supersedes all other relationships, although the client has no insights into the existence of the transference and denies its presence. Psychotic transference requires repetitive, concrete reality testing to separate the nurse from significant others in the client's life. In addition, psychotic transference may be minimized by decreasing the frequency and/or duration of contact with the client. Both negative transference and psychotic transference problems require consistent supervision and cautious management.

UNANALYZED COUNTERTRANSFERENCE Unanalyzed countertransference is almost always a problem, because it inhibits client understanding and may be acted out. One purpose of clinical supervision is to help the mental health care professional develop an awareness of individual countertransference reactions. Chessick (1974) highlights the following signs of countertransference in waking life or while dreaming:

- Anxiety reactions.
- Reactions of irrational concern about and irrational kindness toward the client.
- Reactions of irrational hostility toward the client.

The following are more specific signals that countertransference may be a problem:

- Uneasy feelings during or after meetings.
- Being late or extending the agreed-on duration of meetings for no apparent reason.
- Dreaming about the client.
- Preoccupation with the client during the nurse's leisure time.

It is reassuring that most countertransference problems can be resolved by self-assessment with professional supervision. Once the countertransference process is identified, the nurse can consciously develop therapeutic, goal-directed responses. In rare instances, however, referral to another nurse is appropriate when the first nurse cannot control the disturbed attitudes and emotions.

Conflict Between Caretaker and Therapist Roles

Nurses may erect rigid defenses aimed at denying their personal feelings because of the emotional demands of nursing. For example, some procedures actually require the nurse to violate a client's emotional or physical state (injections, dressings). Defending against feelings becomes one way for the nurse to cope with inflicting pain on another person. Yet you can deal effectively with the feelings of clients only to the extent that you explore your own personal feelings.

Continued assumption of the caretaker role also undermines your therapeutic effectiveness. The caretaker role tends to involve sympathy rather than empathy. The difference between these two responses is significant to therapeutic outcomes.

A one-to-one relationship requires that you help the client actively explore the meaning underlying the client's personal pain, distress, or discomfort. Avoid the caretaker role in which you alleviate pain. Rather, encourage clients to develop ways to do so for themselves. Similarly, the caretaker role requires nurses to make decisions for clients. It does not encourage clients to be accountable for their own decisions.

Critical Distance

It is important for the nurse to observe how the client uses physical space. Hall (1966) asserts that people need to keep a critical distance between themselves and others to maintain their well-being. That specific distance depends on the relationship between the individuals. Nurses may allow physical distance between themselves and clients, especially early in therapy. This distance promotes verbal communication and minimizes any existing anxiety and hostility. Moving rapidly toward closeness, especially in establishing the nurse-client relationship, may overwhelm the client and increase anxiety.

The physical distance between the psychiatric nurse and the client can be indicative of other therapeutic processes. For example, a client may sit in a chair at a great distance from you during initial meetings but move closer and closer as the working relationship is established. Assess the possible interpersonal implications of proximity (nearness) for each client. As the relationship progresses, assess whether physical distance or proximity reduces client anxiety. The client's need for critical distance during the therapeutic process usually increases as the client experiences panic or near-panic levels of anxiety.

Self-Disclosure

Self-disclosure means being open to personal feelings and experiences, being "real" as opposed to hiding behind a professional facade or being a technician of various communication skills. If the nurse reveals personal feelings when appropriate, the client learns it's OK to explore feelings in the therapeutic setting. How much should a nurse share with a client? Under what circumstances is it appropriate?

It may be helpful to view self-disclosure on a continuum. One end represents underdisclosure; the other, overdisclosure. When evaluating any self-disclosure at a given time, ask yourself these questions:

1. What is the purpose of the revelation; who is this self-disclosure for?
2. Does this self-disclosure meet the client's therapeutic goals, or does it meet my needs?
3. Does this self-disclosure foster the development of a more productive therapeutic relationship?

Facilitative self-disclosure must be used within the context of the therapeutic relationship, where attention is given to its timing, appropriateness, and degree. For example, the nurse must use self-disclosure cautiously with a severely dysfunctional client with poor ego boundaries. This client may not be able to separate thoughts and feelings that belong to the client from those that belong to the nurse. The client might misinterpret the nurse's self-disclosure or might not be able to make sense of the disclosure. The client may also fear engulfment by the nurse; that is, the nurse's feelings might be perceived as so threatening that they overwhelm the client. Facilitative self-disclosure fosters the development of the therapeutic relationship rather than threatening its continuance.

When the nurse chooses to disclose personal information in a given instance, nursing evaluation must follow. If the "flow" of the work together was enhanced, the nurse suspects the self-revelation was facilitative. If the nurse is unsure of the outcome, a frank inquiry may be in order. For example, "How did you feel when I told you my age?" The client's reaction and subsequent exploration together can be a gauge for measuring how this client perceives and responds to self-disclosures by the nurse. As the nurse expresses feelings about the evolving relationship, the client may feel free to reciprocate. At times, the nurse may choose to role-model emotive expression.

When the nurse chooses to avoid self-disclosure in a given instance, several communication techniques may be helpful. For instance, a client might ask the nurse to disclose marital status, home address, religious affiliation, or a pressing personal problem. Auvil and Silver (1984) offer these ways to deflect a request for self-disclosure:

- *Use honesty.* "I don't want to share my home address with you."
- *Use benign curiosity.* "I wonder why you're asking me this today?"
- *Use refocusing.* "You were talking about how your father treats you. I wonder why you changed the topic? You were saying that . . ."
- *Use interpretation.* "I notice that every time you talk about your father, you change the subject and ask me a question." (pause)
- *Seek clarification.* "You keep asking me my home address. I wonder what concerns you might have about me today."
- *Respond with feedback and limit setting.* "I'm really uncomfortable when you ask me who pays my tuition. Talking about my finances isn't part of our agreement to work together." Adding "the last time we met, you were deciding if you were going to call your boss on the phone . . ." helps restructure the situation.

Use these communication techniques in the context of the therapeutic relationship, and assess and evaluate client responses in an ongoing manner.

Gift Giving

The giving of gifts may be a special concern in therapeutic relationships. Gift giving may take various forms: a fleeting social amenity (the purchase of a cup of coffee), a gesture (the loan of a favorite book), or the presentation of a valued object (the giving of an original painting). Like self-disclosure, gift giving in any instance must be met with ongoing nursing assessment and evaluation to determine its form, intent, appropriateness, and meaning in the context of the therapeutic relationship. No rule covers all instances of gift giving. Rather, several broad guidelines can help you evaluate the particular situation.

THE CLIENT AS GIFT GIVER During the orientation phase of a therapeutic relationship, the client may overtly offer or ask for a gift. This gesture may be as incidental as offering you (or asking for) a cigarette. Examine this overture, keeping in mind several possible motivations. The client may seek to bribe or manipulate you, thereby seeking to control the direction of the therapeutic relationship. (Chapter 16 deals with manipulation.) The client may seek to "buy" your time and attention. The client may ask for small gifts to reinforce a helpless, "take-care-of-me" interpersonal stance. Of course, the client may have no covert intent and may simply need a cigarette. In the orientation phase, it may be helpful not to accept or give any gift you feel uncomfortable about. Explore the client's intent. Often this mutual exploration not only clarifies the client's intent but also helps define the pa-rameters of the evolving relationship and models the exploratory process for the client.

During the working phase, particularly after the client has shown positive growth, the client may offer a gift in the form of a craft or skill. As in the orientation phase, the intent of the gift needs to be made explicit. Encourage this exploration by asking questions such as, "How is it that you're sharing this gift with me?" or "What feelings might you want to share with this gift?" A client might give a gift during the working phase for several reasons. The client may wish to acknowledge the mutual work that has taken place. The client may wish to show appreciation for being allowed to share concerns with another person. A gift may be a smoke screen to block further exploration of a major dynamic. A gift may outwardly cover up anger or frustration felt inwardly. Finally, a gift may indicate the client's perception that the therapeutic work is finished. In every instance, assess the intent of the gift, as well as its timing and appropriateness, in the context of the therapeutic relationship.

Gifts are most often given during the termination phase of one-to-one relationships. In this phase, a gift may have several overt and covert meanings. The client may wish to give a token of appreciation for any positive personal growth that occurred in this mutual learning endeavor. The client may desire to change the therapeutic relationship into a social one. The client may wish to prolong sessions to avoid the final goodbye. Some nurses accept a small gift from a client at the time of termination if feelings regarding the gift have been explored and clarified. (The gift may be an appropriate remembrance of a mutual and positive growth experience.) You may find receiving a gift at times awkward and "artificial." Yet such a situation gives you the opportunity to help the client toward further self-expression and self-knowledge.

THE NURSE AS GIFT GIVER The nurse is an infrequent and judicious gift giver. Most often, you relate to the client by the therapeutic use of self rather than through objects, such as gifts. There are possible exceptions. For instance, you may give a gift to establish initial contact with a severely dysfunctional client. During the working phase, you may share a resource (a book or article) about some facet of the client's therapy or growth. During the termination phase, you may give the client a small gift to acknowledge growth during therapeutic work. In every instance, evaluate the client's response and the meaning assigned to this gift. Also evaluate personal motives and the personal meaning of the gift.

The Use of Touch

Physical contact is used cautiously in therapeutic work. It is best to avoid unplanned physical contact without therapeutic rationale. Clients with poor ego boundaries may become intensely threatened and feel overwhelmed by physical contact. For example, a client may lose the ability to distinguish self from the nurse during simple hand contact. Such contact may be perceived as a hostile or sexual gesture, although not intended as such by the nurse. In contrast, an acutely grief-stricken client, too distraught to focus on words, might receive needed support from being held.

When considering any use of touch, ask:

1. Does touch meet the client's therapeutic goals, or does it meet my needs?
2. Does touch foster a more productive therapeutic relationship?

Evaluate the use of touch, like self-disclosure, in the context of the therapeutic relationship, paying attention to its timing, appropriateness, and type. For example, a client is thrilled to achieve an on-the-job goal that has taken much personal time and effort. You determine that a firm handshake and a statement of congratulations are facilitative in this instance and at this working phase of the relationship. If you are unsure of the effect of such a gesture, a frank inquiry may be in order: "How did you feel when I shook your hand a few moments ago?" Again, the client's reaction and subsequent exploration can be a gauge for measuring how the client perceives and responds to the use of touch.

Values

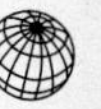

It is crucial for psychiatric nurses to be aware of their personal value system because the therapeutic relationship may be a vehicle for value transmission. In this process, the client may change cultural, religious, and personal values, usually in the direction of the nurse's value system. Such transmission may be helpful or detrimental, and it requires consistent nursing assessment and evaluation (Herron and Rouslin 1982).

Nurses must also address client values and beliefs that interfere with adaptive functioning. The following people hold cultural values and beliefs that may interfere with constructive change:

- The abusive spouse who believes the partner should be subservient, and, conversely, the partner who defers personal needs to preserve the relationship.
- The abusive parent who believes that to "spare the rod" is to "spoil the child."
- The child raised with the family injunction that family problems should not be discussed outside the home, who may view the nurse's actions as an invasion of privacy.

It is possible that religious beliefs, too, may become delusions or at least interfere with change:

- The client who believes that God takes care of His people, and so there is no need to solve personal problems.
- The client who believes that divorce is a sin and therefore will never be forgiven (or forgive self).

Initially, you should become aware of the specific values and beliefs that influence the immediate relationship work. It is often useful to label the value or belief with the client, exploring its history, importance, cultural context, and impact. Nonjudgmental, alternative values may be discussed if the client initiates such an exploration. The humanistic nurse respects the client's values and beliefs, and the client's ultimate choices regarding personal value systems.

The Nursing Process and the Orientation (Beginning) Phase: Establishing Contact

The primary goal of the orientation phase is to establish contact, to begin developing a working relationship with the client. Establishing contact includes the initial encounters between nurse and client—how they approach and interact with each other, both verbally and nonverbally. You and the client meet to discuss how you will work together toward a common goal. You are aware of having impact on the client and acknowledge the client's personal impact as a unique individual. A sensitive and systematic consideration of the client's cultural and ethnic background is important at each phase of the one-to-one relationship.

In informal relationships, contact usually begins when the nurse seeks out the client. Establishment of contact may involve developing client awareness of your presence, followed by working to communicate with the client verbally.

The time required for each phase depends on the severity of client dysfunction, the nurse's skills, the number and types of problems surfacing during treatment, and the type of therapeutic contract negotiated between nurse and client. Although these phases are presented here in their entirety to develop a comprehensive theoretic framework, nurses rarely experience them in such detail and sequence. You are more likely to experience the development of several short-term goals and to experiment with several subsequent interventions in any phase of relationship work. Nevertheless, an exploration of each phase will increase your familiarity with the flow—that is, "what comes next"—and may also provide a framework in which you can see client and nurse behaviors as partial expressions of a specific phase. Finally, an understanding of each phase of a one-to-one relationship may help you select interventions appropriate to that phase. Nursing interventions appropriate in the orientation phase may be very different from those appropriate in the working phase.

In addition to being familiar with significant phases of one-to-one relationships, you must develop an awareness of and effectiveness in using numerous processes that occur in any one-to-one relationship work. The beginning nurse often attends carefully to the *content* of the client sessions—what the client says—and only after considerable experience becomes actively attuned to *process.* Process here does not mean nursing process but rather a complex communication skill that enables the nurse to focus on several aspects of the nurse-client relationship at the same time. Process involves attention to all nonverbal and verbal client behaviors. It involves responding to client "themes," such as anger, hopelessness, and powerlessness. The experienced nurse is simultaneously aware of both content and process, interweaving both for maximum therapeutic effectiveness.

In formal relationships, contact may begin when the client inquires about services or when the psychiatric nurse contacts the client following referral. Settings may include an inpatient unit, an outpatient clinic, or community settings, including the home and private practice facilities. In formal relationships, the sense of working together in a therapeutic alliance enables the client to endure anxiety and deal with resistance to change, which inevitably surface during the course of one-to-one relationships. This phase of the therapeutic relationship concludes with mutual agreement on a therapeutic contract, which may be verbal and quite simple. The contract spells out the client's goals for treatment and the nurse's professional responsibilities.

Issues of trust and confidentiality arise during the orientation phase, for both the client and the nurse. Another concern for the nurse is how best to develop a verbal contract with the client. Initial verbal therapeutic contracts are discussed below. More formal (sometimes written) therapeutic contracts are explored in the section on the working phase.

Issues During the Orientation Phase

Trust Concerns about trust surface in this first phase of the relationship. Trust between nurse and client evolves over time as the client tests the emotional climate of sessions, risks self-disclosure, and observes the nurse's follow-through on responsibilities delineated in the therapeutic contract. You can promote trust by responding to all the client's feeling states without being judgmental or attempting to control emotive expression. The following interventions enhance initial trust:

- Listening attentively to client feelings.
- Responding to client feelings.

Planning and Implementing Interventions

MAKING A THERAPEUTIC CONTRACT Client assessment and nursing diagnoses are the basis on which the psychiatric nurse formulates a plan of action. This plan is a **therapeutic contract** negotiated in a one-to-one relationship. The therapeutic contract evolves to become the client's definition of personal goals for treatment plus the nurse's professional responsibilities. As stated earlier, the goal of the orientation phase of one-to-one work is to establish contact and begin a working relationship with the client. The therapeutic contract is a concrete, detailed, and mutually negotiated expression of this working relationship. The therapeutic contract may be modified over time but always serves as a tool for evaluating the benefit to the client and the effectiveness of the nurse. In an informal therapeutic relationship, the therapeutic contract may differ from the usual care plan often developed in outpatient and inpatient settings. For example, an initial contract may begin as a very simple agreement concerning the time and place of subsequent meetings together.

Planning is achieved by arriving at client-centered therapeutic goals, the client's personal goals for treatment. These may be long-term or short-term goals, but they always specify detailed, observable outcomes. The nurse strives for the most concise, detailed, and accurate description of client goals in the beginning phase. Clearly stated goals facilitate subsequent mutual evaluation during the middle and end phases of one-to-one work. Goals may focus on:

- Decreasing or eliminating troublesome behaviors.
- Increasing socialization.
- Increasing living skills.

Client goals most often contribute to the establishment of a working relationship when they are specific, address intrapersonal or interpersonal behavior patterns, and specifically delineate the degree of change necessary for client self-satisfaction.

A frequently overlooked area of goal formation is preventive health education. For example, the psychiatric nurse may provide a client with information or literature regarding health precautions for HIV/AIDS when the client has indicated concern or fear.

The client participates in the formation of a therapeutic contract by determining personal goals. At times, client goals may be long-term or even inappropriate. In this situation, the nurse may help the client define initial steps toward the long-term goal. For example, a readmitted chronically mentally ill client may pinpoint discharge as an important goal. The nurse may then work with this client to identify the steps needed to achieve this goal. One step may be to maintain self-care in the area of bathing/hygiene. When severe dysfunction limits client input into planning, the nursing staff may supplement goals that are determined to be beneficial to the client.

In a formal therapeutic relationship, as in individual psychotherapy, the therapeutic contract is more detailed and generally includes three practical matters:

1. Determination of the place, duration, and time of therapy.
2. Establishment of fees and payment intervals, if any.
3. Consideration of optional referral sources, should the client be unable to negotiate an agreement on the first two matters.

In formal therapeutic relationships, the therapeutic contract may not reflect client problems and strengths in their entirety. At that moment, the client may not determine that an area is, in fact, a problem. Thus, the therapeutic contract in formal relationship work reflects the *client's* definition of personal goals at one moment in time. The psychiatric nurse, in this instance, remains aware of other probable problem areas and assesses these areas with the client in an ongoing manner, as appropriate.

Regardless of the form that goal identification takes, the therapeutic contract serves the following purposes:

- To facilitate humanistic involvement with the client as an individual.
- To involve the client as a full partner in the therapeutic process.
- As a basis for communication in the therapeutic process.
- To provide continuity for the client and everyone involved with the client.

The initial goals of the therapeutic contract may be modified or deleted in subsequent phases of the one-to-one relationship as appropriate or necessary.

ADDRESSING THE CLIENT'S SUFFERING Interventions during the orientation phase are valid and important, even if the nurse does not reach the working phase with a particular client (because of time limitations or because the client is unable to agree on goals). The psychiatric nurse intervenes by directly addressing the client's suffering within the context of the client's cultural and ethnic background. This intervention allows clients to share how they perceive, experience, and manifest the problem. The following example illustrates how the nurse encourages a client to "move outside himself." Assessment has already occurred regarding the severity of the client's depression on the "inside," that is, how it feels to the client in relation to sleep, appetite, and activity level.

INTERVENTION

Goals, Tasks, and Interventions of the Orientation Phase

Goal: Establishing contact and beginning to form a working relationship with the client.

Therapeutic Tasks	*Nursing Interventions*
Clarify the purpose of relationship work, the role of the nurse, and responsibilities of the client.	Provide information regarding purpose, roles, and responsibilities in relationship work to alleviate initial client anxiety. Immediately and explicitly address any misconceptions, fantasies, and fears regarding relationship work and/or the nurse.
Address client suffering directly, offering to work with the client toward its alleviation.	Use facilitative characteristics, especially empathic understanding. Avoid premature reassurance (allow trust to evolve). Be explicit about who has access to client's revelations (degree of confidentiality).
Negotiate therapeutic contract (client's definition of personal goals for treatment and the nurse's professional responsibilities.)	Whenever possible, encourage delineation of goals that are specific, address intrapersonal and interpersonal behavioral patterns, and designate the degree of change necessary for client self-satisfaction. In informal relationship work, the contract generally includes a determination of time and place for working together to the extent that client ability permits. In formal relationship work, the contract generally includes place, duration, and time of therapy; fees and payment intervals, if any; and optional referral sources.

Client: **This depression is like a big log weighing on my chest.**
Nurse: **How might I, or someone else, know that you are suffering in this way?**
Client: **Well . . . I sigh a lot . . . I don't move a lot, only when I have to . . . I wouldn't look at you, or bother to talk to you. I guess when I feel like this, I close people out. Yeah, I close everyone out, even my wife.**
Nurse: **So when you suffer in this way, you "close people out." And what is this like for you?**
Client: **I'm alone and lonely. Not a soul on earth cares for me.**

Clarifying Purpose, Roles, and Responsibilities An additional therapeutic task is for the nurse to intervene directly in clarifying the purpose of the relationship work, the role of the nurse, and the responsibilities of the client. When this preliminary exploration of purpose, roles, and responsibilities is explicit and detailed, each participant better understands how to move within the relationship. It also decreases anxiety and the chance that a client may use the relationship to obtain special privileges. From the first meeting the nurse also intervenes to reinforce effective coping skills and increase client self-esteem. The accompanying Intervention box summarizes the goals, tasks, and subsequent nursing interventions of the orientation phase of one-to-one relationships.

Evaluation and Outcome Criteria

In the orientation phase, evaluation includes the nurse's initial comprehensive evaluation of client behaviors, any initial steps toward the development of client self-evaluation, and the nurse's ongoing self-evaluation. The more specific and goal-oriented the therapeutic contract, the easier it is for the client and nurse to evaluate the effectiveness of the therapeutic relationship.

In addition to evaluating the effectiveness of each

Table 28–3 Signs of a Working Relationship

For Nurse	*For Client*
Sense of making contact with the client.	Nonverbal and verbal evidence of liking the nurse.
Sense that the client is responding well to the relationship.	Sense of relaxation with the nurse.
Sense that the nurse can facilitate client growth regardless of the severity of client dysfunction.	Sense of confidence in the nurse.
Sense of commitment to addressing the client's problems.	Nonsuperficial (in nature and depth) problems addressed.

therapeutic task, the nurse must evaluate the important goal of the orientation phase: Has a working relationship evolved between the client and nurse, and, if so, to what degree? The working relationship in this initial phase is the framework on which the client constructs behavioral change in the next phase. Table 28–3 highlights common signs of a working relationship. These signs are predicated on trust and a sense that the nurse can be helpful.

Evaluation of specific goals and outcome criteria generally occurs in the working and termination phases. Crucial to any evaluation is the need for the nurse to engage in consistent clinical supervision to maximize the therapeutic use of self and constructive outcomes. Clinical supervision is addressed later in the chapter.

The Nursing Process and the Working (Middle) Phase: Maintenance and Analysis of Contact

Once contact is established, attention turns to maintenance and analysis of contact in the working phase. *Analysis of contact* refers to an in-depth exploration of how the client relates to others as manifested in the nurse-client relationship. In this working phase, the client may address developmental and situational problems, as well as interpersonal problems. It is called the working phase because during this phase, the nurse and client actively and systematically identify, explore, link, modify, and evaluate specific behaviors, especially those determined to be dysfunctional for the client.

The client's clearly stated goals in the therapeutic contract are now explored with the nurse. The nurse has the following two therapeutic goals:

- *Behavioral analysis.* The nurse and client determine the dynamics of the client's response patterns, especially those considered to be dysfunctional. Such analysis also addresses dysfunctional thought and emotive patterns, because these inevitably alter the client's behavior. This analysis flows from the therapeutic contract, in which the client identified specific goals for the one-to-one relationship.
- *Constructive change in behavior.* This applies particularly to dysfunctional response patterns.

Thus, the psychiatric nurse and client work together to analyze behavior and institute behavioral change in this essential phase of the one-to-one relationship.

Assessment

Assessment is continued, detailed, and expanded upon. The nurse builds on the data obtained during the orientation phase. Your observations of nonverbal, verbal, and environmental responses continue to have vital importance as the client begins to address personal response patterns. In addition, you continue to assess emotive, cognitive, cultural, and behavioral aspects. Filling in gaps of information not obtained in the orientation phase, you may now acquire a detailed assessment about a subject the client was unable to share or ignored earlier. The following example illustrates that what was not said (that is, what was avoided, blocked, rejected) by the client may have more significance than what the client shared.

During initial sessions, 18-year-old Maureen avoided any inquiries about her parents, other than to say that she lived alone. After several sessions, the nurse again asked about the parents. Maureen replied softly with tears welling in her eyes. "They're dead. They died in a car crash 2 years ago." She slowly related how, since their deaths, she has spent so much energy trying to survive that she has barely felt much of anything. Subsequent sessions dealt with her apparent delayed grief reaction.

The new data caused the nurse to revise and update the tentative nursing diagnoses and make a marked change in the direction of the sessions. Such shifting is not uncommon in one-to-one relationships. When a change in direction occurs, the nurse assesses if the sudden change indicates the need to avoid a certain topic, or indicates a move toward a deeper level of emotive expression.

In the working phase, you facilitate many aspects of assessment with the client. First, collaborate with the client in identifying important behavioral trends and patterns. Once a pattern is identified, explore it in elaborate detail to determine its origin, causes, operation, and effects on the client and the people in the client's world. Environmental factors (familial, political, economic, or cultural) are separated from intrapersonal factors (depression or anxiety) contributing to the pattern. The client figuratively holds the pattern to the light to examine and make sense of its every aspect. The elements of one pattern will inevitably link with others, so that the major life patterns gradually unfold. The first part of the accompanying Intervention box summarizes the therapeutic tasks undertaken to achieve this objective and offers specific nursing approaches to helping the client.

There are two noteworthy considerations regarding therapeutic tasks of the first goal, behavioral analysis:

1. As clients begin to describe and reexperience conflict, they consciously or unconsciously use defenses to ward off the anxiety this awakens. The development of a good working relationship enables clients to tolerate increased anxiety in the working phase.
2. As clients become familiar with self-assessment, they may modify original personal goals, or develop additional goals, in keeping with what they have learned.

It is important during the working phase to encourage client self-assessment of growth-facilitating and growth-inhibiting behaviors. After assessing one specific response, the client is often able to transfer this skill to begin assessing other aspects of life as well. A realistic self-assessment process is perhaps the most valuable skill that the client can "take home." It is often thrilling to experience the client "taking over" and further applying realistic assessment skills developed in one-to-one work. As the above discussion indicates, assessment is an ongoing process for both the client and the nurse in the working phase of the relationship.

The initial goal of behavioral analysis of the client's response patterns continues throughout the working phase. The goal is achieved when the client has an awareness of, an understanding of, and insight into the causes and manifestations of patterns in the current personality structure and can assess these major trends.

Nursing Diagnosis

In the working phase, nursing diagnoses may be revised, expanded, or deleted to more accurately reflect a central pattern of concern in the evolving one-to-one relationship. As the working phase proceeds, the priority assigned to a nursing diagnosis may change, for example, when the client is able to implement positive change in some areas. Those nursing diagnoses designated as "potential problems" may move up or down on the priority list, depending on what interventions, if any, have been effective. A potential diagnosis may decrease in priority after preventive health education, if both the client and the nurse evaluate this intervention as beneficial.

Planning and Implementing Interventions

In the working phase, planning is ideally done collaboratively between client and nurse. Such planning involves frequent consideration of the client's initial goals. When planning has been systematic and thorough, there is hardly a moment to worry about "what to do." The short-term and long-term treatment goals in the form of the therapeutic contract are a map indicating the direction, momentum, and the steps that are needed to reach a designated point.

There is, however, a potential danger in the implementation of the planning component: moving too quickly and incompletely through an exploration of the client's feelings and thoughts in an attempt to reach a designated goal. *Slowness* and *thoroughness* are all-important here. Change needs to take place in the client's feelings, thoughts, and behaviors. If change does not occur in all aspects, then it is destined to be short-lived and ineffectual in the long run and may contribute to client discouragement.

When the client is working on an issue that is unresolved at the end of a meeting, it is often helpful to summarize the unfinished work for the next meeting. This technique may help the client anticipate, plan, or prepare to tackle this area of concern again. Personal experiments, such as trying out new behaviors in real situations, may be encouraged between sessions. Some clients may be able to continue working through a problem on their own between meetings.

Active intervention is especially important to achieve the second goal of the working phase, constructive changes in behavior, particularly in self-defeating, growth-inhibiting behavior patterns. Behavioral change flows from the first goal of behavioral analysis. The objectives are interrelated and essential for successful therapeutic work. Understanding and insight need to be complemented by behavioral implementation. This statement deserves much attention, because particular clients may consistently generate and thrive on sophisticated insights while continuing to assume a powerless stance about implementing constructive change in their condition. The accompanying Intervention box highlights therapeutic tasks and specific nursing interventions for the second goal in the working phase.

The nurse also uses active experimentation to test the effect of new behaviors. The introverted male client who resolved to establish relationships with women may assume various postures (cavalier, paternal, seductive) with a female nurse to determine the appropriateness of these behaviors before displaying them outside of sessions. Permission to "try on" or role-play new behaviors must also include the freedom to make mistakes. Errors and blunders are rich sources of additional learning and occasional

INTERVENTION

Goals, Tasks, and Interventions of the Working Phase

Goal: Behavioral analysis (mutual determination of dynamics of response patterns identified by client, especially those considered dysfunctional).

Therapeutic Tasks	*Nursing Interventions*
Identify and explore important response patterns in detail.	Explore response pattern in depth, including origin, causes, operation, and effect of pattern (intrapersonally and interpersonally).
	Separate environmental factors (familial, political, economic, cultural) from intrapersonal factors.
	Link elements of one response pattern to other patterns as appropriate, for a gradual unfolding of central life patterns.
Analyze, with the client, client's mode of conflict resolution.	Encourage a detailed exploration of how the client reacts to reduce anxiety associated with conflict.
	Increase awareness of defenses employed to ward off anxiety awakened by such exploration.
Facilitate client self-assessment of growth-producing and growth-inhibiting response patterns.	Encourage client to evaluate each response pattern to determine which are self-defeating and/or thwart gratification of basic needs.

Goal: Constructive change in behavior, especially in dysfunctional response patterns identified by the client.

Therapeutic Tasks	*Nursing Interventions*
Address forces that inhibit desired change (troublesome thoughts, feelings, and behaviors).	Help the client challenge personal resistance to change.
	Use problem-solving strategies, active decision making, and personal accountability.
	Help the client learn and apply problem-solving strategies.
	Encourage the client to assert own needs when external environmental conditions (group, agency, institution) are an inhibiting force.
Create an atmosphere offering permission for active experimentation to test and assess the effectiveness of new behaviors.	Allow freedom to make and assess mistakes and blunders.
	Avoid parental judgment of any behavioral experimentation; encourage client self-assessment instead.
Facilitate the development of coping skills to deal with anxiety associated with constructive changes in behavior.	Address, rather than avoid, anxiety and its manifestations.
	Strengthen existing growth-promoting coping skills, especially regarding unalterable conditions (terminal illness, physical deformity, loss of significant other by death).
	Encourage the development of new coping skills and their application to actual life experiences.

fun. Clients who can see humor in errors in a nondefeatist manner have acquired a new skill. Encourage them to apply this skill, and any other coping skills learned in relationship work, to normal maturational and situational crises encountered throughout life.

In inpatient settings, work with other staff members to make the whole team aware of the meaning of the client's behavior as positive actions that may be exaggerated at first. For example, some staff members may encourage a depressed client to verbalize anger and begin by shouting. If there is no staff collaboration, the client may receive negative feedback (room restrictions) for testing out new coping skills.

PROBLEM-SOLVING STRATEGIES **Problem-solving strategies,** as a mode of intervention, are particularly important in the working phase. Problem-solving strategies are essential after the client has identified, explored, and assessed important behavioral patterns. The nurse can help the client use the sequential problem-solving strategies discussed below.

- *Observation.* Observation as a problem-solving strategy involves gathering and analyzing facts about a potential problem area. It eliminates opinions and impressions and emphasizes facts. (Observation as an aspect of assessment is discussed earlier in the chapter.)
- *Definition.* Definition is perhaps the most significant and far-reaching problem-solving strategy. It involves an initial specification of a problem, followed by a question. Starting a problem-solving exploration with the word "How" ("How is it?" "How does it manifest itself?" "How has this come about?") focuses on the process regarding a specific problem. It is generally more useful than asking "Why," which emphasizes rationale. (Questioning as a communication technique is explored in Chapter 7.)
- *Preparation.* Preparation involves collecting additional pertinent data related to the basic problem that may prove useful in later stages of problem-solving strategies. This enables the nurse and client to anticipate which data might be most useful.
- *Analysis.* As a problem-solving strategy, analysis involves breaking down the relevant material into subproblems so that each subproblem may be assessed separately.
- *Ideation.* Ideation involves accumulating alternative ideas on how to resolve the basic problem.
- *Incubation.* Incubation is used when the problem-solving process or one aspect of it is set aside for a period of time to allow for illumination.
- *Synthesis.* As a problem-solving strategy, synthesis involves putting together all elements of the basic problem, subproblems, and possible alternatives.
- *Evaluation.* Evaluation consists of making judgments about the resultant ideas.
- *Development.* As a final problem-solving strategy, development involves planning the implementation of these ideas.

Problem-solving abilities usually improve with time and experience.

CHALLENGING THE CLIENT'S RESISTANCE TO CHANGE The nurse also assists the client by challenging the client's resistance to change. There are two major categories of forces that inhibit desired change:

1. Intrapersonal forces, which may arise from troublesome thoughts, feelings, or behaviors. Examples include thoughts that hamper the client's sense of worth, the client's inability to control and express emotion appropriately, or the client's inability to relate to others in a meaningful manner.
2. The client's personal resistance to change, which is the greatest inhibiting force. In fact, the client's challenge to this resistance constitutes the major work in one-to-one relationships.

Problems of resistance and general intervention strategies are discussed earlier in the chapter. Of equal significance is the previous discussion of transference and countertransference phenomena, as these may require careful, planned nursing interventions. Sometimes transference and countertransference are so intense that they become a problem for the beginning psychiatric nurse.

Evaluation and Outcome Criteria

Several levels of evaluation occur simultaneously in the working phase. First, do an ongoing evaluation of the client's various levels of intrapersonal and interpersonal functioning. Feedback from family, community agencies, or the client's employer may enhance any current comprehensive evaluation. For example, does the client seem to be facing an impending crisis? If so, you may choose to switch from intrapersonal exploration to a crisis intervention strategy. Second, encourage client self-evaluation, as explored in previous discussion. Finally, constantly perform self-evaluation as a helping person growing in skill and experience. Nursing self-evaluation is done by informal discussions with staff and other mental health care personnel and by formal clinical supervision.

"On-the-spot" evaluations of relevant short-term and long-term goals can occur during any meeting with the client. For example, as the client talks about increasing socialization skills, the nurse may reflect: "Let's look at our contract together. You originally wanted to date a woman of your choice for two hours during an evening without leaving the situation. How do you think this compares with what you're now saying has happened?" The nurse supports any effort at evaluation on the part of the client and explores what else needs to happen for the client to achieve the short-term goal. An additional area of evaluation involves the client's "trying on" alternative behaviors to determine whether these new behaviors may work for the client.

The client and nurse should mutually evaluate the appropriateness of goals in any one of the following areas in the light of current functioning:

- Degree of the client's success in achieving specific goals.
- The client's growth-producing and growth-inhibiting behavior patterns.
- Unfinished business that must be resolved to achieve a desired goal.

The working phase may also involve ongoing evaluations of the status, characteristics, and depth of the nurse-client relationship. The client may view the nurse in different ways (parent, sibling, friend) at various times. It is only when the client makes these views explicit that the nurse may intervene to clarify roles and responsibilities in a facilitative manner.

The psychiatric nurse and the client have moved through the first two phases of therapeutic relationships when:

- They have established a working relationship.
- They have analyzed the dynamics of the client's behavioral patterns.
- The client has effectively instituted behavioral changes in keeping with the therapeutic contract.

In informal relationship work, the nurse may touch on only one or two aspects of the working phase. Even the advanced psychiatric nurse rarely addresses all therapeutic tasks in this phase of relationship work.

The Nursing Process and the Termination (End) Phase

During the termination phase of one-to-one relationships, the psychiatric nurse and client discontinue contact. This phase is as important as the previous two phases, although both the nurse and the client frequently avoid it because of past difficulties with separation.

The goal of the end phase is termination of the one-to-one relationship in a mutually planned, satisfying manner. Remind the client that termination was first addressed in the orientation phase, when the duration of the relationship was discussed. Also emphasize the growth and positive aspects of the relationship, rather than focusing exclusively on separation.

A smooth and complete termination sometimes occurs in actual practice. In informal relationship work in inpatient settings, termination more often occurs with the client's abrupt departure or planned medical discharge. Even in formal relationship work in community settings, contact often ceases without explanation after a series of missed appointments, or with a phone call by the client to inform the therapist of the client's decision to terminate, or with the client abruptly leaving a session and failing to resume subsequent contact. In these instances, the nurse can call or write the client and suggest an additional session to deal with either the therapeutic good-bye or a willingness to continue the relationship work. Termination requires careful preparation, adequate time for the client to work through the feelings about ending, and an opportunity for the nurse to explore personal reactions with a clinical instructor, colleague, supervisor, or consultant.

Assessment

Assessment as a component of the nursing process in the resolution phase deals primarily with determining when the client may be ready to terminate, how the client deals with termination, and how the nurse deals with termination. The following criteria may be useful to determine whether the client is ready to terminate:

- *Relief from the presenting problem.* Symptoms no longer interfere with the client's comfort.
- *Achievement of treatment goals.* These ideally are planned goals included in the therapeutic contract between the nurse and client.
- *Improvement in social functioning.* The client experiences increased satisfaction in interpersonal relationships.
- *Acquisition of adaptive coping strategies.* Ideally, these strategies include the client's use of effective problem-solving strategies on a daily basis.
- *Acquisition of more effective defense mechanisms.* A client who cannot achieve adaptive coping strategies should develop more effective defense mechanisms to ensure stabilization.
- *Attainment of identity.* The client experiences self-satisfaction and no longer needs to depend on the nurse for a sense of well-being.
- *Disruption due to a major impasse in the one-to-one relationship.* Stubborn resistances may surface and persist on the part of the client. Uncontrollable countertransference may develop on the part of the nurse.

Many factors influence how the client reacts to termination. These factors include:

- *Degree of client involvement.* The greater the degree of client involvement, the more intense the client's reaction to termination.

- *Length of treatment.* In general, the longer the nurse-client relationship lasts, the more time should be spent in exploring all aspects of termination.
- *Client's past history of significant losses.* A client who has lost significant others may reexperience past conflicts and emotional responses.
- *Ability to separate from others.* The reaction to termination is influenced by how well the client has mastered the early separation-individuation phase of development.
- *Degree of success achieved.* Reaction to termination depends on how successful and satisfying the relationship has been for the client.
- *Degree of transference in the relationship.* The greater the transference in the nurse-client relationship, the more intense the client's reaction to termination.

The psychiatric nurse must be alert to client responses during termination. Any number of responses—repression, regression, anger, denial, sadness, withdrawal, avoidance, acceptance, joy—may surface, and it is not unusual for several to surface at once. When repressing, the client shows no emotional response. Regression on the part of the client is an extremely common response to termination. Regressive behavior may range from statements of abandonment and hopelessness to an inability to tend to personal hygiene. The central message conveyed is: "See? I can't make it without you!"

Finally, assessment involves how the nurse personally manages separation in the one-to-one relationship. Like the client, the nurse can have any number of responses. Some common responses are:

- Regret that the client did not achieve more than the client actually did.
- Hesitation to give up the dependence elements of the relationship.
- Collusion with the client to prolong sessions to avoid the inevitability of separation.

Nursing Diagnosis

Nursing diagnoses during termination should reflect the termination behaviors manifested by the client. A wide variety of nursing diagnoses may be relevant. Potential nursing diagnoses that stem from regression during the termination phase may be: self-care deficit, hopelessness, powerlessness, and ineffective individual coping. Nursing diagnoses should be modified as necessary, as the client moves through the termination experience.

Planning and Implementing Interventions

Planning involves preparing for the final good-bye and mutual planning about where the client may seek future help if the need arises. When a referral is made (to another nurse or therapist, self-help group, community agency, or job training program), it is often wise for the client to have an initial contact with the referred person or agency before termination. In this way, you can immediately deal with any initial misconceptions. The shift to dependence on other support systems (referrals, family, friends) is a therapeutic task requiring your full awareness of planning and intervention strategy.

Intervention strategies vary according to the client's behaviors. You may respond to the client who is repressing the reality of termination by repeatedly observing that he or she is not addressing the issue of the impending separation. You may then attempt to explore this avoidance with the client. Useful interventions for clients who are regressing in response to termination include the following:

- Addressing the possible underlying fears of abandonment.
- Emphasizing the growth achieved by the client.
- Continuing to focus on the realities of separation.

The acting-out client may protest termination in numerous ways before the termination date, such as attempting suicide, psychiatric hospitalization, quitting a job, or rejecting the therapist. In general, the underlying feelings, fears, and fantasies need ventilation, exploration, and working through, as do reactions of anger, depression, and grief. An exception to this general guideline is the client who uses distraction maneuvers to prevent termination, such as introducing explosive new material in final sessions. In this situation, you may use limit setting rather than exploration because of time constraints. In other words, there may be "unfinished business" despite planning and effort.

The nurse has the final task of participating in an explicit and therapeutic good-bye with the client. Nursing responsibilities in this final phase include anticipating your own personal reaction to separation and, optionally, expressing this reaction in a manner that does not burden the client. In addition, you may share a special wish for the client, based on the client's particular assets within the therapeutic relationship. A therapeutic good-bye gives the client a sense of freedom to move on to other relationships. The end phase may take from one meeting to several months of meetings, depending on the duration of the one-to-one relationship. In general, the longer the duration of the relationship, the longer the time needed to deal explicitly with the termination of contact. The accompanying Intervention box summarizes the goal, therapeutic tasks, and specific nursing interventions of the termination phase. Ideally, the client can completely work through feelings regarding separation so that there is no unfinished business between nurse and client. The

INTERVENTION

Goals, Tasks, and Interventions of the Termination Phase

Goal: Termination of contact in a mutually planned, satisfying manner.

Therapeutic Tasks	Nursing Interventions
Help the client evaluate the therapeutic contract and the therapeutic experience in general.	Encourage the client's realistic appraisal of personal therapeutic goals (motivation, effort, progress, outcome) as these evolved in treatment.
	Provide appropriate feedback regarding the appraisal of goals.
	Review the client's assets and therapeutic gains.
	Review areas for further therapeutic work.
Encourage the transference of dependence to other support systems.	Encourage the client to develop reliance on others in client's immediate environment (spouse, relative, employer, neighbor, friend) for empathic, emotional support.
Participate in explicit therapeutic good-bye with the client.	Be alert to the surfacing of any behavior arising on termination (repression, regression, acting-out, anger, withdrawal, acceptance).
	Help the client work through feelings associated with these behaviors.
	Anticipate own reaction to separation and share in a manner that does not burden the client.
	Allow time and space for termination; the longer the duration of the one-to-one relationship, the more time is needed for the termination phase.

nurse-client relationship has given the client the opportunity to depend on another in a realistic and mature manner. Assessment of the experience helps the client practice self-assessment skills and may help set the stage for additional relationship work in the future. The direct, explicit good-bye is frequently the first such experience for the client. It is usually a moment of unique humanness for both the nurse and the client.

Evaluation and Outcome Criteria

Evaluation is a vital component of the nursing process during the termination phase. You have the task of helping the client evaluate the therapeutic contract. The criteria for evaluation are the goals formulated in the orientation and working phases of the one-to-one relationship. Each goal is evaluated in terms of measurable, observable behavior. Were the goals appropriate, practical, and specific to the client? Did the goals actually help evaluate motivation and effort? Did the goals enable the client and nurse to evaluate progress and outcome? What are the therapeutic gains? What are the areas for possible further therapeutic work? How does the client evaluate motivation, effort, progress, and outcome?

You will also help the client evaluate the therapeutic experience in general, which may set the stage for future psychotherapeutic work. Would the client seek a similar experience in the future, if deemed necessary? You may also invite feedback from the client about your impact on the therapeutic relationship.

The nurse's own personal, ongoing self-evaluation also warrants emphasis here. It is essential to continuously evaluate which of your own behaviors consciously or unconsciously promote, inhibit, or actively block growth-producing client abilities. Clinical supervision is essential if the one-to-one relationship is to be effective. Professional supervision helps you, the nurse, use transference effectively and recognize countertransference phenomena. The supportive function of supervision may be used to monitor your own needs, thereby minimizing the likelihood of severe clinical stress and burnout. There are various methods of evaluation: process recordings, videotapes, client evaluations, audiotapes, didactic instruction, and referral to specific clinical readings. There are several kinds of supervision available, such as intradisciplinary supervision with a psychiatric clinical nurse specialist, or interdisciplinary supervision by another mental health care professional (psychologist, psychiatrist, psychiatric social worker). An ethnic consultant can help to evaluate the influence of transcultural issues, including specific culture-bound syndromes. All of these people can be helpful, depending on the skills and availability. Supervision helps the psychiatric nurse effectively define, initiate, use, and evaluate client and self in any therapeutic relationship.

Chapter Highlights

- A therapeutic one-to-one relationship may evolve in any nursing situation.
- The one-to-one relationship between psychiatric nurse and client is a mutually defined, mutually collaborative, goal-oriented professional relationship.
- Characteristics of a humanistic one-to-one relationship include openness, negotiation, commitment, responsibility, and authenticity.
- Client abilities that tend toward successful therapy outcomes include awareness and ownership of feelings, the desire to change, and the ability to differentiate feelings, concerns, and problems.
- The establishment of a therapeutic alliance is an essential ingredient of formal one-to-one relationship work.
- Psychiatric nurses need to be aware of both content and process in a one-to-one relationship.
- Resistance is best understood as the client's struggle against change; the humanistic stance is that the client has a right to resist the therapeutic process.
- One-to-one relationships may be organized around the nursing process.
- The three phases of a therapeutic relationship are the orientation (beginning), working (middle), and termination (end) phases.
- The orientation phase of a one-to-one relationship is characterized by the establishment of contact and the formation of a working relationship.
- The working phase of the relationship is characterized by behavioral analysis and constructive behavioral change.
- The termination phase of the therapeutic relationship is characterized by the termination of the relationship in a mutually planned, satisfying manner.

References

American Psychiatric Association: *Diagnostic and Statistical Manual of Mental Disorders,* ed 4. American Psychiatric Association, 1994.

Arieti S (ed): *American Handbook of Psychiatry,* vols 1–7. Basic Books, 1974–1981.

Auvil CA, Silver BW: Therapist self-disclosure: When is it appropriate? *Perspect Psychiatr Care* 1984;22:57–61.

Baylis F: Therapist-patient sexual contact. *Can J Psychiatr* 1993;38:502–506.

Chessick R: *The Technique and Practice of Intensive Psychotherapy.* Jason Aronson, 1974.

deShazer S: *Clues: Investigating Solutions in Brief Therapy.* Norton, 1988.

Dilonardo JD, Kendrick KA, Vivaldi KB: Chronic or long-term psychiatric patients: Potential subjects for longitudinal research. *Issues Ment Health Nurs* 1993;14:109–118.

Forchuk C, Brown B: Establishing a nurse-client relationship. *J Psychosoc Nurs* 1989;27:30–34.

Gutheil TG, Simon RI: Between the chair and the door: Boundary issues in the therapeutic "transition zone." *Harvard Rev Psychiatr* 1995;2(6):336–340.

Hall E: *The Hidden Dimension.* Doubleday Anchor Books, 1966.

Heifner C: Positive connectedness in the psychiatric nurse-patient relationship. *Arch Psychiatr Nurs* 1993;7(1):11–15.

Herron WG, Rouslin S: *Issues in Psychotherapy.* Brady, 1982.

Hoeffer B, Murphy S: The unfinished task: Development of nursing theory for psychiatric and mental health nursing practice. *J Psychosoc Nurs Ment Health Serv* 1982;20:9–14.

Kaplan HI, Sadock BJ, Grebb JA: *Kaplan and Sadock's Synopsis of Psychiatry,* ed 7. Williams & Wilkins, 1994.

Kemper, BJ: Therapeutic listening: Developing the concept. *J Psychosoc Nurs* 1992;30(7):21–23.

Lamb H: One-to-one relationships with the long-term mentally ill: Issues in training professionals. *Commun Mental Health J* 1988;24(2):328–337.

Lego S: The one-to-one nurse-patient relationship, in Huey F (ed): *Psychiatric Nursing 1946–1974: A Report on the State of the Art.* American Journal of Nursing, 1975.

Lego S: Point/counterpoint: A psychotherapist is a psychotherapist . . ." *Perspect Psychiatr Care* 1980;18:27,39.

Lego S, Pawlicki C: How does parallel process manifest itself in psychiatric nursing practice? *J Psychosoc Nurs Ment Health Serv* 1993;31(10):41–44.

Lindholm L, Eriksson K: To understand and alleviate suffering in a caring culture. *J Adv Nurs* 1993;18:1354–1361.

Longo, MB: Facilitating acceptance of a patient's decision to stop treatment. *Clin Nurs Spec* 1993;7(3):116–120.

Loomis M: Levels of contracting. *J Psychosoc Nurs* 1985;23 (3):8–14.

Mason WH, Breen RY, Whipple WR: Solution-focused therapy and inpatient psychiatric nursing. *J Psychosoc Nurs Ment Health Serv* 1994;32(10):46–49.

Nezu AM, Nezu CM: Identifying and selecting target problems for clinical interventions: A problem-solving model. *Psychol Assessment* 1993;5:254–263.

Peplau H: Future directions in psychiatric nursing from the perspective of history. *J Psychosoc Nurs* 1989;27(2):18–21, 25–28, 39–40.

Peplau H: *Interpersonal Relations in Nursing*. Putnam, 1952.

Peplau H: Interpersonal techniques: The crux of psychiatric nursing. *Am J Nurs* 1962;62:50–54.

Robitaille-Tremblay M: A data collection tool for the psychiatric nurse. *Can Nurse* 1984;81:26–31.

Schuable P, Pierce R: Client in therapy behavior: A therapist guide to progress. *Psychotherapy* 1974;11:229–234.

Sifneos, PE: Brief dynamic and crisis therapy, in Kaplan HI, Sadock BJ: *Comprehensive Textbook of Psychiatry,* vol 2, ed 5. Williams & Wilkins, 1989.

Ursano R, Hales R: A review of brief individual psychotherapies. *Am J Psychiatry* 1986;143(12):1507–1517.

Witherspoon V: Using Lakovic's system. Countertransference classifications. *J Psychosoc Nurs Mental Health Serv* 1985;23:30–34.

Wolberg L: *The Technique of Psychotherapy,* vols 1 and 2. Grune and Stratton, 1988.

CHAPTER 29

STRESS MANAGEMENT

Carol Ren Kneisl

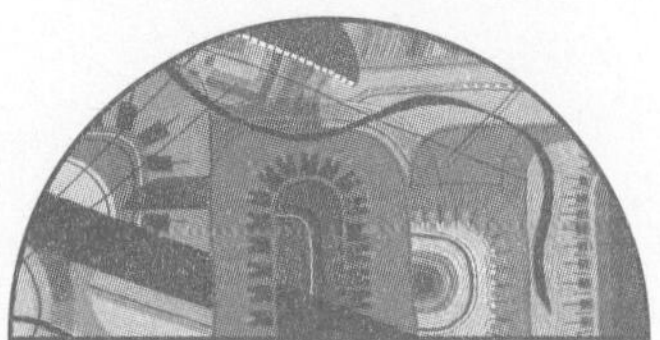

COMPETENCIES

- *Discuss the bases on which stress-management techniques appear to be effective.*
- *Enumerate the therapeutic uses of each of the stress-management techniques discussed in this chapter.*
- *Describe the stress-management techniques discussed in this chapter.*
- *Practice stress-management strategies before using them with clients.*
- *Apply stress-management strategies to the care of clients in any health care or community setting.*
- *Apply stress-management techniques at a personal level to enhance personal and professional functioning.*
- *Teach clients and their families how to use stress-management techniques to promote, maintain, and restore emotional well-being.*

Cross-References

Other topics relevant to this content are: Anxiety disorders, Chapter 16; Psychophysiologic disorders, Chapter 22; Psychotropic medications that may cause hypotension during stress-reduction exercises, Chapter 33; Role of stress, anxiety, and coping, Chapter 4; Sleep disorders, Chapter 19.

Critical Thinking Challenge

Stress is, and will continue to be, a part of your nursing life regardless of your area of clinical practice. Living and working in a high-tech, low-touch environment may cause you to feel apprehensive and to worry about your ability to live your life to its fullest potential. The term existential anxiety *applies to this condition of lacking a sense of purpose or meaning. Connecting with your own spirituality will help you rediscover purpose and meaning in your life. Reflect on how this chapter can help you to cope with the stresses in your nursing life.*

Helping clients manage stress creatively and helping nurses manage their own stress creatively are the subjects of this chapter. Although no one can escape all the stresses of life completely, one can learn to counteract habitual counterproductive responses to them. Being able to relax decreases the alarm response to stress and returns the body to a more normal or balanced state.

Although we do not know exactly how stress-reduction techniques work, research shows that most people find them helpful in gaining control of their lives and easing tension before it becomes unmanageable. As a result, the quality of their lives is enhanced.

Nurses in any setting can and should use the techniques described in this chapter. Certain stress-management techniques, such as autogenic training, self-hypnosis, and biofeedback, require additional training or equipment and are discussed only briefly. To learn more about these techniques, refer to the references at the end of the chapter. This chapter explores stress-reduction techniques that go beyond the everyday ways to cope with stress that were discussed earlier in Chapter 4.

The Nursing Role in the Creative Management of Stress

Stress management is a creative and powerful tool as long as clients learn to use the methods properly. Unfortunately, many clients do not reduce the stresses in their lives because they do not realize that they are at the mercy of involuntary *fight-or-flight* responses. Many fail to identify environmental, physiologic, or cognitive sources of stress.

Like clients in any other health care setting, psychiatric clients must endure time pressures, weather, noise, crowds, interpersonal demands, job performance demands, and various threats to security and self-esteem. And, perhaps more than clients in many of the other settings in which nurses practice, psychiatric clients experience cognitive stress because of how they interpret and label their experiences. For instance, a client might interpret the boss's facial expression as amused rather than pleased or as disgruntled rather than quizzical. This interpretation is likely to provoke anxiety. Dwelling on one's concerns and anxieties causes physical tension in the body, which in turn creates the subjective feeling of uneasiness and leads to more anxious thoughts.

The nurse should begin with the assessment phase of the nursing process to identify clients who might benefit from stress-management techniques. (Assessment of stress and anxiety are discussed in Chapters 4 and 16.) Once assessment has been accomplished, nurses can play a significant role in making clients aware of these methods and facilitating their effective use. Of course, if planning to use these techniques to help others who are experiencing stress, nurses must first develop their own familiarity with them.

Selecting Appropriate Clients and Monitoring Physical Problems

Most stress-management techniques require that a client is motivated to participate in the interventions, is able to concentrate, and can follow directions, some of which may be quite complex. Assess clients to see if they meet these criteria.

Relaxation techniques, especially those that are lengthy and introspective or meditative, should probably not be used with clients who are severely depressed, hallucinating, delusional, or have loss of contact with reality. Introspective techniques may lead to an increased loss of contact with reality, withdrawal, or increased rumination. Brief and externally focused techniques would be better for these clients.

Clients who have multiple problems or are in extremely stressful situations may not have the time or energy to focus on or learn relaxation techniques. Avoid adding another stressor to these clients' lives.

Anyone undergoing a stress-reduction program should first discuss the program with the health care provider monitoring any physical problems. Because these techniques lower the blood pressure, decrease the heart rate, and reduce pain and anxiety, clients beginning a stress-reduction program should have their medications closely monitored. Monitoring is particularly important for psychiatric clients receiving psychotropic medications that may cause hypotension.

Clients with cardiac problems may be at increased risk for cardiac dysrhythmia because of vasovagal stimulation. Caution these clients not to tightly tense muscles if using active progressive relaxation. When clients cannot help in their own treatment or if they have physical problems, psychiatric problems, or medication regimens that make them inappropriate candidates for relaxation techniques, the passive anxiety reduction technique of therapeutic touch may be helpful (see the Research Note).

Experimenting with What Works

It is not necessary to use every suggestion or technique in this chapter. If a particular technique for stress reduction or relaxation doesn't seem to help, move on to another one. What is important is to give each a fair trial and to experiment to find out what works in each person's individual situation.

Enhancing the Chances of Success

Stress management is not magical; one has to work at it and enhance the chances of success through regular practice. It is unrealistic to expect that simply reading about these techniques is all that is required to use them in times of stress. It is also unrealistic to expect that everyone will be able to make a commitment to daily practice. The following nursing actions help clients make the commitment and follow through:

- Recommending stress-reduction strategies to clients and their families.
- Providing information about stress-reduction strategies that are likely to meet clients' specific needs.
- Encouraging clients to make the decision to practice relaxation.
- Encouraging clients to devote this time to themselves alone.
- Enlisting the support of family members, fellow workers, and friends in meeting clients' need for uninterrupted time in a quiet setting.
- Encouraging family members, fellow workers, and friends to lend verbal support to the client.

RESEARCH NOTE

Citation

Gagne D, Toye RC: The effects of therapeutic touch and relaxation therapy in reducing anxiety. *Arch Psychiatr Nurs* 1994;8(3):184–189.

Study Problem/Purpose

Client anxiety is increased and recovery can be delayed by the stress of illness and hospitalization. The purpose of this study was to compare the effects of two noninvasive procedures on psychiatric inpatients.

Methods

Thirty-one inpatients in a federal psychiatric facility were randomly assigned to therapeutic touch, relaxation therapy, or a mimic therapeutic touch placebo condition. Clients completed an anxiety self-report measure. The behavioral measure consisted of rating motor activity before and after each of two 15-minute treatment sessions. Subjects also reported on their belief in the efficacy of the treatment.

Findings

Therapeutic touch significantly decreased reported anxiety. Relaxation therapy significantly reduced reported anxiety and motor activity. Subjects' expectations of the efficacy of the treatment did not correlate with outcome.

Implications

The results suggest that both relaxation therapy and therapeutic touch can be effective interventions in psychiatric settings. It also suggests that therapeutic touch can be used in situations in which relaxation therapy is inappropriate. This study is unique because it was carried out in a psychiatric setting. The study needs to be replicated with a larger number of subjects under more carefully controlled conditions.

- Reminding family members, fellow workers, and friends that because they are also under stress, they too may find relaxation techniques helpful.

Enhancing Relaxation with Music

Many people find that listening to certain kinds of music is relaxing. Dentists use music to help their clients relax and to mask the sounds of the drill. Several health care facilities use soothing music in conjunction with guided visualizations on audiotape or videotape as a substitute for or adjunct to pain medication and tranquilizers when the client chooses. Tapes may be used before or during surgery, during chemotherapy or kidney dialysis, and during recovery from spinal injury or burns.

The therapeutic use of music has led to a new health-related career. Music therapists use a combination of visual imagery and music to teach clients to lower their blood pressure 10–20 points. Music with 60 beats per minute can help those with cardiac dysrhythmias achieve a more relaxed heart rate.

How does music achieve its relaxing effect? One theory is that music produces endorphins in the brain, the same "feel-good" chemicals that running and meditation produce. These natural opiates, secreted by the hypothalamus, reduce the intensity with which pain is felt.

Because people vary in their response to music, encourage clients to experiment with different kinds of music to discover which has positive effects and then to develop their own personal library. A quicker but more expensive way is for clients to purchase tapes and CDs specifically for stress reduction sold in bookstores and through catalogs. They are often available through the public library. Recommend that clients pay attention to their breathing as they listen to music. Slow and deep breathing enhances the relaxing effect of music.

Body Scanning to Assess Body Tension

Many people fail to recognize stress in themselves. They direct their attention externally rather than internally. Because stress and body tensions are simultaneous, one of the first steps in recognizing stress and anxiety is recognizing tension in the body. **Body scanning** helps increase awareness of muscular tension.

Make sure that the spine is straight before beginning body scanning or any of the other exercises described in this chapter. Stand, sit, or lie on the floor, whichever is most comfortable, while maintaining good posture.

Begin by closing your eyes and turning your attention to your own internal world, focusing on your body. Focus on your toes and move up slowly. As you do this, ask yourself: Where am I tense? Become aware of all of the muscles in your body and especially the parts of your body that feel tense or tight. Notice the location of the tenseness and talk to yourself about it, reminding yourself that muscular tension is self-induced. Perhaps you might say: "The muscles in the back of my neck feel tight. This means that I'm creating tension in my body. Tension causes me problems."

Body scanning should be a prelude to the stress-reduction techniques that follow. Use the body-scanning method to determine where tension collects in your body.

The importance of body states and their relationship to stress have been emphasized by Eastern philosophies such as yoga and Zen. In this century, Western psychiatrists were persuaded to study this interaction by Wilhelm Reich, originally a student of Freud. Two contemporary therapies that focus on the body and its relationship to emotional stress are the bioenergetic therapy of Alexander Lowen and the gestalt therapy of Fritz Perls. Both emphasize the notion that the body registers stress long before the conscious mind does.

According to Lowen, body tension is an inevitable response to stress. Once stress is removed, tension goes away. In Lowen's theory, specific muscle groups are tightened by specific attitudes. For example, chronic neck tension and pain can occur in a person who believes that it is bad to express anger.

According to Perls, it is important to differentiate between external awareness (stimulation of the five senses from the outside world) and internal awareness (physical sensations or emotional discomfort or comfort within the body). This distinction helps people separate the world from one's physical reaction to it. Perls believes that we fail to feel the tension in our bodies because we direct most of our awareness to the outside world. Being able to recognize the tension in our bodies is the first step we can take in reducing stress.

Keeping a Stress-Awareness Diary

Most people find that some parts of the day are more stressful than others, and that some events produce more physical and emotional symptoms than others. Keeping a stress-awareness diary helps people identify how particular stresses result in predictable symptoms. Some people react to interpersonal confrontations with a stomach upset or with diarrhea. Feeling rushed or overloaded with tasks or responsibilities may result in vasoconstriction and cause headache or hypertension.

Clients can keep a stress-awareness diary to discover and chart their own personal stressful events and characteristic reactions. In the sample stress-awareness diary in Figure 29–1, a gasoline station manager records the events of a Friday. Notice that it indicates the time that a stressful event took place as well as any physical or emotional reactions that could be related to the stressful event. Clients should keep a stress-awareness diary for at least 2 weeks, tracking this information daily.

Stress-Management Techniques

The stress-management techniques that follow are based on the belief that mind and body are interrelated and that the condition of one will eventually affect the condition of the other. A relaxed body is incompatible with anxiety. If the body is relaxed, the mind will feel relaxed as well. These stress-management techniques teach you how to relax in order to enhance your personal life and your professional life as a nurse. You can then teach these relaxation techniques to clients in any type of health care setting.

Breathing Exercises

Under most circumstances, people take breathing for granted as an automatic body function. They usually become aware of their pattern of breathing only when it has gone awry, such as when they are out of breath. Nurses notice the apneic client or the client with Cheyne-Stokes respirations because they know something has gone wrong and that breathing is essential to life. Breathing properly can, by itself, reduce stress. Psychiatric nurses and maternal health nurses who prepare expectant women for labor have long recognized that breathing exercises can reduce tension. Unfortunately, breathing techniques are virtually ignored in other clinical areas.

Breathing calmly and deeply keeps the blood well oxygenated and purified. It helps remove waste materials from the blood and clears thinking. Poorly oxygenated blood may contribute to fatigue, mental confusion, anxiety, muscular tension, and feelings of depression. The following exercises are designed to facilitate proper breathing.

Awareness of Breathing Do you breathe properly, or does your breathing actually deprive you of oxygen? Take time to pay attention to your own breathing. Begin by placing one hand just below your rib cage and taking a deep breath. Notice what happens when you inhale. Does your hand move in? Does your hand move out? Does your hand move at all? If your hand moves out, you are breathing properly. But if your hand moves in or doesn't move at all, it's probably because you learned, as most did, to hold your stomach in and push your chest out while breathing. People who breathe this way do not fill the lungs to full capacity; they fill only the top third or top half.

Deep Breathing During **deep breathing**, you move the diaphragm downward and fill the lower part of the lungs with air. The chest expands as the middle part fills with air, and the shoulders move upward as the upper part fills. To teach yourself or a client how to take deep, healthful breaths, follow the directions in the Client/Family Teaching box on page 701.

Deep breathing becomes easier with practice. It may become almost automatic. This is an exercise few resist—it's easy to do, it's inconspicuous, and it yields fast results.

Ten-to-One Count This exercise is also quick and simple. Inhale, taking a deep breath, while saying the number 10 to yourself. Then exhale slowly, letting out all the

Stress Awareness Diary

Date 5/6/96 Day of the week Friday

Time	Stressful Event	Physical and Emotional Reactions
6 50 AM	Alarm didn't go off; rushing to get to work	
7 45 AM	Late to relieve night clerk; he threatened to quit	
9 30		Slight headache; took aspirin
10 00		Headache pounding; aspirin not helping
11 00	Customer backs into gas pump & dents pump	Anger
2 30	Teenager drives away without paying for gas	Anger
3 30		Headache back
4 00	Employee calls in sick; have to call in relief worker	
5 30	Commute traffic heavy; twice as long to get home	Indigestion
7 00	Argument with son	
7 05	Wife defends son	
7 10	Argument with wife	
7 30		Indigestion worse
8 30		Went to bed

Figure 29–1 A sample stress-awareness diary.

CLIENT/FAMILY TEACHING

Deep-Breathing Guidelines

- Sit, stand, or lie with your spine straight.
- Scan for body tension.
- Place one hand on your chest and the other on your abdomen.
- Inhale slowly and deeply so that your abdomen pushes your hand up.
- Visualize your lungs slowly filling with air. Your chest should move only slightly as you inhale, but you should be aware of the movement of your abdomen.
- Exhale through your mouth, making a soft, whooshing sound by blowing gently. Keep your face, mouth, and jaw flexed.
- Be aware of what it feels like and what you sound like when you breathe properly.
- Continue to take long, slow, deep breaths for at least 10 minutes at a time, once or twice a day.
- Increase the frequency if you wish, once you have mastered the technique.
- Scan your body for tension again, comparing the tension to what it was like before you began the deep-breathing exercise.

air in your lungs. Inhale again, saying the number 9 to yourself. As you exhale, tell yourself: "I feel more relaxed than I did at number 10." With your next breath, say the number 8 to yourself. As you exhale, remind yourself: "I feel more relaxed than I did at number 9." Continue counting down and experience increasing calmness as you approach the number 1. Some people use an abbreviated version and begin counting at the number 5; others require the full count of 10 to feel calm.

ALTERNATE-NOSTRIL BREATHING Although somewhat more difficult, **alternate-nostril breathing** also helps reduce tension and sinus headaches. First, close off your right nostril by lightly pressing it with your right thumb. Now inhale through your left nostril as slowly and quietly as possible. Remove your thumb from the right nostril and use your forefinger to close off the left nostril. Now exhale slowly through your right nostril. Inhale through your right nostril as slowly and quietly as possible and follow the same procedure outlined above, closing your right nostril with your right thumb while exhaling through your left nostril.

The basic cycle for alternate-nostril breathing should begin with 10 breaths and can be increased up to 25 breaths. It may be easier to breathe through the right nostril at certain times of the day and through the left nostril at other times. The reason is that people breathe primarily through one nostril for approximately 4 hours, then breathe primarily through the other for the next 4 hours.

Progressive Relaxation

Progressive relaxation has its roots in a theory developed in 1929 by Chicago physician Edmund Jacobsen. The technique of progressive relaxation is based on the premise that muscle tension is the body's physiologic response to anxiety-provoking thoughts. Muscular tension increases the feeling of anxiety and reinforces it. Deep muscle relaxation, by contrast, decreases physiologic tension and blocks anxiety.

Progressive relaxation decreases pulse and respiratory rates, blood pressure, and perspiration. In addition, it helps reduce anxiety. Clients with muscle spasms, lower-back pain, tension headaches, insomnia, anxiety, depression, fatigue, irritable bowel, hypertension, or mild phobias are among those who can achieve positive results using this technique.

It may take longer to master progressive relaxation than the deep-breathing stress-reduction techniques discussed earlier. With practice, however, one can learn to relax faster and easier.

ACTIVE PROGRESSIVE RELAXATION **Active progressive relaxation** helps people identify which muscles or muscle groups are chronically tense by distinguishing between sensations of tension (purposeful muscle tensing) and deep relaxation (a conscious relaxing of the muscles). Each muscle or muscle grouping is tensed for 5–7 seconds and then relaxed for 20–30 seconds. This cycle is repeated. Four major muscle groups are covered in this order: hands, forearms, and biceps; head, face, throat, and shoulders; chest, abdomen, and lower back; thighs, buttocks, calves, and feet.

Begin active progressive relaxation by tightening the right fist and paying attention to the tension. Allow the muscles of the right fist to relax, while noticing the pleasant difference. Do the same with the left fist—tensing, relaxing, and noticing the difference. Progress through the other muscle groups as indicated above, remembering to compare the difference in sensation between tensed and relaxed muscles.

Practice progressive relaxation while lying down or seated in a chair with feet firmly on the floor. Remember to return to muscle groups that are only partially relaxed to bring about deeper relaxation.

Counsel clients to observe some cautions while carrying out this technique. To avoid soft-tissue and spinal injury, the muscles of the neck and back should not be excessively tightened. Tightening the muscles of the toes and feet too vigorously could also result in uncomfortable muscle cramps. Postoperative clients should probably avoid active progressive relaxation, a practice that could increase pain in the postoperative period (Good 1995). Teach these clients passive progressive relaxation instead.

PASSIVE PROGRESSIVE RELAXATION In **passive progressive relaxation,** the muscles are not tensed. The goal is to relax the muscles without first tightening them. The sequence in which body parts are relaxed differs from that of the active progressive method. Begin with muscles easiest to relax (in the toes) and progress to muscles most difficult to relax (in the head). The sequence is as follows: feet, lower legs, knees and upper legs, hips and buttocks, lower back, lower arms and hands, chest and diaphragm, abdomen, pelvis and genitals, neck, forehead and upper face, mouth and jaw.

Some clients report feeling less alert after either active or passive progressive relaxation. When alertness is important, one of the other exercises is probably better.

Visualization

A French pharmacist, Emil Coue, began to use the power of imagination with clients around the turn of the century. Carl Jung used it in his psychiatric practice during the early part of the century. Most recently, Carl Simonton and Stephanie Matthews Simonton have had remarkable success in the use of visualization to treat cancer clients. Author Norman Cousins has written of his control over serious illness by using the healing power of his own imagination.

Positive **visualization**, or guided imagery, uses a person's own imagination and positive thinking to create powerful mental pictures or images to reduce stress or promote healing. It was Coue who asked his clients to repeat this now-famous phrase twenty times to themselves on awakening: *"Every day in every way I am getting better and better."* He believed that predicting failure or success in advance was bound to make it happen. Thus, positive visualizations anticipating success reduce stress. Visualization should be used in conjunction with the body-scanning and deep-breathing exercises discussed earlier.

Not everyone finds using the imagination in this way easy, and the technique may not work for everyone. Constructing a detailed, effective visualization requires time, patience, and practice.

VISUALIZATION FOR RELAXATION Relaxing through visualization is enhanced by constructing in one's own mind a relaxing environment. Some find the soothing sounds of a seashore calming; others prefer to imagine themselves floating above the world on a soft cloud or a magic carpet. Still others relax as they imagine themselves descending on a slow-moving escalator into a calmer and more relaxed state.

If visualization seems difficult (and if a warm bath, hot tub, or swimming pool is relaxing) try constructing a visualization while in warm water, combining the physiologic effects of the warm water with the products of the imagination (see the accompanying Client/Family Teaching box).

VISUALIZATION FOR SYMPTOM CONTROL OR HEALING Although visualization techniques for symptom control or healing are practiced in a variety of health care settings, they should be part of a well-rounded health program. For example, visualization can be used with conventional medical treatment for cancer clients and with preoperative clients to control postoperative pain and enhance tissue healing. Clients with vascular problems—migraine headache, hypertension, or Raynaud's disease—benefit from visualization. Allergies, asthma, rheumatoid arthritis, gastritis, colitis, peptic ulcer, insomnia, depression, and chronic pain all respond to visualization.

A visualization for pain relief might use the imagery of orange or red lights in areas of pain or tension in the body. The goal of changing the orange lights to blue lights would signify a change to pain-free or calm areas. Another visualization involves attaching a symbolic visual image to the pain (a lump in the throat, a hammer pounding the head) and then imagining the symbol becoming weakened as the pain or symptom lessens.

Meditation

Meditation is a kind of self-discipline that helps one achieve inner peace and harmony by focusing uncritically on one thing at a time. Meditation has been associated with various religious practices and philosophies for thousands of years. It is seen as a way of becoming one with God or the universe, finding enlightenment, and achieving such virtues as selflessness. However, the person who practices meditation need not associate it with religion or philosophy. It can be practiced as a means of reducing inner discord and increasing self-knowledge.

EFFECTS OF MEDITATION The state of meditation is equivalent to a state of deep rest. The heart rate slows, the body uses less oxygen, and blood lactate—a waste product of metabolism—decreases sharply. Alpha brain waves, present during states of calm alertness, increase.

Meditation seems to have long-lasting effects as well. Stress-related problems such as insomnia and asthma diminish. Natural killer lymphocyte production increases (Borysenko 1993). It has been used successfully in the

CLIENT/FAMILY TEACHING

Visualization for the Bath

In a warm bath, it is difficult to worry or to sustain an anxiety attack. The body feels lighter, muscles are relaxed by the heat and movement of the water, and circulation is increased. Being in warm water for a half-hour will lower the blood pressure and slow down your breathing. Though the effects will be the opposite for the first 2 minutes and you may feel stimulated, the calming properties of warm water will soon soothe you.

This visualization can be used in a bathtub, hot tub, heated swimming pool, or any warm body of water. The temperature should not be over 103F (39C), and you should not stay in the water for longer than 30 minutes. If you are alone, ask someone to call you on the phone after a half-hour, or set a music alarm to rouse you. Turn out the lights and light a candle, or use a small night light.

Get into a comfortable position, either reclining or sitting. Be sure that your back is supported and your breathing unconstricted. Take a full, deep breath and exhale fully and completely. Slowly close your eyes and feel your heart beating strongly and then begin to slow down. Let your thoughts just drift through your consciousness, as you allow them to leave with the warm air. Imagine that with each and every breath, you can breathe away tension or anxiety, as you allow yourself to relax more and more. All the day's burdens, worries, and expectations are leaving your consciousness and evaporating with the hot, moist steam. Feel your arms floating on the water, and the warm, soothing water gently lifting and caressing your body. As you continue to breathe slowly and naturally, let go of any thoughts still remaining in your mind. Watch as your thoughts flow through you and out of you, and see them disappear into the air, leaving your mind clear and calm.

Gently turn your attention to your body, and scan your body for any tension that you might still be holding. Allow it to leave with the next exhalation, as the warm water evaporates into steam. As you continue to breathe slowly and calmly, turn your awareness to your feet and your legs. The water tenderly massages your legs and your feet, as the tension flows through you and out of you. With your next breath, breathe away any tightness still remaining in your feet. Move your attention to your abdomen and your chest, allowing the muscles to just let go, and the tension to melt away from your body. Feel your abdomen and your chest relax, as you gently loosen all the muscles and just breathe away any remaining tension. Focus on relaxing your arms and your hands, letting the muscles go completely loose and limp. Relax your fingers, and your hands, and let the feeling of deep relaxation spread up into your arms. Breathe away any tension still remaining.

Now, relax the muscles of your shoulders and your neck, and feel the heaviness gradually increase throughout your musculature, as all your muscles just let go. The muscles in your back go loose and limp, as the water gently supports your whole body. Allow the relaxation to spread to your head and your face, and the muscles around your eyes, in your jaw, your tongue, and in your forehead. Let yourself drift deeper into a dreamlike state of calm relaxation.

Imagine that the blue water becomes the sky, and the soft clouds gently support you as you drift up above the trees. You no longer feel the weight of your head upon your shoulders, and gravity no longer ties you to the earth. The warm, soft, billowy, pink clouds support you as the sun's gentle heat penetrates through any remaining tension. As you peacefully float through the warm air, the golden sun fills your body with warming heat and light. This golden light penetrates through any tension still remaining in your body. As you free-float in space, your body is becoming lighter and lighter.

When you have floated as high as you wish, you become still, and the clouds gently cradle you in the warmth of the sun's golden rays. The golden sun finds any tension still remaining in your body, and dissolves it in the warm, glowing light. Whenever you are ready, you may return. Feel the warm, pink clouds transform into water, and become aware of the water gently cradling you. Take a few, deep breaths, becoming more and more aware of your surroundings. When you are ready to become fully alert, take a full, deep breath and gently open your eyes on the exhalation. Take a few more deep breaths, and slowly get out of the water, gently drying yourself and feeling the relaxation throughout your body.

Source: Adapted from Mason 1986, pp. 61–63, with permission.

prevention and treatment of hypertension, heart disease, and stroke. Meditation has also helped people decrease their consumption of food, alcohol, tobacco, and drugs and curtail obsessive thinking, anxiety, depression, and hostility. It also improves concentration and attention.

Some theorists believe that meditation quiets the brain, as the person makes contact with more orderly and coherent levels of the mind. The left hemisphere, thought to be responsible for rational and logical thinking, comes into electrical balance with the underdeveloped right hemisphere, thought to modulate intuition, holistic comprehension, and artistic qualities.

MEDITATION EXERCISES Meditation exercises can be relatively easy to learn. Some people experience immediate relief and pleasure in only one session. To experience deeper effects, the person needs to practice meditation regularly for at least a month.

These are the four major requirements for successful meditation:

1. A quiet place.
2. A comfortable position.
3. An object or thought to focus on.
4. A passive attitude.

The environment for meditation should be one that minimizes distractions—a quiet place set aside as a haven from the urgencies of everyday life. A comfortable position that can be held for 20 minutes without stress facilitates meditation. Some possible positions are the yoga lotus position or sitting back on the heels.

Something to focus on—a repeated word, an object or symbol to look at or think about, or a specific thought or feeling—helps keep distracting thoughts from entering the mind. A passive attitude requires understanding that thoughts and distractions will occur and can be cleared from the mind. If they occur, they should be noted and released without concern about their interference. It is counterproductive to worry about how well you are doing at meditating.

Some of the stress-management techniques discussed earlier—body scanning, the breathing ten-to-one count, and visualization—can satisfy the requirement of an object to focus on. Many people who meditate prefer to use a **mantra**, a syllable, word, or name that is repeatedly chanted aloud. Some teachers of meditation insist that each person have a special mantra with a specific meaning and vibration to achieve individual effects. Others recommend the use of any word or phrase the individual is drawn to, such as *peace, love,* or *calm*. Some popular Eastern mantras are *om* (I am), *so-ham* (I am he), and *sa-ham* (I am she). Avoid chanting too loudly or too vigorously. After about 5 minutes, shift to whispering the mantra as you relax more deeply. When it is not possible to chant aloud, some people chant silently.

The best results from meditation are achieved by meditating 15 minutes a day, 5–7 days a week for 2 weeks. After this period of time, the length of the sessions may be increased to 30 minutes if desired. Because digestion interferes with the ability to relax, avoid meditating within 2 hours after eating a heavy meal.

Therapeutic Touch

Therapeutic touch was developed by Dolores Krieger (1979) as a nursing activity, although the "laying on of hands" to help heal is as old as history. It is defined as the specific transfer of energy in a therapeutic manner; that is, some of the excess energies of the healer are directed to the client, or energy is transferred from one place to another within the body of the client. This technique is based on the concept of illness as an imbalance of energies in the body. *Prana* is the subsystem of energy that Krieger believes is the basis of the energy transfer in therapeutic touch. Healthy people usually have an excess of prana, and since each person is an open system, energy can be transferred to another person. This transfer of energy is not a cure but provides an infusion of energy for people who have been depleted by struggles with illness. This energy benefits them until their own healing processes take over.

Therapeutic touch is a conscious, deliberate act composed of three steps called centering, scanning, and rebalancing. The healer first prepares for the procedure through *centering,* the discovery of an inner physical and psychologic stability in which the healer achieves a sense that all faculties are under command. This gathers and focuses the healer's energies on the client and excludes extraneous thoughts from the mind, a process that is akin to meditation.

The healer then *scans* the client from head to foot without actually touching the client's body, attempting to sense temperature changes or feelings of pressure. These areas indicate a static condition, an imbalance, or congestion in the client's energy field.

Intervention consists of mobilizing or *rebalancing* these congested areas. The healer places the hands, with palms facing away from the client, in the area where pressure is felt and moves the hands away from the client's body in a sweeping gesture while consciously directing a flow of energy to the client, a process called *unruffling the field.* Therapists report relief of the sense of pressure they feel in problem areas of the client's body and consider the treatment complete when they no longer perceive an imbalance in the person's symmetry.

Clients report a sense of relaxation and relief from pain. Krieger (1979) has demonstrated experimentally that therapeutic touch has produced a significant change in the hemoglobin component of red blood cells. Advocates of therapeutic touch have found that, although the freeing of bound energy is not long-lasting, it does seem to facilitate the repatterning of energy necessary for healing. Recent research indicates that therapeutic touch can reduce pain, accelerate the healing process, and result in a person's emotional and spiritual growth (Mackey 1995).

Rolfing

Rolfing, or structural integration, is based on the belief that psychologic conflicts are recorded and perpetuated in the body. Ida Rolf (1977), the founder of this therapy, viewed the body as an area of energy within the earth's gravitational field. To function properly, a person must be in correct alignment with the forces of gravity. When the body is in an incorrect position, the myofascia, or connective tissue that supports the body weight, shortens and undergoes metabolic changes that decrease its energy and interfere with free movement.

Many people are not in proper relationship to gravity because they have become alienated from their own bodily sensations. At different points in their development, they have responded to inner and outer threats by contracting the muscles that are related to the impulse that is being blocked. For example, if the impulse is aggressive, they may contract arm muscles. Repeated inhibition and the resulting muscular contractions produce chronically spastic muscles that inhibit motility. The musculature acts as a repository of stored feelings. Energy that would otherwise be available for conscious use is expended internally to keep these muscles tense.

As people age, their posture becomes a reflection of accumulated unresolved feelings. When people become aware of how they contract their muscles in traumatic situations, they can begin to take responsibility for their own physical structure by experimenting with alternative responses. Gracefulness and unitary movement are signs of personal integration. When a body is coordinated and balanced physically, there is a corresponding emotional balance.

Rolfing is a method of working with the body to achieve a realignment of the body structure. The basic therapy consists of ten 1-hour sessions. The rolfer massages and manipulates the client's deep connective tissue. Once this tissue is freed, the body is able to realign itself with gravitational forces. The emotional release and physical healing that often accompany rolfing are not the major goal of therapy. However, they are proof that emotional and physical problems are related to the body's misalignment. Many clients who have been rolfed report they have changed so much that they have difficulty relating to their past environment and must alter their work, interpersonal relationships, and values.

Bioenergetics

Alexander Lowen (1976), founder of the Institute for Bioenergetics, also emphasizes body work. **Bioenergetics** offers techniques for reducing muscular tension through the release of feelings. It makes less use of direct body contact (between client and therapist) than other body therapies, guiding the client instead through a series of exercises and verbal techniques. Stressor and releaser exercises are used to increase the client's awareness of body defenses. The exercises begin with deep breathing and progress to stretching and kicking the limbs, enabling the client to break through muscular rigidity and express feelings previously trapped in habitual postural modes. These modes, called *muscular armoring,* prevent the free flow of energy.

Lowen also thinks that the study of *auras,* or energy fields around the body, can be used to diagnose disturbances in body functioning. In the energy field of a person with schizophrenia, for example, a trained observer can see characteristic alterations, such as interruptions of energy flow or color changes. Different parts of each person's body radiate different kinds of feelings. When chronic muscle tension blocks energy, negative feelings result. The head, neck, and shoulders can radiate openness and affirmation or express hostility and holding back. The abdomen can radiate pleasure and laughter or suffering. The legs can radiate security and balance or instability. When there are no constrictions that disturb energy flow, the feeling is positive, the personality is integrated, and the aura is bright and intense.

People excite and depress each other through their energy fields. People with strong energy fields influence others in a positive way. We are in touch with others only when our energy contacts and excites their energy. Bioenergetics attempts to facilitate this free flow of energy.

Autogenic Training

Autogenic training is used across the country in stress-reduction and holistic health centers to teach self-regulation of the autonomic nervous system. It has its origins in the research done by Oskar Vogt, a neurophysiologist who worked in Berlin in the last decade of the nineteenth century. Johannes Schutz, a Berlin psychiatrist, combined Vogt's research into the effects of hypnosis on the brain with some yoga techniques and published his first work on autogenic training in 1932. Wolfgang Luthe brought autogenic training to the United States in 1969. In its contemporary form, autogenic training does not require a hypnotist. Most individuals can learn autogenic exercises in 4–10 months through a systematic training program or a written course of study.

Autogenic training is based on the achievement of the following six physiologic outcomes:

1. Heaviness in the extremities.
2. Warmth in the extremities.
3. Regulation of the heartbeat.
4. Regulation of breathing.
5. Abdominal warmth.
6. Cooling of the forehead.

Once clients learn to perform the six standard exercises designed to achieve these results, they may go on to learn meditative exercises specifically developed for each client or neutralization exercises to promote abreaction and verbalization.

Autogenic training has proved helpful for the following problems:

- Hyperventilation and asthma.
- Gastrointestinal problems (constipation, diarrhea, gastritis, ulcer, and gastrointestinal spasm).
- Cardiovascular problems (cardiac dysrhythmias and hypertension).
- Some thyroid conditions.
- Headaches and insufficient circulation to the body's extremities.
- Anxiety, irritability, and fatigue.
- Pain.
- Sleep disorders.

It is not recommended for children under 5 years of age or for psychotic clients. People with serious physical health problems should be under the supervision of a health care provider while in autogenic training. Any trainees who experience distress, uncomfortable symptoms, or changes in blood pressure during autogenic training should continue only under the supervision of a qualified instructor.

Self-Hypnosis

Milton Erickson is generally recognized as a leading proponent of the use of hypnosis in medical and psychotherapeutic contexts. Erickson redefined hypnosis as an experience originating in the client in order to cope with a problem overwhelming to the conscious mind.

People practice **self-hypnosis**—hypnosis accomplished by oneself without the help of a second party as hypnotist—to achieve significant relaxation, to make positive suggestions for change (to lose weight, to stop smoking, to overcome fear of the dark or insomnia), to increase learning and remembering, and to uncover significant but forgotten events. Table 29–1 gives examples of some life problems and hypnotic suggestions that can be used to overcome them. Contrary to popular belief, even the most inexperienced of self-hypnosis practitioners cannot harm themselves.

Most people can achieve significant relaxation within two days with self-hypnosis. Self-hypnosis can be self-taught through books on the subject (see the references at the end of this chapter). Community adult education programs or holistic health centers often offer courses on self-hypnosis. Self-hypnosis is clinically effective in relieving insomnia, low to moderate levels of chronic pain, tics and tremors, and low to moderate levels of anxiety. It is a well-established treatment for chronic fatigue.

Thought Stopping

Thought stopping is a behavior-modification technique that is particularly useful in helping a person control obsessive and phobic thoughts. It involves concentrating on the unwanted thoughts and, after a short time, suddenly interrupting the thought and emptying the mind. Thought stopping is based on the belief that negative and frightening thoughts invariably precede negative and frightening emotions. Controlling these thoughts can reduce stress. Some of the obsessive and phobic thought processes that can be interrupted by thought stopping are color naming, counting, rechecking, hypochondriasis, sexual preoccupation, recurring thoughts of failure, and simple phobias, among others. Thought stopping is more successful with phobias than it is with compulsive ritualistic behavior.

Thought stopping begins by using the command "Stop," a loud noise, or a distracter such as pinching oneself, snapping a rubber band, or pressing the fingernails into the palm of the hand to interrupt the unpleasant thoughts. Once the individual has mastered interrupting the unpleasant thought, the next step involves *thought substitution* (replacing the obsessive or phobic thought with a positive assertive statement that is appropriate to the situation). For example, the person who is afraid to drive across a bridge might say to himself or herself, "This is a gorgeous view from up here."

To be effective, thought stopping should be practiced conscientiously throughout the day for 3–7 days. At first the thought will return, but with practice it will return less frequently, and in many instances the thought eventually ceases to recur.

Refuting Irrational Self-Talk

Self-talk is intrapersonal communication, the thoughts with which we describe and interpret the world to ourselves. Irrational or untrue self-talk causes stress and mental disorder. Two common forms of **irrational self-talk** are statements that "awfulize" (catastrophic, nightmarish interpretations of an event or experience) or "absolutize" (words such as *should, must, always,* etc. that imply the need to live up to a standard). These ideas are based on the rational-emotive therapy formulated by Albert Ellis (1975).

Table 29–1 Life Problems and Related Hypnotic Suggestions

Life Problem	*Hypnotic Suggestion*
Fear of coming into the dark house at night	I can come in tonight feeling relaxed and glad to be home.
Anxiety that prevents working or studying to meet deadlines	I can work steadily and calmly. My concentration is improving as I become more relaxed.
Insomnia	I will gradually become more and more drowsy. In just a few minutes I will be able to fall asleep and will sleep peacefully all night.
Chronic fatigue	I can wake up feeling refreshed and rested.
Obsessive and fearful thoughts about death	I am full of life now. I will enjoy today.
Minor chronic headache or backache	As I become more relaxed, my headache (backache) lessens. In just a few minutes, it will go away. Soon my head will be cool and relaxed. Gradually I will feel the muscles in my back loosen, and in an hour, they will be completely relaxed. Whenever these symptoms come back, I will simply turn my ring a quarter of a turn to the right and the pain will relax away.
Feelings of inferiority	The next time I see ___, I can feel secure in myself. I can feel relaxed and at ease because I am perfectly all right.
Anxiety about an upcoming evaluation or test	Whenever I feel nervous, I can say to myself . . . (insert your own special key word or phrase here) . . . and relax.
Chronic anger (or chronic guilt)	I can turn off anger (guilt) because I am the one who turns it on. I will relax my body and breathe deeply.
Worry about interpersonal rejection	Whenever I lace my fingers together, I will feel confidence flowing through me.
Chronic tension in a particular part of the body	I will think about my ___ every hour and let it relax.

Rational-emotive therapy emphasizes human values as the important component of personality. Healthy functioning is possible only when the values we believe in are rational ones. Absolutist, perfectionist attitudes are irrational. Ten basic irrational ideas described by Ellis are discussed in the box on page 708.

According to Ellis, emotional reactions are not caused by events or by our emotional reaction to events but by belief systems. Being insulted, for instance, does not cause us to withdraw from others. Our *beliefs* about being insulted are what cause us to withdraw. Though it is rational to feel angry about insults because they are destructive, withdrawal is irrational because it indicates that an individual has defined being insulted as a frightening event to be avoided. Ellis defines beliefs as rational when they help the individual accept reality, live in intimate relationships with others, work productively, and enjoy recreational pursuits. Irrationality is self-destructive behavior.

Both emotions and behavior depend on the cognitive mediating process that occurs in relation to every experience. Rational-emotive therapy helps people dispel their disturbing beliefs by explaining what irrational beliefs are and how they cause emotional difficulty. After they have logically analyzed their irrational beliefs, clients see how unnecessary they are and eliminate them.

Rational-emotive therapy frequently uses reinforcing techniques to help people change. Clients are taught to reward themselves for working on self-defeating ideas and to penalize themselves if they do not. Clients are also shown how to speak and think more objectively and give up the use of vague terms and overgeneralizations in order to define their own problems in specific terms. For example, the client is shown that the statement "I have some characteristics that are irritating to others" is more precise than "I am an irritating person."

Rational-emotive therapy narrows the focus for change to specific traits and behavior. Because people create most of their own psychologic symptoms, they can eliminate these symptoms by changing their values.

Biofeedback

Biofeedback, or visceral learning, is a technique for gaining conscious control over such involuntary body functions as blood pressure and heart rate, which are mediated by the autonomic nervous system. The clinical appli-cation of biofeedback was pioneered by Alyce and Elmer Green of the Menninger Foundation in the late 1960s. Many other researchers have followed them in exploring this method of treatment. Certified biofeedback

Albert Ellis' Ten Basic Irrational Ideas

1. *It is an absolute necessity for an adult to have love and approval from peers, family, and friends.* In fact, it is impossible to please all the people in your life. Even those who basically like and approve of you will dislike some behaviors and qualities. This irrational belief is probably the single greatest cause of unhappiness.

2. *You must be unfailingly competent and almost perfect in all you undertake.* The results of believing you must behave perfectly are self-blame for inevitable failure, lowered self-esteem, perfectionistic standards applied to mate and friends, and paralysis and fear at attempting anything.

3. *Certain people are evil, wicked, and villainous, and should be punished.* A more realistic position is that they are behaving in ways that are antisocial or inappropriate. They are perhaps stupid, ignorant, or neurotic, and it would be well if their behavior could be changed.

4. *It is horrible when people and things are not the way you would like them to be.* This might be described as the spoiled-child syndrome. As soon as the tire goes flat, the self-talk starts: "Why does this happen to me? Damn, I can't take this. It's awful, I'll get all filthy." Any inconvenience, problem, or failure to get your way is likely to be met with such awfulizing self-statements. The result is intense irritation and stress.

5. *External events cause most human misery; people simply react as events trigger their emotions.* A logical extension of this belief is that you must control the external events in order to create happiness or avoid sorrow. Since such control has limitations and we are at a loss to completely manipulate the will of others, there results a sense of helplessness and chronic anxiety. Ascribing unhappiness to events is a way of avoiding reality. Self-statements *interpreting* the event caused the unhappiness. While you may have only limited control over others, you have enormous control over your emotions.

6. *You should feel fear or anxiety about anything that is unknown, uncertain, or potentially dangerous.* Many describe this as, "a little bell that goes off and I think I ought to start worrying." They begin to rehearse their scenarios of catastrophe. Increasing the fear of anxiety in the face of uncertainty makes coping more difficult and adds to stress. Saving the fear response for actual, perceived danger allows you to enjoy uncertainty as a novel and exciting experience.

7. *It is easier to avoid than to face life's difficulties and responsibilities.* There are many ways of ducking responsibilities: "I should tell him/her I'm no longer interested—but not tonight." "I'd like to get another job, but I'm just too tired on my days off to look." "A leaky faucet won't hurt anything." "We could shop today, but the car is making a sort of funny sound."

8. *You need something other or stronger or greater than yourself to rely on.* This belief becomes a psychologic trap in which your independent judgment, and the awareness of your particular needs, are undermined by reliance on a higher authority.

9. *The past has a lot to do with determining the present.* Just because you were once strongly affected by something does not mean that you must continue the habits you formed to cope with the original situation. Those old patterns and ways of responding are just decisions made so many times they have become nearly automatic. You can identify those old decisions and start changing them *right now.* You can learn from past experience, but you don't have to be overly attached to it.

10. *Happiness can be achieved by inaction, passivity, and endless leisure.* This is called the Elysian Fields syndrome. There is more to happiness than perfect relaxation.

Source: Adapted from Davis, Eshelman, and McKay 1982, pp. 106–107.

practitioners can be found in almost any large city, and training is available at most large universities.

Biofeedback treatment is based on the ability to voluntarily control some autonomic functions to a degree once thought impossible. It has been shown, for instance, that migraine headaches can be relieved by increasing blood flow to the hands.

The technique is based on giving continuous feedback about the results of each consecutive attempt at control. In a typical session, a person might be given this feedback by equipment that amplifies body signals and translates them into a flashing light or a steady tone. Once people can "see" a heartbeat, for instance, and observe when it slows down or speeds up, they have the information they need to control their heart rate. They are instructed to change the signal as they observe it. They are not told to slow the heart rate, but to slow the flashing light. If they can do this, their heart rate will be modified.

Inexpensive monitoring equipment for home use has been developed within the past few years. The drawback is that these systems usually measure only temperature, heart rate, or the alpha activity of the brain, thus giving feedback on only a single system. Single-system feedback often isn't enough to achieve total relaxation.

Biofeedback has been found to be useful in treating a variety of problems, including tension or migraine headaches, insomnia, muscle or colon spasm, pain, hypertension, anxiety, phobias, asthma, stuttering, bruxism (grinding of the teeth), and epilepsy. The psychologic states achieved through biofeedback can be beneficial in decreasing tension and reactions to unpleasant stimuli.

Chapter Highlights

- There are environmental, physiologic, and cognitive sources of stress. Psychiatric clients may experience more cognitive stress than most other people do because of how they interpret and label their experiences.
- Most people, including clients and nurses, find stress-reduction techniques helpful in counteracting habitual and counterproductive responses to the stresses of life.
- Nurses who plan to use stress-management techniques with clients must first develop their own personal familiarity with them.
- Anyone participating in a stress-reduction program should be sure that any physical problems and medications are closely monitored by a health care provider.
- Psychiatric clients taking psychotropic medications that may cause hypotension should be closely monitored when they do stress-reduction exercises.
- Regular practice enhances the chances of successfully using stress-management techniques.
- People should use the relaxation and stress-management techniques that work best in their individual situations.
- Body tension is an inevitable response to stress; once stress is removed, tension goes away.
- Keeping a stress-awareness diary helps clients identify how particular stresses result in predictable symptoms.
- Breathing calmly and deeply keeps the blood well oxygenated and purified. Breathing properly can, by itself, reduce stress.
- Progressive relaxation teaches clients to decrease physiologic tension and block anxiety by achieving deep muscle relaxation.
- Positive visualizations use a person's own imagination and positive thinking to reduce stress or promote healing.
- The state of meditation is equivalent to a state of deep rest. It helps a person to focus uncritically on one thing at a time to achieve inner peace and harmony.
- Therapeutic touch is the "laying on of hands" to help or heal. It is based on the ability of a healer to transfer excess energy to a client, or to transfer energy from one part of the client's body to another.
- In rolfing, the structural realignment of the body to the forces of gravity is accompanied by a corresponding emotional balance.
- Bioenergetics offers techniques for reducing muscular tension by releasing feelings through physical exercises and verbal techniques.
- Autogenic training is a structured program of exercises that have been found to be effective in the treatment of numerous physical symptoms. It is also used to reduce anxiety, irritability, and fatigue; to modify the reaction to pain; and to reduce or eliminate sleep disorders.
- Self-hypnosis is clinically effective in relieving insomnia, low to moderate levels of chronic pain, tics and tremors, and low to moderate levels of anxiety. It is a well-established treatment for chronic fatigue.
- A behavior-modification technique, thought stopping helps control phobic and obsessional thoughts.
- Irrational self-talk creates stress and mental disorder. Changing irrational beliefs can reduce or eliminate emotional difficulty.
- People can learn to control involuntary body functions through biofeedback, thereby reducing or eliminating stress-related conditions.

References

Bandler R, Grinder J: *Patterns of the Hypnotic Techniques of Milton H. Erickson,* vol 1. Meta Publications, 1975.

Borysenko J: *Fire in the Soul: A New Psychology of Spiritual Optimism.* Warner Books, 1993.

Borysenko J: *Guilt Is the Teacher, Love Is the Lesson.* Warner, 1989.

Borysenko J: *Minding the Body, Mending the Mind.* Addison-Wesley, 1987.

Carlson CR, Hoyle RH: Efficacy of abbreviated progressive muscle relaxation training: A quantitative review of behavioral medicine research. *J Cons Clin Psychol* 1993; 61(6):1059–1067.

Clark PE, Clark MJ: Therapeutic touch: Is there a scientific basis for the practice? *Nurs Res* 1984;33(1):37–41.

Cousins N: *Head First: The Biology of Hope.* Dutton, 1990.

Davis M, Eshelman ER, McKay M: *The Relaxation and Stress-Reduction Workbook,* ed 2. New Harbinger Publications, 1982.

Dossey L: *Healing Words: The Power of Prayer and the Practice of Medicine.* Harper San Francisco, 1993.

Ellis A: *A New Guide to Rational Living.* Prentice-Hall, 1975.

Gagne D, Toye RC: The effects of therapeutic touch and relaxation therapy in reducing anxiety. *Arch Psychiatr Nurs* 1994;8(3):184–189.

Godbey KL, Courage MM: Stress-management program: Intervention in nursing student performance anxiety. *Arch Psychiatr Nurs* 1994;8(3):190–199.

Good M: A comparison of the effects of jaw relaxation and music on postoperative pain. *Nurs Res* 1995;44(1):52–57.

Good M: Relaxation techniques for surgical patients. *Amer J Nurs* 1995;95(5):38–42.

Hahn YB, Ro YJ, Song HH, Kim NC, Kim HS, Yoo YS: The effect of thermal biofeedback and progressive muscle relaxation training in reducing blood pressure of patients with essential hypertension. *Image: J Nurs Scholarship* 1993; 25(3):204–207.

Jacobson E: *Progressive Relaxation.* University of Chicago Press, Midway Reprint, 1975.

Kahn S, Saulo M: *Healing Yourself: A Nurse's Guide to Self-Care and Renewal.* Delmar, 1994.

Kaplan KH, Goldenberg DL, Galvin-Nadeau M: The impact of a meditation-based stress-reduction program on fibromyalgia. *Gen Hosp Psychiatr* 1993;15:284–289.

Keegan L: *The Nurse as Healer.* Delmar, 1994.

Krieger D: *Accepting Your Power to Heal.* Bear & Co., 1993.

Krieger D: *The Therapeutic Touch.* Prentice-Hall, 1979.

Larson D: Helper secrets: Internal stressors in nursing. *J Psychosoc Nurs* 1987;25(4):20–27.

LeShan L: *How to Meditate.* Bantam Books, 1974.

Lowen A: *Bioenergetics.* Penguin Books, 1976.

Luthe W (ed): *Autogenic Therapy,* 6 vols. Grune and Stratton, 1969.

Mackey RB: Discover the healing power of therapeutic touch. *Amer J Nurs* 1995;95(4):26–32.

Mason LJ: *Guide to Stress Reduction.* Celestial Arts, 1986.

Miller NE: Rx: Biofeedback. *Psychol Today* 1985;19:54–59.

Morris F: *Self-Hypnosis in Two Days.* Intergalactic, 1974.

Randolph GL: Therapeutic and physical touch: Physiological response to stressful stimuli. *Nurs Res* 1984;33(1):33–36.

Rolf I: *Rolfing: The Structural Integration of Human Structure.* Rolf Institute, 1977.

Stokols D: A congruence analysis of human stress. *Issues Ment Health Nurs* 1985;7:35–41.

Stroebel CF: *The Quieting Reflex: A Six-Second Technique for Coping with Stress Anytime, Anywhere.* Putnam, 1982.

Tache J, Selye J: On stress and coping mechanisms. *Issues Ment Health Nurs* 1985;7:3–24.

Thompson MB, Coppens NM: The effects of guided imagery on anxiety levels and movement of clients undergoing magnetic resonance imaging. *Holistic Nurse Prac* 1994; 8(2):59–69.

Toivanen H, Helin P, Hanninen O: Impact of regular relaxation training and psychosocial working factors on neck-shoulder tension and absenteeism in hospital cleaners. *JOM* 1993;35(11):1123–1130.

Toivanen H, Lansimies E, Jokela V, Hanninen O: Impact of regular relaxation training on the cardiac autonomic nervous system of hospital cleaners and bank employees. *Scand J Work Environ Health* 1993;19:319–325.

Troesch LM, Rodehaver CB, Delaney EA, Yanes B: The influence of guided imagery on chemotherapy-related nausea and vomiting. *ONF* 1993;20(8):1179–1185.

Vandereycken W, et al.: Body-oriented therapy for anorexia nervosa patients. *Am J Psychother* 1987;41(2):252–259.

Wilson LK: High-gear nursing: How it can run you down and what you can do about it. *Nurs Life* 1986;6:44–47.

Wolinski K: Self-awareness, self-renewal, self-management: Learning to deal effectively with stress. *AORN J* 1993; 88(4):721–730.

Wolpe J: *The Practice of Behavior Therapy.* Pergamon Press, 1969.

CHAPTER 30

CRISIS INTERVENTION

Carol Ren Kneisl
Elizabeth A. Riley

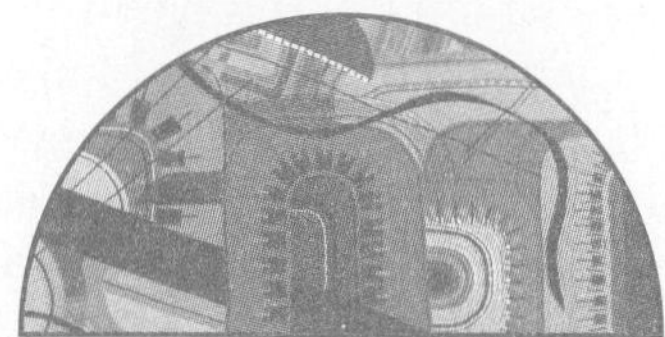

COMPETENCIES

- *Define crisis, crisis intervention, and the types of crises a person may experience.*
- *Trace the sequence of a crisis, and discuss its significance for the nursing care of clients in crisis.*
- *Recognize the DSM-IV diagnostic criteria for acute stress disorder.*
- *Explain the importance of crisis origins and balancing factors in the assessment phase of crisis management.*
- *Discuss three crisis intervention modalities for a person in crisis.*
- *Explain why you may feel overwhelmed in caring for clients who are experiencing a crisis.*

Cross-References

Other topics relevant to this content are: Anxiety, stress, and coping, Chapter 4; Depression, Chapter 15; Ethics, Chapter 10; Nursing intervention in anxiety and panic, Chapter 16; Posttraumatic stress disorder, Chapter 16; Stress management, Chapter 29; Suicide and lethality assessment, Chapter 24; Violence and abuse, Chapters 23 and 34.

Critical Thinking Challenge

You are a nurse working in the emergency department when a client who is a frequent user of emergency services returns for yet another crisis visit. You overhear another staff member say, "Not him again. What is the deal with that person? I can't believe how often he comes in. Can't he work out his problems himself? Besides, I can't tolerate a man crying—how weak!" Do you agree with the staff member? Are there unstated personal or cultural premises involved in those statements? How might the staff member's attitude affect the care the client receives?

What is a crisis? What is stress? What is a trauma? Over the past two decades, there has been a dramatic surge of interest in the impact of stress, stressful life events, and disasters on individuals. Traumatic events are relatively common. However, the impact of the event on an individual is as unique as each individual.

Although stress is not harmful in and of itself, it may precipitate a crisis state if the anxiety accompanying it exceeds the individual's ability to adapt. Anxiety that paralyzes or seriously interferes with usual functioning propels a person into crisis. It is impossible to predict who will or will not experience a crisis as a result of stress.

This chapter explores the period of time when an individual experiences an intolerable stressful event exceeding his or her usual coping resources and resulting in disorganization. This state of crisis has great potential for growth and change for the individual or family. This chapter also explores the variables that affect how an individual will respond.

Nurses are intimately connected with crises. We often interact with people who are faced with new, frightening, and troublesome situations. Because of who we are, where we work, and our accessibility to individuals and families, we are in a position to offer supportive and therapeutic interventions that can change people's lives.

Crisis intervention is not the specialty of any one professional group, however. People who intervene in crises come from the fields of nursing, medicine, psychology, social work, and theology. Police officers, teachers, school guidance counselors, rescue workers, and bartenders, among others, are often on the spot in moments of crisis. Crisis intervention can be the business of many different people.

Biopsychosocial Theories of Crisis

Two events in the 1940s can be said to have provided the starting point for contemporary crisis theory and intervention. One was the report by psychiatrist Erich Lindemann of the crisis response many people had in their direct or indirect experience with the tragic Cocoanut Grove nightclub fire in Boston, in which hundreds of people lost their lives (Cobb and Lindemann 1943; Lindemann 1944). Lindemann's observations and theoretic developments were a landmark in understanding the behavior of people facing emergency situations and the grieving behavior of people who lose loved ones in such situations.

The other event was the observation and treatment by military psychiatrists of battle-weary and emotionally upset military men. In most instances, men who received immediate help at the front lines were able to return to duty rather than being sent to inpatient psychiatric facilities. Later studies and observations during the Korean War added to the knowledge of the behavior of people under stress.

James Tyhurst (1957) contributed further to the understanding of people's responses to natural disasters. He also studied transition states such as parenthood and retirement. Gerald Caplan (1965), who is best known for his work in preventive psychiatry and anticipatory guidance, had similar interests. Many of his methods were tested in the early days of the Peace Corps.

The report of the Joint Commission on Mental Illness and Health (1961) was an important development in crisis work. Soon after publication of the report, large amounts of federal funding were made available for community-based mental health programs. One result was the establishment of suicide prevention and crisis services throughout the country. Crisis telephone counseling services, known popularly as *hotlines,* became common. So did the use of both paid and volunteer nonprofessional crisis workers. As community-based mental health programs became more firmly established and organized, many of them took on these crisis intervention functions.

Norris Hansell (1976) developed a more recent approach to people in crisis. Hansell's work with those in distress is based on findings of the theorists and researchers discussed earlier. In Hansell's social framework approach, the reestablishment of severed social attachments is necessary for successful crisis resolution. In this view, the emphasis is on social factors as the sources of problems.

The importance of evaluating stress, including catastrophic stress and crisis, and its impact on mental health has been clearly recognized. Psychiatry took an important step in this area in 1980. The third edition of the *Diagnostic and Statistical Manual,* published by the American Psychiatric Association in 1980, provided for the first time a system to measure the severity of psychosocial stressors and to reflect that severity within the psychiatric diagnosis (as recorded on Axis IV). The intent was to evaluate the severity of the stressor based on the clinician's assessment of how the stress would affect an average person with similar sociocultural values in a similar situation. Axis V required an overall assessment of how the person functioned in accordance with the stress. This important step demonstrated psychiatry's acceptance and recognition of the link between stress and mental illness.

Crisis Defined

The word *crisis* stems from the Greek *krinein,* "to decide." In Chinese two characters are used to write the word; one is the character for *danger* and the other the character for *opportunity.* A **crisis** is an acute, time-limited state of disequilibrium resulting from situational, developmental, or societal sources of stress. A person in this state is temporarily unable to cope with or adapt to the stressor by using previous methods of problem solving.

To understand the concept fully, we must differentiate among levels of distress to illustrate what a crisis is not. Stress is not crisis. Everyone feels stress at various times, in a variety of forms. Stress is pressure and tension. Stressful situations may demand our attention and may be exhausting, but they are not crises. An emergency is a situation that often demands an immediate response to ensure the survival of an individual. Although an emergency is not itself a crisis, an emergency can ultimately precipitate a crisis. A crisis is not a mental disorder. A crisis can happen to someone who never had a mental disorder or to someone who is currently experiencing a mental disorder.

Crisis situations are turning points or junctures in a person's life. Successful negotiation of a crisis leads either to a return to the precrisis state or to psychologic growth and increased competence. Unsuccessful negotiation of a crisis leaves the person feeling anxious, threatened, and ineffective. Individuals may also respond to a crisis event with disturbed personal coping or with frankly psychotic behavior.

Because a state of disequilibrium is so uncomfortable, a crisis is self-limiting. However, a person experiencing a crisis alone is more vulnerable to unsuccessful negotiation than a person working through a crisis with help. Working with another person increases the likelihood that the person in crisis will resolve it in a positive way.

Factors that place individuals at high risk for crisis are:

- Intensity of exposure to the situation.
- Low educational level.
- Preexisting psychiatric symptoms and diagnosis.
- Prior history of traumatic exposure.
- Family history of psychiatric problems.
- Early separation from parents.
- Family history of anxiety and/or antisocial behavior.
- Childhood abuse.
- Poverty.
- Cultural expectations that prohibit asking others for help.
- Degree of threat to life involved in exposure to the situation (being on a plane that crashes versus watching a plane crash from a distance).

Common characteristics of crises are as follows:

- All crises are experienced as sudden. The person is usually not aware of a warning signal, whether or not others could "see it coming." The individual or family may feel that they have little or no preparation for the event or trauma.
- The crisis is often experienced as ultimately life-threatening, whether this perception is realistic or not.
- Communication with significant others is often decreased or cut off.
- There may be perceived or real displacement from familiar surroundings or significant loved ones.
- All crises have an aspect of loss, whether actual or perceived. The losses can include an object, person, a hope, a dream, or any significant factor for that individual.

In the contemporary view, the origin of a crisis is as important as the type of crisis. Hoff (1989) points out that if we know how the crisis began, we have a better opportunity to intervene effectively. The three categories of crisis origins are:

1. Situational (traditional term: unanticipated).
2. Transitional (traditional terms: maturational, anticipated).
3. Cultural/social.

Situational Crisis

Situational crises can originate from three sources: material or environmental (fire or natural disaster); personal or physical (heart attack, diagnosis of fatal illness, bodily disfigurement); and interpersonal or social (death of a loved one or divorce). These situations are usually unplanned and unexpected. Because the event leading to the crisis is usually unexpected, one generally cannot do anything directly to prevent it. In a more indirect sense, an individual can attempt to keep healthy and focus on the most effective methods of interacting with others. However, the complexity of the experience influences the ability of the individual to resolve the trauma. For instance, a person coping with one traumatic incident is more likely to resolve the experience than someone faced with multiple traumas or factors.

An example of a situational crisis (in which the origin of the crisis is the husband's diagnosis of terminal cancer) follows:

Sally, age 52, is a social worker at a local mental health clinic, who is feeling increasingly less able to function. She learned 3 days ago that her husband has a terminal form of cancer that is inoperable. They were married approximately a year ago. Many arrangements need to be made, including finding adequate medical treatment and doing appropriate evaluations on her husband. Sally has been unable to work for 2–3 days and now tells a psychiatric nurse that she can no longer function and doesn't know what to do. Sally has been unable to make any of the required phone calls, despite knowing she is the person who must coordinate all of this. She says she can't "think straight" and that she is becoming more frightened of talking to the doctors. She shakes her head and says, "Can you believe it, I do this all the time for others, but I can't do it now. Isn't that a joke?" She speaks of being overwhelmed. "What am I going to do without him?"

Transitional Crisis

This category consists of two types, universal and nonuniversal transition states. *Universal transition states* are life cycle changes or normal transitions of human development. These are the traditional stages of human development that include infancy, childhood, puberty, adolescence, adulthood, middle age, and old age. During each stage, the individual is subject to unique stressors. Each stage of development is characterized by developmental tasks the individual must accomplish to progress to the next level. A failure at any one level compromises the next stage of development.

People in transition usually experience increased anxiety and tension as they move through each successive stage. For every stage, there are changes in expectations, roles, sense of self, body image, and attitudes toward others. Thus, the stages are predictable, and the nurse can help with preventive, educative techniques.

The second category of transition states, termed *nonuniversal transition states,* includes such changes as marriage, retirement, and the transition from student to worker. Crises associated with these states arise when the individual enters a new area of development or functioning and cannot adapt to functioning at that level. Crises originating from these sources differ from situational crises. Nonuniversal transition states are like developmental transition states in that they can usually be anticipated and prepared for. Unlike developmental events or transitions, however, they are not experienced by everyone. An individual in a transitional state is at risk for experiencing a crisis. If the person experiences additional trauma or change, the risk increases. Whenever people experience more than two life changes or traumatic events, their coping capacity may be strained, and the potential for crisis becomes greater.

An example of a transitional crisis (where the origin of the crisis is a decision to divorce) follows:

Jennifer, age 31, is currently married with three children. Over the past 3 months, her husband has been drinking excessively. Over the same period, they have been evicted from two apartments, her husband has lost his job, and there is often little food available for the children. Jennifer has decided to divorce her husband. Two nights ago she took her clothes and belongings, put them in the car with her three children, and left home. Although she was hoping to drive to her sister's home in the next state, she was exhausted last night and fell asleep in the car for a few hours. Jennifer awoke when her husband pulled her out of the car, threw her into the street, and beat her with a bat. He threatened that if she did not come home, he "would finish the job." Jennifer has just come into the crisis unit after having been found by the police, crying, sobbing, and mumbling incoherently. Jennifer's children accompany her to the crisis unit and remain mute.

The following clinical example demonstrates how multiple stressors may overwhelm a client:

Bernie is a 62-year-old man. For 40 years, he has carried a diagnosis of schizophrenia, paranoid type. For the last 20 years, he has avoided repeated hospitalizations and exacerbations of his illness because he and his wife Alice have been alert for beginning signs of problems, and he has continued to take his medication. In October their apartment caught fire and burned. Bernie and Alice were upset about losing their home but thankful that they and their dog escaped without injury.

Neighbors rallied around them and helped Bernie and Alice find and furnish a new apartment. Things appeared to return to normal. Then in November, Alice died after a stroke. Bernie was very sad but continued to live in the new apartment. He increased his visits to the mental health clinic, and his widowed sister visited daily. Bernie's medication remained at the same level, and he did not experience additional symptoms. In December, Bernie's dog died. Shortly after that, he experienced a mild heart attack. Bernie felt lost and alone. Because of the cardiac problems, Bernie's former medication, which he believed kept him from hallucinating, was now contraindicated. Bernie became increasingly depressed and stated that he had nothing to live for. He began to experience auditory hallucinations, which were not immediately controlled by the new medications. In January, Bernie took an overdose of his cardiac and neuroleptic medications. The next day his sister found him dead.

Crises that originate from situational and transitional states can be less complex and more easily treated than cultural/social crises.

Cultural/Social Crisis

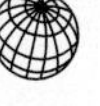

Crises with cultural and social sources include the loss of a job stemming from discrimination, being the victim of deviant acts of others, and behavior that violates social norms, such as robbery, rape, incest, marital infidelity, and physical abuse. These crises are never expected, but they are still somewhat predictable. Crises arising from sociocultural sources are less amenable to control by individuals. There is often a stronger component of community control or influence. Very often, cultural views or government action may be a component of either the identification or the resolution of these crises.

An example of a cultural/social crisis follows. There is a threefold origin to this crisis:

1. The community's concern about the children who were abducted.
2. The blaming of an African-American male.
3. Subsequent information that the mother killed the children herself.

In late October 1994, the entire nation watched and worried with a young mother in South Carolina when she reported that her two children had been abducted during a carjacking. The mother described an African-American male as the person responsible for this terrible event. Worry and sadness turned to anger, shock, and disbelief within the community when 9 days later, the mother confessed to allowing the car with the children in it to roll into a lake. The children drowned in the submerged car. African-Americans expressed anger and outrage because allegations had been made against a black male. The small, close-knit community experienced two sources of disequilibrium: that one of their "own" people had killed her own children, and that racial tensions had further divided the community.

Community and church leaders arranged for memorial services for the children and began the crucial task of restoring equilibrium in the community. All agree it will be a long time before things return to the way they were before the crisis occurred.

Crisis Sequencing

A crisis typically has these three stages: precrisis, crisis, and postcrisis. One assumption in crisis theory is that all individuals are in a state of dynamic equilibrium with their environment. We try to maintain equilibrium by adapting or coping with the events of daily living.

At times in everyone's life, situations occur that have the potential to disrupt the equilibrium and may result in a crisis. Factors that influence whether or not an individual enters a crisis state are called balancing factors. These are described in a later section. Myths about crisis are contrasted with realities about crisis in the accompanying box below.

Precrisis Stage

The *precrisis stage* is the stage of maintaining or attempting to maintain equilibrium. If successful, the person avoids a crisis and reverts to a state of dynamic equilibrium. If the problem(s) are too severe or if the balancing factors are inadequate, equilibrium is not maintained, the problem is not solved, and a crisis results.

Crisis Stage

The *crisis stage* is the reaction to the event, problem, or trauma, not the event itself. Reactions to such events or traumas are highly individual. In this stage, the balancing

Myths and Realities About Crisis

Myth	*Reality*
People in crisis are suffering from a form of mental illness.	Not everyone who is in crisis is "mentally ill"; however, people who are in crisis may have had a prior emotional problem. Inadequate resolution of a crisis may result in more chronic emotional problems.
People in crisis cannot help themselves.	Many who work with people in crisis mistakenly believe this myth. This belief often leads to an incomplete or compromised resolution of the crisis. It also leaves people who work with those in crisis at risk for rescue fantasies, feeling overwhelmed and burned out.
Only psychiatrists or highly trained therapists can effectively help people in crisis.	A great deal of crisis work has been done by volunteers, police, ministers, and front-line workers. Many mental health care professionals have not completed courses in crisis training.
Crisis intervention is merely a stopgap or Band-Aid, a trivial approach in comparison with "real therapy" given by professionals.	This myth is slowly fading as more people become acquainted with crisis intervention techniques. Crisis intervention may be the preferred treatment, especially if the individual was functioning at a high level prior to the crisis.
Crisis intervention is a form of psychotherapy.	While crisis intervention is not a Band-Aid, it is also not psychotherapy.
Crisis intervention happens only as a "one-time shot" and produces changes for a short time.	Crisis intervention is often done in two to eight sessions over a 6-week period. Crisis intervention has been shown to have long-lasting benefits.

Source: Adapted from Hoff 1989, pp. 6–8.

factors have failed, and the individual is in a full crisis state. In this state of disequilibrium, the individual cannot apply previous methods of reducing tension and anxiety. Inner turmoil and intrapersonal conflict are great, as are anxiety and tension. The person may make erratic attempts to solve the problem. Significant others may observe a disorganization that is uncharacteristic of that person.

The crisis stage is so disruptive that an individual cannot maintain this state for long. Crisis stages are time-limited and do not last longer than 6 weeks.

Postcrisis Stage

Because the crisis stage is time-limited, everyone who experiences a crisis enters the *postcrisis stage.* During this stage, the individual arrives at or develops a new equilibrium. This new equilibrium may be close to that of the precrisis state, or it may be a more positive or more negative state. If the new equilibrium is more positive, the person experiences growth and may now have a better social network, newfound problem-solving abilities, or an improved self-image. If the new equilibrium is more negative, it is possible that the individual may lose skills, adopt a regressive stance, or develop socially unacceptable behaviors.

Not all people who are exposed to stress (even extreme stress) experience serious or prolonged problems. Approximately 80% of all people who are confronted with serious life experiences are able to work through these situations themselves with support from significant others. The remaining 20% have difficulties that require intervention and assistance.

Some applicable psychiatric diagnoses for people who experience a mental disorder following a crisis are:

- Acute stress disorder
- Major depressive disorder

DSM-IV Diagnostic Criteria for Acute Stress Disorder

A. The person has been exposed to a traumatic event in which *both* of the following were present:
   1. The person experienced, witnessed, or was confronted with an event or events that involved actual or threatened death or serious injury, or a threat to the physical integrity of self or others.
   2. The person's response involved intense fear, helplessness, or horror.

B. Either while experiencing or after experiencing the distressing event, the individual has *three (or more)* of the following dissociative symptoms:
   1. A subjective sense of numbing, detachment, or absence of emotional responsiveness.
   2. A reduction in awareness of his or her surroundings (e.g., "being in a daze").
   3. Derealization.
   4. Depersonalization.
   5. Dissociative amnesia (i.e., inability to recall an important aspect of the trauma).

C. The traumatic event is persistently reexperienced in at least one of the following ways: recurrent images, thoughts, dreams, illusions, flashback episodes, or a sense of reliving the experience; or distress on exposure to reminders of the traumatic event.

D. Marked avoidance of stimuli that arouse recollections of the trauma (e.g., thoughts, feelings, conversations, activities, places, people).

E. Marked symptoms of anxiety or increased arousal (e.g., difficulty sleeping, irritability, poor concentration, hypervigilance, exaggerated startle response, motor restlessness).

F. The disturbance causes clinically significant distress or impairment in social, occupational, or other important areas of function or impairs the individual's ability to pursue some necessary task, such as obtaining necessary assistance or mobilizing personal resources by telling family members about the traumatic experience.

G. The disturbance lasts for a *minimum of 2 days* and a *maximum of 4 weeks* and occurs *within 4 weeks* of the traumatic event.

H. The disturbance is not due to the direct physiological effects of a substance (e.g., a drug of abuse, a medication) or a general medical condition, is not better accounted for by Brief Psychotic Disorder, and is not merely an exacerbation of a preexisting Axis I or Axis II disorder.

Source: American Psychiatric Association 1994, pp. 429–430.

- Adjustment disorder with depressed mood
- Adjustment disorder with anxiety
- Adjustment disorder with disturbance of conduct
- Adjustment disorder NOS
- Posttraumatic stress disorder
- Adjustment disorder with mixed disturbance of emotions and conduct
- Adjustment disorder with mixed anxiety and depressed mood

Acute stress disorder is a common postcrisis diagnosis when symptoms occur within 1 month after exposure to an extreme traumatic stressor. The DSM-IV diagnostic criteria are given in the accompanying box.

Although not every person experiencing a life change needs psychotherapy, most people benefit from information, support, and advice. An individual's resiliency and vulnerability to stress are important (see Chapter 4).

Balancing Factors

Who will enter a crisis state, since not everyone does? Many factors determine whether a person faced with a life change or traumatic event will enter a crisis period. The nature of the trauma or experience is one influence on the resolution of the crisis. In addition, the greater the number of balancing factors, the more effective the resolution. Aguilera (1994) indicates that these three balancing factors are important to the successful resolution of a crisis:

- *Perception of the event:* how individuals perceive and understand the event/crisis in their lives. Are they being punished? Is this happening only to them and never to anyone else? How will the event affect their future? Do they see the situation realistically, or is it distorted?
- *Situational supports:* the availability of people who can help individuals in crisis solve the problem. Meaningful relationships with others give support and assistance during the crisis. Individuals with inadequate support are likely to experience a decrease in self-esteem. In turn, lowered self-esteem may make an event appear more threatening.
- *Coping mechanisms.* All people use mechanisms to cope with anxiety and tension. Because the individual has used these coping mechanisms with success in the past, they become part of the coping repertoire. These tension-relieving mechanisms can be obvious or subtle (see the discussion in Chapter 4).

If all these balancing factors are present when an individual experiences a state of disequilibrium, it is unlikely that a crisis will result. Figure 30–1 illustrates how these balancing factors affect the outcome of a stressful event.

The Nursing Process and Crisis Intervention

Crisis intervention as a therapeutic strategy is strongly humanistic. People are viewed as capable of personal growth and as having the ability to influence and control their own lives. According to these concepts, the task of the person who intervenes in the crisis is to help the individual understand what combination of events led to the crisis, and guide the individual toward a resolution that will meet the person's unique needs and foster future growth and strength. Especially during the acute phase, the goal of crisis intervention is to restore the person to the pretrauma level of functioning as quickly as possible. This can be accomplished by taking advantage of rapid therapeutic gains that are possible when the person's normal defenses are relatively permeable or weakened. As the disequilibrium subsides, reorganization takes place. This state is generally seen as adaptive and integrative. However, it can also be maladaptive, and might result in further crises or even be destructive. Intervention prior to a maladaptive response is the goal of crisis intervention. The traditional steps of the nursing process correspond closely to the steps of crisis intervention.

Assessment

Assessment of the individual is the first phase of crisis intervention. The nurse or helper must focus on the person and the problem. Collect data about the client, the client's coping style, the precipitating event, the situational supports, the client's perception of the crisis, and the client's ability to handle the problem. This is an essential and critical step of crisis intervention. This information is the basis for later decisions about how and when to intervene, and whom to call.

Also assess and evaluate the client's suicide potential. (See Chapter 24 for lethality assessment.) During this time, a client may need to be hospitalized to ensure safety, and a referral to the psychiatrist or emergency room of the local hospital may be necessary. Part of the overall assessment is to determine what is necessary to return this client to a state of equilibrium; this may be different from what is necessary to solve the problem.

Often the "symptom bearer" or "identified patient" may really be seeking help for the entire family. The crisis may be a response to a family problem.

Kristen, age 13, was referred to the school nurse after talking openly in the classroom about suicide. Kristen lived with her mother, and she had changed schools three times during this school year because of her mother's recent hospitalization. Initially, it appeared that Kristen was reacting to the

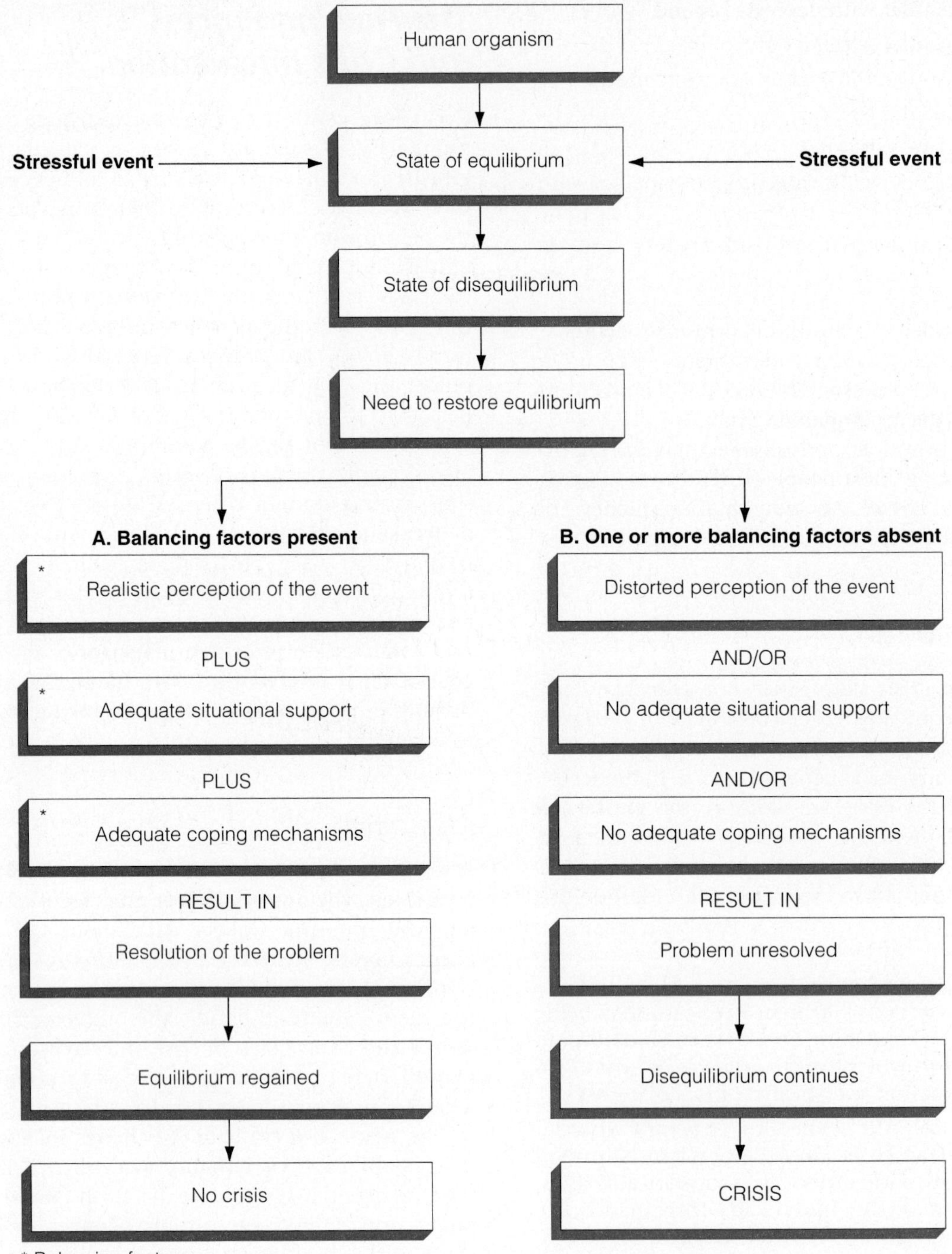

Figure 30–1 The effect of balancing factors in a stressful event. Source: Aguilera 1994, p. 66.

multiple moves and her mother's hospitalization. However, after further interviews with both mother and Kristen, the problem became much clearer. Kristen's father had not been able to see her despite her recent attempts to connect with him. He had been a source of support during her mother's absence. Kristen later said she was frightened that her mother would be rehospitalized and that no one would be there for her. Her parents continued to have a stormy relationship after their divorce, and often arguments would end in cold silences. Kristen said she was frightened and that she wanted and needed some attention. She mentioned being "terrified that I might be all alone." She thought her talk of suicide might make her parents stop fighting and bring them back together.

Some common family crises are the death of a family member, the terminal illness of a family member, single parenting, divorce, drug/alcohol dependence, family violence, infidelity, remarriage, mental illness, incest, and "empty nest syndrome." These usually come under the heading of situational or transitional crises. To intervene effectively, meet with as many family members as possible to assess family resources, coping skills, and interpersonal styles. Very often these crises accompany role changes or additional stress in families that do not have the resources to meet the challenge.

A critically important source of the meaning of an individual's response to stress or trauma is the broader sociocultural context in which the person lives. Lebowitz and Roth (1994) defined this sociocultural context as the ideas, beliefs, and metaphors that emerge from our cultural productions and institutions (literature, media, religion, law, etc.), which can form a recognizable and coherent ideology and are relevant for a particular event. To be effective in sociocultural assessment, you must become aware of the influences and beliefs from your own experiences and be knowledgeable about other cultures. If you are not familiar with a client's culture, ask respectful questions to help the client to fully express his or her distress. For example, "I want to understand how all of this might affect you. Can you tell me more about how you feel about this situation? Tell me how your neighbors might feel about it."

Children and Adolescents Because the coping repertoire of children and adolescents is usually limited—their defenses are immature and they lack life experiences—they are particularly vulnerable to stress and stress responses. The reactions of children to disaster and to crisis are as varied as children themselves and may range from talking frankly about the crisis, complaining of somatic problems without a physical cause, having frightening nightmares, or becoming mute. A wide range of interventions is required. For the child who is in a crisis episode, the home and school are strong supports because of the child's dependence on family members and other adults to provide guidance. When assessing a child or an adolescent in crisis, review the individual factors as well as the resources of the family and the support network.

Webb (1991) points out that there are five factors that comprise the assessment of the child or adolescent.

1. *Age and developmental level.* Specific developmental stages have corresponding expectations about a child's level of cognitive and moral development. Interventions will be quite different for a 12-year-old than a 4-year-old. Precrisis adjustment is an important factor in the assessment of children and adolescents. Information about how the children had been getting along at home and at school with peers prior to the crisis helps gauge the impact of the stress on the child.
2. *Coping style and ego assessment.* This area relates to the child's precrisis adjustment and temperamental style. It assesses particularly the individual's current level of anxiety, ability to separate from parents, and ability to discuss the problem or crisis situation in the presence of symptoms. It also requires an assessment of the child's use of defenses.
3. *Past experience with crisis.* A review of the child's history helps the crisis evaluator understand and evaluate the current level of anxiety.
4. *Global assessment of functioning.* This is the DSM-IV Axis V combined with the specific meaning of the crisis to the child. There may be differences in how the child can clarify the personal meaning of the crisis. When the conflict is close enough to the surface, the child might acknowledge it openly. At other times, it is not possible or desirable to seek information if it might be too threatening. However, it is understood that the underlying meaning of the crisis must be understood by the nurse so that the treatment goals can be appropriately established.
5. *Elements in the support system.* Elements in the support system of a child or adolescent include the nuclear and extended family, the school family, and community supports. Information about these areas makes it easier to incorporate potential resources in the child's network of church, friends, school, health care, and other institutions. It is important to note that with children and adolescents, as with adults, individual characteristics ultimately may determine how, or even whether, supports are used. Even though supports might be available, an individual who is in a vulnerable state or has had multiple past crises may be unable to cope.

Nursing Diagnosis

People in crisis may have a variety of problems and symptoms. They may appear overwhelmed, calm, or agitated. They may speak clearly or be psychotic. An individual's perception of the event and personal response will determine the nursing diagnoses. The most common nursing diagnoses for people in crisis are:

- Ineffective Individual Coping
- Ineffective Family Coping
- Altered Family Process
- Impaired Adjustment
- Anxiety
- Spiritual Distress
- Knowledge Deficit
- Impaired Verbal Communication
- Post-Trauma Response
- Altered Role Performance
- Risk for Violence: Self-Directed
- Risk for Violence: Directed at Others

- Self-Care Deficit
- Hopelessness
- Fatigue
- Fear
- Chronic (or Situational) Low Self Esteem
- Rape-Trauma Syndrome

Planning and Implementing Interventions

Effective planning for crisis intervention must be:

- Based on careful assessment.
- Developed in active collaboration with the person in crisis and the significant people in that person's life.
- Focused on immediate, concrete, contributing problems.
- Based on an understanding of human dependence needs.
- Appropriate to the person's level of thinking, feeling, and behaving.
- Consistent with the person's lifestyle and culture.
- Time limited, concrete, and realistic.
- Mutually negotiated and renegotiated.
- Organized to provide for follow-up.

CRISIS COUNSELING **Crisis counseling** is a type of brief therapy. Unlike therapies that focus on bringing about major personality changes, crisis counseling focuses on solving immediate problems. It lasts five or six sessions and involves individuals, groups, or families. The following techniques are used:

- Listening actively and with concern.
- Encouraging the open expression of feelings.
- Helping the client gain an understanding of the crisis.
- Helping the client gradually accept reality.
- Helping the client explore new ways of coping with problems.
- Linking the client to a social network.
- Engaging in decision counseling or problem solving with the client.
- Reinforcing newly learned coping devices.
- Following up the case after resolution of the crisis.

TELEPHONE COUNSELING Suicide prevention and crisis intervention centers rely heavily on telephone counseling by volunteers who have professional consultation available to them. Also known as hotlines and often available around the clock, they allow callers to remain anonymous and test what it feels like to ask for assistance. No appointment, travel time, or money is necessary, and help is immediately available. The volunteers usually work within a protocol that indicates what information they need from the client to assess the crisis. Their goal is to plan steps to provide immediate relief and then long-term follow-up if necessary.

The calls made to a hotline usually fall into one of four categories: crisis calls, ventilation calls, combinations of ventilation and information calls, or information-only calls. Calls that request information and ventilation are handled by supportive listening and the giving of information. Crisis calls need special techniques. An example of a step-by-step protocol that volunteers might use on a hotline follows.

1. Always remain calm. Anxiety on your part can make the client's anxiety worse.
2. Assess the safety of the caller. Ask questions like:
   a. Are you in a safe place to talk?
   b. Are you free of injury at this time?
   c. Do you need any emergency assistance?
3. Attempt to get the name, phone number, and address of the caller.
   a. Ask specific questions about whether guns or weapons are involved or available close by. Ask specific questions about the level and extent of prior violence in the home and with the individuals involved.
   b. Assess the involvement of vulnerable people or children.
      - Ask specific questions: Have the children been abused, threatened, harmed in any way?
      - Remember that you may need to make a report to Child Protective Services if there is any abuse or danger to a child.
   c. Use counseling tools to deepen the connection.
      - Use active listening skills.
      - Ask open-ended questions that allow the caller to give you more information.
      - Paraphrase what the caller has said to ensure that you understand what has been stated.
      - Allow feelings to emerge and be expressed.
      - Validate feelings.
4. Help the individual form an action plan.
   a. Determine whether direct action is needed, for example, to call the police or to get somebody to an emergency room.
   b. Develop a safety plan that will incorporate actions to take in the event that the danger reemerges.
   c. Give education and information about the particular problem the person is calling about. For example, if the call is about being physically abused, give specific information about abuse and the cycle of violence.
   d. Help the caller prioritize what he or she needs to do next.
   e. Set realistic goals with the caller about what is possible to be done. For example, if there are multiple needs (financial or social support), remind the

caller that it is going to take some time to get those needs fulfilled and goals accomplished.

f. Provide referrals to resources or individuals who have the potential to assist the person.

The following points are also important to consider in telephone counseling:

- If the caller is reluctant to give a name and location, do not press for this information. The caller may feel threatened and hang up.
- Listen for background noises that may give clues to the caller's location.
- Use a note pad to write messages to coworkers so that the conversation is not interrupted.
- Keep the caller talking. This gives you time to begin to develop a relationship, to trace the call, or to contact relatives or the police if necessary.
- Emphasize that you are available to talk as long as the caller needs to do so.
- Reinforce positive responses and actions, such as the fact that the caller is talking instead of acting-out hopeless feelings.
- Acknowledge that the caller feels distress but explain that he or she does not need to inflict self-harm to emphasize it.
- Do not overuse reflection of feelings, which, in this setting, may sound uncaring or superficial. Instead, offer direction and solutions to problems.
- If the caller is threatening immediate harm to self or to others, notify the police, an area mental health crisis unit, or family members to intervene with the caller. Most hotlines have the ability to trace phone calls.
- To fully assess the client for suicide risk, perform a lethality assessment (see Chapter 24).

This type of intervention can be very stressful for the nurse/counselor. It is important to remember that despite our efforts to communicate concern, the ultimate decision maker is the caller.

Home Crisis Visits Home visits are made when telephone counseling does not suffice or when the crisis workers need to obtain additional information by direct observation or to reach a client who is unobtainable by telephone. Home visits are appropriate when crisis workers need to initiate contacts rather than waiting for clients to come to them—for example, when a telephone caller is assessed to be highly suicidal or when a concerned neighbor, physician, or clergyman informs the agency of clients in potential crisis.

Often these clients are too disorganized or distraught to seek help by themselves. The police may arrange for a home crisis visit to avoid imprisoning or hospitalizing a client. Problems commonly encountered are spousal abuse, child abuse, psychiatric emergencies, and medical emergencies.

The crisis workers are usually a team consisting of a man and a woman who are highly skilled and experienced in crisis intervention. The male-female team is generally perceived as less threatening than two men, two women, or a single person. Their goal is to defuse the situation with as little disruption and violence as possible and to engage the clients in longer-term treatment. They may also be members of mobile crisis units.

There are others who intervene in community crises as well. The public health nurse is in an excellent position to identify, assess, and intervene with clients experiencing a life crisis. Public health nurses often have access to community resources as well as informal communication lines, and they usually maintain contact with families and clients for longer periods of time than nurses in other settings. They are often recognized by the community as knowledgeable experts who are available for immediate assistance.

Emily, age 78, and her sister Frances, age 84, lived in a rundown part of town. Frances became seriously ill with pneumonia and became progressively weaker. Emily became more anxious about Frances's health when her sister refused to see a doctor. Emily was afraid her sister would die or need to go to a nursing home. Emily felt paralyzed and didn't know what to do. When the visiting nurse came by to visit Emily's neighbor, Emily asked the nurse to see Frances. Together they were able to persuade Frances to get medical care so that she could stay home.

Other Interventions One-to-one interventions are important to an individual in crisis. However, nurses who work with people in crisis often need to use many nontraditional interventions, which can be as important as any verbal interventions. Nurses who work successfully with people in crisis must have a flexible, open view of what may be therapeutic with different individuals. They must have a full repertoire of skills and interventions that can be individualized to help all types of clients in crisis. Some examples of these interventions follow.

Assisting with Environmental Changes

- Finding shelter for a homeless person.
- Obtaining shelter for an abused woman and her children.
- Arranging for a home health aide to care for a family member.

Assisting with Planned Events

- Discussing methods of contraception with adolescents or young men and women.

- Preparing a child for a tonsillectomy.
- Arranging for a volunteer from the Reach for Recovery Program to visit a woman who has had a mastectomy.

Helping Develop Social Supports

- Introducing a woman whose husband is an alcoholic to Al-Anon groups in her community.
- Referring a family with a terminally ill member to a local hospice.
- Giving a rape victim the telephone number of the rape crisis hotline.

Evaluation and Outcome Criteria

Nurses in acute care or short-term settings may not see the long-term effects of their interventions. Typically, nurses in these settings need to evaluate the crisis, set up the plan, and begin implementing it.

In long-term settings, the nurse can evaluate the client or family response to the intervention by determining whether clients have resumed their precrisis level of functioning or show evidence of increased functioning (growth). A nurse in either a long-term or short-term setting may also have an opportunity to evaluate whether a similar problem might lead to another crisis for the client.

The Nursing Process and Natural and Human-Made Disasters

Over the past two decades, natural disasters have killed 3 billion people worldwide, adversely affected the lives of 800 million more people, and resulted in immediate economic damage exceeding 23 billion U.S. dollars (World Health Organization 1988). Federal aid designated for reconstruction has been available for many years, and crisis intervention services have been provided through the National Institute of Mental Health (NIMH) since 1972. Yet we have only recently begun to study the psychologic impact of a disaster. Weisaeth (1993) notes that in the past there was a general tendency to only consider the basic needs (shelter, food, sanitation, and immunization) of disaster victims. Psychologic needs were considered secondary and did not attract the attention of relief workers and agencies. Although disasters occur worldwide, it is the smallest and poorest countries that are affected most severely by them. Therefore, their populations are most at risk for greater psychologic impact.

Because disasters represent a major public health priority in most developing countries, WHO's role has gradually shifted from providing emergency relief to disaster preparedness and response. As a result, the United Nations General Assembly adopted a resolution in 1987 to designate the 1990s the decade for natural disaster reduction (World Health Organization 1988). They have established a goal that by the end of the 1990s, 70% of all countries participating in that organization will have developed an emergency disaster master plan that will incorporate both physical and mental health components.

Nurses as citizens are often at the scene of natural disasters or may be called upon to help. Nurses can be particularly helpful during the initial stage of the crisis because they have skills needed to perform physical assessments, provide care to the injured, and assess psychologic distress. Nurses will also have their own personal reaction to the disaster. These reactions are outlined later in the chapter.

Assessment

There are many typologies about how people experience disaster and the stages of a disaster response. The classic work was done by James Tyhurst. More contemporary researchers have expanded some stages to reflect additional steps. It is important and useful to understand Tyhurst's stages to recognize how an individual may respond and what the most effective tools for intervention may be. It is important to note that as with any other theoretic formulation, individuals do not always progress through the stages in a neat, orderly fashion. Individual differences will account for each person's ability to process information, to be reassured, and to resolve the experience.

Tyhurst (1951, 1957) identifies three overlapping stages in response to disaster. The first stage, *impact,* is stimulated by the catastrophe. The victims recognize what is happening to them and are concerned mainly with the present. During this acute phase, the victim's major concern may be staying alive. According to Tyhurst, about 75% of the victims experience shock and confusion. Although they appear dazed, they also exhibit the physical signs of fear. Another group of people, up to 25%, remain coherent. They logically and rationally assess the situation and develop and implement a plan for dealing with the immediate problems brought on by the catastrophe. A third group, also up to 25%, may panic or become immobilized with fear. They may behave hysterically, or they may be overlooked because they sit and silently stare into space.

In *recoil,* the second stage, the initial stress of the disaster has passed, and victims may no longer find their lives in immediate danger, although injuries and other discomforts come to their awareness. Emergency shelter, food, and clothing become available. Their behavior is usually dependent—they want to be taken care of. Weeping is common as survivors begin to realize all that has happened to them.

The full impact of the losses the victims have experienced comes in the third, or *posttrauma,* period. Grief is a predominant response to the losses in their lives. Disturbed and psychotic responses may occur.

Many people essentially "relive" the experience in their dreams by having recurrent nightmares. Other sleep disturbances, including insomnia, often occur. Victims may feel a psychic numbing or emotional anesthesia in relation to other people, previously enjoyed activities, and in response to intimacy, tenderness, and sexuality. They may have difficulty concentrating and remembering. The survivors of mass trauma may also feel guilty about having survived or about behavior that helped them survive. When victims are exposed to situations that resemble or in some way symbolize the traumatic event, their symptoms may increase, and they may feel even greater distress.

Assistance that is given as soon as possible, preferably during the acute phase, often prevents a longer-lasting trauma response. This is why crisis intervention is sometimes referred to as primary prevention for posttraumatic stress disorder (PTSD).

Interventions to address the longer-lasting effects of a traumatic incident are more complicated than interventions in the acute phase of crisis intervention. These principles are indicated for intervention in the posttrauma response:

- Establishing the therapeutic trust relationship.
- Education regarding the trauma recovery process.
- Stress management and stress reduction.
- Possible regression back to or a reexperiencing of the trauma.
- Integration of the trauma experience.

The brief examples below illustrate the posttrauma experience.

In October 1994, an airplane crashed in the Midwest. All 68 people on board were killed, although luckily no one on the ground was injured or killed. During the gruesome search to identify the deceased, family members and body handlers were distressed that bones and parts of extremities were found, but very few people's bodies were left intact. For the first time, psychologic assistance was given to body handlers at the site to help them cope with the psychologic difficulties of their job.

At Cape Canaveral, Florida, on January 28, 1986, the space shuttle *Challenger* exploded seconds after launching. All seven astronauts aboard were killed. The entire nation grieved. Each replaying of the videotape of the explosion renewed the grief of the families and of the nation.

In a heavy Colorado snowstorm, over 100 people were involved in a 60-car pile-up on a major interstate highway. Ten people died as a result of injuries sustained during the crash. One month later, people who live nearby are startled whenever they hear car brakes or horns. Eight people involved in the crash still will not drive.

Nursing Diagnosis

The nursing diagnoses for these clients depend on their individual responses. The nursing diagnoses listed earlier in this chapter are also appropriate in natural disasters.

Planning and Implementing Interventions

The type of help needed by disaster victims changes as the disaster unfolds. Initially, people need information about evacuation plans, rescue efforts, and the location of food, shelter, and medical care. The media can provide this information, especially when there is time to plan and anticipate need (as with floods or hurricanes). Table 30–1 outlines the process of assistance during natural disasters.

After acute needs are met at the disaster scene, in makeshift hospitals, or in emergency rooms, morgues, and shelters, more far-reaching interventions are necessary. People need housing, jobs, and help in reconstructing their emotional lives. These are the psychologic needs of victims both during and after a disaster:

- Talking about the experience and expressing their feelings of fear, panic, loss, and grief.
- Becoming fully aware and accepting of what has happened to them.
- Resuming concrete activities and reconstructing their lives with the social, physical, and emotional resources available.

To guide victims through the crisis, crisis workers should:

- Listen with concern and sympathy, and ease the way for them to tell their tragic story, weep, express feelings of anger, loss, frustration, and despair.
- Help them accept in small doses the tragic reality of what has happened. This means staying with them during the initial stages of shock and denial. It also may mean accompanying them back to the scene of the tragedy and being available for support when they are faced with the full impact of their loss.
- Help them make contact with relatives, friends, and other resources required for beginning the process of social and physical reconstruction. This could mean making telephone calls to locate relatives, accompanying someone to apply for financial aid, or giving information about social and mental health care agencies for follow-up services.

Table 30–1 Assistance During Three Stages of Natural Disaster

	Help Needed	*Help Provided by*	*Possible Outcomes If Help Is Unavailable*
Stage I: Impact	Information on source and degree of danger	Communication network: radio, TV, public address system	Physical injury or death
	Escape and rescue from immediate source of danger	Community rescue resources: police and fire departments, Red Cross, National Guard	
Stage II: Recoil	Shelter, food, drink, clothing, medical care	Red Cross	Physical injury
		Salvation Army	Delayed grief reactions
		Voluntary agencies such as colleges used as mass shelters	Later emotional or mental disturbance
		Local health and welfare agencies	
		Mental health and social service agencies skilled in crisis intervention	
		Pastoral counselors	
		State and federal assistance for all of the above services	
Stage III: Posttrauma	Physical reconstruction	State and federal resources for physical reconstruction	Financial hardship
	Social reestablishment	Social welfare agencies	Social instability
	Psychologic support concerning aftereffects of the event itself; bereavement counseling concerning loss of loved ones, home, and personal property	Crisis and mental health services	Long-lasting mental, emotional, or physical health problems
		Pastoral counselors	

SOURCE: Adapted from Hoff 1989, pp. 316–317.

People who are panicked should receive prompt attention, to minimize the potential for contagious panic that sometimes occurs in large groups. One strategy to help a panic-stricken person is to give the person a small, structured task that focuses energies constructively. Remember, however, that assigning tasks beyond the person's capabilities at that time will add to the person's anxiety and feeling of helplessness. Nurses in disaster situations also incorporate concepts and intervention strategies related to death and loss.

Immediate and effective community responses to disaster or crisis situations help victims and survivors resolve their experiences satisfactorily. The example below demonstrates how a community crisis or disaster can be successfully managed.

In a small upstate New York community, four teenage boys were killed in a freak automobile accident. They were well-liked members of the varsity football team who had lived in the community all their lives. A group of concerned community members that included nurses, therapists, and counselors set up a crisis intervention center where they met with students, family members, faculty members, and others. The local church held a memorial service and several area businesses closed for the day so that all could attend. A small work group, with the backing of the entire community, began an investigation into the cause of the accident 1 month later. They are determined that this will never happen again.

Evaluation and Outcome Criteria

It is difficult to evaluate the effectiveness of disaster intervention because of the large numbers of people involved and the disruptive nature of a disaster. Evaluation can take place at many different levels. Nurses can evaluate their work with individual clients; mental health care

text continues on page 729

CASE STUDY

A Client in Crisis

Identifying Information

Peter is a 65-year-old male who has been married to his wife Emile for 45 years. He is of Italian descent, and his wife is of Irish descent. They are both active in their religion. He is employed as the executive director of a local community agency. He has not attended work in the last 4 days. After his 24-year-old son William found him in his cellar with a loaded rifle, with a suicide letter to his family and friends nearby, he was brought to the emergency room by his wife and son. Peter is mute, his wife is sobbing, and his son looks very distressed.

Client's Description of the Problem

At the time of admission, Peter states, "I can't believe it, it's all over now. I can't believe it." He is unable to give any additional information. Peter's wife and son say they are frightened, "especially because of the gun." They report that Peter has seemed more agitated and irritable, but "he won't tell us what's bothering him." Peter will be admitted to an inpatient psychiatric unit.

Peter's problems began approximately 3 weeks ago when he found out that his organization was about to be audited by an outside financial consultant. Peter had worked with this community group for 15 years and is a highly respected community leader. Peter and his wife had experienced financial problems approximately 3 months prior, and Peter took a substantial amount of money from agency funds. He had planned to return it within the next 2 months after he received money from stocks he is selling. The audit is to take place before the money can be replaced. Peter started to ruminate about being "found out" and "they'll know I'm a fraud." Emile reports that he has been driving erratically and came close to a bridge abutment 2 days ago. When she asked her husband what was bothering him, he responded, "You'll never understand." Over the last week he has only slept in 1-hour intervals and has not eaten a complete meal. He has not spoken of his problem to his family or friends.

Psychiatric History

Peter and his family report that he has never had prior treatment for psychiatric problems. His wife and son have both seen counselors for depression in the past. They report that at the time they saw counselors, Peter joked with them about being "so weak" that they needed to "see a shrink."

Family History

Peter was born the twelfth of thirteen children to Italian immigrants. Peter speaks of his family as being proud that he was able to make "something of myself" even though he was quite poor. His wife has had several chronic health problems since her early twenties that have resulted in long periods of hospitalization throughout their marriage. He has children who are married, with their own children. He is the grandfather of 3.

Social History

Peter describes himself as a hard worker, who doesn't always have the "brains" to be a success, but has made up for it with "hard work." He denies alcohol use, but his wife did drink abusively during her own periods of illness. He has always been a religious man—"I go to church every day." "Now even God's given up on me." Peter's three children, William, Marilyn, and Megan, are "good kids" and are prominent in the community themselves. He reports a good relationship with his grandchildren. His parents have been deceased for many years. Peter says that he never "really made it" and "all of me is fake. I'm a fraud." He reports the following as evidence: He entered the military only a few weeks before the end of World War II. "Everyone else was a hero. I played basketball for 3 weeks on Guam." He feels he has never accomplished any of his goals fully. He reports he "faked his way through college" and "I had a chance to make it big several times in my life, but I always wimped out. Look at me now." Peter says that killing himself was "the only way I can solve this problem."

Health History

Peter reports ongoing health problems with adult-onset diabetes. He reports that this illness has not been problematic because "I take care of myself." He appears to have lost weight (he refuses to get on the scale, but his clothes do not fit quite right), his lips are cracked, and he appears dehydrated.

Current Mental Status

Peter's hygiene is poor. He has not shaved in several days, and his clothes are rumpled. After several hours on the unit he appears more dejected but is more willing to talk about his problems. He is pacing and clenching and unclenching his fists.

→

CASE STUDY *(continued)*

A Client in Crisis

Peter is oriented to person, place, and time. He states that "nothing really matters" and "who cares what day it is . . . it's all over anyway." Remote and recent memory are intact and retrievable judging by reports that are consistent with his wife's reports. No obvious impairment. Peter appears to be sad, alternating with angry outbursts; also, he is agitated. He is unable to tolerate talking to anyone except in short intervals. His speech ranges from agitated and irritable to sad and mute. There is no evidence of rambling. Many of his responses are sarcastic; he seems to have little tolerance and is irritable. Cognitively, Peter is preoccupied and ruminating. He admits to having a suicide plan ("What did you think the gun was for . . . I wasn't kidding"). He denies homicidal ideation.

Peter's thoughts are clear and coherent. There is clear evidence that he seems paralyzed with his current situation. He is only able to speak with others for short periods of time, and then leaves to pace again in the day room.

Peter is overwhelmed and unable to mobilize a defense, which is the reason for his high degree of suicide risk during this crisis period. Peter has awareness of his problem, but has little insight at this time about possible alternatives to his state.

Other Subjective or Objective Clinical Data

Suicide potential high. Medications included use of an oral hypoglycemic. A urine specimen to test for changes (spilling ketones) and blood for lab work to determine glucose level were obtained.

Diagnostic Impression

Nursing Diagnoses

Ineffective Individual Coping
Hopelessness
Situational Low Self-Esteem
Sleep Pattern Disturbance
Potential for Self-Directed Violence
Spiritual Distress
Altered Nutrition, Less than Body Requirements

DSM-IV Multiaxial Diagnosis

Axis I: Acute stress disorder, 308.3; R/O major depression, single episode, severe, 296.33
Axis II: Deferred
Axis III: Adult-onset diabetes mellitus
Axis IV: Psychosocial stressors: Problems related to social environment; problems related to legal system; problems with primary support group
Axis V: GAF = 30 (current); GAF = 78 (highest level in past year)

NURSING CARE PLAN

Nursing Diagnosis

Risk for Self-Directed Violence related to suicidal ideation and suicide plan.

Expected Outcome

Client will not harm himself while he is an inpatient. Client will describe a plan to prevent self-harm in the future.

Nursing Interventions

- Institute one-to-one observation and suicide precaution protocol; provide safety on unit.
- Explore in one-to-one discussion with client his feelings about suicide. Speak frankly and directly about his thoughts and plans.
- Explain observation precautions and unit routines, including unit guidelines about sharps and contraband.
- Encourage interaction with other clients and provide frequent staff interventions.
- Monitor need to change level of precautions depending on reassessment of client.
- Encourage ventilation of feelings; expect anger, frustration, helplessness and hopelessness.

Outcome Met If

- Client does not harm self.
- Client verbalizes thoughts and feelings of suicide.
- Client expresses feelings and fears about current situation.
- Client agrees to and does seek out staff when feeling self-destructive.

NURSING CARE PLAN *(continued)*

Nursing Diagnosis

Hopelessness related to financial and legal problems.

Expected Outcome

Client will discuss alternatives to his current situation.

Nursing Interventions

- Explore with client his understanding of his current situation.
- Explore his recall of crisis points in his life.
- Encourage client to discuss his concerns; offer a nonjudgmental environment.
- Encourage and provide opportunities for client to discuss his situation with an objective person (lawyer, clergyman).
- Encourage client to seek out additional information on other ways to resolve this situation.
- When client is able to do so, encourage him to reconnect with family members.

Outcome Met If

- Client verbalizes agreement to discuss situation and examine alternatives.
- Client verbalizes an alternative plan (other than suicide) to cope with the situation.
- Client is able to reconnect with his supports in the community.

Nursing Diagnosis

Ineffective Individual Coping related to the discovery of his involvement in missing funds.

Expected Outcome

Client will verbalize and demonstrate a decrease in anxiety and ability to use three new coping strategies.

Nursing Interventions

- Explore with client past coping skills.
- Explore with client his understanding of current situation and how usual methods to cope have not been effective.
- Provide information to client about crisis states, anxiety, and hopelessness.
- Explore exercise, relaxation techniques, and journaling as three strategies to decrease anxiety.
- Teach skills about recognizing anxiety and teach intervention strategies.

Outcome Met If

- Client verbalizes his understanding of how coping skills can assist his functioning.
- Client verbalizes and demonstrates ability to use at least one new coping skill.
- Client verbalizes confidence in his ability to cope outside of the hospital.

Nursing Diagnosis

Altered Nutrition, Less than Body Requirements, related to depression.

Expected Outcome

Client will verbalize importance of maintaining adequate nutrition.

Nursing Interventions

- Encourage client to eat small, high-calorie meals within his dietary restrictions (due to type II diabetes).
- Discuss with client the impact of crisis situation on his usual sleep and appetite.
- Explain the importance of adequate nutrition and fluid intake.
- Refer client to nutritionist if problems persist with appetite or intake disturbance.
- Ask family to bring in special foods that the client enjoys.
- Stay with client during mealtimes to provide support.

Outcome Met If

- Client expresses understanding of how crisis state can affect his appetite pattern.
- Client returns to usual pattern of eating three meals a day.

Nursing Diagnosis

Sleep Pattern Disturbance related to anxiety.

Expected Outcome

Client will verbalize importance of maintaining adequate rest and sleep.

Nursing Interventions

- Offer client relaxation tapes or music to help decrease anxiety.
- Encourage client to limit intake of foods, beverages, and substances that are CNS stimulants and may increase anxiety.
- Administer medication as needed (includes teaching about intended therapeutic effects and side effects) to help decrease agitation and promote return to usual pattern of sleep.

Outcome Met If

- Client expresses understanding of how crisis state can affect his sleep pattern.
- Client returns to usual pattern of sleeping 6–7 hours daily.

RESEARCH NOTE

Citation

Hodgkinson PE, Shepherd MA: The impact of disaster support work. *J Traumatic Stress* 1994;7(4): 587–600.

Study Problem/Purpose

This study was designed to examine the impact of disaster-related stress on workers offering psychologic support to victims in two major British disasters. The study also examined potential moderating factors for those workers. The literature routinely identifies disaster workers as those who may be at higher risk to have psychologic difficulties after a disaster.

All disaster workers involved in this study had provided psychologic support to either the primary victims of the Piper Alpha North Sea oil production platform explosion, in which 167 people died and 62 were injured, or the Clapham Rail Crash, which killed 35 people and injured 118 more. The workers had provided debriefment/assessment, counseled individuals or families, and facilitated group counseling for survivors and bereaved relatives.

Methods

Sixty-seven workers were sent a detailed questionnaire designed to measure the workers' psychologic distress and ability to function after intervening in the disasters. Established measures to examine mood, coping style, and level of psychologic symptomatology were used. The majority of items required a rating on a 4-point visual-analogue scale, although there were also a number of open-ended questions. The sections covered Demographic Data, Experience, Caseload, Stress and Coping, Immediate Predisaster Life Events, Psychologic Symptoms, Mood, Social Support, Role Issues, and Coping Style. Twelve months after the initial questionnaire was distributed, a brief follow-up questionnaire was sent to all workers.

Findings

The aftereffects and psychologic response of the workers varied across a spectrum of symptoms. The individual responses appear to be determined by a complex interaction between personality characteristics, worker-related factors (such as the impact of client contact and role issues involved in knowing what to do and who is in charge during the disaster), and the prior life events of the individual.

Most of the workers experienced significant levels of symptoms during the first year after the disaster. Follow-up data suggested that this level of symptoms was maintained 12 months after the initial survey. The symptoms most frequently reported were cognitive difficulties, symptoms of depression, and interpersonal sensitivity, such as feelings of inadequacy and insecurity.

Of significant interest is the identification of role problems as a powerful predictor of psychologic symptoms; that is, not knowing what to do or being confused about how to intervene in a disaster is markedly distressing. A high degree of identification with clients who have been injured is also a predictor of subsequent symptoms and illness. Workers who identified closely with clients ruminate on the clients' experience to a greater degree, resulting in a higher degree of cognitive disturbance. The major moderating factors appear to be linked to the coping style of the individual.

Implications

This study reinforces some past concepts of what is known about who is at risk for developing symptoms after a crisis. Perhaps the greatest value of the research is in giving some guidance on how to prepare disaster relief workers for the tasks they face. Effective support would begin with preparing workers before a disaster occurs. The need to identify a defined task and to provide clear management structures is also indicated. Training focusing on both personal and professional issues needs to be provided to help workers negotiate the level of their engagement with clients. Information should be provided to normalize the workers' responses and offer a cognitive framework for their tasks and experiences. Finally, in selecting field workers, it is important to select those who are the least vulnerable to becoming secondary victims.

agencies can monitor statistics on groups of clients; government agencies can assess the numbers of unemployed and homeless; public health departments can measure the extent of disease and disability.

In evaluating the aftereffects of a disaster, it is important to note that there may be an impact on those who are not direct victims of the disaster (see the Research Note). A disaster can affect the mental health of various groups. The groups most commonly at increased risk are identified in the list below. Those individuals who are most affected are listed first:

1. Next-of-kin.
2. Injured survivors and their close ones.
3. Uninjured survivors.
4. Onlookers (the helpless helpers, who are at particularly high risk).
5. Rescuers.
6. Body handlers.
7. Health personnel (many mass injury situations may demand difficult prioritizing).
8. People responsible for the disaster.
9. Coworkers in workplace disasters.
10. Evacuees.

The most important aspect of evaluation is to review how the interventions were implemented and the effectiveness of the relief work. Disaster preparedness is needed to effectively intervene when the unthinkable—a disaster—occurs. Many hospitals and clinics have ongoing drills to prepare for the possibility of a disaster. Nurses must understand their role and the tasks and functions for which they are responsible.

Evaluation of the actual disaster itself offers an opportunity for reflection on whether or not the disaster was avoidable or could have been modified. Disaster experiences afford the survivors better preparation for the future.

The Impact of Crisis Work on Nurses

Working with individuals in crisis is stressful work. Nurses who work with clients in the highly disorganized crisis period or those who work with victims of rape, violence, or disaster may see the results of humankind at its worst.

As a nurse, it is important that you develop increased awareness of yourself and are able to handle your feelings so that you can intervene in a tense situation (see the accompanying Nursing Self-Awareness box). People in crisis will expect you to help them regain control of themselves, *not* to control them. Self-assurance and composure will assist the client. You will become more skilled as you handle each new situation.

NURSING SELF-AWARENESS

Working with People in Crisis

Ask yourself:

- Do I believe that people who are in crisis are helpless?
- How do I feel about providing help to people for short periods of time?
- Can I contain my own anxiety when I am working with someone who makes me anxious?
- How do I feel about not being in control in certain situations?
- How do I react to people who are frightened? Angry? Threatening to me?
- How do I feel about people who don't seem able to handle their own problems?
- How does my experience of my culture influence my thinking?
- Do I have ideas that will hinder my ability to help others? For example, do I believe any of the following: That women who are raped are asking for it; that men should be strong and not show emotions; that children should be seen and not heard?

Walker (1991) identified a number of attitudes and strategies that can help you succeed in your role:

- Strive for balance between your professional life and your personal life.
- Support people who have been victimized.
- Search for new knowledge, and challenge myths about victimization, trauma, and coping.
- Appreciate natural support systems.
- Be willing to create new support systems.
- Be willing to help unskilled clients.
- Be able to collaborate with other professionals.
- Develop support networks with coworkers and other professionals.
- Be willing to tolerate frustration.
- Respect each person's own unique timetable.
- Allow clients to make their own choices, even if you believe them to be misguided or wrong.

- Allow people to make mistakes without becoming angry with them.
- Receive regular supervision.

To remain effective in your work, and to continue to grow personally and professionally, you should also pay attention to these important areas:

- Respect and believe in a person's capacity to grow and change.
- Be aware of the impact of repeatedly listening to horrible stories.
- Formulate your own outlet for stress and anger.
- Be willing to be a role model.
- Deal with your own fears about violence and your own vulnerability to stress and conflict.
- Develop realistic expectations of what can be done for others.
- Involve administrative/supervisory individuals when making extensive intervention plans that call for more than the usual effort.

Chapter Highlights

- Everyday living brings expected and unexpected changes that result in stresses and tensions with the potential for becoming crises.
- A crisis is a self-limiting situation in which an individual's usual problem-solving coping skills are inadequate to successfully resolve the situation.
- A crisis offers the opportunity for growth and change.
- Working with a helping person increases the likelihood that a crisis will be solved in a positive way.
- Nurses are often in key positions to help clients cope with and grow through the crisis experience.
- Crises may originate from three sources: situational experiences (stressful life events that are usually not anticipated), transitional states (usually anticipated maturational experiences), and cultural/societal sources (such as discrimination).
- The crisis episode may be understood as a sequence that involves three stages: precrisis, crisis, and postcrisis.
- Crisis intervention as a therapeutic strategy is strongly humanistic in that people are viewed as capable of personal growth and able to control their own lives.
- Intervention strategies such as individual crisis counseling, crisis groups, family crisis counseling, telephone counseling, and home crisis visits are appropriate modes for dealing with either internal or external crisis.

References

Aguilera DC: *Crisis Intervention: Theory and Methodology,* ed 7. Mosby, 1994.

Allodi FA: Post-traumatic stress disorder in hostages and victims of torture. *Psychiatr Clin N Am* 1994;17(2):279–288.

American Psychiatric Association: *Diagnostic and Statistical Manual of Mental Disorders,* ed 4. American Psychiatric Association, 1994.

Bowler RM, Mergler D, Huel G, Cone JE: Psychological, psychosocial and psychophysiological sequelae in a community affected by a railroad chemical disaster. *J Traumatic Stress* 1994;7(4):601–624.

Britton JG, Mattson-Melcher DM: The crisis home: Sheltering patients in emotional crisis. *J Psychosoc Nurs* 1985; 23(12):18–23.

Burgess AW, Hartman CR, Wolbert WA, Grant CA: Child molestation: Assessing impact in multiple victims (part 1). *Arch Psychiatr Nurs* 1987;1(1):33–39.

Caplan G: *Principles of Preventive Psychiatry.* Basic Books, 1965.

Cobb S, Lindemann E: Neuropsychiatric observations after the Cocoanut Grove fire. *Ann Surg* 1943;117:814.

Gil T, et al.: Cognitive functioning in post-traumatic stress disorder. *J Traumatic Stress* 1990;3(1):29–45.

Green BL: Psychosocial research in traumatic stress: An update. *J Traumatic Stress* 1994;7(2):341–362.

Green BL, Lindi JD: Post-traumatic stress disorder in victims of disasters. *Psychiatr Clin N Am* 1994;17(2):301–309.

Hansell N: *The Person in Distress.* Human Services Press, 1976.

Hardin SB, Weinrich M, Weinrich S: Psychological distress of adolescents exposed to Hurricane Hugo. *J Traumatic Stress* 1994;7(3):427–440.

Hayes G, Goodwin T, Miors B: After disaster: A crisis support team at work. *Am J Nurs* 1990;90(2):61–64.

Herman JL, Perry JC, Van der Kolk B: Childhood trauma in borderline personality disorder. *Am J Psychiatry* 1989; 146(4):490–495.

Hodgkinson PE, Shepherd MA: The impact of disaster support work. *J Traumatic Stress* 1994;7(4):587–600.

Hoff LA: *People in Crisis: Understanding and Helping,* ed 3. Addison-Wesley, 1989.

Joint Commission on Mental Illness and Health. *Action for Mental Health.* Basic Books, 1961.

Karl GT: Survival skills for psychic trauma. *J Psychosoc Nurs Ment Health Serv* 1989;27(4):15–19.

Klingman A, Kupermintz H: Response style and self-control under Scud missile attacks: The case of the sealed room situation during the 1991 Gulf War. *J Traumatic Stress* 1994; 7(3):415–426.

Lebowitz L, Roth S: "I felt like a slut": The cultural context and women's response to being raped. *J Traumatic Stress* 1994;7(3):363–390.

Lindemann E: Symptomatology and management of acute grief. *Am J Psychiatry* 1944;101:101–148.

Lundin T: The treatment of acute trauma: Post-traumatic stress disorder prevention. *Psychiatr Clin N Am* 1994; 17(2):385–391.

Maslow A: *Motivation and Personality,* ed 2. Harper & Row, 1970.

McCann IL, Pearlmann LA: Vicarious traumatization: A framework for understanding the psychological effects of working with victims. *J Traumatic Stress* 1990;3(1): 131–149.

Mitchell J, Bray G: *Emergency Services Stress: Guidelines for Preserving the Health and Careers of Emergency Services Personnel.* Prentice-Hall, 1990.

Murphy SA: Perceptions of stress, coping, and recovery one and three years after a natural disaster. *Issues Ment Health Nurs* 1986;8:63–77.

Orr E, Westman M: Does hardiness moderate stress and how? A review, in Rosenbaum M (ed): *Learned Resourcefulness on Coping Skills, Self-Control and Adaptive Behavior,* Vol 24 of *Behavior Therapy and Behavior Medicine*. Springer, 1990.

Peebles-Kleiger MJ, Kleiger JH: Re-integration stress for Desert Storm families: Wartime deployment and family trauma. *J Traumatic Stress* 1994;7:173–193.

Phifer JF: Psychological distress and somatic symptoms after natural disaster: Differential vulnerability among older adults. *Psychology and Aging* 1990;5(3):412–420.

Puskar KR, Obus NL: Management of the psychiatric emergency. *Nurs Pract* 1989;14(7):9–15.

Sullivan-Taylor L: Policemen and nursing students: Crisis intervention team. *J Psychosoc Nurs* 1985;23:31–33.

Tyhurst JS: Individual reactions to community disaster. *Am J Psychiatr* 1951;107:764–769.

Tyhurst JS: The role of transition states—including disasters—in mental illness. Paper read at the Symposium on Preventative and Social Psychiatry, Walter Reed Army Institute of Research and the National Research Council, Washington, D.C., April 15–17, 1957.

Van der Kolk BA: *Psychological Trauma.* American Psychiatric Press, 1987.

Vernberg EM, Vogel JM: Psychological responses of children to natural and human-made disasters: Interventions with children after disasters 1993;22(4):485–498.

Waigandt A, et al.: The impact of sexual assault on physical health status. *J Traumatic Stress* 1990;3(1):93–102.

Walker L: PTSD in women: Diagnosis and treatment of the battered woman syndrome. *Psychother* 1991;28(1):21–27.

Webb NB: *Play Therapy with Children in Crisis: A Casebook for Practitioners.* Guilford Press, 1991.

Weinrich S, Harden SB, Johnson M: Nurses respond to Hurricane Hugo victims' disaster stress. *Arch Psychiatr Nurs* 1990;4(3):195–205.

Weisaeth L: Disasters: Psychological and psychiatric aspects, in Goldberger L, and Breznitz S (eds): *Handbook of Stress: Theoretical and Clinical Aspects.* Free Press, 1993.

World Health Organization. *Resolution on the International Decade for Natural Disaster Reduction.* WHO, 1988.

CHAPTER 31

GROUP PROCESS AND GROUP THERAPY

Carol Ren Kneisl

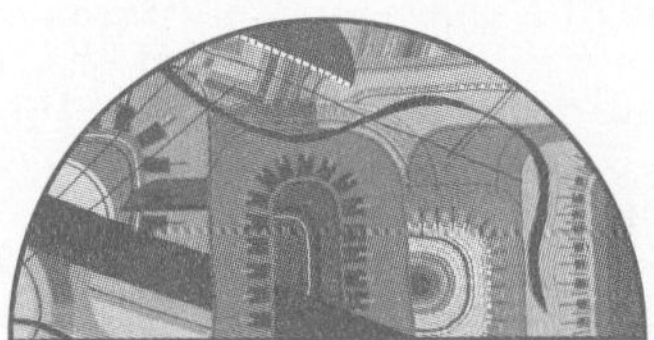

COMPETENCIES

- *Develop an appreciation for the influence of group dynamics in people's lives.*
- *Describe two frameworks for the assessment and understanding of therapy groups.*
- *Assess small groups in terms of their functional, structural, and interactional characteristics.*
- *Describe the process of creating and maintaining a group.*
- *Identify the stages of therapy group development.*
- *Discuss the application of here-and-now activation and process illumination to psychotherapy groups.*

Cross-References

Other topics relevant to this content are: Client government groups and community meetings, Chapter 9; Group therapy with adolescents, Chapter 37; Group therapy with children, Chapter 36.

Critical Thinking Challenge

You are present at a multidisciplinary case conference presentation. The client who is the focus of the discussion is a young man named Mark, a 21-year-old outpatient at the community mental health center. Mark has been alienated from his parents and his brothers and sisters since he was 17 years old and declared an emancipated minor. Some staff members believe that Mark should remain in individual therapy based on the rationale that his family will not agree to participate in family therapy. You are preparing to suggest group therapy as a possibility. What is your rationale?

People live most of their lives in groups. They depend on others for much of their sense of personal fulfillment and achievement. The activities they undertake toward personal fulfillment are, more often than not, activities that they carry out in the company of others.

Why are groups so important? Most people are born into a group—the family—and our survival from the moment of birth depends on relationships formed with other human beings. The sense of self, of being, of personal identity derives from the ways in which we are perceived and responded to by the other members of the groups to which we belong. We interact with others at all stages of our lives in various groups—family groups, peer groups, work groups, play groups, worship groups.

Many of the goals we set for ourselves cannot be achieved without membership in groups. Other people are important to each of us, just as we are important to others. Through cooperation and coordination in groups, we can achieve objectives and reach goals that we could not through individual effort alone. In this way, groups help us improve the quality of our lives.

Much of the nurse's professional life is spent in groups—groups of clients and groups of colleagues with whom the nurse plans and implements the delivery of health care services. To use groups rationally and effectively, nurses must understand the forces that underlie small group interactional processes and recognize their own patterns of participation. Group intervention is one way that psychiatric nurses can provide psychoeducation for their clients. Therapy through the group process gives clients the opportunity to seek validation, give and receive interpersonal feedback, and test new and different ways of being that may improve the quality of life. Mental health can be preserved, maintained, and restored through interaction with others in productive groups.

Nurses have long been involved in working with clients and their families in small groups brought together for health teaching, psychoeducation, or supportive purposes. All nurses, regardless of level of education, can lead therapeutic groups or psychoeducation groups, as long as they understand and apply small group dynamics in their group work. The role of the psychiatric nurse as group therapist, however, is relatively recent. It first received professional endorsement by the American Nurses Association (ANA) in 1967. Qualifications of group therapists are identified later in this chapter. The characteristics of various types of groups are compared in Table 31–1.

Small Group Dynamics

To be effective, any group must perform three main functions:

1. Accomplishing its designated goals.
2. Maintaining its own cohesion.
3. Developing and modifying its structure to improve its effectiveness.

Table 31–2 on page 736 lists some factors that influence these functions. These are useful in evaluating the effectiveness of a given group. They constitute the major characteristics generally observable in effective and ineffective groups and illustrate different ways of dealing with the dynamic forces in every group.

Several forces modify and shape groups, influencing their effectiveness. These forces, as well as several frameworks for analyzing and understanding group process, are discussed in the sections that follow.

Physical Environment

Groups exist in complex environmental settings that strongly influence the group process. The building, room, and chair and table arrangements are aspects of the environmental setting that influence the operation of the group. Superimposed on the physical structure are the influences of territoriality, personal space, and cultural background. As you read about these influences, try to visualize the specific and peculiar features of outpatient clinics, day treatment centers, hospital units, nurses' stations, and ward versus private accommodations for hospitalized clients.

TERRITORIALITY Most people at some time have experienced violating an unspoken and unwritten rule by sitting in someone else's chosen seat. This assumption of proprietary rights to space is but one example of the notion of territoriality. **Territoriality** is the assumption of a proprietary attitude toward a geographic area by a person or a group. People defend their right to the designated territory against invasion by others, despite the absence of legal sanction. People do not really "own" their territory but rather occupy it, permanently or intermittently, and act as if the property belonged to them.

Avoidance of intragroup conflict depends in part on the degree to which group members respect one another's territorial rights. Intergroup conflict may result when one group fails to respect the territorial rights of another group; in fact, this is how most wars between nations begin. In addition, territoriality provides a modicum of privacy for the individual or the group. It may also serve as a method of dominance by an individual or a group over others. The head nurse's chair, or the unit chief's chair at the head of the conference table, are concrete examples.

PERSONAL SPACE **Personal space** is an invisible bubble of territory around a person's body into which intruders may not come. It differs from territoriality in that it is space maintained and carried around with the person, rather than a specific geographic location.

A common defensive response to unwanted intrusion is selecting a position that is as inaccessible as possible. Another common response is flight. The need to defend personal space may also interfere with group functioning. Unwanted intrusion of one member into another's personal space creates discomfort, unease, and other negative feelings. These feelings affect the group dynamics and interfere with group progress.

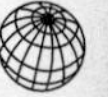

CULTURAL BACKGROUND Cultural background is a strong influence on territoriality and personal space. An American who wants to be alone goes into a room and shuts the door, relying on architectural features for screening. English people have never developed the habit of using space to protect themselves from others. They use other barriers, such as "the silent treatment," which they expect others to recognize and respect. When an Englishman becomes silent in the company of an American man, the American is likely to expend extra effort to break through the barrier to assure himself that all is well.

Table 31–1 Characteristics of Different Types of Groups

Characteristic	*Task Groups*	*Self-Awareness/ Growth Groups*	*Therapy Groups*	*Social Groups*
Purpose, goals	Performance of specific job or task explicitly agreed on by all members at initiation of group. Member participation is determined by task.	Development or use of interpersonal strengths. Broad objectives, such as studying group process, communication patterns, or problem-solving are usually apparent at initiation of group.	Clearly defined: to do the work of therapy. Individual works toward self-understanding, more satisfactory ways of relating, handling stress, etc.	Recreation, relaxation, and comfort promoted through mutual pleasure and enjoyment among friends and acquaintances in a social situation such as a party at someone's home.
Shared aim	To achieve group's task goal.	To improve functioning of group one returns to (job, family, community) through translation of one's own interpersonal strengths or to improve perception of members.	To improve perception of members and to improve individual health.	To experience fun, companionship, and satisfying relationships with friends.
Format	Defined at outset by leader and/or members. Method is specific to task to be performed.	Specific format, if any, and methods defined throughout group process by all members and leader/trainer. Lack of agenda and structure may produce some difficulty.	Defined by therapist within context of some psychotherapeutic orientation. Definition is apparent through implementation of therapeutic principles.	Usually spontaneous. May be defined by members in case of planned recreational activities.
Focus	Completion of specific task.	Interpersonal concerns around current situations.	Member-centered. Past experiences may be just as relevant as current concerns, depending on therapist's orientation.	Member-centered toward enjoyment and mutual meeting of needs.
Role of leader	To establish exchange of information among members and direct group toward task accomplishment, adhering to agenda.	To establish group interaction at emotional level among group members, and to serve as resource person guiding group by calling attention to certain events or processes and facilitating problem solving, mutual understanding, communication.	To establish group interaction between self and individual members and among group members. To facilitate members' interactions in work of therapy.	To meet basic requirements for social companionship, providing place, planning activity, preparing food, drink, etc.
Title of leader	Usually called chairperson.	Usually called trainer.	Usually called therapist.	Usually called host or hostess.
How leader differs from members	Chairperson identifies specific task, clarifies communication, and assists in expressing opinions and offering solutions.	Trainer differs from members by having superior skills in specialized area (understanding and facilitating group process). Trainer's superiority diminishes as group continues and members learn and implement similar skills.	Therapist differs from members by having superior skills in specialized area (group psychotherapy). Therapist never truly becomes member but may at times take on members' roles.	Host or hostess is member of group and works toward own as well as others' pleasure and enjoyment.

Table 31–1 *(continued)*

Characteristic	*Task Groups*	*Self-Awareness/ Growth Groups*	*Therapy Groups*	*Social Groups*
Requirements of leader	Qualified background and expertise in area of task emphasis. Must be accepted by members as an appropriate leader.	Sufficient preparation, experience, and skill to maintain effective control of interpersonal tensions.	Sufficient preparation and skill to undertake psychotherapy within context of situation.	Willingness to take steps to initiate social interaction.
Orientation of group work	Reality-oriented in terms of adhering to explicit work goal. If group deviates into interpersonal realm, task is not accomplished most efficiently.	Reality testing with here-and-now emphasis. Assumption is that members can correct inefficient patterns of relating and communicating with each other. Members learn group process experientially through participation and involvement.	Oriented toward having members gain insight as basis for changing patterns of behavior toward health.	Oriented toward having fun, seeking pleasure and relaxation, releasing tension.
Selection of members	Selection made possibly in terms of individual's functional role, not usually in terms of personal characteristics, often in terms of employment status.	Selection criteria range from simply expressed desire to become more self-aware to mixture of criteria based on personality characteristics.	Selection usually based on extensive consideration of constellation of personalities, behaviors, and needs and identification of group therapy as treatment of choice.	Selection based on considerations of friendship or social obligation. Host or hostess chooses whom to invite.
Title of members	Known as committee members.	May be called trainees.	Known as clients or, in some settings, patients.	Known as guests.
Interviewing of prospective members	Usually not interviewed before entry into group.	May or may not be interviewed and/or requested to complete questionnaires on personal data and personality characteristics before entry into group.	Extensive selection interview(s) required before entry into group.	Not interviewed. Usually known through prior social acquaintance.
Length of group life	Target date usually set in advance.	Tends to be short-term, with target date set in advance.	Usually not set. Termination date usually determined mutually by therapist and members.	May be set in advance or spontaneously determined.

Americans believe that geographic nearness is an acceptable basis for interaction. Living next door to a family entitles a neighbor family to socialize with the members, borrow a cup of flour from them, and have its children play with theirs. To others, nearness is not enough, especially when social status rather than space governs relationships.

Most Europeans perceive Americans as loud. They see this as an intrusive trait, because being overheard interferes with the privacy of others. Americans perceive their "loudness" as an expression of openness or having nothing to hide. They perceive the quiet or hushed conversations of others as sly or secretive.

Conditions that people in the United States perceive as crowded, others (Latinos and those from Mediterranean cultures) may perceive as spacious. A North American in Latin America or the Middle East is likely to feel crowded and hemmed in. In this person's view, people come too close and touch too much. The Middle Easterner or Latino may experience the North American as cold. But, in English and Scandinavian cultures, it is the North American who perceives the others as aloof.

Influences from the various cultures carry over from generation to generation. For satisfactory functioning, a group must pay attention to the cultural factors that influence the individual member. In a large hospital or

Table 31–2 Comparative Features of Effective and Ineffective Groups

Factor	*Effective Groups*	*Ineffective Groups*
Atmosphere	Informal, comfortable, and relaxed. It is a working atmosphere in which people demonstrate their interest and involvement.	Obviously tense. Signs of boredom may appear.
Goal setting	Goals, tasks, and objectives are clarified, understood, and modified so that members of the group can commit themselves to cooperatively structured goals.	Unclear, misunderstood, or imposed goals may be accepted by members. The goals are competitively structured.
Leadership and member participation	Shift from time to time, depending on the circumstances. Different members assume leadership at various times, because of their knowledge or experience.	Delegated and based on authority. The chairperson may dominate the group, or the members may defer unduly. Member participation is unequal, with high-authority members dominating.
Goal emphasis	All three functions of groups—goal accomplishment, internal maintenance, and developmental change—are emphasized.	One or more functions may not be emphasized.
Communication	Open and two-way. Ideas and feelings are encouraged, both about the problem and about the group's operation.	Closed or one-way. Only the production of ideas is encouraged. Feelings are ignored or taboo. Members may be tentative or reluctant to be open and have "hidden agendas" (personal goals at cross-purposes with group goals).
Decision making	By consensus, although various decision-making procedures appropriate to the situation may be instituted.	By the highest authority in the group with minimal involvement by members, or an inflexible style is imposed.
Cohesion	Facilitated through high levels of inclusion, trust, liking, and support.	Either ignored or used as a means of controlling members, thus promoting rigid conformity.
Conflict tolerance	The reasons for disagreements or conflicts are carefully examined and the group seeks to resolve them. The group accepts basic disagreements that cannot be resolved and lives with them.	Attempts may be made to ignore, deny, avoid, suppress, or override controversy by premature group action.
Power	Determined by the members' abilities and the information they possess. Power is shared. The issue is how to get the job done.	Determined by position in the group. Obedience to authority is strong. The issue is who controls.
Problem-solving ability	High. Constructive criticism is frequent, frank, relatively comfortable, and oriented toward removing obstacles to problem solving.	Low. Criticism may be destructive, taking the form of either overt or covert personal attacks. It prevents the group from getting the job done.
Self-evaluation as a group	Frequent. All members participate in evaluation and decisions about how to improve the group's functioning.	Minimal. What little evaluation there is may be done by the highest authority in the group, rather than by the membership as a whole.
Creativity	Encouraged. There is room within the group for members to become self-actualized and interpersonally effective.	Discouraged. People are afraid of appearing foolish if they put forth a creative thought.

metropolitan mental health center, where members of many cultures come together, these differences may lead to misunderstandings and thwart effective group functioning.

Material Aspects of the Setting The material aspects of the physical environment influence the functioning of groups in interesting ways. For example, color and noise have been found to influence people's perceptions and performance. Workers complain of feeling uncomfortably cold in a room painted a cool blue. The same workers feel too warm at the same temperature when the room is painted in warm yellows and restful greens. Recent research indicates that a specific shade of pink initially decreases aggressive behavior. In response, some prison administrators have painted their jail cells pink. Unpredictable noise has been found to evoke feelings of frustration and lead to a decrease in performance. Sound conditioning of work areas has been found to reduce worker discomfort and annoyance.

Likewise, workers in an ugly room report more headaches, monotony, fatigue, hostility, discontent, and room avoidance than workers in a beautiful room. Studies about the material aspects of a setting indicate that elements of the environment are important in determining group and individual behavior. Productivity, interpersonal behavior, and intrapsychic experiences are all affected by a particular setting.

SPATIAL ARRANGEMENTS Seating arrangements have been methodically studied since the 1950s. Researchers have found that adults prefer a side-by-side arrangement for cooperation and a direct face-to-face arrangement for competition. This knowledge can be helpful in understanding the interaction among members of a psychotherapy group, a nursing team conference, or an interdisciplinary clinical conference at a community mental health agency.

There is also a relationship between spatial arrangement and leadership. Because the person who sits at the head of the table is usually perceived as the leader, the spatial position a person occupies in a group has important consequences for that person's chances of emerging as a group leader or for undertaking significant leadership responsibilities. Round tables tend to enhance the development of leadership traits among the membership rather than to invest certain members with authority because of their spatial position. It is for this reason that therapeutic groups usually use movable chairs that are set in a circle.

Leadership

Leadership functions within a group can be fulfilled by the person designated as the leader, and by members who engage in leadership behavior. This distinction is an important one for understanding the emergence of leadership within groups.

Leadership is an influence relationship that occurs among mutually dependent group members attempting to achieve the group's goals. Group members influence one another, and each member exerts leadership at some time in the group's life. This approach to understanding leadership behavior is called the *distributed functions approach.*

The distributed functions approach to group leadership is based on two major beliefs:

1. Any member of a group may become a leader by taking actions that serve group purposes.
2. Different members may perform various functions.

Each member may play more than one role during a meeting of the group and a wide range of roles in successive participations. Any member may play any or all of the roles. The various functional roles may be grouped in two categories:

1. Task roles are related to the task of the group. The job of people assuming these roles is to facilitate and coordinate group efforts in the selection, definition, and solution of a group problem. Examples of task roles are *information seeker, information giver, elaborator, procedural technician, coordinator, opinion seeker,* and *opinion giver,* among others.
2. Maintenance roles are oriented toward building group-centered attitudes among the members and maintaining and perpetuating group-centered behavior. Members who function as *encourager, compromiser, standard setter, follower, group observer,* or *harmonizer* carry out some of the maintenance roles possible in groups.

Sometimes members of a group satisfy individual needs that are irrelevant to the group task. These self-serving roles (the *recognition seeker, blocker, aggressor, dominator, self-confessor,* and *playboy,* for example) may also be negatively oriented to group maintenance functions. If a group is to function effectively, it must perform a self-diagnosis to determine what the needs of the group are, and how they can be met, so that the self-serving roles no longer present obstacles to effective functioning.

Distributing leadership functions among group members is important because it teaches people the diagnostic skills and behaviors needed to accomplish the group's goals and maintain good interpersonal relationships. The distributed functions approach can be best described through its main assumption: *Responsible membership is the same thing as responsible leadership.* Of course, in psychotherapy groups, some functions or activities may be largely, or even solely, the province of the therapist.

Decision Making

A group that makes sound decisions is a group that functions effectively. The purpose of group decision making is to construct well-conceived, well-understood, and well-accepted realistic actions toward the goals agreed on by the group.

EFFECTIVE DECISIONS Following is a list of the five major characteristics of effective decisions:

1. The resources of the group members are well used. The group listens to any member who has ideas or input that helps them make decisions.
2. The group's time is well used. The group concentrates on the task at hand and keeps interruptions and digressions to a minimum.
3. The decision is correct or of high quality. The alternative the group picks to execute is appropriate, reasonable, and error-free.
4. The decision is put into effect fully by group members. Members feel committed to the decision and responsible for its implementation.
5. The problem-solving ability of the group is enhanced. Members feel satisfied with their participation, and the positive group atmosphere increases the members' perception of themselves as adequate problem solvers.

Decision Methods A group can arrive at decisions in several ways:

- When decisions are reached by *consensus,* the group arrives at a collective opinion after each member has had a fair chance to exert influence. Consensus decisions are not always unanimous. However, members support the decisions and are willing to give it a try.
- Sometimes group decisions are made by the person selected as the *group expert.*
- *Averaging members' opinions* is another method for arriving at decisions. It means that the most popular opinion becomes the group decision. Nonetheless, fewer than half the members may hold that opinion.
- *Decision by majority vote,* 51% or more of the members, is the most common method used.
- Decisions can be made through *minority control* of a group. Executive committees of groups with many members exercise minority control over the whole group. A small minority may also quickly and forcefully "railroad" decisions (force the group to accept them by exerting intense pressure).
- In decision making by an *authority after discussion* with the members, the designated leader makes the final decision but first discusses the issue with the members to get their ideas and views.
- In decisions by *authority rule without discussion,* the designated leader makes decisions without consulting the group.

Each of these decision-making methods is appropriate at certain times. In psychotherapy groups, certain decisions (such as whether to add a new member) should be made by the group expert—in this case, the group therapist—who has the clinical expertise. A group that has to make a decision must take several factors into account before selecting a method. Questions such as these should be raised: What type of decision has to be made? How much time can be spent in the decision-making process? What resources are available to the group? What is the past history of the group? What is the task to be worked on? How does the setting influence the method that should be chosen? What are the consequences of the particular method for the group's future operation?

Indecisiveness Sometimes a group has a hard time making decisions. Members cannot agree about what the decision should be. These are some reasons for indecisiveness:

- Fear of the consequences of the decision.
- Conflicts among members that make cooperative activity difficult.
- Choice of a decision-making method inappropriate to the immediate situation.
- Member loyalty to other groups that makes it difficult to commit to making good decisions in this group.

Once the reasons for indecisiveness have been identified and put on the table, a group can work to remove the obstacles in its way. It may be necessary for the group to rearrange its membership, redefine its task, select another decision-making method, or work at resolving the conflicts among its members before continuing its work on the identified task.

Trust

Many theorists and researchers have studied the complex phenomenon of trust. Some of the better-known work is by Morton Deutsch (1949, 1958). In this view, trusting behavior comes about through the following four steps:

1. The person realizes that the decision to trust another may result in either positive or negative consequences for the self. The person realizes the risk involved in trusting another.
2. The person realizes that the future behavior of the other determines whether trusting will bring positive or negative consequences for the self.
3. The person will suffer more if the trust is violated than the person will gain if the trust is fulfilled.
4. The person feels reasonably confident that the other will behave in ways that will bring the beneficial consequences.

The person who decides to have minor elective surgery of little consequence is engaging in the four steps of trusting behavior. The person (1) recognizes that the choice could lead to either beneficial or harmful consequences, (2) realizes that the consequences of the choice depend on the behavior of the surgeon, (3) would suffer much more if the trust is violated and the surgeon does a bad job, and (4) feels relatively confident that the surgeon will make sure that beneficial consequences result.

Trust develops in relationships when people disclose more and more of their thoughts, perceptions, attitudes, and reactions to one another. The group member who makes a suggestion; discloses an attitude, feeling, experience, or perception; gives feedback; or confronts another also engages in trusting behavior and assumes the risks inherent in trusting. Trusting and being trusted are intimately linked to risk taking. The level of trust among the members of a group determines the extent of risk-taking behavior in the group.

Cohesion

"Hanging together" is the aspect of group life generally referred to as group **cohesion.** Groups that hang together or cohere possess a certain spirit of common purpose. The members have a yen for mutual association. Groups in which cohesion is minimal seem always on the verge of breaking up or falling apart. Cohesion is the primary factor keeping a group in existence and working effectively.

ATTRACTION TO THE GROUP A group is cohesive when its members are attracted to it. People are attracted to a group for a wide variety of reasons. The group may meet their needs for affiliation, interpersonal security, or financial security. It may have admired members who not only are available for human interaction but also have important shared attitudes, values, interests, and beliefs. An attractive group has explicit, mutual, and attainable group goals with clear paths to goal attainment. Its members engage in an interdependence that is cooperative rather than competitive. The activities the group undertakes are satisfying and successful, and there is a high degree of member participation in a democratic structure. Communication networks are open, central, and flexible in a warm and friendly atmosphere.

This implies that cohesive groups are not born but developed. Although some features of attraction may account for a "love-at-first-sight" phenomenon, others do not become evident until the group has come together long enough to have shared experiences that provide the basis for attraction.

EVALUATING COHESION What indicates that the spirit of cohesion exists in a given group? How do groups with sufficient cohesion differ from groups with minimal cohesion? The Assessment box on the next page identifies the characteristics of highly cohesive groups and compares them to those of minimally cohesive groups.

BUILDING COHESION How can a group's tendency to cohere be enhanced? Some methods are increasing the trusting and trustworthy behavior of members, the affection expressed among members, the expressions of inclusion and acceptance among members, and the influence that members have on one another. Two other methods for building cohesion are promoting group norms and structuring cooperative relationships among the group members.

Promoting Group Norms **Norms** are the set of unwritten rules of conduct or prescriptions of behavior established by members of a group. They derive from the common beliefs of the group about appropriate behavior. In other words, they tell how members are expected to behave. Norms prevent chaos because they lay out the expectations of members. They help members predict the behavior of others and anticipate the actions that they should take themselves.

Norms are evaluative. They tell members what ought and ought not be done. They represent value judgments that establish accepted standards for behavior. The following characteristics of norms influence group behavior:

- Norms are developed about situations that are important to the group. Groups do not establish norms for every conceivable situation.
- Norms may apply to every member of a group, or to certain members in specific roles only. For example, skiers are expected to wait their turn in the chair lift line, but a member of the Ski Patrol may cut in at the head of the line without challenge.
- Norms vary in the degree to which they are accepted by group members. Most people accept the norm that the driver of a vehicle should not pass a stopped school bus, but many violate the norm that drivers of slow-moving vehicles should stay in the right lane.
- Norms vary in the extent to which people can permissibly deviate from them. Violating a norm that members arrive for the meetings on time is a more acceptable transgression than violating the norm against physically attacking another group member.
- Norms differ in the sanctions applied for their violation. Members who arrive late may be subjected to mild disapproval, whereas the member who slaps or hits another member may be barred from the group.

The importance of norms in the power, influence, and conformity aspects of group life is discussed more completely later in the chapter.

Dealing with Hidden Agendas It takes cooperative action on the part of members to achieve group goals. In addition to group goals, members have individual goals. When the personal or individual goals of group members differ from the group goals, competitive relationships may develop that destroy the effectiveness of group relationships. For example, it is common for members who are in disagreement with the group goals to acquire

ASSESSMENT

High-Cohesion Versus Low-Cohesion Groups

Characteristics of High-Cohesion Groups	Characteristics of Low-Cohesion Groups
Members like one another.	Members seem uncaring or may actively dislike one another.
Members are friendly and willing to interact.	Members seem unfriendly and unwilling to become involved.
Members enjoy interacting with one another and interact readily.	Members get little pleasure from interaction and interact reluctantly.
Members receive support on issues from one another.	Members do not give one another active support.
Members praise one another for accomplishments.	Members do not praise one another's accomplishments or belittle them.
Members share similar opinions and attitudes.	Members have dissimilar or mutually exclusive opinions and attitudes.
Members are likely to influence one another and are willing to be influenced by other members.	Members make few influence attempts and are unwilling to be influenced by other members.
Members accept assigned tasks and roles readily.	Members are reluctant or refuse to accept assigned tasks and roles.
Members trust one another.	Members do not trust one another.
Members are loyal to the group and defend it against external criticism and attack.	Members do not defend the group and may criticize it to others.
Members stay.	Members drop out.
Group goals are valued.	Group goals are not valued.
Group goals are consistent with goals of individuals.	Group goals and individual goals are not consistent.
Group goals best handled by group action.	Group goals best handled by individual action.
Group goals difficult to achieve are met by persistent efforts.	Group goals difficult to achieve are given up.
Attendance is high, and members arrive on time.	Attendance is low or uneven, and members may arrive late or leave early.
Efforts are directed toward maintaining, strengthening, and regulating the group.	Efforts are not directed toward maintaining, strengthening, and regulating the group.
Risk taking and participation are high.	Risk taking and participation are low.
Commitment to group goals increases.	Commitment to group goals is minimal.
Communication is high.	Communication is low.
"We" is frequently heard in discussions.	"I" is frequently heard in discussions.
Leadership is democratic.	Leadership is autocratic.
Group action is interdependent and cooperative.	Group action is independent and competitive.
Group output and productivity are high.	Group output and productivity are low.
Group norms are kept and protected.	Group norms are violated.
Members experience an increase in security and self-esteem and a reduction in anxiety.	Members experience a decrease in security and self-esteem and an increase in anxiety.
Satisfaction with members and work of the group is high.	Satisfaction with members and work of the group is low.

hidden agendas that interfere with group functioning. A **hidden agenda** may be defined as a personal goal, unknown to the other group members, which is at cross-purposes with the dominant group goals.

To structure cooperative relationships around group and individual goals, members need to review and discuss group goals thoroughly when the group is formed, even though goals may have been prescribed for the group by others. Discussion clarifies members' understanding of the goals and the tasks necessary to reach them. The group goals should be recognized and rephrased during the discussion, encouraging members to feel a sense of "ownership" toward the goals. The accompanying Intervention box provides suggestions for dealing with hidden agendas.

Cooperative relationships to achieve goals are extremely important for group effectiveness. When hidden agendas structure a group competitively, members strive for individual goal accomplishment in a way that blocks others from obtaining the group goal.

Power and Influence

Power is a potent force that explains a good deal about the nature, operation, and patterns of interpersonal behavior. It is impossible to discuss group dynamics without discussing power because it is impossible to interact without influencing, and being influenced by, others. This process constantly occurs within groups, forcing members to adjust to one another and modify their behavior. In some instances, attitudes and beliefs are modified as well. *Power* is defined as the ability to do or act, to have possession of command or control over others, to achieve the desired result. The terms *power* and *influence* are used interchangeably in this chapter.

Some people perceive power and influence as negative forces. These people are frequently unaware of the influence they themselves exert on others, or they confuse the judicious use of power in building effective groups with the use of power to control, manage, and manipulate others. Psychiatric–mental health nurses are only now

INTERVENTION

Steps for Dealing with Hidden Agendas

Suggestion	*Rationale*
Look for the presence of hidden agendas.	The group cannot diagnose or solve a problem until its presence is recognized.
Once the presence of hidden agendas has been pinpointed, judge whether or not they should be brought to the surface and rectified.	Sometimes hidden agendas should be left undisturbed, if the consequences of bringing them to the attention of the entire group may be negative, rather than facilitating the work of the group.
Determine whether group members are willing and able to deal with hidden agendas. Suggest that perhaps not all there is to say has been said, but do not force members to disclose their hidden agendas.	Disclosing hidden agendas may be harmful to group attempts to reach cohesion and may result in premature rejection of the member with the hidden agenda.
Accept members whose hidden agendas have been revealed, without rejecting or criticizing them.	Hidden agendas are common and legitimate group occurrences. They should be worked on in the same way that group tasks are.
Devote group time to working on the hidden agendas of members.	Hidden agendas impede group progress. The attention given to hidden agendas should be determined by the extent of the effect on group effectiveness.
As a group, evaluate the group's ability to deal with hidden agendas.	Learning better ways of handling hidden agendas more openly will result from evaluation and reduce the need for keeping agendas hidden.

becoming aware of how it is possible for them to employ power and influence in the service of their clients and their profession.

Power Sources According to power theorists, there are six possible sources of a person's power. People have *reward power* if they can deliver positive consequences or remove negative ones in response to the behavior of group members. They have *coercive power* if they can deliver negative consequences or remove positive ones in response to the behavior of group members. When group members believe a person ought to have influence over them because of the person's position in the group or organization, that person can be said to have *legitimate power.* A person has *referent power* when group members identify with or want to be like that person. Members do what that person wants out of liking, respect, and the desire to be liked themselves. The person with *expert power* is seen by the group as trustworthy and having some special knowledge or skill. When a person has *informational power,* group members believe that person has access to useful information for accomplishing their goal.

The Problem of Unequal Power A group in which certain members have much power and others have little power is likely to be in trouble. The unequal distribution of power affects both the task and the maintenance functions of a group. Members who believe they have little influence within the group are unlikely to feel committed to group goals and to the implementation of group decisions. Their dissatisfaction with the group decreases its attractiveness and reduces its cohesion.

High-power people often are the most popular or have the most authority. Neither circumstance is satisfactory for high-quality decision making. High-quality decision making results when power is based on expertise, competence, and relevant information, not on popularity or authority.

Because much of the role socialization of the nurse emphasizes "following orders," nurses must be especially critical of an unquestioning tendency to behave in concert with the wishes of those in authority. Psychiatric nurses need to find a balance between a submissive role and an autocratic role, seeking instead to temper autonomy with reason and sensitivity. The autocratic and powerful persona of such motion picture nurse figures as the icily dictatorial Miss Davis in *The Snake Pit* and the ruthlessly punitive Nurse Ratched in *One Flew Over the Cuckoo's Nest* are examples of misdirected autonomy.

Theories of Group Development

Two basic theories are discussed in this section. They can be used to understand the development, dynamics, and functioning of small groups, from self-help groups, to psychoeducation groups, and to psychotherapy groups.

The Interpersonal Needs Approach

The basic assumption of the interpersonal needs approach known as FIRO (Fundamental Interpersonal Relationship Orientation) theory is that people need people. In addition, people need to establish some equilibrium between themselves and the people in their environment. This equilibrium is determined by the interaction of certain interpersonal needs, and it appears to be synonymous with interpersonal compatibility (Schutz 1958b).

Three Basic Interpersonal Needs An interpersonal need is one that can be satisfied only through relationships with people. Schutz reasoned that every individual has three interpersonal needs: inclusion, control, and affection.

Inclusion The interpersonal need for **inclusion** is the need to establish and maintain relationships with others that offer interactions and associations satisfying to the individual. The following characterize a satisfying position in terms of inclusion:

- A psychologically comfortable relationship with people somewhere on a continuum that ranges from initiating or originating interaction with all people to not initiating interaction with anyone. In other words, this dimension is *expressed* toward others.
- A psychologically comfortable relationship with people in regard to wanting others to initiate interaction somewhere on a continuum from always initiating interaction with you to never initiating interaction with you. In other words, this dimension is *wanted* from others.

To put this another way, *expressed inclusion* is the ability to take an interest in others to a satisfactory degree, and *wanted inclusion* is the ability to allow other people to take an interest in you to a satisfying degree to yourself. This need determines whether a person is outgoing or prefers privacy.

Control The interpersonal need for **control** is the need to establish and maintain a satisfactory relationship between oneself and other people with regard to power and influence. The following characterize a satisfactory position in terms of control:

- A psychologically comfortable relationship with people somewhere on a continuum from controlling all the behavior of other people to not controlling any behavior of others.
- A psychologically comfortable relationship with people in regard to their control behavior on a continuum from always wanting to be controlled by them to never wanting to be controlled by them.

Stated another way, *expressed control* is the ability to take charge to a satisfactory degree, and *wanted control* is the ability to establish and maintain a feeling of respect for the competence and responsibleness of others to a satisfying degree to yourself.

Affection The interpersonal need for **affection** is the need to establish and maintain a satisfactory relationship between the self and other people with regard to love and affection. The following characterize a satisfactory position in terms of affection:

- A psychologically comfortable relationship with others somewhere on a continuum from initiating close, personal relationships with everyone to originating close, personal relationships with no one.
- A psychologically comfortable relationship with people in regard to their affection behavior on a continuum from wanting everyone to originate close, personal relationships toward you, to wanting no one to originate close, personal relationships toward you.

Put another way, *expressed affection* is being able to love other people or to be close and intimate to a satisfactory degree, and *wanted affection* is having others love you or to be close and intimate with you to a satisfactory degree.

Figure 31–1 illustrates the dimensions of the interpersonal needs approach.

GROUP DEVELOPMENT The interpersonal needs approach asserts that any group, given enough time, moves through three interpersonal phases—inclusion, control, and affection, in that order—that correspond to the three basic interpersonal needs.

Inclusion Phase The first or inclusion phase is concerned with the problem of *in or out.* People attempt to find their place in the group and are concerned with learning whether they will be acknowledged as individuals or left behind and ignored. Because these concerns give rise to anxiety, this phase is dominated by behavior centered around the self. Overtalking, withdrawal, exhibitionism, and sharing other group experiences and biographies are some examples.

Frequently, *goblet issues* predominate. These are issues of minor importance to the group that help people get to know one another and test each other. They are a vehicle for sizing people up. Goblet issues may revolve around the weather, sports, rules of procedure, and so on.

Control Phase The second or control phase is concerned with the problem of *top or bottom,* which becomes salient after problems of inclusion have been resolved. Concern about decision-making procedures predominates, and the problems that emerge involve the sharing of responsibility and the distribution of power and influence. There are struggles for leadership and about the

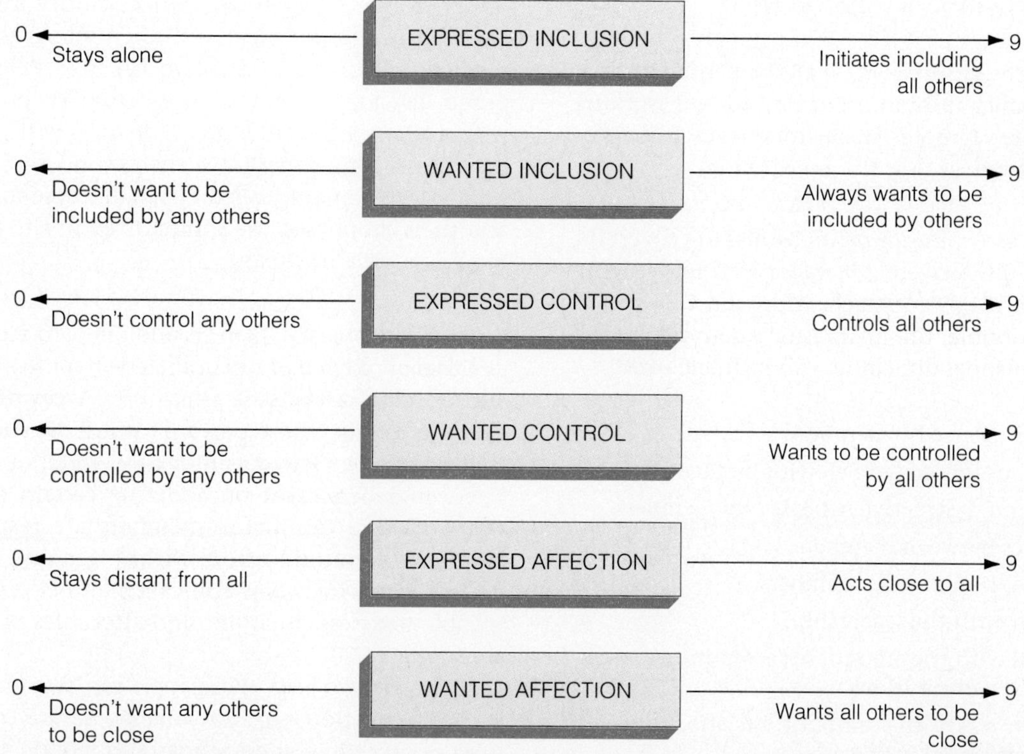

Figure 31–1 The dimensions of the FIRO theory or interpersonal needs approach.

structure, rules of procedure, and methods of decision making. Members are attempting to establish comfortable positions for themselves in terms of responsibility and influence.

Affection Phase The third or affection phase is concerned with the problem of *near or far,* and it follows satisfactory resolution of the preceding two phases. Individual members are now faced with the problem of becoming emotionally integrated. Concerns about not being liked by, being too close to, or not being close enough to others become relevant. The behavior in this phase is generally characterized by high emotion—positive feelings, jealousy, hostility, and pairing are some examples. Schutz (1958a) describes this phase as one in which, like porcupines, people attempt to get close enough to receive warmth, yet avoid the pain that sharp quills can inflict.

Interweaving of Phases None of these phases is distinct, since all three problem areas are present at all times, even though only one predominates. Schutz uses a tire-changing analogy, what he calls *tightening the bolts,* to describe the sequence of the phases:

> When a person changes a tire and replaces the wheel, he first sets the wheel in place and secures it by tightening the bolts one after another just so the wheel is in place and the next step can be taken. Then the bolts are tightened further, usually in the same sequence, until the wheel is firmly in place. Finally each bolt is gone over separately to secure it (1958a, p. 130).

The leader helps the group work on all three interpersonal need areas in similar fashion, returning to and working over each area to a more satisfactory level than was reached the last time.

APPLYING THE THEORY *Clearing the air* by making covert interpersonal difficulties overt is a major step in applying the interpersonal needs approach. Although this step is initially uncomfortable, the final result is rewarding. The following interpersonal difficulties can be made overt:

- Withdrawal or silence by members.
- Inactivity and unintegrated behavior by members.
- Overactivity and destructive behavior by members.
- Power struggles between members.
- Battles for attention among members.
- Dissatisfaction with the leadership.
- Dissatisfaction with the amount of recognition a member receives for contributions.
- Dissatisfaction with the amount of affection and warmth demonstrated in the group.

A group that is relatively compatible can function smoothly with minimal discussion of its problems. Groups in which the interpersonal problems are extremely minor can usually ignore them (or, if problems exist between two members, work them out outside the group) without hampering group effectiveness. A group that is basically incompatible has to spend much time and energy resolving its interpersonal problems so that it can function effectively.

The interpersonal needs approach of Schutz is based on the belief that the way to attack problems within groups is by investigating what is going on among the individuals in the group and attempting to improve their interpersonal relations.

The Authority Relations/ Personal Relations Approach

Two major areas of internal uncertainty or stress in groups are dependence (authority relations) and interdependence (personal relations) (Bennis and Shepard 1956). The first area has to do with group members' orientations toward authority—the handling and distribution of power within the group. The second area has to do with group members' orientations toward one another. A central assumption in this theory is that the principal obstacles to a valid group communication (and hence to group effectiveness) derive from the members' orientations toward authority and intimacy.

A new group is highly concerned with authority and power. Earlier experiences with authority influence and partially determine members' orientations toward other members. Bennis and Shepard call this Phase I. As the group develops, it moves away from its preoccupation with authority toward a preoccupation with personal interactions. This constitutes the second major phase in group development, called Phase II. These major phases, and their subphases, are summarized in the accompanying box on the next page.

MEMBER PERSONALITY Bennis and Shepard view members as either conflicted or unconflicted about the dependence and personal aspects of group life. A **conflicted group member** is one whose posture toward dependence or intimacy may be viewed as inflexible, rigid, or compulsive. These members insist on adopting certain roles despite the situation. Conflicted members are responsible for confused communication within groups. An **unconflicted group member**, also called an *independent,* is better able to assess situations and alter roles of behavior as appropriate.

There are two ways that people can be conflicted about authority relationships. Members who are comforted by rules of procedure and agendas and rely on the decisions

The Bennis and Shepard Model

Phase I: Dependence-Power Relations

Subphase 1: Dependence-Submission

This subphase is characterized by dependence and flight. Members discuss problems external to the group. Assertive or aggressive members play dominant roles. Self-oriented behavior and subgrouping are evident.

Subphase 2: Counterdependence

This subphase is characterized by counterdependence and fight. Members discuss the organization and structure of the group. Assertive counterdependent and dependent members play dominant roles. The group searches for what to talk about and how to make decisions. Uncertainty causes anxiety.

Subphase 3: Resolution

This subphase is characterized by involvement in the group tasks. Assertive independents play dominant roles. The group unifies to pursue the task, and members take over some leadership roles.

Phase II: Interdependence-Personal Relations

Subphase 4: Enchantment

This subphase is characterized by a high level of solidarity, fusion, camaraderie, and suggestibility. Members talk about the positive aspects of the group and its members. For the first time, there is general distribution of participation. Overpersonal members play dominant roles. Laughter and joking are common, as is planning social events outside of the group.

Subphase 5: Disenchantment

This subphase is characterized by fight or flight, evidenced in distrust and suspicion of various group members. The content themes in Subphase 1 are revived. The most assertive counterpersonal members play dominant roles; overpersonal members are also active. The group may divide on the basis of shared attitudes toward intimacy. The group may be disparaged by the members in a variety of ways.

Subphase 6: Consensual Validation

This subphase is characterized by understanding and acceptance. Assertive independent members play dominant roles. The group views itself and its accomplishments in realistic terms. Consensus on important issues is easier to achieve.

Source: Adapted from Bennis and Shepard 1956.

of others (who are viewed as experts) are said to be *dependent.* Members who are uncomfortable with structure and authority are *counterdependent.* Counterdependents manifest their dissatisfaction with authority by opposing it regardless of its style or intent. Nothing the authority or leader does is acceptable. The counterdependent views failure to design an agenda as evidence of the authority's lack of ability. Paradoxically, designing an agenda may be viewed as too controlling. The counterdependent takes a "damned if you do, and damned if you don't" stance toward authority.

Members can be conflicted about personal relations in two ways as well. People who direct uninterrupted efforts toward reaching a high degree of intimacy with all other group members are termed *overpersonal.* Members who expend great amounts of energy in avoiding intimacy and maintaining distance are said to be *counterpersonal.*

People who are unconflicted in terms of either the authority relationships or the personal relationships in the group are responsible for major movements in the group's development toward valid communication. These unconflicted members who move the group on to the next phase are called **catalysts.** They reduce the internal uncertainty or stress in the group. Actions of these unconflicted members that move the group forward into the next phase are called *barometric events.*

RELATIONSHIP TO GROUP STRATEGIES The Bennis and Shepard model demonstrates group development along a continuum from an emphasis on power to an emphasis on affection. The activities of Phase I are concerned with such things as social class, ethnic background, and personal and professional interests. Concern with personality and feelings, such as warmth, anger, love, and anxiety, arise in Phase II. Bennis and Shepard believe that group therapies should be based on an adequate understanding of the group dynamic barriers to communication.

Interactional Group Therapy

There are great diversity and flux in the field of group therapy. Many types of groups are found in mental health care settings or in communities at large. People may belong to encounter groups, sensitivity training groups, gestalt groups, transactional analysis groups, psychodrama groups, psychoanalytic groups, nonverbal groups, body movement groups, nude swimming therapy groups, and so on. This list is certainly incomplete—a wide and sometimes bewildering array of group approaches is available.

Certain common principles seem to apply to all therapeutic groups, although specific methods and techniques may vary according to the purpose of the group or the skills and theoretic orientation of the therapist. Irvin Yalom (1985) uses the term *interactional group therapy* to describe a process of group therapy in which member interaction plays a crucial role. The common principles that apply to interactional group therapy are discussed below.

Advantages of Group Over Individual Therapy

The advantages of group therapy stem from one major factor: the presence of many people, rather than a solitary therapist, who participate in the therapeutic experience. Specifically, group therapy provides the following:

- Stimuli from multiple sources, revealing distortions in interpersonal relationships so that they can be examined and resolved.
- Multiple sources of feedback.
- An interpersonal testing ground that allows members to try out old and new ways of being in an environment specifically structured for that purpose.

Table 31–3 Curative Factors of Group Therapy

Factor	*Definition*
THERAPIST	
Instilling hope	Imbuing the client with optimism for the success of the group therapy experience.
Universality	Disconfirming the client's sense of aloneness or uniqueness in misery or hurt.
Imparting information	Giving instruction, advice, or suggestions.
Altruism	Finding that the client can be of importance to others; having something of value to give.
CLIENT	
Corrective recapitulation of the primary family group	Reviewing and correctively reliving early familial conflicts and growth-inhibiting relationships.
Development of socializing techniques	Acquiring sophisticated social skills, e.g., being attuned to process, resolving conflicts, and being facilitative toward others.
Imitative behavior	Trying out bits and pieces of the behavior of others and experimenting with those that fit well.
Interpersonal learning	Learning that one authors one's interpersonal world, and moving to alter it.
Group cohesiveness	Being attracted to the group and the other members with a sense of "we"-ness rather than "I"-ness.
Catharsis	Being able to express feelings.
Existential factors	Being able to "be" with others; to be a part of a group.

SOURCE: *Adapted from Yalom 1985.*

Qualified Group Therapists

Mental health care professionals may believe, in error, that group therapy is less complex and therefore "easier" than individual therapy, for example, because the presence of more people makes interactions between therapist and client less intense. Although it is true that the interactions between any one member and the therapist may be less intense because interactions are dispersed among others, it *does not follow* that anyone can be an effective group therapist.

To be effective, the group therapist should have the following special preparation:

- Education in small group dynamics.
- Education in group therapy theory.
- Clinical practice with groups.
- Expert supervision of the clinical practice (with ongoing supervision and/or consultation, depending on level of expertise).

The ANA 1994 Standards of Psychiatric–Mental Health Clinical Nursing Practice identify the group psychotherapist role as appropriate for clinical specialists prepared at the master's level (see Chapter 1). Experienced therapists report that it is also valuable to have been a member of a therapy or sensitivity training group, before becoming a group leader.

The Curative Factors

Yalom (1985) contends that eleven interdependent curative factors or mechanisms of change in group therapy help people. These factors are the framework for an effective approach to therapy, because they constitute a rational basis for the therapist's choices of tactics and strategies. They are identified and defined in Table 31–3 on the previous page.

Types of Group Leadership

Groups can be led by a therapist working alone or by cotherapists working together in a variety of ways. Each approach is reviewed in the following sections.

THE SINGLE THERAPIST APPROACH Groups led by a single therapist are common. They have an economic advantage in that only one therapist need be involved. A disadvantage is that the therapist cannot compare analyses of the group process with a cotherapist or get instant feedback or validation from a peer. Therapists working alone, however, do not have to direct their energies toward creating and maintaining a relationship with a colleague.

Recorders or observers may be used to help the solitary therapist be aware of the multiple complexities of any one group session. Nonparticipant observer/recorders are especially useful for giving the therapist feedback and focusing on the nonverbal aspects of the session. If they are truly to be nonparticipants, recorder/observers must be very careful not to react on a nonverbal level to the content or process of the session, in order to minimize, as much as possible, the effect that their presence might have on the group.

THE COTHERAPY APPROACH Groups led by two therapists, who share responsibility for leadership of the group to varying degrees, are gaining in popularity. The two models seen most often are the junior-senior and the egalitarian styles of cotherapy.

Junior-Senior Cotherapy In the junior-senior approach, the therapists have unequal responsibilities toward the group. The senior member of the team is usually the more experienced or educated. Besides having major responsibility for the success of the group, the senior therapist is responsible for training the junior member of the team. This approach is commonly used in agency settings, because it provides in-service training of new personnel and nonprofessionals under the guidance and watchful eye of an experienced group leader. However, relationship problems frequently surface when the roles of the leaders are not clear, or when one or both leaders are unable, or unwilling, to remain in the designated roles. The members of the group may also be unclear about the subordinate/superordinate roles and unsure of how to deal with and respond to leaders of unequal abilities and responsibilities.

Egalitarian Cotherapy In the egalitarian approach to cotherapy, two therapists of relatively equal ability and status share equally in responsibility for the group. The method is also used for training, with both cotherapists working under clinical supervision. It is preferable to the junior-senior approach for many reasons, which are set forth in Table 31–4. The egalitarian position is not without certain potential disadvantages, however. These are listed in Table 31–5. Overall, the advantages of the egalitarian approach outweigh its potential disadvantages. Cotherapists who arrange for supervision or consultation for themselves find that potential disadvantages can be turned in their favor. Identification and analysis of

Table 31–4 Advantages of the Egalitarian Cotherapist Approach

Advantage	*Rationale*
Facilitates group development	Two therapists of similar abilities can monitor and facilitate group development better than one alone.
Facilitates dealing with heightened affect	One therapist can relate more directly to the member experiencing heightened affect, while the other therapist assumes responsibility for assisting the group members with their responses. When one therapist is involved in an interaction with a member or members, the other can take an observer stance, helping those involved to become more aware of the interaction and their participation in it.
Enhances therapists' personal and professional development	Egalitarian cotherapists can provide each other with corrective feedback and help each other analyze group process and plan intervention strategies.
Provides a synergistic effect	This is another way of saying "two heads are better than one." It is likely that two people working together will make better decisions than one person working alone. The synergistic effect is similar to that of making decisions by consensus.
Provides an opportunity for modeling	Group members observe the acceptance and respect for each other that egalitarian cotherapists demonstrate. The therapists tolerate differences and disagreements between them in an atmosphere of mutual trust.
Reduces dependence	Because leadership is shared, the problem of dependence is somewhat dissipated.
Promotes appropriate pacing	Cotherapists check each other's timing, thus allowing the process to emerge. The presence of a cotherapist provides a respite from being continually "on guard" in relation to group process.

Table 31–5 Potential Disadvantages of the Egalitarian Cotherapist Approach

Potential Disadvantage	Rationale
Creates conflict if therapists have different orientations	Although there is room for uniqueness and difference, radically different styles or beliefs about group therapy between cotherapists may hinder therapeutic work within the group.
Requires extra energy and time	Each therapist must spend time and energy maintaining an effective working relationship with the other, since the quality of the relationship between them determines their effectiveness in the group setting.
May make members feel overloaded	If the style of the therapists turns out to be "two-on-one" (both working at once with one group member), members may feel overwhelmed or "overtherapized."
May suffer from the fact that the therapists share blind spots	Therapists who are very similar in style and personality may have the same blind spots and fail to give each other corrective feed back.
May provide the opportunity for misleading modeling	The model the therapists provide may be negative if their relationship is tense, mistrustful, closed, competitive, or threatening.

disadvantages that arise can lead to learning and behavior change in the cotherapists.

Two nurses considering an egalitarian cotherapy relationship with each other need to engage in preliminary work to determine whether such a relationship is feasible for them. Exploration should include a discussion of each therapist's theoretic approaches, intervention styles, past experiences with groups, background, and personality characteristics. The therapists should consider and resolve such issues as how and when feedback is to be given, how disagreements between them are to be handled in the session, and the general conditions under which they will work together.

Decisions on client selection, length and number of sessions, time, and place are made together. Decisions of an emergency nature made by one therapist in the absence of the other should be based on mutually agreed-upon procedures for just such situations.

Obviously, egalitarian cotherapists must establish and maintain clear channels of communication. Not only must they expend a great deal of time and energy in preparation for the group experience, they must also plan for presession and postsession meetings, joint analysis of data, and joint supervision or consultation.

Creating the Group

The effectiveness of a group depends greatly on the conditions under which it is created. Much as architects design buildings, therapists design groups with certain functions and characteristics in mind.

Selecting Members

Selecting the members is one of the most important functions of the therapists, since the quality of the interpersonal relationships among the members constitutes the core of successful group treatment. This is one of the major differences between group and individual therapy.

Inclusion Criteria It is more difficult to identify the characteristics of people who make good candidates for group therapy than those of people who do not make good candidates. We know that a person's motivation for therapy in general, and group therapy in particular, is of primary importance. Inclusion in a therapy group should also be at least partially determined by the effect a prospective member will have on the others, in terms of the prospective member's ability to bring the curative factors into play. Inclusion is also determined by the balance, in terms of behavior or characteristics, a prospective member will bring to the group. Will the person's subdued presentation prevent a member with similar behavior from being marginal and alone in the group? Does the person's age, occupation, or sex match another's so that the member will not feel singled out as different or deviant? The factor that appears to be most important, however, is that members be homogeneous in terms of their vulnerability or ego strength. Highly vulnerable members retard the progress of the less vulnerable, and vice versa.

Exclusion Criteria There have been a number of studies of group therapy dropouts. Dropouts significantly reduce the effectiveness of a group. They tend to have a demoralizing effect on the remaining group members. Group members see the act of dropping out as a comment on the worth of the group. For this reason, therapists should gear selection to avoid taking on members who are likely to terminate prematurely. Yalom (1985) identified several reasons for premature termination, listed in Table 31–6. Yalom's research has also demonstrated that people who drop out are likely to have some of the following characteristics:

- They use denial to a significant extent.
- They somatize frequently.
- They are less motivated than those who continue.
- They are less psychologically oriented than those who continue in the group.

Table 31–6 Client Reasons for Premature Termination of Group Therapy

Reason	*Rationale*
External factors	
Physical reasons	Distance, commuting, transportation, or scheduling problems may arise.
High external stress	An extremely stressful life may make it difficult or impossible for a client to expend energy participating in the group.
Group deviance	Members who differ significantly from others may wish to terminate; however, deviance that is unrelated to the group task is irrelevant.
Problems of intimacy	Isolated and withdrawn people, or those with a pervasive dread of self-disclosure, are threatened by group therapy.
Fear of emotional contagion	Members may find they become highly upset on hearing the problems of others.
Early provocateurs	Members may create a nonviable role for themselves in the group; they plunge in with behavior that provides the main focus, are furiously active, then wish to withdraw.
Problems in orientation to group therapy	If pretherapy tasks have not been properly undertaken, the member may not be realis tically prepared for the group.
Complications arising from subgrouping	Subunits that split up the group may disrupt therapeutic work if not understood and handled appropriately.
Complications arising from concurrent individual and group therapy	The member's two therapies may work at cross-purposes; members may "save" their affect and experiences in the group for exploration in an individual session.

SOURCE: *Adapted from Yalom 1985.*

- They have more severe psychiatric pathology.
- They are less likable (by group therapists).
- They are lower in socioeconomic status than those who continue.
- They are less effective socially than those who continue.
- They have lower IQs than those who continue.

It is also not uncommon to find that group therapy dropouts are people who used the group for crisis resolution. They drop out once the crisis has passed.

THE SELECTION INTERVIEW The pregroup interview session has two major purposes: selecting the members and establishing the initial contract. Cotherapists should always interview potential members jointly, and both should make all decisions regarding membership. The interview session gives members and therapists the opportunity to be exposed to one another. The therapists should accomplish the following tasks in the selection interview:

- Determine the motivation of the potential member.
- Determine the presence and extent of any exclusion criteria.
- Identify the presence of any external crisis that may have propelled the person into treatment.
- Encourage the client to ask questions about the group.
- Correct erroneous prejudgments or misinformation the client has about group therapy.
- Inquire about any major pending life changes that may prevent the client's full and continued participation in the group.
- Inquire about what hurts; what the client sees as a need to work on.
- Establish and clarify the initial group contract.

During this period, therapists and members have a chance to decide whether they can work together in the specific group under consideration. Clients as well as therapists can choose whether they will participate or not.

THE GROUP CONTRACT The group contract identifies the shared rights and responsibilities of therapists and members. It is a negotiated set of rules or arrangements for the structure and functioning of the group. It may be written or verbal, and it should cover the following elements:

- Goals and purposes of the group
- Time and length of meetings
- Place of meetings
- Starting and ending dates
- Addition of new members
- Attendance
- Confidentiality
- Roles of members and therapists
- Fees

Goals and Purposes The purpose of the group must be clear to all involved. In interactive group psychotherapy, the purpose is to bring about enduring behavioral and character change. The interactive group psychotherapy experience takes place largely in the here-and-now.

Goals may be long-term or short-term and are both group-oriented and individualized. Some goals may be identified as early as the selection interview, and others may be added as they emerge during the life of the group. Goals may be altered as appropriate.

Time, Length, and Frequency of Meetings The time, length, and frequency of meetings should be determined by the therapists after consideration of the clients' needs. Most outpatient clients find one 80- to 90-minute session per week useful. Shorter periods may not allow adequate time for discussion. Longer periods generally tax the endurance and alertness of both members and therapists. Inpatient groups are generally held more than once per week and frequently last for 50–60 minutes, although they may be longer or shorter depending on the anxiety and tolerance levels of the particular clients.

Place of Meetings The physical environment is important and influences the interaction among members. It is best to choose a pleasant room with comfortable chairs, preferably placed in a circle. The room should be private and free from external distractions.

Starting and Ending Dates If the group has a predetermined life span and the inclusive dates are known, members should be told the dates. Groups without fixed termination dates usually plan termination individually as each member is ready to move away from the group.

Addition of New Members Open groups accept members after the first session; closed groups begin with a certain number of members and do not add new members. Open groups maintain their size by replacing members who leave the group. They may continue indefinitely or have a predetermined life span. Closed groups are more common in settings where the stability of membership is likely. Such settings include residential facilities of various types, long-term psychiatric inpatient settings, and prisons. A major problem with the closed group is that it runs the risk of extinction as members leave the group for various reasons.

Attendance It is important that members make a commitment to attend every session. Absences hinder the establishment of cohesion and have a demoralizing effect, especially when perceived as evidence that a member lacks interest or that the group is not attractive and valuable to its members. Stability of membership and high attendance have been demonstrated to be critical factors in the successful outcome of group therapy.

Confidentiality Some rules regarding confidentiality should be established, and clients' concerns about which people will have access to information concerning them should be explored. Many therapists like to use tape recorders so that their work can be evaluated afterward by supervisors. They must obtain client agreement to use of a tape recorder.

Rules about confidentiality and access may be determined by the therapists' employing agency. In some instances, therapists may be required to make regular notes concerning each member's participation. Therapists may also wish to establish with group members guidelines on confidentiality that allow the therapists to share content with professionals who provide clinical supervision to the therapist, or when clients are dangerous to themselves or others. A good rule of thumb is: *Promise only what you can safely deliver.* Members should also be held accountable for maintaining the confidentiality of the group.

Roles of Members and Therapists Therapists and clients should reach an understanding about the responsibilities of participants. Humanistic psychotherapy involves the full and informed participation of the client in the therapeutic process. Participants should share their expectations about the behavior and functions of clients and therapists and should clearly understand the modes of participation.

Fees Fees should be determined in advance and arrangements for payment made. Most mental health care agencies have a sliding fee scale determined by the client's income and ability to pay. Clients should know whether fees will be charged for missed sessions.

Stages in Therapy Group Development

There is comfort in being able to predict, to some extent, the behavior of members at specific points in the group's life. Therapists organize predictions around stages or phases in the therapeutic experience, hoping to be prepared for expressions of behavior. They must bear in mind, however, that human experiences are dynamic and fluid and do not always progress as neatly as predicted.

The Schutz and Bennis and Shepard frameworks, presented earlier, give clear indications of how group life develops. This section focuses on the characteristics of member behavior and therapist interventions in the beginning, middle, and termination phases of interactional group therapy. As members' problems in living are revealed, group life becomes richer and more complex. Therefore, there is no "cookbook" method that a therapist can follow to respond to every situation. The accompanying Intervention box is simply a guide for identifying some common member behaviors and therapist interventions at various points in the life of the group.

The Here-and-Now Emphasis

The core of interactional group therapy is the here-and-now. According to Yalom (1985), the here-and-now work of the interactional group therapist occurs on two levels:

1. Focusing attention on each member's feelings toward other group members, the therapists, and the group.

INTERVENTION

Characteristic Member Behaviors and Nursing Interventions in Phases of Group Therapy

Member Behavior	Nursing Interventions
Beginning Phase	
Anxiety is high.	Move to reduce anxiety; avoid making demands until group anxiety has abated.
Members are unsure of what to do or say; need to be included.	Be active and provide some structure and direction; suggest members introduce themselves; work to sustain therapeutic rather than social role; include all members and encourage sharing but limit monopolizing.
Members are unclear about contract.	Clarify contract; give information to dispel confusion or misunderstandings.
Members test therapists and other members in terms of trustworthiness, value stances, etc., often through goblet issues.	Capitalize on opportunity to "pass" tests by proving trustworthy and by being open to and accepting the values of others.
Beginning attempts at self-disclosure and problem identification are made.	Focus on related themes; begin exploration; begin to focus on here-and-now experiences in session.
Members have sense of "I"-ness, little sense of "we"-ness.	Encourage involvement with others through curative factor of *universality*.
Middle Phase	
Sense of "I"-ness is replaced by "we"-ness.	Encourage cohesion; provide opportunity for expression of warm feelings.
Self-disclosure increases.	Encourage exploration and move to problem solving.
Members are more aware of interpersonal interactions in the here-and-now.	Encourage members to participate in observing and commenting on the here-and-now; make process comments.
Additions and losses of members evoke strong reactions.	Prepare members for additions and losses where possible; provide opportunity to talk about addition and loss experience.
Ability to maintain focus on one topic increases.	Encourage exploration of topic area in depth.
Termination Phase	
Feelings about separation may run the gamut (anger, sadness, indifference, joy, etc.).	Provide adequate time in as many sessions as necessary to work through affective responses; be sure members know the termination date in advance; help members leave with positive feelings by identifying positive changes that have occurred in individual members and in the group.
Members may feel lost and rudderless.	Explore support systems available to individual members; bridge the gap where possible (to another agency, another therapist, etc.); keep in focus the task of resolving the loss.

2. Illuminating the process (the relationship implications of interpersonal transactions).

Thus, group members need to become aware of the here-and-now events—*what* happened—and then reflect back on them—*why* it happened. Yalom has called this the *self-reflective loop*.

The first task of the therapist is to steer the group into the here-and-now. As the group progresses and becomes comfortable with awareness of the here-and-now, much of the work is taken on by the members. Initially, however, a primary task of the therapist is to actively steer the group discourse in an *ahistoric* direction. In other words, events in the session take precedence over those that occur outside or have occurred outside.

If the group is to engage in interpersonal learning, the therapist must illuminate the process. This is the second task of prime importance. The group must move beyond a focus on content toward a focus on process—the how and the why of an interaction. The process can be considered from any number of perspectives. The perspective chosen should be determined by the mood and needs of the group at that particular time. The group must recognize, examine, and understand the process. The task of illuminating it belongs mainly to the therapist.

Process commentary is anxiety-producing for new or inexperienced therapists and group members because there are so many injunctions against it in social situations. For example, commenting on someone's nervousness at a party is generally taboo. It not only makes the nervous person uncomfortable but also puts the process commentator in a high-risk situation. The comment may well be taken as criticism or viewed as inappropriate to the social context, and the commentator is vulnerable to retaliation from others. It is essential to educate members about this difference and to prepare them to hear, respond to, and eventually initiate process commentary.

Focusing on the here-and-now experience differentiates interactive group psychotherapy from many other group therapies or therapeutic groups such as those discussed later in the chapter.

Outpatient Versus Inpatient Groups

There are several essential differences between outpatient and inpatient groups that should be taken into consideration when planning for these groups. The selection criteria discussed earlier in this chapter are more likely to apply to outpatient groups. Inpatient groups have little prior selection. Clients may be admitted to an inpatient group on the basis of being hospitalized on a particular unit or being assigned to a particular therapist. Therefore, they tend to have a more heterogeneous composition; that is, the members may vary significantly in terms of their vulnerability or ego strength.

Because clients in outpatient groups have the choice of being a member of the group or not, they tend to be motivated to learn and to change. Inpatients, on the other hand, may be members of the group because the unit rules determine that group therapy is compulsory for all clients. They tend to be more ambivalent about group therapy.

Inpatient groups usually have rapid turnover because membership is limited to the extent of time the client is hospitalized. Once the client leaves the inpatient setting, membership in the group ends. This has several effects. For one, it means that since most hospitalizations are of 1–3 weeks' duration, there is little time for cohesion to develop. The rapid turnover also works against the development of cohesion. Cohesion develops in outpatient groups because of their length—1 or more years in duration, and 52 or more meetings.

The length of time per session is also different. Outpatient groups generally meet once a week for approximately 90 minutes. Inpatient groups generally meet several times per week, or even daily for about 45–60 minutes, depending on the tolerance level of its members.

Members in outpatient groups are discouraged from having relationships with other members outside the meetings. This is impossible in inpatient groups because the members may have 24-hour exposure to one another on the hospital unit and may also interact with the group therapist while the therapist is functioning in other roles. In fact, interaction with one another is encouraged.

It is important for the inpatient group therapist to provide significantly more structure for the group and to take on a more active role than would be necessary in an outpatient group. Hospitalized inpatients are likely to be in crisis and to be more dysfunctional than outpatients. Passivity on the therapist's part would be destructive to the group and could increase a client's distress. Yalom (1985) suggests the following protocol for structuring an inpatient group:

1. 3–5 minutes of orientation, warm-up, or preparation.
2. 20–30 minutes for an agenda go-around in which each member may share their personal concerns or problems.
3. 20–30 minutes in which the therapist attempts to fit the members' agendas together by finding commonalities or threads to work on.
4. 3–5 minutes to review the work of the group and to identify the issues or concerns that remain up in the air.

Both the inpatient and the outpatient group therapist can use the here-and-now approach of Yalom (1985) discussed earlier.

Other Group Therapies and Therapeutic Groups

Analytic Group Psychotherapy

Analytic group psychotherapy stems from psychoanalysis and shares its goal of personality reconstruction. In this process, there is an intensive analytic focus on the individuals in the group. It is sometimes described as treatment of one person in front of an audience of many. Dream material and fantasies are explored in the group, and the technique of free association is used. The interpersonal interactions of the members are of secondary importance and are explored in terms of how they demonstrate unresolved conflicts in the individual members' earlier relationships.

Psychodrama

Psychodrama is chiefly concerned with problems unique to the individual. It provides a medium through which catharsis can be achieved on both the nonverbal action and gesture level and the verbal level. In psychodrama groups, members act out real or imagined situations, while alter egos (other members) attempt to add what they think the actor may be feeling or thinking. The participants are encouraged to change roles. The practice of role reversal offers them the opportunity to "get into the other person's skin." The psychodramatist (therapist) is called a "director" whose responsibility is to direct the drama toward the goal of achieving catharsis and reaching for insight.

The psychodramatic stage may be quite complex. It sometimes consists of a series of tiers where different parts of the drama are acted out. Complex lighting and mood music may also be used to achieve the desired effect.

Transactional Analysis

Eric Berne's (1960) **transactional analysis (TA)** is a method of group therapy as well as a method of communication analysis. Transactional analysis is concerned with the changes in a person's posture, verbalization, voice, attitude, and feeling. Transactional analysis is both quick and easily understood. It is useful in understanding brief contacts with clients or colleagues when there is little time to establish a rewarding relationship. Nurses can use transactional analysis concepts in understanding their own behavior as well.

STRUCTURAL ANALYSIS Before beginning TA it is important to carry out a structural analysis of an individual's personality. Each person has three main sources of behavior, or ego states: the Parent, the Adult, and the Child. The **Child ego state** is manifested through childlike behavior similar to that of a child less than 7 years old. Giggling, coyness, naïveté, charm, boisterousness, and whining are characteristics of the Child ego state. So are "I want," "gosh," "golly," "me," "mine," and "I dunno."

By the time children become adults, they learn that they must adapt the spontaneous and free expression of feelings in their natural state, the *Natural Child ego state,* to meet the demands and expectations of parents and the culture in which they live. Their adaptive behavior results in the *Adapted Child ego state,* which has one of two common manifestations: compliance with parents or other authority figures, or rebellion and refusal to follow orders. Most people's Child ego state falls somewhere between the two extremes.

Objective appraisal of reality and the capacity to process data are the domain of the **Adult ego state.** The Adult is manifested in accomplishments beyond those of children, such as accurate analysis of complex realities and realistic manipulation of concepts. Perceptive skill, data processing, sociability, and communicativeness are attributed to the Adult. So are "it appears," "I think," "why," "what," "where," "when," and "how."

The **Parent ego state** incorporates the feelings and behaviors learned from parents or authority figures. A Parent ego state can be identified when the person's behavior includes the language, intonations, attitudes, postures, and mannerisms of one or both parents. All-wise, all-knowing, benevolent, prim, critical, or righteous attitudes are some examples. So are "if I were you," "how many times have I told you," "poor dear," "disgusting," "now what," and "do it this way." The *Nurturing Parent ego state* cuddles, protects, and cares for, while the *Critical Parent ego state* corrects or condemns.

Berne postulated that an individual exhibits a Parent or an Adult or a Child ego state, and that shifts can occur from one ego state to another. A nursing student, new to a day treatment unit of a community mental health center, reported her ego state switches in the following situation:

When I walked into the TV room to pick up the pen that I had left there, I saw one of the group members pacing the floor; he was angrily muttering a string of obscenities. I don't mind telling you that I was plenty scared. I was afraid that he might hurt me (Child ego state). I told myself that I should do something about reducing his anxiety and stress (Parent ego state). But I felt so helpless and dumb (Child ego state). Then I decided that I really didn't know how to handle this situation and remembered something you said in class—that it's OK to ask for help—and I didn't feel scared or dumb any more. This has really turned into a good learning situation for me (Adult ego state).

These ego state switches are illustrated in Figure 31–2.

In TA theory, structural analysis determines which ego state controls a person's behavior at a particular time.

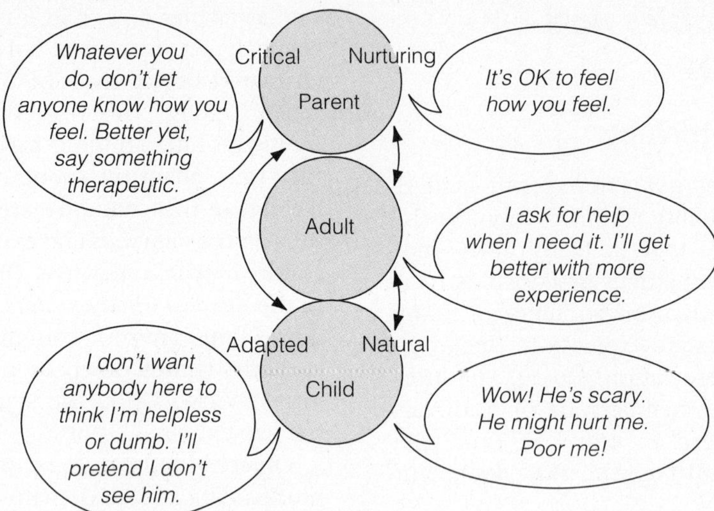

Figure 31–2 Ego state shifts.

Spontaneity, charm, creativity, and enjoyment reside in the Child. The Adult not only is necessary for survival in dealing effectively with the outside world but also regulates and mediates the activities of the Parent and the Child. The Parent enables an individual to act effectively as a parent and makes many automatic responses that free the Adult from routine, trivial decisions. Each of the three ego states performs vital functions.

EGO STATES IN WELLNESS/ILLNESS Most of the time, people who are dysfunctional or disordered are in a Child ego state. A stereotype is the "problem client" who is demanding, becomes extremely dependent, or refuses to follow a prescribed medical regimen. These problem clients are using the Adapted Child to cope with unfamiliar or frightening situations. The overly cheerful, overly friendly, or overly helpful client is less often identified as a problem but is also using the Adapted Child ego state to cope. The Child ego state is also at work in the client who is confused, disoriented, and enraged; who screams or strikes at others; or who withholds information because of fear of retaliation.

Sick people in their Parent ego state may be critical of staff or suspicious of their intentions. Sometimes they nurture and protect other clients or even the staff. People in a Parent ego state are critical of themselves for being ill or unable to cope with the stresses of life. Such people berate themselves for bothering staff, family, and friends. Some even hallucinate figures or voices that criticize them for their real or imagined transgressions.

The client in the Adult ego state contributes to wellness by deciding when to sleep or rest, whether to visit with friends or family, and what steps to take to decrease stress. People in this ego state are able to accept the temporary limitations imposed by illness or stress, to care for themselves within the imposed limitations, and to seek partnership in decisions about the direction of their health care.

Obviously, the sick person in the Adult ego state is in the best possible situation under the circumstances. However, other ego states can also contribute to both illness and wellness. For example, people in the Nurturing Parent ego state can allow themselves to be taken care of by others and may give themselves "permission" to be sick or to feel depressed. They are more likely to return quickly to a state of well-being than those who constantly berate themselves for being ill or succumbing to life's stresses. The Child ego state is helpful in achieving wellness, because it allows for the natural expression of feelings that can then be handled.

TRANSACTIONAL ANALYSIS Whereas structural analysis is directed toward the analysis of the individual's personality, transactional analysis is broadened to focus on what occurs between two or more people.

Complementary Transactions In a **complementary transaction**, the transactional stimulus and the transactional response occur on identical ego levels. A transaction is complementary when a message sent to an ego state is responded to from that ego state. Complementary transactions can go on uninterrupted until one or the other of the participants changes ego state. Most of the time, productive communication occurs in complementary transactions, because the participants behave according to their perceptions of, and their predictions about, the ego state of the other. However, continuing, or locked, complementary transactions—for instance, from Critical Parent to Adapted Child—result in uninterrupted but uncomfortable, nonfacilitative communication. The Parent-

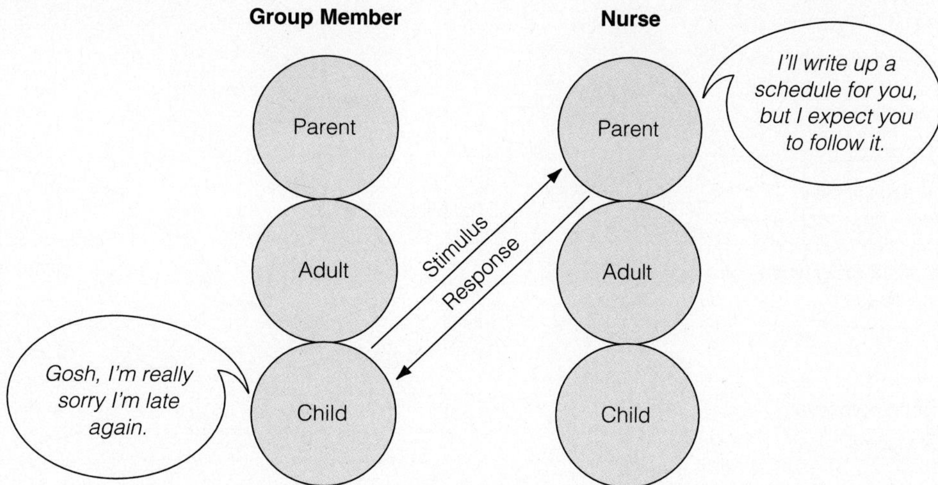

Figure 31–3 A complementary transaction.

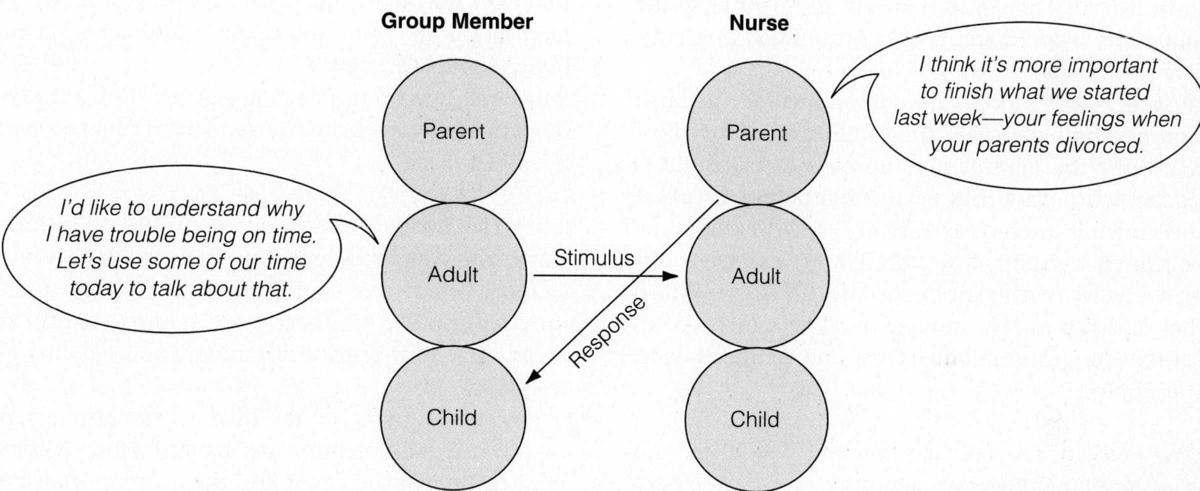

Figure 31–4 A crossed transaction.

Child transaction of nurse and group member in Figure 31–3 limits the client's growth. It encourages dependence and discourages responsibility.

Crossed Transactions **Crossed transactions** result from changes in ego states that terminate the complementary relationship. Figure 31–4 illustrates one such crossed transaction: The client tries to relate to the nurse on an Adult-to-Adult level, but the nurse responds on a Parent-to-Child level. In crossed transactions, communication is usually not smooth or satisfactory and is soon terminated. When complementary transactions become locked (and interpersonally uncomfortable), it may be useful to cross ego states to move the communication forward. For example, if a nurse is aware of having behaved like a Critical Parent to a client who responds from the Adapted Child state, the nurse can alter communication behavior by switching to the Adult ego state. The client will probably follow this lead, resulting in a better nurse-client working relationship.

Ulterior Transactions and Games **Ulterior transactions** are complex phenomena that occur on two levels—social (the surface, or overt one) and psychologic (the hidden, or covert one). **Games** are series of ulterior transactions with concealed motivations. Figure 31–5 shows an ulterior transaction as it occurs in the "Why don't you . . . Yes, but . . ." game. In this game, one person presents a problem to another person or to members of a group, who offer solutions to the problem. The first player, however, rejects all solutions. The gimmick, or concealed motivation, is that, although this is supposedly

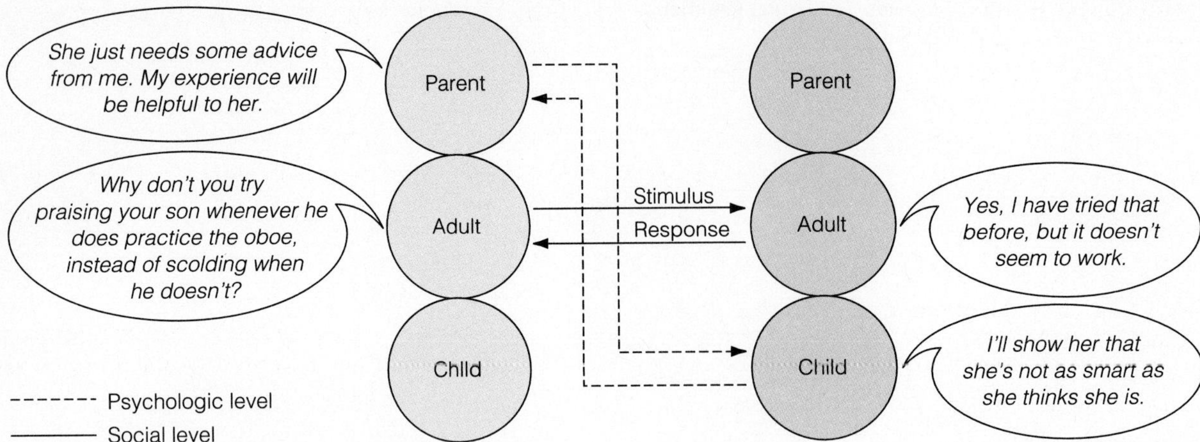

Figure 31–5 An ulterior transaction in the "Why don't you . . . Yes, but . . ." game.

an Adult request for information, the psychologic level is Child to Parent. The Child is always the winner, while the supposedly "wise" Parents are confounded and confused one after another.

Because the interactions are complementary at both social and psychologic levels, the game can be played indefinitely until the Parents give up or a more sophisticated person who recognizes what is happening breaks it up. The following interaction is typical of how this game might occur in a group. Rose, the client, has been discussing her view of the problems she has experienced since her mother-in-law moved in. The nurse group leader and other group members respond to Rose's overt request for help.

Nurse: The problem seems to be that you give in to your mother-in-law all the time. How about trying to talk to her?
Rose: If I talk to her, it won't do any good. She'll just continue to act the same way.
Ben: How about getting your husband to help?
Rose: I'd ask him to talk to her, but he says that it's my house, so I should give the orders and there should be no problem.
Nurse: You mentioned that she has another son. Do you think that you could talk to him and work out some plan to have her live by herself?
Rose: No. We haven't talked to him in a long while, and anyway she doesn't have enough money to live on her own.
Marilyn: How about a nursing home?
Rose: We can't afford to send her to a nursing home.

Apparently giving up on finding a solution for the client's "mother-in-law problem," the group begins to work on other tangentially related household problems.

Anne: You said that taking care of six children is quite a job. Do you think you could hire a baby-sitter to watch them in the afternoon?
Rose: There's nobody in the neighborhood who I can get to sit. Either they're too young or they don't want to.
Marilyn: Do you think you could hire someone to clean the house one day a week?
Rose: Well, we could afford it, but my husband says that I don't need anyone to help me and that I could do everything by myself.

After the nurse assessed her own and the group's ego states, the game broke up, and the participants moved on to more productive communication. The nurse did so by moving into her Adult ego state, figuring out the dynamics and her contributions to them, and then changing her responses.

"Why don't you . . . Yes, but . . ." can also take place in one-to-one relationships, particularly when it is a behavioral pattern of the client and the nurse is unaware of the psychologic level.

Self-Help Groups

The major operating principle in self-help groups is that the help given to members comes from members. A professional mental health care worker is viewed as unnecessary. In fact, many of these groups were developed because of the failure of programs planned and implemented by professionals. In most, leaders are former members. Alcoholics Anonymous is a well-known example of this principle.

There is a wide variety of self-help groups. Some are:

- Recovery Incorporated, Schizophrenics Anonymous, and Neurotics Anonymous, concerned with mental illness.
- Overeaters Anonymous, concerned with overeating.
- Gamblers Anonymous and Gam-Anon, concerned with compulsive gambling.

- Five-Day Plan and Smoke Watchers Anonymous, concerned with smoking.
- Child Abuse Listening Mediation, Inc. (CALM) and Parents Anonymous, concerned with child abuse.
- La Leche League, concerned with breast-feeding.
- Al-Anon and Al-a-Teen, concerned with the families of alcoholics.

Self-help groups are proliferating rapidly. Groups for divorced, widowed, or single people, for parents of runaways and troubled adolescents, for parents who abuse their children, and for the recently bereaved are a common part of the scene in most major cities throughout the world. Client clubs for people who have had a colostomy, ileostomy, laryngectomy, mastectomy, or amputation are also popular.

The role of the nurse in self-help groups is that of a resource person. Nurses need to be informed about such groups so that they can refer potential members to groups appropriate to their needs, or to provide consultation when invited to do so.

Psychoeducation Groups

Psychoeducation groups have the sharing of mental health care information as a primary goal. They also have the secondary benefit of facilitating the discussion of feelings such as isolation, helplessness, sadness, stigmatization, and/or anger and possible strategies for dealing with these feelings (see the Research Note). Some examples of psychoeducation groups follow.

Medication Teaching Groups Studies have shown that the causes of medication noncompliance are related to a lack of insight and understanding by clients of their illness and of their drug treatment (Forman 1993). In addition, drug side effects such as dry mouth, blurred vision, sedation, and akathisia can be difficult to tolerate. Medication teaching groups provide an opportunity for psychiatric nurses to educate clients about medications, their side effects, the nature and course of their mental disorder, the possibility of relapse without continued drug treatment, and the positive effect medications have on their lives.

Family Education Groups Family members can also benefit from psychoeducation groups designed specifically to help family members cope with their loved one's illness. Much like medication teaching groups, family education groups educate family members about the specific mental disorder including its signs and symptoms, the medications the client takes, the symptoms and stages of relapse, the fluctuating course of mental illness. They also learn about life events that cause stress for the seriously and persistently mentally ill, how to prevent relapse, and how to manage behavior that is disturbing to others.

Family therapy is another form of group therapy. It differs from the group therapy described in this chapter because the family is a naturally formed group with a history. Family therapy is discussed in detail in Chapter 32. Psychoeducation and interventions with family members of people with schizophrenia are discussed in Chapter 14.

Remotivation Groups Remotivation and reeducation groups were developed to help people who had under-

RESEARCH NOTE

Citation

Maynard C: Comparison of effectiveness of group interventions for depression in women. *Arch Psychiatr Nurs* 1993;7(5):277–283.

Study Problem/Purpose

The purpose of this study was to test the efficacy of a structured cognitive-behavioral group intervention designed by Verona Gordon.

Methods

Twenty women between the ages of 18 and 65 were assigned either to 12 weekly 1.5-hour group intervention sessions based on Gordon's structured approach, or to a support group. Fourteen women who were unable to attend sessions were assigned to a control untreated group. All participants were administered the Beck Depression Inventory, Coopersmith Self-Esteem Inventory, Beck Hopelessness Scale, and Speilberger's State-Trait Anxiety Inventory, before and at the end of the 12 weeks.

Findings

Subjects who participated in Gordon's structured approach had a significant decrease in depression, hopelessness, and state anxiety. There was a corresponding significant increase in self-esteem. There were no significant changes in the support group or the control group.

Implications

The structured group approach is a less expensive way to manage depression, and it also serves to increase self-esteem. In this milieu of cost-consciousness and health care reform, substantial savings are important.

gone long-term institutionalization become less isolated and more socially adept. Long-term institutionalization produces apathy and isolation. Clients ready for release are often unaware of accepted norms or socially appropriate behavior and therefore are ill-equipped to live outside a totally protected environment. Remotivation groups help prepare these people to live beyond the confines of the institution. The groups bring members up to date with contemporary society. They can be led effectively by people with minimal preparation in group work. In many psychiatric hospitals, this role falls to the psychiatric aide. Nurses are more likely to supervise than to lead remotivation groups.

Groups of Medical-Surgical Clients and Their Families Groups composed of medical-surgical clients are increasingly common, as psychiatric nurses move into general medical-surgical settings offering liaison and consultation services to clients and staff. Group work is useful for chronically ill or disabled clients, preoperative and postoperative clients, clients with regulative medical problems (such as diabetes, cardiac disease, or kidney disease), dying clients, elderly clients, and clients with psychophysiologic disorders, among others.

Such groups generally focus on the stress of hospitalization and illness and have as their goal the reduction of stress. Groups may be composed of clients alone, family members alone, or a combination.

Activity Therapy Groups

Activity therapies are manual, recreational, and creative techniques to facilitate personal experiences and increase social responses and self-esteem. Activity therapies are generally the province of health and recreation specialists.

Some activity therapies, such as the creative arts therapies discussed below, are organized and conducted in groups. Although there are specifically educated creative arts therapists, their numbers are small. Nurses may lead such groups or use their principles to reach beyond the ordinary realm of verbal communication with clients.

Poetry Therapy Groups The goal of poetry therapy groups is to help members get in touch with feelings and emotions through the use of poetry. Poems that are read aloud provide the stimulus for understanding and catharsis. They are selected as the therapeutic medium because they are powerful but not explicit avenues of communication. It is not necessary to be able to write poetry to be a member or leader of a poetry therapy group, although some members or leaders may be stimulated to write poems of their own.

Art Therapy Groups Painting offers many people a comfortable opportunity for social exchange. In art therapy groups, the art produced by each member gives the art therapist or group leader a personal insight into the artist's personality. The art is produced during the session and is used as the basis for discussion and for exploring members' feelings.

Music Therapy Groups Music therapy consists of singing, rhythm, body movement, and listening. It is designed to increase group members' concentration, memory retention, conceptual development, rhythmic behavior, movement behavior, verbal and nonverbal retention, and auditory discrimination. It is also used to stimulate members' expression and discussion of affect.

Dance Therapy Groups Dance therapy combines movement and verbal modes. In dance, members find it easier to express nonverbally the feelings and emotions that have been difficult to realize and communicate by other means. The person's inner sense is often reflected in body movements, and dance therapists work to help members integrate their experiences verbally as well as nonverbally.

Bibliotherapy Groups In bibliotherapy, literature is the means for achieving a therapeutic goal. The purpose of a bibliotherapy group is to assimilate the psychologic, sociologic, and aesthetic insights books give into human character, personality, and behavior. Literature provides a stimulus for group members to compare events and characters with their own interpersonal and intrapsychic experiences.

Community Client Groups

Psychiatric nurses in community settings are involved with different kinds of community groups. These settings include schools, youth centers, industries, neighborhood centers, churches, prisons, summer camps, single-room occupancy boarding houses, transitional facilities (halfway houses), apartments for the elderly, and residential facilities for delinquent youths, runaways, and unwed mothers. Clients may also be people who have direct contact with these groups, such as teachers, youth counselors, prison guards, police officers, and camp counselors.

Groups with Nurse Colleagues

There is increasing interest among nurses who work together in forming discussion and counseling groups to help reduce their job-related stress and to help them deal with problems of interpersonal relationships in more satisfying ways. Nurses in various intensive care and other high-pressure settings identify with increasing frequency the need for group work services that the psychiatric nurse can provide. The psychiatric nurse may also identify the need and offer this opportunity to colleagues.

Chapter Highlights

- Most people's lives are spent interacting with other people in groups. An individual's sense of being arises through membership in groups that help achieve goals they set for themselves.
- Nurses interact with groups of clients and colleagues in a wide variety of settings. To use groups rationally and effectively, nurses must understand the forces that underlie small group interactional processes and recognize their own patterns of participation.
- Effective groups accomplish their goals, maintain cohesion, and develop and modify their structure in ways that improve effectiveness.
- The most effective group leadership is based on the assumption that responsible membership is the same thing as responsible leadership. In this distributed-functions approach, both the leader and the members engage in leadership behavior.
- The hallmark of a group that functions effectively is sound decision making that leads to well-conceived, well-understood, and well-accepted realistic actions toward the agreed-upon goals of the group.
- The existence of trust in groups enables members to make suggestions; disclose attitudes, feelings, experiences, and perceptions; give feedback; and confront one another.
- Cohesion in groups is the spirit of "we"-ness that develops when a group has had shared experiences that provide a basis for attraction—the primary factor that keeps a group in existence and working effectively.
- Power and influence in groups operate constantly and force members to adjust to one another and modify their behavior.
- Nurses can provide humanistic care to clients in a variety of settings through group intervention by offering them opportunities to seek validation, give and receive interpersonal feedback, and test new and different ways of being that may increase their quality of life.
- Group development occurs in identifiable stages and has implications for member behavior and therapist intervention.
- Curative factors, or mechanisms of change that constitute a rational basis for the therapist's choices of tactics and strategies, are unique to the group therapy process.
- Critical considerations in designing a group are the selection of members and the establishment of a group contract.
- In interactive groups, member interaction plays a crucial role in change, which is achieved through the use of the here-and-now to illuminate group process.

References

Agazarian YM: Contemporary theories of group psychotherapy: A systems approach to the group-as-a-whole. *Int J Group Psychother* 1992;42:177–201.

Alonso A, Swiller HI: *Group Therapy in Clinical Practice.* American Psychiatric Association, 1993.

Becu M, Becu N, Manzur G, Kochen S: Self-help epilepsy groups: An evaluation of effect on depression and schizophrenia. *Epilepsia* 1993;34(5):841–845.

Bennis W, Shepard HA: A theory of group development. *Hum Relations* 1956;9:415–437.

Berne E: *Transactional Analysis in Psychotherapy.* Grove Press, 1960.

Clark WG, Vorst VR: Group therapy with chronically depressed geriatric patients. *J Psychosoc Nurs Ment Health Serv* 1994;32(5):9–13.

Corey MS, Corey G: *Groups: Process and Practice,* ed 4. Brooks/Cole, 1992.

Deffenbacher JL, Thwaites GA, Wallace TL, Oetting ER: Social skills and cognitive-relaxation approaches to general anger reduction. *J Cons Psychol* 1994;41(3):386–396.

Deutsch M: The effects of cooperation and competition upon group process. *Hum Relations* 1949;2:129–152, 199–231.

Deutsch M: Trust and suspicion. *J Conflict Resolution* 1958; 2:265–279.

Echternacht MR: Day treatment transition groups. *J Psychosoc Nurs* 1984;22(10):11–16.

Elbirlik K, Apprey M, Moles K: Individual and group therapies as constructive continuous experiences. *Am J Psychother* 1994;48(1):141–154.

Evans M, Marad G: A triage model of psychotherapeutic group intervention. *Arch Psychiatr Nurs* 1993;7(4):244–248.

Feldman JS: An alternative group approach: Using multidisciplinary expertise to support patients with prostate cancer and their families. *J Psychosoc Oncol* 1993;11(2):83–93.

Forester B, Kornfeld DS, Fleiss JL, Thompson S: Group psychotherapy during radiotherapy: Effects on emotional and physical distress. *Am J Psychiatr* 1993;150(11):1700–1706.

Forman L: Medication: Reasons and interventions for noncompliance. *J Psychosoc Nurs* 1993;31(10):23–25.

Gallagher-Thompson D, DeVries HM: "Coping with frustration" classes: Development and preliminary outcomes with women who care for relatives with dementia. *Gerontologist* 1994;34:548–552.

Gans JS: Hostility in group psychotherapy. *Int J Group Psychother* 1989;39:4–11.

Gilbert CM: Sexual abuse and group therapy. *J Psychosoc Nurs* 1988;26(5):19–23.

Gordon VC, Gordon EM: Short-term group treatment of depressed women: A replication study in Great Britain. *Arch Psychiatric Nurs* 1987;1(2):111–125.

Hamilton JD et al.: Quality assessment and improvement in group psychotherapy. *Am J Psychiatr* 1993;150(2):316–320.

Harpaz N: Failures in group psychotherapy: The therapist variable. *Int J Group Psychother* 1994;44(1):3–19.

Hierholzer R, Liberman R: Successful living: A social skills and problem-solving group for the chronically mentally ill. *Hosp Commun Psychiatr* 1986;37(9):913–918.

Hunka CD, O'Toole AW, O'Toole RW: Self-help therapy in parents anonymous. *J Psychosoc Nurs* 1985;23(7):24–32.

Johnson DW, Johnson FP: *Joining Together: Group Therapy and Group Skills,* ed 3. Prentice-Hall, 1987.

Kane CF, DiMartino E, Jimenez M: A comparison of short-term psychoeducational and support groups for relatives coping with chronic schizophrenia. *Arch Psychiatr Nurs* 1990;4(6):343–353.

Kaplan HI, Sadock BJ: *Comprehensive Group Psychotherapy,* ed 3. Williams & Wilkins, 1993.

Kaplan KL: *Directive Group Therapy: Innovative Mental Health Treatment,* Slack, 1988.

Kelly KK, Sautter F, Tugrul K, Weaver MD: Fostering self-help on an inpatient unit. *Arch Psychiatr Nurs* 1990;4(3):161–165.

Kipper DA: Psychodrama: Group psychotherapy through role playing. *Int J Group Psychother* 1992;42:495–521.

MacKenzie KR: *Effective Use of Group Therapy in Managed Care.* American Psychiatric Association, 1994.

MacKenzie KR: *Introduction to Time-Limited Group Psychotherapy.* American Psychiatric Association, 1990.

Madison TS: *Psychoanalytic Group Therapy and Therapy.* International Universities Press, 1991.

Maestri B, Carruth AK: When the CNS needs help establishing a woman's support group: Getting the most from the consultation process. *Clin Nurs Specialist* 1993;7(5):281–285.

Maynard C: Comparison of effectiveness of group interventions for depression in women. *Arch Psychiatr Nurs* 1993;7(5):277–283.

Maynard C: A psychoeducational approach to depression in women. *J Psychosoc Nurs Ment Health Serv* 1993;31(12):9–14.

McHale M: Getting the joke: Interpreting humor in group therapy. *J Psychosoc Nurs* 1989;27(9):24–28.

Miller CR, Eisner W, Allport C: Creative coping: A cognitive-behavioral group for borderline personality disorder. *Arch Psychiatr Nurs* 1994;8(4):280–285.

Moreno JL: *Psychodrama.* Beacon Press, 1946.

Pollack LE: Do inpatients with bipolar disorder evaluate diagnostically homogeneous groups? *J Psychosoc Nurs* 1993;31(10):26–32.

Pollack LE: Improving relationships: Groups for inpatients with bipolar disorder. *J Psychosoc Nurs* 1990;28(5):17–22.

Prehn RA, Thomas P: Does it make a difference? The effect of a women's issues group on female psychiatric inpatients. *J Psychosoc Nurs* 1990;28(11):34–38.

Pringer P, Agana-Defensor R, Mullen NM, Lee L: A model for the development and implementation of a patient support group in a medical-surgical setting. *Holistic Nurse Prac* 1993;8(1):16–26.

Scheidlinger S: An overview of nine decades of group psychotherapy. *Hosp Commn Psychiatr* 1994;45(3):217–225.

Schutz WC: Interpersonal underworld. *Harvard Business Review* 1958a;36:123–135.

Schutz WC: *The Interpersonal Underworld: FIRO.* Science and Behavior Books, 1958b.

Selander JM, Miller WC: Prolixin group: Can nursing intervention groups lower recidivism rates? *J Psychosoc Nurs* 1985;23(11):16–20.

Shields JD, Lanza ML: The parallel process of resistance by clients and therapists to starting groups: A guide for nurses. *Arch Psychiatr Nurs* 1993;7(5):300–307.

Stewart NJ, McMullen LM, Rubin LD: Movement therapy with depressed inpatients: A randomized multiple single case design. *Arch Psychiatr Nurs* 1994;8(1):22–29.

Urbancic JC: Resolving incest experiences through group therapy. *J Psychosoc Nurs* 1989;27(9):4–10.

Vannicelli M: *Group Psychotherapy with Adult Children of Alcoholics.* Guilford Press, 1989.

van Servellen G, Poster EC, Ryan J, Allen J: Nursing-led group modalities in a psychiatric inpatient setting: A program evaluation. *Arch Psychiatr Nurs* 1991;5(3):128–136.

Vinogradov S, Yalom ID: *A Concise Guide to Group Psychotherapy.* American Psychiatric Association, 1989.

Wenckus EM: Storyteling: Using an ancient art to work with groups. *J Psychosoc Nurs Mental Health Serv* 1994;32:30–32.

Wolfe M: Group modalities in the care of clients with drug and alcohol problems, in Naegle MA (ed): *Substance Abuse Education in Nursing,* Vol. III. National League for Nursing, 1993.

Yalom ID: *Inpatient Group Psychotherapy.* Basic Books, 1983.

Yalom ID: *The Theory and Practice of Group Psychotherapy,* ed 3. Basic Books, 1985.

CHAPTER 32

FAMILY PROCESS AND FAMILY THERAPY

Carol Ren Kneisl

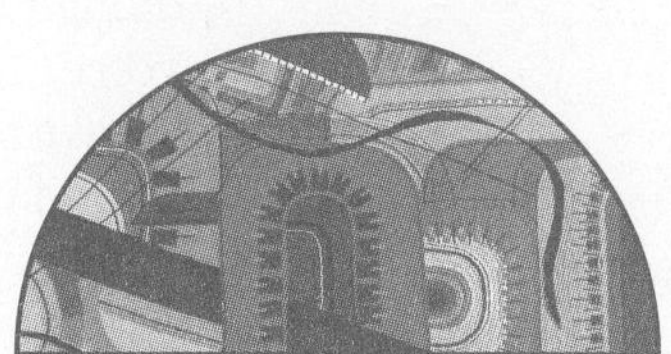

COMPETENCIES

- *Identify the diverse forms of family life.*
- *Identify the developmental tasks that confront couples and families.*
- *Describe the family in terms of the relationships, associations, and connections that occur in a dynamic, interacting whole.*
- *Describe relationship and communication complexities in functional families and families in difficulty.*
- *Discuss strategies for family assessment and intervention.*
- *Apply understandings of family process and family therapy in promoting and maintaining family mental health.*

Cross-References

Other topics relevant to this content are: Codependence, Chapter 26; Communication skills, Chapter 7; Intrafamily physical and sexual abuse, Chapter 23; Psychoeducation, Chapters 14 and 31.

Critical Thinking Challenge

Mark James, your 22-year-old client, is being discharged after his first hospital admission to the home he shares with his parents and two sisters. The mental health care team has recommended family therapy to the James family. You perceive what you think is annoyance on Mr. James' face, and one of Mark's sisters appears embarrassed. Although you will not be the James family therapist because you are not a clinical specialist, you recognize how important Mark's family can be to his progress. What actions can you take to address the family's unspoken concerns and needs?

The family is the context in which most people develop their first relationships with other people. Their view of the larger social world outside their own unique family is molded by the events that happen within families and that influence the development of the individual.

Nurses encounter families in many areas of their practice—in the emergency room, the intensive care unit, the school, the cancer hospital, the community health setting, and the mental health care setting. Preventive approaches to family mental health, assessment of families in trouble, and intervention on their behalf must be based on an understanding of how families grow and interact and how family coping patterns develop. This chapter describes those processes and offers strategies for intervention into dysfunctional family systems.

Family Structures

Today's family is:

- Mom, dad, and 2.2 kids.
- A couple with eight kids: three of hers, three of his, and two of theirs.
- A 32-year-old electrical engineer and his three foster children.
- A divorced woman and her infant child.
- A widowed man, his two children, and his parents.
- A grandmother raising her two grandchildren.
- Two lesbian mothers and their children.
- Two couples sharing an apartment neither could afford alone.
- Three gay men who live and work together.
- Four couples and their children in a remote commune.

The *nuclear family*—mom, dad, and 2.2 kids—is the family structure people refer to when they speak of "strengthening the family."

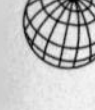

Is it true that the family is dying out or needs strengthening? Actually, constant transformation or change is the one permanent quality of the family. Many family forms have appeared, disappeared, reappeared, and coexisted within and across cultures. Families have been defined by blood relationships, tribes, households, kinship systems, clans, and language alliances. They have been called *blended, extended, conjugal,* and *communal.* The American family is changing, but not dying: It is simply becoming different. Sensitive psychiatric nurses reject a narrow definition of family and adapt their clinical practice to the wide variety of family constellations that exist in contemporary society.

The Traditional Nuclear Family

The traditional **nuclear family** is a two-parent, time-limited, two-generation family consisting of a married couple and their children by birth or adoption. Despite its name, it is a relatively recent development in human history. It evolved as societies became more urban and industrialized in the move away from agrarianism. It is time-limited because, in most instances, the members of the younger generation begin their own families soon after they are 20 years of age.

Shortly after its development, the traditional nuclear family became known as the *isolated nuclear family.* Ties to the **extended family**—all people related by birth, marriage, or adoption to the nuclear family—were weakened. This diminished the basic support system that formerly surrounded families. The isolated nuclear family had less contact with the adults' **families of origin** (the families from which they came).

The Single-Parent Family

A *single-parent family* is also two-generational and occurs when a lone parent and offspring live together as a nucleus. It is a more common family form than most people believe. The number of single-parent families has been steadily increasing since 1970. The current prevalence in the United States is one in five.

Although most single-parent families result from death or divorce, increasing numbers of women are bearing children with the intention of rearing them alone. Single women and men are also adopting children with increasing frequency, something that was not done or even permitted only a few years ago. And more often than ever before, single-parent families are headed by men.

The Blended Family

The **blended family**, an increasingly common phenomenon, is one in which one or both marital partners bring with them their children from a former relationship. Various types of blended families exist. The loosest structure is a weekend blending that occurs when the children from one parent's previous marriage visit that parent's later family for a brief time. In a more permanent blend, the children from a previous marriage live with one parent and a later spouse, forming the new nucleus. In a third type of blended family, the children from previous marriages of both spouses are included in the same household. A "mine, yours, and ours" variety also includes children who are the offspring of the new marriage.

Alternative Family Forms

Alternative families consist of people with or without blood or conjugal (marriage) ties who live and interact together to achieve common goals. Two or more adults, of the same or opposite sex, and their children, or adults without children, may choose to live together. Unlike the family constellations described earlier, alternative families may be one-generational, consisting of adult members of a single generation.

Communal families, in which many people band together, are found both in sophisticated metropolitan centers and in more remote rural areas. The commune is further defined by how members have negotiated the privileges and responsibilities associated with their roles, material possessions, economic concerns, sexual activities, and parenting activities. The Israeli kibbutzim are among the best known of the communes. Another type of communal arrangement is that of the religious cult.

Households of homosexual (gay) people are another alternative family form. Gay people who live together in the same household are choosing to be open about their sexual preference. Not all segments of society recognize homosexuality as an acceptable alternative, and gays still face restrictions that often prevent them from adopting children or gaining custody of children from their previous heterosexual marriages that ended in divorce.

Chosen kinship is yet another family form. Even the well-known phrase, "You can choose your friends but you can't choose your relatives," is becoming obsolete, according to Lindsey (1982), who wrote a book on chosen kin. In her view, two factors in contemporary life are important. The first is economics. Because many single people and older adults can no longer afford to live alone, there is a trend toward communal, familial living among these groups. The second factor is geography. Because the average American moves once every 3 years, an individual who lives on the East coast may have family on the West coast. Friends, chosen to recreate the extended family, become kin.

Family Theories

Developmental Tasks Confronting Families

Families, like individuals and groups, are confronted with developmental tasks. The family sociologist Evelyn Duvall (1985) lists the following developmental tasks of American families:

- *Physical maintenance:* providing food, shelter, clothing, health care.
- *Resource allocation (both physical and emotional):* meeting family expenses; apportioning material goods, space, and facilities; and apportioning emotional goods, such as affection, respect, and authority.
- *Division of labor:* deciding who does what in relation to earning money, managing the household, caring for family members, and so on.
- *Socialization of family members:* guiding members in mature patterns of controlling aggression, elimination, food intake, sexual drives, sleep, and so on.
- *Reproduction, recruitment, and release of family members:* giving birth to or adopting children, rearing them for release from the family at maturity, incorporating new members, and establishing policies for including others, such as in-laws, stepparents, and friends.
- *Maintaining order:* ensuring conformity to family and/or societal norms.
- *Placing members in the larger society:* interacting with the community, school, church, and economic and political systems to protect family members from undesirable outside influences.
- *Maintaining motivation and morale:* rewarding members for achievements; developing a life philosophy and sense of family loyalty through rituals and celebrations; satisfying personal needs for acceptance, encouragement, and affection; confronting personal and family crises.

These developmental tasks are a considerable undertaking. It is the families who do not succeed very well at accomplishing them who come to the psychiatric nurse's attention most often.

The Family as a System

In a general systems theory framework, a family can be seen as a system of interrelated parts forming a whole. A family system includes not only the family members but also their relationships, their communication with one another, and their interactions with the environment.

Wholeness Because a system functions as a whole, its parts are interdependent, and a change or movement in any part of the system affects all other parts. For example, an accomplishment by one member of the family affects all the other members in the family system. Dysfunction in one member also changes the whole system. This concept of *wholeness* is important in understanding families. It means that counseling one family member will change all members in some way.

Homeostasis Another important characteristic of a system is that it strives to maintain a dynamic equilibrium, or balance, among the various forces that operate within and on it. This process is referred to as *homeostasis.* All systems need to balance themselves within a range of functioning in which the work of the system can be accomplished. The mental image of a seesaw may help show what happens in the attempt to achieve balance. Too much weight on one end brings it to the ground. It is no longer in balance. However, before that point, balance can be achieved at any of several points, even though the seesaw is not perfectly horizontal. When a family member behaves in a way not prescribed within the family system, other members react with attempts to minimize the disruption, always trying to maintain a steady state.

Jackson (1957) introduced the concept of *family homeostasis* based on his observations that the families of psychiatric clients often experienced depression or psychophysiologic disorders when the client improved. He postulated that these behaviors of family members and the psychologic disruptions of the client were homeostatic mechanisms that operated to bring the disturbed system back into its delicate balance. When a family has to use most of its energy to maintain balance, little energy is left for the growth of the family or its individual members.

Subsystems Elements in the system may also be parts of another system. Billy may be simultaneously the oldest child in the family, a catcher for the Little League baseball team, and a member of the debate team. Billy's family is a member of other larger systems as well—the extended family, the city, the nation, and so on. The family itself has *subsystems,* such as dyads (Billy and his father), triads (Billy, his brother, and his sister), and other groups of family members who are linked together in some special association.

Openness Systems can also be viewed as *open* or *closed,* although these are actually the extremes of a continuum. Some family systems are more open than others, while some are more closed. Openness requires that a system be flexible in adapting to the changes demanded by the environment. Adaptation takes energy to maintain homeostasis in the face of outside information or new input. Families whose systems are more closed tend to shut out or distort information from the environment so as not to upset the balance.

Boundaries Family systems have *boundaries* as well. Boundaries define who participates in the system. They also tell family members the extent of differentiation permitted (among members and between members and outsiders), the amount or intensity of emotional investment in the system, the amount and kind of experiences available outside the system, and particular ways to evaluate experiences in terms of the family system. Boundaries may be clear, rigid, diffuse, or conflicting. These critical factors in family systems are referred to throughout the chapter.

Relationship Strains or Conflicts Relationship strains or conflicts can occur between subsystems in the family or between various systems in the family or outside of it. A strain can exist between the individual members of a family—for instance, between two siblings with differing views on an issue. Conflict or strain can also occur between a member of the family and the rest of the family, or between a minority of family members and the other members. This commonly occurs when a previously and unanimously held family view is challenged by one or more members. Strain can also exist between a family and the community when a family view differs from that of the community at large. On a broader level, strain can exist between communities when one community's priorities differ from those of another.

Family Characteristics and Dynamics

Whether they are functional or dysfunctional, families have certain characteristics and dynamics. The functional family is distinguished from the dysfunctional one by the amount and quality of the energy used to maintain the family system.

Family Roles Members of a family must determine how to accomplish the family developmental tasks listed earlier. They do so by establishing roles, patterns of behavior sanctioned by the culture. Jackson (1968a) believes that families set roles by operating as a rule-governed system, an ordered format designed so that members may be aware of their positions in relation to one another. Although a family system engages in a multitude of behaviors, a relatively small set of rules is sufficient to govern family life. Roles are assigned according to family rules. Families decide which roles will exist within the system, socialize members into the roles, and then expend energy maintaining members within their roles.

When members are unable or unwilling to perform assigned roles, the family experiences stress. For example, the roles of mother and father have long been stereotyped in American society. Mothers were the family nurturers and caretakers, whereas fathers were the family decision makers and wage earners. These roles are not completely satisfying to many American families, and many women and men have moved to negotiate their roles differently. The trend in society is now toward dual-earner families with two working parents and families in which fathers share, or assume, the nurturing role. For the health of the family system, roles often must be negotiated in other than stereotyped ways. When the roles are not negotiated satisfactorily, family disequilibrium results.

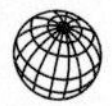

Power Structure Most families have a hierarchical power structure in which the adults wield power, usually in an authoritarian manner. The power structure is often developed in this way because it creates a safe environment in which young children can grow and develop, and because it is easy to operate. However, stress develops when disagreements exist about who holds the power.

Tom, the 17-year-old son in the M family, always used the family car without permission. Although some serious arguments ensued between Tom and his father, no restrictions were placed on Tom's behavior, and the car keys continued to hang on a key rack in the front hall. Tom's paternal grandfather, who lived with the M family, took Tom's side in his arguments with his father. Grandfather M adopted a fond "boys-will-be-boys" stance. One evening when the family car was in a repair shop for some minor work, Tom "borrowed" his grandfather's new car. Tom was involved in a collision about an hour later. Although no one was injured, Grandfather M's car had to be towed away, extensively damaged. Later that night, the adults of the M family managed to come together to agree on a stance concerning Tom's use of the family car that they could mutually support.

Once the adults in the M family were able to acknowledge their internal power struggle and come to an agreement on what rules were to be set and by whom, the family system was was subject to less stress.

Grandparents residing with a family are not the only causes of disagreements. Disagreements between husband and wife about who holds the power are also common. In some dysfunctional families, there is chronic discord about power.

When children mature and become capable of assuming greater responsibility for their own functioning, power is often diffused among all members of a family system in a more democratic fashion. Certain families, however, do not allow power to be redistributed, thus hindering the individual development of the members who have less power.

Family System Behavior In the systems view of a family, the family interaction system has four important qualities. The first, *wholeness,* is discussed earlier in this chapter. It refers to the interrelationship of all the elements in the system.

Synergy, the second characteristic, refers to the fact that the whole is greater than the sum of its parts. In other words, combined efforts produce a greater effect than the sum of individual actions. Two young children at play in their mother's cosmetics exemplify the effects of synergy. They encourage one another gleefully and enthusiastically to open and use the various jars, pots, and tubes they have discovered. Before long, the children and the environment have been thoroughly decorated. To their angry mother, each child blames the other, believing that without the other they would not have been in trouble. The effects of synergy can also be seen in families distinguished by open affection. Open affection stimulates more open affection, which cycles back into the system to stimulate even more of this particular distinguishing characteristic.

Circularity and *feedback* also characterize family system behavior. Each member engages in behavior that influences the other members. The process has been described as an uninterrupted sequence of interchanges. The usual way people think about relationships does not allow for circularity. In a teenage daughter's view, for example, if her mother would only trust her, they would get along better. The mother's view is that the problem lies with her adolescent's uncooperativeness. Both mother and daughter are stopping the circular process by seeing one behavior as a cause and the other as an effect. The circular view is that each person's behavior is both cause and effect at the same time. Mother and daughter are caught up in a cycle, as they monitor and influence each other.

RESEARCH NOTE

Citation

Uttaro T, Mechanic D: The NAMI consumer survey analysis of unmet needs. *Hosp Commun Psychiatr* 1994;45(4):372–374.

Study Problem/Purpose

The purpose of this study was to survey people with mental illness in families associated with the National Alliance for the Mentally Ill (NAMI) to determine what they identify as their unmet service needs.

Methods

A telephone survey was conducted of a representative sample of 1722 families of NAMI membership lists. A structured interview was used to obtain information about consumers' perceived needs in 15 areas related to housing, finance, employment, personal relationships, and other aspects of daily living.

Findings

The highest levels of unmet needs were reported in the areas of role restoration (keeping busy, recognizing and controlling symptoms, and maintaining friendships) and behavior (recognizing and managing symptoms and controlling anger).

Implications

Both role restoration and behavior are areas that lend themselves well to psychoeducation. These are areas in which psychiatric nurses can focus their psychoeducation activities.

Family Therapy

Nurses work with families and family problems in many different settings. Most often, nurses encounter family members while in a health teaching role. While caring for the diabetic client, the client who has undergone major surgery, or the client who has had a myocardial infarction, the nurse teaches the client's family how to care for the person physically and what lifestyle changes the illness might impose on the family. Psychiatric nurses have a psychoeducation role with families especially in relation to role restoration and behavior, as described in the Research Note. The family therapy role, however, is still a relatively new one for nurses. Nurse family therapists should be prepared at the master's level.

Family therapy is a different way of viewing problems. In general, family therapists believe that the emotional symptoms or problems of an individual are an expression of emotional symptoms or problems in a family. Therefore, family therapists view the family system as a unit of treatment. Their concerns are basically with the relationships between the family members, not with the intrapsychic functioning of Mom, Dad, Kevin, or Susan.

Various therapeutic strategies have emerged from these shared beliefs. Family therapists do not have as fixed a set of procedures for interventions as psychoanalysts do. However, certain intervention strategies and therapeutic postures seem to flow naturally from the basic beliefs family therapists hold.

Qualifications of Family Therapists

Family therapists should be specially educated in the practice of family therapy and strongly committed to a belief in the importance of the family. Increasing numbers of psychiatric nurse clinical specialists are being prepared in graduate programs that provide both theory and supervised clinical practice in this specialized area. Although undergraduate nursing programs focus on the importance of relating to families in all settings, they (rightfully) do not prepare nurses as family therapists. (Refer to the ANA Standards in Chapter 1.)

Relationship and Communication Intricacies in Families

People negotiate their views of themselves and others according to their perceptions. Perceptions also influence how people interact with one another on both content and relationship levels. In a family system, each person's behavior is contingent on the behavior of the others. This creates some interesting and complex turns in family relationships.

Functional families allow for individuation and growth-producing experiences. Rigidity within a family system makes it difficult for the family to adapt to change and easier for the family to become dysfunctional. Some of the relationship complexities described below exist in all families, but dysfunctional families handle them differently than functional families do. Other factors arise only in family systems that are dysfunctional.

Although some of the factors discussed below may be easily categorized as communicational, it is important to recognize their relational aspects. Other communication factors (discounting, disconfirming, disqualifying, symmetry, complementarity, congruity, and incongruity) are discussed in Chapter 7.

THE SELF-FULFILLING PROPHECY AND LIFE SCRIPTS A **self-fulfilling prophecy** is an idea or expectation that is acted out, largely unconsciously, thus "proving" itself. In families, self-fulfilling prophecies are often seen in the guise of family **life scripts.** Steiner (1974) calls a script "the blueprint for a life course." It is a plan decided not by the fates, but by experiences early in life. In Steiner's words, "Human beings are deeply affected by and submissive to the will of the specific divinities of their household—their parents—whose injunctions they are impotent against as they blindly follow them through life, sometimes to their self-destruction" (p. 54). People with life scripts are following forced, premature, early childhood decisions. Steiner notes that, although not everyone has a script, script-free living is typically the exception rather than the rule.

There is an endless variety among life scripts. The Miss America script is decided for the 5-year-old girl whose parents enroll her in the Little Miss New York State (or Kansas or Colorado) competition. There are My Son the Doctor, Delinquent, Alcoholic, and Drug Addict scripts. A person with a script, either "good" or "bad," is terribly disadvantaged in terms of autonomy or life potentials. Unless people recognize what the script is and take steps to change it, they are prevented from living to their potential.

FAMILY MYTHS, LIFESTYLES, AND THEMES Family myths, lifestyles, and themes help families maintain balance by permitting them to resist change. **Family myths** are well-integrated beliefs, shared by all family members, about each other and their positions in family life. The beliefs are unchallenged, even though family members may have to resort to distortions to maintain the myth. The family myth is related to the family's inner image—how the family appears to its members.

A myth in the Lundqvist family was that the father had the ability to make wise decisions. Individual members in this family participated to maintain the myth of the father as a Solomon by gearing interactions with him in such a way that he appeared to make high-level family decisions single-handedly.

The concepts of family theme and family lifestyle are alike in their focus on the family's ways of relating to the outside world. The **family theme** is the family's perception of its development and history.

The Weber family had a theme constructed around second-generation grandparents of Austrian descent, who were able to provide their oldest son with a law school education through their hard work. This family conceived of people on welfare as "lazy," thus reaffirming its view of the value of working hard and becoming educated.

Determining the salient themes in a family's life is important because they shape the fates of individual members and determine the pressures with which each person must contend.

The **family lifestyle** has to do with the family's biased perception of the outside world and its automated means of coping with this world. Family lifestyles are designed to uphold particular images of the family—as the most popular, talented, financially successful, nonconformist, or whatever. The lifestyle is the front the family strives to present to others.

Coalitions, Dyads, and Triangles Of all the forms of communicative exchange, dyadic communication is the most common. In fact, a family begins with a dyad, the marital couple. The natural alliance, or coalition, of this dyad presents a united front to the world—to deal with one member, people have to deal with them both. However, if one partner does not actively support the other, severe strain results.

The presence of a third person always has an effect on an existing dyad. When the marital couple gives birth to a child, the relationship becomes triadic. A triad is not a stable social situation, because it actually consists of a dyad plus one. Shifting alliances characterize triads; mother and father may unit to discipline the child, mother and child may unite to argue for a family vacation, or father and child may join forces to go fishing together. The process of forming a triad is called **triangulation.** Triangulation becomes dysfunctional when issues are solved in families by shifting the intimacy among members, rather than by working the actual issue through. Such coalitions always result in someone feeling "left out" (Bowen 1978).

Coalitions arise basically to affect the distribution of power. By joining forces, two people can increase their influence over a third. A husband and wife frequently pair up to discipline their child better. However, the child may also attempt to pair up with one parent to avoid discipline. In families with a number of children, typical coalitions involve children closest in age, or children of the same sex.

Pseudomutuality and Pseudohostility A family in which **pseudomutuality** occurs functions as if it were a close, happy family. This pattern of relating has the following characteristics:

- Persistent sameness in the structuring of roles.
- Insistence on the desirability and appropriateness of the role structures within the family, despite evidence to the contrary.
- Intense concern over deviations from the role structure or emerging autonomy.
- Marked absence of spontaneity, enthusiasm, and humor in participating together.

In these families, the members do not form intimate bonds with one another as individuals. Instead, an inordinate amount of energy is expended in maintaining ritualized and stereotyped ways of behaving and relating. There is a desperate struggle to maintain harmony. Wynne et al. (1958) give a perfect example in one mother who said: "We are all peaceful. I like peace if I have to kill someone to get it." Such a family requires its members to give up their sense of personal identity.

Pseudohostility exists in families characterized by chronic conflict, alienation, tension, and inappropriate remoteness. As in pseudomutuality, family members deny the problems in an attempt to negate the hostility. Family members view their differences as only minor ones. Both pseudomutual and pseudohostile family environments are stifling milieus.

Deviations in the Parental Coalition In some families, problems develop from the parents' inability to form a satisfying coalition in terms of intimacy and control. Several common deviations within the family are examined in the sections that follow.

Schism **Schismatic families** are those in which the children are forced to join one or the other camp of two warring spouses. The constant fighting in these families is most likely a defense against intimacy or closeness. In schismatic families, spouses devalue and undercut each other. This makes it difficult for the children to want to be like either of them.

Skew **Skewed families** are those in which one spouse is severely dysfunctional. The other spouse, who is usually aware of the dysfunction of the partner, assumes a passive, peace-making, submissive stance to preserve the marriage. The passive partner is caught between effectively responding to the view of "reality" of the outside world and giving up this view within the home, accepting the dysfunctional mate's view. On the surface, a skewed couple may appear to be complementary. Their relationship is actually lopsided and unsuited to many basic family tasks, however.

Enmeshment **Enmeshed families** are characterized by a fast tempo of interpersonal exchange. Interactions within the family are of high intensity and are directed more toward issues of power than toward issues of affection. In enmeshed families, one parent, usually the mother, is often overcontrolling and becomes anxious over the possibility of losing control over the children. The mother appears to be trying to prevent herself from becoming helpless. Adult males are often absent in these families, or, if present, are controlled in much the same way the children are.

Disengagement **Disengaged families** move to the other extreme from enmeshment—abandonment. Family members seem oblivious to the effects of their actions on one another. They are unresponsive and unconnected to each other. Structure, order, or authority in the family may be weak or nonexistent. Assuming control and guidance increases the anxiety of the parent, who may feel overwhelmed and depressed. In these families, a child often assumes the parental role.

SCAPEGOATING **Scapegoating** is a social process that has been written and talked about since the time of the ancient Greeks. A scapegoat is one who is made to bear the blame for others or to suffer in their place. In families, a disturbed member may play the role of family scapegoat, thus acting out the conflicts in the system and stabilizing it. For example, one or both parents may blame the child when things go wrong, rather than blame themselves or one another. This allows the parent to declare, "Our marriage would be fine if it weren't for that kid." Children are not the only ones who may be scapegoated within the family. Adults, or whole groups of people, may also be scapegoated.

PARADOXES AND DOUBLE BINDS A **paradox** is a self-contradictory communication. An example is the paradoxical bumper sticker: "Individualists Unite!" Paradoxes are common in everyday communication. The client who says, "Tell me what to do, so I can be independent," creates a paradox for the nurse. The nurse who says, "I think you should find a new job, but it's not my place to say so," creates a paradox for the client.

A **double bind** is a complex series of paradoxes. The example of a double-bind situation classically cited is from Gregory Bateson et al. (1956, p. 259):

> A young man who had fairly well recovered from an acute schizophrenic episode was visited in the hospital by his mother. He was glad to see her and impulsively put his arm around her shoulders, whereupon she stiffened. He withdrew his arm and she asked, "Don't you love me anymore?" He then blushed, and she said, "Dear, you must not be so easily embarrassed and afraid of your feelings." The client was able to stay with her only a few minutes more. Following his mother's departure from the hospital, the young man assaulted an aide and was put in the tubs.

The conditions necessary to produce the double bind are present in the above example:

- Two people, one of whom is the victim (the young man).
- A repeated experience, so that the double bind becomes a habitual expectation.
- A primary negative injunction, carrying a threat of punishment (the mother stiffens).
- A secondary injunction conflicting with the first injunction, but at a more abstract level. Like the primary injunction, the second threatens punishment ("Don't you love me anymore?").
- A tertiary negative injunction prohibiting the victim from escaping from the field ("Dear, you must not be so easily embarrassed and afraid of your feelings.").

It is theorized that repeated exposure to double binds in families produces schizophrenia. The evidence, however, is not convincing. Although people labeled schizophrenic are victims of double binds, not all victims of double binds are, or become, schizophrenic. In addition, the theory does not allow for a biologic basis.

The Treatment Unit and the Treatment Setting

Most family therapists recommend that all people in the family constellation participate in the assessment phase of family therapy. Not all agree on which people make up the family constellation or the treatment unit. Some include all members of the nuclear family; others include members of the extended family; and still others, large numbers of people in the family's social network. Different coalitions may be seen together at different times to accomplish specific goals. For example, mates are often seen together for the first few sessions.

Children 4 years of age and younger are often not included in ongoing family therapy sessions. They may misinterpret, or be frightened by, the dialogue. In addition, small children tend to be disruptive. Some therapists, however, make it a point to bring all the children into therapy for at least two sessions to see how the family as a whole operates.

Family therapists often reverse the traditional territorial control of the professional by engaging the family system in therapy in its own milieu—the home. There are several reasons these therapists see families on their own ground:

- The interactions of the family system are more natural in their usual environment.
- Customary roles are more spontaneously played out on home ground.
- Family members reluctant to participate in therapy tend to be less so in the home than in a formal office or mental health care setting.

Family Assessment

Family therapy consists of four major components: assessment, contract or goal negotiation, intervention, and evaluation. The first phase of a therapeutic process involves the initial assessment of the family. Family assessment involves gathering data in several different areas.

DEMOGRAPHIC INFORMATION Data pertaining to gender, age, occupation, religion, and ethnicity should be ob- 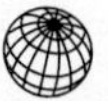

tained. In addition to gathering discrete bits of information (the father is a 39-year-old Latino, physician's assistant, and a member of St. Ann's Roman Catholic parish), it is important to gather more detailed information that will give insight into family functioning. How actively does the family pursue religious/spiritual activities? What is the link of religion/spirituality to the family's value system, norms, and practices? What is the family's racial, cultural, and ethnic identification in relation to sense of identity and belonging? Who in the family is employed? What are their attitudes about employment?

Past Medical and Mental Health History Here, substantive information should also be gathered. The family therapist will want to know about past medical and mental health treatment; past and present illnesses; pertinent health facts in the family of origin, the extended family, and in the family history; and the identity of the "identified patient."

Gather information about the developmental stage of the family—what were (are) the problems in transition from one developmental level to another? How has the family solved problems at earlier stages? What shifts in role responsibility have occurred over time? Let the developmental tasks of American families listed earlier in the chapter guide you in gathering information in this area.

Family Interactional Data This is probably the most complex data to obtain. For example, you will want to gather information about family rules. What family rules foster stability in the family? What rules foster maladaptation? How are rules modified? What happens when all members do not agree about the family rules?

You will also need to determine the roles of family members. What are the formal roles for each member? What are the informal roles (scapegoat, controller, decision maker, and so on)? Do the roles seem to have a good fit in the family?

How do family members communicate? What are the channels of communication—who speaks to whom? Are the messages clear? What is the extent of unclear or ambiguous messages, mixed messages, or missed messages? Do members "hear" one another?

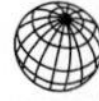

Family System Data How does the family interact with other social units? How permeable or rigid are its boundaries? Find out the extent to which the family fits into the larger culture of which it is a part. To what degree could the family be considered deviant from the larger culture?

Within the family, what are the family alliances—who supports whom? Which members are in conflict with one another, or with the family as a whole?

Needs, Goals, Values, and Aspirations Determine whether essential physical needs are met. At what level does the family meet social and emotional needs? Are the family needs shared among the individual members? What are the individual needs of family members, and how do they fit with the family needs? Is the family willing or able to meet the individual needs of its members?

Determine the extent to which individual family members' goals and values are articulated and understood by the other members. Are the goals and values shared by all? Do some members compromise? Do other members simply give up and give in? Does the family as a whole allow individual members to pursue individual goals and values?

Family assessments may be accomplished in a variety of ways. Some suggestions are given below. Others are discussed in the later section on intervention.

Taking a Family Life Chronology Virginia Satir, in a classic family therapy work (1967) suggests that the family therapist should structure at least the first two sessions of therapy by taking a family life chronology. Her rationale is based on the following factors:

- The family therapist enters a session knowing little more than who the "identified patient" (IP) is and what symptoms that person manifests. The therapist does not have clues about the meaning of the symptoms—how the pain that exists in the marital relationship is expressed, how the mates have attempted to cope with their problems, or what models have influenced each mate's expectations about being a mate or parent.
- The therapist knows that the family has a history but does not know what the history is—what events have occurred and which members were influenced (directly or indirectly) by those events.
- Family members are fearful about embarking on family therapy. Structuring early sessions with a family life chronology helps decrease the threat. Members can answer relatively nonthreatening questions, and they tend to relax as the therapist demonstrates an ability to take charge and keep things under control.
- Family members are often despairing when they enter therapy. The therapist's structure tells the family that they can take specified directions to accomplish goals. The questions also provide family members with the opportunity to review success as well as failures.
- The family life chronology is a nonthreatening way to change the focus from a "sick" family member to the family system and marital relationship.
- Taking the chronology gives the family therapist the opportunity to be a model of effective communication and provides the framework within which change can take place.

Figure 32–1 shows the structure of the family life chronology recommended by Satir.

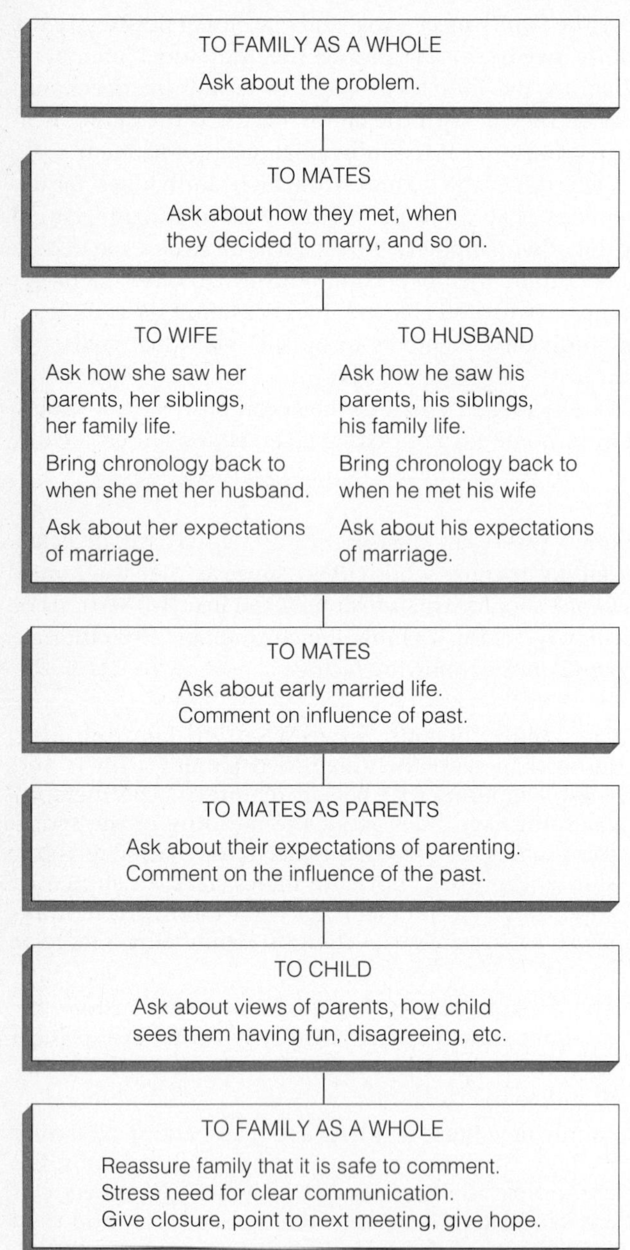

Figure 32–1 Main flow of a family life chronology. *Source: Adapted from Satir 1967.*

Family Genealogy or Time Line Walter Toman's family constellation theory (1976) is a useful basis for constructing a family genealogy or timeline.

From the study of families in detail, it becomes apparent that patterns are spread over generations. At first Bowen (1978) believed that a schizophrenic child could be produced after psychologic impairment in 3 generations. He now believes that the level of impairment in schizophrenia is the result of 8–10 generations of impairment. An intrinsic difficulty in analyzing generational transmission is that only a minute slice of a family generation—3 generations out of at least 4000—can be studied. Few people are able to do what one university professor can. He can trace his paternal ancestry in China back to 2255 BC—an incredible 4000 years and 131 generations.

Each generation, according to Laing (1972), projects onto the next the following elements:

- What was projected onto it by prior generations.
- What was induced in it by prior generations.
- Its response to this projection and induction.

This process, which Laing calls *mapping,* is endless. Since it is impractical and impossible to understand the effect of 4000 earlier generations on a family, the time line can serve a therapist and a family as a more limited means for understanding the family's roots.

The timeline is highly effective as a visual representation. By drawing it on a long, narrow piece of paper and taping it to the wall during the family's sessions, the therapist can use it repeatedly as therapy progresses. Colored lines can differentiate individual family members. Colored flags, pins, or asterisks can identify and call attention to significant events in the family history. Births, deaths, marriages, and leavetakings should be noted. The therapist can use any of several family tree or genealogic tracing formats for the family timeline.

The Structured Family Interview A structured family interview (Watzlawick 1966) has elements similar to Satir's family life chronology. In addition, the family members are asked to participate in demonstrating the system's operation. The structured interview is composed of the following segments:

- *The main problems:* Each member is asked separately to identify what he or she considers the main problems in the family. The therapist assures the family member that the answer will not be divulged. Family members are then brought together to discuss this topic. The therapist leaves the room after telling the family members that their conversation will be recorded and they will be observed through a one-way screen. This task undermines the myth that the IP is the only "problem" in the family and paves the way for future work.
- *Planning something together:* The family is asked to plan something together, as a family, in the 5 minutes during which the therapist leaves the room. The important things to notice are whether and how a decision was reached. The content, while revealing, is of secondary importance.
- *How the mates met:* This task is for the mates only. With the children in another room, the mates are asked how, out of all the millions of people in the world, they got together. The parents share their views of the past and reveal their predominant patterns of interacting in the present.

- *The meaning of a proverb:* The parents are asked to discuss the meaning of a proverb, such as "A rolling stone gathers no moss." At the end of 5 minutes, they are to call the children in and teach them the meaning of the proverb. This proverb has two valid but mutually exclusive interpretations: that *moss* (roots, stability, friends) is valuable, or that *rolling* (not stagnating, being alert, moving) is desirable. This task reveals how the mates handle disagreements and how they explain things to their children.
- *Blaming:* The entire family and the therapist are together for this task. The father sits to the left of the therapist followed at his left by the mother and the children, from the oldest to the youngest, in a clockwise direction around the table. Each family member is asked to write down, on an index card, the main fault of the person to the left. (The youngest child writes what he or she sees as the main fault of the father.) The therapist writes two cards, which state "too good" and "too weak." The therapist collects the cards and reads them out loud, beginning with the two the therapist has written. The therapist then asks to which two family members these cards apply. The other cards are read aloud in random order, and the authors are not revealed. This task reveals such processes as scapegoating, favoritism, and self-blame. This assessment tool may actually serve a therapeutic function and be used as an intervention technique if it helps family members achieve spontaneous understanding of the patterns and relationships in their family.

Contract or Goal Negotiation

The negotiation phase of family therapy is begun by identifying what each member would like changed in the family. When each family member and the therapist have identified important goals, they begin negotiating a set of attainable goals that everyone is willing to work on. Compromise is needed to achieve a working goal. At this time, the family therapist may also identify the means—tasks, strategies, and so on—that will be used to reach the negotiated goals.

Written and verbal contracts for work with individuals are discussed in Chapter 28. These can be modified for family work.

Intervention

Therapy for a family system involves understanding and use of the here-and-now, of the basic processes that occur in the system. General guidelines for using the here-and-now process with families are in the Intervention box on the next page. Some of the wide variety of specific strategies and tasks are also discussed.

Structured Family Tasks Structured family tasks are used for joint assessment and intervention purposes. They provide historical data and, in some cases, relate the data to present behavior. They give family members the opportunity to collaborate actively in changing the family system.

Role Playing In her practice, Satir (1967) uses *role playing* with families. The simulated family experience is used to teach families about themselves. Family members may simulate each other's behavior or their conceptions of it. They may also play themselves in a simulated situation. Videotape feedback helps family members become acquainted with their own behavior. In addition, systems games and communication games are used to help families communicate more effectively and congruently. These role-playing experiences are also effective educational tools in the preparation of family therapists.

Family Photostudy and Other Tasks Sedgwick (1978) suggests *photostudy of the family album* as a means of providing tangible, longitudinal evidence to raise questions, validate or invalidate hunches, and developmentally examine the individual and the family. Sedgwick suggests that the family picture album is one of the most obvious, and most overlooked, tools for understanding family dynamics. The photographs and the process of selecting them give insights into decision making, themes, interaction patterns, patterns of development, and power and influence relationships within the family. The therapist and family discuss and analyze the photographs together.

Other interesting *family tasks* suggested by Sedgwick include writing a family autobiography; comparing and contrasting family members with one another and with selected families from the neighborhood, the school, or the church; drawing a family picture; writing a family news article or a family epitaph; dispelling a family myth; weaving a family dream; or writing a family play. Such tools are helpful in examining histories, prophecies, scripts, and myths. They are limited only by the imagination and ingenuity of the therapist.

Therapeutic Rituals *Therapeutic rituals* can help families mobilize their resources for healing, growth, and change. The rationale for the creation of a family ritual is that family rituals facilitate life cycle transitions. Conversely, their lack inhibits family development. Bright (1990) constructs therapeutic rituals to help families resolve conflicts or resentments, to negotiate new roles or relationship boundaries, and to develop new, shared meanings about their life together. She cautions that rituals must be constructed around an understanding of the family's culture, values, and needs; for example, a healing forgiveness ritual constructed in the language of a sacramental rite for a couple from a strong Roman Catholic background, a celebration ritual to mark a family transition such as a birth or an adoption, a graduation, or an anniversary or a letting-go ritual following a divorce.

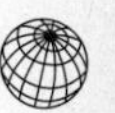

text continues on page 774

INTERVENTION

The Role of the Family Therapist

Satir (1967) offers the following standard guidelines for the role of the family therapist:

1. Creating a setting in which members can risk looking at themselves and their actions.
   a. Reducing their fears.
   b. Giving direction.
   c. Helping them feel comfortable and hopeful about the therapy process.
   d. Accepting the "expert" label and being comfortable in the role.
   e. Structuring questions to gain important data.
2. Being unafraid but open.
   a. Framing questions to help members be less afraid.
   b. Validating members' assumptions and questioning personal assumptions.
   c. Eliciting the facts about planning processes, loopholes in planning, perceptions of self and others, perceptions of roles, communication patterns and techniques, sexual feelings and activities.
   d. Responding with a belief in the integrity of the members.
3. Helping members see how they look to others.
   a. Sharing observations of how members manifest themselves.
   b. Teaching members how to share their observations with one another.
   c. Playing back tape recordings (or video tapes).
4. Asking for and giving information in a matter-of-fact, nonjudgmental, light, congruent way.
   a. Verbally recreating situations (with imagination) in order to collect pertinent facts.
   b. Being easy about giving and receiving information, thereby making it easier for family members to do so.
5. Building self-esteem.
   a. Making constant "I value you" comments.
   b. Labeling assets.
   c. Asking questions that family members can answer.
   d. Emphasizing that the therapist and family members are equals in learning from therapy.
   e. Responding as a person whose meaning or intent can be checked on.
   f. Noting past achievements.
   g. Accentuating the family's "good" intentions but "bad" communication.
   h. Asking each family member what he or she can do to bring pleasure to another family member.
   i. Being human, clear, and direct (and recognizing that warmth and good intentions are not enough in themselves).
6. Decreasing threat by setting rules for interaction.
   a. Seeing to it that all members participate.
   b. Making it clear that interruptions are not tolerated.
   c. Emphasizing that acting-out or making it impossible to converse is not allowed.
   d. Making sure that no one speaks for anyone else.
   e. Helping everyone speak out clearly so that each can be heard.
   f. Using humor appropriately.
   g. Connecting silence to covert control.
7. Decreasing threat by structuring sessions.
   a. Announcing concrete goals and a definite end to the therapy or deadlines for reevaluation.
   b. Viewing the family as a family and not taking sides.
   c. Seeing units or subsystems of the family alone to accomplish specific work or because this is feasible or practical (other members are not available), with the knowledge and understanding of all members.

INTERVENTION *(continued)*

8. Decreasing threat by reducing the need for defenses.
   a. Discussing anger and hurt openly, thus decreasing fears about showing anger or hurt.
   b. Interpreting anger as hurt.
   c. Acknowledging anger as a defense and dealing with the hurt.
   d. Showing that pain and the "forbidden" are safe to look at.
   e. Burlesquing basic fears—painting a picture exaggerated to the point of absurdity—to decrease overprotectiveness and feelings of omnipotence.
9. Decreasing threat by handling loaded material with care.
   a. Using careful timing.
   b. Moving from the least loaded to the most loaded.
   c. Switching to less loaded material when things get hot (to another subject or to the past rather than the present).
   d. Generalizing about what a therapist expects to see in families (hurt, anger, fear, fighting, and so on).
   e. Relating feelings to facts (events, circumstances).
   f. Using personal idioms, slang, profanity, or vulgarity when appropriate, and avoiding pedantic words and psychiatric jargon.
   g. Preventing closure on episodes or complaints; assuring that things will become clearer as learning continues.
10. Reeducating members to be accountable.
    a. Reminding members of their ability to be in charge of themselves.
    b. Identifying global pronouns.
    c. Dealing openly with tattletales, spokespersons, and acting-out members.
    d. Highlighting problems of accountability in the relationship with the therapist.
11. Helping members see the influence of past models on their expectations and behavior.
    a. Reminding members that they are acting from past models.
    b. Openly challenging expectations.
    c. Highlighting expectations by helping members verbalize the unspoken.
    d. Highlighting expectations by exaggerating them.
12. Delineating family roles and functions.
    a. Recognizing roles by calling the parents "Mom" and "Dad" when referring to them as parents and "Jane" and "Bill" when addressing them as individuals or as husband and wife.
    b. Including members in history taking in the order of their entrance into the family.
    c. Questioning members about their roles.
    d. Teaching explicitly about role responses and role choices.
13. Completing gaps in communication and interpreting messages.
    a. Clarifying the content and relationship aspects of messages.
    b. Separating comments about the self from comments about others.
    c. Pointing out significant discrepancies, incongruities, or double-level messages.
    d. Spelling out nonverbal communication.

Interestingly, the brief ecstatic change that occurs during a ritual results from changes in neurologic activity. Routinely, either the sympathetic or the parasympathetic nervous system is in a state of excitation. This excitation of the one system inhibits the other. During rituals, however, both divisions of the CNS are simultaneously stimulated (Bright 1990). This neurobiologic event is responsible for the intensely pleasurable experience of ecstasy, and the sense of union and oneness with others and life itself that occurs during a ritual.

Criteria for Terminating Treatment

Reid (1985) suggests that termination in family therapy should occur in a flexible way, helping families achieve realistic goals and end therapy with a feeling of accomplishment. Satir (1967) developed criteria for determining when to terminate family therapy. Termination is appropriate when family members can

- Complete transactions, check, and ask.
- Interpret hostility.
- See how others see them.
- Tell one another how they appear.
- Tell one another their hopes, fears, and expectations.
- Disagree.
- Make choices.
- Learn through practice.
- Free themselves from the harmful influences of past models.
- Give clear messages.

Family Psychoeducation

Although not every family is a candidate for family therapy, almost every family can participate in family psychoeducation. Psychoeducation is important for families in which there is a member who is seriously ill. According to a recent survey by NAMI (the National Alliance for the Mentally Ill), many families receiving mental health care services have unmet needs that can be substantially met by psychoeducation (see the Research Note). Psychoeducation for families is discussed in greater detail in Chapters 14 and 31.

Chapter Highlights

- The family is the context in which people develop their first relationships with others. How one views the world is molded by the events that happen within the family.
- Family forms in the United States are changing and becoming more diverse; a wide variety of family constellations exists in contemporary society.
- The family can be viewed as a system in terms of the relationships, associations, and connections that occur in a dynamic, interacting whole.
- The family system includes not only family members but their relationships, communications, and interaction with the environment.
- A change or movement in any part of the family system affects all other parts of the family system.
- The family seeks to maintain a dynamic balance, or homeostasis, among various forces that operate within and upon it.
- Just as individuals and groups are confronted with developmental tasks, so are families.
- The functional family is distinguished from the dysfunctional one by the amount and quality of energy used to maintain the family system and to perform the developmental tasks.
- Family therapists believe that an individual's emotional symptoms or problems are an expression of emotional symptoms or problems in that person's family. In family therapy work, the family system is the unit of treatment.
- Nurses at all levels and in all areas of nursing work with families and family problems in many settings. To function as a family therapist, however, the psychiatric nurse needs graduate-level preparation.
- The family therapist may use structured family tasks and therapeutic strategies for both assessment and intervention.
- The family therapist helps family members look at themselves in the here-and-now and recognize the influence of past models on their behavior and expectations.

References

Attala J, Oetker D, McSweeney M: Partner abuse against female nursing students. *J Psychosoc Nurs Ment Health Serv* 1995;33:11–16.

Aponte H: If I don't get simple, I cry. *Fam Process* 1986; 25(4):531–548.

Bartol GM, Moon E, Linton M: Nursing assistance for families of patients. *J Psychosoc Nurs Ment Health Serv* 1994; 32(12):27–29.

Bateson G, Jackson DD, Haley J, Weakland JH: Toward a theory of schizophrenia. *Behav Sci* 1956;1:251–264.

Beavers W, Hampson W. *Successful Families*. Norton, 1991.

Bishop SM: *Family Psychiatric Nursing*. Mosby, 1991.

Black EI (ed): *Secrets in Families and Family Therapy*. Norton, 1993.

Bowen M: *Family Therapy in Clinical Practice.* Jason Aronson, 1978.

Bright MA: Therapeutic ritual: Helping families grow. *J Psychosoc Nurs* 1990;28(12):24–29.

Brock G, Barnard C: *Procedures in Family Therapy.* Allyn & Bacon, 1988.

Butler MK, Harper JM: The divine triangle: God in the marital system of religious couples. *Fam Process* 1994;33(3): 277–286.

Carter B, McGoldrick J: *The Changing Family Life Cycle.* Gardiner Press, 1988.

Clement JA: Psychiatric nursing phenomena and the construct of family boundaries. *Arch Psychiatr Nurs* 1991; 5(4):236–243.

Doherty W, Burge S: Attending to the context of family treatment: Pitfalls and prospects. *J Marriage Fam Ther* 1987; 13(1):37–47.

Drake R, Oscher F: Using family psychoeducation when there is no family. *Hosp Commun Psychiatr* 1987;38(3):274–277.

Duvall E: *Family Development.* Lippincott, 1985.

Edwards AP: Catch 22: Manipulative family members. *Nurs Manage* 1993;24(10):33–38.

Forchuk C, Park J: Hildegard Peplau meets family systems nursing: Innovations in theory-based practice. *J Adv Nurs* 1995;21(1):110–115.

Griffith J: Employing the God-family relationship in therapy with religious families. *Fam Process* 1986;25(4):609–618.

Haber J: A family systems model for divorce and the loss of self. *Arch Psychiatr Nurs* 1990;4(4):228–234.

Haley J: *Problem Solving Therapy.* Jossey-Bass, 1987.

Imber-Black E: *Families and Larger Systems.* Guilford Press, 1988.

Jackson DD (ed): *Communication, Family, and Marriage.* Science and Behavior Books, 1968a.

Jackson DD: The question of family homeostasis. *Psychiatr Q* 1957;[Suppl]:79–90.

Jackson DD (ed): *Therapy, Communication, and Change.* Science and Behavior Books, 1968b.

Kaufman BA: Training tales in family therapy: Exploring the Alexandria Quartet. *J Marital Fam Therapy* 1995;21(1): 67–75.

Kiecolt-Glaser J, et al.: Marital quality, marital disruption, and immune function. *Psychosom Med* 1987;49(1):13–34.

Knudson-Martin C: The female voice: Applications to Bowen's family systems theory. *J Marital Family Ther* 1994; 20(1):35–46.

Kurdek LA: Conflict resolution styles in gay, lesbian, heterosexual nonparent, and heterosexual parent couples. *J Marriage Family* 1994;56(3):705–722.

Laing RD: *The Politics of the Family.* Vintage Books, 1972.

Lesser E, Comet J: Help and hindrance: Parents of divorcing children. *J Marriage Fam Ther* 1987;13(2):197–202.

Lindsey K: *Friends or Family.* Beacon Press, 1982.

McGoldrick K, Rohrbaugh M: Researching ethnic family stereotypes. *Fam Process* 1987;26(1):89–99.

McGoldrick M, Anderson C, Walsh F (eds): Women in families: A framework for family therapy. Norton, 1989.

McGoldrick M, Gerson R: *Genograms in Family Assessment.* Norton, 1985.

Onnis L, et al.: Sculpting present and future: A systemic intervention model applied to psychosomatic families. *Fam Process* 1994;33(3):341–356.

Palazzoli MS, Cirillo S, Selvini M, et al.: *Family Games: General Models of Psychotic Processes in the Family.* Norton, 1989.

Pam A, Pearson J: The geometry of the eternal triangle. *Fam Process* 1994;33(2):175–190.

Pruchno R, Burant C, Peters ND: Family mental health: Marital and parent-child consensus as predictors. *J Marriage Family* 1994;56(3):747–758.

Reichelt S, Sveaass N: Therapy with refugee families: What is a "good" conversation? *Fam Process* 1994;33(3):247–252.

Reid W: *Family Problem Solving.* Columbia University Press, 1985.

Satir V: *Conjoint Family Therapy,* rev ed. Science and Behavior Books, 1967.

Sedgwick R: Photostudy as a diagnostic tool in working with families, in Kneisl CR, Wilson HS (eds): *Current Perspectives in Psychiatric Nursing: Issues and Trends,* vol 2. Mosby, 1978.

Steiner C: *Scripts People Live.* Grove Press, 1974.

Toman W: *Family Constellation,* ed 3. Springer, 1976.

Uttaro T, Mechanic D: The NAMI consumer survey analysis of unmet needs. *Hosp Commun Psychiatr* 1994;45(4): 372–374.

Watzlawick P: A structured family interview. *Fam Process* 1966;5:256–271.

Watzlawick P, Beavin JH, Jackson DD: *The Pragmatics of Human Communication.* Norton, 1967.

Wood BL: Beyond the "psychosomatic family": A biobehavioral family model of pediatric illness. *Fam Process* 1993; 32:261–278.

Worthington E: Treatment of families during life transitions: Matching treatment to family response. *Fam Process* 1987; 26(2):295–308.

Wright LM: When clients ask questions: Enriching the therapeutic conversation. *Family Therapy Networker* 1989; 13:15–16.

Wynne L, Ryckoff IM, Day J, Hirsch SI: Pseudo-mutuality in the family relationships of schizophrenics. *Psychiatry* 1958;21:205–220.

CHAPTER 33

PSYCHOPHARMACOLOGY

Eileen Trigoboff

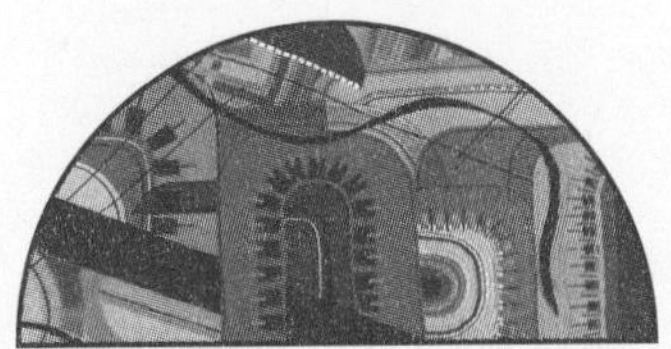

COMPETENCIES

- Define psychopharmacology from the information in this chapter.
- Describe a psychopharmacologic problem that does not exist for nurses in other specialty areas.
- List three categories of psychiatric medication.
- Recognize the positive and negative impacts of psychiatric medications on behavior.
- Explain how you would feel if you had to take these medications for an indefinite period of time.
- Discuss three factors that affect the extent to which clients will comply with prescribed medication treatment regimens.
- Describe major side effects associated with broad categories of psychotropic medications, and formulate nursing interventions to address them.

Cross-References

Other topics relevant to this content are: Anxiety disorders, Chapter 16; Drugs, Appendix A; Historical perspectives, Chapters 1 and 2; Mood disorders, Chapter 15; Philosophic perspective, Chapter 2; Psychobiology, Chapter 3; Recidivism among the chronically mentally ill, Chapter 21; Schizophrenia, Chapter 14.

Critical Thinking Challenge

You have been a psychiatric nurse for 2 years and have recently taken a position in a newly established psychiatric intensive treatment unit. Clients admitted to this unit are acutely ill with various psychiatric disorders. Although treatment regimens vary, medications play a key role in almost every treatment plan. Over the past year, one client has assaulted female staff members, but he has not acted out in 3 months. During group he became angry and was trying to express his anger about a perceived slight by one of the staff. He was yelling and got up to pace. The female nurse coleading the group with you (who has been a staff member 4 years and has been assaulted by this client) leaves the group room and returns with a syringe of Ativan 1 mg for an IM. She insists he take the injection to control his anger, and other staff members arrive to help. The injection is given and the client goes to his room for some "quiet time." What do you think happened in this situation?

The twentieth century has witnessed many great pharmacologic discoveries, including most of the drugs used in psychiatry today. The earliest medication discovery was made in 1949 by an Australian physician, John Cade. Cade found that lithium worked to subdue wild behavior in animals. To the astonishment of his colleagues, he went one step further and gave lithium to humans. Since then, of course, lithium has become the drug of choice for the treatment of bipolar mood disorder.

Portions of this chapter were contributed to the fourth edition by Geoffry McEnany.

In the 1950s **antipsychotic**, **antidepressant**, and some **anxiolytic medications** were discovered. Before then, the care of psychiatric clients had consisted mainly of behavioral interventions, seclusion, and various forms of restraint. Suddenly many clients were suffering less, getting better, and returning to the mainstream of life. This chapter explores the various medications used in psychiatric–mental health nursing practice today.

Psychopharmacology and Nursing

The area of psychopharmacology has grown considerably in recent years. Psychiatric–mental health nursing has similarly grown, and our responsibilities to recipients of mental health care services involve, to a large degree, psychopharmacologic expertise. Our national professional organization, the American Nurses Association (ANA), examined this issue, and the ANA's Task Force on Psychopharmacology set forth guidelines for this aspect of our nursing practice (ANA 1994). The guidelines delineate three areas that unite the practice of psychiatric–mental health nursing with expertise in psychopharmacology. We must:

1. Integrate current data from the neurosciences.
2. Demonstrate knowledge of psychopharmacologic principles.
3. Provide safe and effective clinical management of clients taking these medications through assessment, diagnosis, and treatment.

Prescribing practices now involve more than physicians. The word *prescriber* is used for the person who is writing the prescription for the medication. This use is deliberate because it addresses current psychiatric caregiver skills; the word includes advanced practice nurses (clinical specialists and nurse practitioners) and physicians. While various states have different restrictions and eligibility requirements for prescriptive privileging, advanced practice nurses are involved in many areas, including prescribing medications and providing comprehensive care to recipients of mental health services (Talley and Brooke 1992).

Psychiatric–mental health nurses must understand current advances in psychobiology, to maintain an updated knowledge base for clinical work. The goal of merging nursing and psychopharmacologic interventions is to promote clients' physiologic stability, so they can achieve psychologic, social, and spiritual growth—recipes for enhancing the quality of life (Beeber, Clement, and Simmons-Alling 1994).

The word *drugs* conjures up a variety of powerful positive and negative images. Television coverage of the devastating effects of crack cocaine exemplifies the negative image. Another image leaps from the pages of nursing and medical journals; pharmaceutical advertisements show people leading productive lives or smiling nurses, allegedly grateful for a medication that controls psychiatric symptoms. Yet another drug-related image is that of schoolchildren being inoculated against diphtheria, polio, and pertussis. All these images are powerful, and each is backed by truth.

Assessment of the Client Taking Psychiatric Medications

Our responsibilities as nurses to clients receiving psychotropic medications are very different from the responsibilities of nurses in other settings. A nurse working with clients having cardiac difficulties, for example, may have clear physiologic indicators for the administration of drugs such as isosorbide dinitrate or nitroglycerin, but psychiatric nurses rarely have comparable consistent complexes of symptoms on which to base clinical judgments. In psychiatric work, nurses must often observe client behaviors closely to be aware of the sometimes subtle nature of the presenting symptom. Pacing, mild diaphoresis, slight increases in blood pressure or pulse, heightened muscle tone, and hypervigilant posture may be indicative of escalating anxiety, but they may also point to other problems such as caffeine toxicity or excessive use of tobacco. Accurate nursing assessment of client behavior is crucial if medications are to be given effectively and appropriately. Psychiatric nurses must also be attuned to determining instances of polypharmacy (taking several different medications at the same time). See the Research Note on the following page for a discussion of polypharmacy in the elderly.

Assessment is not a static process. It takes shape over time and includes a wide range of nursing knowledge. Conflicting sources of similar behaviors often exist with psychiatric clients. A sleepy, isolated client with schizophrenia may be experiencing paranoid ideation, may have negative symptoms of the illness, may be having sedating side effects of the antipsychotic medication, or may be depressed as well as schizophrenic. Your assessment of this client and your clinical judgment will direct the nursing care. Whether you decide to administer a PRN antipsychotic, hold the next dose of antipsychotic, develop a treatment plan that includes motivational aspects, or discuss the possibility of depression with the other treatment team members depends upon your assessment of this client.

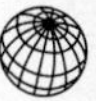

THE CLIENT'S CULTURAL PERSPECTIVE Another vital aspect to appropriate assessment is accounting for the client's cultural perspective or meaning behind the behavior. Refusing to take medication may be more than paranoia or misunderstanding; it may be intrinsically representative of a cultural standard—for example, the belief that illness

RESEARCH NOTE

Citation

Pollow RL, Stoller EP, Forster LE, Duniho TS: Drug combinations and potential for risk of adverse drug reaction among community-dwelling elderly. *Nurs Res* 1994;43(1):44–49.

Study Problem/Purpose

Relatively large numbers of medications are used concurrently by older adults, increasing the chances of interactions, drug-specific adverse effects, and other problems with this population. Three categories of psychopharmacologic substances (antidepressants, sedative-hypnotics, and tranquilizers) are among those linked to adverse drug reactions in elderly clients. The researchers uncovered combinations of medications that place people at risk for hypotension and cognitive impairment. Awareness of both drug-use patterns and the risk of adverse drug reactions is promoted by this research.

Methods

Participants were 667 people, age 65 years or older, living in a community setting in northeastern New York state. Most were in relatively good health. Fewer than 10% needed help with activities of daily living. The personal interview included questions about their use of prescription and OTC medications during the last month. Lists of these medications were provided. Alcohol consumption was also determined, along with exercise, eating patterns, and smoking. A list of possible drug-drug and drug-alcohol combinations that could produce adverse reactions was developed. Drug-alcohol combinations were coded only if the participant drank "sometimes" or "regularly" as opposed to "never" or "rarely."

Findings

Of the 667 participants, 65.8% took at least one potentially risky combination, and 10.6% were taking psychiatric medications (71 people). Of those individuals, 98.6% were taking the medication at a possible risk to themselves. Seventy of the 71 participants taking psychiatric medications were at risk for a possible adverse drug reaction. Also of note were the groups with larger numbers of participants, taking antihypertensives (182 people) and diuretics (162 people) in combinations that pose a possible risk.

Prescription or OTC analgesics were the most frequently reported combination involving psychiatric medications, a combination reported by 80% of those participants exposing themselves to potential risk. Other potentially adverse combinations (in descending percentages) included diuretics, antihypertensives, OTC antacids, laxatives, antiarthritics, and alcohol.

Of the entire sample of older people, including those not taking any medications, 20.2% were at risk for hypotension and 15.9% were at risk for cognitive impairments.

Implications

Concerns about polypharmacy are routinely examined in the older psychiatric population. However, when we think about older clients in the community, basically healthy people, polypharmacy is of primary importance. Striking in this research is the number of people taking psychiatric medications who are at risk for having an adverse reaction of some kind because of the combination of medications and/or alcohol. A thorough knowledge of interactions and counterreactions among various medications is imperative for the effective treatment of all clients. Teaching and learning about psychiatric medications is critical so the transition from inpatient to outpatient is smooth, or community living is not endangered by an adverse drug reaction.

is caused by a supreme being, and that prayer and good wishes from others are the only acceptable routes to healing. Nurses often act as liaisons between the health care system and the culture of clients. Jezewski (1993) calls this "culture brokering," making a bridge between the health care system and the client's belief system. This can be accomplished by being open and nonjudgmental about the cultural practice while promoting healthy aspects of its use. Psychiatric nurses may be especially challenged by certain cultural differences, however. A client's native language may provide a more detailed, or a more restricted, description of events than the English language. For example, the Japanese language enforces politeness, so it is difficult to be direct or confrontational in Japanese (Tierney, Minarik, and Tierney 1994).

It has been argued that it is difficult to incorporate non-Western sensibilities into our present psychiatric classification system because it is an ethnocentric system based on Western culture (Farrington 1993). Your recognition of the validity of cultural backgrounds other than Western will promote client rights and afford clients legitimate entry into health care delivery systems. An awareness of the issues relating to culture helps minimize the problem and is necessary for providing quality mental health care.

Biologic Impact on Ethnically Distinct Groups In addition to assessing for cultural impacts on behavior, you must also assess for the biologic impacts of medications on ethnically distinct groups. Factors such as benefits received from drug treatment, drug toxicity levels, and addiction liabilities are not the same for all groups of individuals (Kudzma 1992).

One important factor is the variation in metabolic rates among ethnic groups (an important point in evaluating the effectiveness of a medication). A high metabolic rate may produce effects below the optimal level, resulting in ineffective treatment. A low metabolic rate increases side effects. Because Asians have low metabolic rates, almost all Asians (95%) experience extrapyramidal side effects (EPS), as compared to European- and African-Americans, two-thirds of whom experience EPS (Lin, Poland, and Nakasaki 1993). Also because of metabolic differences, the therapeutic range for lithium differs among Asian, African American, and Caucasian groups. The determination of effective lithium levels must take ethnicity into account.

Antipsychotics may be overprescribed for African-Americans and Latinos because these groups are at greater risk for being misdiagnosed as schizophrenic rather than as having bipolar affective disorder (Jones and Gary 1986). Worthington (1992) recommends a thorough cultural assessment to avoid potential misdiagnosis and subsequent treatment errors.

Recognizing the ethnic differences in response to drugs promotes the provision of culturally competent care (Campinha-Bacote 1991). How ethnicity affects the expression of abnormal biologic processes is a growing field of study. Exploring the related literature will help you to incorporate this expanding knowledge base into your psychiatric nursing practice and promote your cultural competence.

Drug Administration

Administering psychiatric medications demands more than the right medication, the right dose, the right route, the right time, to the right client. These aspects of medication administration in psychiatry are confounded by the psychiatric illness. Knowing the side effects of the medication, in addition to the interactive effects with other psychiatric and medical-surgical medications, is another facet to psychiatric nursing.

The right medication in a psychiatric setting depends on the nursing assessment skills of the nurse. The right medication may be one of a number of choices. A medication may be ordered by mouth (PO) for routine administration, but the client may refuse the medication. Assessment skills come into play here as well; the nurse must determine whether the client needs a liquid or a pill, or whether a PRN injection is necessary. Client identification regarding medication administration is different than in medical-surgical settings because clients usually do not wear wristbands. They may be confused or have psychiatric symptoms that encourage them to spontaneously assume the identity of another client in order to please the staff.

Documenting the rationale for the effect of medications is an important nursing responsibility. Follow-up documentation on a medication that was given as a PRN will simplify treatment decisions for the client. Did the PRN work? How did you determine the value of the PRN's effect? What behavioral indicators are you using in your evaluation of a medication's effectiveness?

Medication Teaching

Nursing responsibilities include educating clients about their medication. Compliance with medication regimens is often an issue for psychiatric clients, and nurses have explored the efficacy of teaching as a way of improving client adherence to medication regimens after discharge. Variables related to compliance include socioeconomic status, marital status, number of concurrent medications, diagnosis, side effects, health benefits, and health values. Although the data vary on the degrees of influence of these variables, compliance is thought to be better among people who are upper middle class, married, taking more than four types of medication, and diagnosed as having a bipolar disorder with reported mild or nonexistent side effects from medications. Clients' individual differences must be addressed in the course of the teaching-learning process.

An issue of great concern to many nurses is the planning of teaching-learning experiences for clients who suffer from chronic mental illness. Although this population has learning needs concerning care and treatment, teaching is often difficult, depending on the severity and chronicity of the illness.

Recidivism, the tendency to relapse into a previous mode of behavior requiring readmission to a treatment program, is believed to be linked to a psychiatric client's psychoeducation (Polk-Walker et al. 1993). Helping a client change health-related behavior in a stage-and-process model can enhance client learning (Conn 1994). Interventions designed to match the readiness-for-change stage makes a client's learning, and your teaching endeavors, more effective.

Another concern for nurses working with psychiatric clients is the need to assess their learning capacity at different points in their disorders. For example, when clients are first admitted to an inpatient unit, they may be too disorganized to focus on specific learning tasks. Depressed clients may be so psychomotorally slowed, because of hormonal shifts and dysfunctional neurotransmission, that they may be unable to learn. Given appropriate treatment and care, however, a client's psychobiologic disequilibrium may be corrected, making learning possible.

Even when a nurse perceives that a client is ready to learn (cognitive abilities are intact), learning will not necessarily occur. Many nurses conduct medication groups on an acute psychiatric unit to address the importance of not only assessing cognitive abilities but also exploring affective and social issues that may contribute to effective learning experiences. After considering the client's readiness, knowledge, background, environment, beliefs, preferences, and lifestyle, involving the client and significant others in the design and implementation of the medication treatment plan will help ensure the client's active collaboration in his or her care (ANA 1994).

In many ways, psychiatric clients are no different from other learners. When presented with material that is clearly beneficial to them, they are likely to be more interested in the learning process. An evaluation of teaching efforts is essential to completing the teaching-learning process. This part of the process can be as informal or formal as the nurse chooses or deems necessary to check the client's knowledge of information taught. You will not be able to evaluate a client's understanding of information unless, at minimum, the client verbally reiterates information or performs a return demonstration of the skill. A change in behavior over time is a powerful indication of learning. A nurse desiring a more extensive evaluation may consider using a paper-and-pencil "pretest/posttest" format. In this case, the nurse develops a written test to cover the content of the teaching and has the client complete the test *before* the nurse begins teaching. This provides a written measure of the client's learning needs. After the nurse implements the teaching plan, the client completes the same examination (a posttest). Comparison of the pretest and posttest results yields a documented measure of how much learning has occurred as a result of the nurse's teaching intervention.

Antipsychotic Medications

The discovery of the first antipsychotic drug, chlorpromazine (Thorazine), is a prime example of the role chance has played in the history of psychopharmacology. Chlorpromazine was initially synthesized as an antihistamine and was not tried as a tranquilizer for clients with schizophrenia until 1952. Its effects on the behavior, thinking, affect, and perception of schizophrenic clients were so profound that knowledge of its properties was rapidly disseminated, and it became widely used within 3–4 years. Chlorpromazine's effects on the hospital practice of psychiatry were staggering. Its use contributed to reversing a steadily increasing population in U.S. mental institutions, and that population has progressively decreased ever since. One might say that chlorpromazine gave birth to the modern notions of psychiatric treatment—unlocked wards, milieu treatment, occupational and recreational therapy, and halfway houses. The entire field of community mental health is ultimately linked to its discovery, because it enabled clients to return to their homes.

Psychobiologic Considerations

Understanding the psychobiology of antipsychotic medications requires a basic knowledge of the functions of the central nervous system. An extended discussion of how these drugs work to reduce symptoms is beyond the scope of this chapter, but here is a brief overview of the basic mechanisms of action.

Generally, neuroleptics work by blocking a variety of CNS receptors. Drugs such as antipsychotics do not work only on the neurotransmitter system. Therefore, it is likely that several types of neurotransmitters and neuromodulators are affected by the administration of a single medication. While most neuroleptics have an affinity for several types of neurotransmitters others are more specific and work more selectively. These differences account for the effects of the various neuroleptic medications.

Major Effects

The beneficial effects of antipsychotic medications in all psychotic states have been demonstrated beyond question. Multiple and varied criteria have been used to measure improvement. These drugs have been used successfully in clients with delusional thinking, confusion, motor agitation, and motor retardation. Antipsychotic drug treatment also decreases formal thought disorder, blunted affect, bizarre behavior, social withdrawal, hallucinations, belligerence, and uncooperativeness.

The most common disintegrative condition treated with antipsychotic drugs is the group of symptoms traditionally labeled schizophrenia. (See Chapter 14 for information on evaluating schizophrenic clients and the diagnostic criteria in *DSM-IV*.) The problem of assessment is complicated by the fact that many diseases can cause syndromes with features like those of schizophrenia. For example, delusions may indicate a variety of *DSM-IV* conditions, including schizophrenia and vascular dementia with delusions. The finer points of differentiation between these two conditions include assessments of cognitive functioning and the client's presenting history.

(Chapter 12 provides a detailed discussion of delirium, dementia, and related disorders.) All clients manifesting psychotic symptoms should give a thorough medical history and take a physical examination, to rule out treatable "medical" illnesses, many of which are accompanied by behaviors considered psychotic or "psychobiologic."

The Choice of a Specific Drug

There are many antipsychotic medications on the market, and you may have noticed the recent expansion of this class of drugs. Claims are made for the greater effectiveness of one over another, especially by the respective drug companies. Controlled studies, however, have failed to demonstrate substantial differences in antipsychotic effects among the various available drugs (Ayd 1994). The choice of a particular medication, then, depends on knowledge of the pharmacologic properties and side effects, the client's or a family member's history of drug response, and the prescriber's experience with various compounds. Important client variables are past successes with specific drugs, a history of allergies, and a history of serious or intolerable side effects. Some medications may have side effects with certain clients, which while not necessarily desired by the prescriber, may nevertheless prove to be helpful in treatment. Expect a certain amount of trial and error with each clinical application.

Table 33–1 summarizes the characteristics of the major antipsychotic medications. The list is extensive and growing, and it makes sense for each member of the treatment team to become familiar with just a few representative drugs, their predictable effects, and their common side effects. The characteristics covered in the table are discussed in the sections that follow (see also Appendix A).

There are now seven distinct chemical classes of antipsychotic medications commonly used in the United States. (One class, the phenothiazines, is subdivided into three different types of medications.) Thus, there is a broad choice in terms of side effects and potential client responsiveness. A client who is unresponsive to one class may well respond to another that circumvents a problem in absorption, accumulation at neurotransmitter receptor sites, or metabolism.

Table 33–1 shows the wide range among these medications in milligram-per-milligram potency. This fact has most relevance when treating clients who require large doses. In such cases, a potent medication is best.

Clozapine and Risperidone The antipsychotic drugs clozapine (Clozaril) and risperidone (Risperdal) have been introduced in the United States recently. These medications provide new options for the care and treatment of clients suffering from psychotic conditions. And the search continues for psychopharmacologic treatments

Table 33–1 Antipsychotic Medications

Class	Generic Name	Trade Name	Potency (mg equivalent to 100 mg chlorpromazine)	Usual Dosage Range (mg/day)	Sedative	SIDE EFFECTS	
						Extra-pyramidal*	Anti-cholinergic*
Phenothiazines							
Aliphatic	chlorpromazine	Thorazine	100	150–1500	Very strong	Moderate	Strong
Piperidine	thioridazine	Mellaril	100	150–800	Moderate	Minimal	Moderate
Piperazine	trifluoperazine	Stelazine	5	10–60	Weak	Strong	Weak
	fluphenazine	Prolixin	2	3–45	Weak	Strong	Weak
	perphenazine	Trilafon	10	12–60	Weak	Strong	Weak
Butyrophenones	haloperidol	Haldol	2.5	2–40	Weak	Strong	Weak
Thioxanthenes	thiothixene	Navane	5	10–60	Weak	Strong	Weak
	chlorprothixene	Taractan	100	40–600	Strong	Moderate	Strong
Dihydroindolones	molindone	Moban	10	15–225	Weak	Moderate	Weak
Dibenzoxazepines	loxapine	Loxitane	20	10–100	Moderate	Strong	Moderate
Dibenzodiazepines	clozapine	Clozaril	50	12.5–900	Moderate	Weak	Strong
Benzisoxazole derivatives	risperidone	Risperdal	Not established yet	4–16	Weak	Weak	Weak

Extrapyramidal and anticholinergic side effects are discussed later in this chapter.

for psychoses. Medications are being researched and tested every day, and if they provide relief from symptoms without undue side effects, they will enhance our psychopharmacologic arsenal.

Clozapine is an antipsychotic drug with an unusual pharmacologic and clinical profile. It was used in Europe for several years and is generally used in the U.S. with clients who cannot tolerate the EPS of other antipsychotics, or who have a treatment-resistant or treatment-refractory psychosis, as is the case with certain schizophrenic clients (Medical Letter 1993). Reviews of studies regarding the effectiveness of clozapine have demonstrated its decided impact on both negative and positive symptoms, with improvement evident on follow-up as well (Miller et al. 1994; Safferman et al. 1992).

Despite its capacity to ameliorate symptoms of some very recalcitrant clients, clozapine has some serious side effects. The most serious is agranulocytosis (a marked decrease in granulated white blood cells), which occurs in approximately 1–2% of clients taking this medication. The risk period for the emergence of this side effect is highest between 4 and 18 weeks after starting clozapine (Krupp and Barnes 1989), but it can occur later during the course of treatment. It is essential to monitor white blood cell (WBC) counts of clients taking clozapine. Immediately discontinuing the medication when agranulocytosis is detected and before signs of an infection develop will usually resolve the episode. If a client experiences agranulocytosis as a result of using clozapine, the drug cannot be reinstituted. Another serious side effect is the potential for seizure, which seems to be dose-related. Less acute but nonetheless important side effects include sedation, tachycardia, sialorrhea (drooling), weight gain, and hypotension.

Risperidone (Risperdal) was introduced in the U.S. in the spring of 1994. It is the first of a new class of antipsychotics, benzisoxazole derivatives, that does not clinically relate to any existing antipsychotic drug. Its unique feature is the relative absence of EPS. It addresses the positive, negative, and affective symptoms of schizophrenia and may also alleviate depression and anxiety (Ayd 1994). Risperidone has demonstrated an ability to suppress tardive dyskinesia without increasing parkinsonism, somewhat like clozapine (Chouinard and Arnott 1993).

Dosage of this new medication has been described as "the 1-2-3" regimen, in which the client receives 1 mg BID, the next increase is to 2 mg BID, and the next increase after that is to 3 mg BID. This places the client at 6 mg/day, which is in the therapeutic window of 4–8 mg/day currently recommended. Risperidone can be administered up to 16 mg/day, but the absence of EPS fades over 10 mg/day. Response within 1–10 weeks gives the drug a fair trial. Dosage for older clients is lower, generally cutting the initial dosage in half (0.5 mg BID, 1 mg BID, and 1.5 mg BID) and taking a full week between dosage changes.

This medication has been very popular in some areas, and the clinical knowledge gained from using it regularly has been valuable. Plans for an IM form of risperidone and eventually a depot form are being considered.

Dosage

Dosage ranges of antipsychotic medications vary widely among clients. Medications must be titrated against the psychotic target symptoms and the appearance of side effects. Most clients are initially given a relatively low dose of an antipsychotic to test for adverse effects for 1–2 hours. Let's consider chlorpromazine, with an initial dose of 20–50 mg orally (PO) or 25 mg intramuscularly (IM). Then the medication is typically given in a starting dose of 300–400 mg (or IM equivalent) per day, and gradually increased by 25–50% each day until maximum improvement is noted or intolerable side effects are encountered. You will see this type of progression with the various antipsychotic medications.

The treatment setting frequently influences the drug regimen. In a crowded hospital emergency room, for example, hourly doses of medication may be given until a client is sedated. In more completely staffed, private inpatient units, a client may be observed for several days before medication is given. However, in terms of long-term outcome and length of eventual remission, neither approach can claim documented superiority (Gaebel 1993).

Clients who are extremely agitated, violent, severely withdrawn, or catatonic require significant doses during the first few days of treatment, delivered by injection to ensure rapid relief. Chlorpromazine, 50–100 mg IM, may be used, particularly if sedation is required. The nurse must be aware that this is an irritating drug; injections must be deeply intramuscular in either the buttocks or upper arms, and sites must be rotated. Substantial IM doses of the more potent antipsychotics, such as haloperidol 10 mg or trifluoperazine 10 mg, may be given to agitated clients. This approach frequently avoids some of the more troublesome side effects while ameliorating behavioral and cognitive symptoms.

Because antipsychotic medications have a rather long biologic half-life and many have significant sedative effects, there is little reason to give divided doses of medication after the initial days of treatment. It is recommended that the drugs, particularly the sedative ones such as chlorpromazine, be given in substantial doses at bedtime. In addition to promoting sleep, decreasing the chances the client will forget to take a dose after discharge, and saving nursing time in the hospital, this method saves money because large-dose capsules or tablets cost less than an equivalent amount of medication prepared in smaller doses.

After maximum clinical improvement has been obtained, antipsychotic medications are generally reduced gradually. Continuing to give a client modest doses of an antipsychotic following a psychotic episode lowers the chances of relapse and rehospitalization. Psychotherapy with schizophrenic clients may not be particularly effective without maintenance medications in conventional treatment settings, but it does improve psychosocial functioning in clients who are also taking maintenance medications. It is generally believed that clients should be kept on doses of antipsychotics sufficient to suppress symptoms for 3 months to 1 year following an acute episode. After such an interval, the client's course and life situation must be considered and treatment individualized. Some clients recover from a psychotic episode completely within 6 months. These clients, with schizophreniform disorder, should not receive long-term maintenance drug treatment. For individuals who have already experienced recurrent episodes of psychosis and demonstrate a deteriorating course, it is clearly advantageous to prevent relapses with drugs if possible.

The Decision to Use a Drug

Today, these general principles govern antipsychotic drug use:

- Drugs are given to treat target symptoms of schizophrenia or other psychotic disorders.
- Initial treatment may require parenteral doses. These are changed to oral pill or concentrate forms as the behavior disturbance subsides.
- Total dosages are tailored to individual needs; wide variations exist among clients.
- As soon as practical with drugs having sedating side effects, divided doses are changed to a single dose given at bedtime to maximize use of the drug's sedative properties.
- Most clients with a chronic course require maintenance doses for sustained improvement (Schooler 1993).

Special Considerations

These special considerations apply to the use of antipsychotic medication:

A UNIQUE ROUTE OF ADMINISTRATION The phenothiazines fluphenazine (Prolixin) and haloperidol (Haldol) are available in long-acting intramuscular injectable forms that behave like timed-release capsules. These medications are gradually released over a long period of time, 2–3 weeks. Long-acting fluphenazine and haloperidol are available in decanoate (long-acting **depot injection**) preparations. The main advantage of decanoate forms is that they reduce clients' ambivalence about taking medication and eliminate the need for constant pill taking. The treatment team must also honor the clients' civil liberties; truly involuntary treatment can be performed only according to due process, as required by a particular state's mental hygiene laws.

The psychiatric nurse in a community setting may frequently have occasion to administer the long-acting fluphenazine or haloperidol. With a client whose treatment will include a long-acting medication, a dose of regular fluphenazine or haloperidol is usually taken first to rule out the possibility of allergic reactions. Such reactions can be devastating if discovered after a 2- or 3-week supply of medicine has been given as a depot treatment. If no adverse reactions are noted within 1 hour, the long-acting form is injected, usually in the upper outer quadrant of the buttocks.

Another administration issue you will encounter is the manner in which you deliver these types of medications. The Z track method is a particular IM procedure described in Figure 33–1. Implementation of the Z track technique

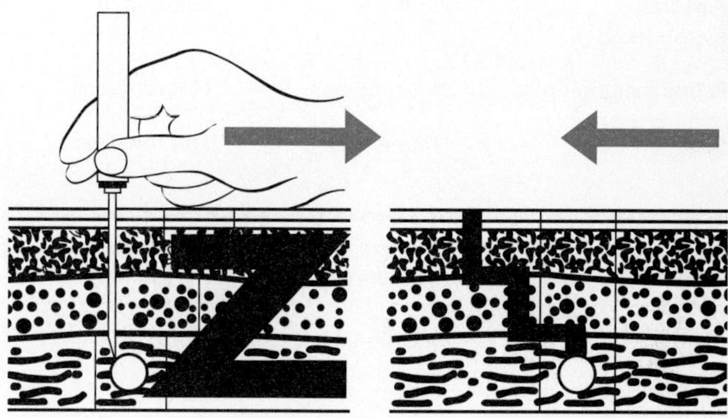

Figure 33–1 The Z Track Technique Decanoate, or long-acting depot, medications are injected into the gluteal muscle mass of the gluteus maximus, the upper outer quadrant of a buttock. Rotate the sites of injection so that one area does not get overused. Procedure for Z track injections: Draw up the medication into the syringe and then change the needle, to avoid having viscous materials such as depot medications cling to the needle, interfering with a smooth injection process; and to reduce depositing the medication into the subcutaneous and adipose tissues. Z tracking when you inject minimizes the leakage of medication back out the injection track into nonmuscle tissue and onto the surface of the skin. Choose your injection site. Before injecting, with a push-and-slide motion, pull the skin at your chosen site to one side, to change the angles of the skin, fatty tissue, and muscle in relation to each other. Inject at a 90° angle to the skin, deeply penetrating the gluteal muscle. Check muscle placement by aspirating (no blood on aspiration assures you have not struck a blood vessel). Slowly depress the syringe's plunger to administer the depot medication. Wait about 10 sec before withdrawing the needle and releasing your hold on the skin. Apply light pressure to the injection area.

Table 33–2 Side Effects of Antipsychotic Medications

Effect	*Chlorpromazine (Thorazine)*	*Haloperidol (Haldol)*	*Loxapine (Loxitane)*	*Molindone (Moban)*	*Risperidone (Risperdal)*	*Clozapine (Clozaril)*
Akathisia	Occasional	Frequent	Occasional	Frequent	Occasional	Occasional
Allergic skin reactions	Occasional	Rare	Rare	Rare	Rare	Occasional
Anticholinergic effects	Frequent	Not reported	Rare	Occasional	Occasional	Rare
Blood dyscrasia	Occasional	Occasional	Not reported	Rare	Not reported	Occasional
Cholestatic jaundice	Occasional	Rare	Not reported	Not reported	Not reported	Not reported
Dystonias	Occasional	Frequent	Rare	Occasional	Rare	Occasional
Impotence	Occasional	Not reported	Not reported	Not reported	Rare	Rare
Parkinsonism	Occasional	Frequent	Frequent	Occasional	Rare	Rare
Photosensitivity	Occasional	Rare	Not reported	Not reported	Not reported	Not reported
Postural hypotension	Frequent	Occasional	Rare	Rare	Occasional	Frequent
Retinitis pigmentosa	Not reported	Not reported	Not reported	Not reported	Not reported	Not reported
Sedation	Frequent	Not reported	Occasional	Rare	Rare	Frequent

Effect	*Thioridazine (Mellaril)*	*Thiothixene (Navane)*	*Trifluoperazine (Stelazine)*	*Fluphenazine (Prolixin)*
Akathisia	Occasional	Occasional	Frequent	Frequent
Allergic skin reactions	Not reported	Rare	Rare	Rare
Anticholinergic effects	Frequent	Occasional	Frequent	Frequent
Blood dyscrasia	Rare	Rare	Rare	Rare
Cholestatic jaundice	Rare	Rare	Rare	Rare
Dystonias	Occasional	Occasional	Frequent	Frequent
Impotence	Occasional	Not reported	Occasional	Occasional
Parkinsonism	Occasional	Occasional	Frequent	Frequent
Photosensitivity	Occasional	Rare	Occasional	Occasional
Postural hypotension	Frequent	Occasional	Rare	Rare
Retinitis pigmentosa	Occasional	Not reported	Not reported	Not reported
Sedation	Frequent	Frequent	Not reported	Occasional

prevents or minimizes leaking of the medication or the formation of abcesses (Middlemiss and Beeber 1989; Reinke and Wiesert 1992).

Medication Requirements of Certain Age Groups In elderly clients, the agitation often associated with delirium, dementia, and related disorders is markedly responsive to phenothiazines. Other sedatives, such as barbiturates and benzodiazepines, may further compromise cerebral functioning, further depressing the level of awareness and concentration and thereby worsening the disorder. Doses of phenothiazines are generally reduced for older adults. Trifluoperazine (Stelazine) 5–20 mg/day or haloperidol 1–6 mg/day might constitute adequate treatment.

Antipsychotic medications are effective in treating childhood psychoses and in managing the behavior problems associated with mental retardation. The general principle of reduced dosage is again applicable. The upper limit of the usual daily dosage for children under 12 might be 200 mg/day of chlorpromazine (Thorazine) or thioridazine (Mellaril) or 20 mg/day per day of trifluoperazine. Amounts of individual IM injections of chlorprom-azine must also be kept at 0.25 mg per pound of body weight every 6–8 hr, or not over 40 mg/day for up to 50 lb and not over 75 mg/day for children weighing 50–100 lb.

Potential Side Effects of Antipsychotic Medications Continuous contact with clients gives nurses an advantage over physicians, who may see a client only every other day or, at best, once a day at the same time. Both the dangerous and the more uncomfortable side effects frequently have a rapid onset and need attention promptly.

The side effects of antipsychotic medications that nurses must recognize can be divided into these classes:

- Autonomic nervous system
- Extrapyramidal
- Other central nervous system (CNS)
- Allergic
- Blood
- Skin
- Eye
- Endocrine

Table 33–2 lists the side effects of various antipsychotic medications.

Autonomic Nervous System Effects The antipsychotics all possess **anticholinergic side effects** and antiadrenergic side effects; that is, they interfere with the normal transmission of nerve impulses by acetylcholine and epinephrine, in both central and peripheral nerves. The most common side effects are the anticholinergic ones. These include dry mouth, blurred vision, constipation, urinary hesitance or retention, and, under rarer circumstances, paralytic ileus.

Orthostatic hypotension, also known as postural hypotension, is a common antiadrenergic effect. The primary danger here is injury from a fall. Clients receiving parenteral medications, such as chlorpromazine intramuscularly, must have their blood pressure monitored lying and standing before and a half hour after each dose. Clients should be advised to rise from a supine position gradually and to sit down if they feel faint. Support stockings and a large intake of fluids may be indicated. This problem is much less significant with oral administration of the drug. However, nurses working with clients receiving oral antipsychotic medications should take both baseline and routine vital sign readings at regular intervals. This practice establishes the client's tolerance for medications without the untoward side effects of orthostatic hypotension and subsequent falls. The accompanying box provides guidelines for measuring orthostatic blood pressure.

INTERVENTION

Guidelines for Measuring Orthostatic Blood Pressure

1. Instruct the client to lie down for approximately 5 minutes. This allows for an equilibration of the blood pressure in the supine position and gives a precise supine reading. *Do not substitute a supine reading for a sitting reading!* Take the client's blood pressure and pulse.
2. Instruct the client to stand. Wait for approximately 30 sec to 1 min and retake the blood pressure and pulse. Waiting this brief period allows for a full evaluation of the initial orthostasis.
3. Wait 2 more minutes and retake the vital signs once again. This third set of measurements allows for an evaluation of the client's body mechanisms to compensate for the presence of any orthostasis that may be present.

Extrapyramidal Side Effects Another common and sometimes frightening group of adverse reactions results from the effects of antipsychotics on the extrapyramidal

ASSESSMENT

A Comparison of Akathisia and Agitation or Psychotic Relapse

Akathisia	Agitation or Relapse
Relieved by reducing phenothiazine dosage.	Worsened by reducing phenothiazine dosage.
Worsened by increasing phenothiazine dosage.	Improved by increasing phenothiazine dosage.
Responsive to antiparkinsonian agents.	Unresponsive to antiparkinsonian agents.
Motor restlessness predominant.	Verbalization predominant.

tracts of the central nervous system, which are involved in the production and control of involuntary movements. These **extrapyramidal side effects (EPS)** can be broken down into four types, each with distinguishing clinical characteristics and times of onset after the initiation of drug therapy.

The earliest and most dramatic reactions are the *acute dystonic reactions,* forms of dystonia. These occur in the first days of treatment, sometimes after a single dose of medication. They involve bizarre and severe muscle contractions usually of the tongue, face, or extraocular muscles, producing **torticollis** (twisting of the neck), **opisthotonos** (spasms of the neck and back, forcing the back to arch and the neck to bend backward), and **oculogyric crisis** (a fixed gaze, often upward). Of particular importance to the nurse is that dystonic reactions may also lead to laryngeal spasm. This spasm may begin as a scratching feeling in the back of the client's throat, leading to a coughing fit, and advancing to respiratory distress. The respiratory distress may lead to respiratory arrest, which necessitates mechanical ventilation. These reactions can be physically painful and are almost always frightening to the individual. They are readily reversible with one of the antiparkinsonian agents—benztropine 1–2 mg or diphenhydramine 20–50 mg, intravenously (for immediate relief), intramuscularly (for rapid action), or orally (for relief within hours).

Parkinsonian syndrome, so named because of its striking resemblance to true Parkinson's disease, commonly occurs after a week or two of the therapy. It is the result of dopamine blockade, caused by the neuroleptic drugs. The hallmark signs include masklike facies, resting tremor, general rigidity of posture with slow voluntary movement, and a shuffling gait. This syndrome is treatable with the antiparkinsonian agents amantadine (Symmetrel), benztropine (Cogentin), biperiden (Akineton), diphenhydramine (Benadryl), procyclidine (Kemadrin), and trihexyphenidyl (Artane). Oral medication is usually sufficient, since urgency is seldom a consideration in the management of this syndrome.

A third reversible extrapyramidal side effect is known as **akathisia.** This characteristically is a motor restlessness perceived subjectively by the client and experienced as an urge to pace, a need to shift weight from one foot to another, or an inability to sit or stand still. Akathisia is generally a later complication of drug treatment, occurring weeks to months into the course of therapy. It responds to oral antiparkinsonian agents.

Accurate observation of the course of therapy by the psychiatric nurse can promote prompt recognition and proper interpretation of EPS. If care is not taken, the health care provider may misinterpret the increasing withdrawal, emotional blunting, apathy, and lack of spontaneity as increasing schizophrenic behavior. This error in interpretation may lead to a mistaken increase in dosage of antipsychotic medication, which will aggravate the condition. Akathisia can also be confused with psychotic agitation, and this error also prompts an increase in medication. For a comparison of the two conditions, see the accompanying Assessment box. Clients with akathisia require a reduction in the dosage of phenothiazines or other offending agents and/or treatment with an antiparkinsonian drug. You can save the client many uncomfortable and worrisome days by being aware of the frequency with which these syndromes complicate treatment and by reporting any suspicious sign or symptom to the physician, while reassuring the client of the reversibility of the syndrome in almost all cases.

Whether clients should be treated prophylactically with antiparkinsonian agents, in view of the relatively high incidence of EPS, is open to debate. Some argue that the use of antiparkinsonian agents eventually leads to relatively higher antipsychotic doses, thereby increasing the probability of serious side effects. Another argument is that antiparkinsonian agents also pose risks and thus should be used only to counteract EPS, not to guard against their possible emergence. Moreover, a great many clients never develop the syndromes. If the likelihood of an extrapyramidal reaction is high (if, for example, the client has a history of them) and the possible consequences significant (the client may discontinue medication or drop out of treatment altogether), antipsychotic and antiparkinsonian agents are frequently initiated simultaneously.

Nursing assessment of extrapyramidal side effects is important to the quality care of clients receiving psychotropic medications. One difficulty is *consistency* of assessment among caregivers. For example, nurses usually assess for the presence of cogwheeling or muscle rigidity in clients receiving psychotropic drugs. However, the reliability among those assessments is sorely lacking; what one nurse may consider moderate to severe side effects may be assessed as mild to moderate by another nurse.

Two assessment tools are the Simpson Neurological Rating Scale for the assessment of extrapyramidal side effects and the Abnormal Involuntary Movement Scale (AIMS) for the assessment of iatrogenic movements resulting from particular psychotropic drugs. See Figures 33–2 and 33–3 for sample forms. They are helpful in quantifying EPS prior to administering a medication to counteract the side effect. Readministering the instruments after the medication is given helps the nurse assess the amelioration of the side effect. These data chart the course of a client's side effects and the effectiveness of medications to decrease them. This information is critical to quality nursing care.

The last EPS to emerge in the course of treatment is also the most severe because it can be largely irreversible. This is **tardive dyskinesia (TD),** a disorder characterized by involuntary movements of the face, jaw, and tongue that produce bizarre grimaces, lip smacking, and protrusion of the tongue. There may also be jerky choreiform movements of the upper extremities, slow writhing athetoid movements of the arms and legs, and tense, tonic contractions of the neck and back. TD frequently appears after years of antipsychotic drug treatment, although it can occur earlier. It usually occurs after a maintenance dose is discontinued or reduced, and it can be masked—but not treated—by reinstituting the medication or the dosage or by switching to another drug.

Current estimates put the incidence of TD at 5% per year for young adults and as high as 30% after 1 year in elderly clients (Benjamin and Munetz 1994). Early detection through regular examinations (at least every 6 months) is recommended by the American Psychiatric Association Tardive Dyskinesia Task Force (APA 1992).

There is no known cure for TD. The recommended intervention is to stop all medication to see if the syndrome resolves spontaneously. This course of action must be weighed against the client's need for medication and the likelihood of relapse into psychosis. Reserpine, deanol, and several other drugs have been used experimentally to treat tardive dyskinesia, with equivocal results.

With the emergence of antipsychotic medications such as clozapine and risperidone, which can have an effect on TD and are not likely to cause a significant number of TD cases, the choices in this area are expanding. As noted above, both of these antipsychotics have been known to reduce tardive dyskinesia.

For an overview of EPS, see the Assessment box on page 792. Table 33–3 on page 793 lists the commonly used antiparkinsonian medications for addressing EPS.

Other Central Nervous System Effects CNS side effects of antipsychotic medications are sedation and reduction of the seizure threshold. Because antipsychotic drugs vary in their sedative effects, this side effect is troublesome, but it can be managed by changing to a less sedative agent. Seizures are not a contraindication for the drugs, but they do require close observation.

Allergic Effects The principal allergic manifestation of the antipsychotics is cholestatic jaundice. This occurs much less frequently than in the early days of psychopharmacology, and it is usually a benign and self-limiting condition.

Blood, Skin, and Eye Effects Among the other side effects, agranulocytosis is the most serious. It is both potentially fatal and, fortunately, extremely rare. Usually the person gets an infection and deteriorates rapidly or begins to bleed spontaneously, requiring emergency medical attention.

Skin eruptions, photosensitivity leading to severe sunburn, blue-gray metallic discolorations over the face and hands, and pigmentation changes in the eyes are all potential side effects. Clients are generally advised to avoid prolonged exposure to sunlight or to use a sunscreen agent when outdoors. These conditions usually remit. One serious and permanent eye change is retinitis pigmentosa. This condition may occur in clients on dosages of thioridazine (Mellaril) exceeding 800 mg/day. The condition may lead to blindness. Therefore, doses exceeding 800 mg per day are contraindicated.

Endocrine Effects Lactation in females and gynecomastia and impotence in males lead a list of endocrine changes that can occur with antipsychotic drug treatments. You should be alert to any changes in body functions reported by clients taking these medications.

Neuroleptic Malignant Syndrome **Neuroleptic malignant syndrome (NMS)** is a severe and potentially life-threatening side effect of all psychotropic medications. This extreme condition occurs in clients who are severely ill and is believed to be the result of dopamine blockade in the striatum of the brain. NMS occurs in 0.5–1% of clients taking neuroleptic medications. Men are affected more than women, approximately twice as much, and younger clients appear to be more susceptible than older ones (Thornberg and Ereshefsky 1993). NMS is typically seen within the first 2 weeks of treatment with a different medication or a dosage increase, but cases have been reported months after a new medication regimen has begun. Nurses are in the best position to assess for this condition because its symptoms are muscle rigidity, hyperpyrexia, altered consciousness, and diaphoresis. If cooling and rehydration are not achieved quickly, the

text continues on page 792

DEPARTMENT OF HEALTH AND HUMAN SERVICES
PUBLIC HEALTH SERVICE
Alcohol, Drug Abuse, and Mental Health Administration
NIMH Treatment Strategies in Schizophrenia Study

NEUROLOGICAL RATING SCALE
(Simpson)

PATIENT NUMBER	DATA GROUP	EVALUATION DATE
__ __ __ __	**eps**	__ __ - __ __ - __ __ M M D D Y Y

PATIENT NAME

RATER NAME

RATER NUMBER	EVALUATION TYPE (*Circle*)			
__ __ __	1 Baseline 2 2-Week minor 3	4 Start double-blind 5 Major evaluation 6 Other	7 Start open meds 8 During open meds 9 Stop open meds	10 Early termination 11 Study completion

The examination should be conducted in a room where the patient can walk a sufficient distance to allow him/her to get into a natural rhythm, e.g., 15 paces.

Each side of the body should be examined; if one side shows more pronounced pathology than the other, record more severe pathology.

Cogwheel rigidity may be palpated when the examination is carried out for items 3,4, 5, and 6. It is not rated separately and is merely another way to detect rigidity. It would indicate that a minimum score of 2 would be mandatory.

1. **GAIT:** The patient is examined as he walks into the examining room—his gait, the swing of his arms, his general posture, all form the basis for an overall score for this item.
   - 1 = Normal
   - 2 = Mild diminution in swing while the patient is walking
   - 3 = Obvious diminution in swing suggesting shoulder rigidity
   - 4 = Stiff gait with little or no armswing noticeable
   - 5 = Rigid gait with arms slightly pronated; or stooped-shuffling gait with propulsion and repropulsion
   - 9 = Not ratable
2. **ARM DROPPING:** The patient and the examiner both raise their arms to shoulder height and let them fall to their sides. In a normal subject, a stout slap is heard as the arms hit the sides. In the patient with extreme Parkinson's syndrome, the arms fall very slowly.
   - 1 = Normal, free fall with loud slap and rebound
   - 2 = Fall slowed slightly with less audible contact and little rebound
   - 3 = Fall slowed, no rebound
   - 4 = Marked slowing, no slap at all
   - 5 = Arms fall as though against resistance; as though through glue
   - 9 = Not ratable
3. **SHOULDER SHAKING:** The subject's arms are bent at a right angle at the elbow and are taken one at a time by the examiner who grasps one hand and also clasps the other around the patient's elbow. The subject's upper arm is pushed to and fro and the humerus is externally rotated. The degree of resistance from normal to extreme rigidity is scored as detailed. The procedure is repeated with one hand palpating the shoulder cuff while rotation takes place.
   - 1 = Normal
   - 2 = Slight stiffness and resistance
   - 3 = Moderate stiffness and resistance
   - 4 = Moderate rigidity with difficulty in passive movement
   - 5 = Extreme stiffness and rigidity with almost a frozen joint
   - 9 = Not ratable
4. **ELBOW RIGIDITY:** The elbow joints are separately bent at right agles and passively extended and flexed, with the subject's biceps observed and simultaneously palpated. The resistance to this procedure is rated.
   - 1 = Normal
   - 2 = Slight stiffness and resistance
   - 3 = Moderate stiffness and resistance
   - 4 = Marked rigidity with difficulty in passive movement
   - 5 = Extreme stiffness and rigidity with almost a frozen joint
   - 9 = Not ratable

Page 1

Figure 33–2 The Simpson Neurological Rating Scale.

→

5. **WRIST RIGIDITY:** The wrist is held in one hand and the fingers held by the examiner's other hand, with the wrist moved to extension, flexion and ulner and radial deviation or the extended wrist is allowed to fall under its own weight, or the arm can be grasped above the wrist and shaken to and fro. A "1" score would be a hand that extends easily, falls loosely, or flaps easily upwards and downwards.
   1 = Normal
   2 = Slight stiffness and resistance
   3 = Moderate stiffness and resistance
   4 = Marked rigidity with difficulty in passive movement
   5 = Extreme stiffness and rigidity with almost a frozen wrist
   9 = Not ratable
6. **HEAD ROTATION:** The patient sits or stands and is told that you are going to move his head from side to side, that it will not hurt and that he should try and relax. (Questions about pain in the cervical area or difficulty in moving his head should be obtained to avoid causing any pain.) Clasp the patient's head between the two hands with the fingers on the back of the neck. Gently rotate the head in a circular motion 3 times and evaluate the muscular resistance to this movement.
   1 = Loose, no resistance
   2 = Slight resistance to movement although the time to rotate may be normal
   3 = Resistance is apparent and the time of rotation is shortened
   4 = Resistance is obvious and rotation is slowed
   5 = Head appears stiff and rotation is difficult to carry out
   9 = Not ratable
7. **GLABELLAR TAP:** Subject is told to open eyes wide and not to blink. The glabellar region is tapped at a steady, rapid speed. Note number of times patient blinks in succession. Take care to stand behind the subject so that he does not observe the movement of the tapping finger. A full blink need not be observed; there may be contraction of the infraorbital muscle producing a twitch each time a stimulus is delivered. Vary speed of tapping to assure that muscle contraction is related to the tap.
   1 = 0-5 blinks
   2 = 6-10 blinks
   3 = 11-15 blinks
   4 = 16-20 blinks
   5 = 21 and more blinks
   9 = Not ratable
8. **TREMOR:** Patient is observed walking into examing room and then is re-examined for this item with arms extended at right angles to the body and the fingers spread out as far as possible.
   1 = Normal
   2 = Mild finger tremor, obvious to sight and touch
   3 = Tremor of hand or arm occurring spasmodically
   4 = Persistent tremor of one or more limbs
   5 = Whole body tremor
   9 = Not ratable
9. **SALIVATION:** Patient is observed while talking and then asked to open his mouth and elevate his tongue.
   1 = Normal
   2 = Excess salivation so that pooling takes place if mouth is open and tongue raised
   3 = Excess salivation is present and might occasionally result in difficulty in speaking
   4 = Speaking with difficulty because of excess salivation
   5 = Frank drooling
   9 = Not ratable
10. **AKATHISIA:** Patient is observed for restlessness. If restlessness is noted, ask: "Do you feel restless or jittery inside; is it difficult to sit still?" Subjective response is not necessary for scoring but patient report can help make the assessment.
   1 = No restlessness reported or observed
   2 = Mild restlessness observed, e.g., occasional jiggling of the foot occurs when patient is seated
   3 = Moderate restlessness observed, e.g., on several occasions, jiggles foot, crosses and uncrosses legs or twists a part of the body
   4 = Restlessness is frequently observed, e.g., the foot or legs moving most of the time
   5 = Restlessness persistently observed, e.g., patient cannot sit still, may get up and walk
   9 = Not ratable

Page 2

Figure 33–2 (continued)

DEPARTMENT OF HEALTH AND HUMAN SERVICES
PUBLIC HEALTH SERVICE
Alcohol, Drug Abuse, and Mental Health Administration
NIMH Treatment Strategies in Schizophrenia Study

ABNORMAL INVOLUNTARY MOVEMENT SCALE (AIMS)

PATIENT NUMBER	DATA GROUP	EVALUATION DATE
— — — —	**aims**	__ __ - __ __ - __ __ M M D D Y Y

PATIENT NAME

RATER NAME

RATER NUMBER	EVALUATION TYPE (*Circle*)			
— — —	1 Baseline	4 Start double-blind	7 Start open meds	10 Early termination
	2 2-Week minor	5 Major evaluation	8 During open meds	11 Study completion
	3	6 Other	9 Stop open meds	

INSTRUCTIONS: Complete Examination Procedure (reverse side) before making ratings.
MOVEMENT RATINGS: Rate highest severity observed.

Code: 1 = None; 2 = Minimal, may be extreme normal; 3 = Mild; 4 = Moderate; 5 = Severe

	Item	(Circle One)				
FACIAL AND ORAL MOVEMENTS:	**1. Muscles of Facial Expression** e.g., movements of forehead, eyebrows, periorbital area, cheeks; include frowning, blinking, smiling, grimacing	1	2	3	4	5
	2. Lips and Perioral Area e.g., puckering, pouting, smacking	1	2	3	4	5
	3. Jaw e.g., biting, clenching, chewing, mouth opening, lateral movement	1	2	3	4	5
	4. Tongue Rate only increase in movement both in and out of mouth, NOT inability to sustain movement	1	2	3	4	5
EXTREMITY MOVEMENTS:	**5. Upper** *(arms, wrists, hands, fingers)* Include choreic movements, (i.e., rapid, objectively purposeless, irregular, spontaneous), athetoid movements (i.e., slow, irregular, complex, serpentine). Do NOT include tremor (i.e., repetitive, regular, rhythmic)	1	2	3	4	5
	6. Lower *(legs, knees, ankles, toes)* e.g., lateral knee movement, foot tapping, heel dropping, foot squirming, inversion and eversion of foot	1	2	3	4	5
TRUNK MOVEMENTS:	**7. Neck, shoulders, hips** e.g., rocking, twisting, squirming, pelvic gyrations	1	2	3	4	5

	Item	Response	Score
GLOBAL JUDGEMENTS:	**8. Severity of abnormal movements**	None, normal	1
		Minimal	2
		Mild	3
		Moderate	4
		Severe	5
	9. Incapacitation due to abnormal movements	None, normal	1
		Minimal	2
		Mild	3
		Moderate	4
		Severe	5
	10. Patient's awareness of abnormal movements Rate only patient's report	No awareness	1
		Aware, no distress	2
		Aware, mild distress	3
		Aware, moderate distress	4
		Aware, severe distress	5
DENTAL STATUS:	**11. Current problems with teeth and/or dentures**	No	1
		Yes	2
	12. Does patient usually wear dentures?	No	1
		Yes	2

Figure 33–3 The Abnormal Involuntary Movement Scale (AIMS).

→

EXAMINATION PROCEDURE

Either before or after completing the Examination Procedure observe the patient unobtrusively, at rest (e.g., in waiting room.)

The chair to be used in this examination should be a hard, firm one without arms.

---

1. Ask patient to remove shoes and socks.
2. Ask patient whether there is anything in his/her mouth (i.e., gum, candy, etc.) and if there is, to remove it.
3. Ask patient about the current condition of his/her teeth. Ask patient if he/she wears dentures. Do teeth or dentures bother patient now?
4. Ask patient whether he/she notices any movements in mouth, face, hands, or feet. If yes, ask to describe and to what extent they currently bother patient or interfere with his/her activities.
5. Have patient sit in chair with hands on knees, legs slightly apart, and feet flat on floor. (Look at entire body for movements while in this position.)
6. Ask patient to sit with hands hanging unsupported. If male, between legs, if female and wearing a dress, hanging over knees. (Observe hands and other body areas.)
7. Ask patient to open mouth. (Observe tongue at rest within mouth.) Do this twice.
8. Ask patient to protrude tongue. (Observe abnormalities of tongue movement.) Do this twice.
9. Ask patient to tap thumb, with each finger, as rapidly as possible for 10-15 seconds; separately with right hand, then with left hand. (Observe facial and leg movements.)
10. Flex and extend patient's left and right arms (one at a time.) (Note any rigidity.)
11. Ask patient to stand up. (Observe in profile. Observe all body areas again, hips included.)
12. Ask patient to extend both arms outstretched in front with palms down. (Observe trunk, legs, and mouth.)
13. Have patient walk a few paces, turn, and walk back to chair. (Observe hands and gait.) Do this twice.

Figure 33–3 (continued)

ASSESSMENT

Extrapyramidal Side Effects (EPS)

Dystonia

- Usually occurs within 48 hr after beginning treatment.
- Described by the client as "Sometimes my back tightens up," or "I get tongue-tied when I try to talk."
- Characterized by abnormal tonic contractions of muscle groups.
- Characterized by odd posturing and strange facial expressions.
- More common in young males.
- Prophylactically treated by anticholinergics.

Drug-Induced Parkinsonism

- Usually occurs after 3 or more weeks of treatment.
- Characterized by rigidity (cogwheeling), tremor, or regular rhythmic oscillations of the extremities, particularly the distal parts, and in the hands, by a pill-rolling movement of the fingers.
- More common in elderly clients.
- Clients are more susceptible to aspirate food or incur injury by falling.
- Treatment is decreasing the medication dosage or administering anticholinergics.

Akathisia

- Usually occurs after 3 or more weeks of treatment.
- Described by the client as "My nerves are jumping," or "I feel like jumping out of my skin."
- A subjective need or desire to move, not a type of pattern or movement.
- *Mild akathisia:* vague feelings of apprehension and irritability.
- *Severe akathisia:* an inability to sit for more than a few seconds, resulting in running, rocking, or agitated dancing.
- Not always responsive to anticholinergics; it may necessitate lowering the medication dosage.

Akinesia

- Usually occurs after 1–2 weeks of treatment.
- Described by the client as "There's nothing that interests me anymore," or "I feel blah."
- Characterized by slowed movement, a shuffling gait, an absence of spontaneous muscular movement, and a lifeless appearance.
- Sometimes gives rise to suicidal rumination.
- A frequently missed side effect that readily responds to antiparkinsonian medications.

Dopamine-Acetylcholine Imbalance in the Extrapyramidal System

- Characterized by hallucinations, dry mouth, blurred vision, decreased absorption of antipsychotics, decreased gastric motility, tachycardia, and urinary retention.

Tardive Dyskinesia (TD)

- Late onset during the course of treatment with antipsychotics, with frequently irreversible abnormal movements or a neurologic syndrome.
- Characterized by coordinated, rhythmic, involuntary movements, lip smacking, tongue protrusion, rocking, foot tapping.
- Complications include an inability to wear dentures, impaired respirations, weight loss, and impaired gait and posture.
- Treatment is primary prevention through careful initial assessment of the client's needs, as well as continual evaluation of the course of treatment.

client may die. Because NMS often occurs in clients whose presentations are already complex, the nursing assessment can be difficult. The clinical example below illustrates this serious side effect.

Alicia is a 22-year-old woman admitted to the inpatient psychiatric unit of a general hospital for treatment of bipolar disorder, manic. Prior to her admission, she had been taking 600 mg of lithium carbonate twice daily, which adequately controlled her symptoms. Two weeks ago her father was killed in an automobile accident. Since the funeral, Alicia has had a sleep disturbance evidenced by a need for only 3 hours of sleep per night. Her thoughts began racing 5 days prior to admission, and 2 days ago she began hearing the voice of

Table 33–3 Antiparkinsonian Medications

Generic Name	Trade Name	Maximum Daily Dosage	Available in Injectable Form
amantadine	Symmetrel	300 mg	No
benztropine	Cogentin	8 mg	Yes
biperiden	Akineton	8 mg	Yes
diphenhydramine	Benadryl	100 mg	Yes
procyclidine	Kemadrin	15 mg	No
trihexyphenidyl	Artane	15 mg	No

her father "telling me to join him by jumping out of a fourth-story window."

On admission to the unit, the physician prescribed lithium at the above noted dosage, with orders for a lithium level to be drawn the next day. In addition, the physician ordered haloperidol (Haldol), 5 mg orally twice daily, and alprazolam (Xanax), 0.5 mg every 4 hours orally as needed for agitation. On the fourth day of her hospitalization, Alicia began to demonstrate increasing agitation and psychotic thought. Nurses working with her administered the maximum number of doses of alprazolam allowed under the physician's orders. Recognizing that the psychotic agitation was becoming worse despite the medication, the physician increased the haloperidol dosage to 8 mg twice daily. A day later the agitation was still worsening, and the haloperidol dosage was again increased to 10 mg twice daily. On the eighth day of the hospitalization, nursing staff recognized that Alicia had extrapyramidal side effects. They reported this to the physician, who in turn ordered benztropine mesylate (Cogentin), 2 mg orally twice daily. The side effects worsened, as did the client's mental status. At this point, she rambled incoherently, drooled, was extremely diaphoretic, exhibited significant muscle rigidity, and had a fever of 103.1F (39.5C) (treated symptomatically). The hyperpyrexia led the treatment team to believe that Alicia had developed neuroleptic malignant syndrome.

All neuroleptic medications were stopped immediately. An intravenous line provided Alicia with needed hydration and some calories, as she was unable to eat. She required total nursing care for 72 hours, at which time her mental status began improving and she reengaged in her own care.

Treatment for NMS includes discontinuing all psychotropic medication immediately and supporting the client medically through the crisis. Caution in follow-up care is, of course, critical. The pathology of NMS is complex and not completely understood at this time beyond the knowledge that the major symptoms of NMS are caused by the neuroleptic blockade of the dopamine receptors.

Clinical Implications

Nurses have many responsibilities to clients receiving neuroleptic drugs. To ensure the bioavailability and effectiveness of neuroleptic medications, it is important to understand the relationships between the medication and the liquid (or substance) you administer it with, as well as the relationships between medications. Some medications are not compatible with all substances. For an overview of the compatibility of drugs and typical liquids, see Table 33–4.

Client Teaching

As with any medication, client teaching is essential for clients receiving neuroleptic medication. A medication teaching plan for antipsychotics is presented in the Client/Family Teaching box on page 795.

Antidepressant Medications

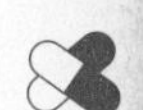

Like antipsychotic drugs, the major antidepressant medications were discovered accidentally. Four classes of antidepressants currently exist: tricyclic antidepressants (TCAs), monoamine oxidase inhibitors (MAOIs), selective serotonin reuptake inhibitors (SSRIs), and phenethylamine antidepressants. In the case of imipramine (Tofranil), the first of the tricyclic antidepressants, investigators were actually searching for effective antipsychotics similar to chlorpromazine. Iproniazid, a MAOI, was discovered when tuberculous clients regularly treated with a similar drug, isoniazid, became less depressed. The antidepressants have shed considerable light on the biochemical mechanisms of the brain in both normal and abnormal emotional expression.

Psychobiologic Considerations

Knowledge about the pharmacology of antidepressant medications has led to a theory of the biochemistry of depression. Basically, all the true antidepressants make the neurotransmitters norepinephrine (NE) and serotonin (5-HT) more available to the synaptic receptors in the central nervous system. Tricyclics block the reuptake of these substances into the neuron after their release, thereby postponing their degradation. MAOIs interfere with the enzymes responsible for the actual breakdown of the neurotransmitter molecules. Since both are antidepressants, these observations have led to the theory that NE and 5-HT shortages in the brain cause depression, at least the type of depression that responds to drug therapy. The Client/Family Teaching box on page 797 details a teaching plan to be used with clients undergoing the dexamethasone suppression test (DST), an examination of

Table 33–4 Antipsychotic Medication and Lithium Compatibility with Liquids and Other Drugs

Liquid	*Chlor-promazine*	*Fluphenazine*	*Haloperidol*	*Loxapine*	*Mesorid-azine*	*Thioridazine*	*Thiothixene*	*Trifluo-perazine*	*Lithium Citrate*
Water	C	C	C		C	C	C	C	C
Saline	C	C	X			C		C	C
Milk	C	C	X			X	C	C	C
Coffee	U	X	X	C		X	X	U	C
Tea	U	X	X			X	X	C	C
Apple juice/cider	X	X	C			X	X	X	X
Apricot juice	C	C				U	C	C	C
Cranberry juice	X			C	C	C	C		C
Grape juice	X		X		C	X		X	C
Grapefruit juice	C	C	X	C	C	C	C	C	C
Lemonade						C			C
Orange juice	C	C	C	C	C	C	C	C	C
Pineapple juice		C		C		X	C	C	C
Prune juice	U	C				X	C	C	C
Tang	X			C					C
Tomato juice	C	C	C			X	C	C	C
V-8	C	C				X	X	C	C
Cola	U	X	C	C		X	X	C	C
Ginger ale		C				C			
Mellow-Yellow		X				C		C	C
Orange soda	C	C				X		C	C
7-Up/Sprite	C	C		C		C		C	C
Soups/Pudding	C	C	C				C	C	C
Drug									
Chlorpromazine						X			X
Haloperidol									X
Lithium citrate	X	C	U	C	C	X	C	X	
Thioridazine	X	X	X	X	X		X		X
Trifluoperazine									X

C = compatible; X = incompatible; U = unconfirmed, conflicting data; blank = no data available.
SOURCE: Department of Pharmacy, Buffalo Psychiatric Center, Buffalo, New York, 1994.

CLIENT/FAMILY TEACHING

Medication Teaching Plan: Antipsychotics

Trade Name: ______________________________

Generic Name: ______________________________

Administration: Your medication is taken by mouth or injection.

Purpose: Your medication provides relief from your symptoms so you are able to participate in activities, use therapy more effectively, and take better care of yourself.

Target Symptoms: Your medication will decrease some symptoms you are having, such as: ______________________________

Report any sore throat, fever, increased fatigue, vomiting, diarrhea, skin rash, or unusual body movements to your nurse and doctor. If you are pregnant, or think you may be pregnant, discuss this with your doctor. Sudden stoppage of your medication may result in a return of symptoms or other side effects. Discuss any decision about stopping medications with your doctor.

Other special instructions (if any): ______________________________

The material, on both sides of this form, has been presented to me and discussed with me by: ______________

Client's Signature ______________________________ Date ______________

Air, Food, Fluid

Dry mouth

- Rinse mouth with water.
- Brush teeth more frequently.
- Chew sugarless candy/gum.
- Apply lip balm to your lips and nostrils.

Nasal stuffiness

- Avoid using OTC nasal sprays/drops.

Weight gain

- Eat less sugar, starch, and fats.
- Increase protein intake.
- Exercise daily.
- Follow a diet prescribed by your doctor.

Elimination

Difficulty urinating

- Drink 6–8 glasses of fluid each day.
- Notify your nurse and doctor.
- Do relaxation exercises to promote urination.
- Apply warm water to genital area.
- Take a lukewarm shower.
- Listen to running water.

Constipation

- Drink 6–8 glasses of fluid each day.
- Eat green vegetables and bran each day.
- Exercise daily.
- Eat prunes or raisins.
- Take laxative medication only with your doctor's advice.
- Notify your nurse and doctor.

Personal Hygiene and Body Temperature

Decrease of normal bacteria in mouth may result in infection

- Avoid foods high in sugar.
- Observe your tongue for signs of thick white coating.
- Increase mouth care, including brushing tongue and gargling with mouthwash.

Increased sensitivity to the heat and decreased sweating

- Shower in lukewarm water.
- Avoid exertion in hot weather.
- Dress appropriately for environmental conditions.

→

CLIENT/FAMILY TEACHING *(continued)*

Medication Teaching Plan: Antipsychotics (continued)

- Take own oral temperature.
- Avoid temperature extremes such as hot tubs.

Personal Hygiene and Body Temperature

Greater chance of a bad sunburn

- Use sunscreen and lip balm when out in the sun.
- Wear clothes that protect skin, including a hat.
- Wear sunglasses.

Vaginal dryness

- Use a lubricant such as K-Y jelly.

Menstrual period may stop

- Notify your nurse and doctor.
- Continue to use birth control.

General changes in interest in sex

- Notify your nurse and doctor.

Decreased moisture around eyes

- Use extra caution if you wear contact lenses to avoid eye irritation.

Rest/Activity

Dizziness

- Lie down and rest.
- Get up slowly from lying position; dangle legs over edge of bed.
- Have nurse check blood pressure.

Drowsiness

- Drive your car or other vehicles with extra care.
- Avoid alcoholic beverages or street drugs.
- Plan for extra rest time.
- Avoid other medications unless approved by your doctor.

Muscle tightness/cramping in arms, legs, neck, or face

- Notify your nurse and doctor.
- Take medications for side effects.

Compulsion to keep moving and inability to sit down; restlessness

- Notify your nurse and doctor.
- Take medication for side effects.

Blurred vision

- Use a magnifying glass for reading.

Eye pain in sunlight

- Wear sunglasses when outside.

Solitude/Socialization

Understanding of illness and medications

- Talk with your nurse and doctor to identify symptoms that are part of your illness or side effects from your medication.

Decreased interest in surroundings and usual activities

- Discuss this feeling with your nurse and doctor.

Source: Adapted from Langley Porter Psychiatric Institute Hospital and Clinics, 1984. University of California, San Francisco.

psychoendocrine function in light of depressive behavior. Chapter 15 provides an overview of the current psychobiologic theories of depression.

The initial distinction to be understood in the psychopharmacology of depression is between true antidepressants and stimulants or euphoriants. TCAs and MAOIs are not stimulants and will not induce euphoria in healthy people, but in a single dose, they have a sedative effect. Amphetamines and methylphenidate (Ritalin), on the other hand, are stimulants but not antidepressants in the pharmacologic sense. They can induce an increased sense of well-being in certain individuals, but do nothing to combat depression on a lasting basis.

MAOIs are the "first generation" of antidepressant medications. This means they were among the first medications identified as effective in the treatment of depression.

Bupropion, a second-generation antidepressant, is a nonsedating drug with few anticholinergic side effects and essentially no important cardiovascular effects and has not so far seemed to cause postural hypotension. Of note, however, is that this drug lowers the seizure threshold. This effect is dose-related. Nurses must keep this in

CLIENT/FAMILY TEACHING

Dexamethasone Suppression Test Information

For: ____________ Date: ____________

Therapists often order a test called the *dexamethasone suppression test (DST)*. The results of this test are useful to staff in making decisions about medications to control depressive symptoms. Some forms of depression are associated with a hormonal imbalance in the body that may respond favorably to certain antidepressant medications. Your therapist has ordered the DST for you. This sheet tells you what you can expect during the two-day period required to complete the test.

On the first day of the test, a technician will draw a small amount of your blood at 4:00 PM. The purpose of this test is to measure a hormone in your blood known as *cortisol*. On the evening of the first day at 11:30 PM, you will receive a very small dose (1 mg) of *dexamethasone*. The 1 mg of dexamethasone should not cause any side effects, but may cause a *decrease* in your blood level of cortisol. On the day after you receive the dexamethasone, your blood level of cortisol will be measured two separate times—once at 4:00 PM and again at 11:00 PM. The results of this test will be used, along with other information about you, by your therapist and the treatment team to plan your treatment with you.

If you have further questions about the DST or depression, ask your primary care nurse or primary therapist. Your primary therapist will let you know the results of your test.

1. *Cortisol test:* Blood drawn at 4:00 PM on (date) ____________
2. *Dexamethasone:* 1 mg at 11:30 PM on (date) ____________
3. *Cortisol test:* Blood drawn at 4:00 PM on (date) ____________
4. *Cortisol test:* Blood drawn at 11:00 PM on (date) ____________

This was explained to me by ____________

Source: Adapted from Langley Porter Psychiatric Institute and Clinics, 1985. University of California, San Francisco.

Table 33–5 Antidepressant Medications

First Generation	*Second Generation*	*Third Generation*	*Fourth Generation*
imipramine (Tofranil)	maprotiline (Ludiomil)	fluoxetine (Prozac)	venlafaxine (Effexor)
amitriptyline (Elavil)	amoxapine (Asendin)	sertraline (Zoloft)	
desipramine (Norpramin)	trazodone (Desyrel)	paroxetine (Paxil)	
nortriptyline (Aventyl)	bupropion (Wellbutrin)		
protriptyline (Vivactil)			

mind during assessment especially of clients with seizure disorders. Since these drugs appeared, two more generations of antidepressant medications have become available (see Table 33–5).

Nursing Responsibilities When Clients Receive Uncommon Drug Combinations

In the early 1980s, physicians began to prescribe combinations of antidepressants for clients who had received no relief from depressive symptoms with a single antidepressant medication. In a qualitative study of the biologic learning needs of practicing psychiatric nurses (Trygstad 1994), nurses said their practice often included giving several different psychiatric medications to the same client. Knowing the interactive effects of medications is an important feature of effective psychopharmacologic nursing.

As drug combinations and innovative psychobiologic therapies become more commonplace in the practice of psychiatry, psychiatric nurses must be observant for idiosyncratic responses among clients. Planning and implementing care for this specialized client subpopulation are likely to be challenging, and nurses need to be aware of the underlying psychobiology to recognize potential drug-related behaviors among clients who are on multiple drug regimens.

Clinical Considerations

The most important clinical consideration in the use of medications to treat depression is that antidepressant drugs are not effective in all cases of depressed mood. Evidence from research and clinical practice indicates that only a portion of depressive disorders respond to this category of drugs. For example, TCAs, MAOIs, and amphetamines are generally contraindicated in depression resulting from what commonly has been referred to as grief reaction or pathologic grief. Other types of depression, described in the *DSM-IV,* may be more amenable to psychopharmacologic intervention. Thus, accurate diagnosis is necessary to ensure maximum effectiveness.

Clients for whom antidepressants are indicated usually suffer from characteristic symptoms: a severely depressed mood, loss of interest, an inability to respond to normally pleasurable events or situations, a depression that is worse in the morning and lessens slightly as the day goes on, early morning awakening (and an inability to fall asleep again), marked psychomotor retardation or agitation, anorexia and weight loss, and excessive or inappropriate guilt. The *DSM-IV* calls this melancholia. In fact, the symptoms of melancholia are the features that most reliably predict response to drug therapy. A significant, and commonly overlooked, clinical consideration is that antidepressants have a delayed-reaction onset. A client will not show lessening of depressed mood until 2–3 weeks after the institution of an adequate dose of tricyclic antidepressants, for example.

Tricyclic Antidepressants (TCAs)

By far the most important and most commonly used class of antidepressant drugs is TCAs. These compounds are close in chemical structure to phenothiazines and have many similar side effects, but they have profoundly different effects on mood, behavior, and cognition. Tricyclic antidepressants are not antipsychotic agents when given to schizophrenic clients and may in fact aggravate a disintegrative pattern or precipitate overt symptoms in a client with latent disintegrative behavior. Imipramine (Tofranil) and amitriptyline (Elavil) are the two prime representative TCAs. Desipramine (Norpramin, Pertofrane), nortriptyline (Pamelor), and protriptyline (Vivactil) are compounds prepared in simpler forms (similar to the conversions made in normal metabolism) that are reported to reduce the incidence of side effects.

Dosage What constitutes an adequate dose of tricyclics is a matter of debate. Using imipramine and amitriptyline as examples, most clinicians agree that most of the responsive clients with a major depression need doses of 150–250 mg/day. Some clients with depression may respond to as little as 75 mg and some require 400 mg, but these are exceptional doses. Dosages of other tricyclics, such as nortriptyline (Pamelor) are not recommended above 150 mg/day.

A client is ordinarily started on 25 mg of imipramine or amitriptyline three times a day for 2 days, and the dosage is increased by 25–50% every other day, until 200 or 250 mg is reached or intolerable side effects are encountered. Common clinical practice is to use imipramine in the presence of motor retardation and amitriptyline with agitated clients because it has a more sedative effect. Once the client's dosage is established, it can be converted to a single bedtime dose. This practice frequently precludes the need for insomnia medication. The onset of action takes 7–10 days. Although full improvement may take 4 weeks, a gradual lessening of symptoms will be apparent in those who are going to respond.

After remission of the symptoms, clients who are put on a reduced maintenance dosage (perhaps 50% of the acute dosage) show less likelihood of relapse. Therefore, most clients are continued on treatment for 6 months to 1 year following a major depressive episode. Clients who have had repeated episodes may require longer drug maintenance or should be considered for lithium carbonate treatment because of its prophylactic effects on recurrent major depression and the depressive episodes of bipolar disorder.

Most depressive clients who do not respond to TCAs have a form of illness that is not of the melancholic type. These may include so-called neurotic or characterologic depressions, termed dysthymic disorder in the *DSM-IV.* Other clients do not reach or maintain effective blood levels of the drugs even when given adequate daily doses because of idiosyncrasies in their metabolic processes. However, tricyclic blood levels can be measured and doses increased until an effective blood level is obtained.

Side Effects Many of the common side effects of the tricyclic drugs are autonomic due to the anticholinergic characteristics of the medications. These side effects include dry mouth, blurred vision, constipation, palpitations, and urinary retention. Clients with glaucoma must be treated with caution. Some allergic skin reactions have been observed. TCAs also cause changes in the normal electrical conduction of the heart, which is particularly significant in treating clients with a history of cardiovascular disease, especially heart block. Sudden death has occurred during tricyclic treatment. Clients with known heart disease and most elderly clients require EKGs before, and periodically during, the course of tricyclic therapy. Several other CNS effects may occur, including tremor, twitching, paresthesias, ataxia, and convulsions.

Overdose Effects One aspect of TCA treatment that deserves attention is the consequences of an overdose. Significant overdoses may cause delirium; hyperthermia;

convulsions; and even coma, shock, and respiratory failure. A lethal dose of an antidepressant such as amitriptyline is estimated at between ten and thirty times the usual daily therapeutic dose. Drug intake deserves close attention, because many clients treated with these drugs are severely suicidal. Serious overdosing is a medical emergency and may require resuscitative measures. When the nurse reports delirium and peripheral autonomic symptoms of anticholinergic poisoning due to mild overdose, the psychiatrist can intervene with intravenous or intramuscular physostigmine (0.2 or 0.4 mg), an anticholinesterase that will reverse the delirium and other symptoms at least transiently.

Client Teaching The Client/Family Teaching box on page 800 outlines the main side effects of TCAs and self-care measures to counteract the side effects that are experienced by the client.

Monoamine Oxidase Inhibitors (MAOIs)

Clients who do not respond to tricyclic antidepressants may respond to the other major class, MAOIs. These drugs generally are not as effective as tricyclics and are somewhat slower to act, sometimes requiring a month of treatment before improvement shows. Isocarboxazid (Marplan) is considered the most effective, with phenelzine (Nardil) and tranylcypromine (Parnate) slightly behind. Complicating the decision to use MAOIs is their association with several very severe side effects. Hepatic necrosis, commonly fatal, and **hypertensive crisis** leading to intracranial bleeding are among the most threatening. The latter reaction, heralded by severe headache, stiff neck, nausea, vomiting, and sharply increased blood pressure, follows the ingestion of foods that contain the amino acid tyramine and of sympathomimetic medications.

Client Teaching The MAOI antidepressants require an especially strong, concerted teaching effort from nurses. These medications have many drawbacks that directly affect nursing intervention. For example, clients on MAOIs *must* avoid foods that contain even moderate amounts of tyramine; failure to do so will result in hypertensive crisis. The Client/Family Teaching box on page 802 outlines the low-tyramine diet and shows a teaching plan for clients taking MAOIs.

The principles guiding the use of MAOI and TCA medications are as follows:

- Drug treatment does not preclude psychotherapy, electroconvulsive therapy, or behavioral treatments if they are also indicated.
- Other antidepressant treatment should be given first unless there are contraindications, clinical indications for MAOI, or a past history of unresponsiveness to other antidepressants.
- The usual therapeutic range is 150–300 mg/day. Dosage may vary and may be limited by significant side effects.
- A response is seen 2–3 weeks after the therapeutic dose is reached.
- Clients with recurrent major depressive episodes with melancholia may require long-term maintenance treatment, although doses are usually lower than those needed in acute episodes.

Second-Generation Antidepressants

The second-generation antidepressants were the result of a scientific search for drugs with fewer toxic side effects and greater biologic predictability in the treatment of depression. They are believed to be more neurotransmitter–specific and better able to treat conditions related to dopamine, serotonin, or nonadrenergic dysfunctions. The following medications exemplify the second-generation drug classification:

- Trazodone (Desyrel): triazolopyridine derivative.
- Maprotiline (Ludiomil): tetracyclic.
- Amoxapine (Asendin): tricyclic dibenzoxazepine.

The side effects of these medications are generally less than those of the first-generation antidepressants. However, nurses must continue assessing clients for signs of anticholinergic activity, cardiovascular effects, and the inability to perform psychomotor tasks.

Third-Generation Antidepressants

There are disadvantages with first-generation and second-generation antidepressants. Uncomfortable and sometimes intolerable side effects, and a number of use restrictions with certain populations, combined with the dietary restrictions of the MAOIs, make these drugs for depression inappropriate for many people.

The third generation of antidepressant medications are the SSRIs. A profound difference with this group of drugs is their minimal side effects. While all chemically different, SSRIs inhibit the reuptake (and thus the deactivation) of the neurotransmitter serotonin, allowing for the increased availability of serotonin at synapses. You may have heard a great deal about the first third-generation antidepressant, fluoxetine (Prozac). It is a potent and highly specific reuptake blocker of serotonin, and the only other medication that had a similar action when fluoxetine was marketed was trazodone (Desyrel).

Side Effects Although the side effects of SSRIs are less severe than those of other antidepressants, some may be

CLIENT/FAMILY TEACHING

Medication Teaching Plan: TCAs

Trade Name: ______________________________

Generic Name: ______________________________

Administration: Your medication is taken by mouth.

Purpose: Your medication provides relief from your symptoms so you are able to participate in activities, use therapy more effectively, and take better care of yourself. Initially you may experience some sedation. The antidepressant effects occur in about 7–28 days.

Target Symptoms: Your medication will decrease some symptoms you are having, such as: ______________________________

____

Report any sore throat, fever, increased fatigue, vomiting, diarrhea, skin rash, or unusual body movements to your nurse and doctor. If you are pregnant, or think you may be pregnant, discuss this with your doctor. Sudden stoppage of your medication may result in a return of symptoms or other side effects. Discuss any decision about stopping medications with your doctor.

Other special instructions (if any): ______________________________

____

____

____

____

The material, on both sides of this form, has been presented to me and discussed with me by: ______________

Client's Signature ______________________________ Date ______________

Air, Food, Fluid

Dry mouth

- Rinse mouth with water.
- Brush teeth more frequently.
- Chew sugarless candy/gum.
- Apply lip balm to your lips and nostrils.

Nausea, vomiting, poor appetite

- Eat crackers, toast, drink tea.
- Drink protein supplement to maintain weight.

Weight gain

- Eat less sugar, starch, and fats.
- Increase protein intake.
- Exercise daily.
- Follow a diet prescribed by your doctor.

Elimination

Difficulty urinating

- Drink 6–8 glasses of fluid each day.
- Notify your nurse and doctor.
- Do relaxation exercises to promote urination.
- Apply warm water to genital area.
- Take a lukewarm shower.
- Listen to running water.

Constipation

- Drink 6–8 glasses of fluid each day.
- Eat green vegetables and bran each day.
- Exercise daily.
- Eat prunes or raisins.
- Take laxative medication only with your doctor's advice.
- Notify your nurse and doctor.

→

intolerable for certain clients. Activation, a more energized state including decreased sleep and akathisia, has been reported. Special care must be taken with clients who have hypomania or mania in their histories. SSRIs may precipitate a relapse.

An important consideration with clients taking SSRIs is the proximity of the administration of MAOIs. Fluoxetine and a MAOI together may cause serious and fatal interactions. The half-life of fluoxetine is such that there must be a 5-week gap between taking fluoxetine

CLIENT/FAMILY TEACHING *(continued)*

Personal Hygiene and Body Temperature

Decrease of normal bacteria in mouth may result in infection

- Avoid foods high in sugar.
- Observe your tongue for signs of thick white coating.
- Increase mouth care, including brushing tongue and gargling with mouthwash.

Increased sensitivity to the heat and decreased sweating

- Shower in lukewarm water.
- Avoid exertion in hot weather.
- Dress appropriately for environmental conditions.
- Take own oral temperature.
- Avoid temperature extremes such as hot tubs.

Greater chance of a bad sunburn

- Use sunscreen and lip balm when out in the sun.
- Wear clothes that protect skin, including a hat.
- Wear sunglasses.

Vaginal dryness

- Use a lubricant such as K-Y jelly.

Menstrual period may stop

- Notify your nurse and doctor.
- Continue to use birth control.

General changes in interest in sex

- Notify your nurse and doctor.

Decreased moisture around eyes

- Use extra caution if you wear contact lenses to avoid eye irritation.

Rest/Activity

Dizziness

- Lie down and rest.
- Get up slowly from lying position; dangle legs over edge of bed.
- Have nurse check blood pressure.

Drowsiness

- Drive your car or other vehicles with extra care.
- Avoid alcoholic beverages or street drugs.
- Plan for extra rest time.
- Avoid other medications unless approved by your doctor.

Muscle tightness/cramping in arms, legs, neck, or face

- Notify your nurse and doctor.
- Take medications for side effects.

Compulsion to keep moving and inability to sit down; restlessness

- Notify your nurse and doctor.
- Take medication for side effects.

Blurred vision

- Use a magnifying glass for reading.

Eye pain in sunlight

- Wear sunglasses when outside.

Solitude/Socialization

Understanding of illness and medications

- Talk with your nurse and doctor to identify symptoms that are part of your illness or side effects from your medication.

Decreased interest in surroundings and usual activities

- Discuss this feeling with your nurse and doctor.

Source: Adapted from Langley Porter Psychiatric Institute Hospital and Clinics, 1984. University of California, San Francisco.

and taking a MAOI, and vice versa. Sertraline (Zoloft) and paroxetine (Paxil) have shorter half-lives, and there must be a 2-week gap (both directions) with these medications and MAOIs. Table 33–6 on page 804 lists the common side effects of SSRIs.

Figure 33–4 on page 805 illustrates the process of serotonin neurotransmission, so important to the effectiveness of this new class of medications. Imagine the movement of the neurotransmitters back and forth across the synapse. This is the movement that SSRIs affect.

text continues on page 804

CLIENT/FAMILY TEACHING

Medication Teaching Plan: MAOIs

Trade Name: ______________________

Generic Name: ______________________

Administration: Your medication is taken by mouth.

Purpose: Your medication provides relief from your symptoms so you are able to participate in activities, use therapy more effectively, and take better care of yourself. It may take several days to a few weeks for you to feel less anxious, more optimistic, and more in control.

Target Symptoms: Your medication will decrease some symptoms you are having, such as: ______________________

Report the following symptoms to your doctor: rapid heartbeat, frequent headaches, yellowing of eyes or skin, severe increases or decreases in blood pressure. If you are pregnant or think you may become pregnant, report this to your doctor.

In general, tell any doctor who is prescribing medication for you that you are taking this medication and check over-the-counter medications with your therapist. If a severe, sudden, or unusual headache develops, it may be a symptom of a rise in blood pressure. Notify your doctor immediately.

Other special instructions (if any): ______________________

The material, on both sides of this form, has been presented to me and discussed with me by: ______________

Client's Signature ______________________ Date ____________

Air, Food, Fluid

Dry mouth

- Rinse mouth with water.
- Brush teeth more frequently.
- Chew sugarless candy/gum.
- Apply lip balm to your lips and nostrils.

Nausea, vomiting, poor appetite

- Eat crackers, toast, drink tea.
- Drink protein supplement to maintain weight.

Weight gain

- Eat less sugar, starch, and fats.
- Increase protein intake.
- Exercise daily.
- Avoid using OTC reducing pills.
- Follow a diet prescribed by your doctor.

Limitations on over-the-counter drug use

- Avoid cold/hay fever medications.
- Avoid weight-reducing medications.

Severe, sudden, or unusual headache due to increased blood pressure

- Follow attached diet to prevent problem.
- Report headache to your doctor immediately.

Limitations on certain foods

- Discuss diet limitations with nurse or doctor.
- Refer to the low-tyramine diet for foods to avoid.
- Determine substitute food choices.
- Continue food and drug limits for 10 days after stopping the medication.

Elimination

Constipation

- Drink 6–8 glasses of fluid each day.
- Eat green vegetables and bran every day.
- Exercise every day.
- Take laxative medications only with your doctor's advice.
- Notify your nurse and doctor.

CLIENT/FAMILY TEACHING *(continued)*

Personal Hygiene and Body Temperature

Flushing/sweating

- Take lukewarm showers.

Rest/Activity

Dizziness

- Lie down and rest.
- Get up slowly from lying position; dangle legs over edge of bed.
- Have nurse check blood pressure.

Drowsiness

- Drive your car or other vehicles with extra care.
- Avoid alcoholic beverages or street drugs.
- Plan for extra rest time.
- Take medication at bedtime.

Swelling in legs or feet

- Eat less salt, salty foods.
- Sit with feet raised.
- Practice careful skin care.

Solitude/Socialization

Confusion/poor memory

- Discuss this with your doctor or nurse.

Understanding of your illness and medication

- Talk with your nurse and doctor to identify symptoms that are part of your illness or side effects from your medication.

Low-Tyramine Diet

MAOIs combine with certain foods and medications to produce a significant increase in your blood pressure, which can be a health problem. In general, foods that can cause a reaction are ones that have been pickled, fermented, smoked, or aged. The list below includes the main foods and medications to avoid while you are taking this medication and for 2 weeks after discontinuing this medication.

Food and beverages to avoid completely:

Meats and fish:
- Pickled herring
- Dried fish
- Unrefrigerated fermented fish
- Caviar
- Fermented sausage (bologna, salami, pepperoni, summer sausage)

Sauce:
- Hoisin (fermented oyster sauce used in Oriental dishes)

Vegetables:
- English broad beans
- Chinese pea pods
- Fava beans

Dairy products:
- Most cheeses (exceptions listed below)
- Yogurt

Beverages:
- Chianti, aged red wines
- Imported, aged beers

Combination foods
- Pizza
- Lasagna
- Souffles
- Macaroni and cheese
- Quiche
- Pate (liver)
- Caesar salad
- Eggplant parmesan

Also:
- All yeast extracts (e.g., Marmite) and all yeast preparations (e.g., brewer's yeast)

Food and beverages to avoid taking in large amounts:

Dairy products:
- Processed American Cheese

Fruits:
- Raisins
- Prunes
- Bananas
- Avocados
- Plums
- Canned figs

Caffeine sources:
- Coffee
- Chocolate
- Colas

Beverages:
- Domestic jug red wines
- Domestic beers, ales, and stouts
- Sherry

CLIENT/FAMILY TEACHING *(continued)*

Medication Teaching Plan: MAOIs

(continued)

Food and beverages that may be taken without problems:

Dairy products:

Cottage cheese
Cream cheese
Milk, cream, and ice cream

Beverages:

White wines

Also:

Any baked goods raised with yeast

Medications to avoid:

Cold medications
Nasal decongestants (tablets, drops, or sprays)
Hay fever medications
Weight-reducing preparations, "pep pills"
Antiappetite medications
Asthma inhalants

Source: Adapted from Langley Porter Psychiatric Institute Hospital and Clinics, 1984. University of California, San Francisco.

Table 33–6 Side Effects of SSRIs

	Fluoxetine (Prozac)	*Sertraline (Zoloft)*	*Paroxetine (Paxil)*
Anticholinergic	0	1	1
Sedation	1–2	1–2	0–1
Activation	1–2	1–2	1–2
Hypotension	0	0	0
GI activation	1–2	1–2	1–2
Seizures	+	+	0
Compare this with a typical tricyclic antidepressant (amitriptyline [Elavil]):			
Anticholinergic	4		
Sedation	3		
Activation	0		
Hypotension	3		
GI activation	0		
Seizures	+		

0 = low; 4 = high; + = present

Phenethylamine Antidepressants

Venlafaxine (Effexor) is the newest antidepressant. It is the first in a new class of medications called phenethylamine antidepressants. It has two mechanisms of action: inhibiting the reuptake of both serotonin and norepinephrine. There is no affinity for muscarinic, histaminergic, or adrenergic receptors with this medication.

Side Effects Anticholinergiclike side effects may occur with venlafaxine. There are also reports of sustained increases in blood pressure with some clients. This last side effect seems to be dose-related, so nursing management of clients taking venlafaxine should include regular blood pressure monitoring. There is also a need for a time buffer regarding MAOIs: a 14-day gap after discontinuing a MAOI before starting venlafaxine, and at least a 7-day gap after discontinuing venlafaxine before starting a MAOI.

The side effects of this new medication include nervousness and anorexia. Medications, such as this one, that have an activation component can cause nervous feelings. Anorexia may be a difficult side effect for underweight individuals. Other reported side effects include:

- Nausea
- Somnolence
- Dry mouth
- Dizziness
- Constipation
- Nervousness
- Sweating
- Asthenia
- Abnormal ejaculation/orgasm
- Anorexia

Dosage The recommended starting dosage for venlafaxine is 75 mg/day, administered in divided doses and taken with food. The dose may be increased to 150 mg/day according to clinical needs, and even further increased to 225 mg/day (P&T 1994). It is recommended that clients who have been taking venlafaxine (Effexor) for more than 1 week taper the dose when discontinuing the medication. Clients taking it for 6 weeks or more should time this taper over a 2-week period to minimize the risk of symptoms caused by discontinuing the medication.

Because this is a new medication, long-term, widespread use has yet to give us the full spectrum of information about it. Studies have shown that it has response rates comparable to other antidepressants (Cunningham

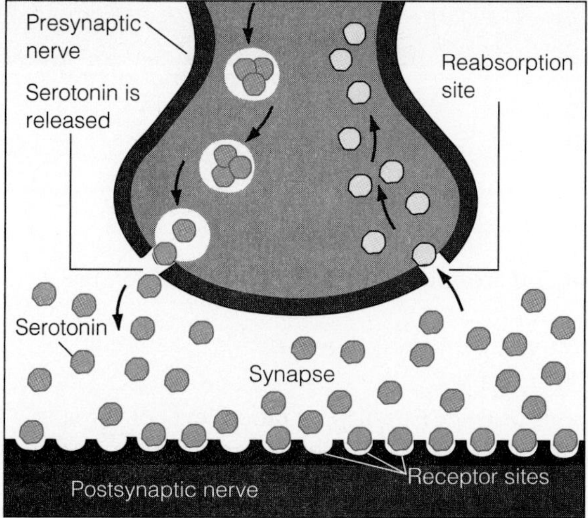

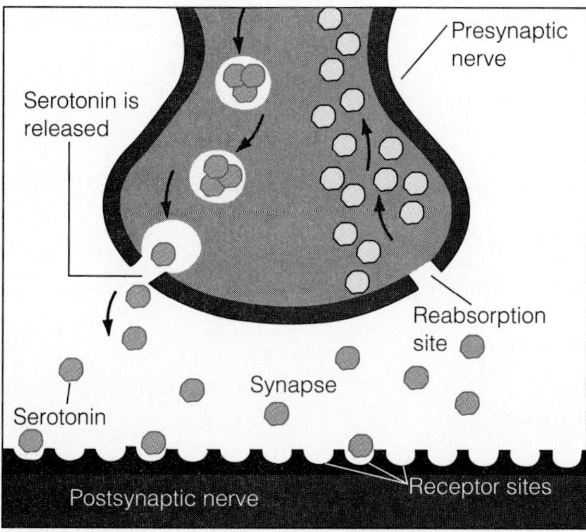

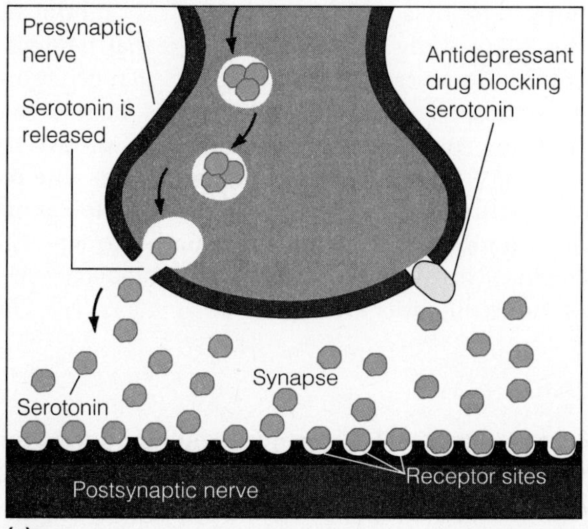

Figure 33–4 Serotonin neurotransmission. (a) A highly schematic model of normal serotonin (5-HT) neurotransmission. (b) In depression, there may be a shortage of 5-HT in the synapse. (c) The action of an antidepressant drug blocking 5-HT reabsorption (reuptake).

et al. 1994; Schweizer et al. 1991), and research continues. The new information we derive from these substances will be incorporated into our psychopharmacologic knowledge base.

Other Drugs

Stimulants, such as amphetamines and methylphenidate (Ritalin), and the phenothiazines are less commonly used antidepressants. Stimulants are not a proven treatment. Phenothiazines may be particularly useful in the presence of agitation. Some clinicians and researchers believe that major depressive episodes with psychotic features (delusional depressions) respond better to a combination of an antidepressant and an antipsychotic agent or to electroconvulsive therapy (ECT) than to antidepressants alone. Others simply recommend higher-than-usual doses of antidepressants.

Antimania Medications

The psychopharmacologic treatment of conditions collectively labeled mania has become virtually synonymous with lithium carbonate therapy in the United States. Many well-controlled clinical studies indicate unequivocally that lithium is the most effective agent for treating the vast majority of acute manic and hypomanic episodes. In addition, because of the absence of sedative side effects, the client feels much more related to the environment and able to function normally while under the influence of lithium.

In the last few years, several drugs have been added to the list of pharmacologic treatments for bipolar disorder. Of special interest is the use of carbamazepine (Tegretol) as a treatment to control bipolar symptoms in people who either cannot take lithium or do not respond therapeutically to it.

Recent reports address a psychobiologic phenomenon known as kindling, and relate this process to aberrant activity in the limbic system, often considered the emotional brain. Some psychobiologists believe that the characteristic behaviors of bipolar disorder are reflective of underlying limbic system dysfunction. Carbamazepine is chemically similar to the tricyclic imipramine, and it blocks the return of the neurotransmitter norepinephrine. Such action may be the psychobiologic reason that carbamazepine has the potential effect on behaviors of

CLIENT/FAMILY TEACHING

Medication Teaching Plan: Carbamazepine

Trade Name: ______________________________

Generic Name: ______________________________

Administration: Your medication is taken by mouth.

Purpose: Your medication provides relief from symptoms so that you are able to participate in activities, use therapy more effectively, and take better care of yourself.

Target Symptoms: Your medication will decrease some symptoms you are having, such as: ______________________________

____

Other special instructions: The following drugs may cause increases or decreases in your blood level of carbamazepine: troleandomycin (Tao), warfarin (Coumadin), erythromycin (Robimycin), phenytoin (Dilantin), isoniazid (INH), propoxyphene (Darvon, Wygesic, Unigesic), and nicotinic acid (Nicobid, Nicolar). Before taking any of these medications, be sure that the prescribing physician is aware that you are taking carbamazepine.

Do *not* stop taking this drug without the assistance or advice of your doctor. Carbamazepine is a medicine that must be slowly withdrawn.

If any of the following symptoms occur, report them immediately to your nurse or physician: fever, sore throat, mouth ulcers, easy bruising.

The material, on both sides of this form, has been presented to me and discussed with me by: ______________

Client's Signature ______________________________ Date ______________

Air, Food, Fluid

Dry mouth

- Rinse mouth with water.
- Brush teeth more frequently.
- Chew sugarless candy/gum.
- Apply lip balm to your lips and nostrils.

Nausea/vomiting, poor appetite

- Eat soda crackers, toast; drink tea.
- Notify your nurse or physician.

Elimination

Difficulty urinating or increase in frequency of urination

- Notify your nurse or doctor.

the bipolar spectrum. See the accompanying Client/Family Teaching box for a description of the use of this medication.

Recognizing the potential effectiveness of carbamazepine in certain mood disorders, other physicians prescribe another seizure medication, valproic acid amide, to treat clients with diagnoses of bipolar mood disorder or schizoaffective disorder. Valproic acid and verapamil, both calcium channel blockers, are also currently used to control affective symptoms. Possibly such innovative uses of various medications will yield valuable information concerning the underlying psychobiology of behavioral disturbances, especially affectively related conditions.

Antipsychotic medications are also an effective treatment for mania (Chou 1991), and the dosage is currently being studied (Rifkin et al. 1994). Haloperidol (Haldol) is reported to be effective; just as effective as lithium and superior to chlorpromazine, with a more rapid onset than lithium. Prophylactic benztropine was administered in the Rifkin study because of the EPS that haloperidol can cause. However, that study suggests that giving more than 10 mg/day of haloperidol offers no advantage in treating mania. Despite the advances in antipsychotic medications, lithium continues to be the first-line pharmacologic intervention for the treatment of bipolar mood disorder and, more recently, cyclic unipolar depressions or "rapid cycling," a condition in which bipolar cycles occur at unusually brief intervals.

Dosage

The management of an acute manic episode involves rapid initiation of lithium, increased to substantial doses during the first week of treatment. Usually 1500–2100 mg/day are needed by clients of average size during an

CLIENT/FAMILY TEACHING *(continued)*

- Drink 6–8 glasses of fluid each day.
- If you are having difficulty urinating, try the following:
- Apply warm water to genital area.
- Take a lukewarm shower.
- Listen to running water.

Diarrhea

- Maintain fluid intake.
- Notify your physician and nurse.

Personal Hygiene and Body Temperature

Possible inflammation of the tongue and lining of the mouth

- Notify your physician or nurse immediately.
- Use a soft bristle toothbrush.
- Rinse mouth frequently.
- Avoid foods that contain spices such as pepper, nutmeg, or vinegar.

Possible rash/itching skin

- Notify your nurse or doctor.
- Apply lotions to skin.
- Do not use soaps that dry the skin.

Rest/Activity

Dizziness

- Lie down and rest.
- Get up slowly from a lying position; dangle legs over edge of bed for 5 minutes before standing up.
- Have nurse check your blood pressure.

Drowsiness

- Drive car or other vehicles with extra care.
- Avoid alcoholic beverages or street drugs.
- Plan for extra rest time.

Blurred vision

- Notify your nurse or physician.
- Use a magnifying glass for reading.

Solitude/Socialization

Understanding your illness and medication

- Talk with your nurse or physician to identify symptoms that are part of your illness or side effects of your medication.

Source: Adapted from Langley Porter Psychiatric Institute Hospital and Clinics, 1984. University of California, San Francisco.

acute period. Lithium is available only in oral form in 250, 300, and 450 mg capsules and time-release tablets or as a liquid known as lithium citrate. Because lithium is an ion, its concentration can be measured in the blood. In the acute phase the blood level must usually attain a concentration of 1.0–1.5 mEq/L. After 1 week to 10 days, as the bipolar symptoms subside, the dosage of lithium can be decreased to 900–1200 mg/day, with the blood level maintained in the range of 0.6–1.2 mEq/L for continuing control of symptoms.

The basic principles for antimania drug therapy are as follows:

- Lithium is indicated and effective in the treatment of acute manic episodes and in the prevention of recurrent manic or depressive episodes, cyclic unipolar depression, or "rapid cycling."
- Lithium is usually given in divided doses with increases in daily dosage until the blood level reaches 1.0–1.5 mEq/L in acute phases of the disorder. Blood levels must be monitored after each increase.
- Antipsychotic medications may be necessary early in the course of treatment for behavioral control.
- Blood levels are checked every 2–3 months or when there is a behavioral reason to suspect a change.

Length of treatment with lithium for bipolar disorder is a debated issue. A recent study agrees with clinical prac tice that prophylactic use of lithium last at least 2 years (Goodwin 1994). If the client has no intention of taking the medication that long, there may be a premature recurrence of the mania from lithium withdrawal (Post, Leverich, and Altshuler 1992).

The following clinical example illustrates the appropriate use of lithium in the case of a client suffering from bipolar disorder.

CLIENT/FAMILY TEACHING

Medication Teaching Plan: Lithium Carbonate

Trade Name: ______________________________

Generic Name: ______________________________

Administration: This medication is taken by mouth.

Purpose: This medication should provide relief from symptoms so that you are able to participate in activities, use therapy more effectively, take better care of yourself and work more productively. It may take 1–3 weeks before improvement is felt.

Target Symptoms: This medication should decrease some symptoms you have, such as: ______________________________

____

Report the following symptoms to your physician or nurse: diarrhea, vomiting, chills, fever, infection, dizziness, slurred speech, weak muscles, unsteadiness when walking, twitching muscles, sleepiness and/or blurred vision. If you are pregnant, or think you may be, report this to your physician. Follow up with appointments for blood tests to check lithium levels. Do not discontinue taking this medication without the assistance and advice of your physician.

Other special instructions: ______________________________

____

____

The material, on both sides of this form, has been presented to me and discussed with me by: ______________

Client's Signature ______________________________ Date ______________

Air, Food, Fluid

Initial symptoms of nausea

- Take lithium with meals or with food in the stomach.
- Drink tea or broth and eat soda crackers.

Worsening of symptoms of nausea or vomiting

- Notify nurse and physician.
- Do not take your next dose of lithium until you speak with your nurse and physician.

Dry mouth

- Rinse mouth with water.
- Brush teeth more frequently.
- Chew sugarless candy/gum.
- Apply lip balm to lips and nostrils.

Need to maintain food/fluid intake

- Drink 6–8 glasses fluid each day.
- Eat usual foods including foods containing salt (ham, pickles, tomato juice).

Walt, a 23-year-old musician, came for treatment after losing his job in a Broadway show. His producer had fired him because he was irritable and argumentative and seemed to refuse to concentrate on his pieces during rehearsals, instead roaming around the stage giving unsolicited advice to others. His wife had called the mental health center in desperation, claiming that Walt was pacing the apartment talking out of his head, and that he seemed totally unconcerned about losing his job. The previous day he had been admitted and discharged against medical advice from a local hospital, where he had received chlorpromazine.

On observation, Walt exhibited pressured speech with grandiose ideas, an irritable mood, and an inability to sit in the chair in the interviewing room. His family history revealed that his father had lost many jobs and had been taking lithium for the past 5 years. Walt was told that he had bipolar disorder with a genetic basis, and he was started on lithium carbonate 300 mg BID. This was raised by 300 mg every third day, with a blood level sample drawn and tested after each increase, until Walt was on 1500 mg/day and showed a blood level of 1.3 mEq/L. Walt was asymptomatic 1 week later, without hospitalization, and returned to work.

Side Effects

Lithium has a significant number of side effects that can be troublesome and, in some cases, quite dangerous. Significant side effects are usually correlated with blood lev-

CLIENT/FAMILY TEACHING *(continued)*

- Do not diet unless specifically prescribed by your physician.

Elimination

Increased urination

- Drink 6–8 glasses of fluid each day.
- Notify nurse and/or physician.

Diarrhea

- Maintain fluid intake.
- Notify nurse and/or physician.

Personal Hygiene and Body Temperature

Skin breakdown due to swelling

- Elevate legs when swelling is present.
- Maintain good personal hygiene.

Sweating may affect the lithium level

- Avoid exposure to changes in temperature.
- Wear clothes appropriate to the temperature.
- Maintain fluid and salt intake.

Rest/Activity

Increased sweating due to exercise

- Wear clothes appropriate to the temperature.
- Maintain fluid and salt intake.
- Do not change exercise habits without discussion with nurse and physician.

Muscle weakness

- Operate your car and other vehicles with care.
- Plan for extra rest time.
- Do not use alcoholic beverages or street drugs.

Tremor/shakiness

- Notify nurse and/or physician.
- Lie down and rest.
- Get up slowly from lying position and dangle legs over edge of bed.

Solitude/Socialization

Understanding your illness and medication

- Talk with nurse and physician to separate symptoms that are part of your illness from side effects of medication.
- Learn the material presented in this Teaching Plan.
- Take medication correctly/as prescribed.
- Report response to medication accurately and promptly.

Source: Adapted from Langley Porter Psychiatric Institute Hospital and Clinics, 1984. University of California, San Francisco.

els of lithium above 1.5 mEq/L. Common side effects include tremor, nausea, thirst, and polyuria. Thyroid goiter has also been seen as a side effect. Severe lithium poisoning is a potential medical emergency. Early signs include vomiting and diarrhea, lethargy, and muscle twitching. These may progress to ataxia and slurred speech. The client may become semiconscious or comatose; seizures may occur; and electrolyte imbalances may lead to cardiac arrest. This syndrome of severe toxicity ordinarily occurs only when the client has a blood lithium level of 2–3 mEq/L. The client may have overdosed or severely restricted food or salt intake (or taken diuretics) to induce this state.

Occasionally very violent, agitated, or paranoid individuals with mania require phenothiazines or phenothiazine/benzodiazepine combinations at the beginning of their treatment. These can be started simultaneously with the lithium, raised to whatever level is required to control the disintegrative behavior, then gradually reduced, and eliminated after therapeutic lithium levels have been effective for about 1 week.

Client Teaching and Nursing Considerations

The accompanying Client/Family Teaching box outlines a teaching plan for the client receiving lithium therapy, and the previous box outlines an additional medication teaching plan for the client who is undergoing a trial of carbamazepine to control affective symptoms.

The Psychobiology of Lithium

Although the specifics of bipolar disorder are difficult to delineate, much can be said about the psychobiology of lithium. Lithium, not unlike the antidepressants, affects neurotransmitters, especially norepinephrine and serotonin. In short, lithium aids in the reduction of neurotransmitter release into the synapse and enhances its return, yielding a lower overall amount of the neurotransmitter in the synapse. Behaviorally, these biologic changes can be observed as an absence of mania or depression. What is unclear at this time is why lithium takes up to a few weeks to be fully effective, when the drug's effects can be observed on synaptic activity almost immediately. Also, why do some people with bipolar disorder *not* respond at all to lithium therapy? Many psychobiologists believe that lithium's effects are likely to be based on neurocellular changes that occur over weeks or months after a client begins lithium therapy. A similar explanation may hold true concerning the effectiveness of carbamazepine.

Anxiolytic Medications

Effects

The anxiolytic or antianxiety agents—sedatives and hypnotics—have very similar pharmacologic attributes. All can be used in small or moderate doses to relieve anxiety and in larger doses to induce sleep. Although they share the major clinical effect of tranquilization or **disinhibition** of fear-induced behavior, their side effects, including their addictive potentials and overdose sequelae, make certain representations of this category of medications more suitable for routine use and others better to reserve for limited, special circumstances.

Antianxiety medications are sometimes called "minor tranquilizers," but this is a misleading term. Their effects on anxiety are qualitatively, not quantitatively, different from those of the "major tranquilizers" or antipsychotic medications.

Drug Classification

MEPROBAMATE Meprobamate (Miltown, Equanil) was the first antianxiety agent to gain popularity in the 1960s. The result of controlled studies of the effects of meprobamate compared to placebos are generally favorable but not overwhelmingly convincing. This, and the addictive and fatal overdose potentials of the drugs, prompted investigators to develop more effective and safer medications that have all but made meprobamate obsolete.

BENZODIAZEPINES The major class of drugs today in the management of anxiety is the benzodiazepines. This group, represented by chlordiazepoxide (Librium), diazepam (Valium), and others, accounts for a very high percentage of all the psychoactive medications prescribed in the United States. This fact usually evokes a mixed response in professional circles. The easy distribution of drugs for such a ubiquitous human phenomenon as anxiety fosters the development of a pill-oriented and pill-dependent society, say critics. Sympathizers focus on the proved effectiveness of the drugs, which help people achieve higher levels of functioning, more pleasurable experiences, and even more productive psychotherapies in some instances.

NEW DRUGS In the last decade, anxiety-related research has expanded tremendously, and several new anxiolytic drugs have been introduced. The newer benzodiazepines give prescribers a wider range of therapies to target the often idiosyncratic manifestations of anxiety. Some of the new drugs have more rapid onsets and shorter half-lives (triazolam [Halcion], quazepam [Doral]), while others have a usual benzodiazepine onset time and an extended half-life (clonazepam).

With the psychobiologic knowledge explosion, a great variety of benzodiazepine drugs have been used in the treatment of a number of disorders. According to Hollister et al. (1993), benzodiazepines are used for many reasons:

- Anxiety disorders
- Sleep disorders
- Mood disorders
- Anxiety associated with medical illness
- Psychotic symptoms and disorders
- Convulsive disorders
- Involuntary movement disorders
- Spastic disorders and acute muscle spasms
- Intoxication and withdrawal from alcohol and other substances
- Preanesthesia
- Nausea and vomiting associated with chemotherapy
- Anxiolytic, sedative, and amnestic effects in a wide range of stressful diagnostic procedures

For a list of currently available benzodiazepines, see Table 33–7 on page 811.

New drugs and new uses for existing drugs are accompanied by new side effects and the need for new teaching plans developed by nurses for use in client education. The assessment skills of nurses must be finely tuned to detect unusual behaviors in relation to benzodiazepine therapy.

Use in Reducing Anxiety

There is no question that benzodiazepines offer a rapid, effective, and safe treatment for the emotional state commonly known as anxiety. In contrast to all other sedatives with proved effectiveness, benzodiazepines do not inter-

Table 33–7 Generic and Trade Names of Benzodiazepines

Generic Name	*Trade Names*
adinazolam	Deracyn
alprazolam	Xanax
bromazepam	Lexotan, Lexotanil, Lexomil
brotizolam	Lendormin
camazepam	Albego
chlordiazepoxide	Librium, Elenium
clobazam	Frisium
clonazepam	Klonopin
clorazepate	Tranxene
clotiazepam	Clozan, Trecalmo
cloxazolam	Enadel
diazepam	Valium
estazolam	ProSom, Nuctalm
ethyl loflazepate	Meilax, Victan
etizolam	Depas
flunitrazepam	Rohypnol
flurazepam	Dalmane, Dalmadorm
halazepam	Paxipam
ketazolam	Anxon, Unakalm
loprazolam	Dormonoct
lorazepam	Ativan
lormetazepam	Loramet
medazepam	Nobrium
midazolam	Versed, Dormicum
nitrazepam	Mogadon
oxazepam	Serax
oxazolam	Tranquit
pinazepam	Domar
prazepam	Centrax
quazepam	Doral, Oniria, Dormalin, Quazium
temazepam	Restoril
tetrazepam	Musaril, Myolastan
tofizopam (tofisopam)	Grandaxin, Seriel, Tavor
triazolam	Halcion

fere with or accelerate the metabolism of medications taken concurrently. Caffeine, however, interferes with the effectiveness of these drugs.

The effects are evident within the first days of treatment. These medications are absorbed much more rapidly and completely from the gastrointestinal tract than from intramuscular injection and are almost always administered orally. An exception is the use of intravenous diazepam to induce sleep before anesthesia or to manage status epilepticus. Peak levels of chlordiazepoxide are reached in the bloodstream 2–4 hours after oral ingestion, and peak levels of diazepam are reached in 1–2 hours.

The major side effects of benzodiazepines are related to their sedative qualities. Clients may complain of excessive drowsiness and must be cautioned against driving a car or operating other machinery.

Other drugs used to treat anxiety but generally less effective include the antihistamines diphenhydramine (Benadryl) and hydroxyzine (Vistaril, Atarax), the beta-blocker propranolol (Inderal), and methaqualone (Quaalude), a synthetic nonbarbiturate sedative. Methaqualone has been a much-abused drug, probably because of the intense euphoria associated with peak blood levels.

Another common use of benzodiazepines, especially Valium (diazepam) and Librium (chlordiazepoxide), is in the detoxification of individuals addicted to alcohol. Given adequate doses of benzodiazepines to induce sedation (usually starting at 30–40 mg/day of diazepam or 150–350 mg/day of chlordiazepoxide), alcoholic clients can be smoothly withdrawn by stepwise reductions in chlordiazepoxide dose over a 1- to 2-week period, without encountering alcohol withdrawal delirium or grand mal seizures.

Client Teaching and Nursing Considerations

Client teaching is an especially important element in the care of clients taking antianxiety medications. As most people know, anxiety is a generally uncomfortable experience. Self-medication often becomes the relief-seeking behavior used by many with severe anxiety. Such a psychopharmacologic approach is *temporarily* helpful in the restoration of a person's capacities and internal comfort. When the client is able and ready to learn, however, other means of anxiety control *must* be taught. Many of the anxiolytic drugs (especially benzodiazepines) carry a potential for dependence and tolerance. Therefore, nurses have a responsibility to help clients control anxiety in the most effective and safest way possible. The Client/Family Teaching box on page 812 outlines a teaching plan for clients receiving benzodiazepines.

The Psychobiology of Anxiolytic Medications

Antianxiety drugs probably work through a process of synaptic activity involving the neurotransmitter gamma-aminobutyric acid (GABA) in the brain and spinal cord.

CLIENT/FAMILY TEACHING

Medication Teaching Plan: Benzodiazepines

Trade Name: ______________________

Generic Name: ______________________

Administration: Your medication is taken by mouth.

Purpose: Your medication provides relief from symptoms of anxiety so you are able to participate in activities, use therapy more effectively, and take better care of yourself.

Target Symptoms: Your medication will decrease some symptoms you are having, such as: ______________________

Other special instructions: Do not stop taking this drug without the assistance and advice of your physician. ______________ is a medicine that must be slowly withdrawn. Drugs in this category are not intended for long-term use as physical and psychologic dependencies are possible.

Report the following symptoms to your therapist or primary care nurse: marked drowsiness, weakness, staggering gait, tremor, feeling of drunkenness.

The material, on both sides of this form, has been presented to me and discussed with me by: ______________

Client's Signature ______________________ Date ______________

Air, Food, Fluid

Food in your stomach will slow the absorption of this medicine.

- Do not take medication with meals.
- If stomach upset is present, drink tea and broth and take soda crackers.
- Notify your nurse or physician if other stomach problems arise.

Effectiveness of this drug is lessened with excessive intake of caffeine or heavy tobacco smoking.

- Drink decaffeinated beverages; avoid caffeinated colas, chocolate, or tea.
- Keep smoking to a minimum, if possible.

Alcohol increases the sedating effects of this drug.

- Alcohol intake is not permitted during your hospitalization on this unit.
- Do not use alcohol after discharge, if you continue with this medication.

Personal Hygiene and Body Temperature

Possible rash/itching skin

- Notify your nurse or physician.
- Apply lotions to skin.
- Do not use soap that dries skin.

Source: Adapted from Langley Porter Psychiatric Institute Hospital and Clinics, 1984. University of California, San Francisco.

Rest/Activity

Dizziness

- Lie down and rest.
- Get up slowly from lying position; dangle legs over edge of bed.
- Have your nurse check your blood pressure.
- Notify your physician or nurse.

Drowsiness

- Drive your car or other vehicles with extra care.
- Plan for extra rest time.
- Do not take other medications unless approved by your physician.

Blurred vision

- Notify your nurse or doctor.
- Use a magnifying glass for reading.

Solitude/Socialization

Unusual irritability or nervousness

- Notify your physician or nurse.
- Ask your nurse for assistance in selecting an appropriate relaxation exercise.

Understanding your illness and medications

- Talk with your nurse and physician to identify symptoms that are part of your illness or side effects from your medication.

Benzodiazepines most likely potentiate GABA, producing muscle relaxation. This mechanism involves a complex process of presynaptic and postsynaptic receptor activity. Recent research has yielded information about the presence of a postsynaptic receptor called the *benzodiazepine receptor.* As the term implies, benzodiazepines bind perfectly and with great specificity to these receptors, allowing for the sensation of relaxation.

Sedative-Hypnotic Medications

The pharmacologic management of insomnia presents an interesting and challenging clinical problem. Many of the truly hypnotic drugs tend to have undesirable effects, including physiologic addiction, fatal overdose potential, and dangerous interactions with other medications because of liver enzyme induction. The first principle of treatment is to assess whether the insomnia is related to one of the major mental disorders, such as schizophrenia or major depression. If so, the insomnia can and should be treated as part of the larger problem, and sedative antipsychotics or antidepressants may be given at bedtime for this purpose.

Benzodiazepines

In the management of simple insomnia without an associated major mental disorder, the benzodiazepine compound flurazepam (Dalmane), 15–30 mg at bedtime, is the drug of choice. This drug is as free of toxicity as others in its class and therefore is both effective and safe. It is the one sleeping medication that does not seem to interfere with REM sleep and therefore can be used on consecutive nights for about 1 month. Other benzodiazepine compounds that are used for their hypnotic qualities include triazolam (Halcion) and lorazepam (Ativan).

Barbiturates

Barbiturates are less commonly prescribed for their hypnotic effects. Their only advantage over benzodiazepines is their low cost. Barbiturates, especially the short-acting types, such as secobarbital, are powerfully addicting substances. They are frequently used in successful suicide attempts, since overdoses can cause severe CNS and respiratory depression. Barbiturates suppress REM sleep, leading to the phenomenon of REM deprivation and REM rebound—that is, after a week or two of treatment, they help induce the insomnia they were intended to control. Barbiturates also speed up the metabolism of anticoagulant and other drugs because they induce enzyme synthesis in the liver. This effect can be fatal. Long-acting barbiturates (phenobarbital) are very useful, however, in the detoxification of barbiturate addicts and the management of epilepsy.

The following groups of hypnotic preparations are commonly prescribed:

- Chloral derivatives (such as chloral hydrate)
- Piperidinediones (such as Doriden, Noludar)
- Alphatic alcohols (such as Placidyl)
- Antihistamines (such as Benadryl)

Client Teaching and Nursing Considerations

As with benzodiazepines, sedative-hypnotic preparations are generally intended for either occasional or short-term use. These medications are appropriate for clients newly admitted to a psychiatric inpatient unit or for clients in outpatient therapy who develop sleep disorders. As other medications (antidepressants, lithium, antipsychotics) start to yield a therapeutic effect, however, the need for sedative-hypnotic medication should almost, if not completely, abate.

Nurses working with clients in these situations need to help them regulate their sleep patterns. Here are some strategies to reinstitute regular sleep patterns:

- Avoid caffeine and nicotine.
- Exercise several hours before bedtime.
- Use relaxation techniques, including white noise.
- Avoid alcoholic beverages before bed.
- Take warm baths.
- Eat tryptophan-rich foods.
- Follow a regular routine of retiring and rising.
- Avoid bright light before sleep.

It is essential that the nurse teaching relaxation techniques assess the client's sleep patterns and presleep routines, to prescribe the correct technique to meet the client's needs. Ongoing evaluation of the effectiveness of the relaxation intervention allows for a change in approach if necessary.

Chapter Highlights

- Uniting the practice of psychiatric–mental health nursing with expertise in psychopharmacology requires integrating current data from the neurosciences, demonstrating knowledge of psychopharmacologic principles, and providing safe and effective clinical management of clients taking psychotropic medications.
- Psychotropic medications primarily affect the mind by exerting an effect on the cells of the CNS.
- Psychiatric nurses rarely have consistent complexes of symptoms on which to base clinical judgments

regarding the administration of psychotropic medications. In psychiatric work, nurses must often observe client behaviors closely because of the sometimes subtle nature of the presenting symptom.

- Psychiatric nurses may be especially challenged by certain cultural differences such as the client's cultural perspective, language and behavior subtleties and differences, biologic impacts of medications on culturally distinct groups, and ethnic differences in response to psychoactive medications.
- Educating clients about their medication is an important nursing responsibility.
- Medication compliance is often an issue for psychiatric clients. Client compliance can often be improved by providing the client with a teaching guide that discusses how to handle side effects and how to tell if the medication is effective.
- The major classes of psychotropic medications include antipsychotics (neuroleptics); antidepressants (TCAs, MAOIs); anxiolytics (benzodiazepines, etc.); antimania drugs (lithium, carbamazepine, valproic acid); and sedative-hypnotic medications (chloral derivatives, barbiturates, etc.).
- New psychotropic medications such as benzisoxazole, SSRIs, and phenethylamines are being developed and clinically applied.

References

American Hospital Formulary Service, American Society of Hospital Pharmacists, 1994.

American Nurses Association: *Psychiatric–Mental Health Nursing Psychopharmacology Project,* American Nurses Association Task Force on Psychopharmacology, Guidelines for Psychiatric–Mental Health Nurses. American Nursing Association, 1994.

American Psychiatric Association: *Diagnostic and Statistical Manual of Mental Disorders,* ed 4. American Psychiatric Association, 1994.

American Psychiatric Association: Tardive dyskinesia: A task force report of the American Psychiatric Association. American Psychiatric Association, 1992.

Ayd FJ: Risperidone (Risperdal): A unique antipsychotic. *International Drug Therapy Newsletter* 1994;29(2):5–12.

Beeber LS, Clement JA, Simmons-Alling S: Guiding principles in the clinical management of psychopharmacology. *Psychiatric–Mental Health Nursing Psychopharmacology Project,* American Nurses Association Task Force on Psychopharmacology. American Nursing Association, 1994.

Benjamin S, Munetz MR: CMHC practices related to tardive dyskinesia screening and informed consent for neuroleptic drugs. *Hosp Commun Psychiatr* 1994;45(4):343–346.

Buchwald D, Caralis PV, Gany F, et al.: Caring for patients in a multicultural society. *Patient Care* 1994;28(11):105–123.

Campinha-Bacote, J: *The Process of Cultural Competence.* Transcultural C.R.R.E. Associates Press, 1991.

Chou JCY: Recent advances in treatment of acute mania. *J Clin Psychopharmacology* 1991;11:3–21.

Chouinard G., Arnott W: Clinical review of Risperidone. *Canadian J Psychiatr* 1993;38(Supplement 3):S89–95.

Computerized Clinical Information System, Micromedex, 1994.

Conn VS: A staged-based approach to helping people change health behaviors. *Clin Nurse Specialist* 1994;8(4):187–193.

Cunningham LA, Diamond BI, Fischer DE, Hearst E: A comparison of venlafaxine, trazodone, and placebo in major depression. *J Clin Psychopharmacology* 1994;14(2):99–106.

Farrington A: Transcultural psychiatry, ethnic minorities and marginalization. *Brit J Nurs* 1993;2(16):805–809.

Gaebel W: The importance of non-biological factors in influencing the outcome of clinical trials. *Brit J Psychiatr* 1993;163(Suppl 22):45–50.

Goodwin GM: Recurrence of mania after lithium withdrawal. *Brit J Psychiatr* 1994;164:149–152.

Guze BH, Gitlin M: New antidepressants and the treatment of depression. *J Fam Prac* 1994;38(1):49–57.

Hollister LE, Muller-Oerlinghausen B, Rickels K, Shader RI: Clinical uses of benzodiazepines. *J Clin Psychopharmacology* 1993;13(6):1S–169S.

Jezewski MA: Acting as a culture broker for culturally diverse staff. Aspens Advisor for Nurse Executives 1993;8(10):6–8.

Jones BE, Gary BA: Problems in diagnosing schizophrenia and affective disorders among Blacks. *Hosp Commun Psychiatr,* 1986;37:61–65.

Krupp P, Barnes P: Leponex-associated granulocytopenia: A review of the situation. *Psychopharmacology* 1989;99: S118–S121.

Kudzma E: Drug response: All bodies are not created equal. *Amer J Nurs* 1992; 48–51.

Lefley H: Culture and chronic mental illness. *Hosp Commun Psychiatr* 1990;41(3):277–286.

Levy R: *Ethnic and Racial Differences in Response to Medication.* National Pharmaceutical Council, 1993.

Lin K, Poland RE, Nakasaki, G: *Psychopharmacology and Psychobiology of Ethnicity.* American Psychiatric Press, 1993.

Medical Letter on Drugs and Therapeutics, Vol. 35. 1993;(890): 16–18.

Medical Letter on Drugs and Therapeutics, Vol. 36. 1994;(924).

Middlemiss MA, Beeber LS: Issues in the use of depot neuroleptics. *J Psychosoc Nurs* 1989;27(6):36–37.

Miller DD, Perry PJ, Cadoret RJ, Andreasen NC: Clozapine's effect on negative symptoms in treat-refractory schizophrenics. *Comp Psychiatr* 1994;35(1):8–15.

Nursing94 Drug Handbook. Springhouse, 1994.

P&T: *Pharmacy & Therapeutics,* New Drugs/Drug News, Aug 1994:746.

Physician's Desk Reference, ed 48. Medical Economics Company, 1994.

Polk-Walker GC, Chan W, Meltzer AA, Goldapp G, Williams B: Psychiatric recidivism prediction factors. *Western J Nurs Res* 1993;15(2):163–176.

Pollow RL, Stoller EP, Forster LE, Daniho TS: Drug combinations and potential for risk of adverse drug reaction among community-dwelling elderly. *Nurs Res* 1994;43(1): 44–49.

Post RM, Leverich GS, Altshuler L: Lithium discontinuation-induced refractoriness: Preliminary observations. *Am J Psychiatr* 1992;149:1727–1729.

Reinke M, Wiesert K: Incidence of haloperidol decanoate injection site reactions (letter). *J Clin Psychiatr* 1992;53:415.

Rifkin A, Doddi S, Karajgi B, Borenstein M, Munne R: Dosage of haloperidol for mania. *Brit J Psychiatr* 1994;165: 113–116.

Safferman A, Lieberman JA, Kane JM, Szymanski S, Kinon B: Update on the clinical efficacy and side effects of clozapine. *Innovations and Res* 1992;1(3):3–14.

Guide to Psychotropic Medications

A psychiatric nurse's ability to recognize some common psychotropic drugs can be essential for client and family teaching about medications. This guide includes color reproductions of some commonly prescribed major psychotherapeutic drugs. While these photographs are accurate, remember that the appearance of psychotropic medications varies according to different dosages and manufacturers.

Antabuse disulfiram 250mg*	***Dalmane*** flurazepam HCl 30mg*	***Eskalith*** lithium carbonate 300mg	***Mellaril*** thioridazine 50mg*
Ativan iorazepam 1mg*	***Desyrel*** trazodone HCl 50 mg*	***Halcion*** triazolam 0.25mg*	***Methadone HCl Disket*** methadone HCl 40mg
Buspar buspirone HCl 5mg*	***Effexor*** venlafazine 50mg*	***Haldol*** haloperiodol 5mg*	***Nardil*** phenelzine sulfate 15mg*
Clozaril clozapine 100mg*	***Elavil*** amitriptyline HCl 50mg*	***Klonopin*** clonazepam 1mg*	***Navane*** thiothixene 10mg*
Compazine prochlorperazine 10mg*	***Endep*** amitriptyline 50mg*	***Librium*** chlordiazepoxide HCl 10mg*	***Nembutal*** pentobarbital sodium 50mg*

*Other dosages available; check directly with the manufacturer.

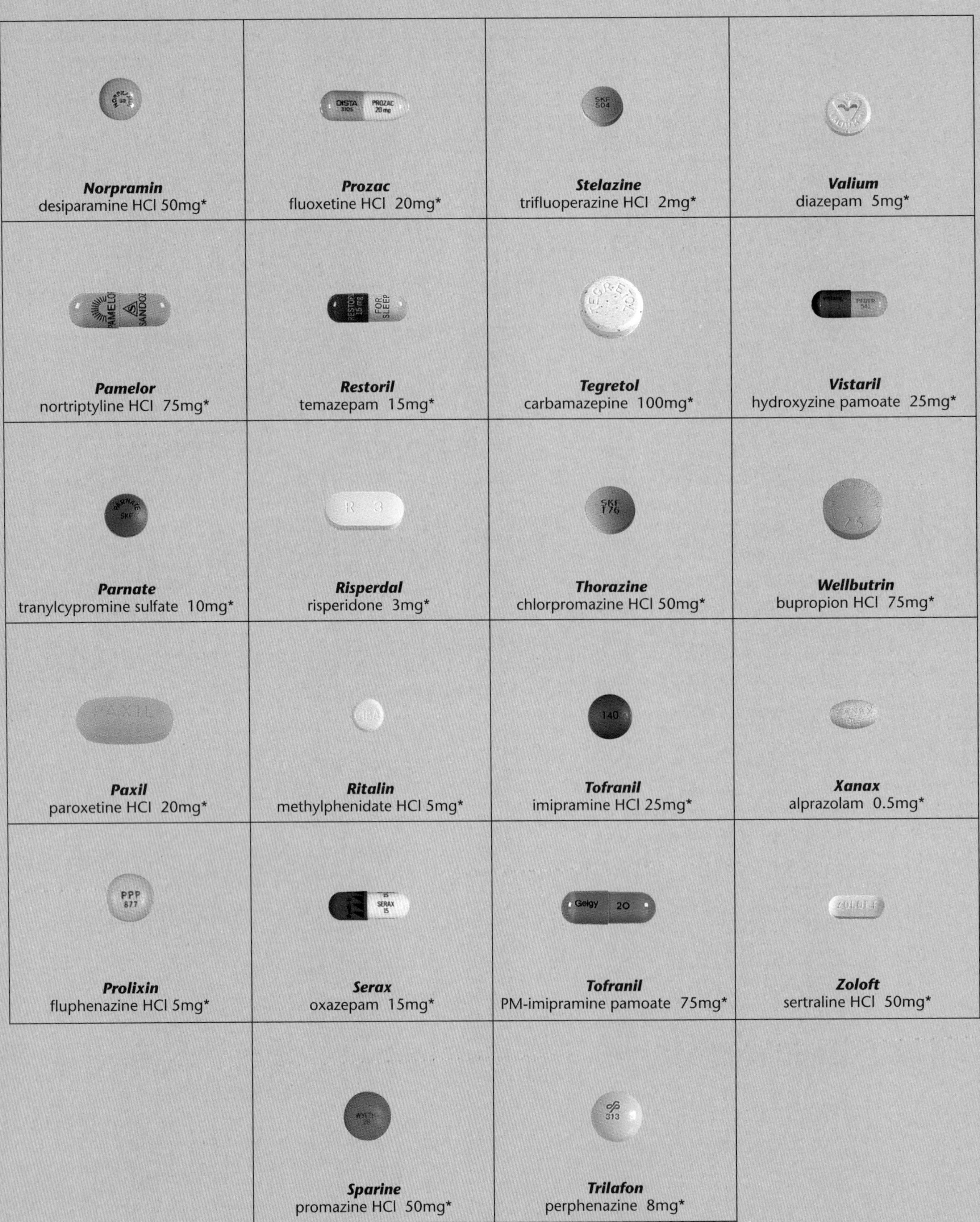

*Other dosages available; check directly with the manufacturer.

Schooler NR: Reducing dosage in maintenance treatment of schizophrenia: Review and prognosis. *Brit J Psychiatr* 1993;163(Suppl 22):45–50.

Schweizer E, Weise C, Clary C, Fox I, Rickels K: Placebo controlled trial of venlafaxine for the treatment of major depression. *J Clin Psychopharmacology* 1991;11:233–236.

Stinson SM, Kerr JC: *International Issues in Nursing Research.* The Charles Press, 1986.

Talley S, Brooke PS: Prescriptive authority for psychiatric clinical specialists: Framing the issues. *Arch Psychiatr Nurs* 1992;6(2):71–82.

Thornberg SA, Ereshefsky L: Neuroleptic Malignant Syndrome associated with clozapine monotherapy. *Pharmacotherapy* 1993;13(5):510–514.

Tierney MJ, Minarik PA, Tierney LM: Ethics in Japanese health care: A perspective for clinical nurse specialists. *Clin Nurse Specialist* 1994;8(5):235–240.

Trygstad LN: The need to know: Biological learning needs of practicing psychiatric nurses. *J Psychosoc Nurs* 1994;32(2): 13–18.

Worthington C: An examination of factors influencing the diagnosis and treatment of black patients in the mental health system. *Arch Psychiatr Nurs* 1992;6(3):195–204.

Zito, JM: *Psychotherapeutic Drug Manual,* ed 3, revised. Wiley, 1994.

CHAPTER 34

INTERVENING IN VIOLENCE IN THE PSYCHIATRIC SETTING

Anastasia Fisher

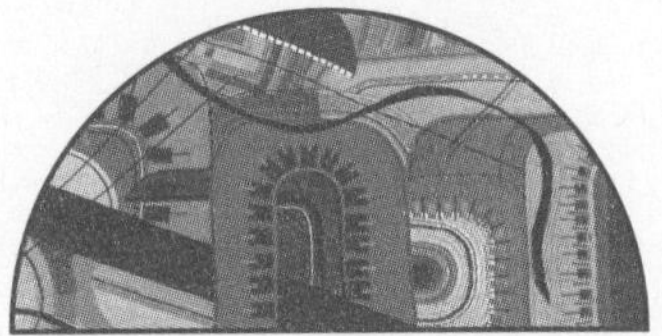

COMPETENCIES

- *Define psychiatric violence, aggression, and dangerousness.*
- *Define four theoretical perspectives useful in understanding violence.*
- *Identify and describe three strategies for managing violent behavior, including at least one verbal strategy.*
- *Explain two frequent staff responses to violent assault.*
- *Explain your concerns about working with clients who have a potential for violent behavior.*

Cross-References

Other topics relevant to this content are: Ethics, Chapter 10; Legal issues, Chapter 11; Milieu therapy, Chapter 9; Rape and abuse, Chapter 23; Suicide, Chapter 24; Psychopharmacology, Chapter 33.

Critical Thinking Challenge

Clients assessed to be dangerous to others can be involuntarily hospitalized, medicated against their will, secluded and restrained, confined for prolonged periods of time, and denied placement in community facilities at the time of discharge. The rationale for these decisions is protection of society, yet research suggests that predictions of dangerousness remain inaccurate. Do you think that danger to self or others is an appropriate basis for involuntary hospitalization? What other options, besides dangerousness, do you think might be considered? How might the treatment decisions noted here affect clients?

There is increasing recognition in society and nursing that violence is a significant public health problem, requiring attention by the community and the profession (American Academy of Nursing 1993; Campbell 1994; Morrison 1990). In the United States, the rates of homicide; physical and sexual abuse toward women, children, and the elderly; and the incidence of assault injuries in adults have reached monstrous proportions (Fulmer and Ashley 1989; U.S. Department of Health and Human Services 1989). Although it remains difficult to assess the actual incidence of violence by individuals with serious mental illness, there is disturbing evidence that violence is escalating within psychiatric hospitals (Adler, Kreeger, and Ziegler 1983; Davis 1991; Miller et al. 1993; Morrison 1990; Snyder 1994; Torrey 1994). The reasons for this escalation include hospital downsizing; the change in the skill level of staff members, which include increased numbers of paraprofessionals; and the severity of psychiatric symptoms among a small group of very aggressive clients. These trends, and the fact that nurses are the most frequent victims of psychiatric assault, magnify the need for psychiatric nurses to learn to accurately assess and intervene with their clients in order to maintain safety (Carmel and Hunter 1989).

This chapter introduces the concepts of violence, aggression, and dangerousness and explores a variety of theoretic perspectives useful in understanding psychiatric violence. It also identifies a number of management strategies that can be implemented by psychiatric–mental health nurses, and suggests several staff and institutional responses to violence.

John is a 25-year-old unemployed, homeless dishwasher who was brought to the psychiatric emergency room by the police because he has been unable to sleep, has not been eating or bathing regularly, and has been keeping other shelter residents awake at night by his loud praying. He spent yesterday hiding in the basement of the building where he resides, threatening to hurt the shelter manager when he approached to offer John his help. He was disheveled, muttering to himself, and screaming, "Don't touch me," to the emergency room staff as they attempted to talk to him. He was unable to answer the staff's questions, would not allow himself to be searched, and could not agree to control his behavior in the psychiatric emergency setting. He was restrained and medicated prior to being admitted to the inpatient psychiatric unit.

Christine, a 44-year-old woman, was admitted to the inpatient unit from the city jail. In the jail she had been loud and unable to sleep. In addition, she had exposed herself to the security staff and had physically assaulted another inmate. Christine was brought to the city jail after her arrest for striking a stranger when he refused to give her the spare change she demanded.

Harold, an 80-year-old retired jeweler, was admitted to the inpatient unit after striking a nursing assistant at the Ocean Breeze Rest Home, where he has resided for 10 years. On admission he is mute, not eating, wanders in and out of others' rooms, and is easily frustrated. He has started to strike out at the nursing staff when they attempt to assist him with routine self-care activities. The staff has requested a case conference to develop a new approach to his care.

Biopsychosocial Theories

The examples above depict the variety among clients who exhibit violent behavior prior to or during a psychiatric admission. It is generally acknowledged that violence is an interactive phenomenon; aspects of the environment, including space and the presence of others, affect individual behavior (Davis 1991; Whittington and Wykes 1994). Because of the diversity of individuals, situations, and interpersonal discourse, no single theoretic framework can sufficiently explain or predict violence. It is, therefore, more valuable to approach psychiatric violence from a variety of perspectives. For the purpose of this chapter, **psychiatric violence** is defined as behavior by a psychiatric inpatient that threatens or actually harms or injures others or destroys property (APA 1974). There is debate in the literature about whether violence and aggression represent the same phenomenon (Morrison 1992b) and evidence that the terms are often used interchangeably (Monahan 1984). Here, psychiatric violence is being distinguished from the concept of aggression, because customarily **aggression** refers to a broad range of behaviors, including conduct necessary for success and creativity, as well as destructive actions characterized, in the extreme, by actual violence (Sheard 1984). Another important distinction in this chapter is the difference between violence and assault. Assault is a legal (rather than clinical) term that applies to behavioral incidents in the following categories: simple assault, assault and battery, and aggravated assault. Each of these types of assault carries specific legal definitions and sanctions.

Biologic Perspective

Numerous studies have explored the biologic basis of aggression, using both animal models and human subjects. While it is likely that violence may be influenced by many biologic variables—genetic factors, hormonal factors, neurotransmitters, and neurophysiological factors—the relationship between these factors and violent behavior remains uncertain and the subject of ongoing research (Burrowes, Hales, and Arrington 1988; Garza-Trevino 1994; Krakowski and Czobor 1994).

Genetic Factors Many of the human studies on the genetic basis of aggression have focused on sex chromosome abnormalities. Studies in this area determined that men possessing the abnormal XYY chromosome were overrepresented in prisons and correctional facilities (Burrowes, Hales, and Arrington 1988). Research also revealed an association between this chromosomal configuration and high impulsivity, poor decision making, and low intelligence (Schiavi, Theilgaard, and Owen 1984). In his review of this research, Tardiff (1987) concludes that no specific genetic link to violence has yet been determined, and that rather than violence, these studies suggest a genetic link to economic property crime.

Hormonal Factors Violent behavior has been linked to abnormal plasma testosterone levels in males and to hormonal fluctuations in females. Although a number of studies have explored the link between testosterone levels and violence, their results have been contradictory, leaving the specific role of androgens in violent behavior elusive (Burrowes, Hales, and Arrington 1988; Tardiff 1987).

More recently, premenstrual syndrome (PMS) has become the focus of attention in determining criminal responsibility in cases involving violence (Dalton 1980). Although methodologic questions have plagued this research, Reid and Yen (1981), in their extensive review of the literature, conclude that there is a lack of evidence supporting the role of excess estrogen or progesterone deficiency in violent behavior. As with the genetic research, the evidence that androgens or PMS are factors in violence remains inconclusive.

Neurotransmitters The last decade has seen an increasing number of studies exploring the relationship between aggression and neurotransmitters, chemicals that transmit impulses between nerve cells (Garza-Trevino 1994). Early studies in this area implicated increased levels of norepinephrine (NE) and dopamine (DA) in aggressive behavior, but the more recent and promising work involves gamma-aminbutyric acid (GABA) and serotonin (5-HT), both of which have been associated with impulsivity and aggression (Burrowes, Hales, and Arrington 1988). Recent work exploring low levels of CSF-5HIAA, metabolite of serotonin, in highly violent, aggressive, and suicidal clients has yielded rather consistent results. Although some of the findings have suggested that low CSF-5HIAA levels may be more closely associated with irritability than overt aggression, researchers are optimistic about this line of inquiry in biologic psychiatry (Burrowes, Hales, and Arrington 1988; Tardiff 1987).

Neurophysiologic Factors Brain abnormalities due to lesions, trauma, or electrical malfunction may play a significant role in violent behavior (Burrowes, Hales, and Arrington 1988; Garza-Trevino 1994; Krakowski and Czobor 1994). Clients with temporal lobe epilepsy and those with complex-partial seizures have received particular attention from researchers. It is hypothesized that repetitive hypothalamic-limbic stimulation, such as is found in temporal lobe epilepsy, results in chronic changes in the threshold of excitability in this system, thereby contributing to aggression in these individuals (Burrowes, Hales, and Arrington 1988; Garza-Trevino 1994; Tardiff 1987). Some researchers suggest that individuals with epilepsy have other conditions present, such as reduced impulse control, that may have more to do with their violent behavior (Tardiff 1987). In addition to seizure disorders, intense rage reactions have also been associated with lesions in the orbital lobe, head trauma, and hemorrhage (Garza-Trevino 1994).

To date, these biologic markers are nonspecific in the way they contribute to violence. Tardiff (1987) suggests that rather than a direct relationship to violence, these mechanisms may predispose individuals toward violence by increasing their impulsivity, irritability, and irrationality in dealing with stressful situations.

Individual Perspective

This perspective reflects the idea that the client brings or imports certain values, attitudes, and behavior patterns conducive to violence into the treatment setting. Most of the literature on violence supports this perspective, identifying such client characteristics as sociocultural factors, psychiatric diagnosis, personality traits, and demographic characteristics.

Sociocultural Factors The sociocultural conditions often associated with violent behavior include:

- Low socioeconomic status.
- A history of childhood abuse.
- Life experiences from a subculture condoning or expecting the use of violence to resolve conflicts.
- A history of violent behavior.

Psychiatric Diagnosis Research findings on the role of psychiatric diagnosis in producing violent behavior are conflicting and unclear. Violent behavior has been observed across the entire spectrum of diagnoses, but violent clients are more likely to have a diagnosis of schizophrenia, personality disorder, dementia, delirium, or mental retardation (Lion, Snyder, and Merrill 1981; Tardiff and Sweillam 1980, 1982). Most current thinking suggests that the degree of psychopathology, or severity of the illness, is the more significant contributor to violent behavior, not the specific diagnostic classification.

Personality Traits A central psychodynamic theme repeatedly described in the literature is that violent clients perceive themselves to be hopeless and powerless (APA 1974; Lion, Snyder, and Merrill 1981). Violent clients are also three to four times more likely than nonviolent clients to have attempted suicide at least once (Tardiff 1983).

Demographic Characteristics Age and gender are the demographic characteristics typically included in research on psychiatric client violence. Young males tend to be overrepresented in the samples. Whether this reflects a subculture that condones violence or the frustration associated with a deprived status is not clear.

Of all the characteristics noted, the only one found to be predictive of future violence is a history of violent behavior. This generalization requires some modification because a past episode of violent behavior in the community appears to be the best predictor of future violence in the community, and a past event of violent behavior in the hospital setting is a good indicator of a future event in the same setting (Steadman 1981).

If one were to use the individual perspective to construct *a profile of a client most likely to exhibit violent behavior,* it might look like the following:

- He would be a young male (under age 44) from a subculture or minority group that condones the use of violence to resolve conflicts.
- He would be poor, have little formal education, and possess few employment skills and poor verbal communication skills.
- He would come from a home in which there was violence or parental deprivation.
- His parents would have had problems with alcoholism, and he would have experienced abuse as a child.
- He would have engaged in some expression of violent behavior in the recent past.
- His psychiatric diagnosis would be anything from psychiatric conditions such as schizophrenia or dementia or delirium to a severe personality disorder.
- He would exhibit severe psychopathology and impairment in function.
- He would see himself as helpless and powerless.
- He would have a history of at least one previous suicide attempt.

Factors Associated with Risk for Violence

These characteristics are associated with people at risk for violence:

- Early age of onset of psychiatric symptoms
- Presence of a psychotic disorder with severe psychopathology, including persecutory delusions and hallucinations
- Male gender
- Low socioeconomic status
- Limited formal education
- History of suicide attempts
- Previous history of violent behavior
- Feelings of hopelessness to change his situation
- Use of drugs and alcohol
- Past history of arrests
- Presents with hostility and suspiciousness
- Presents with agitation and excitement

The case of Mr G highlights some of these characteristics.

Mr G, a 40-year-old single Latino male, was brought to the acute psychiatric emergency unit by the police. They had received a call from Mr G's mother, who was terrified by her son's behavior. Mr G had been pounding on the door of his mother's home, screaming obscenities and wielding a knife.

Staff at the psychiatric emergency room recognized Mr G immediately; he has been hospitalized there over 100 times over the past several years. Mr G was first diagnosed with paranoid schizophrenia at age 18. Early in his illness he responded well to the supportive hospital environment and medications but did not follow up with day treatment, residential care, or medication when released from the inpatient hospital.

Mr G is tormented with delusions and hallucinations that frighten him and lead him to strike out at others in the belief that they are trying to hurt him. He has a history of assaults toward his mother and the nursing staff. Assaults on the staff occur early in his hospitalizations; once stabilized on medications he adapts well to the hospital environment. Mr G is often homeless and has been arrested numerous times for public disturbance and threatening to hurt other people. When his acute symptoms are under control with medications and supportive care, he reports feeling hopeless to change his situation and has attempted to commit suicide numerous times.

On admission to the psychiatric emergency room, Mr G is disheveled, unable to cooperate with the staff, and is screaming and flailing. The staff assess Mr G's risk for imminent violence to be high and administer Droperidol 10 mg IM and place him in a seclusion room where they hope he will rest and feel safer; Mr G has responded positively to these interventions in the past when he presented with similar symptoms.

See the accompanying box for an outline of the characteristics of people at risk for violence.

Knowing the numerous individual characteristics that are the basis of this perspective has not helped in predicting psychiatric client violence. Despite the popularity of the individual perspective, the characteristics identified are not descriptive of all clients who are violent, and not all clients fitting this profile exhibit violent behavior. The frameworks below address dimensions excluded by the individual perspective and explain the problem of violence in terms of the environment or the interpersonal process as components contributing to violence.

Environmental Perspective

The environmental perspective proposes that violence is a response to the unique, coercive, and regimented hospital environment in which the client feels devalued and dehumanized (Armstrong 1978). Research conducted in this area suggests that the environmental elements contributing to the violence process on inpatient psychiatric units include space and location, time of day, architectural design, staffing patterns, activity levels, and client population composition.

Space and Location Space and location factors include territoriality, privacy, overcrowding, and place of the incident (Depp 1983; Dietz and Rada 1983; Kinzel 1970). The concept of territoriality involves defending physical objects or the space a client has identified or "staked out" as personal space. For example, a client often "claims" a special chair on the unit, and a new client comes along and sits in it. The resulting conflicts over special territory also raise the issue of privacy.

Overcrowding Overcrowding is also related to the issue of privacy. Evidence suggests that assaultive clients have unusual and consistent difficulty tolerating people near them or touching them (Depp 1983; Kinzel 1970).

Place on the Unit Observation of the location or place on the unit where assaults take place can be instructive. For instance, one study of assaults on a forensic service revealed that most assaults occurred in the dining room during mealtime (Dietz and Rada 1983). In another study, the highest number of incidents occurred in the corridors or in clients' rooms, with fewer assaults occurring in the dining room (Quinsey and Varney 1977). The difference in results appeared to be related to institutional policy. In the first example, all clients except those in seclusion were required to go to the dining room for meals, while in the second instance, access to the dining room was obtained only after the client had demonstrated the ability to handle that social environment.

Time of Day The above examples indicate that the time of day may be closely linked to the location of violent incidents. Although the times of assaults vary across research studies, assaults appear to occur with greatest frequency at the times and places with the highest level of interaction among clients (Dietz and Rada 1983).

Architectural Design Another reported precondition for violence is architectural designs that create blind spots and opportunities for nonobservation. Research suggests, however, that rather than a lack of staff monitoring contributing to violence, fights between clients occur around scarce items that require sharing, often creating an atmosphere of competition (Depp 1983). Placement of the radio, telephone, piano, or washer and dryer in out-of-the-way places (to decrease noise on the unit) often contributes to incidents. Mirrors have been used effectively to cope with particular architectural design problems in psychiatric units. But how a unit and staff choose to handle scarce items is far more complex and is related not only to institutional policy and unit philosophy but also to individual clinical judgment. Many units monitor these items, by using sign-up procedures or by locking them up and distributing them at the discretion of the staff or a member of the client government. The significant issue is developing an awareness that location of these items often creates areas where violence occurs. Sometimes the simple installation of one additional client telephone or a minor structural alteration on a unit can significantly reduce the number of incidents.

Staffing Patterns The relationship between staffing patterns and violence is not well understood. The notion of optimal staffing, often cited as a prerequisite for achieving treatment objectives, is ambiguous and appears more complex than "more staff equals less violence." Whether a given hospital environment has sufficient staff to manage potentially violent clients depends on the amount of care required by the total client population at that period of time. Most units are prepared to deal with a certain amount of acting-out, disorganized, agitated, or violent behaviors, but beyond that, staff members may become overwhelmed.

Although a number of researchers have attempted to clarify the relationship between staffing patterns and violence, they report conflicting results. Some have found increased numbers of assaults on days with higher staffing levels (Depp 1983; Kalogerakis 1971). The researchers attribute this finding to activity level (see below) or the potential for physical coercion that occurs with an increased presence of staff authority. Other researchers exploring the problem of understaffing and its relationship to psychiatric violence have found that the presence of one or two staff members is associated with a significant decrease in violent episodes (Rogers, Ciula, and Cavanaugh 1980). In this case it is not clear whether staff passively provide an audience that inhibits violent behavior or whether staff actively model more acceptable role behaviors (Cobb 1984). In addition to confusion over optimum numbers of staff, there is controversy over the relationship between client violence and nursing staff gender. It has been suggested that female staff are less likely to provoke violence than male staff (Levy and Hartocollis 1976).

Because of the difficulty of comparing studies that represent differences in unit and staffing compositions, the relationship between staffing and violence remains unclear. It is likely that the staffing question will not be answered by studying such survey characteristics as number or gender of staff members, but by pursuing an understanding of the quality, content, and variations in staff to client interactions.

ACTIVITY LEVEL Activity level refers to the requirement that clients participate in therapeutic activities. As mentioned previously, peak times for violent incidents tend to be mealtimes and periods of concentrated treatment programming. In both situations, there is a high concentration of clients, and performance and participation are demanded. Ways of handling the problems suggested by activity level include scheduling, coordinating, and withdrawing. Scheduling staff breaks and mealtimes during client meals can create a situation of temporary understaffing on the unit. Whether this contributes to staff anxiety that is communicated to clients is not clear, but staggering mealtimes for clients and staff is a simple alternative and may prevent violent behavior. Coordinating client activities with the nursing staff schedule, although a tedious process, is an important consideration.

Staff who are expected to cajole or coerce clients into participation often create a situation in which the client feels trapped, and striking out becomes the only defense. Sometimes the most valuable intervention with any client—but particularly with one who is agitated, angry, and frightened—is temporary withdrawal. This allows the client quiet time free from the anxiety of interpersonal demands. Making frequent, short, individualized contact with the client is more reassuring and does more to de-escalate a situation than forcing the client to attend a community meeting or other activity where the client's behavior is likely to be the focal point of discussion. Individualizing the milieu activities of clients may be as important to advancing their treatment and preventing violence as the proper medication regimen.

CLIENT POPULATION COMPOSITION The last element in the environmental perspective is the composition of the client population, which involves the risks and benefits of segregating violent clients or establishing special units for them. This raises clinical as well as ethical issues. On the one hand, designating one unit for "assaultive clients," while creating a homogeneous treatment unit, may actually create an assaultive unit. On the other hand, admitting violent clients to all units contributes to an increased risk from assault for more vulnerable clients. Although the latter is by far the most popular and pragmatic approach, the danger of serious injury to other clients by unit violence is a concern in many hospitals.

It has been suggested that much of the violent and disruptive behavior within settings reflects the success with which the institutional environment conveys the message that clients are expected to act violently (Dietz and Rada 1983). This is particularly true in forensic services, but every treatment unit contributes to these messages, either implicitly or explicitly. Physical characteristics, such as the notice "High Assault Risk" on the door of the unit or the storage of leather restraints in plain view, alert clients as well as staff to potential problems.

While it is important to attend to issues such as space and location, time of day, and architectural design, their contribution to psychiatric violence is not well understood. However, the environmental perspective provides an additional framework from which to understand violence and generate assessment data. These data can then be used to plan individual interventions that take into account the environmental component of violent behavior. The major limitation of this perspective is that it fails to account for the vast majority of clients in these settings who do not engage in violent behavior. Like the individual perspective, this perspective fails to address the complexity of psychiatric violence. The framework discussed next emphasizes interpersonal interaction as a contributing element in psychiatric violence.

Interpersonal Perspective

Emphasizing the interpersonal process as the trigger or cue for violent assault, this perspective concentrates on client and staff interaction. The specific interactional processes identified as cues to violence between staff and clients tend to cluster around three elements: provocations, expectations, and conflicts. While the emphasis here is on client-staff violence, and these elements have been noted typically in relation to this specific interactional pattern, they may also be important in understanding client-client violence.

PROVOCATION It has been suggested that provocative styles of interaction contribute to violence (Morrison 1992a). These provocations include frustrating clients by not granting requests regarding hospitalization or medications and making clients do something they were unwilling to do, such as attend group activities.

Individual therapist behaviors that increase the likelihood of assault are irritability, a tendency to speak up when angry, and a tendency to fight when confronted with physically threatening situations (Ruben, Wolkon, and Yamamoto 1980). Although nurses may not know what part they play in the violent encounter, repetitive incidents of assault or threats of assault on the same nursing staff member may provide clues. A tendency to take a controlling, rigidly authoritarian, intolerant stance toward clients increases vulnerability to assault (Soloff 1983). Such attitudes are often communicated unwittingly through tone of voice, physical demeanor, or choice of language. Abusive language or actual assault on clients may provoke a violent defense. Provocations and abusive interactions increase a nurse's vulnerability to violent assault. Strategies for providing supervision and

RESEARCH NOTE

Citation

Whittington R, Wykes T: Violence in psychiatric hospitals: Are certain staff prone to being assaulted? *J Adv Nurs* 1994;19:219–225.

Study Problem/Purpose

This study explored the following questions: Were certain staff members in psychiatric hospitals more prone to being assaulted than others? Was their susceptibility to assault due to fixed personality attributes (age, gender)? Were staff and clients with certain attributes more likely to be involved in violent incidents?

Methods

The investigation was conducted on 13 units (general and specialty) of two psychiatric teaching hospitals in London. Subjects were nurses and clients present on the units during the 14-week study period. Sixty-five nurses who were assaulted during this period were compared with 136 others who were not assaulted during the 14 weeks. Twenty-two clients who committed violent assaults during the study period were also included in the sample. A comparison group of nonassaultive clients was not included. Data were collected on 100 consecutive violent incidents. Information about individual characteristics (age, height, weight, ethnicity) was collected on self-rating forms from nurses after being involved in an assaultive incident. The same information was obtained for the nonassaulted nurses from their personnel records and from clients via interview or from their medical records. In addition, as a measure of personality, assaulted nurses completed an Impulsivity Questionnaire.

Findings

There was significant variation between staff and clients in the frequency of involvement with assault. Clients had a higher rate of assault toward the staff than the staff had of being assaulted. No significant differences were found between the characteristics of the assaulted nurses and those who were not assaulted. However, charge and staff nurses were nearly twice as likely to be assaulted as nurses from other grades (enrolled nurses or nursing assistants). It was noteworthy that the most repeated assaults involved the same nurse-client pair.

Implications

The lack of difference in personality factors between assaulted and nonassaulted subjects, combined with the finding that those who were repeatedly assaulted were assaulted by the same client, suggests the possibility of a problematic relationship between two people rather than a problematic staff member. In addition, contextual conditions on the unit may have contributed to repeated assaults on staff and indicates an area for further research. The authors also note that the factors contributing to assaults on staff may be different from those contributing to assaults on clients and recommend that the two events be studied as separate phenomena.

staff support are discussed later in the chapter. At this point, it is important to suggest that some nurses may not be able to work successfully with certain types of clients at certain times. For an interesting study examining this issue, see the Research Note.

Nurses working with the violent need to monitor themselves and each other with regard to the following:

- Their ability to use anger constructively and not to take clients' anger personally.
- Their capacity for clear verbal communication.
- Their capacity for self-analysis.
- Their capacity to listen.
- Their capacity to both establish and maintain empathic linkages with clients, and to disengage.
- Their capacity to understand their fears and anxieties about violence.
- Their belief that violent clients are treatable.

Nurses with long-standing difficulties in these areas and the previously mentioned controlling interpersonal style may be more successful in other clinical settings.

In addition to the behavior styles and provocations that increase vulnerability to violence, two major staff expectations have been associated with increased psychiatric violence:

1. Expectations that clients will act violently.
2. Expectations that clients are hopeless and cannot be treated.

EXPECTATIONS Within the hospital setting, persistent expectations and fears of assault may set up a self-fulfilling prophecy (Levy and Hartocollis 1976; Straker et al. 1977; Whitman, Armao, and Dent 1976). Seeing the danger of being assaulted as part of the work hazard in psychiatric nursing and expecting to be assaulted at work are related but separate experiences (Duvall 1984). A greater need for staff vigilance in recognizing that they work with assaultive individuals is necessary, but this does not require that assaultive behavior be expected or acceptable. Clients may interpret such attitudes to mean that violence is not serious (Madden 1983).

Staff hopelessness about clients has also been associated with psychiatric violence. It is believed that communications by staff members supporting perceptions that clients are hopeless and powerless provide another interpersonal cue to violence (Depp 1983).

CONFLICTS It has long been suggested that conflicts between staff members can become the basis for acting-out behavior in clients. As a result of philosophic splits or competitive rivalries among staff, clients can be scapegoated into behaving violently to release tension on the unit (Straker et al. 1977).

In conjunction with provocations, expectations, and staff conflicts, it is important to consider the concept of timing; knowing when to engage in interaction is as crucial as knowing how to engage. Single episodes of provocation, assault expectations, or staff conflicts may have no adverse effects, but repeated interactions involving these dynamics may culminate in violence.

Assessment

Assessing psychiatric clients for their violence potential is an ongoing process and occurs throughout hospitalization or clinic visits. The prediction of who in a given setting poses a risk for violence, and the perception that someone is more likely to be violent, is known as **dangerousness.** An assessment that someone is dangerous determines fundamental decisions about the need for hospitalization, special supervision, emergency psychopharmacologic intervention, and community placement options. The prediction of danger is the result of an assessment. Learning to assess and predict is, therefore, essential for guiding treatment decisions.

Predictions of client danger have a long history in psychiatry but there is minimal research about how nurses in particular make these decisions, and little information about how these decisions are made on inpatient psychiatric units, along with continued problems with the accuracy of the predictions (Lidz, Mulvey, and Gardner 1993). Psychiatric nurses' definitions of danger are variable and idiosyncratic (Finnema, Dassen, and Halfens 1994; Fisher 1989).

Because of the inaccuracies associated with violence prediction, several authors (Fenn 1990; McNiel and Binder 1994) suggest that we begin to conceptualize the process as an assessment of the *risk* of violence rather than the *prediction* of violence. These authors believe that this position better reflects actual clinical practice which requires that practitioners gather available information to make an assessment of the risk for violence and intervene to reduce that level of risk.

Research on the association between demographic variables, psychiatric symptoms, and short-term risk for violence presents a mixed picture. Studies with community samples suggest that demographic variables (such as age and gender) are more important indicators of risk than clinical indicators (such as diagnosis and severity of symptoms). Studies of acutely disturbed patients evaluated just before or during hospitalization suggest that clinical variables are better predictors of risk for violence than demographic variables (McNiel and Binder 1991, 1994; Miller et al. 1993).

An increased risk for violence among acutely disturbed clients has been clearly associated with the following variables:

- Severity of psychopathology.
- Higher levels of hostility-suspiciousness, thinking disturbance, and agitation-excitement [as measured on the Brief Psychiatric Rating Scale (BPRS)].
- Length of time in the hospital.
- Early age of onset of psychiatric symptoms.
- Frequency of admission to psychiatric hospitals.

Hostility is used to describe the type of aggression that is oriented to do purposeful harm because of anger or provocation. **Suspiciousness** includes behaviors such as hypervigilance and hyperalertness to the environment. The box on the next page provides a profile of characteristics associated with short-term risk for violence among clients recently admitted to a psychiatric facility.

The four frameworks presented previously provide us with areas for assessment. It is important to remember that each person will bring unique characteristics to the culture of your clinical setting, thus making it impossible to provide a list of cues that will give you an accurate assessment of client danger. It is more important that you learn how to assess each client in the setting, to reason about each situation, and to make sound clinical decisions based on the frameworks presented.

History Taking

It is important to begin your assessment by taking comprehensive violence histories on admission. In taking the history, think of each acute violent episode as an event in

Short-Term Risk Factors for Violence

These characteristics are associated with short-term risk for violence among acutely ill clients recently admitted to a psychiatric facility.

- Psychiatric diagnosis (schizophrenia, mania, organic psychotic disorders)
- The presence of severe psychopathology and functional impairment
- High levels of hostile-suspiciousness, thinking disturbance, and agitation-excitement (as measured on the BPRS)
- Length of hospitalization (total time in the hospital)
- Early age of onset of psychiatric symptoms
- Frequency of admission to acute services

a life history, and establish a longitudinal picture of violence in and out of the hospital. The goal of history taking is to find patterns or trends in the violent behaviors, to understand the conditions under which an individual is likely to act violently.

Figure 34–1 is a comprehensive violence assessment tool addressing individual, environmental, and interpersonal factors to help you collect and organize data. Information from the assessment tool can be used to plan meaningful, individualized interventions for decreasing the incidence of violent behavior.

Clients and their families are important sources of information. Interview questions about the violent client's history should be open and direct, as if you were questioning a suicidal individual. Ask, "How much have you thought about violence?" "What have you done about it?" "What weapons are available to you, and what preparations have you made?" "How close have you come to being violent, and what is the most violent thing you have done?" (Monahan 1981). Do not, however, rely on client responses as the sole basis for your assessment. Review the client's history and past records. Consider the individual profile characteristics.

Use this assessment tool to gather data throughout the hospitalization or during multiple hospitalizations, adding data with each admission. Do not become discouraged if the data prove difficult to obtain. At this time, few practitioners use such a comprehensive framework when assessing for violence. Document your efforts to obtain this information, and communicate it to your colleagues.

Planning

After obtaining a comprehensive history and assessment data, planning treatment and setting goals with the client are the next steps. You can begin to address and minimize the coercive regimentation of the hospital environment by developing a sensitivity to the person's habits, strengths, and perceived needs. A treatment plan reflecting an awareness of the client's capacity and tolerance for participation in therapeutic activities, as well as specific "cues" to violent behavior, is the goal.

When planning the client's treatment, be cautious in using catharsis as a way of handling violent feelings. Encouraging clients to hit punching bags and pillows may actually increase emotions and lead to violent acts. Consult with the therapist involved in the client's treatment before recommending or initiating this technique. Teaching the client how to talk about violence and develop optional actions to the violent behavior is often a more useful intervention.

Approaches to Intervening and Managing Violence

A holistic approach to the assessment of violence is essential if the problem is to be adequately managed. This approach requires attention to the interactions of the participants (including the violent client), the environment, and the others involved (Monahan 1981). Capitalizing on this perspective, the inpatient management strategies presented here cluster around three considerations: the client, the unit, and the staff. These strategies emphasize negotiation, collaboration, and sensitivity to the multiple meanings each person brings to the situation. This emphasis on negotiation is important, since there is evidence that coercive and problematic interactions between nurses and clients contribute to violent behavior (Morrison 1992a; Whittington and Wykes 1994).

When considering these approaches to violent behavior, it is important to recognize the need for differential treatment of violent behavior in psychiatric inpatients, since different psychopathologic processes may be involved (Garza-Trevino 1994). In other words, there is much variation in the client population exhibiting violent behavior. This variation requires us to understand the meaning of violence on an individual basis, and to develop our approaches to management accordingly. Table 34–1 on page 827 outlines some of the psychiatric conditions associated with violence.

Client-Centered Strategies

Client-centered strategies are targeted to individuals who are currently violent or who require intervention to pre-

I. Clinical history

A. Diagnosis at discharge
Axis I: ______________
____
Axis II: ______________
____

B. Age: ________
C. Sex: __ M __ F
D. Admitting status
__ 72-HR hold __ Vol.
__ 14-DAY cert. __ Other
__ Temp conservatorship
E. Previous experience in seclusion/restraint
__Yes __ No
Reaction to seclusion/restraint
____
____
____

F. Age at onset: ____________________
G. Psychotropic medications:
__ Taking prior to admission
__ Not taking prior to admission

Medications:
____
____
____
____

Previous criminal history
__Yes __ No
____
____

I. Use of ETOH/street drugs
__Yes __ No
____
____
____

II. Violence history

A. Previous institutional violence __ Yes __ No

Type of institution: ________________ Date(s): ________ ________
Number of incidents: ________________ ________ ________

Type of violence:				
	Against person	__Yes	__No	Date ______________
	Family	__Yes	__No	Date ______________
	Stranger	__Yes	__No	Date ______________
	Inmate/client	__Yes	__No	Date ______________
	RN/LPT/MD	__Yes	__No	Date ______________
	Other	__Yes	__No	Date ______________
				Who ______________
	Weapon used	__Yes	__No	Date ______________
	Against property	__Yes	__No	Date ______________
	Type	______________		
	Verbal threat (only)	__Yes	__No	Date ______________
Situational factors:	Time of day	______________		
	Location	______________		
	Engaged in therapeutic activity	__Yes	__No	
	Type of activity	______________		

Other factors ______________________________
____
____

Interactional factors: Engaged in interaction with victim __Yes __ No
Type of interaction ______________________
____
With whom: ______________________
Content of conversation, request:
____
____

Figure 34–1 A violence assessment tool.

vent violence. They are also common in the long-term management of violent behavior. The overall goal of these strategies, whether considered individually or used in combination, is to strengthen clients' ability to control themselves. Implementation of client-centered management strategies must be considered within the context of the principle of least restrictiveness. This principle requires that staff demonstrate attempts to use less restrictive measures of control before resorting to more restrictive interventions. For example, *staff members must document their efforts to intervene with a client using verbal strategies before they intervene physically.*

Response to violence: Medications __Yes __No
Type and dose: ____________________

Seclusion only __Yes __No
Seclusion/restraint __Yes __No
Milieu management __Yes __No
Combination __Yes __No
(list) ____________________

Client's response to intervention(s): ____________________

B. Community violence
Previous violence: __ Yes __ No
Number of incidents:______ Date(s): ______ ______

Type of violence: Against person __ Yes __No Date ________
Family __ Yes __No Date ________
Stranger __ Yes __No Date ________
Inmate/client __ Yes __No Date ________
RN/LPT/MD __ Yes __No Date ________
Other __ Yes __No Date ________
Who ________
Weapon used __ Yes __No Date ________
Against property __ Yes __No Date ________
Type ____________________
Verbal threat (only) __ Yes __No Date ________
Situational factors: ETOH __ Yes __No Amount ________
Street drugs __ Yes __No
Type ____________________

Time of day ________ Activity ____________________

Location ________ ____________________
Other factors ____________________

Interactional factors: Engaged in interaction with victim __Yes __No
Type of interaction: ____________________

Others present: ____________________

Content of conversation, request, argument, or dispute: ____________________

Figure 34–1 *(continued)*

VERBAL INTERVENTIONS Forming a verbal alliance with the potentially violent client is often the first step to containing the violent behavior. Two common errors occur during the initial efforts to intervene with the potentially violent or violent client (Nigrosh 1983):

1. Confusion between strategies for control and perceived confrontation.
2. Overemphasis on supportive concern characterized by statements such as, "I know how you feel and I'm here to help."

Table 34–1 Psychiatric Conditions Associated with Violent Behavior

Condition	*Precipitant to Violence*	*Characteristics of Violence and Treatment*
Paranoid delusions	Violence precipitated from fear and misperception of the environment, usually in response to internal factors rather than external cues.	Violence is usually transient, occurring prior to or early in an admission. Treatment of the underlying psychiatric condition with antipsychotic medications and provision of a safe setting generally reduce risk for violence.
Neurologic impairment	Violence is the result of a neurologic disability and is stimulated by frustrating experiences.	Violence is often persistent and repetitive. Treatment includes structured behavior-modification programs and pharmacologic regimens.
Personality disorders	Violence reflects an inability to meet needs through more socially acceptable means.	Violence may be both impulsive and chronic. Treatment includes basic social skills training including cognitive, behavioral, and affective components, to give clients an increased repertoire of behaviors.
Drug and/or alcohol intoxication	Violence reflects reduced impulse control with accompanying cognitive impairment from substance intoxication.	Violent behavior is associated with intoxication. Treatment for the substance abuse is primary in managing the violence.

It is important to convey control in the situation by using clear, calm statements and a confident physical stance rather than through remarks or cues that can be interpreted as challenging the client. A confrontational, aggressive, or threatening manner or a tendency to overidentify with the client's experience can make the staff member a target of violence and actually precipitate violence.

Several strategies are suggested as guidelines for establishing quick rapport and alliance with the potentially violent client. Clinical judgment and the situation itself must dictate the appropriateness of their use. Some violent behavior occurs impulsively and without warning. Most episodes, however, involve an escalation of behavior and are therefore more appropriate for verbal intervention. Examples of verbal interventions and positional strategies for working with potentially violent clients are provided in the Intervention box on the following page. The overall goals are to establish a relationship that minimizes the client's projection on the caregiver, and to protect the client's already damaged self-esteem as much as possible, thereby decreasing the potential for violent behavior.

Sometimes verbal interventions are insufficient to contain the situation, particularly when the violent behavior occurs impulsively. In these instances, additional interventions—including medications, behavioral techniques, and seclusion and restraint—can be used with or instead of the verbal strategies.

PHARMACOLOGIC INTERVENTIONS At this time no medication has been approved by the Food and Drug Administration (FDA) for the treatment of violence (Corrigan, Yudofsky, and Silver 1993). Although daily use of neuroleptic medication is the most widely used treatment for the control of violent behavior in institutional settings, it is important to recognize that pharmacologic agents alone are not the answer to violence (Corrigan, Yudofsky, and Silver 1993). Whether these medications are being prescribed in response to the degree of psychotic symptomatology or in response to the violent behavior remains an issue for future research.

Choice of medication is often a function of the clinician's preference and medication history. Among those medications routinely used are haloperidol (Haldol), chlorpromazine (Thorazine), thioridazine (Mellaril), and thiothixene (Navane). Long-acting injectable fluphenazine (Prolixin) and haloperidol are used with clients discharged to the community to be followed as outpatients, as well as with clients who have histories of noncompliance. Dosages vary for each medication.

Current medication practice involves the combination of antianxiety and antipsychotic medications. The benzodiazepine lorazepam (Ativan) is commonly prescribed with one of the medications mentioned above. This combination reduces anxiety and permits the use of a lower dose of the neuroleptic, thereby reducing the potential of developing tardive dyskinesia (see Chapter 33). Other medications used in the treatment of clients who exhibit violent behavior include lithium, carbamazepine (Tegretol), and propranolol (Inderal). Younger clients with previously documented histories of violent behavior tend to receive higher doses of neuroleptic medications. See the box on page 829 concerning psychopharmocologic agents for treating chronically violent clients.

INTERVENTION

Verbal Interventions and Positional Strategies for Potentially Violent Clients

Technique	*Rationale*
Approach the client from the side, symbolically facing what the client faces. Do not stand face-to-face with a potentially violent person.	Decreases the tendency of the violent person to project and externalize the assault.
Leave plenty of space between yourself and the client.	Reduces anxiety and the opportunity for assault.
Speak slowly, directly, in a normal tone of voice, using simple statements like, "Mr. Jones, put the chair down," or "Mrs. Clark, let's sit down and talk about what's bothering you."	Reduces anxiety, communicates control, increases the client's self-esteem, and models negotiation. Encourage the client to sit down. If the client is pacing and can't sit down, pace with the client.
Center your statements on the issues concerning the client. For example, if the client states, "The nurse said I'm too sick to leave the hospital," a response such as, "You're upset at this big disappointment" will likely be more effective than "I can see how you must be upset by that."	Deflects attention away from the staff member who has become the target for the violent behavior.
When responding to the client's anger at not being allowed to leave, try saying, "I'm interested in understanding how terrible that is for you, Mr. Lewis."	Avoids challenging the client and expresses interest in the client's perspective.
Express clear expectations of control. For example, "I expect you can control yourself."	Communicates clarity and emphasizes the client's ability to control own behavior.
It is probably best to not touch clients when they are upset and posing an immediate danger.	Communicates respect for the client and maintains a comfortable distance, thereby reducing the client's sense of threat.
Acknowledge nonviolent behavior. When the client sits down to talk, try stating, "Thank you for sitting with me, I can listen better this way."	Focuses on the client's strength and maintains the client's self-esteem.

Behavioral Interventions Various behavioral strategies established around the principle of progressive isolation are often attempted before initiation of seclusion and restraint. The therapeutic intent is to reduce disruptive stimulation and provide the client with a contained, well-defined space for reassurance, protection, and defense. Depending on unit construction, the client can be encouraged to seek quiet refuge at the back of the unit or in a private room. Isolation can progress from the back of the unit, to the client's room, to open seclusion or a quiet room as indicated. These strategies are typically used in conjunction with the medications previously mentioned and to avoid the more aggressive and restrictive procedures of seclusion and restraint.

When efforts to contain the client's behavior using verbal techniques separately or in combination with the administration of medications and behavioral techniques do not prevent the violent behavior, or if an assault occurs without warning, staff must intervene to restrain the client and protect the therapeutic environment.

Seclusion and Restraint Seclusion and restraint are techniques used to contain violent clients who do not respond to less restrictive interventions. Using seclusion or restraint as punishment, divorced from the treatment interests of the client, cannot be justified and represents a serious mismatch between the needs of the client and those of the treatment setting (Soloff 1983).

Psychopharmacologic Agents for Treating Chronically Violent Persons

Antipsychotics

A range of antipsychotic agents are used in the management of violent persons with psychotic symptoms. These include the following drugs with approximate typical dosage:

- Navane (thiothixene): 10 mg IM or 20 mg concentrate
- Haldol (haloperidol): 5 mg IM or 10 mg concentrate
- Loxitane (loxapine): 10 mg IM or 25 mg concentrate
- Inapsine (droperidol): 5–10 mg IM

These are often given in combination with:

- Ativan (lorazepam): 2–4 mg IM

Anticonvulsants

These medications are used when the violence is thought to be related to organic brain disorders, partial seizure disorder, or excitement secondary to bipolar or schizoaffective disorder. The most frequently used agents and approximate typical dosages are:

- Tegretol (carbamazepine): 600–1200 mg per day (divided doses)
- Depakene (valproic acid): 750–3000 mg per day (divided doses)

Lithium

This medication is used when violence is related to irritability characteristic of manic excitement or a cyclic affective disorder. The approximate typical dosage follows:

- Lithium: 300 mg TID

Beta Blocker

Prescribed for patients with chronic or recurrent violence related to organic brain disease or injury; an approximate typical dosage follows:

- Inderal (propranolol): 200–800 mg per day in divided doses

Seclusion and restraint represent two of the most restrictive interventions available to psychiatric treatment staff. Their use in psychiatry has a long and controversial history (Strumpf and Tomes 1993), as these interventions have the potential to be abusive, to adversely affect clients' relationships with treatment teams, and to contribute to their negative view of the entire treatment process (Norris and Kennedy 1992; Stilling 1992). In addition, there is evidence that many staff injuries occur during the seclusion and restraint process, thus contributing to short-term and long-term trauma among staff members, loss of time at work, and increased financial burden on the institution.

Seclusion is a type of limit setting that provides security, containment, safety, and boundaries for a client (Baradell 1985). **Restraint** is the application of devices to contain and restrict clients who do not respond to seclusion. These interventions raise important moral-ethical questions about the use of behavior control techniques as treatment (see Chapter 10). Learning to apply these interventions and the rationale for their use are important psychiatric nursing responsibilities.

Facilities using seclusion and restraint as a means of controlling violent behavior generally require staff attendance at assault training programs. These programs teach hospital policies and procedures for dealing with assaultive clients, including legal and clinical documentation requirements, as well as appropriate physical contact skills for use with violent psychiatric inpatients. While all courses in contact skills emphasize the concept of team building, variations do exist. Some courses emphasize situation-specific skills, such as standard therapeutic holds and "release from hair pull," while others provide practice for more general strategies such as evasive techniques and deflection and neutralization of blows.* The most comprehensive programs provide analysis and opportunities to role-play interview situations, as well as other noncontact techniques, in addition to specific contact skills training. Evidence indicates an association between participation in staff training programs and not being assaulted. In other words, nursing personnel who participate in staff training workshops are less likely to be assaulted than staff who do not participate (Infantino and Musingo 1985). The following evasive self-defense guidelines are presented with a word of caution:

**L. Holpit, MSN, RNC, Director of Staff Development and Quality Improvement, Psychiatric Nursing Division, San Francisco General Hospital Medical Center, personal communication, July 14, 1994.*

Physical Intervention Techniques

Possible physical intervention techniques are presented below. Remember, don't try using these techniques unless you have been trained. As a student, you have lots of choices about who you work with in psychiatric settings. You can move away from clients who are beginning to lose control, attending to the other clients on the unit who will become anxious because of the impending violence. Yelling for help is an important and acceptable intervention.

Technique	*Description*
Back choke release	Quickly throw your hands in the air and pivot clockwise using a "windmill" movement.
Front choke release	Make a fist with both of your hands. Quickly and with force bring your clasped hands up and through the attacker's hands, "windmilling" (back and away) from the attacker.
Hair pull release	Do not pull away! Place your hands directly on the attacker's hands and push them against your head, or drift with the attacker. Keep your hands on those of your attacker.
Arm grab release	Make a fist out of the hand that's been grabbed, and roll your arm toward the attacker's thumb (the weakest point of the grab). Use your other hand to help.
Bite release	Push into the bite. Use the same principle as with the hair pull. Pushing into the bite, move the attacker's head back and upward, using your other hand as needed.

At no time should students or other untrained personnel intervene using these techniques, because they involve actual physical contact with clients, thereby increasing the risk of personal injury. One of the most widely used programs of verbal and physical intervention techniques for managing violence is the Physical Assault Training Program (PART). See the accompanying box for some of the frequently used physical contact techniques for defending yourself against chokes, hair pull, arm grab, and bites.

Whichever type of program is offered, it is desirable to provide monthly on-unit reviews for each shift. These reviews, emphasizing the team orientation, provide opportunities for practice, role modeling, and performance evaluation. In addition, it is important to integrate these physical contact skills into a larger training program that places the physical interventions into proper clinical perspective.

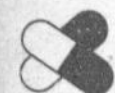

The decision to use medication, seclusion, or restraint to control violent behavior depends on an understanding of the individual client. For example, the use of repetitive doses of neuroleptic medication to control violent behavior in an organically impaired client may not be as desirable as using restraint or seclusion or a time-out as the interventions. On the other hand, emergency involuntary medication administration may be preferred to the use of seclusion and restraint in the case of a schizophrenic client whose violent behavior is a response to paranoid delusions.

Techniques of Seclusion and Restraint Psychiatric nurses have a major responsibility in the decision to isolate and restrain as well as in caring for the client while in seclusion and restraints. Once the decision has been made to seclude and restrain a potentially violent client, a "leader" is chosen from among the available staff. The leader is responsible for designating roles to be played by the remaining staff and for directing the steps in the seclusion and restraint procedure. Choice of the leader is important and can be based on various factors, including familiarity with the client. Remember that the goal is to gain maximum cooperation from the client and minimize violence. For example, one would not choose a large male staff member to confront a psychotic client in homosexual panic (Tardiff 1984a).

After a leader is chosen, a sufficient number of personnel must be gathered. This support staff should convey confidence and calm, reflecting a detached, professional approach to a familiar procedure. Staff members should avoid intimidating language and physical stances, since these behaviors may provoke the client's potential for violence. It is often sufficient to have the support staff gather around the leader the first time the client is approached. This **show of force** may be interaction enough, and the client may comply without further escalation. It is important for the client to perceive that sufficient strength is available to control his or her behavior. From the staff's perspective, the show of force provides confidence with minimal physical risk to staff, client, and the others who are present in the therapeutic environment (Tardiff 1984a).

One staff member is assigned responsibility for managing the unit environment and other clients. This person is responsible for supporting and calming the other clients, who may become anxious during the procedure. In addition, the area near the seclusion room must be cleared of clients or physical obstructions to minimize the potential of injury.

Once the unit environment is safe, the team approaches the potentially violent client. The leader offers a clear, brief statement of the purpose and rationale for seclusion or restraint. For example, the client is told that his or her behavior is out of control and that time in seclusion is required to help him or her regain control. The other team members position themselves around the client for easy access to the client's limbs. The leader then asks the client to walk into the seclusion room accompanied by staff. At this point, further discussion or negotiation should be avoided as it frequently aggravates the situation. The behavioral options given to the client must be kept simple, clear, and minimal. Time allowed for client cooperation must be brief, measured in seconds rather than minutes, in order to avoid an escalation of the behavior into an uncontrolled episode of violence (Tardiff 1984a).

If the client does not begin to walk toward the seclusion room, on cue from the leader, the team members positioned around the client move in to restrain the client physically. Using practiced techniques, the team brings the client to the ground and restrains each limb at the joint.

Once the client is safely controlled on the ground, additional staff may be needed to transport the client to the seclusion room where mechanical restraints can be applied. These clients can be carried in the recumbent position with arms pinned to sides, legs held at the knees, and head controlled. Other clients may be walked into the seclusion room with staff maintaining adequate control over both arms.

In the seclusion room, the client is positioned on the bed on his or her back. Street clothes are removed, and the client is placed in a hospital gown. Belts, shoes, jewelry, and glasses are usually removed to avoid self-injury. The client should be searched for items such as matches or lighters. In situations of high risk, elastic bras, shoe laces, and the like may also be removed. If the client is to be restrained, one limb at a time is secured in the restraint, while a staff member announces as each limb is secured and pressure released. The client's head should be secured until all staff members have withdrawn their holds, to reduce the chance of a staff member being bitten. Medications are frequently injected at this time. Once the client is safely restrained and medicated, the leader reassures the client that he or she will be carefully monitored and the staff will assess his or her capacity for control. Then the team can exit one at a time, with the final member moving backward out of the seclusion room door, which is then quickly locked.

The final step in the seclusion or restraint process is a rehash of the procedures and techniques used. A **rehash** is a group review, during which staff members can express their emotional reactions to the episode. The client community should also be given an opportunity in community meetings or other forums to ventilate their feelings and verbalize their concerns about the seclusion and restraint procedure. Clear therapeutic rationales for the use of seclusion or restraint should be openly discussed with the client community (Tardiff 1984a).

Care of the Client in Seclusion and Restraint Once a client is placed in seclusion or restraint, observations of the client's behavior are required every 15 minutes by nursing staff. These checks include a description of the client's behavior, as well as routine care activities, including meals, circulation checks, and toileting. When the client is quiet, these checks should be conducted by nursing staff entering the seclusion room and participating in a verbal exchange with the client. The nurse should document content of these dialogues, paying particular attention to a reduction in the client's symptoms, responsiveness to limits, capacity to discuss options, and increased capacity to tolerate frustration. Documentation of these behavioral checks and routine physical care activities are required and can be done in checklist format. A sample of a nursing care checklist is presented in Figure 34–2.

Release from Seclusion and Restraint Clients may be released from seclusion and restraint when the goals of the intervention have been accomplished—that is, when the client's behavior is under control and no longer poses a danger to self, others, or the environment. The decision to release from seclusion or wean from restraint and seclusion is based on an assessment of data gathered while the client is in seclusion. The ability of the client to control his or her behavior has been observed many times during the course of seclusion or restraint and is the basis for the decision to release. Each time nursing staff enter the seclusion room for the purpose of feeding, bathing, or toileting the client, responsiveness to verbal direction can be assessed. If a client has been secluded and not restrained, the first entries into the seclusion room should always be preceded by specific behavior requests. For example, the nurse should ask the client to sit on the bed before entering. The capacity of the client to follow simple directive statements is a first step in gathering assessment data for making a decision to release (Tardiff 1984a).

The release process follows a behavioral course that can be outlined in the nursing care plan. The initial step

Date ______ Time in ______

Renew R/S order at ______

Seclusion only ______

Type of restraint ______

Client I.D.

Level of search:
I. Clothing and belongings ______
II. In hospital gown ______
III. Body search ______

Time every 15 minutes	Check circulation q 15 min.	Fluids offered every hour	Exercise/limb massage q hour	Hygiene needs assessed q 2°	Need for elimination assessed q 2°	Observations (include client behavior, sleep, etc):	Staff Initials

CRITERIA FOR RELEASE MET

Time	Accepts limits	Tolerates frustration	Contracts	Other	Staff initials

Initials	Staff signatures/title	Initials	Staff signatures/title

Figure 34–2 A nursing care checklist for clients in seclusion or restraint.

Removal from Seclusion and Restraint

Weaning clients from seclusion and restraint follows a set of strict behavioral guidelines established in each clinical setting. The following represents some general principles.

Step 1
Starts with opening the seclusion room door for brief periods of time. During the open-door period, the client is expected to remain within the room and converse with staff across the open door. Deviation from this behavior can lead to closing the door and starting the weaning process again.

Step 2
Once clients have demonstrated cooperation with the open seclusion process, they can be transferred to their own room (preferably a single room in a quiet area on the unit). Since clients may benefit from spending varying periods of time in that room to titrate the stimulation from the unit environment, some consideration might be given to this negotiation.

Step 3
Release from restraints moves gradually. This is frequently achieved by moving clients from four-point restraint (two ankle, two wrist), to three-point (two ankle, one wrist), to two-point (opposite ankle and wrist). During this gradual release process, staff are continually assessing the client's capacity to follow directions, listen and comply with requests, make requests of, and converse with staff. These can include such activities as medications, hygiene and toileting needs, and meals. Inability to demonstrate control during these activities suggests that clients may be moving too quickly toward release and, as in the first step, the weaning of the restraints should not continue.

Step 4
It is important that the plan for the weaning process involve the entire team, including the client. Consultation should be obtained at any point in the process and particularly when there are questions, uncertainties, or unexpected behavioral manifestations.

may be opening the seclusion room door for brief periods of time and monitoring the client's tolerance. With the door open, the client is expected to remain in the room and converse with staff members across the open door. Deviation from stated staff expectations leads to a relocking of the door and a requirement to begin the process again. Once the client has demonstrated cooperation with medications, meals, hygiene care, and interaction with staff from an open seclusion setting, staff can consider a return to the client's room and the milieu.

The client in restraints should be released from restraints gradually. There are many different types of restraints, from cloth camisoles and posey vests to locked leather restraints. Locked leather restraints are frequently used in acute psychiatric facilities. These restraints are secured to the frame of a bed that is often bolted to the floor of the seclusion room. A restraint is applied to each limb of the client and locked. With this type of restraint it is possible to vary the placement based on an assessment of the client's need for external control. It is common when assessing the client's capacity for control to move gradually from a condition of four-point restraints (two ankle, two wrist), to three-point restraints (two ankle, one wrist), to two-point restraints (opposite ankle and wrist). This strategy allows the staff a margin of safety while providing the client gradual release. The accompanying box summarizes the principles to keep in mind. Once released from restraints, clients require the same assessment as indicated above for individuals in seclusion (McCoy and Garritson 1983; Soloff 1983; Tardiff 1984b).

Rehashing Violent Episodes If a violent act occurs on the unit, use a rehash format for witnesses to the violence, as well as with the individual client(s) involved if possible. In a rehash, a small, spontaneous group led by staff members discusses what happened, the outcome, and the feelings of the community members about the incident. The goal is to decrease anxiety, increase understanding about violence and its management, and reduce the potential for others in the client group to behave violently.

Reintegration If a client assaults another client or a member of the staff, it is important to gradually reintegrate that client with the assaulted individual and the milieu (Baradell 1985). If the client has been secluded after the incident, reintegration can begin after the client has regained control but before release from the seclusion room. Understanding the reasons for an assault is important, but it is early in the process of reintegration to begin that discussion. Instead, your attention might focus on helping the client perform specific tasks within a schedule for the shift, such as participating in meals, showering, and meeting with the treatment team (Baradell 1985). Successful completion of these tasks may be an indication that the client is ready to discuss the details of the assault. Failure to reintegrate the individuals involved in the violent act can result in lingering anxieties for them and the larger milieu.

Unit-Centered Strategies

The six strategies below provide nurses with additional management strategies and focus on the unit environment.

Unit Philosophy Nurses can help develop a unit philosophy of preventing violent behavior. No single professional discipline can assume responsibility for the prevention of violent behavior. It is important to articulate a unit philosophy that identifies shared responsibility among all disciplines for the maintenance of acceptable client behaviors.

Unit Policies Nurses can also help establish and regularly evaluate unit policies regarding the management of violent incidents. The policies should include client consequences for violent behavior and a careful delineation of areas of responsibility among the disciplines in the management of violence in the milieu.

Team Approach Staff members should develop a unit attitude of collaboration and negotiation and a team approach to prevention and violence management. Developing a consensus about the unit's position on violent behavior and its consequences decreases arguments and anxieties among staff and clients.

Although no one can be expected to prevent and manage violent behavior alone, nurses who have responsibility for milieu management must have the authority for decisions regarding violence management. This authority must be clearly articulated and supported by unit leaders and departmental administrators.

Record Keeping Comprehensive unit record keeping of violent incidents is important. In addition to the formal unusual occurrence reports with their administrative orientation, it is useful to collect clinical documentation on incidents, which provides a basis for structured clinical audits. Contents of the clinical documentation include identification of the who, what, where, when, and how of a violent act. These notations are behavioral rather than interpretive and serve multiple purposes, including:

- Increasing understanding of violence by looking for patterns among episodes.
- Teaching and clinical supervision.
- Establishing and revising policy.
- Conducting research.

Review Committee A unit-based committee could be established for a periodic review of incidents, policies, and mechanisms for handling client and staff issues about violent incidents. All the disciplines on the unit should be represented, with nursing as chair.

Unit Redesign Additional management strategies suggested by this approach include options such as structural enlargement of communal areas, or diversion of some clients to alternative unit areas at times of highest use (Dietz and Rada 1983). The frequency of dining room incidents might be reduced by staggering mealtimes, seating fewer clients at a table, or increasing selectivity over which clients go to the dining room. On units where assaults are highest in client rooms, consideration might be given to issues of negotiating ward census, structural changes providing a higher proportion of single rooms, and flexibility in moving clients to decrease density or establish a better match of roommates.

Staff-Centered Strategies

The following staff-centered strategies are suggested as the last element in the intervention and management of psychiatric inpatient violence. These strategies are compatible with and complementary to the client-centered and unit-centered strategies already discussed.

Supervision The department should provide ongoing clinical supervision with an expert in the management of inpatient violence.

In-Service Education Continuous in-service training on violence helps staff members:

- Understand ways in which they increase their vulnerability to assault.
- Develop provocation profiles of themselves to increase their sensitivity and awareness.
- Role-play conversations with violent clients.
- Practice teamwork for physical restraint procedures.
- Promote a safe, nonblaming environment to discuss their experiences of working with violent clients.
- Develop sensitivity to the effects their own experiences of violence have in their daily work.

These discussions are not a license to act in abusive or punishing ways toward clients or other staff members.

Research Nursing staff should encourage and participate in nursing research in the area of psychiatric violence and

NURSING SELF-AWARENESS

Working with Violent Clients

To increase self-awareness about your own ability to manage stress and effectively work with violent clients, ask yourself:

- How much stress am I under today?
- What is the source of my stress?
- Why am I letting things get to me?
- What can I do about my stress?
- Am I afraid of this client?
- Why am I afraid?
- Is my fear keeping me away from the client?
- How is my fear affecting the client?
- What else can I do with my fear and anxiety?
- Do I think this client should be here?

establish contact with doctoral programs in nursing, inviting interested researchers to discuss their studies and providing them access to the unit.

INCIDENT REVIEW Nurses can encourage and ritualize the use of reviews after each incident to understand, not blame, those involved in the episode. These sessions can focus on identifying precipitants to the violence, reinforcing the client's own control, and working together as a team. The overall goal of the review sessions is improved competence and confidence for the staff.

CRISIS INTERVENTION Staff victims of violence need a safe, supportive environment. When nursing staff are assaulted on the unit, establishing a "buddy system" with another nursing staff member may decrease the isolation and denial of the incident (Dawson, Johnston, and Kehiayan 1988; Lanza 1983, 1984, 1992). In addition, providing supportive crisis intervention for the staff may decrease the potential for retaliation and long-term negative consequences.

SELF-AWARENESS Although not all nurses can work with the violent mentally ill, most of us can be quite successful working with this client population. Since such work can be frightening and upsetting, it is important for each of us to take the time to reflect on ourselves and assess our reactions to others and events on the unit, in order to remain available and effective to our clients. Self-awareness requires that we think about the things that "push our buttons," the events that increase our stress and anxiety, and the things we can do for relief (see the accompanying Nursing Self-Awareness box). This is particularly important when working with violent clients, since our own stress and anxiety can greatly interfere with our ability to attend to their subtle cues and to initiate sensitive interventions in a timely manner.

Evaluating the Effectiveness of Interventions

There are many elements to consider in evaluating the effectiveness of strategies for violence management. Individual characteristics, biologic factors, conditions in the social environment, and the interpersonal styles of both clients and staff contribute to violent behavior. In spite of our theoretic understandings of violent behavior and efforts to implement management strategies to decrease the likelihood of its occurrence, we are not yet able to predict with certainty when someone will act in a violent manner. The fact is that violence occurs in our health care settings and that psychiatric nurses are victims of assault from psychiatric inpatients.

Staff and Institutional Reactions to Violence

The study of victims of violent assault, whether from psychiatric inpatients or other sources, is called **victimatology.** The literature on client-nurse violence is increasing (Lanza 1992). Research results suggest that:

- Nurses are frequent victims of inpatient assault.
- Assault rates are high and remain grossly underreported.
- Nurses have short-term and long-term biologic, social, psychologic, and cognitive reactions to the assault.

Staff Reactions

Lanza's classic 1983 study reported two interesting and contradictory findings:

1. Reactions of staff members who have been assaulted can last much longer than the time they are away from work.
2. Staff members often report having no reaction to the assault.

Research suggests that client-nurse assaults result in acute or immediate responses as well as long-term sequelae for the staff member (Carmel and Hunter 1989; Ryan and Poster 1989). In addition, denial of any reaction may be the most frequent immediate response to the assault, possibly due to fear of being overwhelmed by the event if it were acknowledged or of being blamed by colleagues.

Among the emotional reactions reported by staff who were assaulted are anger, anxiety, irritability, depression, shock, disbelief, apathy, self-blame, fear of returning to work and of other clients, disturbed sleep patterns, and other somatic symptoms, as well as a change in their relationships with coworkers and feelings of professional incompetence (Engel and Marsh 1986). In one study of psychiatric nurses, physical violence in the workplace was most frequently cited by the respondents as the reason for leaving the psychiatric nursing profession (Melick 1982). Whether these responses are typical of members from other disciplines or across different work settings is a subject for further research. It is apparent, even from the scarce information available, that for many nursing personnel, being assaulted on the job has serious personal and professional ramifications.

Institutional Implications

Violence in the context of the work environment has an impact on the setting. Although it is difficult to draw clear distinctions between the consequences for the individuals and the impact on the institution, there are several identifiable implications for the work setting. When either physical or emotional injuries occur, staff often lose time from work. The need to hire a temporary worker strains the budget. Morale is often lower among the remaining staff, who frequently share guilt and a sense of responsibility for the incident. Other staff members can feel afraid and vulnerable after an incident, and their effectiveness decreases as a result.

An incident of violence often leads to an overemphasis on control among staff members. This attitude of control takes precedence over treatment and sound clinical judgment. These measures and efforts to overcontrol can actually increase the staff's vulnerability to future assaults.

The staff may also limit their interactions with certain clients whom they perceive as likely to be violent. This withdrawal and avoidance, coupled with staff anxiety, can also increase their vulnerability to assaults.

INSTITUTIONAL SERVICES Staff victims of psychiatric assault require a variety of services, as well as emotional support from their unit leaders and coworkers. The employee health service or an employee assistance program can provide these services. Among these are opportunities for medical attention, supportive trauma-crisis counseling, legal advice, and information regarding insurance, workers' compensation, and rights to health and safety in the workplace (Engel and Marsh 1986; Lanza 1992). Because of the number of incidents occurring in health care settings, many institutions have developed a policy and procedure for filing assault charges against a client. While this remains controversial, and nursing personnel report ambivalent feelings about using this option, it is being used more frequently and is considered a major institutional support for the staff (Hoge and Gutheil 1987; Phelan, Mills, and Ryan 1985).

Much of our understanding of staff victims of psychiatric violence is speculative. Recognizing that staff assaults occur and assuming a multidimensional response approach are important first steps. As research studies increase our knowledge about the phenomenon of staff victims, their needs, and the impact on the institutional setting, interventions to help them recover are evolving and are being used (Lanza 1992).

Chapter Highlights

- Violence is a complex human behavior with biologic, individual, environmental, and interpersonal components.
- A theoretic understanding of violence helps staff design management strategies.
- Nurses are frequent targets of inpatient psychiatric violence.
- Comprehensive assessment and treatment planning can decrease the likelihood of violent behavior among psychiatric inpatients.
- Psychiatric nurses are in a key position to contribute a unique perspective on psychiatric violence.
- Not all violence is committed by psychiatric clients, and not all psychiatric clients are violent.

References

Adler W, Kreeger C, Ziegler P: Patient violence in a private psychiatric hospital, in Lion JR, Reid WH (eds): *Assaults Within Psychiatric Facilities.* Grune & Stratton, 1983.

American Academy of Nursing: Violence as a nursing priority: Policy implications. *Nurs Outlook* 1993;2:83–92.

American Psychiatric Association: *Clinical Aspects of the Violent Individual.* Task Force Report No. 8. U.S. Government Printing Office, 1974.

Armstrong B: Conference report: Handling the violent patient in the hospital. *Hosp Commun Psychiatr* 1978;140: 301–304.

Baradell JG: Humanistic care of the patient in seclusion. *J Psychosoc Nurs* 1985;23(2):9–14.

Burrowes KL, Hales ER, Arrington E: Research on the biologic aspects of violence. *Psychiatr Clin N Am* 1988;11(4): 499–509.

Campbell J: Putting violence in context. *Hosp Commun Psychiatr* 1994;45(7):633.

Carmel H, Hunter M: Staff injuries from inpatient violence. *Hosp Commun Psychiatr* 1989;40:41–46.

Cobb BA: *A Descriptive Correlational Study Exploring the Relationship Between Adult Psychiatric Patient Role Strain and Violence in an Inpatient Setting,* thesis. University of California, San Francisco, 1984.

Corrigan PW, Yudofsky SC, Silver, JM: Pharmacological and behavioral treatments for aggressive psychiatric inpatients. *Hosp Commun Psychiatr* 1993;44(2):125–133.

Dalton K: Cyclical criminal acts in premenstrual syndrome. *Lancet* 1980;2:1070–1071.

Davis S: Violence by psychiatric inpatients: A review. *Hosp Commun Psychiatr* 1991;42(6):585–590.

Dawson J, Johnston M, Kehiayan N: Responses to patient assault: A peer support program for nurses. *J Psychosoc Nurs* 1988;26(2):8–15.

Depp FC: Assaults in a public mental hospital, in Lion JR, Reid WH (eds): *Assaults Within Psychiatric Facilities*. Grune & Stratton, 1983.

Dietz PE, Rada RT: Interpersonal violence in forensic facilities, in Lion JR, Reid WH (eds): *Assaults Within Psychiatric Facilities*. Grune & Stratton, 1983.

Duvall J: Violence is hazard for psych nurses. *Am Nurse* (June) 1984:4.

Engel F, Marsh S: Helping the employee victim of violence in hospitals. *Hosp Commun Psychiatr* 1986;37:159–162.

Fenn, H: Violence: Probability versus prediction. *Hosp Commun Psychiatr* 1990;41(2):117.

Finnema EJ, Dassen T, Halfens R: Aggression in psychiatry: A qualitative study focusing on the characterization and perception of patient aggression by nurses working on psychiatric wards. *J Adv Nurs* 1994;19:1088–1095.

Fisher A: The process of definition and action: The case of dangerousness. Unpublished doctoral dissertation. University of California, San Francisco, 1989.

Fulmer T, Ashley J: Clinical indicators which signal neglect. *Applied Nurs Res* 1989;2:161–167.

Garza-Trevino ES: Neurobiological factors in aggressive behavior. *Hosp Commun Psychiatr* 1994;45(7):690–699.

Hoge SK, Gutheil TG: The prosecution of psychiatric patients for assaults on staff: A preliminary empirical study. *Hosp Commun Psychiatr* 1987;38:44–49.

Infantino JA, Musingo S-Y: Assaults and injuries among staff with and without training in aggressive control techniques. *Hosp Commun Psychiatr* 1985;36:1312–1314.

Kalogerakis MG: The assaultive psychiatric patient. *Psychiatr Q* 1971;45:372–381.

Kinzel AF: Body-buffer zones in violent prisoners. *Am J Psychiatr* 1970;127:99–104.

Krakowski MI, Czobor P: Clinical symptoms, neurological impairment, and the prediction of violence in psychiatric inpatients. *Hosp Commun Psychiatr* 1994;45(7):700–705.

Lanza ML: A follow-up study of nurses' reactions to physical assault. *Hosp Commun Psychiatr* 1984;35:492–494.

Lanza ML: Nurses as patient assault victims: An update, synthesis, and recommendations. *Arch Psych Nurs* 1992;6(3): 163–171.

Lanza ML: The reactions of nursing staff to physical assault by a patient. *Hosp Commun Psychiatr* 1983;34:44–47.

Levy P, Hartocollis P: Nursing aids and patient violence. *Am J Psychiatr* 1976;133:429–431.

Lidz CW, Mulvey EP, Gardner W: The accuracy of predictions of violence to others. *Hosp Commun Psychiatr* 1993;269(8): 1007–1011.

Lion JR: Special aspects of psychopharmacology, in Lion JR, Reid WH (eds): *Assaults Within Psychiatric Facilities*. Grune & Stratton, 1983.

Lion JR, Snyder W, Merrill GL: Underreporting of assaults on staff in a state hospital. *Hosp Commun Psychiatr* 1981;32: 497–498.

Madden DJ: Recognition and prevention of violence in psychiatric facilities, in Lion JR, Reid WH (eds): *Assaults Within Psychiatric Facilities*. Grune & Stratton, 1983.

Maier G et al.: A model for understanding and managing cycles of aggression among psychiatric inpatients. *Hosp Commun Psychiatr* 1987;38:5:520–524.

McCoy SM, Garritson SH: Seclusion: The process of intervening. *J Psychosoc Nurs Ment Health Serv* 1983;21:8–15.

McNiel DE, Binder RL: Clinical assessment of the risk of violence among psychiatric inpatients. *Amer J Psychiatr* 1991;148(10):1317–1321.

McNiel DE, Binder RL: The relationship between acute psychiatric symptoms, diagnosis, and short term risk of violence. *Hosp Commun Psychiatr* 1994;45(2):133–137.

Melick ME: *Factors Associated with Psychiatric Nurse Turnover: A Report on an Exit Survey and Some Recommendations*. Manpower Programs for a Changing Mental Health System, National Institute of Mental Health, January 1982.

Miller JR, Zadolinnyj K, Hafner JR, Phil M: Profiles and predictors of assaultiveness for different psychiatric ward populations. *Am J Psychiatr* 1993;150(9):1368–1373.

Monahan J: *Predicting Violent Behavior: An Assessment of Clinical Techniques*. Sage, 1981.

Monahan J: The prediction of violent behavior: Toward a second generation of theory and policy. *Am J Psychiatr* 1984; 141:10–15.

Morrison EF: A coercive interactional style as an antecedent to aggression in psychiatric patients. *Res Nurs Health* 1992a; 15:421–431.

Morrison EF: A hierarchy of aggressive and violent behaviors among psychiatric inpatients. *Hosp Commun Psychiatr* 1992b;43(5):505–506.

Morrison EF: Violent psychiatric inpatients in a public hospital. *Scholarly Inquiry for Nursing Practice: An International Journal* 1990;4(1):65–82.

Nigrosh BJ: Physical contact skills in specialized training for the prevention and management of violence, in Lion JR, Reid WH (eds): *Assaults Within Psychiatric Facilities*. Grune & Stratton, 1983.

Norris MK, Kennedy, CW: The view from within: How patients perceive the seclusion process. *J Psychosoc Nurs* 1992;30(30):7–13.

Phelan LA, Mills MJ, Ryan J: Prosecuting psychiatric patients for assaults. *Hosp Commun Psychiatr* 1985;36:581–582.

Poster EC, Ryan JA: Nurses' attitudes toward physical assaults by patients. *Arch Psychiatr Nurs* 1989;3(6):315–322.

Quinsey VC, Varney GW: Characteristics of assaults and assaulters in a maximum security hospital unit. *Crimes and Justice* 1977;5:212–220.

Reid RL, Yen SSC: Premenstrual syndrome. *Am J Obstet Gynecol* 1981;139:85–104.

Rogers R, Ciula B, Cavanaugh JL: Aggressive and socially disruptive behavior among maximum security psychiatric patients. *Psychol Rep* 1980;46:291–294.

Ruben I, Wolkon G, Yamamoto J: Physical attacks on psychiatric residents by patients. *J Nerv Ment Dis* 1980;168: 243–245.

Ryan JA, Poster EC: The assaulted nurse: Short-term and long-term responses. *Arch Psychiatr Nurs* 1989;3(6):323–331.

Schiavi R, Theilgaard A, Owen D: Sex chromosome anomalies, hormones and aggressitivity. *Arch Gen Psychiatr* 1984;41:93–99.

Sheard MH: Clinical pharmacology of aggressive behavior. *Clin Neuropharmacology* 1984;7(3):173–183.

Smith P: Professional Assault Response Training: A Manual. State Department of Mental Health, Sacramento, CA, 1983.

Snyder W: Hospital downsizing and increased frequency of assaults on staff. *Hosp Commun Psychiatr* 1994;45(4): 378–380.

Soloff PH: Seclusion and restraint, in Lion JR, Reid WH (eds): *Assaults Within Psychiatric Facilities*. Grune & Stratton, 1983.

Steadman HJ: Special problems: The prediction of violence among the mentally ill, in Hays JR, Roberts TK, Soloway

KF (eds): *Violence and the Violent Individual.* Spectrum, 1981.

Stevenson S: Heading off violence with verbal de-escalation. *J Psychosoc Nurs* 1991;29(9):6–10.

Stilling L: The pros and cons of physical restraints and behavior controls. *J Psychosoc Nurs* 1992;30(3):18–20.

Straker M et al.: Assaultive behaviors in an institutional setting. *Psychiatr J Univ Ottawa* 1977;II:185-190.

Strumpf NE, Tomes N: Restraining the troublesome patient: A historical perspective on a contemporary debate. *Nurs History Rev* 1993;1:3–24.

Tardiff K: Determinants of human violence, in Hales R, Francis A (eds): *American Psychiatric Association Annual Review 6,* 451–464, American Psychiatric Press, 1987.

Tardiff K: *The Psychiatric Use of Seclusion and Restraint.* American Psychiatry Press, 1984a.

Tardiff K: A survey of assault by chronic patients in a state hospital system, in Lion JR, Reid WH (eds): *Assaults Within Psychiatric Facilities.* Grune & Stratton, 1983.

Tardiff K: The use of medication for assaultive patients. *Hosp Commun Psychiatr* 1981;33:307–308.

Tardiff K: Violence: The psychiatric patient, in Turner JT (ed): *Violence in the Medical Care Setting.* Aspen, 1984b.

Tardiff K, Sweillam A: Assaultive behavior among chronic psychiatric inpatients. *Am J Psychiatr* 1982;139:212–215.

Tardiff K, Sweillam A: Assault, suicide and mental illness. *Arch Gen Psychiatr* 1980;37:164–169.

Torrey FE: Violent behavior by individuals with serious mental illness. *Hosp Commun Psychiatr* 1994;45(7):653–662.

U.S. Department of Health and Human Services: Education about adult domestic violence in the U.S. and Canadian medical schools, 1987–1988. *Morbidity and Mortality Weekly* 1989;38(2):17–19.

Whitman RN, Armao B, Dent OB: Assault on the therapist. *Am J Psychiatr* 1976;133:426–429.

Whittington R, Wykes T: Violence in psychiatric hospitals: Are certain staff prone to being assaulted? *J Adv Nurs* 1994;19:219–225.

CHAPTER 35

MANAGED MENTAL HEALTH CARE

Lorraine M. Wheeler

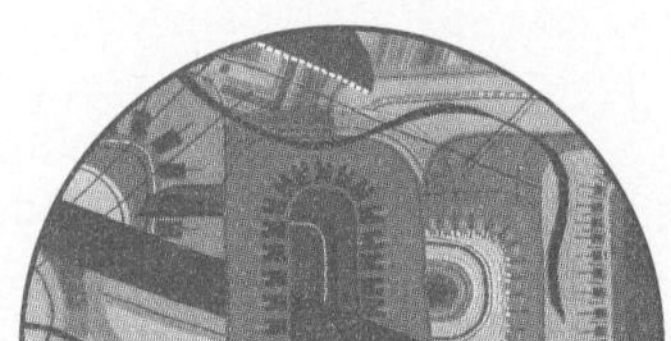

COMPETENCIES

- *Compare and contrast major differences in types of managed-care plans.*
- *Describe managed mental health care.*
- *Explain the role of the nurse in mental health triage.*
- *Identify ways psychiatric nurses can enlarge their scope of practice in managed-care organizations.*
- *Explain the role of the psychiatric nurse as a case manager.*
- *Describe the importance of ethical considerations for psychiatric nurses in managed-care settings.*
- *Recognize continuous quality improvement (CQI) as an emerging aspect of managed mental health care.*
- *Project implications for the future of psychiatric–mental health nursing practice in managed-care organizations.*

Cross-References

Other topics relevant to this content are: Chronically mentally ill, Chapter 21; Families, Chapter 32; Family burden in schizophrenia, Chapter 14; Legal issues, Chapter 11.

Critical Thinking Challenge

As this decade began, many considered the U.S. health care system to be in crisis and in need of a complete overhaul. Consider these statistics: 25 million Americans choose to go without health insurance each year; 60% of these people have jobs; 80 million Americans are locked into current jobs or are unable to get health insurance at new jobs because they have preexisting medical conditions (Gannett News Service 1994). Given this disparity between the majority of Americans with insured access to medical services and a growing minority without, or at risk of losing, insured access, how should the risk of providing and paying for health care for Americans be redistributed to gain full coverage? How would your approach affect the traditional roles of health care providers? What new opportunities emerge for nursing?

Managed mental health care, a method for capping the rate of increase in the cost of mental health care, while ensuring access to quality mental health care services, has become an increasingly important force in psychiatric–mental health nursing. As a service delivery system, managed mental health care creates a rich climate for nurses to become actively involved in primary prevention and education.

Managed health care and health care reform share a common element—the shift in economic risk. In the fee-for-service system of medical care, health care providers deliver services ordered by physicians. These services are paid for largely by employer-funded indemnity insurance plans, with the employer (or government, in the cases of Medicare and Medicaid) bearing the risk of the costs incurred. By contracting with health plans on a prepaid basis for care, an employer can shift some of the economic risk to the providers.

The more providers are at risk, the more attention they pay to controlling the use of services. Incentives operate to influence the choice of the least costly, appropriate setting for services. Those incentives directly affect the environment of the practicing psychiatric–mental health nurse.

Initial federal efforts at reforming the health care system are based on broad principles, including:

- Guaranteeing every American private health insurance.
- Giving people a choice of plan and physician.
- Providing security with coverage that can never be taken away.
- Mandating employers to share the cost of coverage.
- Preserving Medicare.
- Extending coverage for prescription drugs and long-term care (Health Security Plan 1993).

With or without federal reform, market forces are continuing to transform the health care industry, and health care delivery systems are restructuring in response.

Managed Competition

As the government, employers, and insurers all change the way they buy health care services, competition intensifies among institutions and providers seeking to serve consumers. Hospital mergers, the formation of large physician group practices, and the rise of specialty service companies create many new opportunities for nursing practice. Nurses can develop new roles, enrich the scope of nursing practice, become economically independent, and increase their entrepreneurial skills. Change calls upon all of us to operate outside our customary levels.

Rapid Change and Health Care Delivery

The information age of the 1990s has accelerated the rate of change. The information superhighway has created an atmosphere of intensity and urgency unknown in previous decades. What used to be done in days is now expected to be done in hours. Crisis theory teaches that rapid change catapults systems into crisis and disequilibrium (see Chapter 30). The ancient Chinese thought of crisis as opportunity. This opportunity now exists in our health care delivery system. The belief is that energies of opposites work together to achieve harmony and balance. In the health care crisis, the creative and innovative nurse emerges with an opportunity to gain more autonomy over psychiatric nursing practice.

Change affects mass consciousness. Your consciousness as a nurse is a part of the total health care consciousness of our nation's communities. Whenever a small but significant number of individuals move to a new level of awareness and change their beliefs and attitudes, behavior also changes. Others then move in the same direction. The whole process may have started with one person taking the first step. Eastern philosophy may state it as, "As I transform the world, I am transformed." Nursing positions you to act as a powerful change agent as the health care paradigm shifts. First, however, you must thoughtfully consider the questions and statements posed in the Nursing Self-Awareness box.

Employer-Employee Partnerships

Employers must bring their costs down to remain competitive, and they are enlisting their employees in this effort. By keeping employees and their families healthier, using services only when needed, and guiding workers in smart purchasing decisions, employers are reducing their spending on health insurance. Employees often prefer this approach to salary rebates, schedule reductions, or job loss.

Managed Care

Managed care is an organized approach to health care delivery, which controls the cost of care, measures the quality of care, and ensures access to care (United Health Care Corporation 1992). The basic elements of managed-care systems include:

- A panel of contracted providers.
- Limits on benefits to subscribers who use noncontracted providers; thus, subscribers pay more for noncontracted or "out-of-system" providers.
- Some type of authorization system.

The goal of managed care is to maximize value for the consumer while judiciously using available resources. Quality and cost need to be kept in balance while delivering service to a defined population. The **managed-care organization (MCO)** has evolved as the umbrella term that describes all types of managed care delivery systems. For clarity in this chapter, MCO will be used when referring to managed-care delivery systems. Managed care is a spectrum of services, ranging from Open Panel (members do not need a referral from an approved physician; they may self-refer) and Closed Panel (referrals must be made by approved primary care providers within the plan), **Health Maintenance Organizations (HMOs), Preferred Provider Organizations (PPOs),** and **Point of Service Organizations (POSs).** As hybrid models of managed care

NURSING SELF-AWARENESS

Your Attitude About the Health Care Crisis

Looking ahead to the year 2000, what impact do you believe the health care crisis will have on you as a nurse in your practice setting? Consider the indicators of the health care crisis listed below.

- National health care expenditures are projected to be more than $1 trillion in 1995, up from $900 billion in 1993. What does this mean to you as a citizen and taxpayer?
- Medicare spending is expected to increase by 18% by the end of the decade, costing an estimated $4308 billion in the year 2000. Medicaid is expected to grow by 15%, strapping state budgets. What impact might this have on your practice setting?
- People who don't believe there is a crisis say that American health care is the best system in the world. Do you agree or disagree with this statement? Why?
- More people have health insurance than don't. Polls show that most people are satisfied with their health care. In your mind, does this justify leaving the system alone?
- Despite the cost, no one is denied care for lack of money. Do you believe we need to share the burden of responsibility for both the haves and the have-nots?
- It is a certainty that the nursing role will have to change in response to the health care crisis. Do you think there will be more or less stress for nurses? How will you adapt to such stress in your practice?

develop, a whole new lexicon of terms and acronyms associated with MCOs emerges. Table 35–1 on page 842 defines and summarizes the basic types of MCOs. As you will see in the table, the key difference among various plans is the amount of choice or flexibility the consumer is given when choosing providers and facilities for specific services.

Historical Roots

The earliest HMO, Kaiser Permanente, began in California in the 1930s. While workers built the Hoover Dam, a need arose for their health care coverage. There were no health care services available, and the response was to develop a prepaid, employer-sponsored health care system. Over the next several decades, the growth in HMOs was modest.

By the 1970s, Dr. Paul Ellwood and others began to describe a health care system that focused on the promotion of health and the prevention of illness. Since then, we have seen an explosion in multiple, hybrid organizations that have developed in response to the need to contain spending. The current generation of MCOs have broadened their purpose to include the following objectives:

- To analyze the process and results of medical treatment.
- To develop and communicate practice guidelines and protocols for efficient and cost-effective care.
- To build networks of providers to improve the cost-effectiveness of health care delivery.
- To seek continuous quality improvement.
- To facilitate access to preventive services and early treatment.
- To support consumers and their families in finding the most appropriate treatments available.
- To play a coordinating role among the complex network of payers, providers, and consumers to enhance communication and continuity of care.

These objectives are met using tools such as utilization review, case management, **provider contracting**, and information technology.

How Is Service Delivered?

Each type of MCO is organized differently to deliver services cost effectively. Table 35–2 on page 843 compares four HMO models—staff, group, network, and independent practice association (IPA). Each is described by percentage of enrollees, structure, incentives, utilization review mechanisms, and advantages and disadvantages. As you review the table, think of yourself as a consumer attempting to choose between plans, and consider which plan you might choose. What factors enter into your decision? What changes in lifestyle, geography, or family structure might influence your choice? If you were helping clients decide which health care coverage to choose, what would you tell them?

Table 35–1 Types of Managed Care Organizations

Plan Type	*Definition*	*Enrollees*
Health Maintenance Organization (HMO)	An entity that provides, offers, or arranges for coverage of designated health services for a fixed, prepaid premium. There are four basic HMO models: Staff, Group, Network, and Independent Practice Association (IPA).	Companies with a strong need to control medical costs and to provide consumers the least degree of choice among medical care providers. Younger, healthier workers/families without strong specialist ties may choose this option for the least out-of-pocket cost and lowest levels of copayment for services.
Preferred Provider Organization (PPO)	A health care plan in which contracts are established with "preferred" providers of medical care. The benefit contract provides significantly better payment for services of preferred providers, thus encouraging members to use these providers who may be, but are not necessarily, paid on a discounted fee-for-service basis.	Allows the worker/family a choice from a panel of contracted providers. Panels are often widespread geographically and may contain specialists with whom the client has an established relationship.
Point of Service (POS)	A health care plan that allows the covered person to choose to receive a service from a participating or nonparticipating provider, with greater benefit levels associated with the use of participating providers.	Employers choose this hybrid between HMO and PPO plans with limits on provider choice and free choice indemnity plans. Clients with established specialist relationships may favor this plan, which is slightly less costly, and accept certain, but not all, limits on choice.
Indemnity Insurance	An insurance program in which the insured person is reimbursed for covered expenses under a cash or cost-of-services payment arrangement. This plan offers the largest degree of choice among providers.	Traditionally, employer-paid group plans were indemnity-based with enrollment of employees and their families. Protection for costs incurred means that older, more frequent users of medical services will favor this plan, even if premium costs are higher. This is called adverse selection, because higher-use rates of service incur greater cost and increase premiums.

Managed Mental Health Care

Behavioral Health Care

Trends toward managed competition, focus on employer and employee needs, and prevention/education have brought into use the term **behavioral health care.** This idea, that behaviors can be measured and presumably changed, indicates the dramatic impact managed care is having on the field of psychiatry. While psychiatry will continue to treat true, biologically based disorders, behavioral health care is a term rooted in pragmatism. The controversial question is: What is treatment success? For employers, the answer is helping a client to continue effective day-to-day functioning. Employers ask the mental health team an extremely practical question: How quickly can you get this employee back to work?

Primary Mental Health Care

We are challenged to address mental health care problems at opposite ends of the health care continuum. We focus on biologic psychiatry at one end of the spectrum as we treat psychoses and other severe forms of mental illness. On the other end of the health care continuum, we have the opportunity to expand our presence in primary care models, with a focus on education and prevention. MCOs have created a new practice arena where primary prevention and tertiary mental health care exist side by side in daily practice.

Practice in a Wide Variety of Settings

The shift in practice settings from inpatient to ambulatory care presents new challenges to you as a psychiatric–mental health nurse. Nursing is responding to pressures to use health care resources more efficiently. Clients are admitted to hospitals in later stages of disease or illness, or perhaps not admitted at all. Criteria for hospitalization are based on medical necessity. For instance, the once standard 28-day program for sub-

Table 35–2 Four Models of Health Maintenance Organizations

	Staff	*Group*	*Network*	*IPA*
Distribution by type	10.3%	13.5%	15.1%	61.1%
Percentage of enrollees	12.4%	29.9%	14.9%	42.8%
Structure	Salaried MDs; owned/capitated (covering health care services for an agreed-upon per-person cost) facilities; HMO underwrites risk.	Contract MD services from single multispecialty group; payment to group at negotiated rate/cap.	Contract MD services from many groups; payments to groups at negotiated rates/caps.	Contract MD services from solo/small groups; payment on discounted fee-for-service schedule.
Incentives	Hospital use not incented; capped MDs control utilization.	Members of group share risk of costs exceeding payments.	Contracting groups share risk of costs exceeding payments.	Physicians at risk for costs above rate; some plans have withholds.
Utilization review	Peer MD review within group.	Peer MD review within groups.	Peer MD review at plan level.	Peer MD review at plan level.
Advantages	Smaller number of MDs have same practice culture; owned facilities managed efficiently.	Services available from full range of MDs in group; may be more quickly organized.	Ability to recruit established MD practices; ability to provide better access and distribution of services; little capital investment.	Access large number of MDs over wide area; escape large capital facility investment; adapts fee-for-service system.
Disadvantages	Requires facilities; less choice of MD and/or site allowed to the consumer.	Degree of control over MDs is less than staff plan.	Time required to build network; less control over MDs than group.	Least control over utilization; larger number of MDs to oversee.

Source: *Group Health Insurance Association of America 1990.*

stance abuse treatment has given way to innovative and shorter models for detoxification services and outpatient treatment that meet the lifestyle needs of clients and their employers. Employer demands, coupled with cost containment, have created an entire range of ambulatory care services that at one time would have been considered ineffective. Substance-abusing clients may have options of day, evening, or weekend partial hospitalization programs. Some programs adhere to a Monday through Friday schedule of 4–6 hours per day or evening. Weekend programs are usually 8 hours on Saturday and 8 hours on Sunday. These programs provide individual, group, and family rehabilitation classes and twelve-step meetings.

Inpatient Settings

Shorter, More Intense Stays Clients admitted to inpatient settings must meet the admission criteria established by MCOs. The admitting diagnosis is often one that is life-threatening. Overall effectiveness of functioning using the *DSM-IV* Axis V global assessment of functioning scale determines the acuity of the illness. Impairment in functioning must be in the 10–50 range to qualify for admission, in most instances. Clients experiencing this degree of discomfort require intense, skilled nursing care to provide for safety needs. For example, a GAF score of 30 indicates that behavior is considerably influenced by delusions or hallucinations or serious impairment in communication or judgment, or an inability to function in almost all areas. Some MCOs have designed their own criteria that require ratings of functioning, physical impairments, family support, and other elements as part of the preadmission assessment.

You can easily see how your role as a nurse in the inpatient setting is similar to the role of the critical care nurse. Clients who are admitted to the psychiatric unit with active suicidal ideation, who are psychotic, or who are experiencing withdrawal symptoms require intensive nursing care and case management. Critical pathways, or road maps of expected outcomes, are valuable tools for helping nurses in delivering care within managed-care frameworks.

Critical Pathways **Critical pathways** are clinical management tools that organize, sequence, and time the major interventions of the multidisciplinary team for a particular DSM-IV diagnosis. The critical pathway represents standards of anticipated interventions and length of stay. The critical pathway provides an outline of needed interventions and time frames. When a client "falls off the map" or fails to meet the desired outcomes, this information can be fed to a quality-improvement program to avoid such deviations in the future.

To illustrate the shortness and intensity of nursing care required, consider the critical pathways in Chapters 12, 13, 15, 16, and 18. Note that the treatment approaches in the critical pathways are more specific and more aggressive than the treatment planning conferences and scheduling practices of the past, which addressed clients in order of admission. Psychiatric–mental health nurses have lagged behind medical-surgical nurses in integrating critical pathways as part of the inpatient treatment program. It is often said we cannot measure or standardize psychiatric care. This thinking is being challenged by MCO principles and practices.

Primary Care Centers

Alternatives to hospitalization and accelerated discharge to ambulatory care settings create a demand for sophisticated, comprehensive, and well-coordinated services in the primary care setting. We think of primary care as:

> a mode of service delivery that is initiated at the first point of contact with the mental health care system. It involves the continuous and comprehensive mental health services necessary for promotion of optimal mental health, prevention of mental illness, and intervention, health maintenance, and rehabilitation (American Nurses Association 1994, p. 7).

Managed care sites can offer rich concentrations of resources to meet client needs. Such a setting is conducive to delegating responsibility to the most cost-effective, medically appropriate provider. For example, nurses assessing alcoholic clients for hospitalization can use medical records, laboratory services, medical consultation, and benefit data before making a decision. This setup also enables the use of internal consultants and provides a collaborative atmosphere in which to meet client needs. The ambulatory care facilities of MCOs are ideal settings for psychiatric nurses to function in the role of primary mental health care provider.

Generally, psychiatric nurses in MCOs perform mental health assessments, monitor chronic illness, provide direct care for acute problems, and facilitate health-promotion groups. Examples of the health-promotion activities nurses can initiate in primary care settings are stress management, parenting education, violence prevention, bereavement counseling, suicide prevention, and teen pregnancy prevention.

TRIAGE Psychiatric nurses provide effective **triage** services in the ambulatory care setting. As defined by the United Health Corporation (1992), triage is "the classification of sick or injured persons according to severity [of illness] to direct care and ensure the efficient use of medical and nursing staff and facilities" (p. 64). In the triage role, you often act as the **gatekeeper** of the system. You essentially decide who will use the system and at what level of care.

Many factors need to be considered in the role of triage nurse. The common denominator in all instances is allocation of resources for ensuring quality and cost-effectiveness. You may be performing face-to-face assessments or telephone triage. One of the most important required skills is good listening ability, coupled with an ability to collect information for making a decision about appropriate intervention. Information may be fragmented, and interviews with several people may be required to provide a comprehensive view of the client's presenting problem.

In MCOs, employee-assistance counselors may have initiated the referral and be actively involved in client care. In a child's case, you may gather data from teachers and counselors and also coordinate with the primary pediatric provider. Triage nurses use protocols, designed to ensure that appropriate guidelines are followed. These protocols do not substitute for a comprehensive assessment. They provide a mechanism by which the triage clinician is afforded a second opinion.

Triage Process Triage clinicians in mental health care settings provide short-term, episodic intervention to members enrolled in the plan and simplify access to appropriate points of service in the system. Figure 35–1 depicts the triage process and the complexity of options available to clinicians in managed care. Collaboration and consultation are important processes nurses use when performing this first-point-of-contact service.

When triaging, you use a variety of nursing skills to evaluate the client's presenting problem. Using listening skills, you combine verbal and nonverbal data with information available in the client's medical record. Clients in managed-care settings may refer themselves or be referred through primary care providers or other resources. A unique and valuable feature of some types of MCOs, especially the closed panel type, is immediate access to a member's medical record. This access enables you to assess how the client uses the health care system and add this information to your assessment.

Margaret, a 35-year-old woman, is referred after several visits for minor medical problems. You note from the record a pattern of medication refills for antianxiety medication from the primary care provider. You also notice she has been referred for mental health care on two other occasions but has failed to keep these appointments. This information is valuable as you begin your assessment.

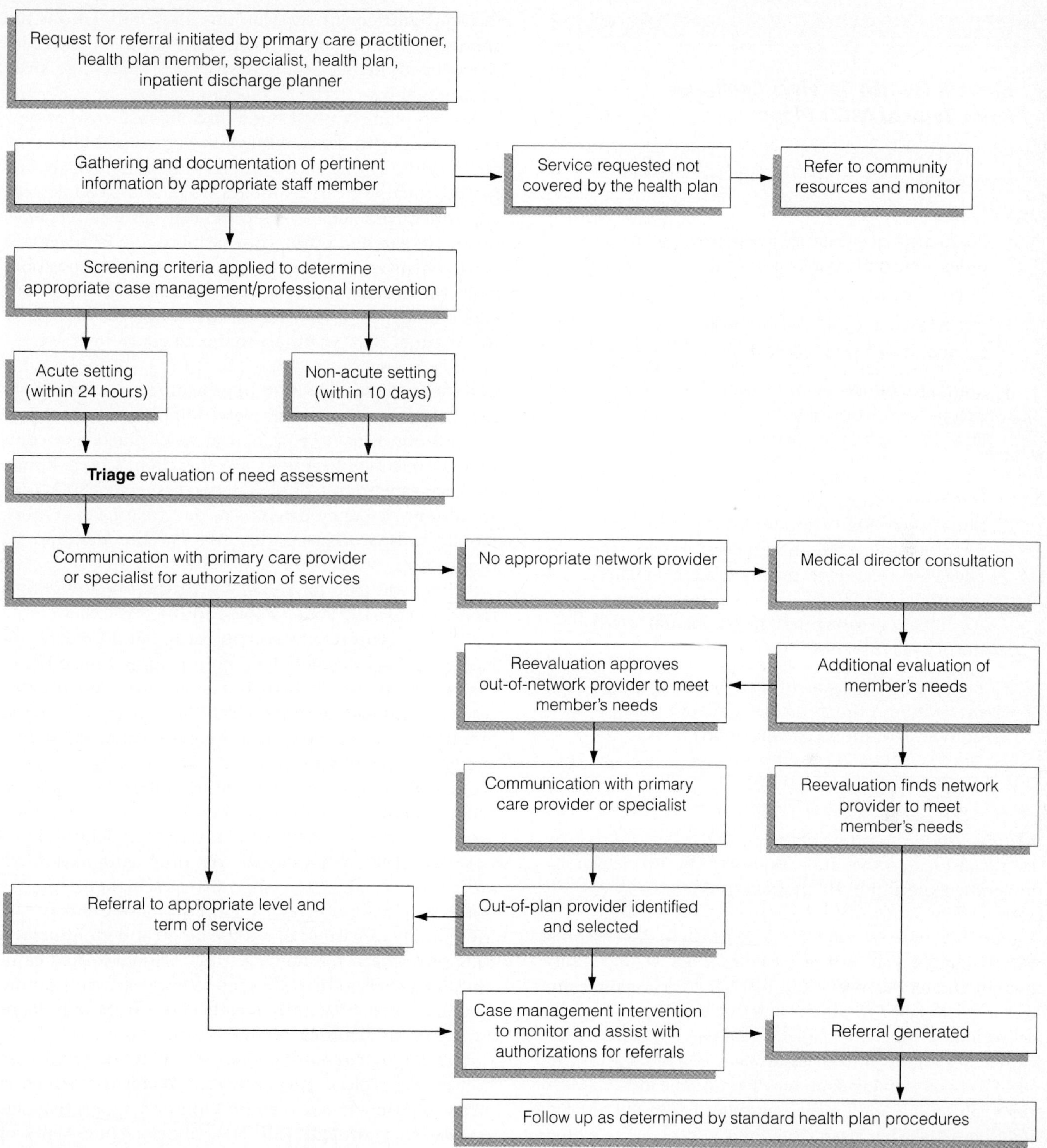

Figure 35–1 Psychiatric nursing triage process.

After completing the assessment, your next step is to decide a course of action. Using the nursing process, you begin to plan appropriate interventions. Choices include no intervention, immediate intervention, intervention within 24 hours, or routine appointment. Your further options include a private office, a public clinic, or a hospital emergency room.

Limit Setting In a managed-care setting, you will be challenged to resolve unrealistic member expectations.

Mental Health Services Excluded from Typical MCO Plans

Following are some examples of mental health services that are not included in typical MCO plans:

- Psychiatric or substance abuse therapy on court order, unless plan-approved as medically necessary.
- Psychologic testing, except for diagnosis or treatment of a psychiatric disorder.
- Marriage counseling or treatment for stress, except when connected to treatment for a DSM-IV psychiatric disorder.
- Smoking cessation, obesity, weight reduction, aversion therapy, custodial care, V code conditions (non-DSM-IV conditions that may be a focus of clinical attention such as noncompliance with treatment, malingering, age-related cognitive decline, etc. discussed in Appendix A), autism, learning disabilities, mental retardation, congenital disorders.
- Experimental treatment (psychosurgery, megavitamin therapy, codependence therapy, or treatment for sexual addiction).

Members' understanding of the managed care philosophy is crucial for effective and responsible health behaviors, including expectations of available services.

You are the nurse on call for a large HMO. At 2:00 AM on a Saturday night you receive a call from Ms M. She is distraught and tearful, explaining that her 15-year-old daughter, Amy, has failed to come home that evening. She relates an argument with Amy earlier in the day regarding Amy's curfew. As you begin your assessment, Ms M interrupts to say, "You don't understand. Amy has become incorrigible. I can't control her and I want you to put her in the hospital right now. Make her listen to us." As you continue to gather assessment data, Ms M becomes angry and tells you she is going to report you to the medical director and to her employer for not providing the services she expects. She ends with, "I've already paid for this care, and I want you to authorize it now!"

This is a clear example of unreasonable member expectations. The member's entitlement expectations is the member's understanding of the care he or she expects to receive. Entitlement expectations often differ from the specific provisions of the health plan contract. Examples of excluded mental health services of several large MCO contracts appear in the accompanying box.

Health plan members often do not consider what type of mental health benefits they have purchased until they are in crisis. The memory of television commercials suggesting inpatient care as the only solution to adolescent adjustment problems is often the first point of reference for many parents. While your primary role in triage is a comprehensive assessment and appropriate disposition, your role as consumer educator is crucial to helping your clients understand how to use their managed-care plans in a manner that is satisfactory for all concerned.

COMMUNITY CARE The shift to providing care in the community in recent years has created opportunities for psychiatric nurses to develop new areas of practice in community settings. Examples are the client's own home, personal care homes, prisons, schools, shelters, SROs (single-room-occupancy dwellings), day treatment centers, mobile vans, workplace sites, homes, churches, and senior centers.

When you care for the client in the home environment, you expand your database and view the client more realistically. This provides a rich background for data collection and is extremely helpful in planning meaningful interventions. Working in home settings, you provide teaching and counseling services that help the client and family adapt to the increasingly sophisticated technological health care environment.

As clients are discharged from hospitals more quickly, the nurse who is providing home care may be providing services that traditionally would have been delivered in a hospital setting. For example, the drug clozapine (Clozaril), used to alleviate symptoms of schizophrenia, requires frequent blood tests to monitor for side effects. The MCO home care nurse draws the blood and monitors the drug protocol in the home setting. Alcohol-related complications such as diabetes may require extensive family teaching to enable family members to successfully manage a chronic alcoholic family member.

You might encounter your clients in personal care homes or hospices. Clients with AIDS-related dementia often require extensive counseling and supportive services as they struggle with their illness. These types of clients are often quite medically ill, and you may collaborate with another nurse provider in meeting their needs.

In some personal care homes, you may be the only professional who visits an elderly client. In these instances, part of your teaching plan is to work with ancillary staff members who are responsible for running the personal care home. The importance of medication compliance for a severely, persistently mentally ill person cannot be overemphasized. Your method of ensuring that clients in personal care homes receive their medication as ordered is often to teach the managers of these facilities about the medication and its effects on behavior.

If you encounter your clients in retirement complexes, your teaching emphasis may be with an aging spouse. This person may not be able to carry out instructions and may require repetitive teaching plans and other aids to ensure that your client follows treatment protocols. In these instances, your skills in family systems will be useful aids in planning appropriate interventions.

Employer-Based Clinics As managed health care continues to develop new models, employers are becoming increasingly sophisticated in developing systems to meet the needs of their employees. Employers may establish on-site clinics with an MCO. The office is staffed with MCO employees. Here the psychiatric nurse might be asked to serve as a consultant, counseling at the site a day or two per week, seeing clients referred through the primary care providers in the employer-based clinic. While you might maintain a small caseload for follow-up, leave adequate space on your schedule to see new clients each week. It is always necessary to establish a method for responding to emergencies, because one of the quality assessment measures in MCOs is that clients are seen in a timely manner.

Enlarging the Scope of Practice

Managed mental health care and nursing may have mutually beneficial goals. Nurses provide cost-effective care, and managed care provides nurses practice settings to expand their role. Nursing priorities for changing the mental health care system include:

- Primary mental health services.
- Managed care.
- Universal access to a basic mental health benefits package.
- Structure and financing of the public mental health system for continuous care (Krauss 1993).

For psychiatric nurses, the shift to managed care as the delivery system of choice creates opportunities to find new roles, practice more autonomously, and become economically independent. Nurses who are entrepreneurial can expand their practice in the following areas:

- Prevention and education services.
- Direct-care provider companies.
- Case management services companies.
- Total quality management services.
- Consultation services.
- Outcomes measurement products; client satisfaction surveys, provider profiling.

Collaborative Practice

When you practice psychiatric nursing in an MCO, you engage in collaborative practice with other members of the health care team. In closed panel HMOs, you often practice side by side, while in network MCOs, fax machines and telephones are your tools for communicating with others on the team. Studies have shown that nurses, particularly at the advanced practice level, can provide cost-effective primary care while improving quality and client satisfaction (Safreit 1992). Such studies have shown members to be receptive to the care delivered by nonphysician providers.

In states where prescriptive authority for advanced practice nurses has been enacted in law, collaborative relationships with physicians become even more crucial when adhering to standards of practice. As a psychiatric nurse in an MCO, you must have established relationships that allow you to call for consultation and, if needed, referral for those cases that may be beyond your realm of expertise.

One pitfall inherent during referral is the potential "loss" of an established client. One way to prevent this from happening is to develop an open, honest working relationship with the provider upon whom you depend for consultation. You must be comfortable enough to confront such situations as they arise. In addition, preparing the client for the consultative visit by explaining the nature and intent of your referral allows the client to remain in a therapeutic alliance with you and prevents misunderstandings. The importance of a safe, trusting consultative relationship cannot be overemphasized as nurses expand their scope of nursing practice to include nontraditional settings.

Advanced Practice Role

The likely partnership of psychiatric nurses and MCOs is further enhanced by the skill mix of the advanced practice nurse. The clinical specialist and advanced practice roles are discussed in Chapter 1.

Advanced practice nurses are prepared to manage medication and provide primary mental health care services. Nurse practitioners, nurse midwives, and others have pioneered roles for nurses in MCOs, demonstrating nursing expertise and competence as well as high levels of consumer satisfaction.

Nurses in advanced practice may also be asked to serve on administrative committees. Duties might include:

- Developing treatment protocols with a multidisciplinary team.

- Establishing credentialing criteria.
- Reviewing statistics and trend analysis.
- Individual case review for high-risk situations.
- Developing total quality management (TQM) standards and compliance with National Committee for Quality Assurance (NCQA) criteria.

MCOs as a Practice Environment

We have already discussed the unique aspects of MCO practice when describing the gatekeeper role in triage and the importance of the therapeutic alliance in client education and partnering. There are several other aspects of practicing in managed care settings in mental health that are unique to this delivery system. These include boundaries, legal issues, treatment and medication compliance, and continuity of care.

Boundaries Boundaries are personal limits we use to differentiate between one event and another. Working as a clinician in the managed-care arena exposes one to demands, crises, time pressures, schedules, and other stressful events inherent in any health care delivery system. It is crucial for you to maintain adequate boundaries to prevent burnout, maintain objectivity, and be comfortable setting limits with consumers.

Therapists working in MCOs need orientation to the structure, goals, and operating philosophy to become part of the culture of the practice setting. Therapists whose own values are congruent with the MCO will be less susceptible to burnout and able to feel satisfied in practice. Burnout can be prevented by:

- A reasonable caseload (maximum of 6 hours of therapy per day).
- Supportive administrative, collegial, and staff relations.
- Library access and clerical support.
- Manageable on-call schedules and adequate medical backup.
- Availability of research opportunities.
- Weekly supervision meetings and peer consultation.
- Financial support for continuing education and opportunities to present professional work.
- A balance of therapy hours with other professional activities, and work time with personal time.
- Available part-time opportunities to extend job life expectancy, and job rotation for variety.

Legal Issues In traditional fee-for-service practice when a judge mandates treatment, there is usually acceptance of the client into the system for service. Service is delivered on demand, and then a charge is issued to the client. In MCOs, court-ordered treatment is negotiated on a case-by-case basis. What this means is that not every person who presents with a request for court-ordered treatment will automatically receive this service.

A transportation worker who has received his third DUI (driving under the influence) citation requests service. The member has already received two previous episodes of treatment and is not covered for services in the current calendar year.

A decision must then be made about how to respond to this request. These sometimes thorny and difficult legal cases are often referred for individual case review to the medical director.

A decision may be made to allow for a "flexing" of benefits or authorization of out-of-plan services. In flexing, an outpatient mental health care benefit may be converted to an inpatient benefit to allow for the needed hospitalization. The psychiatric nurse is sometimes in the role of client advocate, helping negotiate uncharted territory in these unusual circumstances.

Treatment Compliance Compliance issues are more readily observed in MCOs, particularly in closed panel systems where appointment clerks, clinicians, and pharmacists may work side by side. Perhaps because services are prepaid, MCO consumers find it easier not to keep scheduled appointments. This is sometimes referred to as DNKA (did not keep appointment). In mental health care, this behavior has clinical and administrative significance. It is important to note that different MCOs deal with this problem in various ways. One alternative is to set strict limits and not allow future appointments to be scheduled until the client makes copayment for all missed appointments. Another is to require clients to wait their turn in line for the next available appointment. Finally, the DNKA must be handled as a therapeutic issue in the therapy.

The problems created for the clinician with missed appointments are particularly troublesome. You are often juggling a full schedule, an impending emergency, and a two-week wait for your next open appointment. Some MCOs "double-book" appointments, relying on no-shows to balance out the schedule. When these missed appointments occur following hospitalization for a major psychiatric episode of illness, the clinician must aggressively maintain contact with the client. The importance of adhering to an after-care plan to avoid relapse is crucial. Phone calls, letters, or catching clients while they are visiting another department in the facility are all useful interventions. Some MCOs have developed transportation systems such as a free bus to ensure that clients keep appointments and follow after-care plans.

Medication Compliance Medication compliance follows many principles used in other settings. Nurses in MCOs 

Table 35–3 Comparative Dominant Values of Long-Term and Short-Term Therapists

Long-Term Therapist	*Short-Term Therapist*
Seeks change in basic character.	Prefers pragmatism, parsimony, and least radical intervention, and does not believe in the notion of "cure."
Believes that significant psychologic change is unlikely in everyday life.	Maintains an adult developmental perspective from which significant psychologic change is viewed as inevitable.
Sees the presenting problem as reflecting basic pathology.	Emphasizes client strengths and resources; presenting problems are taken seriously (although not necessarily at face value).
Wants to "be there" as client makes significant changes.	Accepts that many changes will occur "after therapy."
Sees therapy as having a "timeless" quality.	Does not accept timelessness as essential.
Unconsciously recognizes the fiscal convenience.	Fiscal issues are often muted, either by the nature of the therapist's practice or by the organizational structure of payment.
Views psychotherapy as almost always benign and useful.	Views psychotherapy as being sometimes useful and sometimes harmful.
Considers the client's being in therapy as the most important part of the client's life.	Considers being in the world as more important than being in therapy.

SOURCE: *Adapted from Budman 1991, p. 234.*

often work in collaborative relationships with other providers to ensure compliance. When medication copayments are low, appointments are available, and transportation is accessible, the likelihood of compliance is increased. In the MCO setting, the primary care provider is an ally of the mental health care team. **Primary care providers** who see clients for routine medical problems are in a position to reinforce the importance of staying on psychotropic drugs. Often a discussion of side effects eliminates confusion and increases understanding of the medicine's effect. Managed-care pharmacists can also help the mental health team ensure that clients comply with their medication regimens.

CONTINUITY OF CARE AND TREATMENT BREAKS Some MCOs are seamless delivery systems. In other words, consumers can move from one level of care to the next while remaining in the same delivery system. In this sense, members of an MCO can be considered to be in continuous therapy. This has clinical implications that require new conceptual frameworks for treatment. Table 35–3 distinguishes key differences between the orientations of therapists who practice in an MCO setting from those therapists who practice in more traditional fee-for-service models of care.

A short-term episodic framework, introduced by Bennett (1992), is based on the following ideas. Psychopathology has its roots in the biologic and psychologic makeup of the individual. People react in the present based on biologic and psychosocial events from the past. As one moves through life, there is a tendency to reach impasses. These impasses, which have agendas specific to each human being, reflect both present problems and current expressions of underlying developmental obstacles. Impasses harness energy and push the individual toward healthy coping through the agendas presented. Bennett (1992) calls these *problem-driven interventions,* as opposed to problem-centered interventions. Primary care services tend to focus on the present impasse, while secondary care services are geared to examine the underlying obstacle. It is essential to the healing process that both are coordinated.

When care is delivered in the problem-driven model, it is most likely to be brief rather than extended, discontinuous rather than ongoing, and incremental rather than circumscribed. The problem-driven model, with its belief in the person's natural tendency toward health, is in direct contrast to the illness model. In the illness model, treatment is often lifelong, highly specialized, and costly, and creates an unavoidable dependence on the caregiver. Integrating the primary level of care (or primary presenting problem) and the secondary level of care (or impasse), enables the clinician to design a focal intervention that works on both levels simultaneously.

In this framework, the mental health client begins to view the psychiatric clinician as similar to the primary medical care provider. The nurse therapist is viewed as available as needed over the life span, but not as a provider who must be seen for an extended course of long-term psychotherapy. Clients may consider themselves "in therapy" with you even while taking "treatment breaks" due to the nature of the setting.

As a therapist, you can treat a client across all levels of care for consistency and continuity of care.

You have assessed Ms B and found her to be in need of admission for self-mutilating behavior which makes it unsafe for her to function outside the hospital. As Ms B is settling into the unit, you introduce yourself to the staff as her primary therapist. You work collaboratively with Dr C and the inpatient mental health team. Ms B is given a DSM-IV diagnosis of borderline personality disorder. Her anticipated length of stay is 5 days, with the goal of stabilizing her mood and beginning antidepressant medication. As her primary therapist, you meet with the team for treatment planning and spend 45 minutes each day developing a therapeutic relationship with Ms B.

Following her discharge, you see her in the office weekly for 4 weeks, then every 2 weeks for the next 2 months. Following this, you see Ms B monthly for the next 4 months. At this point, you discharge Ms B, labeling this as a treatment break, letting Ms B know she can come back as needed.

The concept of the treatment break decreases dependence, empowers Ms B to take some responsibility for her care, and leaves the door open to return if she is not able to manage.

One year later, on the anniversary of her hospitalization, Ms B telephones. You schedule one or two visits and again suggest a treatment break. Several months go by, and Ms B decides to join a women's support group you are forming.

This type of discontinuous therapy offers many creative options for the innovative clinician.

Case Management in MCOs

Rapid changes in the health care system have contributed to client feelings of being overwhelmed and confused about how to use prepaid services effectively. In many systems, clients no longer rely on a single provider or institution to shepherd them through an episode of illness. The objective of MCOs is outcome-oriented, cost-effective mental health care. To achieve this goal, the process involved in managing the care must be revised. **Case management** is one strategy that has evolved to meet the needs of clients, families, employers, and providers. Case management services are designed to advocate for the client through coordination of care. Assigning clients to case managers before discharge can ease the transition and provide support and continuity of care.

Conceptual Framework

Case Management as a System The fundamental focus of case management is to integrate, coordinate, and advocate for individuals, families, and groups requiring extensive services. The ultimate goal is to achieve planned care outcomes by brokering services across the health care continuum. Case management can simultaneously be described as a system, a role, a technology, and a service. As a system, case management has several elements:

- Assessment and problem identification.
- Planning.
- Procurement, delivery, and coordination of service.
- Monitoring to ensure that the multiple service needs of the client are met.

The central element that differentiates case management from other types of care is the coordination of one episode of care across the multiple settings of the care continuum. The strategy focuses on the effective use of time frames and resources to achieve desired outcomes (Bower 1992).

The Case Manager Role The role of the clinician in an MCO is highly visible and active. Nurses who perform this role must be vested with the authority and accountability necessary to negotiate with complex systems and a wide diversity of providers and populations. Nurses are particularly prepared to function in this role by the very nature of the profession.

This is especially evident in the managed care setting where clients from diverse backgrounds sometimes struggle to negotiate a new system of health care delivery. We know that race and poverty are factors that impede a client's access to mental health services and that race and ethnicity affect how clients use mental health services. For example, Asians are more likely to use individual and outpatient services, while whites are more likely to use emergency, inpatient, and case management services. African Americans are less likely than whites to use case management services, and Latinos are more likely to use them. African Americans are also less likely than whites to use individual outpatient services. Latinos are less likely than whites to use emergency services, while African Americans are more likely to use them (Krauss 1993). Increased use of emergency services is problematic because not only is it more costly to render services this way, but emergency services tend to be discontinuous with minimal or no follow-up. Our racial diversity as a nation is increasing, and case management can help individuals and families who bring

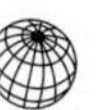

unique needs and cultural experiences to the managed-care setting.

As case managers, nurses can provide the majority of services that social workers offer to clients; however, the reverse is not true. Social workers have few, if any, of the physical assessment or illness-detection skills of the nurse. An additional factor contributing to the natural fit between nurses and consumers is the increased emphasis on psychobiology and pharmacology in helping clients cope with alterations in their mental health.

Case Management as a Technology Nurses who practice as case managers in MCOs use current technological advances to assist with coordination of care. Intense time frames, complex care, and sequencing of multiple events require immediate response. Equipment such as notebook computers, fax machines, local area networks, beepers, and voice-messaging systems are critical tools in the effective use of time and resources. In the not-too-distant future, video-teleconferencing will be added to the toolkit of effective case managers.

The Process of Case Management in MCOs

Like the nursing process, case management as an MCO process focuses on the following elements:

- Assessment
- Outcome development
- Planning
- Intervention
- Monitoring
- Evaluation

In managed-care environments, the process of case management enhances quality by preventing unnecessary hospitalization, focusing treatment goals in least-restrictive settings, and preventing the duplication and fragmentation of services.

Gatekeeping and Facilitating The service you provide as a case manager is one of gatekeeping and facilitating. As gatekeeper, you serve as the client's initial contact for care and referrals. For example, the case manager for a client with bipolar disorder may be contacted as that client presents in the emergency department in a manic state. Because of knowledge of prior history and treatment, you are able to determine if inpatient care is required. You would have access to recent laboratory studies regarding lithium carbonate levels and also have an established relationship with family members. In other words, case management helps clients and their caregivers make informed decisions, such as whether the client needs hospitalization, based on client needs, abilities, resources, and personal preferences.

In a case of recurring substance abuse, the nurse case manager can help a family make informed decisions, taking into consideration the client's health status and diagnosis, treatment plan, payment resources, and health care options. This facilitation aspect of case management assures that clients in a managed mental health care environment receive care that is appropriate, individualized, cost-effective, and has optimal outcomes. Note that not all triage clinicians function as case managers, nor do case managers always provide triage services. In some instances, roles overlap. However, there are important distinctions in each role.

Client Advocacy MCOs must have clear statements regarding client rights and responsibilities. The case manager often refers to these in negotiating with both client and system regarding appropriate referrals and authorizations for treatment.

A statement of rights helps focus our awareness on the most fundamental aspect of the case manager role, that of being a client advocate. While there are many and varied models of case management, the nurse who defines this role as client advocate will have the greatest chance of success. When you carry out your role in this framework, you bring to the multidisciplinary team skills and knowledge that extend beyond biologic or pathologic aspects of care. You view the client through a holistic perspective. You piece together the fragmented pieces of the client's care. This cannot be done in the isolation of an office or simply by telephone. It requires active, on-site presence, interviews, meetings, attendance at treatment planning conferences, and appropriate documentation. It may be necessary for you to obtain hospital privileges for the access that is required to perform the role of a nurse case manager fully.

In the role of case manager the nurse may be caught in the middle of conflicting value systems. For example, clients with alcoholism or bulimia have been treated traditionally with intensive, extended inpatient treatment programs. Managed care plans may authorize this treatment only in an outpatient setting. The nurse must respond to clients' need for autonomy in making decisions regarding treatment as well as negotiate within the limitations of the managed care plan. Case managers must use creativity and flexibility in negotiating among the conflicting needs of several parties. Clients and families who are accustomed to specific treatment models for illnesses with relapse potential often feel confused and misunderstood when new treatment approaches are suggested that appear economically motivated.

This type of case management is an internal process, which differentiates it from other models. In external case management, outside consultants are employed by insurers to coordinate care, usually isolated and geographically distant from the client, family, and care setting.

Other System Issues

Case managers wield informal and formal power in the system. Four types of authority exist in the roles of case manager: administrative, legal, fiscal, and clinical (Schwartz, Goldman, and Churgin 1982). The lines of accountability and authority must be clearly drawn as the case manager enters the delivery system. The client may see the case manager as an advocate of the MCO. The staff may view the case manager as an intruder or an extra set of hands. Finally, physicians may view the case manager as a "snoop." Because this is a new area of practice in some mental health settings, it is important for the nurse to clearly define the role and responsibilities and clarify any misconceptions that may exist.

Nurses who choose this role must have in-depth knowledge and skill in the field of psychiatric–mental health nursing. Case managers are empowered nurses who are decisive and assertive on their clients' behalf. Administrative complexities, financing mechanisms, legal issues, and sequencing of care all require a sound clinician who can think critically and make reasoned judgments. Knowledge of community resources and how to access them are other important considerations for the role of case manager. Other characteristics include experience as a team participant, an ability to take risks and speak assertively, clinical maturity, tenacity, commitment, a sense of humor, and coping mechanisms to avoid burnout.

Assessment Phase Challenges The case manager must be alert to those cases that are not eligible for services. When benefit limits have been met, negotiation for appropriate placement and utilization of community resources is crucial to providing for the safety needs of clients.

Nurses who function as case managers must interact with all members of the health care team. Trust, mutual support, and clear communication among team members is necessary before case management services can be implemented. Meetings with administrative personnel and tactful systems entry strategies must be employed while laying the groundwork for a case management program. Physicians sometimes consider themselves to be case managers. Careful introduction of the role, which differentiates it from medical care management, is necessary in clarifying role responsibilities. Other members of the team may feel threatened by the addition of a case manager and view it as an indictment of their own role performance. When system administration can orient its members to the case manager's role, there is a higher level of acceptance of the service as augmenting client care rather than interfering with it.

Planning Phase Challenges In this phase of care, the nurse can bring valuable information concerning benefits, limits, family resources, employer expectations, and other pertinent data to the treatment planning table. Using the formal and informal support systems, the treatment team is able to set mutually agreed-upon goals with desired outcomes and can begin to plan action steps using intended time frames or critical pathways as a guide.

Implementation Phase Challenges The next phase of the case management process is to ensure that the client gets needed care. In some systems the case manager may be asked to deliver care. However, this approach is not in the best interest of the client because the case manager's role is to remain the objective, internal consultant, looking at the whole picture. When pulled into delivering the care, the case manager loses perspective and may find important issues clouded. For example, a case management nurse who is asked to function as the client's primary therapist because the primary nurse is overloaded will sacrifice time and resources needed to monitor the quality of care delivered and perhaps lose objectivity.

Keep in mind during the implementation phase that your role involves conflict resolution. To set limits tactfully, arbitrate differences, and maintain successful outcomes for all, you need patience, maturity, and experience. The case manager is also called on to provide additional data or client/family education where a denial or extension of service is in question. As client advocate, you may identify gaps in care that require action in community, facilities, or nursing systems. Nurse case managers are among the best consultants to nursing departments for improving quality because they view problems in the system from the client's perspective.

Evaluation Phase Challenges The case manager's role in evaluation consists of continuous monitoring of intervention responses and progress toward desired outcomes. This may include medication monitoring for dosage and compliance, as well as monitoring client response to other therapies. You may interview the client directly to gather this information, and then compare it with what is recorded in the medical record. Inconsistent data are always a red flag for intervention by the case manager. Perhaps the process is moving too slowly or the client is not an active participant in the care plan. Once outcomes are achieved and the client is discharged, there must be a mechanism for ongoing quality improvement based on recommended standards of nursing practice. Critical incidents and inconsistencies in the care must be communicated in an ongoing, systematic program of continuous quality improvement. This information is ultimately used to measure provider and facility performance for contract renewal decisions.

The primary functions of the case manager are summarized in the accompanying box. Not limited to this scope, the role of nurse case manager will continue to evolve as mental health care delivery systems respond to

Functions of the Case Manager in Managed Mental Health Care

- Screening the enrolled population for appropriate clients for case management.
- Assessing formal and informal support systems of clients.
- Assessing client goals comprehensively, and determining client status: physical, mental, social, environmental, functional, and financial.
- Analyzing and synthesizing all data for formulating appropriate diagnoses and/or interdisciplinary problem statements.
- Developing, executing, monitoring, and adapting a plan of care through an interdisciplinary, team process.
- Coordinating care delivery by all providers responsible for serving a given client's needs, extending to payment for services.
- Referring the client to the most appropriate resource, at the institutional or community level, or creating options where none exist.
- Securing services, including authorizations and determinations of eligibility for services at the appropriate level.
- Solving problems; facilitating access; providing direct care as indicated; liaisoning with elements of the system.
- Educating the client, family, and support systems and agencies; expediting the goal of self-care by the client and family.
- Monitoring and documenting client progress toward goals; periodic reassessment; monitoring the effectiveness of services within the plan.

Source: Adapted from Bower 1992.

pressures from employers, communities, and government agencies to ensure that the care delivered is affordable, accessible, and appropriate (Bower 1992).

Ethical Considerations

Confidentiality

Health care providers have ethical and legal obligations to maintain the confidentiality of medical records and medical information. A breach of confidentiality can subject a provider to liability to a client.

Confidentiality has always been a significant issue for people seeking mental health services. With the popularity of managed care as a delivery system, confidentiality becomes even more of an issue as a result of the freedom with which information is shared. Because managed care requires tighter controls and accountability and consultation for treatment, clinical information is shared with administrative offices to authorize payment.

Recently, data collection has been expanded to include data reporting. HEIDIS, or the Health Plan Employer Data and Information Set, was developed in response to employers asking, "How do I understand what 'value' my health care dollar is purchasing, and how do I hold a health plan 'accountable' for its performance?" This data set is being developed in stages and will ultimately influence mental health care services. These "report cards" measure five areas of performance of a health plan: quality, access, client satisfaction, membership and utilization, and finance.

While MCOs have internally monitored such activity, what is different is sharing this information with employers. Many questions remain to be answered regarding privacy, sanitizing the medical record, and efforts to protect confidentiality. The handling of sensitive medical information is a major concern of the American public. Consider the findings from a national poll in the Research Note on the next page.

Client Satisfaction

Typical MCO member survey questions include:

- Were you treated courteously and respectfully by the professional who saw you?
- How long did you wait at the office?
- How do you rate the clinician regarding carefulness, competence, and thoroughness?
- Was the location convenient? Was it neat and clean?
- Did you have difficulty getting through on the phone?
- How long did you wait for an appointment?
- Was the treatment process explained to you?

RESEARCH NOTE

Citation

Peck RL (ed): Results from an Equifax Privacy Poll, *Behav Health Man* (July-August) 1994;14(4):10–11.

Study Problem/Purpose

Efforts to reform or change the health delivery system both increase the amount of personal data generated and give more administrative access to these data than ever before. This poll was commisssioned to identify and measure specific public concerns about the privacy of medical information.

Methods

The survey was conducted in communities in 48 states, covering 1000 individuals age 18 or older. In addition, 650 health care "leaders" were interviewed by the study staff.

Findings

Approximately 25% of the subjects believed that their medical information has been improperly disclosed during medical claim transactions. Nearly two-thirds were concerned that their medical information is being seen by organizations other than those providing health care. Nearly two-thirds believed that computers are implicated in the unauthorized release of their medical records. Users of mental health care services exceed nonusers in such concerns. Furthermore, they are the most well-represented among those (approximately 1 in 12) who reported having avoided treatment or making insurance claims in order to protect jobs or careers. More users than nonusers of mental health care services feared loss of insurance upon changing jobs.

Implications

The public has slightly less confidence than health care leaders in the ability of providers to maintain confidentiality, and health care leaders have slightly less confidence than the public that existing privacy standards can be maintained in the changing field of the future. Users of behavioral health care services are among the most sensitive to privacy issues. However, as important as privacy of medical information has been in the past, it is clearly going to be a key factor in the public perception of the effectiveness of managed mental health programs in the immediate future.

Such surveys, along with office inspection visits and monitoring of telephone pick-up times, are becoming commonplace as the managed-care industry begins to set standards.

Quality Standards

The challenge of quality in managed mental health care is the ability to strike a balance between client welfare and economics. As MCOs mature, they must continue to refine quality-improvement programs to meet the expectations of outside interests. An excellent quality-improvement program must contain the following elements: definitions of quality, a method of measuring the quality, and mechanisms for improving quality. The usual basic audits include structure, process, and outcome. For nurses in managed-care settings, peer review mechanisms should be established. Advanced practice nurses must have peer review systems that can provide for growth and support of the practicing professional. Nursing representation on quality review committees is essential when reviewing the credentials of new providers or conducting individual case reviews. Sentinel events that can be monitored in managed mental health care might include:

- Administrative discharges.
- AMA (against medical advice) discharges.
- AWOL (absent without leave) elopements at any level of care.
- Denials of payment.
- Emergency admissions without prior authorization.
- All admissions for attempted suicide.
- Readmissions within 31–90 days.
- Use of restraints and/or seclusion.
- Weekly or daily progress notes by attending physicians.

Limit Setting

Perhaps no other mechanism in the managed-care field has received as much attention and is fraught with as much controversy as limit setting. While limits or exclusions have always existed in mental health care benefit plans, some would have you believe that the standard benefits provided by MCOs will leave us all abandoned. Again, the judicious use of resources, coupled with effective triage and ongoing case management, can do much to provide essential services to an enrolled population while maintaining quality.

National Committee for Quality Assurance (NCQA)

The National Committee for Quality Assurance (NCQA) is a nonprofit organization seeking to improve client care quality and health plan performance in partnership with managed-care plans, purchasers, consumers, and the public sector. NCQA's efforts are complementary to MCOs as they evaluate health plans' internal quality processes and develop plan performance measures. Managed-care plans are accredited through NCQA in the same way hospitals are accredited by the Joint Commission on Accreditation of Healthcare Organizations (JCAHO).

Research Agenda

Very little research has been conducted in managed-care settings, and clearly this needs to occur. However, efforts are beginning, particularly in large, well-established companies, with a focus on quality care, treatment protocols, and outcome measurement. Nursing must participate in such studies and establish a research agenda for managed mental health care.

Implications for the Future

The economic climate and the need for health care reform require that nurses create and implement creative practice strategies. The MCO is one environment where psychiatric–mental health nurses must be willing to aggressively move ahead in developing new roles. Nurses possess the knowledge and skill required in these new practice settings. Our colleagues, other members of the multidisciplinary team, have already embraced this new model of care. We have been slow to rise to the challenge of marketing our services to these new customers. For too long, we have been dependent on the paternalistic system of hospital services to take care of us. These rapidly changing times cry out to the entrepreneurial spirit to move nursing forward and capitalize on the expanding roles possible in managed-care organizations. To ensure that managed care stays on a path that ensures quality cost-effective mental health care, psychiatric nurses must actively endorse the following principles:

- Mental health and psychiatric problems, including chemical dependence, must be addressed by MCOs on a parity with physical health coverage.
- Nontraditional settings (such as home, school, and community-based settings) should be emphasized.
- Authorized services should include a continuum of health promotion and illness prevention services.
- Less restrictive interventions should be encouraged in lieu of more restrictive ones.
- Concepts of quality, cultural sensitivity, access, cost-effectiveness, provider choice, and continuity of care must drive the managed-care system.
- The managed-care industry must be standardized, monitored, and regulated to avoid cumbersome bureaucracy and to prevent abuses (Krauss 1993).

If as a nation we are to achieve the principles of health care reform as outlined in the mid-1990s, then each of us has the obligation to actively participate in improving the mental health of our communities. We need a system based on balanced principles of quality and cost that is comprehensive, well-coordinated, and community-based. We are all part of the interdependent web of humankind—and what affects one of us, affects us all.

Chapter Highlights

- Major efforts to reshape the health care system are based on guaranteed private insurance, choice of provider, security, employer mandate, preservation of Medicare, and coverage for prescription drugs and long-term care.
- The shifting of economic risk, managed competition, information technology, and the rapid rate of change have created a climate that provides opportunities to transform the health care service delivery system.
- Behavioral health care has emerged from trends toward managed competition, employer demands, and a focus on prevention and education in our practice settings.
- Primary mental health care and biologic psychiatry are important conceptual frameworks for nursing practice in managed-care settings.
- Triage services are fundamental to the role of the gatekeeper in primary mental health care.
- The requirement to balance quality and cost have positioned case management services as important models of care coordination.
- Ethical considerations regarding confidentiality, limits, and client satisfaction are being raised as important issues for discussion in MCOs.
- The agenda for the reform of mental health care services has implications for psychiatric–mental health nurses practicing in MCOs.

References

American Academy of Nursing: *Managed Care and National Health Care Reform: Nurses Can Make It Work.* American Academy of Nursing, 1993.

American Nurses Association: *Nursing's Agenda for Health Care Reform,* Executive Summary, American Nurses Publishing, 1992.

American Nurses Association: *A Statement on Psychiatric–Mental Health Clinical Nursing Practice and Standards of Psychiatric–Mental Health Clinical Nursing Practice.* American Nurses Association, 1994.

Are HMO's the answer? *Consumer Reports,* August 1992; 57(8):519–527.

Bennett M: Managed care as a framework for clinical practice. In *Managed Mental Health Care: Administrative and Clinical Issues.* Feldman JL, Fitzpatrick RJ (eds). American Psychiatric Press, 1992, pp 206–208.

Bower KA: *Case Management by Nurses.* American Nurses Publishing, 1992.

Budman S: *Psychotherapy and Managed Care: The Optimal Use of Time and Resources.* American Psychological Press, 1991.

Feldman JL, Fitzpatrick RJ: *Managed Mental Health Care: Administrative and Clinical Issues.* American Psychiatric Press, 1992.

Fitzpatrick PB, Levich D: Patient expectations imperil HMO's. *Health Man Quart.* First Quarter, 1988:24–26.

Gannett News Service: *Who Says What About Health Care.* March 1994.

George Washington University Health Plan: *Member Handbook, The George Washington University Health Plan,* 1993.

Goodman M, Brown J, Deitz P: *Managing Managed Care: A Mental Health Practitioner's Survival Guide.* American Psychiatric Press, 1992.

Group Health Association of America: *Fact Sheet.* Group Health Association of America, 1990.

Health Security Plan: U.S. Government Printing Office, 1993.

Hicks LL, Stallmeyer JM, Coleman JR: *Role of the Nurse in Managed Care.* American Nurses Publishing, 1993.

Hoff LA: Health policy and the plight of the mentally ill. *Psychiatr* 1993; 56:400–419.

Hoge MA et al: Defining managed care in public-sector psychiatry. *Hosp Commun Psychiatr* 1994;45:1085–1089.

Kaplan, HI, Sadock BJ, Grebb JA: *Synopsis of Psychiatry,* ed 7. Williams & Wilkins, 1994.

Kneisl CR: On the brink of health care reform: Vital issues for psychiatric–mental health nurses. *Capsules and Comments in Psychiatric Nursing* 1994;1(2):4–17.

Knollmueller RN: *Prevention Across the Life Span: Healthy People for the 21st Century.* American Nurses Publishing, 1993.

Krauss JB: *Health Care Reform: Essential Mental Health Services.* American Nurses Publishing, 1993.

Leibenluft E, Tasman A, Green SA: *Less Time to Do More: Psychotherapy on the Short-Term Inpatient Unit.* American Psychiatric Press, 1993.

MacKenzie KR: *Effective Use of Group Therapy in Managed Care.* American Psychiatric Press, 1994.

Mechanic D: Mental health services in the context of health insurance reform. *Milbank Q* 1993;71:349–364.

Mundinger M: Community-based care: Who will be the case managers? *Nurs Outlook* 1994;32(6):294–295.

National Advisory Mental Health Council: Health care reform for Americans with severe mental illness: Report of the National Advisory Mental Health Council. *Am J Psychiatr* 1993;150:1447–1465.

Peck R (ed): Results from an Equifax Privacy Poll. *Behav Health Man* (July–August) 1994;14(4):10–11.

Safreit BJ: Health care dollars and regulatory sense: The role of the advanced practice nurse. *Yale J Regulation* 1992;9(2).

Schreter RK, Sharfstein SS, Schreter CA: *Allies and Adversaries: The Impact of Managed Care on Mental Health Services.* American Psychiatric Press, 1994.

Schwartz S, Goldman H, Churgin S: Case management for the chronically mentally ill: Moods and dimensions. *Hosp Commun Psychiatr* 1982;33(12):1006–1009.

United Health Care Corporation: *The Managed Care Resource: The Language of Managed Health Care and Organized Health Systems.* United Health Care Corporation, 1992.

Zach J, Cohen M: Managing mental health costs is a balancing act. *Personnel Journal* (March)1993;107–111.

PART SIX

PSYCHIATRIC–MENTAL HEALTH NURSING ACROSS THE LIFE SPAN

CONTENTS

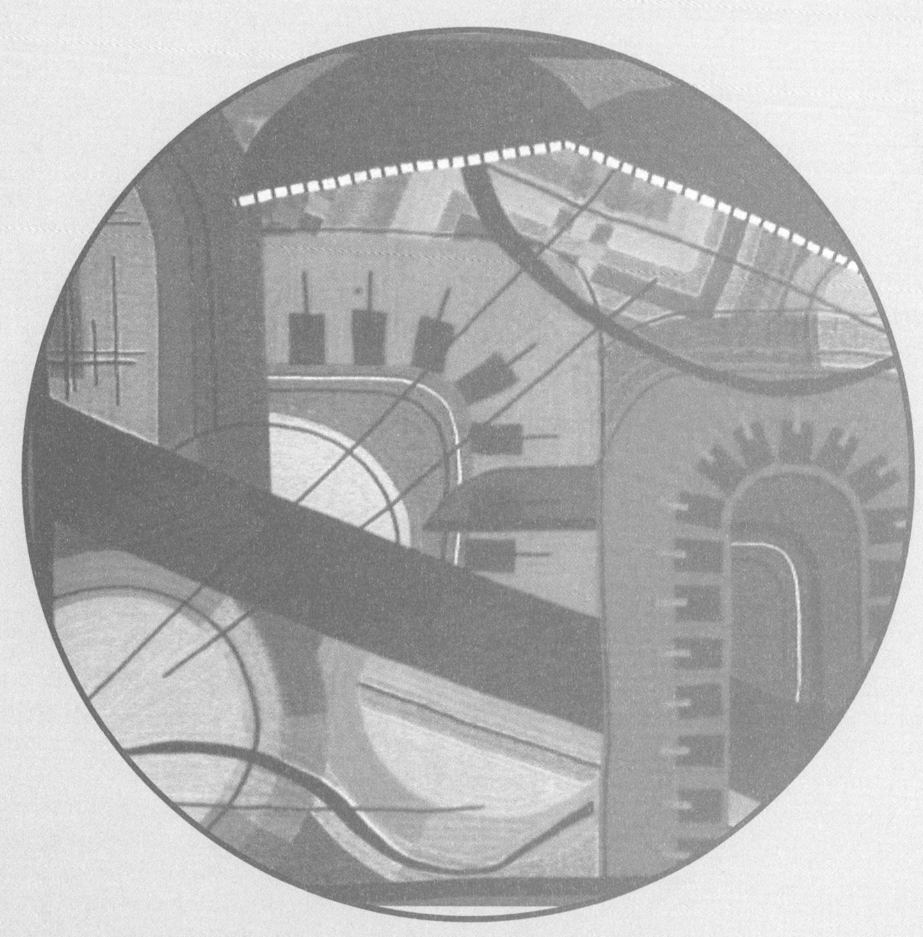

CHAPTER 36

APPLYING THE NURSING PROCESS WITH CHILDREN

Sandra Weiss

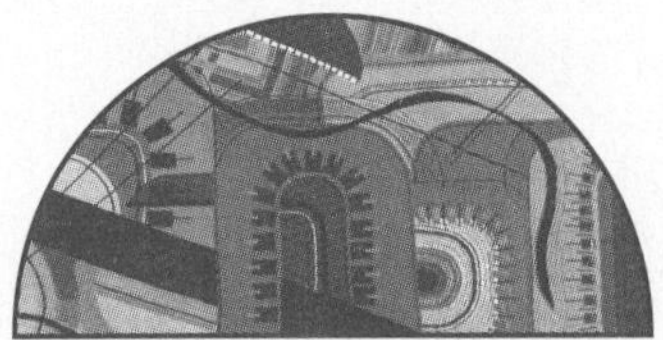

COMPETENCIES

- *Describe the generalist and specialist roles of the nurse in child psychiatry.*
- *Describe major theories underlying the development of childhood psychiatric disorders.*
- *Identify the symptoms of common psychiatric disorders of children.*
- *Discuss the basic methods for assessment and diagnosis of children with mental health problems.*
- *Describe various approaches to planning and treatment that can be used by the child psychiatric nurse.*
- *Discuss how your own attitudes toward a child may affect therapeutic outcomes.*

Cross-References

Other topics relevant to this content are: Schizophrenia, Chapter 14; Mood disorders, Chapter 15; Anxiety disorders, Chapter 16; Eating disorders, Chapter 18; Family assessment and family therapy, Chapter 32; Intrafamily physical and sexual abuse of children, Chapter 23; Suicide, Chapter 24.

Critical Thinking Challenge

There is much controversy regarding the family's role in child mental health problems. Some clinicians think that parental interactions with children contribute substantially to the development of psychiatric disorders in those children, while other clinicians believe that these disorders are primarily biologically determined. Where do you stand on this issue? What factors would you consider in your assessment of the family's contribution to a child's emotional problems? How might your stance on this issue affect the nature of the care you provide to the child?

It is both the best and the worst of times for child psychiatric nursing. On one hand, there are more children in need of psychiatric care than ever before in the history of the field. A growing recognition of the psychobiologic underpinnings of mental illness has resulted in a greater dependence on nurses for a variety of roles that demand knowledge of both mental and physical health. For example, nurses in child psychiatry must assess psychologic and physical symptoms, explain laboratory tests to children, administer medications that require strict and systematic monitoring, and work with children having a dual medical and psychiatric diagnosis (such as diabetes and conduct disorder). Child psychiatric nurses have the knowledge to perform these diverse clinical functions at a reasonable cost to society. However, the resources available for prevention and treatment of mental illness in children are rapidly shrinking. Because of the scarce resources, there is competition from psychiatry, psychology, and social work that limits the positions available for nurses to work with children who have mental health problems.

As a specialty, child psychiatric nursing had its inception in the early 1950s, when graduate programs opened and training funds became available through the National Institute of Mental Health (NIMH). The early child mental health teams did not include the nurse. In some residential programs, the majority of milieu staff were from other disciplines, and only one nurse was included for each shift, primarily to attend to the physical needs of the children and administer medications. As the community mental health movement developed, programs specifically for children began to offer appropriate roles for the child psychiatric nurse, including treatment, consultation, education, and medication supervision. However, these programs had great difficulty sustaining themselves. The small number of professional staff in these programs provided few opportunities and low visibility for the child psychiatric nurse. Because positions in child psychiatry were so limited, many of these nurses were also involved in the care of chronically institutionalized adults.

The contemporary interdisciplinary team consists of child psychiatrists, nurses, social workers, psychologists, occupational therapists, recreational therapists, special educators, pediatricians, and child care workers. Other specialists are used for consultations as indicated, particularly child neurologists, speech and language specialists, child abuse teams, clergy, and physical therapists.

Standards of Practice in Child Psychiatric Nursing

In contrast to many psychiatric professions that focus strictly on disorders, child psychiatric nursing concerns itself with the entire continuum between health and illness. The nurse's role includes the promotion of mental health, prevention and early intervention, and the treatment of children with severe mental illness. Nursing care aimed at promotion and prevention occurs within settings such as schools, community agencies, and pediatric inpatient and ambulatory care centers. Nursing care involving the treatment of psychiatric disorders usually occurs within psychiatric hospitals, day treatment centers, and residential care facilities. However, nurses may also be involved in transitional or follow-up care of more severely disturbed children at community mental health clinics and through school districts or public health departments.

The specific roles assumed by the child psychiatric nurse depend on whether the nurse is a generalist or clinical specialist. The American Nurses Association, in cooperation with Advocates for Child Psychiatric Nursing, developed Standards of Child and Adolescent Psychiatric and Mental Health Nursing to distinguish and advance the quality of nursing care by both generalists and specialists in the field (American Nurses Association, 1985). Generalists are nurses who are educated in basic professional nursing programs. These are some of the roles that child psychiatric nurse generalists assume:

- Milieu therapist who shares the responsibility for providing an atmosphere in which all activities and behaviors are focused on the therapeutic care of the child or adolescent.
- Counselor or teacher of parents who have an emotionally disturbed or mentally retarded child or adolescent.
- Collaborator with other psychiatric–mental health professionals in assessing the needs and planning for the care of a child or adolescent and family.
- Responsible citizen and change agent who provides for the mental health needs of children and adolescents.
- Promoter of mental health with individual children, families, and groups.
- Participant in the research process and consumer of research findings relevant to child and adolescent psychiatric–mental health nursing.

Clinical specialists are nurses who hold at least a master's degree in child and adolescent psychiatric nursing, have had supervised clinical practice at the graduate level, and demonstrate breadth and depth of knowledge, skills, and competence in the field. Certification is highly recommended for the specialist. Specialists may assume any of the generalist roles and may also assume, but are not limited to, these additional roles:

- Psychotherapist for individual children, groups of children, and families.
- Clinical supervisor of client care staff and graduate nursing students.
- Administrator of child and adolescent psychiatric–mental health nursing services.
- Educator of nurses and other child care personnel in a variety of academic and clinical settings.
- Consultant to professional and nonprofessional individuals or groups concerned with the general welfare, education, and care of children.
- Researcher who contributes to the theory and practice of child and adolescent psychiatric–mental health nursing through research in this field or a related field.

The actual standards, presented in the accompanying box, pertain to all settings in which nurses practice. They apply to children at various developmental levels.

ANA Standards of Child and Adolescent Psychiatric and Mental Health Nursing Practice

Professional Practice Standards

Standard I. Theory The nurse applies appropriate, scientifically sound theory as a basis for nursing practice decisions.

Standard II. Assessment The nurse systematically collects, records, and analyzes data that are comprehensive and accurate.

Standard III. Diagnosis The nurse, in expressing conclusions supported by recorded assessment and current scientific premises, uses nursing diagnoses and/or standard classifications of mental disorders for childhood and adolescence.

Standard IV. Planning The nurse develops a nursing care plan with specific goals and interventions delineating nursing actions unique to the needs of each child or adolescent, as well as those of the family and other relevant interactive social systems.

Standard V. Intervention The nurse intervenes as guided by the nursing care plan to implement nursing actions that promote, maintain, or restore physical and mental health, prevent illness, effect rehabilitation in childhood and adolescence, and restore developmental progression.

Standard V-A. Intervention: Therapeutic Environment The nurse provides, structures, and maintains a therapeutic environment in collaboration with the child or adolescent, the family, and other health care providers.

Standard V-B. Intervention: Activities of Daily Living The nurse uses the activities of daily living in a goal-directed way to foster the physical and mental well-being of the child or adolescent and family.

Standard V-C. Intervention: Psychotherapeutic Interventions The nurse uses psychotherapeutic interventions to assist children or adolescents and families to develop, improve, or regain their adaptive functioning, to promote health, prevent illness, and facilitate rehabilitation.

Standard V-D. Intervention: Psychotherapy* The child and adolescent psychiatric and mental health specialist uses advanced clinical expertise to function as a psychotherapist for the child or adolescent and family and accepts professional accountability for nursing practice.

Standard V-E. Intervention: Health Teaching and Anticipatory Guidance The nurse assists the child or adolescent and family to achieve more satisfying and productive patterns of living through health teaching and anticipatory guidance.

Standard V-F. Intervention: Somatic Therapies The nurse uses knowledge of somatic therapies with the child or adolescent and family to enhance therapeutic interventions.

Standard VI. Evaluation The nurse evaluates the response of the child or adolescent and family to nursing actions in order to revise the database, nursing diagnoses, and nursing care plan.

Professional Performance Standards

Standard VII. Quality Assurance The nurse participates in peer review and other means of evaluation to assure quality of nursing care provided for children and adolescents and their families.

Standard VIII. Continuing Education The nurse assumes responsibility for continuing education and professional development and contributes to the professional growth of others studying children's and adolescents' mental health.

Standard IX. Interdisciplinary Collaboration The nurse collaborates with other health care providers in assessing, planning, implementing, and evaluating programs and other activities related to child and adolescent psychiatric and mental health nursing.

Standard X. Use of Community Health Systems* The nurse participates with other members of the community in assessing, planning, implementing, and evaluating mental health services and community systems that attend to primary, secondary, and tertiary prevention of mental disorders in children and adolescents.

Standard XI. Research The nurse contributes to nursing and the child and adolescent psychiatric and mental health field through innovations in theory and practice and participation in research, and communicates these contributions.

**Standards V-D and X apply only to the clinical specialist in child and adolescent psychiatric and mental health nursing.*

Source: American Nurses Association 1985. Reprinted with permission of the American Nurses Association.

Psychiatric Disorders of Infancy and Childhood

A number of mental health problems typically appear in childhood, although they may continue into adulthood, or manifest themselves as other psychiatric disorders in later life. Each type of disorder has a particular constellation of symptoms or descriptive features that sets it apart from others. Remember that the disorders described in this chapter are not the only ones found in childhood, but they represent the disorders first diagnosed or quite commonly found in childhood.

Mental Retardation

The major feature of **mental retardation** is significantly subaverage intellectual functioning (an IQ below 70 in children, or, in infants, clinical judgment based on cognitive tests). The degree of severity of intellectual impairment is described as mild (IQ 50/55–70), moderate (IQ 35/40–50/55), severe (IQ 20/25–35/40), or profound (IQ below 20/25). The child must also show deficits or impairments in adaptive functioning in at least two areas of life; for example, communication, social/interpersonal skills, or safety. The onset of this disorder occurs before the age of 18.

Mental retardation is found in approximately 1% of the population. The major risk factor for retardation is the early alteration of embryonic development as a result of exposure to toxins in utero (maternal drug use, for example) or chromosomal changes (such as Down syndrome). Other predisposing factors include inherited errors of metabolism (such as fragile X syndrome), pregnancy and perinatal problems such as prematurity or trauma, medical conditions acquired in infancy or childhood, and early environmental influences such as deprivation of nurturance or other stimulation.

Learning Disorders

A **learning disorder** may be diagnosed when a child's achievement on standardized tests in reading, mathematics, or written expression is substantially below what is expected for his or her age, schooling, or intelligence level. The problems are so major as to significantly interfere with the child's activities of daily living or academic progress.

Learning disorders affect 2–10% of the population, with about 5% of all public school students identified as having a learning disorder. Reading is the major learning problem.

Motor Skills Disorder

A **motor skills disorder**, marked impairment in the development of motor coordination, occurs in approximately 6% of all children. You may first notice this problem in a child's delay in achieving motor milestones such as walking or crawling, in "clumsiness," and in poor handwriting or sports performance. To be considered a psychiatric disorder, the impairment must significantly interfere with the child's academic achievement or activities of daily living and not be the result of a physical health problem such as cerebral palsy.

Communication Disorders

Communication disorders can be one of four different problems: impairments in language expression, in the understanding of language, in phonology, or stuttering. These impairments must be severe enough to interfere with academic achievement or social communication. Problems in language expression may include a markedly limited vocabulary, errors in tense, or difficulty recalling words or producing sentences with developmentally appropriate length or complexity. Problems in understanding language include difficulty understanding words, sentences, or specific types of words. The symptom of a phonological disorder is the failure to use developmentally expected speech sounds appropriate for a child's age and dialect. For example, the child may substitute one sound for another ("t" for "k") or omit sounds in words. Stuttering is a disturbance in the normal timing and fluency of speech; for instance, frequent repetitions, prolonged sounds, or pauses in the middle of a word. Word substitution is often used by a child to avoid problematic words.

While stuttering occurs in about 1% of prepubertal children, the prevalence of the other communication disorders is somewhat greater: about 3–5% of all children. When considering a diagnosis of communication disorder, remember to evaluate any problems within the cultural and language context of a child, especially if the child is bilingual. The only known predisposing factor for the development of a communication disorder is a family history of the disorder. For stuttering, especially, family and twin studies provide strong evidence of a genetic factor in its etiology.

Pervasive Developmental Disorders

The pervasive developmental disorders include autistic disorder, Rett's disorder, childhood disintegrative disorder, and Asperger's disorder. Each of these psychiatric conditions usually arises in the first years of life and is characterized by severe developmental impairment in several areas.

Autistic, disintegrative, and Asperger's disorders are much more common in boys, with autism having rates four to five times higher for boys. Rett's disorder has been found only to occur in girls. The reasons for these gender differences are not yet understood.

All of these disorders are rare, with autistic disorder having the highest incidence. It occurs in 2–5 children per 10,000. Regardless of the small percentage of children affected by pervasive developmental disorders, their impact on children and families is enormous. They also represent a substantial segment of the families to whom child psychiatric nurses provide care, because the problems these families encounter are severe and require much professional support.

AUTISTIC DISORDER Sometimes referred to as autism, **autistic disorder** involves difficulties in both the quality of a child's social interaction and communication. In social interaction, the child may have problems making eye contact, fail to develop appropriate peer relationships, fail to spontaneously seek out shared enjoyment with other people, or show no social or emotional reciprocity. In communication, the child may have a delay in developing language or a total absence of speech; use language in a stereotyped, repetitive, or idiosyncratic fashion; show deficits in spontaneous, imaginative play; or have a restricted, repetitive repertoire of interests or behaviors (as in folding a facial tissue repeatedly or flapping his or her hands up and down).

There is also a diagnosis of mental retardation in about 75% of children with autism, usually in the moderate range. The onset of autism is prior to age 3. Parents may tell you that their baby does not want to cuddle, has an indifference to touch and affection, does not make eye contact, or is not facially responsive. Children may also have many associated behavioral problems such as hyperactivity, aggressiveness, self-injurious behaviors (such as head banging), temper tantrums, and unusual sensitivities to sensory stimuli (such as an oversensitivity to touch or a high threshold for pain). You may notice abnormal mood or affect as well; for example, either an overreaction or an absence of any emotional reaction by the child to the environment.

RETT'S DISORDER **Rett's disorder** is the accumulation of multiple developmental deficits by a child after there has been a period of normal development during the first 5 months of life. Within the first or second year of life, the baby begins to show deceleration in head growth, loss of previously acquired hand skills and eventual stereotyped hand movements, loss of social engagement, poorly coordinated gait or trunk movements, and severely impaired language development with severe psychomotor retardation. The disorder is lifelong, with persistent and progressive loss of skills. Only modest developmental gains have been noted in a few children later in their childhood or adolescence.

CHILDHOOD DISINTEGRATIVE DISORDER **Childhood disintegrative disorder (CDD)** is quite similar to Rett's disorder except that its period of normal development is much longer, with symptoms not appearing until age 2–10. In addition, there is no head growth deceleration or loss of hand skills. Instead, the losses involve skills in expressive or receptive language, social skills, play, and bowel or bladder control. Some of the abnormalities of functioning that develop are similar to those in autistic disorder, such as impairments in social interaction, communication, and repetitive, restricted, stereotyped behavior. However, in autistic disorder, the abnormalities are usually noticed within the first year of life and do not reflect the pattern of developmental regression found in CDD.

ASPERGER'S DISORDER **Asperger's disorder** has some but not all of the features of autism. Children with this disorder show the same problems with social interaction and restricted, repetitive behavior as in autism. However, there is no delay in language, in cognitive development, in age appropriate self-help and adaptive skills, or in curiosity about the environment. The onset of the disorder is also later than autism, most commonly in the preschool period. In contrast to CDD, there is no loss of previously acquired skills in Asperger's disorder.

Attention Deficit and Disruptive Behavior Disorders

This category of child psychiatric problems includes attention deficit hyperactivity disorder, conduct disorder, and oppositional defiant disorder. While there are certain behavioral symptoms common to all of these disorders, they each have a unique constellation of symptoms.

ATTENTION DEFICIT HYPERACTIVITY DISORDER The most distinctive features of **attention deficit hyperactivity disorder (ADHD)** are the child's inattention to the surrounding environment, and hyperactivity and/or impulsiveness. Both of these symptoms must persist for at least 6 months, be apparent in two or more settings, be inconsistent with the child's developmental level, and cause clinically significant impairment in functioning. In addition, some of these symptoms must have been present prior to age 7. To determine whether inattention exists, look for behaviors such as making careless mistakes in schoolwork, not listening when spoken to, disliking tasks that require sustained mental effort, and being easily distracted by extraneous stimuli. You will see hyperactivity in fidgeting or squirming, running around when the child is asked to stay seated, or talking excessively. Signs of impulsiveness are a child's difficulty waiting for his or her turn in activities, or interrupting others. Most children with this disorder have a combination of symptoms indicating both inattention and hyperactivity-impulsiveness, but some children have predominantly one or the other of the features.

ADHD is most commonly diagnosed in early school years, when demands for sustained attention increase. By late childhood and adolescence, excesses in gross motor activity become less apparent, and symptoms may reflect primarily fidgetiness or even inner feelings of restlessness without any observable signs. A client profile that includes ADHD is in the next section on conduct disorder.

CONDUCT DISORDER **Conduct disorder (CD)** is one of the most frequently diagnosed problems for children. Boys show an incidence of 6–16%, while only about 2–9% of girls have this disorder. The central feature of CD is repetitive and persistent behavior in which the basic rights of others or major age-appropriate societal norms or rules are violated. Look for behaviors that show aggression toward people and animals, destruction of property, deceitfulness or theft, or serious violation of parental or school rules. These symptoms may appear as early as 5–6 years of age, but occur more typically in later childhood or early adolescence. There are two subtypes of this disorder: childhood-onset and adolescent-onset. Childhood-onset must show at least one symptom prior to 10 years of age. In the majority of cases, the disorder remits by adulthood, but those individuals with childhood-onset are more likely to develop adult antisocial personality disorder (ASPD; see Chapter 20) than are those with onset in adolescence. The diagnosis of CD is made only when the behavior is symptomatic of a problem within the child and not a reaction to a social context of war, poverty, high crime, or fear for one's well-being.

Boys with the disorder are more likely to fight, steal, vandalize, or have school problems, whereas girls are more likely to run away, be truant, or show evidence of prostitution or substance use. Girls usually do not show confrontational behavior. While almost all cases of CD in childhood are boys, there is a more even gender balance in adolescent-onset. Children with the disorder may have little empathy toward others, and in ambiguous situations, they often misinterpret the intentions of others as hostile and threatening, responding with aggressive behavior which they view as reasonable and justified. Self-esteem is commonly low but covered up by a facade of toughness.

Rob, a 9-year-old boy, was recently diagnosed with conduct disorder in addition to an earlier diagnosis of attention deficit hyperactivity disorder. Rob has been in numerous fights at school for the past 2 months. His grades have dropped substantially, and he was caught vandalizing school property. At home, he refuses to talk to his parents and hit his mother when she was yelling at him for stealing money from her purse.

Rob's long history of behavioral problems began with temper tantrums at 6 months of age. At the age of 3, he cut up the family sofa. His parents took him out of preschool because the teachers couldn't handle his behavior, especially his shoving other children and running around. During his early school years he had difficulty in concentrating and focusing on an activity for a sustained period of time, and interrupted ongoing activities. He has almost no friends in school.

Rob views his problems as the result of others' hostile and threatening intent. He expresses much anger toward the "school bullies" and all authority figures in his life.

OPPOSITIONAL DEFIANT DISORDER All of the features of **oppositional defiant disorder (ODD)** are usually present in conduct disorder, so it is not diagnosed if it meets the criteria for CD. ODD is a recurrent and hostile pattern of behavior toward authority figures. However, it does not involve the physical aggression, destructive behavior, deceitfulness, theft, or serious violation of rules shown in CD. ODD has a prevalence rate of 2–16%. It is more common in children from families where the child experiences many different caregivers; families in which harsh, inconsistent, or neglectful child-rearing practices are used; where mothers are depressed; or where serious marital discord exists. The disorder is associated with problematic preschool temperaments and a high degree of motor activity by the child. ODD usually becomes apparent before age 8, with symptoms first appearing in the home and then later within other settings. The child may show low self-esteem, minimal frustration tolerance, swearing, mood lability, and precocious use of tobacco, alcohol, or illegal drugs.

Feeding and Eating Disorders

Three disorders in this category are specific to childhood: pica, rumination disorder, and feeding disorder of infancy or early childhood. Anorexia nervosa and bulimia nervosa may also occur during later childhood, but these disorders are discussed in Chapter 18 because they are not unique to childhood, nor do they necessarily first appear in childhood.

PICA **Pica** is a disorder in which the child persistently eats nonnutritive substances (such as paint, plaster, string, hair, cloth, animal droppings, insects, or leaves). The behavior must be inappropriate for the developmental level of the child and not part of a culturally sanctioned practice. This disorder is most frequently seen in preschool children and in individuals who are retarded. Lack of adequate supervision, neglect, and poverty increase the possibility of the problem. Usually the disorder lasts only for a few months, but it can continue into adolescence or adulthood.

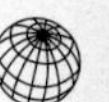

RUMINATION DISORDER **Rumination disorder** is the repeated regurgitation and rechewing of food. It appears after a period of normal eating behavior in an infant or child. The child brings up partially digested food into the mouth, without any evidence of nausea or retching, and then chews and reswallows it. Sometimes the food is spit out. These symptoms are not associated with any medical condition or with any other eating disorder. Rumination disorder is most common in male infants between 3 and 12 months of age. You will see a characteristic straining and arching of the back in these babies, and they make sucking movements with the tongue, appearing to enjoy the process very much. However, between the times of regurgitation, these babies are often irritable and hungry, and they eat a lot when fed. Because they regurgitate immediately after eating, there is common weight loss or failure to gain expected weight. Certain factors place an infant at risk for the disorder, including lack of stimulation, neglect, and problems in the parent-child relationship. In turn, the unsuccessful nature of the feeding experience and the aversive nature of the regurgitation may result in a parent's difficulty in providing responsive or loving care.

FEEDING DISORDER OF INFANCY OR EARLY CHILDHOOD **Feeding disorder of infancy or early childhood** is the persistent failure to eat adequately, accompanied by either a failure to gain weight or significant weight loss. Resulting malnutrition can threaten the baby's life. As with other disorders in this category, there is no medical condition causing the behavior. Babies with this problem are particularly irritable and difficult to console during feeding. At other times, they may appear apathetic or withdrawn. Infants who have preexisting developmental impairments or problems with regulation of the nervous system (for example, sleep-wake irregularities) may be less responsive to the parent, creating difficulties in the feeding process. In addition, parent behavior can make the feeding problem worse. For example, a parent may force the food into a baby's mouth too roughly or at too rapid a pace. There is a high incidence of parental psychopathology as well as child abuse or neglect associated with the condition. Although the disorder is most common in infancy (about 1–3% of all pediatric hospital admissions), it may have its onset as late as age 2–3. Most children eventually achieve improved growth patterns.

Tic Disorders

There are three disorders classified as tics: Tourette's disorder, chronic motor or vocal tics disorder, and transient tic disorder. In each of these conditions, there is a rapid, recurring, nonrhythmic, stereotyped movement or vocalization that occurs suddenly and involuntarily. Tics are worse during stress but occur less frequently when the child is focused intently on an activity such as reading.

Most tic disorders appear to be transmitted through a genetic or constitutional factor, which gives the child a vulnerability to developing the disorder. However, about 10% of children with the disorder have a "nongenetic" form; these children frequently have a dual diagnosis with another mental disorder or a medical condition such as epilepsy. Regardless of type, boys are more likely to develop tic disorders than girls.

TOURETTE'S DISORDER **Tourette's disorder** involves multiple motor tics and one or more vocal tics, which can occur simultaneously or at different periods during the illness. The diagnosis requires that there is never a tic-free period for more than 3 months. Vocal tics are words or sounds such as yelps, barks, snorts, or coughs. **Coprolalia** is a specific type of vocal tic in which obscenities are uttered. *Motor tics* include such behavior as eye blinking, protruding the tongue, sniffing, retracing steps, or twirling when walking. The disorder may begin as early as age 2, but more often it starts during childhood or early adolescence. Tourette's disorder normally lasts for a lifetime with periods of remission, but in most cases the symptoms decrease during adolescence and adulthood.

CHRONIC MOTOR OR VOCAL TIC DISORDER AND TRANSIENT TIC DISORDER **Chronic motor or vocal tic disorder** differs from Tourette's disorder in that it involves *either* motor tics or vocal tics, but not both, as is required for a diagnosis of Tourette's disorder. **Transient tic disorder** differs from all of the above in its duration. While the others require that the problems have occurred for at least a year, transient tic disorder does not last longer than 12 months.

Elimination Disorders

The elimination disorders are encopresis and enuresis. In order to be classified as a mental disorder, these problems must not be due to any medical condition or to the physiologic effects of a laxative, diuretic, or other substance.

Encopresis is the repeated passing of feces by the child into inappropriate places such as clothing or a corner of the room. This is usually involuntary behavior, but it may be intentional in some situations. There are two subtypes of the disorder. The first involves constipation and continuous leakage of feces during the day and during sleep. Incontinence stops once the constipation is treated. The constipation may develop for psychologic reasons, often related to a general pattern of anxious or oppositional behavior that leads the child to avoid defecation. Health problems causing dehydration, or the side effects of medication, may also initially create the constipation, but once it has developed, a child may retain stool because of painful defecation or anal fissure. The second subtype does not involve constipation or incontinence. Feces are normal and soiling is intermittent, with feces usually found in an obvious place. Children with this subtype often have a dual diagnosis of ODD or CD. With either subtype, smearing the feces may result from attempts to clean or hide the feces, or it may be a deliberate effort to make a mess.

Enuresis is the repeated voiding of urine into the bed or clothes, either during the day or at night. The *nocturnal type* is most common and typically occurs during the first part of the night. The *diurnal type* (during waking hours) happens most typically in the early afternoon of school days. This type may be related to social anxiety and a resulting reluctance to use the toilet, or it may be because the child becomes preoccupied with play or other activities. Some children show a combination of both day and night enuresis.

For both encopresis and enuresis, there is a primary and secondary type. With the *primary type,* the child has never achieved fecal or urinary continence. In the *secondary type,* the disturbance develops after a period of continence. Of course, the problem is not diagnosed as a mental disorder unless the child has reached a chronological age where elimination problems should not be apparent (at least age 4 for encopresis and age 5 for enuresis).

Predisposing factors for both disorders include inconsistent or lax toilet training, or psychosocial stressors such as entry to school or a sibling birth. In contrast to encopresis, about 75% of all children with enuresis have a first-degree biologic relative with the disorder.

Both disorders are more common in boys, with prevalence rates for enuresis being higher (3–7% of 5-year-olds) than for encopresis (1% of all 5-year-olds). Neither disorder is typically chronic. Most children become continent by adolescence. The degree of immediate and long-term impairment depends to a great extent on the amount of resulting peer rejection, punishment and rejection by the caregiver, and a child's overall self-esteem.

Anxiety Disorders

Anxiety disorders are discussed in detail in Chapter 16 because in general, their symptoms are similar in both children and adults. Phobias may be seen in children even before age 5. The onset of obsessive-compulsive disorder (OCD) is common for children age 9–11. Generalized anxiety disorder (GAD) and posttraumatic stress disorder (PTSD) are also found in children (see Chapter 16).

SEPARATION ANXIETY DISORDER There is one anxiety disorder that is specific to childhood: **separation anxiety disorder.** This mental health problem involves a developmentally inappropriate and excessive anxiety over separation from home or from attachment figures. Symptoms may include fear and worry about possible harm befalling attachment figures or about being separated from them. There is usually a reluctance or refusal to go to school, be without attachment figures, or go to sleep without them nearby. It is also common for the child to have somatic complaints when separation occurs or is anticipated. Children with this disorder frequently come from close-knit families and are often described as demanding, intrusive, or in need of constant attention. They may also be unusually compliant, conscientious, or eager to please. Depressed mood is typical and may increase over time.

The disorder occurs in about 4% of children and may appear after a stressful life event such as the death of a pet, a family illness, or immigration. There are periods of exacerbation and remission over the course of the disorder that persist for many years, including into adulthood.

Mood Disorders

Mood disorders are discussed fully in Chapter 15, so they will not be covered in detail here. However, a few issues related to mood disorders in children are important to note. One class of mood disorders, bipolar disorders, is very rare in childhood. In contrast, another class, depressive disorders, is quite common in children, with depressive symptoms occurring even in the first year of life. Diagnoses are usually not made during infancy, because developmentally, children often do not have the ability to reflect on their feelings even if the feelings are strongly affecting them. Also remember that children may not be able to accurately report symptoms even if they are experiencing them.

The two types of depressive disorders are major depression and dysthymia. Major depression involves a definite change in behavior from the child's normal functioning. The child begins to show a depressed or sad mood or a lack of pleasure (anhedonia) in almost all activities at least 50% of the time. There are some important differences in how children and adults may manifest these symptoms. Children may describe things as bad, gloomy, blue, or empty when they are depressed. You may see a bland, frozen look on their faces or only fleeting smiles, as if they are smiling because it is socially expected rather than because they feel like smiling. On the other hand, you may see no evidence of sadness in children but rather a persistent irritability around even small matters. Boredom is a common sign of anhedonia in children (50–90% of the time). Another sign is social withdrawal, especially when a child avoids or rejects opportunities to play. Other symptoms of depression in children include unexplained somatic complaints, poor school performance, sleep and appetite changes, and/or psychomotor agitation and increased risk taking. The most common type of depression in children is called *reactive depression,* meaning that it occurs in response to a particular situation, such as the trauma of hospitalization or an extended separation from a parent.

Dysthymia is a chronic disorder in which there are periods of depressed affect interspersed with normal mood. Symptoms of later adult dysthymia often begin in childhood, even if not diagnosed until later. Because of this early and chronic quality, the person is often described as a "depressive personality." Although the symptoms of dysthymia are the same for children and adults, children are likely to show greater evidence of irritability, not simply depressed affect, and may react negatively or shyly to praise. They may respond to positive relationships with testing, anger, or avoidance. Other symptoms of dysthymia are similar to those described for major depression, except that the child may show more evidence of low energy and low self-esteem. A key predisposing factor for childhood dysthymia is the presence of an inadequate, rejecting, or chaotic home environment.

There is strong evidence of a familial pattern for both major depression and dysthymia, with clear support for a genetic, biochemical etiology. Although there is a greater incidence of depressive disorders for women in adulthood, the prepubertal incidence is the same for boys and girls (about 2% of all children).

Other Disorders Specific to Childhood

Three other disorders are usually first diagnosed in childhood: selective mutism, reactive attachment disorder of infancy or early childhood, and stereotypic movement disorder.

SELECTIVE MUTISM **Selective mutism** is the persistent failure to speak in specific social situations, even though the child can speak in other situations. Of course, the failure to speak must not be the result of a lack of normal language skills or knowledge of a certain language. The child can be excessively shy, fearful of embarrassment, withdrawn, clinging, and negative; the child may have temper tantrums or show oppositional behavior, especially at home. Mutism is rare, but slightly more common in girls. Usually, the disturbance lasts for only a few months, but it can continue for several years.

REACTIVE ATTACHMENT DISORDER OF INFANCY OR EARLY CHILDHOOD **Reactive attachment disorder of infancy or early childhood** is a markedly disturbed and developmentally inappropriate way of relating that is presumed to be the result of gross pathologic care. This pathologic care may be any of the following:

- Persistent disregard of the child's basic emotional needs for comfort, stimulation, or affection.
- Persistent disregard of the child's basic physical needs.
- Repeated changes of caregivers that prevent the formation of stable attachments.

However, not all children who experience gross pathologic care will develop the disorder.

Two types of this disorder are distinctly opposite in their symptoms. The *inhibited type* involves a failure to initiate and respond to most social interactions in a developmentally appropriate way. Children show excessively inhibited, hypervigilant, or ambivalent responses. Examples are a look of frozen watchfulness, resistance to comfort, and a mixture of approach and avoidance. In contrast, the *disinhibited type* involves an indiscriminate sociability or lack of selectivity in the choice of attachment figures. The child may be excessively familiar with strangers in demonstrating affection or seeking comfort and affection from a variety of adults who are not well known to the child. The severity and duration of the disorder depend on the degree of psychosocial deprivation and the nature of any intervention. If a supportive environment is provided, improvement does occur. Children with this disorder commonly have a feeding and eating disorder as well.

STEREOTYPIC MOVEMENT DISORDER **Stereotypic movement disorder** is a pattern of motor behavior that is repetitive and nonfunctional and one that the child appears driven to do. Examples of such movements are rocking, twirling objects, head banging, self-biting, picking at skin or body orifices, or hitting parts of one's own body. The specific behaviors may change over time from one type of behavior to another. The disorder can result in tissue damage or be life-threatening, and it is frequently associated with mental retardation. Sometimes children try to restrain themselves from the behavior, for example, by putting their hands in their pockets; but if the restraint is interfered with, the behaviors resume. Onset of the disorder may follow a stressful event.

CHILDHOOD-ONSET SCHIZOPHRENIA Occuring as early as age 5 or 6, **childhood-onset schizophrenia** is rare. Its incidence is about 1 in every 1000 children, mostly boys. The features of schizophrenia (delusions, hallucinations, disorganized speech and behavior, and negative symptoms) are the same in children as adults. (Schizophrenia is discussed fully in Chapter 14.)

Doris, an 11-year-old, described hearing the voice of her mother calling her name and yelling at her, although her mother was not present. At times, she heard her own voice telling her to do things such as chores for her mother. She experienced her mother's voice as coming from outside her head and her own voice as coming from inside her head. She reported seeing a woman who looked like her mother and

she thought was her mother. She also believed that her mother was watching her. Doris described going to the bathroom in the morning and "daydreaming" that objects were weapons (e.g., cotton swabs were sticks to stab people, and washcloths were used to smother people). All these experiences seemed real to Doris as they happened. Doris also believed that the world was coming to an end. She described hearing on the news that a hole was breaking apart pieces of the earth, and she thought this was going to happen. She also expressed concern that a heat wave might result in there not being enough air to breathe.

It is difficult to make the diagnosis in children, however, because delusions and hallucinations are less detailed and more accepted developmentally as normal fantasy or imaginary playmates. Disorganized speech (such as in communication disorders) or disorganized behavior (as in ADHD or autistic disorder) may result in other diagnoses when they are actually symptoms of schizophrenia.

Biopsychosocial Theories

Five major theories guide existing views regarding the etiology of childhood psychopathology and the therapeutic approaches underlying its prevention and treatment. These are psychodynamic theory, object-relations theory, attachment theory, cognitive-behavioral theory, and biologic diathesis theory. Although many specific schools of thought fall within these perspectives, only the central features of these overarching theories will be discussed here.

Psychodynamic Theory

Psychodynamic theory originated with Freud in his conceptualization of psychoanalysis but has evolved substantially since its original formulation. Much of Freud's speculation regarding psychosexual stages of development has been rejected, but many components of his personality theory continue to serve as a foundation for assessment and treatment in child psychiatry.

A central component of this theory is the concept of *psychic determinism,* which proposes that the child's initial perceptions of the world are defined substantially during the first 5–6 years of life and will influence the child's later views and behavior in a causal way. While this stance seems almost a given in today's world, the concept was unheard of when Freud first proposed it. Psychodynamic theory also holds that the child is born with instincts for the gratification of needs to ensure survival. *Libido* is described as the psychic energy that makes the child try to meet these needs. If the needs are not satisfied during development, the child may become so fixated on meeting the needs that they influence much of his or her behavior.

In addition, children attempt to ward off and cope with the anxiety associated with need deprivation through the unconscious mental processes known as defense mechanisms (see Chapter 4). Defense mechanisms commonly employed by children are repression, reaction formation, and projection. The child comes to deal with the world through these distorted views in an attempt to defend against painful unconscious issues. However, the unconscious content continues to influence the behavior and conscious thoughts of the child, often in ways which severely impair his or her ability to function in life. Defense mechanisms are, therefore, considered to be symptoms of mental health problems. The focus of treatment is attempting to bring repressed conflicts and issues into awareness so that they can be addressed and resolved. Refer to the Research Note for a discussion of a study evaluating the effectiveness of psychoanalytic approaches with children.

Object-Relations Theory

Object-relations theory is built upon the foundation of psychodynamic theory and is based in the work of Fairbairn (1962); Winnicott (1965); and others (Greenberg and Mitchell 1983; Stern 1985). In this theory, an "object" is defined as a person or thing in the child's environment that has psychologic significance to the child.

A major assumption of this theory is that rather than being driven simply by physical needs or instincts that enhance survival, infants have an innate biologic need for relationships. These relationships increase in quality and complexity as a child develops. Initially infants are undifferentiated from the object they seek (the primary caregiver) and are in a state of diffuse, unorganized experiences. The child is totally dependent upon the mother to organize the child's different experiences into an understandable whole. As the young child begins to differentiate—that is, separate and develop a sense of his or her own self as an individual—the relationships with interpersonal "objects" in the world of the child are internalized and become the internal mental representations that form the self.

The differentiated self forms the basis for the child's future views of his or her own worth and the availability and responsiveness of others. Ultimately, it determines whether or not the child becomes healthy, strong, and creative. Development of the self is considered to depend primarily on the relationship between mother and child, and how effectively a mother responds to the baby's needs and assists in organizing experience. Object-relations theorists maintain that an individual will repeat in relationships throughout life what is learned about self and others from the individual's initial experience with the primary caregiver.

RESEARCH NOTE

Citation

Target M, Fonagy P: Efficacy of psychoanalysis for children with emotional disorders. *J Am Acad Child Adol Psych* 1994;33:361–371.

Study Problem/Purpose

Although the psychoanalytic approach has been a foundation of child psychotherapy, little evaluation of its effects has been done. The purpose of this study was to determine the impact of psychoanalytic treatment on the improvement of children diagnosed with depression or anxiety.

Methods

Two-hundred fifty-four children received daily analysis, and 100 were treated 1–3 times a week over an average of 2 years. Specific criteria for improvement after treatment included the absence of the original psychiatric diagnosis and a change in overall adaptation as measured by the Children's Global Assessment Scale (CGAS).

Findings

Rates of improvement as a result of treatment ranged from 40% to 71%. Depressed children benefited less from the treatment than did children with anxiety disorders. Younger children did significantly better than those who were older when treated. The intensity of treatment influenced the outcome, since 87% of those given full analytic treatment exhibited reliable change and 86% moved from the dysfunctional group. The strongest predictors of a good outcome were a relatively high CGAS score at the time of assessment, a longer treatment time, and a mother who functioned relatively well psychologically at the time the child was referred.

Implications

The results indicate that "internalizing" disorders in children do improve after psychoanalytic treatment. However, as the authors point out, the improvements are not significantly greater than what occurs through the spontaneous or natural history of most of these disorders. The degree of improvement does seem superior to that found for "general" psychotherapy with children, although it is unclear where the authors acquired the data for this comparison or just what modalities have been combined under the rubric of general psychotherapy.

That most important implication of this study is that intensive treatment (frequent sessions of 4–5 times per week) may be essential for more severely disturbed children, yet may be a waste of time and money for children with only moderate levels of emotional disorder. However, it is possible that treatment with psychoanalysis—or any form of psychotherapy, for that matter—is not the critical factor at all. Perhaps the opportunity for a child to spend one-to-one time with a caring adult 4–5 times a week is what really makes the difference in the recovery of severely mentally ill children. What if the outcomes were the same if the adult were an attentive, sensitive caretaker, with minimal education and no psychotherapeutic training? Such questions must be addressed through future comparative studies, because the answer has significant societal implications for providing effective services to a broader base of children at relatively low cost.

Attachment Theory

Attachment theory builds on the psychodynamic concepts of psychic determinism and the impact of unconscious processes. As in object-relations theory, relationships are viewed as the organizing principle for the development of psychologic well-being in the child. However, the concept of *security* within the relationship is the main focus of attachment theory. Attachment theory was originally described by Bowlby (1969; 1973) and later extended by Ainsworth et al. (1978) and others.

Attachment refers to the socioemotional bond of the child to another person (the attachment figure) who is perceived as strong or powerful and who can be turned to for protection and support in situations of perceived danger or adversity. Infants are viewed as coming into the world with an innate neurobiologic structure called the attachment behavioral system. This evolutionary-based adaptive system monitors and processes information regarding uncertainty, stress, or potential danger; and accessibility of the attachment figure during these situations. The infant appraises both the environmental conditions and his or her emotional state to determine how much proximity or contact is needed in order to feel secure. The child then uses attachment behaviors (proximity or contact-promoting behaviors such as calling, approaching, or clinging) to acquire a sense of security.

The ways the attachment figure responds to the child's attachment behaviors are considered critical to the foundation of the child's internal working models. These models are ways of viewing relationships that will come to guide the child's evaluation of his or her own capacity to handle stress, as well as the responses he or she expects of others in times of need. Four major patterns of attachment have been identified as resulting from the initial experiences with the primary attachment figure.

1. Secure
2. Insecure-avoidant
3. Insecure-resistant
4. Disorganized

While the first three patterns reflect different internal working models, the last pattern is viewed as a lack of any integrated or consolidated model to guide attachment behavior during situations where comfort or felt security is needed.

Secure working models involve a view of the attachment figure as available and responsive, and they encourage the child to seek security through proximity and contact. *Insecure-avoidant* children appear indifferent to stress and uncertainty, although their physiologic responses suggest otherwise. They actively avoid their attachment figure during stressful times and focus on other things, such as play. Research suggests that this pattern results from an insensitivity of the caregiver to the child's needs for comforting and an active rebuffing of the child's attempts to be comforted during distress (Main 1990).

Children with *insecure-resistant* patterns of attachment tend to resist interaction and contact with the caregiver when it is available, yet show proximity-seeking behavior when it is not available. They shift between excessively seeking and monitoring comfort, and being difficult to settle or soothe when contact is acquired. Primary caregivers of these children tend to be unpredictable in their accessibility, less adaptable, hesitant, and occupied with caregiving routines rather than providing tender, sensitive care (Weber, Levitt, and Clark 1986).

Infants with a *disorganized* attachment pattern show unexplainable behaviors toward the attachment figure during distress, seemingly conflicted or disoriented behavior such as frightened expressions and freezing while greeting the parent with raised arms, smiling while forcefully striking the parent's face, or extended rocking or ear pulling. Some parents of these children behave in frightening or threatening ways toward the infant or else reverse roles with the infant, acting timid or deferential to the child even when he or she is very small.

These various patterns can be seen in children by 12 months of age and eventually stabilize into cognitive frameworks that influence all intimate relationships in adulthood. While the primary attachment relationship is seen as central to the development of these life patterns, other significant relationships and the child's own degree of resilience or temperamental vulnerability are recognized as important mediators in developing secure or insecure attachment patterns (Weiss 1994).

Cognitive-Behavioral Theory

The origins of cognitive-behavioral theory stem from the behavioral learning school of thought (Skinner 1976). However, current views integrate more recent cognitive theory and social learning theory traditions. The basis of this theory is the importance of the environment in the child's psychologic development. The environment encompasses everything to which the child is exposed, including the immediate caregiving environment (the family, school, and neighborhood), as well as the larger sociocultural milieu within which values and expectations are developed. Infants are viewed as coming into the world with a relatively "blank slate," and they develop personality by being conditioned to respond in certain ways by others in the environment. Bandura (1977) emphasized the importance of modeling as well, whereby children learn by watching others and what happens to those people as a result of their behavior.

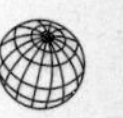

The original views of behavioral theory were that positive and negative reinforcement alone could condition a child's behavior. Bandura (1977) expanded this conceptualization to emphasize the child's ability to deliberate consciously on what occurs and make certain choices about behaviors that are used. He describes this as "reciprocal determinism." In this view, the environment provides information that influences the child in choosing how to behave, but *interpretation* of the environment is the determinant of the child's behavior, not the environment itself. However, without the environment, the child has no stimulus toward growth or development.

Beck (1976) describes the ways in which individuals perceive and make sense of the world through cognitive structures, which he refers to as schemata. Children's experiences with the environment create these schemata, or ways of viewing the world, which then influence what is perceived and how it is processed and understood in all future interactions. Distortions in schemata are considered the central causative factors of mental health problems. Biased or inaccurate ways of thinking or processing information can take a number of forms; for instance, interpreting things as worse than they are, overgeneralization, selective perception, disqualifying the positive, jumping to conclusions, or personalizing events that are not actually related to the child. These distortions are brought about by the irrational beliefs stemming from the child's schemata. External events and relationships set off particular schemata that have been established early in life and that can create major problems in the child's ability to function appropriately, or that are adaptive for the child. Treatment is thus focused on a reeducation or relearning process aimed at the child's irrational beliefs and their related behaviors.

Biologic Diathesis Theory

A *biologic diathesis* is some constitutional predisposition to the development of a disease. There is no single view regarding how a diathesis for mental illness is acquired. Rather, there are many hypotheses regarding the particular biologic characteristics that may make children vulnerable to developing certain psychiatric disorders.

For example, there is considerable evidence for the role of neurobiologic factors in the development of disorders such as autistic disorder and childhood-onset schizophrenia. Children with these disorders have more physical anomalies, neurologic soft signs, and brain abnormalities on EEGs and in CT and MRI scans. These problems are considered potential causes of the mental disorder (Torrey et al. 1994).

There is growing support for the existence of certain abnormalities in neurotransmitter secretion. Serotonin (5-HT) has been of major interest in a number of disorders. For instance, studies suggest that 5-HT levels may be elevated in autism (Anderson and Hoshiro 1987) and depleted in childhood depression (Rutter 1988). However, it is unclear whether the dysfunction in neurotransmitter levels causes the disorder, or whether the disorder may create nervous system changes that cause the neurotransmitter abnormality.

Studies also indicate that problems with nervous system responsiveness may be related to certain psychiatric disorders. For example, children with schizophrenia have unusually high autonomic system reactivity when in baseline or resting states (Zahn 1988), and children with ADHD appear to have a lowered excitability in the reticular activating system of the brain, requiring more stimulation in order to feel optimally aroused (Scatterfield, Scatterfield, and Cantwell 1981).

While the exact relationship between these factors and mental illness is not yet understood, the data suggest three primary factors as the most likely sources of these abnormalities: perinatal complications resulting in CNS injury, a genetic deficiency, and early childhood trauma (McKenna, Gordon, and Rappaport 1994; Pauls 1987). Twin and adoption studies continue to provide evidence in support of genetic etiology for many disorders, including pervasive developmental disorders, schizophrenia, and depression. Adopted children and their biologic parents show much stronger affinity in these disorders than adoptive parents and children. In addition, when one twin has a disorder, the other is much more likely to have the disorder than might be another sibling, parent, or other relative.

Risk Factors for Developing Mental Health Problems in Childhood

- Inherited metabolic deficiencies or abnormalities.
- Injury, or toxic exposure or physical complications in utero or during the perinatal period.
- Medical conditions of infancy or childhood (such as epilepsy, low birth weight).
- Early deprivation of nurturance or stimulation (parental absence or loss, neglect or rejection, large family size, foster placement).
- Family history of a psychiatric disorder.
- A chaotic home environment (family violence or severe marital discord).
- Disadvantaged socioeconomic status (poverty, violence, hopelessness).

Regardless of the genetic evidence, perinatal complications, including perinatal asphyxia, congenital anomalies, and intrauterine exposure to drugs and alcohol have also been found to be associated with psychiatric disorders. Similarly, lead poisoning, CNS trauma, and infections in childhood have all been implicated as possible causative factors.

Integrative, Interactive Theory

While each of the theoretic perspectives just described is often considered in isolation, there is growing acceptance of a multicausal, multidimensional nature in any etiology of mental illness. The accompanying box lists potential risk factors that have been identified for childhood mental illness.

Although various schools of thought may emphasize specific risk factors, as nurses, we need to view mental health in an integrative, interactive way. In this view, the child's biologically based attributes or vulnerabilities are seen to interact with the family and larger social environment to influence mental health outcomes. Many children show tremendous hardiness and resilience in the face of major environmental adversity, while other, more vulnerable children may be severely affected by even a minimally stressful or adverse environment. Not only do the child's characteristics affect how the child will respond to and internalize what is experienced in the environment, but he or she will influence what the environment provides by virtue of a genetically given temperament or biomedical status. Scarr (1987) describes this as children "making their own environments."

It is important to remember that children both:

- Actively elicit and seek out certain responses and experiences, and
- Perceive what is given by the environment through the looking glass of their unique genotype.

These factors interact with what is actually available in the environment to determine the degree to which a child achieves mental health or develops a mental illness. In this theoretic perspective, there is no certain etiology, no predictable set of risk factors, and no specific therapeutic approach having a standard effectiveness. The unique fit between a particular child and a particular environment must be considered to understand the child's mental health problems and develop an appropriate intervention.

The Nursing Process and Child Psychiatric Nursing

The assessment, diagnosis, planning, implementation, and evaluation activities undertaken by the child psychiatric nurse are always in collaboration with the child, the family, and professional colleagues who are part of the child's care. The degree to which these individuals are active partners in the nursing process will influence the resulting quality and efficacy of nursing care.

Assessment

The ability to perform a valid assessment depends on a nurse's knowledge of developmental standards and his or her cultural sensitivity, including gathering pertinent cultural information within which to consider a particular child's behavior.

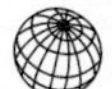

CULTURAL CONTEXT Any nursing assessment must occur within the context of a child's cultural background and developmental stage. What can be defined as "normal or functional" versus "dysfunctional or abnormal" is relative to the meaning certain behaviors have within a culture and the child's developmental capabilities. Lack of attention to cultural beliefs and expectations has resulted in misdiagnosis and mistreatment for many ethnic minority children (Siantz 1993). A comprehensive assessment requires adequate time for full responses to open-ended questions, active listening, and careful observation of patterns of behavior. It also requires that assessment be an ongoing process rather than a one-time session. Do not assume that observations can be generalized to other times and settings.

THE HISTORY-TAKING INTERVIEW WITH PARENTS The most basic assessment includes a history-taking interview with the parent(s) and a clinical assessment of the child. There are four important aspects of history to be acquired from the parents or guardians. First, discuss the history of the child's current problem, including the parents' major concerns or complaints, how long it has been since the problem first began, the specific symptoms they have observed in the child, and their previous and current efforts to address the problem.

Next, talk with the family about their own history and family process. This aspect of the assessment can include a genogram or family time line, discussion of child-rearing beliefs and behaviors, supports and stressors for the family, the history of any separations between parents and the child, and any psychiatric or other illness in the family.

Pay careful attention not only to what the parents say, but to the nonverbal communication among family members. The way in which they interact gives important clues regarding the family's functioning in areas such as closeness, conflict, decision making, and flexibility. See Chapter 32 for specific suggestions on a complete assessment of the family's process.

The maternal grandmother of a suicidal child who was scheduled for admission to an in patient unit tried to block the admission. She told her daughter just to send the child to stay with her for a while. The child psychiatrist and the child psychiatric nurse spent time with the parents discussing the pressure they experienced from the child's grandmother. They reminded the parents that psychiatric services are unfamiliar to the grandmother's generation. They also reviewed the basis for the recommendation of hospitalization. The parents were encouraged to make their own decision based on their experience with their child and their concerns for her safety. Possible explanations for the grandparents were suggested, and the professionals offered to be available to discuss the grandparents' questions and concerns.

The child's medical history is a third area for the interview with the parents. Find out about any childhood illnesses, allergies, medications, and so on. And finally, have the parents describe the child's developmental history. Starting with pregnancy or birth complications, progress through the child's development to identify any lags or events in achieving developmental milestones. Find out the parents' view of the child's temperament, interests, and skills.

An 11-year-old boy with attention deficit hyperactivity disorder and mood disorder was described by his parents as doing poorly on tests in school. The parents were frustrated by their own sense of incompetence and angry at the child for

ASSESSMENT

Assessment Areas During the Mental Status Exam

General Appearance

Grooming, orientation to time and place, alertness, overall demeanor.

Motor Behavior and Coordination

Activity level, gross motor and fine motor control, nature of movements, posture.

Speech and Language

Clarity and articulation, rhythm and organization, appropriateness of word choice.

Thinking and Perception

Ability to understand and express meaning in an age-appropriate way, content, themes in play and talk, threshold and tolerance for sensory input, reality orientation, attention span.

Emotional Status

Overall mood state, manner of expressing feelings, range and intensity of emotions, self-esteem, evidence of dysphoric state (anger, anxiety, sadness).

Interpersonal Style

Eye contact, receptivity versus negativity, independence versus dependence, involvement versus withdrawal.

defeating himself. They generalized their worries to a longitudinal concern that the child would never accomplish anything worthwhile.

During this aspect of the interview, you can also identify the nature of the child's sociocultural environment (home, neighborhood, school) and how it may support or inhibit the achievement of developmental tasks.

CLINICAL ASSESSMENT OF THE CHILD The clinical assessment of the child involves a mental status exam by the nurse and referral of the child for a complete physical and neuropsychologic evaluation. These latter evaluations are important in order to rule out any medical conditions and identify any neurologic or cognitive problems that may be associated with the child's psychiatric symptoms.

A mental status exam consists of both a semistructured interview and an unstructured play session with the child. If the child is nearing adolescence or is ambivalent about unstructured play, try games instead, as a medium through which you can observe the child's way of relating and approaching various situations. For both aspects of the exam, a relaxed, conversational approach is the most effective, where the child has the opportunity to tell you his story about problems he may be having and his relationships with family, peers, and teachers. Frame questions in ways that are developmentally appropriate for the child. Asking children simple, informal questions like what kinds of snacks they like to eat, what they would want if they could have three wishes, or what was the saddest thing that ever happened to them, can provide a great deal of information regarding speech, modes of thinking and perception, and feeling states. Having children draw and discuss pictures of themselves and their family can be very useful for understanding their view of the world. Areas for assessment during the mental status exam are shown in the accompanying Assessment box.

Nursing Diagnosis

Your nursing assessment will provide information for both a medical diagnosis using DSM-IV criteria and nursing diagnoses.

Nursing diagnoses are the critical foundation underlying all planning, implementation, and evaluation activities with a child. West and Pothier (1989) describe a four-step model for formulating nursing diagnoses.

1. Identify the child's responses (both problems and strengths/resources).
2. Group the problems according to common links among them (such as difficulties communicating).
3. Label the groups according to their common theme under various NANDA diagnostic categories, such as Impaired Communication.
4. Prioritize the diagnoses based on either their urgency or their need for attention before other problems can be addressed.

There are no diagnoses specific to children in the NANDA classification system; however, some subcategories address child-related issues, and many family and parent-related diagnoses are quite relevant. In addition, when a nursing diagnosis is written, the second part of the statement, which describes the etiology of the specific problem, helps to identify child-specific issues.

Planning and Implementing Interventions

Each nursing diagnosis provides the basis for planning and implementation of nursing care. The care plan involves identification of specific outcomes that you want to achieve for each nursing diagnosis, along with your nursing interventions for each expected outcome and how you will evaluate whether outcomes have been achieved. The most widely used treatment approaches for children include play therapy, cognitive-behavioral therapy, family therapy, and psychopharmacology.

PLAY THERAPY **Play therapy** builds upon the foundation of the psychodynamic, object-relations, and attachment theories described earlier. Although play therapy is used as part of most assessment protocols and to treat a variety of mental health problems, you may find it quite helpful for nursing diagnoses associated with attention deficit disorders, disruptive behavior disorders, mood disorders, and reactive attachment disorder.

Types of Play There are four major types of play, which are also related to stages of play development in children (Schaefer 1993). During the first year of life, *sensorimotor play* is the child's focus. This play involves attempts to assimilate sensory information and gain control over objects in the environment, by mouthing toys or pulling them around, for instance. During the second year of life, *construction or combinatorial play* becomes the child's focus, as in putting together shapes or stacking blocks. From age 2–6, *symbolic or pretend play* emerges. At this age, the capacity to fantasize and put the self cognitively into other situations or other people's shoes enables play therapy to become a central vehicle for treatment of the child. The themes of the child's play are now motivated by inner psychologic dynamics. At age 5 or 6, children develop the capacity for and interest in *game play.* In games with rules, children are required to assume the perspective of others, remain attentive, and control their impulses. The ways in which children interact with others around the rules and activities provide another base of information regarding their inner world and how they view others.

Nondirective play is normally viewed as the best way to begin play therapy. The symbols and themes that emerge in play provide a core of information for assessment and subsequent treatment. They give us the same type of information that we gather through verbal communication with adults. Remember that symbols (such as aggressive behavior toward a father doll) can have several meanings and should never be interpreted in a standardized fashion. Always consider the way a symbol is used in the play as it may relate to the particular context of the child's life before interpreting a symbol's subjective meaning to a child. Your impressions must be verified or refuted based on a variety of different types of information collected over time.

Twelve-year-old Laura had been sexually molested by her father. Her father was sent to prison for the sexual molestation of another preschooler. During Laura's therapy session, she asked the nurse therapist to go to the playroom. She built a fortress of large multicolored blocks. She put a chair inside the structure and sat down stating, "This is a dungeon. A rainbow dungeon." Her play demonstrated her ambivalent feelings toward her father.

There is a general belief that toys with ambiguous meaning and diverse uses foster symbolic play more effectively because they allow the child to project his or her own identity and function onto the toy. However, there may be times when you want to move the child more directly into specific play themes through structured play. In these situations, toys with an obvious identity or function may be selected for a play session (as in addressing themes of parental separation or abuse). Structured play is rarely used until nondirective play has enabled a full assessment of relevant themes and issues, and the child's trust around anxiety-laden issues has been developed.

Purposes of Play Therapy Play therapy can serve many purposes. A major use is for **catharsis,** the release of strong emotions in order to provide relief from the inner tension they may be causing the child. It is also believed that expressing the themes, even though they may not be conscious for the child, provides some kind of cognitive relief. Catharsis can be facilitated through many forms of play, including drawings, doll play, clay modeling, or the acting-out of certain feelings through pounding toys or punching dolls or bags. Another purpose of play therapy is **abreaction,** the reliving through play of past events and their related feelings. Through abreaction, the child gradually can assimilate previous experiences that have been traumatic or painful. Assimilation occurs through the release of related emotions, as well as through integrating what happened into the child's ongoing view of himself and the world. The basis of this integration is the opportunity, through play, to gain mastery over an experience in which the child most likely had no control. Mastery comes from reenacting the event in the child's own way, working through the feelings that were part of the experience, and modifying, over time, how it happened and what the outcome may have been.

Another frequent use of play therapy is to help the child try out other ways of relating to the world or responding to situations. At about 3 years of age, children have the capacity for role-play. In taking on certain roles, children can learn how others may feel or think (by putting themselves in somebody else's shoes). Role-play can occur through the child's taking on a character himself, or projecting that character onto a puppet or doll.

Therapeutic Interventions Regardless of the specific purpose of play therapy, your interventions involve a combination of reflection and interpretation to help the child gain greater awareness of the unconscious issues becoming apparent. *Reflection* involves simple commenting on what is happening in the child's play—for example, "The boy doll is hitting the father doll again." Such a statement includes no interpretation but has the potential to help the child become more aware of what is happening in the play. Reflection is the major intervention used by more inexperienced clinicians, including the generalist nurse. It is also the mainstay for clinical specialists during their initial work with the child. However, there should be a few sessions of play observation without any reflective comment, to allow the child to gain comfort in the play, before eliciting any anxiety that may arise as a result of reflection.

The use of *interpretation* begins after rapport and trust have been established, and it can range from subtle to very direct. Subtle interpretations are more removed from the child and speak to the potential meaning behind the toy's behavior—for instance, "The boy doll is hitting the father doll because he's very angry at him." More direct interpretations are used over time as the nurse develops greater confidence in the validity of the interpretations for the child—for example, "I wonder if you feel like the boy doll. You seem angry at your dad for leaving." Obviously, these more direct interpretations must integrate anything observed in the play with your total assessment of the child's issues and problems in the real world.

COGNITIVE-BEHAVIORAL THERAPY The approaches used in cognitive-behavioral therapy stem from cognitive-behavioral theory, described earlier. Two major differences exist between this modality and play therapy. First, cognitive-behavioral approaches focus on conscious rather than unconscious issues. Second, emphasis is placed on more effective coping in the present rather than on mastery over unresolved feelings associated with the child's past experiences. Cognitive-behavioral approaches have been particularly successful in treating problems associated with depression, conduct disorder, ADHD, and anxiety in children 9 and older (Kendall 1993). Behavioral techniques, without the cognitive component, are also widely used to address therapeutic goals for children with mental retardation, learning and communication disorders, pervasive developmental disorders, tic disorders, and elimination disorders.

Cognitive Restructuring Cognitive-behavioral treatment is a reeducation and relearning process involving the development of new ways of thinking about life and new behaviors that are more adaptive and more functional for the child. The cognitive aspects of therapy attempt to modify inaccurate or biased ways of processing information that result in distortions of what is actually occurring in the child's world. This process of **cognitive restructuring** involves strategies such as finding out what the child means by statements he makes, teaching him to question the "evidence" he's using to maintain any irrational beliefs, helping him identify other options for what a situation might mean, listing advantages and disadvantages of a particular belief, and teaching the child to use self-talk or directives to himself to help change or reframe a situation—for example, "Stop and wait; don't get angry until you find out more." You can coach the child to reconceptualize problems, thereby helping him more effectively make sense of the world. In this way, the child begins to modify his perceptions of interactions with others and his expectations for the future.

Behavioral Aspects The behavioral aspects of therapy are based to a great extent on classical and operant conditioning techniques. The major classical conditioning technique is systematic desensitization, which involves the pairing of a negative stimulus (such as a feared situation or animal) with a positive stimulus (such as candy or relaxation exercises). The pairing is done in a progressive way, so the child begins to handle situations that are increasingly fearful or aversive. For example, a child may initially look at pictures of a dog that scares him while having a favorite snack, and progress through a series of more frightening situations. Eventually, the child is asked to touch a dog in the context of many positive rewards, which counteract the negative impact.

Examples of operant conditioning techniques are contingency contracting, the use of tokens, modeling, and behavioral role-play groups. *Contracting* involves setting goals with a child, with specific consequences (positive and negative) clearly identified for achieving or not achieving the goals. *Tokens* can also be used in contracting, whereby points are accumulated or lost depending on the child's following through with agreed-upon behavior. These tokens can then be exchanged for various rewards that are important to the child. When a *modeling* intervention is used, children with specific problems are exposed to real or filmed examples of other children who model effective responses to difficult situations. *Behavioral role-play* takes modeling a step further to help the child try out new behaviors before applying them in the real world.

Milieu Approaches Cognitive-behavioral approaches, such as the ones just described, serve as the basis for most milieu therapy in child psychiatric inpatient settings. These settings are for children with more severe mental health problems, who may require around-the-clock assessment to determine the exact diagnosis, or intensive, consistent care for life-threatening or violent conditions. The use of behavioral interventions on inpatient units allows nursing staff to give continuous feedback to the children about the appropriateness of their behavior. The children receive rewards such as verbal praise, a sticker, or points for appropriate behavior. For example, children who have a problem hitting others all the time may receive a sticker and verbal praise for no hits hourly, until they associate their behavior with the reward. At that time, the need for feedback may decrease to a less-frequent schedule, and later to the need for only verbal reminders of the desired behavior.

At the same time staff members are trying to reward children for positive behavior, children also need to know that certain hostile or aggressive behaviors cannot be tolerated. When children cannot behave in acceptable ways, you can have them take a time-out from the activity by sitting in chairs until they are able to pull themselves together. If that does not work, the time-out may be taken in a quiet room free of objects and stimulation. If isolation is also too difficult, you may need to use a restraining hold to help them calm down. As children are able to calm down, help them see why they needed a time-out and what they could do differently next time. The goal is to have children learn what precedes episodes during which they get out of control, and learn ways to avoid the negative consequences of out-of-control behavior such as fights with other children. It is through effective limit setting that we can help children separate their feelings from their behavior and learn more adaptive ways of expressing themselves.

Family Involvement Family involvement in cognitive-behavioral approaches with children is also very common. For instance, you can help parents implement contracting and other behavioral approaches within the home. Involving parents as active members of their child's hospital treatment team has a profound impact on the degree to which the inpatient treatment is carried over into the real world of the child and the family. In both inpatient and outpatient settings, you can work closely with parents to help them understand the use of cognitive-behavioral strategies in their parenting practices. For example, they can learn to apply reward systems and time-outs, as well as help their children use self-talk to better understand situations before they do something impulsively. Remember also to give written and verbal information to parents so that they become truly informed partners in their child's care.

FAMILY THERAPY Family therapy goes beyond family involvement in the child's treatment to focus on treatment of the entire family. This method is selected when interactions among family members need attention in order to address specific problems exhibited by the child. The goal is to increase the likelihood that improvements in the child's mental health will occur and will be supported in the home with consistent and sustained family patterns. Although the focus is on interaction among all family members, the goal of therapy is some beneficial outcome for the child's mental health.

The staff in an inpatient clinic found they needed to help the parents of a 12-year-old boy plan his weekend day passes. The child reported he barely saw his parents while home on pass, and he generally returned early. His mother went to work, and his father had outside activities. The child hung out at the local mall with his friends. This situation interfered with the goal of a transition of the child back into the family. The family therapist and primary nurse worked with the family to structure the passes to meet the goals of reentry and increase availability of the parents to the child.

Family therapy approaches are described fully in Chapter 32, but there are a few issues specific to family therapy when children are included.

If children under age 7 are involved in family therapy, the nurse may choose to alternate having the child present and seeing the parents or other family members only. The child's presence provides information for clinical assessment, allows for direct comment on and discussion of the dynamics that occur among parents and children, and provides opportunities for the nurse to model effective interaction with the child, as well as teach the family about normal development and positive parenting. However, there may be issues for discussion that are beyond the child's capacity to understand and/or inappropriate for discussion in front of the child. Meeting with the parents alone enables these issues to be more openly addressed in a setting with fewer distractions.

Family play therapy is another option with young children that enables their full participation (Griff 1983; Stoddard, Wilberger, and Olafson 1993). Usually, the first half of the family session involves either directive or nondirective play. In the second half, the parents talk with the therapist about family issues that arose during the play, while the child continues to play or engages in discussion as desired or when invited.

Older children can be involved with more typical family therapy approaches. The developmental status of the child's capabilities and the nature of the child's problems should guide the nurse's decisions with the family regarding the specific strategies to use.

PSYCHOPHARMACOLOGY The nature of drug therapy is detailed in Chapter 33. However, there are important considerations in using medications with children. First, one can never assume that the actions and side effects of any drug will be the same for children as for adults. Determining the dosage of a drug by body weight is thus not appropriate. Only recently have studies been undertaken to carefully examine the impact of medications on

children at various developmental stages. Not only do children at various stages have different medication needs in terms of rates of absorption, excretion, sites of action, and toxicity, but these may change for the same child as he or she develops (Shapiro 1985). Children must, therefore, be carefully monitored, with ongoing titration, if they are kept on a drug over extended periods of time.

Second, the developmental impact of a drug on a child must be weighed alongside the potential benefits it has for a specific mental health problem. Medications are often used with children to address a behavioral problem that may be disturbing to their family or teachers, yet their use may interfere with the developmental capacity of the child. For instance, antipsychotic medications such as chlorpromazine may interfere with learning and cause tardive dyskinesia. Stimulants may increase learning potential for children with ADHD, but they can affect the physical growth potential of the child. All the benefits and risks must be balanced against one another in a full and open discussion with the child's family.

Medications Commonly Used with Children Three classes of drugs are most commonly used with children: stimulants, antidepressants, and low-dose antipsychotics. Methylphenidate (Ritalin) and pemoline (Cylert) are the stimulants used most frequently for ADHD. They decrease behavioral agitation and enhance the ability to concentrate and focus. Antidepressants, most commonly the tricyclics such as imipramine (Tofranil), are used for many disorders, including depression, school phobia, ADHD, and enuresis. The Food and Drug Administration (FDA) limits the use of these medications because they have cardiotoxic effects and require the careful monitoring of heart rate and rhythm as well as blood serum levels. Monoamine oxidase inhibitors (MAOIs) are less frequently used antidepressants because they require careful dietary control to prevent untoward interactions, and such control is difficult for children. Antipsychotic medications such as haloperidol (Haldol) are used to sedate children with mental retardation or to reduce behavioral agitation in children with pervasive developmental disorders or childhood-onset schizophrenia. However, these medications may be inappropriately employed as a substitute for careful supervision or intensive behavioral intervention to help modify and control behaviors that may cause self-injury or injury to others. Antipsychotics should be used cautiously with children because of side effects and the many unknowns regarding long-term developmental impact.

Nursing Interventions Nurses play an important role in monitoring the child on medication and educating the child and parents about the medication.

- Monitor side effects daily in inpatient settings and weekly in outpatient settings.
- If the child is being treated in an outpatient setting, work closely with parents and teachers to record the child's behavior.
- Assess the concerns the child has about side effects and stigmatization by peers related to the medication.
- Take time to assess the parents' beliefs and fears about the medications. Parents are often concerned about the potential for the child to become dependent on medication, as well as its side effects. Give parents an opportunity to discuss their worries and questions and become informed about the medication.
- Prepare the child and the parents for a potential increase in symptoms when a medication is removed or decreased. Plan other interventions to help the child and family at this time.

Evaluation and Outcome Criteria

The purpose of evaluation is to determine whether interventions are effective and how you should modify your care if necessary. Be sure that the focus of evaluation is on concrete and observable aspects of the child's behavior or psychophysiologic response. Tangible changes or improvements are more readily assessed than vague statements that cannot be measured or observed in some way. For example, assessing an increase in the child's self-esteem is very difficult, but evaluating specific behaviors indicating esteem (such as positive statements about self or improved grooming) will make your evaluation easier and more useful.

Acquiring input from as many sources as possible is also essential to effective evaluation. Have you obtained information from the child, parents, other nursing staff, or school personnel? Depending on the situation, it may or may not be possible to conduct a comprehensive evaluation, but it should be your goal whenever possible. Finally, outcome criteria for evaluation must be congruent with appropriate developmental and sociocultural expectations. Frustration tolerance, for example, is far different in the 4-year-old than the 14-year-old. For this reason, an accurate evaluation must consider the norms for age-appropriateness. Similarly, expectations should take into consideration the child's sociocultural norms. For instance, a child who exhibits aggressiveness or informality with adults may have had such behaviors encouraged at home, yet they are viewed by the larger society as disrespectful toward authority. Children need to fit in with their own communities and social context as well as society as a whole, so these factors must be weighed as various outcomes are identified for your interventions.

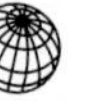

In addition to the outcome criteria you establish to assess the effectiveness of your interventions, another critical feature of evaluation is the ongoing review and evaluation of your own process as a child psychiatric nurse.

Eleven-year-old Luisa had a history of living with extended family and several hospitalizations. Luisa's mother was am-

NURSING SELF-AWARENESS

Promoting Sensitive Child Psychiatric Nursing

To assist you in your own self-growth and in examining your attitudes and behavior toward child psychiatric clients, answer the following:

Attitudes

- What do I like about this child?
- What don't I like about this child?
- Is there anything about this child's personality or problems that reminds me of myself or my own childhood?
- What feelings arise in me when I'm working with this child? What is it about the child or me that might cause these feelings?

Behavior

- How are my views/feelings about this child affecting the way I relate to the child? How are they helping my therapeutic work? How are they hindering my therapeutic work?
- How is the child responding to my interventions?

Self-Growth

- What am I learning about myself as I work with this child?
- Am I fully exploring these issues with my supervisor so that I can improve both my working relationship with this child and my insight as a child psychiatric nurse?

bivalent toward her, often openly rejecting her (such as limited visitations and missed family sessions). Luisa stimulated a lot of feeling among the staff about bad mothers and good mothers, and the staff was protective of the child and angry at the mother. The staff was encouraged to examine the mother's own deprivation by an abusive mother and the difficulties in raising this very troubled child.

Are you aware of your attitudes and behaviors in working with specific children? How are these affecting your interventions with each child? For some key areas to consider in evaluating your potential impact, see the accompanying Nursing Self-Awareness box.

Working with children, particularly children with emotional problems, may activate feelings about your own unresolved issues with your family of origin or current family. You may then react as if the child is feeling or acting in ways that you might have felt or acted, and project your own issues onto the child, rather than responding to the actual therapeutic needs of the child. Nurses may also respond to children or parents with certain stereotyped attitudes or beliefs, rather than being open to each child and parent as individuals. Self-awareness and ongoing self-monitoring are essential skills for child psychiatric nurses to acquire. Without this capacity, we can have little assurance that we will be truly therapeutic in providing nursing care.

Chapter Highlights

- Child psychiatric nurses have responsibilities across the continuum of mental health and illness for children. The specific roles of the nurse depend upon whether the nurse is a generalist or a clinical specialist. Standards for each of these levels of nursing have been identified by the American Nurses Association.
- A number of mental health problems typically appear during childhood, although they may continue into adulthood. These disorders include mental retardation, learning disorders, motor skills disorder, communication disorders, pervasive developmental disorders, attention deficit and disruptive behavior disorders, feeding and eating disorders, tic disorders, elimination disorders, and separation anxiety disorder. Depressive disorders, selective mutism, reactive attachment disorder of infancy or early childhood, stereotypic movement disorder, and childhood-onset schizophrenia are also important childhood mental disorders.
- Five major theories guide our understanding and treatment of childhood psychopathology: psychodynamic theory, object-relations theory, attachment theory, cognitive-behavioral theory, and biologic diathesis theory. Nurses must consider the multicausal nature of mental illness by integrating the contributions of each of these theoretic perspectives.
- Nursing assessment includes a history-taking interview with the parents and a clinical assessment of the child. The clinical assessment includes a mental status exam in which both a semistructured interview and an unstructured play session are carried out.
- Nursing diagnoses are the foundation underlying all planning, implementation, and evaluation activities with a child. The child's problems are grouped according to common themes, which are given various diagnostic labels in the NANDA classification system. These diagnoses are then prioritized in terms of need for attention.

- The most widely used treatment modalities for children are play therapy, cognitive-behavioral therapy (the basis of most milieu therapy in psychiatric inpatient settings), family therapy, and psychopharmacology. The child psychiatric nurse generalist may perform aspects of these as part of a team (in collaboration with or under the supervision of another mental health care professional) or independently, if the nurse is a specialist who has been educated in the use of these interventions.
- Evaluation of interventions helps determine whether nursing care is effective and how it should be modified, if at all. Evaluate both specific outcome criteria related to the changes in the child and your own attitudes and behaviors to assess how they may be influencing the effectiveness of the care.

References

Ainsworth M, Blehar M, Waters E, Walls S: *Patterns of Attachment.* Erlbaum, 1978.

American Nurses Association: *Standards of Child and Adolescent Psychiatric and Mental Health Nursing Practice.* American Nurses Association, 1985.

Anderson G, Hoshiro Y: Neurochemical studies of autism, in Cohen D, Donnellan A (eds): *Handbook of Autism and Pervasive Developmental Disorders.* Wiley, 1987.

Bandura A: *Social Learning Theory.* Prentice-Hall, 1977.

Beck A: *Cognitive Therapy and the Emotional Disorders.* New American Library, 1976.

Bowlby J: *Attachment and Loss, Vol. I: Attachment,* ed 2. Basic Books, 1969.

Bowlby J: *Attachment and Loss, Vol. II, Separation,* ed 2. Basic Books, 1973.

Fairbairn W: Synopsis of an object relation's theory of personality. *Int J Psychoanal* 1962;44:224–225.

Fonagy P, Moran G: Understanding psychic change in child psychoanalysis. *Int J Psychoanal* 1991;72(1):15–22.

Freud S: *An Outline of Psychoanalysis.* Norton, 1949 (originally published 1940).

Greenberg J, Mitchell SH: *Object Relations in Psychoanalytic Theory.* Harvard University Press, 1983.

Griff M: Family play therapy, in Schaeffer C, O'Connor K (eds): *Handbook of Play Therapy.* Wiley, 1983.

Guerney L, Guerney B: Integrating child and family therapy. *Psychotherapy* 1987;24:109–118.

Kendall P: Cognitive-behavioral therapies with youth: Guiding theory, current status and emerging developments. *J Consult Clin Psych* 1993; 61(2):235–247.

Main M: Parental aversion to infant-initiated contact is correlated with the parent's own rejection during childhood: The effects of experience on signals of security with respect to attachment, in Barnard K, Brazelton TB (eds): *Touch: The Foundation of Experience.* International Universities Press, 1990.

McKenna K, Gordon C, Rappoport J: Childhood-onset schizophrenia: Timely neurobiological research. *J Am Acad Child Adol Psychiatr* 1994;33(6):771–781.

Pauls D: The familiarity of autism and related disorders: A review of the evidence, in Cohen C, Donnellan A (eds): *Handbook of Autism and Pervasive Developmental Disorders.* Wiley, 1987.

Rutter M: Depressive disorders, in Rutter M, Tuma A, Lann I (eds): *Assessment and Diagnosis in Child Psychopathology.* Guilford Press, 1988.

Scarr S: Distinctive environments depend on genotypes. *Behav Brain Sci* 1987;10(1):38–39.

Scatterfield J, Scatterfield B, Cantwell D: Three-year multimodality treatment study of hyperactive boys. *J Pediatrics* 1981;90:650.

Schaefer C: What is play and why is it therapeutic? in Schaefer C (ed): *The Therapeutic Powers of Play.* Jason Aronson, 1993.

Shapiro T: Developmental considerations in psychopharmacology: The interaction of drugs and development, in Weiner J (ed): *Diagnosis and Psychopharmacology of Childhood and Adolescent Disorders.* Wiley, 1985.

Siantz ML: Child and family minority research: How are we doing? *J Child Psychiatric Nurs* 1993;6(4):6–9.

Skinner BF: *About Behaviorism.* Random House, 1976.

Sroufe LA, Fleeson J: Attachment and the construction of relationships, in Hartup W, Rubin Z (eds): *Relationships and Development.* Erlbaum, 1986.

Stern D: *The Interpersonal World of the Infant.* Basic Books, 1985.

Stoddard F, Wilberger M, Olafson E: A case of functional urinary retention: The use of family play therapy. *Fam Process* 1993;32:279–289.

Target M, Fonagy P: Efficacy of psychoanalysis for children with emotional disorders. *J Am Acad Child Adol Psych* 1994;33:361–371.

Torrey E, Taylor E, Brache H, Bowler A, McNeil T, Rawlings R, Quinn P, Bigelow L, Rickler K, Sjostrom K, Higgins E, Gottesman I: Prenatal origin of schizophrenia in a subgroup of discordant monozygotic twins. *Schiz Bull* 1994; 20(3):423–432.

Weber RA, Levitt MJ, Clark MC: Individual variation in attachment security and strange situation behavior: The role of maternal and infant temperament. *Child Dev* 1986; 57:56–65.

Weiss S: Attachment theory, in Johnson B (ed): *Child, Adolescent and Family Psychiatric Nursing.* Lippincott, 1994.

West P, Pothier P: Clinical application of human responses classification system: Child example. *Arch Psychiatr Nurs* 1989;3(5):300–304.

Winnicott DW: *The Maturational Processes and the Facilitating Environment.* International Universities Press, 1965.

Zahn T: Studies of autonomic psychophysiology and attention in schizophrenia. *Schiz Bull* 1988;14:205–208.

Zilbach J: *Young Children in Family Therapy.* Brunner/Mazel, 1986.

CHAPTER 37

APPLYING THE NURSING PROCESS WITH ADOLESCENTS

Carol Bradley-Corpuel

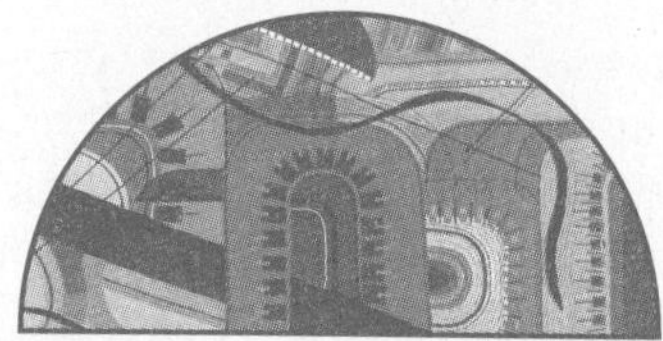

COMPETENCIES

- *Discuss the relevance of biologic and developmental data in the assessment of adolescents.*
- *Relate the importance of using a humanistic interactionist perspective in a comprehensive assessment of adolescent problems.*
- *Describe nursing roles and functions in outpatient and inpatient treatment settings for adolescents.*
- *Describe nursing roles and functions in working with families of adolescent clients.*
- *List at least four functions of the staff nurse working to maintain a therapeutic environment.*
- *Define* acting-out, *and give an example of an adolescent acting out a "life script."*
- *Construct a client contract for use with an adolescent in treatment.*
- *Explain why a keen self-awareness of your own adolescence and unresolved issues is important in working with adolescents.*

Cross-References

Other topics relevant to this content are: ANA Standards of Child and Adolescent Psychiatric–Mental Health Nursing, Chapter 36; Depression, Chapter 15; Eating disorders, Chapter 18; Family assessment and family therapy, Chapter 32; Nurse-client relationship, Chapter 28; Psychobiology, Chapter 3; Suicide, Chapter 24; Theories, Chapter 2; Therapeutic communication, Chapter 7; Therapeutic environment, Chapter 9; Violence in the psychiatric setting, Chapter 34.

Critical Thinking Challenge

Discussions about school-based clinics have become embroiled in the controversy about sex education. Much of the controversy surrounding sex education and family planning services revolves around the belief that providing such services will lead to an increase in sexual activity among adolescents, with a corresponding rise in pregnancy rates and HIV transmissions. Opponents of such clinics exclaim that sex education should be provided by the parents, not the schools. Do you agree with this position? What other considerations are there in attempting to deal with various at-risk behaviors of adolescents?

What is adolescence? Some sources define it simply as the time of physical and psychosocial development between the ages of 12 and 20. Others describe it as a period of "normal psychosis." Still others see it as an attempt by a tyrannical subculture to overtake adult America. It is not necessary to accept the latter two definitions verbatim to understand their implications. Most people recognize the immense stress that occurs during adolescence and the importance that managing the stress has for an adolescent's future.

The role of the nurse in the care and treatment of adolescents has dramatically changed over the past decade. Once regarded simply as a technician who monitored somatic therapies, the nurse is now acknowledged as a professional with numerous capabilities and skills that have a direct bearing on the favorable treatment outcome of adolescents.

The American Nurses Association (ANA) now recognizes child and adolescent psychiatric–mental health nursing as a specialty area of psychiatric–mental health nursing practice. The ANA Standards of Child and Adolescent Psychiatric and Mental Health Nursing Practice (1985) are reproduced in Chapter 36, p. 860.

Whether a generalist or clinical specialist, the nurse in today's health care setting integrates these characteristics and role responsibilities to intervene with adolescents to achieve optimal social, emotional, cognitive, and physical development. Using expertise in identifying relevant deviations in the developmental process, the nurse works closely with the systems (family, school, community, and institution) on which adolescents are emotionally and economically dependent.

Trying to understand adolescents is a challenge to anyone. For the nurse who chooses to work with adolescents, the challenge offers considerable rewards. Nurses who can recollect their own experiences and reactions during this tumultuous time will better appreciate the dilemma of adolescent clients.

Biopsychosocial Theories

A sound theoretic knowledge base helps you differentiate between the "normal" and "abnormal," or the usual and unusual, behaviors of adolescents. In particular, you can do a comprehensive assessment by focusing on the psychologic development of the individual and the evolution of the adolescent as a biopsychosocial being. You can accomplish the first task with an understanding of developmental theory and the second with an appreciation of biologic and humanistic interactionist theories.

Biologic Theory

Psychiatric nursing in the 1990s requires that you integrate a biologic focus into your practice, to accommodate both changing client needs and an expanding biologic knowledge base. An appreciation of hormonal changes, growth spurts, stress and immune function, chronic illness, depression, and other mental disorders can help you evaluate adolescents from a more effective and comprehensive perspective.

More specifically, research in the areas of psychopharmacology and psychiatric disorders, particularly major depression, is increasingly attempted with adolescent populations, whereas a decade or so ago, studies were limited to adult populations. Researchers are exploring the validity of such findings with adolescents in various realms of biologic studies, including abnormalities in basal thyroid hormone levels in depressed and manic adolescents (Sokolov, Kutcher, and Joffe 1994); the role of adverse life events and alterations in the immune system (Birmaher, Rabin, and Garcia 1994); the relationship between biochemical parameters and behavioral problems (Gabel, Stadler, and Bjorn 1994); the use of antipsychotic medications with nonpsychotic children and adolescents (Kaplan, Simms, and Busner 1994); pharmacologic interventions with such disorders as OCD (Apter, Ratzoni, and King 1994), depression (Kutcher, Boulos, and Ward 1994), and schizophrenia (Frazier, Gordon, and McKenna 1994).

Of equal importance in the literature has become the effect of chronic physical illness on the adolescent's mental health (Blanz, Rensch-Riemann, and Fritz-Sigmund 1993; Goldston, Kovacs, and Ho 1994; Howe, Feinstein, and Reiss 1993). In addition, poor immigrant families with a handicapped child or adolescent are at increased risk for disorders because they must cope with a triple set of stress factors: loss of home and familiar surroundings, coping with a physically or psychologically challenged child, and living in an unfamiliar environment that probably includes a complex and confusing health care system (Lequerica 1993).

Developmental Theory

An understanding of developmental theory helps you identify deviations in adolescent growth and development processes and intervene appropriately. The theories of Freud, Erikson, and Sullivan provide considerable insight into the adolescent's struggle to attain adulthood.

The development of an adolescent's sense of identity entails a preoccupation with self-image. It also entails a connection between future role and past experiences. In the search for a new sense of sameness and continuity, many adolescents must repeat the crisis resolutions of earlier years to integrate these past elements and establish the lasting ideals of a final identity. According to Erikson, these crisis periods or stages are reviews of the adolescent's sense of trust, autonomy, initiative, and industry, in that order. Equally important for an adolescent's development is cognition. Piaget's research revealed three stages of cognitive development. The third stage, called formal operations, develops between ages 12 and 14 and results in the adolescent's ability to conceptualize on an adult level. The adolescent has the capacity to think abstractly, to be self-reflective, and to adopt a multidimensional perspective on problems (National Nursing Research Agenda 1993). (For a discussion of developmental theories as they relate to adolescent growth and development, see Chapter 2.)

Humanistic Interactionist Theory

As a nurse, you not only need knowledge about developmental theories and psychobiology, you must also integrate humanistic interactionist principles into assessment and interventions to develop a trusting, caring interpersonal relationship with adolescent clients. The adolescent developmental period is a time in the individual's life when identity, values, and goals are in a state of flux. You should take into account not only the immediate situation but also the impact of the developmental stage; the social, ethnic, and cultural factors; family influences; and psychodynamic conflicts on the adolescent's behavior.

In order to accomplish this, you must explore the meaning of the identified problem or behavior. The following questions can guide this exploration:

- What meaning does this behavior or problem hold for the adolescent?
- What message is he or she conveying through this behavior?
- What impact does this problem have on the client in this developmental stage? Is this a usual or unusual problem or behavior for the adolescent's peer group?
- How have resulting changes, if any, affected the adolescent and his or her relationships with others?
- What goals does the client have for the immediate and distant future?
- What personal strengths does the adolescent have to help deal with this problem?
- What considerations have you and the client given to other developmental, familial, biologic, or sociocultural factors involved?

It is insufficient to base the nursing response to the adolescent's needs and dilemmas solely on behaviors without a more comprehensive evaluation of these other factors. This approach can lead to ineffective treatment, a temporary ceasing of the initial behaviors with an upheaval of symptoms in another area, and possibly a sterile treatment environment without any meaningful therapeutic alliance. Only by considering all aspects of the adolescent client as a biopsychosocial being can you truly understand the meanings of such behaviors to the client and intervene effectively in the situation.

The Role of the Nurse

The nurse can assume numerous roles within a variety of treatment modalities to help maintain the health and well-being of adolescent clients and identify abnormal or problem-causing behavior during this difficult period of development.

In the Outpatient Setting

As a Community Health Nurse In the school, clinic, or community health agency, you have excellent opportunities to observe adolescents engaging in the normal activities of daily living. You have frequent occasions to counsel adolescents in the problems that confront them daily and to advise school or clinic staff members in their encounters with adolescents. The nurse who knows how to deal with normal adolescent problems will also be adept in identifying obstacles to effective resolution of emotional problems and suggesting further treatment.

School is the most influential experience in an adolescent's life outside the home. Adolescents spend more waking time in school activities than in any other activity, and most of their successes, problems, and conflicts are demonstrated in the school setting. Even adolescents who are supposedly truant from school are often on the school grounds, perhaps meeting their friends at lunchtime, playing cards in the library, or "hanging out" on the school steps. Such an "absent" student may suddenly appear at the school nurse's door because of "boredom" or a physical complaint.

Unfortunately, the school nurse's role in the early recognition and treatment of predelinquent individuals has been minimized or has gone unrecognized. There are several reasons for this. One reason is that school administrators and teachers tend to view the school nurse as a person who deals only with physical sickness and medical emergencies. They may not be aware that because of the intimate quality of a nurse-client relationship or the comprehensive and holistic nature of nursing assessments, the nurse may be helpful in exploring an area of conflict in an adolescent's life or intervening with a disruptive student. Such early intervention could prevent more serious problems in later years. Many studies have indicated a direct correlation between the problems of early school life and family dysfunction and the incidence of subsequent juvenile delinquency, depression, and suicidal behavior (Brent, Perper, and Moritz 1994; Pfeffer, Klerman, and Hurt 1991). Here is a list of problems demonstrated by adolescents in the school setting that call for early intervention:

- Antisocial behavior (stealing, setting fires, bullying others).
- Avoidant social behavior.
- Chronic illness.
- Depression.
- Disruptive classroom behavior.
- Substance abuse.
- Excessive daydreaming.
- Hypochondriasis.
- Learning difficulties.
- Poor school performance, or a dramatic shift in school performance.
- Temper tantrums.
- Truancy.

Another reason is that administrators tend to limit the nurse's activities to the school itself. They may see no need for the nurse to make home visits to meet with a sick student's family or view problems first-hand. Many school districts lack the time and money to provide for counseling families or individuals in a formal setting. As the role of the independent nursing practitioner expands, and as legislation for third-party reimbursement for independent practice becomes a reality in more states, nurses will be better able to assume more autonomy and responsibility in meeting student needs more comprehensively and effectively.

Meanwhile, the nurse who is already employed in the school setting or community agency can seize every opportunity to provide an active school health program and to educate school administrators and faculty members about the importance of preventive care. For example, the nurse in a viable school health program can provide preventive counseling not only to troubled adolescents in school but also to their preschool siblings during routine home visits. Nurses can establish productive relationships with teachers, help other faculty members encourage parent-teacher conferences, take an active part in developing the curriculum, and help adolescents on probation or parole return to school.

The many problems encountered by today's youth—substance abuse, teenage pregnancy, family violence, street crime, and school failure—are increasingly being recognized in community, judicial, and social arenas. School-based programs to tackle family dysfunction, substance abuse, and school dropout problems are showing positive results (Eggert, Thompson, and Herting 1994; Uphold and Graham 1994). America's juvenile and family court judges are now committed to providing a center for the coordination and provision of services and resources to youth and families in the community. This includes individual and family assessment, education, and treatment, first. The courtroom is used only when other appropriate avenues of intervention and resolution have failed (National Council of Juvenile and Family Court Judges 1993).

Innovative social programs are attempting to help failing adolescents (and failing families). One such program in Tennessee entitled Home Ties involves professionals working closely in the homes of adolescents who would ordinarily have been cast out by their families as a result of their antisocial disruptive behaviors ("Close-Up: America" 1993). Another short-term program is designed as an alternative to psychiatric hospitalization for children and adolescents. The program uses a team of multidisciplinary professionals and specially trained individuals, or mentors. The adolescent and the adolescent's biologic family work with the mentor in the mentor's home. The findings of the follow-up study indicate a low rate of subsequent psychiatric hospitalizations (Mikkelsen, Bereika, and McKenzie 1993).

With the promise for change that these innovations bring, community health nurses are in a prime position to play a key role in the movement toward proactive partnerships among schools, families, and the community in enhancing the health and ensuring the future of our nation's youth.

As a Nurse Counselor/Therapist Whether in the clinic, home, school, or community health setting, the psychiatric nurse has many opportunities to organize individual, group, or family counseling sessions. Nurses can function within a variety of treatment roles, according to their experience and capabilities.

As an Individual Therapist The nurse's qualifications and role in the clinic, school, or community setting may allow for counseling adolescents on an individual basis. Sometimes the nurse can establish a trusting alliance and facilitate communication with the client. Sometimes, however, the adolescent is too threatened to talk openly with the nurse in this intimate setting. Some adolescents view the nurse as an authority figure and resist all efforts to communicate. You may make more headway with this mode of treatment when it is used in conjunction with group therapy. Unless certified to provide this service, you should counsel the adolescent only for the purposes of identifying the problem area and referring the client to a qualified professional for individual psychotherapy.

As a Group Therapist It is usually more effective to work with adolescents in a group. Because the values, acceptance, and recognition of peers are so important during adolescence, the group can provide the support for dealing with problems and effecting change. In addition, involving the adolescent's peers helps dilute the conflict with adults that may exist in one-to-one work. In the school setting, health education groups can provide an acceptable forum for peer interaction and discussion of difficult topics. Otherwise, the nurse should practice as a group therapist only as a certified individual or with adequate supervision by a certified individual. Knowledge of group dynamics is crucial to be an effective group leader.

As a Family Therapist Being a parent of a "normal" adolescent is difficult, at best. As the child grows into adulthood with all its perplexing questions and problems, parents normally worry about their child's safety and well-being. They may feel rejected because they are no longer needed in the same way. Because many parents of relatively normal adolescents share this plight, they can usually find receptive listeners who will give them comfort and support.

The problems of the parents of emotionally disturbed adolescents are more complicated. Many such parents have a strong sense of failure because their children did not turn out "right." Their feelings of guilt, frustration, and helplessness are likely to increase if their child is institutionalized. They probably felt confused and resentful when experts offered them smug and guilt-provoking advice. Unlike the parents of other adolescents, these parents may have no one in whom to confide, either because they lack the support and understanding of others, or because their own self-reproach prevents them from seeking out such confidants.

Meetings with family members may be indicated if the adolescent's role in the family seems to compound the problems presented in the school or agency setting. An important part of the problem-solving process is organizing initial interviews with parents and family members. Use the information gathered during these meetings to determine whether the problems stem from difficulties posed by the larger system (the family), and, if so, whether family therapy is indicated.

Show compassion and understanding for the parents' dilemma without blaming them or their offspring. Parents will be more receptive to family therapy and to exploring their part in the adolescent's problems if they sense that you will support them, too. Stress and psychologic symptoms evidenced by parents can serve as markers for emotional or behavioral problems in adolescents (Brent, Perper, and Moritz 1994; Pfeffer, Klerman, and Hurt 1991). Any tendency to feel self-righteous or superior to the disturbed adolescent's parents is an obstacle to effective treatment. Such feelings are readily communicated to parents and can only validate their fear of blame and increase their reluctance to participate in therapy with their child. By the same token, resist any temptation to overidentify with the parents, thereby inadvertently perpetuating the family system's problems. The adolescent and the family need a neutral party who can play an objective, knowledgeable, and supportive role in helping them change. The adolescent's chances for resolving the underlying conflicts and maintaining a healthy life are virtually nonexistent if the family system remains unchanged.

Parents, school, and agency staff must understand the objectives and goals of treatment to appreciate the progress the client has made and avoid reinforcing the client's previously maladaptive behavior. The following incident illustrates the problems that arise when parents and school authorities, particularly those who must deal directly with behavior problems in the classroom, lack psychologic sophistication.

Jeremy, a 13-year-old boy, was referred to the school nurse because he was introverted and isolated. He made no contact with either his peers or his teachers and rarely spoke unless addressed directly. After he had spent 3 months in group and individual therapy sessions with the nurse, Jeremy began to come to the grade counselor's office of his own accord to talk about his depression and the problems he had been having in his family. Both the grade counselor and the boy's family believed this to be an indication that his difficulties had worsened, and they began to complain to the nurse about his illness! Not only were Jeremy's parents and counselor ignorant of the goals of treatment and the behaviors expected to come with change, but apparently they were also uncomfortable with the changes in Jeremy's behavior and with the implications of these changes for their relationships with him.

The client's siblings may experience many different feelings. Sometimes they share in the parents' guilt and shame. Sometimes, however, they are pleased and relieved when the "troublemaker" is out of the family and hospitalized. You should extend the same understanding to the siblings as to the parents, helping them see how each member of the family contributes to the problem. If the troubled adolescent is hospitalized, another member of the family, usually a sibling, may assume the role of the "bad" or "sick" person in the family because the identified "bad" person is no longer at home. Be aware of this tendency. If you are not skilled in assessing the need for family therapy or in providing this service, refer the family to a competent family therapist (see Chapter 32).

You may identify a need for all of the above therapies in dealing with a client's problems. In some cases, an informal discussion with you is all that is warranted. In other cases, you may identify problems that require considerable attention. Sometimes a period of unsuccessful treatment is necessary to determine that outpatient therapy is ineffective and that hospitalization is indicated. Before making such a recommendation, you need to establish a trusting relationship with the client and the client's parents.

In the Inpatient Setting

Admission into a hospital or other residential treatment facility may be indicated under the following circumstances:

- If the adolescent lacks sufficient ego strength to control impulsivity.
- If the degree of destructive or antisocial behavior escalates beyond normal limits.
- If the adolescent cannot form meaningful, stable relationships within the everyday environment (as in the case of family dysfunction).

The existence of any of these conditions warrants counseling or professional treatment. A combination of two or more is likely to make treatment on an outpatient basis virtually ineffective, indicating the need for hospital or residential treatment.

Hospitalization of the disturbed adolescent has these possible advantages:

- It provides additional structure within which to handle the physically and psychologically destructive elements of the adolescent's behavior.
- It removes the individual from the stresses of a disturbed family environment.
- It offers opportunities for supporting existing ego strengths and for promoting whatever ability the client has for forming relationships.

Adolescents are sometimes institutionalized because their ideas are strange or threatening to their families, or because the responsible authorities seek to punish the adolescent's unacceptable behavior. The results can be disastrous. Therefore, it is important to make accurate assessments and to implement early treatment when indicated. You can play a crucial role in making such assessments, undertaking appropriate interventions, and educating parents, teachers, and school officials to recognize such needs.

As a Staff Nurse in a General Hospital Setting Adolescents with emotional problems may have symptoms of physical illness and as a result may be admitted to a general hospital setting for evaluation and treatment. Clients with anorexia nervosa, in particular, may be referred for inpatient treatment on general adolescent medical units. As a staff nurse in such a setting, you can take the opportunity to reach out to adolescents in these programs.

As a Consultant in a General Hospital Setting Staff nurses from a psychiatric inpatient unit of a general hospital may be consulted by other nursing staff about emotionally disturbed adolescents who have been admitted to their general medical or surgical units. Some general hospital settings have clinical nurse specialists in psychiatric liaison positions as consultants.

As a Staff Nurse or Clinical Specialist in a Psychiatric Setting In inpatient psychiatric settings, the staff nurse or clinical nurse specialist may assume any of the previously mentioned roles. Nurses in inpatient settings also have numerous opportunities to observe and assess the family dynamics among the adolescent's family members and possibly to intervene. Nurses involved in family therapy sessions can perceive maladaptive ways of relating and take direct steps to work toward change. However, you need not work within the structured format of a therapy hour to have an impact on the family system. The accompanying Intervention box delineates specific parent behaviors and corresponding interventions by the nurse in the therapeutic environment.

Because inpatient nursing entails around-the-clock care, the nurse has the responsibility to maintain the therapeutic environment. The role of the inpatient staff nurse includes the following:

- Maintaining physical and psychologic safety of the unit.
- Setting verbal and physical limits on client behavior.
- Establishing meaningful one-to-one relationships with clients.
- Identifying client strengths and promoting more adaptive coping skills.
- Role-modeling socially acceptable behaviors.
- Participating in group therapies and other structured activities.

As a Milieu Therapist Many authors have described the importance of the therapeutic environment, indicating the strong influence of the treatment environment on the treatment outcome (Tuck and Keels 1992). (For a complete discussion, see Chapter 9.)

Because of adolescents' needs for peer acceptance, their overwhelming uncertainties and fears, and their everchanging behaviors and attitudes about identity, their chances for success in inpatient treatment are increased by a peer group setting. Much has been written about the value of the therapeutic environment in dealing with adolescent problems, including the problems of substance abuse and similar destructive activities. Without the social interaction and living-learning situations provided by the peer group, psychotherapy may be sterile and ineffectual.

The therapeutic environment provides valuable experiences for adolescents for the following reasons:

- Adolescents more readily hear and accept limits from peers than from adults.
- Adolescents more readily respond to feedback, both negative and positive, from peers than from adults.
- Shared goals and objectives facilitate group processes and the development of cohesion among adolescent group members.
- Group interaction allows for the expression of appropriate feelings and identification with peers with similar feelings.
- Group interaction provides opportunities for learning how to develop relationships with others.
- Group structure allows for the testing of new, more adaptive behaviors.
- Adolescents receive feedback from the peer group and have the opportunity to give feedback in a supportive environment.
- The group format provides an opportunity to work out specific issues of conflict with adult group leaders while receiving the support and understanding of peers.

INTERVENTION

Guidelines for Intervening with Specific Parent Behaviors

Parent Behavior

Initiates loud verbal arguments during visits with adolescent.

Nursing Interventions

- Stop the immediate behavior, pointing out the disruptiveness to the unit.
- Refer adolescent and family to family therapist to resolve differences and learn more adaptive ways of relating in supportive atmosphere of family therapy.

  Suggest that family therapist contract with family for one or more of the following:

  Staff will monitor visits.

  Family will bring up potentially volatile topics only within the structure of family meetings and not on the unit during visits.

  Staff will intervene if arguments ensue on unit.

  Staff may limit visiting time on unit.

Parent Behavior

Has history of physical violence against adolescent.

Nursing Interventions

- Upon admission, contract with adolescent and family for no acts of violence against people or property.
- Monitor visits with adolescent on unit.
- Limit or deny passes with parents until progress is demonstrated.
- Depending on abilities with impulse control, refuse visiting privileges with adolescent until progress is seen in family therapy.

Parent Behavior

Is unable to set limits with adolescent during unit visits (is adversely influenced by manipulative attempts, tolerates verbal abuse, etc.)

Nursing Interventions

- Intervene if demands or behavior could lead to physical harm, unit rule breaking, or other negative results.
- Point out problem and refer adolescent and parents to family therapy.
- Role-model appropriate and effective limit setting with adolescent, if necessary.
- Offer to discuss situation with parents and adolescent if desirable in immediate situation.
- Offer emotional support to parent who needs to talk.

Parent Behavior

Has limited interaction with adolescent during unit visits.

Nursing Interventions

- Initiate discussion among adolescent and family members related to visit and treatment goals.
- Refer problem and give observations to family therapist.
- Initiate discussion with parents to allow exploration of difficulty, if desired.
- Suggest that family members and adolescent discuss problem in family therapy.
- Plan outings or special-occasion celebrations to include family, if appropriate.

The Nursing Process and Adolescents

Adolescents present behaviors and problems unique to their developmental stage. Without knowledge and understanding about potentially difficult areas, you may respond with confusion, anger, and even hostility, which will cause feelings of frustration and failure for both yourself and your adolescent clients. The following pages contain numerous examples of either typical behaviors expected of the "normal" adolescent or problem behaviors that may provide the impetus for referral to a treatment setting, or both. In many situations, you may simply need to focus on the difficult issues encountered in working with adolescents. That information is given in the Assessment section. Situations that represent an identified problem necessitating treatment are discussed under Planning and Implementing Interventions.

Assessment

Accurate and comprehensive assessments can be obtained only by viewing the adolescent as a biopsychosocial being. Only by integrating knowledge from biology, psychology, and humanistic interactionist theory can you understand what a particular behavior means to an adolescent. If you can remember your own adolescent experiences—the conflicts and uncertainty as well as the elation and the triumphs—you will better appreciate the adolescent's turmoil. It is equally important that you discover who the individual adolescent is. Meanings of behavior, values, and actions can vary from client to client and may not reflect meanings or values that you hold. For example, the client who has trouble with competitive feelings may be reluctant to accept an invitation to play a game of Jeopardy. And because adolescents are developmentally between childhood and adulthood, they frequently have the feelings and choices of adulthood without an adult's abilities in verbal discourse and impulse control. As a result, adolescents may "act out" feelings and decisions nonverbally, in a childlike way. This is particularly true of the emotionally disturbed adolescent.

ACTING-OUT The concept of **acting-out** is complex. The term has been used to describe a variety of behaviors, ranging from antisocial, destructive acts to unconscious impulses expressed in action rather than in symbolic words or symptoms. Acting-out may, and often does, include destructive actions and seemingly undefinable behaviors. The term describes a recreation of the client's life experiences, relationships with significant others, and resulting unresolved conflicts.

These are all components of what is commonly called the client's **life script,** which unfolds as the client relates, reacts, and behaves in accustomed ways. Through observation of and interaction with the client, you can uncover the meanings that various behaviors and actions hold for the individual. For example, the child who has assumed the "black sheep" role in the family seeks to recreate that familiar role with others outside the home, particularly in the inpatient setting. The following clinical example illustrates one girl's relationship with her parents as replayed with the staff on an inpatient unit.

Liza is 14 years old. She has been on the unit for 6 days. She is an attractive, engaging young person who has been friendly with both staff and clients. Liza has been on the periphery of several rule-breaking incidents but has not been directly involved. She has begun to establish close ties with Jim, a nurse, and engages in frequent lengthy discussions with him about her innermost feelings and fears. One evening she candidly talks to him about the callous way in which she was treated by one of the other nurses, a woman, in regard to a gynecologic problem. Liza says with undisguised fear and embarrassment that she is afraid the situation will repeat itself. She expresses great respect for Jim's knowledge and style and asks him to attend to any subsequent problems himself rather than report her dissatisfaction with Jane, the other nurse.

The implications for treatment are many. The most important factors for Jim to consider are what meaning Liza's behavior has for her and what would be the most therapeutically effective way to deal with the situation. The client's presenting problems and the expectation that the client will act out previous conflicts and life scripts have provided Jim adequate information on which to base an appropriate intervention. The client's attempt to seduce the nurse, and the need for nurses to examine their own behavior and motivations, are discussed in detail later in this chapter.

Jim recognizes the "pull" from Liza to feel that only he can adequately handle the situation. He remembers that Liza's home situation is chaotic. Liza's mother and father frequently fight over who is the better parent. Jim surmises that Liza also plays a part in these fights. The present situation seems to indicate that he is about to be played off against Jane, just as Liza perhaps plays one parent against the other. Jim responds by reiterating his concern for her dilemma and suggesting that Liza speak with Jane about the situation that is causing her concern.

In this example, it is clear that the client is attempting to recreate her home situation, using two of the nurses to reenact the roles of her parents. Had Jim been seduced into playing the father's role in the script, he would have recreated the family's conflict on the unit. The ideal solution is for staff to interrupt this pathologic process by substituting a healthier way of resolving the problem. Thus, Jim does not react with compliance or with anger to Liza's attempts. Instead, he recognizes the significance of her behavior and deals with the situation in a concerned yet healthy way, suggesting a resolution to the immediate problem that demonstrates respect for both Liza's and Jane's abilities to resolve the conflict.

Such situations are commonplace with adolescents. They require nursing staff to evaluate the client's psychodynamics and psychopathology as well as their own inner feelings and behavior. For these reasons, it is imperative to identify transference and countertransference issues and to discuss them with your clinical supervisor. Transference and countertransference are discussed in Chapter 28. But these situations are not limited to the inpatient setting. This fact alone obliges you to be alert in observing and assessing verbal and nonverbal communication and to understand your own feelings and behavior in order to make accurate assessments and appropriate interventions. In this way, you will be most effective when working with adolescents.

COMMUNICATION Communication with adolescents is an art in itself. To become proficient in this area, you must accept and understand the following:

- Adolescents tend to act out feelings and conflicts rather than verbalize them.
- Adolescents have an unconventional language of their own.
- Adolescents, especially disturbed ones, may use profanity frequently.
- Many clues can be obtained simply by observing an adolescent's behavior, dress, or environment.

If you learn the skills of interviewing and the use of nonverbal cues and messages, you can use them comfortably and naturally in communicating with adolescents.

Adolescents give many nonverbal cues to their specific emotional struggles, underlying confusion, or transitory moods. A glance around their rooms or a brief study of their dress can tell you more than several direct questions would elicit. Sometimes adolescents give obvious cues. A client who wears a coat around the unit may be planning to run away. Other less-obvious behaviors, which are often outside the client's conscious awareness or control, can also yield vital information. A sudden escalation of horseplay among the boys around bedtime is an example. You would probably be correct in identifying this behavior as an expression of anxiety related to sexual identity and fears of homosexual feelings. Interactionist theory holds that the adolescent boy's newfound sexual feelings and changing body image provide unfamiliar ways of relating to members of his own sex. As a result, he regresses to preadolescent behavior, which served him well in handling close feelings then but now proves inappropriate. In this instance, firm limit setting is in order. Avoid interpreting the behavior or paying undue attention to the specifics. (Testing and limit setting are discussed later in the chapter.)

Adolescents create a language all their own. This takes some understanding and acceptance. In seeking their identity, adolescents establish a form of communication unique to the group. To gain acceptance into the adolescent world, the adult must accept this need to use ambiguous (to the adult) yet specific (to the adolescent) terms to express themselves. In many cases, you must communicate with adolescents by using their jargon.

This jargon often includes obscene and profane words. This is particularly true of disturbed adolescents, who have an especially difficult time expressing anger and fear appropriately. The words they use often reveal the nature of the emotional conflict. For example, a young male adolescent grappling with his sexual identity and aggressive feelings may resort to sexually graphic words when he feels anxious or afraid. You may sometimes find it productive to use similar words to give explanations or to clarify communication. Understandably, some nurses have difficulty tolerating profane or sexually graphic language. However, you must evaluate your clients' underlying reasons for using such language, to help them understand their feelings. Only then can you encourage clients to use more appropriate means of expression. If clients sense that the reason you want them to speak more appropriately is only to make you, the nurse, feel more comfortable, the end result will not be satisfactory.

The adolescent psychiatric client often presents with symptoms of disturbed communication, which can affect all realms of daily living, particularly in relationships with peers, family members, and nonparental authority figures. Giving information is one way you can help decrease communication deficits and facilitate relationships with others. Other nursing behaviors are outlined in the Planning and Implementing Interventions section. (For the general principles of therapeutic communication, see Chapter 7.)

ANGER AND HOSTILITY Expressions of anger and hostility are common on an adolescent unit. Anger expressed verbally usually takes the form of profanity. How effectively we deal with expressions of anger and hostility depends on how effectively we handle our own angry or hostile feelings. You will compromise your effectiveness as a nurse if you are uncomfortable with expressions of anger or hostility, or view anger and hostility as negative or to be avoided at all costs.

Nurse's Self-Assessment A subject that is rarely considered is anger felt and expressed by the nurse toward the client. The general focus on the client's need for understanding and good care seem to make it unacceptable to display negative feelings toward the client. In the nursing care of adolescents, however, a constant all-giving and all-accepting attitude by the nurse, particularly during times of testing, would be not only nontherapeutic but also illogical and dishonest. Testing behavior is at an all-time high, and adolescents need honest feedback. The adolescent sometimes escalates the provocative behavior to evoke an angry reaction. For you to pretend that you are not angry in such a situation is as undesirable for treatment as it would be to pretend that you are fond of the client. Being honest about your feelings is a prime prerequisite in establishing and maintaining meaningful and

NURSING SELF-AWARENESS

A Self-Awareness Inventory for Working with Adolescents

To increase self-awareness about your own way of dealing with anger:

- What kinds of things make me angry?
- How do I deal with my anger? Do I tend to ignore or hide it, or do I show that I am angry?
- Do I sometimes use profanity or act out my feelings in a physical way? How do I feel about others who do this?
- What do I think about how I handle anger?
- How do I feel about how I handle anger?
- How do I react to others when they are angry?

To increase self-awareness about your tendency to be seduced or manipulated:

- Is this client's friendliness compromising the professional role boundaries between us to "personalize" our relationship?
- Do I feel compelled to respond in a personal rather than a therapeutic way, possibly revealing information about my own life and lifestyle?
- Do I feel uncomfortable with the client's flattering comments or probing questions?
- Do I tend to forget that this person is a client?
- Is the client encouraging me to keep secrets from other staff or to "side" with client against other staff?

To increase self-awareness about your own sexual attitudes and feelings:

- How would I describe my adolescence as it related to my developing sexuality?
- What do I remember about the development and changes in my body?
- How did I feel about these changes?
- How would I describe my adolescent relationships with members of my sex?
- How would I describe my adolescent relationships with members of the opposite sex?
- What events stand out in my mind when I recall my sexual experiences during adolescence?
- How have these past relationships, events, and feelings influenced me today?

productive relationships with adolescent clients. This does not mean that you should give vent to all your thoughts or impulses. Be aware of your reactions, and use good judgment in handling them. The questions in the accompanying Nursing Self-Awareness box will help you assess your own ways of dealing with anger.

Anxiety and Resistance Normal adolescents frequently feel anxious as they experience change and inner turmoil in adapting to a new identity. The anxiety evidenced by disturbed adolescents in treatment can indicate many other things. The changes required of disturbed adolescents are much more threatening than those required of normal adolescents. If treatment is to be successful, clients must look at the meaning of their behavior and must change many of their earlier interactional patterns. This can be frightening. For example, it is more comfortable to play the role of the "bad seed" or "bad kid," with its known pitfalls and expectations, than to attempt a change that entails many uncertainties and unknowns.

Clients feel threatened and anxious when the nurse does not act according to their expectations, because they must then find other ways of handling the situation. They must also deal with the anxiety. Frequently this anxiety is channeled into a game of "cops and robbers," as the client once again assumes a familiar role and maintains the negative or unhealthy image. The anxiety caused by unfamiliar roles is dissipated by further testing and acting-out. Do not take this as an indication that therapy is not working. It may simply indicate that the client needs to move ahead more slowly with insightful discoveries and needs your support in doing so.

Keep in mind that to such adolescents, "opening up" in a trusting way does not hold the same positive promise that it might for you. Adolescents who have been rejected or have experienced loss following close relationships in the past will feel wary of your expressions of interest or concern and will be cautious about repeating such experiences. They may respond to you with testing behaviors, anger and mistrust, or outright rejection. Adolescents who expect rejection assume some control over the relationship if they reject others before being rejected themselves.

Sometimes nurses find it difficult to allow adolescents to grapple with their anxieties and fears. At other times, you may not recognize the client's behavior as a symptom of anxiety or depression. The following clinical example demonstrates the value of a comprehensive assessment, of exploring all possible reasons for a client's resistance to your efforts before implementing action.

Kathy was the quietest and most aloof client on the unit. She had isolated herself from the other clients during the week that followed admission and avoided conversing with staff members outside meetings. One evening she seemed especially receptive to the new nurse, Ellie, who was able to interest her in a sewing project. Ellie, who was a new graduate, felt pleased that Kathy had responded warmly to her during their time together. The next day, Kathy did not speak to Ellie and seemed to avoid her at all costs. Later, Ellie noticed that the dress Kathy had been sewing was torn into shreds and stuffed into the wastepaper basket. Ellie interpreted this quite personally. She felt deeply hurt and rejected. In her discussion with her supervisor, Ellie showed her disappointment and anger. Her supervisor observed that, although the good time and feelings that Ellie and Kathy had shared the evening before were genuine, Kathy had not experienced many such times before with her parents or other adults. She suggested that Kathy was probably angry with Ellie for pointing up what she, Kathy, had missed. The supervisor suggested that Ellie be patient with Kathy. Perhaps later Ellie could reestablish the bond, and they would be able to talk about what had happened.

Fortunately, Ellie did not act on her angry feelings. Had she done so, she might have impulsively assessed Kathy's behavior as "hopeless," interpreting Kathy's anxiety and resistance as an inability to trust, or she may have begun to relate to the client in a vindictive way, withdrawing from Kathy in turn. Instead, she sought advice. Ellie's supervisor recognized that Ellie wanted badly to do well and needed positive feedback. She also realized that Ellie did not understand the nature of giving to emotionally disturbed adolescents. Had Ellie not sought advice, she might have acted on her angry feelings, further alienating Kathy and causing herself more anger and frustration. Without an understanding of Kathy's actions, Ellie would have continued to expect kindness in return for kindness and would have been keenly disappointed.

Seduction and Manipulation of the Nurse In working with adolescents, there is always a risk of seduction of the nurse, or being manipulated into relating in a nontherapeutic way. These factors contribute to the problem:

- The intimate nature of the nurse's involvement with the adolescent client.
- The narcissism inherent in this age group.
- The nurse's all-accepting attitude in working with the adolescent client.

Narcissism in this age group is caused by the child's withdrawal from the parents and their value system. This withdrawal leads to a general self-centeredness, overevaluation of the self, heightened self-perception, decreased ability for reality testing, and extreme self-absorption. The result is that the people to whom adolescents turn become all-important and perfect in their eyes. Nurses may be strongly tempted to respond accordingly.

The dangers inherent in this situation are not simply the two possible extremes: total submission to temptation, resulting in a sexual relationship with the client; or strong denial of temptation by maintaining a rigid, unapproachable stance that makes it impossible to establish a meaningful, trusting relationship. Neither of these extremes is unknown, but the greatest danger is actually intrinsic to the role of the helping professional. It is tempting to respond to the adolescent's idealized view, to be the "savior" who succeeded with this difficult person where everyone else has failed, to feel superior to the imperfect parents, the harassed school teacher, the skeptical juvenile judge, or other members of the staff on the unit. However, you should not give in to such temptations. Complications will most certainly develop that at best will temporarily compromise your effectiveness and at worst will render the treatment program completely ineffective. Liza's example of acting-out demonstrates this. Jim, the evening nurse, could have been seduced by Liza to collude with her against the day nurse, Jane, had he not been keenly aware of the possibility.

Nurses who work intensively with adolescents often face situations in which their own unresolved feelings are aroused. You must choose whether to act on these impulses or to explore their origin. Of course, one is not always conscious of these unresolved feelings. It would be unrealistic to expect you to be totally aware of the meaning of your behavior at any given moment. Nonetheless, the skilled clinician is usually acquainted with the issues or conflicts that have caused problems in the past. In doubtful cases, the knowledgeable nurse will seek consultation from such a clinician. The clinician can help you assess the situation and understand what part you may have played in initiating it. Nurses who wish to explore their personal conflicts further may then seek counseling or therapy. You can use the questions in the Nursing Self-Awareness box to assess the nature of such interactions with clients.

In addition, nursing staff would benefit from establishing one or more of the following to provide a consistent format for assessing and evaluating ongoing situations with adolescent clients:

- Each nurse's own ongoing supervision with preceptor or nurse supervisor.
- A regularly scheduled meeting (perhaps monthly) for all nursing staff to discuss difficult situations and conflicting feelings.

- Staff meetings (perhaps weekly) in which all disciplines identify interpersonal obstacles and plan interventions toward more optimal treatment.

Given the nature of their work, the staff—particularly the nursing staff—undergo considerable stress as adolescents challenge accepted ideas and values (Lego and Pawlicki 1993).

SEXUAL BEHAVIOR OF THE ADOLESCENT The biologic changes that occur in late childhood and early adolescence are rapid and pervasive. Hormones secreted by the adrenal glands and gonads initiate visible primary and secondary sex characteristics. Research now supports decades of speculation that the increase in puberty-related hormones is related to the health and behavior problems of adolescents (National Nursing Research Agenda 1993).

Do not underestimate the importance of the adolescent's experimentation and attitude in sexual matters. Likewise, evaluate your own attitudes and feelings about sexual issues as they relate to past experiences and current activities. Conflicts in such matters or resentments left over from the past will certainly affect your decisions or interaction with clients regarding sexual matters. Again, while it is not necessary for you to resolve all these issues, it is highly desirable to be aware of areas of conflict that might make it difficult to view a situation objectively or set rational limits. Refer again to the Nursing Self-Awareness box to increase your self-awareness about sexual attitudes and feelings.

Until adolescents master their anxieties and fears about their sexual identity and gain control over sexual urges, they will exhibit a variety of behaviors and attitudes that may confuse or trouble you. The national school-based Youth Risk Behavior Surveillance Survey (YRBSS) reports that 54.1% of the students studied had participated in sexual intercourse and 18.7% had four or more sex partners during their lifetime. Female students were significantly more likely to be currently sexually active than males. African-American students reported a significantly higher frequency of intercourse than whites or Latinos. White students had used a contraceptive method (birth control pill, condom, or withdrawal) during their most recent sexual intercourse significantly more often than African-American students or Latino students (Public Health Service 1993).

Heterosexual Behavior Heterosexual activity is normal and desirable during adolescence. However, nurses working with either normal or disturbed adolescents will sometimes see them engage in sexual activities that do not seem healthy or growth-producing. For example, the adolescent girl who seeks punishment rather than true pleasure in her sexual exploits will display them in an overt, exhibitionistic way in a place where a particularly moralistic person will discover her and give her the reprimands she desires. She may be testing a parent's values in an attempt to resolve her own inner conflicts. Adolescents in an inpatient treatment setting where sexual intercourse is forbidden may engage in sexual intercourse where you or another staff member will be sure to discover them. The experience may reinforce their image of sexual behavior as "bad" behavior. Or it may simply provide a means of acting out their defiance of the rules, thereby earning the familiar "bad kid" label. The incident involving the nurse Barbara and the clients Laurie and Bill in the Planning and Implementing Interventions section is an excellent example of this situation.

Homosexual Behavior Preadolescents usually choose a member of the same sex with whom to experience intimate or loving feelings. This does not necessarily mean that a sexual relationship will ensue, although it often does. Homosexual activity may continue into the adolescent years.

Generally, however, adolescents begin to view homosexual feelings as a threat to the development of their identity. As a result, they may ward off such feelings by engaging in frantic sexual activity with a member of the opposite sex. This is particularly true for boys. It is normal for an adolescent boy to be afraid of his own passive wishes and to label them homosexual. He has probably been brought up to identify with physical displays of strength or aggressive displays of power. Thus, an incident in which he feels threatened or powerless would produce feelings of sexual impotence, a fear of castration, a feeling of dependence or weakness, and a greater fear of homosexuality. The adolescent boy in treatment may act out these feelings, or he may attempt to reaffirm his masculinity with inappropriate displays of aggression or destructive behavior.

At the other extreme are adolescents who engage in predominantly homosexual activities. Many of these individuals find relationships with the opposite sex threatening or unrewarding and continue to seek intimacy with people of the same sex. Some feel more comfortable with companions of the same sex and are satisfied with these relationships. Others use their homosexual affiliation to express and act out hostility directed against their parents and their parents' values.

Since nurses who work with adolescents may encounter any of these situations, they must attempt to understand the meaning that homosexual behavior has for the client. The clients may need to explore their feelings and anxieties openly. Open discussion with an understanding yet knowledgeable professional may help resolve many of the concerns and conflicts inherent in adolescent sexual behavior.

Clients who use homosexuality to express hostility toward their parents will undoubtedly act out with the staff as well. Remain objective and relatively nonjudgmental with these clients, allowing them to deal with the feelings of anger or depression that may result from addressing the conflict.

Although homosexual behavior during adolescence does not predict adult sexual preference, some adolescents make a lasting identification as homosexuals during these years. Such adolescents will not experience conflicts about homosexual relationships or need to flaunt them or act out with the staff in an angry or hostile way. In such cases, however, you may have to deal with your own negative feelings about homosexuality, if any exist. It is important for you to consider what their relationships mean to clients and to respect them.

Pregnancy Adolescent pregnancy may reflect social and family expectations and unconscious motivations. Some teenage girls are quite pleased to be pregnant and suffer no emotional consequences from motherhood. In general, however, a conscious, deliberate decision to become pregnant at this age is manipulative. The goal may be to escape a difficult family situation, to express hostility toward parents, or to act out a life script in which the daughter is seen as "bad." The adolescent girl who did not receive adequate nurturing as a child could be acting out dependence needs by giving her baby the love and caring she herself did not receive. In so doing, she feels loved and cared for in turn.

Be sensitive to motivational factors in dealing with emotionally deprived adolescents. Use existing educational tools and interpersonal relationships to help adolescent girls understand their needs and motivations in becoming pregnant. It is also important to educate teenagers of both sexes about sex and birth control. Many high schools are now recognizing this need and providing such information in birth control clinics or through health education classes. Too often parents and professionals alike deny the adolescent's sexual activity until an unwanted pregnancy occurs.

DIETARY PROBLEMS AND EATING DISORDERS The eating habits and food preferences of disturbed adolescents can reveal a lot about the nature of their inner turmoil. A comparison between the client's diet and that of a normal, healthy adolescent may show little difference in variety but probably a great difference in quantity. Teen-agers who have been deprived of early nurturing tend to eat more than others and probably place a higher value on mealtimes and on receiving their "share" of the food. You may notice that adolescents consume more milk than usual during periods of stress or anxiety. In general, girls want to follow food fads or unreasonable dietary regimens to become slim and attractive. This usually gives you an opportunity to engage in health teaching about nutrition and exercise, and to express a cooperative interest in their developing feminine identity. (Eating disorders are discussed in Chapter 18.)

DEPRESSION AND SUICIDE Both depression and suicide are thought to be underreported among adolescents. Research indicates that one out of every four adolescents experiences a major depressive disorder (Lewinsohn et al. 1994). For every successful suicide, some researchers say, there are 200 attempts (Valente 1989). Moreover, there is real concern about a contagion of suicides known as cluster suicides, in which one suicide appears to set off another. Such clusters were reported in several communities in the last decade: In Fairfax, Virginia, eleven youths killed themselves during one school year; in Plano, Texas, seven adolescents died within a year; in Westchester County, New York, five teens killed themselves within one month. The Research Note provides additional data for assessments of depression in adolescents. (See Chapter 24 for a complete discussion of adolescent suicide, including assessment and nursing intervention.)

SUBSTANCE USE AND ABUSE Experimentation with alcohol and drugs among the adolescent population is widespread. Surveys report that 50–90% of adolescent subjects have used drugs or alcohol at least once. The YRBSS revealed that 81.6% of the students had consumed alcohol during their lifetime, and 50.8% did so during the 30 days preceding the survey (Public Health Service 1993).

Adolescents give many reasons for using drugs: to experiment, to get high, to "get inside my head," to have fun, to understand more about life. Adolescents may also use drugs to cope with feelings of worthlessness or loneliness, or to avoid uncomfortable feelings.

According to Cindy, a 15-year-old high school sophomore, her three-year history of substance abuse has involved regular marijuana use 1–2 times a week, occasional use of Valium (which she sneaks from her mother's 5-mg tablet prescription bottle), Seconal ("street reds") on two occasions, and LSD on two occasions.

Cindy describes herself as a "loner" who has few friends and keeps to herself at home and at school. She leaves the house each morning for school before the others are awake "to avoid the hassles with my mother and sisters." She describes one female classmate to whom she feels close but states that their time together is usually brief and usually involves smoking marijuana in the morning just before school. Cindy has recently been suspended from school as a result of the school principal's discovery of Cindy and her friend smoking marijuana outside the cafeteria.

Cindy is lonely and depressed, and has extreme feelings of worthlessness. She characterizes herself as "bored," "bad," and "hopeless." Cindy says that when she uses drugs, her situation doesn't seem as bad.

RESEARCH NOTE

Citation

Lewinsohn PM, Clarke GN, Seeley JR, Rohde P: Depression in community adolescents: Age at onset, episode duration, and time to recurrence. *J Am Acad Child Adoles Psychiatr* 1994;33(6):809–818.

Study Problem/Purpose

The purpose of this study (the Oregon Adolescent Depression Project) was to assess various parameters of major depression in adolescents age 14–18 in the community. Among the areas for assessment are time to onset and recovery and, when applicable, time to recurrence. The importance of time course parameters was affirmed by the *DSM-IV,* but almost all of the characteristics were based on data from adult clinical populations. This paper is one in a series reporting on the project.

Methods

Initial interviews/questionnaires were completed and followed 13.8 months later, with diagnostic interviews of 1508 randomly selected high school students between ages 14 and 18. Education levels and occupations of the parents were assessed. The initial diagnostic interviews consisted of a version of the Schedule for Affective Disorders and Schizophrenia for School-Age Children (K-SADS), the Epidemiologic Version (KSADS-E), and the Present Episode Version (K-SADS-P), with additional items to compare with characteristics of psychiatric disorders as defined by DSM-III-R criteria (data gathered between 1987 and 1989). The follow-up interviews consisted of information from the Longitudinal Interval Followup Evaluation evaluating the course of psychiatric symptoms and disorders and looking at criteria for recovery from a disorder. A second interviewer reviewed audiotaped or videotaped recordings of a randomly selected 12% of the interviews. Additional variables that were assessed and considered include: gender, lifetime comorbidity with dysthymia, anxiety disorders, disruptive behavior disorders and/or substance use disorders, suicide attempts, suicide ideation, depression severity, endogeneity (evaluating classic neurovegetative signs and symptoms of depression), functional impairment, and mental health treatment utilization.

Findings

Three-hundred sixty-two of the subjects had experienced at least one episode of major depression. Mean age at onset of the first episode was 14.9. Early onset was associated with female gender and suicide ideation. Depressive episode duration ranged from 2 to 520 weeks; thus, a mean of 26.4 weeks and a median of 8 weeks. Longer episodes were assessed in those whose depression occurred early, at or before age 15, and whose depression had been accompanied by suicidal ideation. Of those who recovered, 5% relapsed within 6 months, 12% within 1 year, and approximately 33% within 4 years. Those subjects with a shorter recurrence time gave a history of suicidal ideation/attempt and a later first onset.

Implications

Risk of major depression increases substantially with the onset of adolescence. The 24% incidence of a randomly selected community population of this size is significant. It would be beneficial for nurses in any setting to assess adolescents for symptoms of depression and the existence of suicidal ideation or prior attempt. This study demonstrates that although the majority of episodes in a nonpsychiatric adolescent population may be brief, the risk of recurrence is substantial. Suicidal behaviors play an important role in the assessment, intervention, and planning for such individuals. Researchers could profit from these results as well, particularly regarding duration and recurrence. These data could be used to compare and contrast results with other teenage groups, such as teens with bipolar disorder or adolescents treated with a new intervention. Recognizing and treating the depression in one of every four adolescents would be a major accomplishment, not only toward enhancing the quality of life for these adolescents, but toward improving the mental health of a future adult population.

Although the general public may disagree about whether drugs are harmful, the fact remains that using drugs—or at least experimenting with them—is acceptable to most adolescents.

How can you determine when drug *use* becomes drug *abuse*? Generally, the adolescent who abuses drugs or alcohol exhibits at least one of these following characteristics:

- The adolescent's performance at school or work increasingly deteriorates.
- The adolescent is frequently caught high or in the act of getting high by parents or other authority figures.
- The adolescent increasingly resorts to alcohol or drugs in times of stress or boredom.
- The adolescent has seriously deficient interpersonal relationships and can relate only when under the influence of drugs or alcohol.
- The adolescent may lose interest in interpersonal relationships altogether, preferring to be high alone rather than to be with others.

Nurses are most effective when they can determine what the particular drug or high does for the client. A boy with a poor self-image and low-esteem may say that it makes him "feel like a man." A particularly shy or introverted girl may say that it makes her "outgoing and friendly." You may discover that being high helps rid disturbed adolescents of angry or depressed feelings. Indeed, in the treatment setting, the client frequently resorts to smoking marijuana or "popping" uppers or downers to escape uncomfortable feelings.

Nursing Diagnosis

The use of nursing diagnoses with adolescent clients can lend meaning and substance to the clients' behavior that might be overlooked with a DSM-IV diagnosis alone. For example, a DSM-IV diagnosis of conduct disorder, adolescent-onset type, identifies the nature of the adolescent's difficulty. By using the various subsystems provided by nursing diagnoses, you can establish a more comprehensive picture of the client's difficulty and immediately become more goal-oriented in assessing and planning care. Moreover, in many treatment settings, mental health care professionals are reluctant to give adolescents a DSM-IV diagnosis during these formative years to avoid having them be psychiatrically labeled (possibly erroneously). Such labeling may result in inadequate treatment, self-fulfilling prophecy, or both, in subsequent mental health care contacts.

Planning and Implementing Interventions

Planning for Prevention It is estimated that in the United States, as many as 12% of children and adolescents suffer with a mental disorder, with only one-fifth of these 7.4 million children receiving adequate or appropriate treatment (Finke 1994). As nurses in numerous roles and diverse settings, we are in prime positions to recognize and intervene early with pathologic symptoms and behaviors. Figure 37–1 delineates a continuous chain of prevention. By preventing certain factors or circumstances in the early stages of life, health improvements are made possible at later stages (Serrano 1993). As one progresses along the chain from primary prevention and education/self-care, to secondary prevention with its risk factors and early problem recognition and treatment, to tertiary prevention with its more complicated and serious forms of illness and risky behaviors, it is obvious that services become increasingly more technological, expensive, and exclusive.

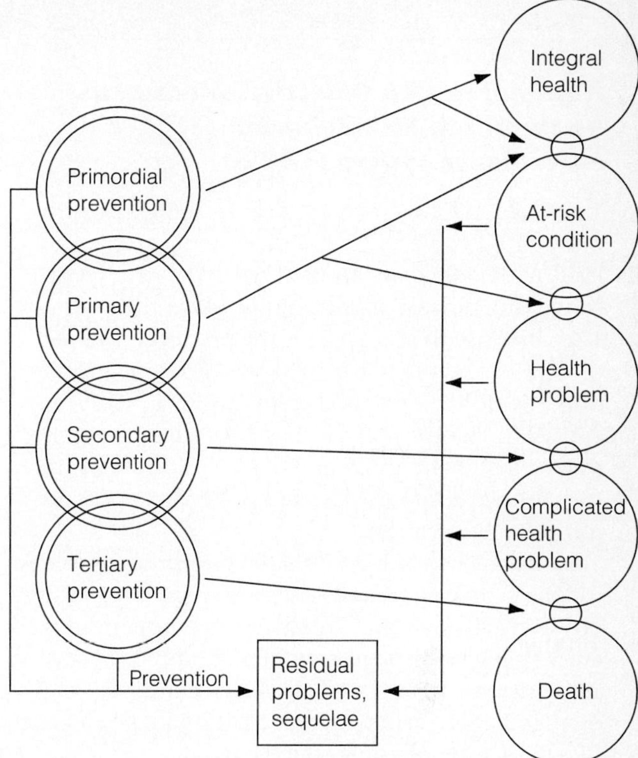

Figure 37–1 The continuous chain of prevention. *Source: Serrano 1993, p. 617.*

The Centers for Disease Control and Prevention (CDC) developed the YRBSS to focus attention on specific behaviors that place adolescents at risk for the most significant health problems: motor vehicle accident injuries, homicide, suicide, heart disease, and cancer (Public Health Service 1993). By reviewing these leading causes of mortality and morbidity on a national scale, the YRBSS looked at the following:

- Unintentional and intentional injury, including wearing a seatbelt in a car or truck; wearing a helmet on a motorcycle; carrying a weapon such as a gun, knife, or club; attempting suicide; having suicidal ideation or plan.
- Tobacco use.
- Alcohol and other drug use.
- Sexual behaviors.
- Dietary behaviors.
- Physical activity.

National Health Objectives Measured by the Youth Risk Behavior Surveillance System (YRBSS)

1.3, 15.11, 17.13 Increase to at least 30% the proportion of people age 6 and older who engage regularly, preferably daily, in light to moderate physical activity for at least 30 minutes per day.

1.4 Increase to at least 20% the proportion of people age 18 and older and to at least 75% the proportion of children and adolescents age 6–17 who engage in vigorous physical activity that promotes the development and maintenance of cardiorespiratory fitness 3 or more days per week for 20 or more minutes per occasion.

1.6 Increase to at least 40% the proportion of overweight people age 6 and older who regularly perform physical activities that enhance and maintain muscular strength, muscular endurance, and flexibility.

1.8 Increase to at least 50% the proportion of children and adolescents in grades 1–12 who participate in daily school physical education.

1.9 Increase to at least 50% the proportion of school physical education class time that students spend being physically active, preferably engaged in lifetime physical activities.

3.5 Reduce the initiation of cigarette smoking by children and youth so that no more than 15% have become regular smokers by age 20.

3.9 Reduce smokeless tobacco use by males age 12–24 to a prevalence of no more than 4%.

4.5 Increase by at least 1 year the average age of first use of cigarettes from 11.6, alcohol from 13.1, and marijuana from 13.4 by adolescents age 12–17.

4.6 Reduce the proportion of young people who have used alcohol to 12.6%, marijuana to 3.2%, and cocaine to 0.6% in the past month.

4.7 Reduce the proportion of high school seniors and college students engaging in recent occasions of heavy drinking of alcoholic beverages to no more than 28% of high school seniors and 32% of college students.

4.11 Reduce to no more than 3% the proportion of male high school seniors who use anabolic steroids.

5.4, 18.3, 19.9 Reduce the proportion of adolescents who have engaged in sexual intercourse to no more than 15% by age 15 and no more than 40% by age 17.

5.5 Increase to at least 40% the proportion of ever sexually active adolescents age 17 and younger who have abstained from sexual activity for the previous 3 months.

5.6 Increase to at least 90% the proportion of sexually active, unmarried people age 19 and younger who use contraception, especially combined-method contraception that both effectively prevents pregnancy and provides barrier protection against disease.

6.2, 7.8 Reduce by 15% the incidence of injurious suicide attempts among adolescents age 14–17.

7.9 Reduce by 20% the incidence of physical fighting among adolescents age 14–17.

7.10 Reduce by 20% the incidence of weapon-carrying by adolescents age 14–17.

9.12 Increase use of occupant protection systems, such as safety belts, inflatable safety restraints, and child safety seat, to at least 85% of motor vehicle occupants.

9.13 Increase use of helmets to at least 80% of motorcyclists and at least 50% of bicyclists.

18.4, 19.10 Increase to at least 50% the proportion of sexually active, unmarried people who used a condom at last sexual intercourse.

18.4a, 19.10a Increase to at least 60% the proportion of sexually active young women age 15–19 who used (by their partners) a condom at last sexual intercourse.

18.4b, 19.10b Increase to at least 75% the proportion of sexually active young men age 15–19 who used a condom at last sexual intercourse.

Source: Adapted from Public Health Service 1993.

Of the 26 national health objectives related to adolescents and measured by the YRBSS, only three objectives—1.3, 15.11, and 17.13, as shown in the accompanying box—had been met by high school students when surveyed in 1991. Achievement of the twenty-three remaining objectives by the year 2000 will require sustained and coordinated efforts by quality health-promotion programs.

Working with Adolescents in Focus Groups To help identify potential strategies for influencing high-risk behaviors, one research study involved focus groups with 160 youth between ages 10 and 18 (Public Health Service 1992). Groups were held with African-American, white, Latino, and Native American youth who were already engaged in high-risk health practices and met at least one of the following criteria:

- Were in alternative school programs or were considered school drop-ins or drop-outs.
- Were involved in the juvenile justice system.
- Were runaways.
- Were in drug or alcohol treatment programs.

In addition, the following characteristics were significant:

- Nearly 50% lived with their mother alone.
- Approximately two-thirds lived in households that received public assistance.
- More than two-thirds were truant or school drop-outs.
- More than 40% were involved with gangs.
- Approximately one-third were engaged in alcohol and drug abuse or had arrest records.

Table 37–1 on page 896 delineates twelve life priorities ranked by ethnic groups. In general, a superficial scan of the responses might reveal relevant differences in value/lifestyle practices for a particular group. More specifically, an appreciation of these differences might "make or break" your intervention with an adolescent. For example, it might be correct to assume that education for its own sake (as in education regarding birth control) could be valued and positively received by an African-American female in this group. Thus, attempting to establish a relationship with her through such an educational channel might be productive if, indeed, she values "learning something" and "being healthy," as the list suggests. On the other hand, initiating such an educational plan with a Native American Indian female from this group could have an adverse response, particularly if "having a family" was highest on her list.

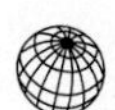

Establishing a Contract with the Adolescent Contracts can be particularly useful with adolescents because they can feel powerless in a treatment setting, especially when "referred" by parents or the legal system. Moreover, with this increased sense of control over their own behavior, adolescents become your collaborators in their treatment rather than objects of your treatment plan.

With most adolescents, a written contract is best, for these reasons:

- The goals and expectations are less easily forgotten.
- The process seems more formal and "serious."
- There is less room for misinterpretation and manipulation.

Contracts seem especially helpful in situations of substance abuse, eating disorders, suicidal behavior, and impulsive or manipulative behaviors (as with some personality disorders). Whether verbal or written, the contract can be simply stated to promote clarity, consistency, and cooperation. Here is an example:

> I will not take drugs or bring drugs into the unit.
>
> I will not call or accept calls from my drug friends while in the treatment program.
>
> I will go directly to my outpatient therapy appointment and return immediately to the unit.
>
> I will not harm myself or others. If I feel like hurting myself, others, or property, I will tell the staff.

If written, the contract is signed by the client, dated, and cosigned by you. The contract is renegotiated at regular intervals (hourly, daily, or weekly), depending on the goals, the severity of the symptoms, and the degree of compliance with the agreement. The form of the contract is less important than the way you and the client jointly set the goals and expectations, carry out the contract, set limits and renegotiate changes, and evaluate the final outcome. Chapter 28 discusses contracting with clients in general, and Chapter 24 discusses no-suicide contracts.

Anger and Hostility Depending on the degree to which the client is experiencing and expressing anger and hostility, you may choose any of a variety of interventions. These range from doing nothing other than observing the client's behavior, to physically restraining someone who is attempting destructive action (see Chapter 34). In some situations, a disturbed adolescent's ability to express anger directly to another person can be a sign of success in treatment. The choice of interventions also depends on your own experiences with such feelings, your knowledge and understanding of this client's life experiences with anger, and the external limits imposed by the mental health agency.

In choosing an appropriate nursing intervention, attempt to discover what meaning anger and hostility have for the client by asking the following questions:

- How has this person handled anger in the past?
- Does the client have a history of aggression toward objects or people?
- If so, what were the consequences of this behavior?
- How does the adolescent feel after such a reaction?
- What kinds of things make this client angry? Which of these would be most likely to occur on the unit or in our setting?

Steve had expressed great interest in building a model airplane. He had saved up his money and had taken a long time to choose "just the right one" at the hobby shop. After spending most of the afternoon constructing and painting it, he was interrupted by a phone call from his mother. She told him that she would not be able to attend the family meeting that week, giving a number of specious-sounding reasons. This was the third consecutive week that she had missed. Each time, she gave questionable reasons for being unable to attend. Steve was disappointed and angry. He

Table 37–1 Life Priorities by Ethnic Group

	AFRICAN AMERICAN		MEXICAN AMERICAN		WHITE		NATIVE AMERICAN	
Rank	***Male***	***Female***	***Male***	***Female***	***Male***	***Female***	***Male***	***Female***
1	Being close to God	Being close to God	Having a family	Having a family	Having some place to call home*	Being loved	Having a family	Being loved
2	Having some place to call home	Being loved	Being close to God	Being close to God	Having enough to eat*	Having some place to call home	Being loved	Having a family
3	Being loved	Having a family	Being loved	Being loved	Being loved	Having a family	Feeling safe	Feeling safe
4	Having a family	Learning something	Feeling safe	Being healthy	Having money	Getting along with others	Having enough to eat	Being close to God*
5	Looking good	Having some place to call home	Having enough to eat	Feeling safe	Feeling important	Feeling safe	Feeling important	Having some place to call home*
6	Feeling safe	Being healthy	Feeling important	Looking good	Looking good	Having money	Being close to God	Getting along with others
7	Having enough to eat	Feeling safe	Being healthy	Having some place to call home	Being close to God	Feeling important	Having some place to call home*	Having enough to to eat
8	Having money	Having enough to eat	Having some place to call home	Feeling important	Having a family	Being healthy*	Being healthy*	Having money
9	Learning something	Having money	Learning something	Having enough to eat	Being healthy	Looking good*	Having money	Feeling important
10	Being healthy	Feeling important	Having money	Learning something	Getting along with others	Being close to God	Getting along with others	Being healthy
11	Feeling important	Getting along with others	Getting along with others	Having money	Feeling safe	Having enough to eat	Learning something	Looking good
12	Getting along with others	Looking good	Looking good	Getting along with others	Learning something	Learning something	Looking good	Learning something

**Tied*
Source: Public Health Service 1992.

slammed down the receiver, yelling obscenities in response to the nurse's questions, and ran into his room. There he began to destroy the plane by throwing it repeatedly against the floor.

In this example, Steve was not hurting himself or another. Although he did destroy property, the plane belonged to him, and he was free to do with it as he chose. The nurse resisted any impulse to stop Steve from damaging his plane. Since it was of significant value to him, he later regretted having taken out his anger on it. However, the situation provided Steve with an opportunity to explore his actions, and he later asked the nurse why he would destroy something that he valued so much after his mother had disappointed and angered him. The parallel between this situation and hurting himself with drugs right after he had argued with his mother was only too apparent.

Incidents in which the nurse bears the brunt of a client's anger or hostility do not offer such obvious solutions. Disturbed adolescents may not think twice about addressing a female nurse as "bitch" and coupling such a greeting with a request for a favor. Adolescents direct insults and hostile remarks at nurses for many reasons, most of which have little to do with the nurses as people but a lot to do with them as adults or authority figures.

There are as many suggestions for intervention as there are people who will be involved in such exchanges. In choosing interventions, consider the meaning behind the client's behavior, your own relationship with this client, your immediate feelings, and the result desired. For example, if the client calls you "bitch" the first time you meet, you may interpret this as a form of testing and may choose to respond immediately with a bewildered look at this unwarranted display of hostility. Later, you may approach the client, expressing a naive curiosity as to the origin of the hostile feelings: "Hey, I don't understand what happened between us a few minutes ago. We just met, and you're calling me a bitch. What's that all about?" This simple question conveys two messages. First, it indicates to the client that you are not accustomed to this kind of salutation. Second, it indicates that you are more interested in the motivation for the remark than in curtailing its use.

If the client resorts to name calling only when angry or under stress, you may decide to ignore the words and deal only with the feelings involved. For example, if a client has angrily left an ongoing family meeting and then calls you a bitch, you can probably assume that the anger is displaced. It is probably a result of overwhelming feelings experienced during the meeting. You may elect simply to say, "I know you're not angry at me right now. It seems like the meeting is pretty heavy, though. Do you want to talk about why you don't want to be in there now?" In neither situation is the name calling intended as a personal affront. However, the way you handle it determines both the outcome of the immediate situation and your chances of furthering your relationship with the client.

The adolescent's reaction to your intervention largely determines its effectiveness. For example, with Steve, the boy who destroyed his plane, the nurse's goal was to help Steve understand the impulsive reaction that destroyed something he loved and to encourage a more appropriate and direct expression of anger at his mother. He was able to do this as well as draw a parallel between anger at his mother and his drug abuse, which hurt himself. If the nurse's goal had been simply to stop the destruction of his property, Steve could have felt even greater anger and frustration, and he might have turned his aggression toward himself, the nurse, or the environment. Certainly if Steve had escalated his destructive behavior, turning his aggression toward himself or others, then direct limit setting, including physical restraints, would have been indicated.

In first-time encounters with any client new to the setting, do not be surprised or dismayed about less-than-optimal success with intervention. It may take some time and trial and error to assess the client's behaviors and choose the most effective interventions.

TESTING AND LIMIT SETTING As young adolescents attempt to adjust to the upheaval in their emotional lives and begin to emancipate themselves from parental figures, a good deal of testing is to be expected. This is normal. However, the meaning that testing holds for the disturbed adolescent is a more complicated matter.

Adolescents who lack early nurturing have difficulty with interpersonal relationships. In many cases, parents were emotionally unable to provide parenting. In other cases, they chose not to impose their values on their children. In either case, the children never developed the internalized values that reduce conflict and avert crisis during adolescence. This causes identity diffusion, which in turn results in emptiness, a lack of basic trust, and difficulties with intimacy on any level.

In the treatment setting, testing for these clients seems to consist of making limitless and absolute demands. Although these clients often react to imposed limits with cries of injustice, they often really seem to be asking for limits as an indication of caring.

Julie had been on the unit only 2 days. During that time she had seen several of the older clients run away from the unit, commonly known as going AWOL, and had witnessed the staff members' attempts to encourage those remaining on the ward to deal with whatever feelings they were experiencing. Toward the end of her second evening, Julie abruptly jumped up from a conversation with a nurse and ran toward the open door. The surprised nurse immediately followed, running down the stairs after her. A smiling Julie was waiting at the bottom step when the nurse arrived, quite breathless and thoroughly confused, and began her barrage of questions. Julie quickly answered, "I just wanted to see if you cared enough to come after me."

In this situation, no further action was necessary.

Sometimes the client may use annoying or destructive behavior to test you. At these times, firm limit setting without further interpretation or exploration may be indicated. In other instances, the client may be reacting to some real threat or uncomfortable situation.

Joanne was quietly playing pool by herself when she noticed her therapist talking to a new female client. Her volatile nature gave way to jealousy and rage, and she immediately began to hit the billiard balls off the table, making a lot of noise and startling everyone around her. The nurse who had been observing her witnessed the change in her behavior and understood the reaction. Without questioning Joanne's apparent anger, she stepped up to the table and challenged her to a game, which Joanne immediately accepted. Since Joanne prided herself on her pool-playing ability, she quickly channeled her energy and competitive feelings into the game and won. She then sought out her therapist and happily announced her victory.

Had the nurse not understood what had triggered Joanne's outburst, she might have become angry with her for making noise. She might have seen this as a form of testing and might even have begun to set limits on Joanne's privilege of playing pool. This would certainly have produced a helpless and even angrier Joanne, who would probably have escalated her behavior. Since the nurse was perceptive and adept in handling such situations, the results were more satisfying to both parties. Because of the nurse's action, Joanne was able to save face by winning at pool and was not forced into a situation where she would feel more helpless.

SCAPEGOATING **Scapegoating** is common in many groups, but particularly in adolescent groups. It occurs in three stages:

1. Frustration generates aggression.
2. Aggression is displaced on other people.
3. Through a process of blaming, projecting, and stereotyping, this displaced aggression is rationalized and finally justified, since the identified scapegoat is "different" in some real way.

The members of a group tend to attack the scapegoat because they are afraid to attack the person on whom their feelings are actually focused. Adolescents readily identify peers who are "different" and project on them their own fears and insecurities about their changing images. The client identified as the scapegoat is the object of much teasing and many hostile remarks. Refrain from attempting merely to rescue the scapegoat, as this may augment the other clients' anger and frustration and encourage an escalation of the hostility. Set limits on the behavior and then ask the group to focus on what is going on, to acknowledge the anxiety or other uncomfortable feeling that preceded the scapegoating incident. If possible, anticipate the occurrence of scapegoating in times of stress and try to circumvent the process before it gets out of control.

Also be aware that identified scapegoats share some responsibility for their predicament by presenting themselves to the other clients in a different or provocative stance. In some instances the scapegoat of choice has an inner need to be punished and meets the group's urgent need to punish as well. You can be valuable to these clients by helping them explore whatever function this role serves for them.

SEXUAL BEHAVIORS With a self-awareness and understanding of feelings and attitudes about sexual issues, you can more readily plan interventions with sexual behaviors of the adolescent client.

Masturbation Masturbation is a normal sexual activity for people of all ages, from the beginning of sexual awareness to senescence. If you have a relatively healthy attitude toward masturbation, it is not likely to cause problems unless the client masturbates in inappropriate places or uses masturbation to express hostility. You may be confronted with an adolescent boy who fondles his genitals when he is anxious or feels threatened. Understanding his behavior as an indication of anxiety, you may elect to ignore the gesture and explore the nature of his anxiety with him. At other times, the boy may make a masturbatory gesture to convey contempt or hostility. In this case it would be ludicrous to feign indifference in response.

Your reaction depends on all the previously mentioned factors, such as the nurse-client relationship and the behavior that preceded the gesture. Generally, however, it is wise to comment on the client's gesture, for example, by mentioning it as an attempt to "make me uncomfortable," and then to allow the client the opportunity to express his feelings verbally. It is unlikely that this intervention will produce a tumultuous outpouring of feeling resulting in immediate resolution. However, it does allow you to acknowledge both the client's and your own feelings, perhaps paving the way for a more appropriate exchange in the future.

Heterosexual Behavior The adolescent often uses sexual behavior as a means of acting-out other conflicts and as a testing ground for the nursing staff's feelings and attitudes.

This is the third time Barbara, a nurse, had gone into Laurie's room to check on two clients, Laurie and Bill, who were an identified couple on the unit. Although there was a rule against clients having sexual intercourse with each other, Laurie and Bill had been discovered in the act each evening Barbara was on duty. Barbara found these discoveries disconcerting. She began to wonder whether she was the only staff member who checked on clients, since no one else had reported any sexual activity. She decided to bring the subject up in the next nursing care plan meeting to find a more effective way of dealing with the situation.

Imagine Barbara's surprise when the group agreed that Barbara was actually partly responsible for Laurie and Bill's

acting-out. While they supported Barbara, they evaluated the problem and gave Barbara feedback regarding her nonverbal messages. It seemed that her frequent checking on clients conveyed her expectation that they were up to something. Barbara acknowledged that she expected that sort of behavior from them and was quite afraid of discovering them in the act of intercourse. The group helped Barbara see that her own expectations were being met. Laurie and Bill were doing exactly what she expected them to do—maybe even wanted them to do. Laurie and Bill were following their scripts of being "bad" and expressing their hostility to Barbara. When Barbara heard how other staff members spent time with the couple to encourage them in indirect ways to join the larger group activities and compared her own behavior to that of her peers, it became apparent to her how obvious her anxiety and unconscious messages actually were. She then began to question her own attitudes about sexual matters and to explore why she feared discovering the couple engaged in sexual intercourse.

In this example, the client couple used sexual behaviors to act out their own underlying feelings. Had Barbara's assessment been limited to the immediate situation, she would have focused only on their unacceptable behavior and would not have been open to the implications for her. By seeking out information and feedback from her peers, she made a discovery about herself and realized more effective ways of anticipating and possibly circumventing such client behaviors rather than having to intervene after the fact. Had Barbara not asked for feedback, the problem would have continued with an increase in the sexual behaviors and in Barbara's frustration. The situation would have then demanded intervention by an astute supervisor or an empathetic colleague.

Homosexual Behavior In situations where homosexual behavior is an expected developmental step or a lifestyle without expressions of anger or hostility toward parents or staff, little or no intervention may be indicated. However, when homosexual behavior is used to act out feelings of impotence, or aggressive behavior is used to counteract feelings of intimacy, limits must be imposed.

Try to anticipate such behavior and provide other ways for the adolescent client to demonstrate his masculinity, perhaps by organizing a game of football or tennis, if he is fairly proficient at these skills, or engaging him in some other activity in which he excels. The point is to reestablish the adolescent's feeling of competence and control. Without such intervention, his feelings of impotence will escalate to the point where he will most certainly act them out in a negative way. The client who uses homosexuality to express defiance against authority figures will most assuredly flaunt homosexual activities and consistently incur the anger, embarrassment, or both, of staff and clients alike.

Substance Abuse You will benefit from self-awareness and an appreciation for the feelings that working with substance abusers can evoke. For example, the nurse who feels angry and punitive with the client who abuses drugs or overidentifies with the client and finds adventure in the client's drug stories cannot establish a therapeutic relationship with the client. Feelings of disdain or envy can compromise nursing care and, indeed, may make the client's treatment ineffective. Only by viewing substance abuse as a symptom of a broader illness can you be effective in dealing with adolescents. Nurses who have contact with adolescents, especially in school or community settings, should familiarize themselves with the general effects of various drugs and the first aid treatment for each (see Chapter 13).

Evaluation and Outcome Criteria

Evaluating nursing interventions with adolescent clients can be tricky for numerous reasons:

- The adolescent client may need to test the limit one more time following a nursing intervention to avoid appearing "too compliant" or to "save face" with the group.
- Although it is important to set limits, it is equally important to be flexible. To set a limit and immediately "draw the line" with the next infraction is to invite the client to step over that line to test its seriousness.
- Quick judgments should not be made if immediate results are not obtained. Persistence and consistency are the keys to success.
- The behaviors that brought the adolescent to psychiatric treatment will continue long after treatment and nursing interventions are begun. Despite a well-designed nursing care plan and client contract, the adolescent will resort to previous maladaptive ways, immature and impulsive acts, or destructive behaviors in the face of change, particularly if this change represents improvement or growth (such as an increase in privileges or an impending discharge). The nurse who thinks the nursing interventions are not effective may feel hopeless about progress and convey that hopelessness to the client and the rest of the treatment team.
- Use of a behavioral contract without understanding the underlying reasons or factors contributing to the adolescent's problems will result in a superficial approach with an equally superficial evaluation.

If the adolescent had the desire or the impulse control simply to "act right" after being given the rules and consequences, then the client would be doing so already, and psychiatric treatment would not have been necessary. The adolescent needs the structure and consistency of a nursing care plan and client contract without the rigidity that can be imposed by a "now or never" behavioral plan with absolute consequences.

You can make a more adequate evaluation if you attempt to be aware of the social context and meaning of the behavior to the adolescent. For example, you may be wrong in determining that an indicator of increased self-esteem for a female client would be to stop dyeing her hair purple. Dyeing one's hair an unusual color may have been an indication of low self-esteem during your adolescent years, but for the client in question, that may or may not be the case. For that adolescent client and her peer group, purple hair may be a well-defined status symbol.

Evaluation is determined to be effective or ineffective by the use of various subjective and objective behavioral criteria reflecting the client care goals.

Chapter Highlights

- Adolescence is a stormy time of conflicting ideas and feelings when identity, values, and goals are in a state of flux. The individual is no longer a child with investment in play or parental approval, but not yet an adult with abilities in verbal discourse or impulse control.
- A comprehensive assessment of this developmental period and the adolescent's problems is possible with the use of principles related to the developmental stage; ethnic, social, and cultural factors; biologic factors; family influences; and psychodynamic conflicts.
- In the home, school, or clinic environment, the general hospital setting, or the inpatient psychiatric setting, nurses can perform a central role in counseling parents and families of adolescent clients.
- Nurses can maintain a therapeutic environment by providing a physically and psychologically safe environment, setting verbal and physical limits on the client's behavior, establishing meaningful relationships with the adolescent, identifying the client's strengths, promoting more adaptive coping skills, role-modeling more socially acceptable behaviors, and participating in therapy groups and structured activities.
- Adolescents can present "normal" behaviors and problems unique to this developmental stage that could give nurses difficulty. To be effective with nursing interventions, nurses must understand typical adolescent behaviors as well as extremes in behavior.
- Specific issues and problems frequently related to the psychiatric nursing care of adolescents include attempts to manipulate the nurse into relating in a nontherapeutic way, use of unconventional language and profanity, testing and limit setting, anxiety and resistance, anger and hostility, scapegoating, adolescent sexual behavior, dietary problems, eating disorders, substance use and abuse, and suicidal behavior.
- Acting-out is often misused to describe antisocial destructive acts. It may include destructive actions, but it is much more than that. The term describes a recreation of the client's life experiences, the relationships with significant others, and the resulting unresolved conflicts.
- Nursing interventions with adolescents may be most effective if designed within the format of a client contract.
- Scapegoating is common to adolescent groups. The key to effective intervention is identifying the need that the scapegoat has to be "different" and setting limits on the scapegoating behaviors.
- To evaluate behavior adequately, nurses should be aware of its social contexts and its meaning to the adolescent. Likewise, a nurse's keen awareness of his or her own unresolved issues can be useful in effectively intervening with difficult adolescent behaviors.

References

American Nurses Association: *Standards of Child and Adolescent Psychiatric and Mental Health Nursing Practice.* American Nurses Association, 1985.

Apter A, Ratzoni G, King RA: Fluvoxamine open-label treatment of adolescent inpatients with obsessive-compulsive disorder or depression. *J Am Acad Child Adoles Psychiatr* 1994;33(3):342–348.

Birmaher B, Rabin BS, Garcia MR: Cellular immunity in depressed, conduct disorder, and normal adolescents: Role of adverse life events. *J Am Acad Child Adoles Psychiatr* 1994;33(5):671–678.

Blanz BJ, Rensch-Riemann BS, Fritz-Sigmund DI: IDDM is a risk factor for adolescent psychiatric disorders. *Diabetes Care* 1993;16(12):1579–1587.

Brent DA, Perper BDA, Moritz G: Familial risk factors for adolescent suicide: A case-control study. *Acta Psychiatr Scand* 1994;89:52–58.

"Close-Up: America," NBC-TV Television News Magazine Broadcast, November 30, 1993.

Eggert LI, Thompson EA, Herting JR: Preventing adoles-cent drug abuse and high school dropout through an intensive school-based social network development program. *Am J Health Promotion* 1994;8(3):202–215.

Finke LM: Child psychiatric nursing: Moving into the 21st century. *Nurs Clin N Am* 1994;29(1):43–48.

Frazier JA, Gordon CT, McKenna K: An open trial of Clozapine in eleven adolescents with childhood onset schizophrenia. *J Am Acad Child Adoles Psychiatr* 1994;33(5):658–670.

Gabel S, Stadler J, Bjorn J: Sensation seeking in psychiatrically disturbed youth: Relationship to biochemical parameters and behavior problems. *J Am Acad Child Adoles Psychiatr* 1994;33(1):123–129.

Goldston DB, Kovacs M, Ho VY: Suicidal ideation and suicide attempts among youth with insulin-dependent diabetes mellitus. *J Am Acad Child Adoles Psychiatr* 1994;33(2):240–246.

Howe GW, Feinstein C, Reiss D: Adolescent adjustment to chronic physical disorders. *J Child Psychol Psychiatr* 1993;34(7):1153–1171.

Kaplan SL, Simms RM, Busner J: Prescribing practices of outpatient child psychiatrists. *J Am Acad Child Adoles Psychiatr* 1994;33(1):35–44.

Kutcher S, Boulos C, Ward B: Response to desipramine treatment in adolescent depression: A fixed-dose, placebo-controlled trial. *J Am Acad Child Adoles Psychiatr* 1994; 33(5):686–694.

Lego S, Pawlicki C: How does parallel process manifest itself in psychiatric nursing practice? *J Psychosoc Nurs* 1993; 31(10):41–44.

Lequerica M: Stress in immigrant families with handicapped children: A child advocacy approach. *Am J Orthopsychiatr* 1993;63(4):545–552.

Lewinsohn PM, Clarke GN, Seeley JR, Rohde P: Depression in community adolescents: Age at onset, episode duration, and time to recurrence. *J Am Acad Child Adoles Psychiatr* 1994;33(6):809–818.

Mikkelsen EJ, Bereika GM, McKenzie JC: Short-term family-based residential treatment: An alternative to psychiatric hospitalization for children. *Am J Orthopsychiatr* 1993; 63(1):28–33.

National Council of Juvenile and Family Court Judges: Children and families first: A mandate for America's courts. *Today: A Publication of the NCJFCJ* 1993;2(3):12–15.

National Nursing Research Agenda: Health promotion for older children and adolescents: A report of the NINR priority expert panel on health promotion. U.S. Department of Health and Human Services, 1993.

Pfeffer CR, Klerman GL, Hurt SW: Suicidal children grow up: Demographic and clinical risk factors for adolescent suicide attempts. *J Am Acad Child Adoles Psychiatr* 1991; 30:609–616.

Public Health Service: Designing health promotion approaches to high-risk adolescents through formative research with youth and parents. U.S. Department of Health and Human Services, Publication No. 282-89-0021, 1992.

Public Health Service: Healthy people 2000: National health promotion and disease prevention objectives—full report with commentary. U.S. Department of Health and Human Services, Publication No. (PHS) 91-50212, 1990.

Public Health Service: Measuring the health behavior of adolescents: The youth risk behavior surveillance system and recent reports on high-risk adolescents. U.S. Department of Health and Human Services, Vol. 108, Supplement 1, 1993.

Serrano CV: A conceptual framework for understanding "problems" in adolescence and youth. *J Adoles Health* 1993;14:613–618.

Sokolov ST, Kutcher SP, Joffe RT: Basal thyroid indices in adolescent depression and bipolar disorder. *J Am Acad Child Adoles Psychiatr* 1994;33(4):469–475.

Trygstad LN: The need to know: Biological learning needs identified by practicing psychiatric nurses. *J Psychosoc Nurs* 1994;32(2):13–18.

Tuck I, Keels MC: Milieu therapy: A review of development of this concept and its implications for psychiatric nursing. *Issues Ment Health Nurs* 1992;13:51–58.

Uphold CR, Graham MV: Schools as centers for collaborative services for families: A vision for change. *Nurs Outlook* 1994;41(5):204–211.

Valente SM: Adolescent suicide: Assessment and intervention. *J Child Adoles Psychiatr Ment Health Nurs* 1989; 2(1):34–39.

Watson L: Maintenance of therapeutic community principles in an age of biopharmacy and economic restraints. *Arch Psych Nurs* 1992;6:183–188.

CHAPTER 38

APPLYING THE NURSING PROCESS WITH THE ELDERLY

Gloria Kuhlman

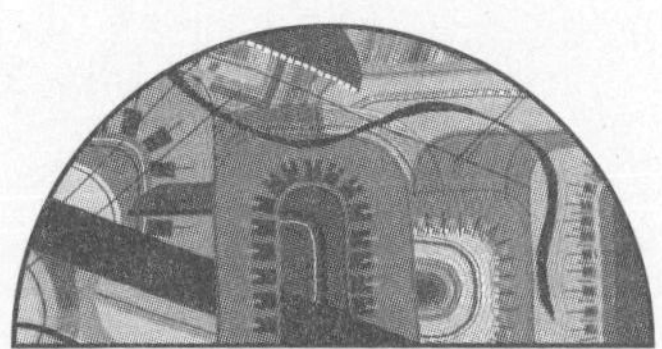

COMPETENCIES

- *Discuss three significant age-related demographic projections and their implications for future health services for the elderly.*
- *Describe the normal physical and psychosocial changes accompanying the aging process.*
- *List the major theories of aging and the main points of each one.*
- *Apply the nursing process to care of older clients.*
- *List the important components of a multifactorial assessment of an older client.*
- *Explain the importance of distinguishing between depression, dementia, and delirium.*
- *Identify the most common DSM-IV mental disorders and associated nursing diagnoses among elderly psychiatric clients.*
- *Explain the feelings you may experience when caring for an elderly psychiatric client.*

Cross-References

Other topics relevant to this content are: Severely and persistently mentally ill, Chapter 21; Elder abuse, Chapter 23; Delirium and dementia, Chapter 12; Psychotropic medications, Chapter 33; Substance-related disorders, Chapter 13; Suicide, Chapter 24; Sleep disorders, Chapter 19.

Critical Thinking Challenge

A recently retired man is brought to your clinic by his wife who states that he "just sits around all day and won't do anything." She reveals that he used to be very active, but seems unable to concentrate. Upon interviewing the client, you find that he had been a successful small business owner with his brother, who had recently died of a heart attack at the office, and that the client had retired soon after at the family's insistence. Upon further examination your client reveals that his memory seems impaired, he has difficulty concentrating and sleeping, and has lost his previously robust appetite. The other members of your treatment team want to have a dementia workup performed, but you are not convinced and would like to gather further data before beginning the assessment. What areas would you assess?

The American elderly population is growing faster than that of the nation as a whole. In 1990, the U.S. Bureau of Census reported that by the year 2050, almost 21.8% of the population will be age 65 and older. The over-65 population, which includes the "middle-old" (75–84) and the "old-old" (85+), reached 30.3 million in 1990, or more than 12% of the U.S. population.

It is important to examine the age distribution of the over-65 population carefully. Grouping the elderly into an aggregate of all those over the age of 65 tends to blur important distinctions between elderly age groups. The "old-old" group tends to have the greatest incidences of depression, delirium and dementia, and chronic disabling illnesses. Of this group, 44% have some limitation in their ability to perform activities of daily living (Rabin 1989). Thus, the stereotypic **frail elderly**, who need many health care and maintenance services, constitute only 5% of the over-65 population. This differentiation by age group indicates that there is a large proportion of healthy older people, particularly older women living alone (who outnumber single elderly men by 2.5 to 1), who will benefit from supportive psychosocial services.

The implications of a growing population of aging individuals are important for projecting needs and planning for social programs and fund allocation. The figures point to a need for greater numbers of health care professionals versed in the multiple requirements of older adults. Nursing's role in geriatrics and **psychogerontology** is expanding as the needs and real numbers of elderly increase (Eliopoulos 1993).

The aim of this chapter is to provide a comprehensive discussion of health promotion, advocacy, and application of the nursing process to mental health care for the elderly. It provides a broad overview of important age-related, biopsychosocial nursing considerations for advocacy and health promotion in later life, discusses the DSM-IV mental disorders commonly seen in later life, and presents guidelines for applying the nursing process to the mental health care of the aged.

Roadblocks to Mental Health Services for the Elderly

The elderly are the most underserved population in need of supportive and tertiary mental health services. This discussion highlights four roadblocks to mental health services—ageism, myths, stigma, and access—and examines the demographic realities that compel us to break down these disabling roadblocks through health promotion and client advocacy.

Ageism

A primary roadblock to mental health services for older people is ageism. In contemporary social environments, aging is often viewed with disdain and contempt. Elderly people are criticized for being unattractive, incompetent, socially irrelevant, and unhealthy. For many years, older adults were considered inappropriate candidates for mental health interventions. Ageism also stems from the belief that the elderly present a financial and emotional drain to the family and society (Ebersole and Hess 1994). Ageist attitudes can be internalized by elderly people, causing decreased self-worth and self-esteem.

When caring for elderly clients, be aware of their feelings and make a conscious effort not to let your personal biases influence clinical assessment and interventions. You can provide invaluable support, in-sight, and feedback to colleagues who are working with older clients. We now know the elderly are as responsive to mental health services as members of any other age group. By modeling positive attitudes toward aging and by advocating quality of life and health care for the aged in all settings and at all levels of function, you can help dispel ageist influences on the health care of the elderly.

Myths

Health care professionals, and elders themselves, often equate growing old with growing sad, disengaged, and depressed. The myths that depression, disengagement, and senility are part of growing old all too often inhibit older people from seeking treatment for feelings and behaviors they think are a "normal" part of aging. Misled by these myths, professionals are less inclined to refer elderly clients for mental health services. We now know that advancing age does not condemn an individual to senility, isolation, loneliness, and depression. Most older adults live independently and contentedly well into late life.

Nurses can serve as elder advocates by educating the public, health care professionals, and the elderly themselves to differentiate between normal and pathologic states in later life. Dispelling the myths surrounding the aging process helps promote the notion that aging itself is not a "problem," so that when problems do arise, they will be identified and treated.

Stigma

Despite recent advances in mental health care, the stigma associated with mental illness remains very real to elderly people who were socialized when psychiatric treatment was less sophisticated than it is today (Ebersole and Hess 1994). The elderly rarely seek mental health services and often deny or hide their psychic pain for fear of being labeled "crazy" or of losing control and being institutionalized. Attitudes toward the aged historically have been more negative than toward younger individuals. Elders with mental illnesses may elicit feelings of vulnerability in people who are near the same age. Generally younger people or those who work regularly with healthy older adults have a positive regard toward the elderly (Ebersole and Hess 1994).

As a nurse, you have tremendous access to people at all levels of the health care and social systems. By educating the public about mental disorders and state-of-the-art mental health care, you can help decrease the stigma associated with mental illness and psychiatric treatment, thereby helping allay the fears of the elderly who require mental health services.

Access

Financial barriers, physical disability, and transportation problems limit older adults' access to health care services. The financing of health care for mentally ill elderly is a very real problem. Medicare, the major form of health care financing for the elderly, covers only a portion of the health care costs of its beneficiaries, and there is a notable lack of long-term care coverage and coverage for chronic problems. Outpatient and home care coverage for mental health services is limited at best. Many mental health services are not covered under Medicare at all. Even when services are reimbursed through Medicare, there is often a large copayment, which is a burden to those without supplementary coverage. Financial problems often add to an older person's psychosocial stressors. Nurses must be active in lobbying for policy changes to improve access to health care through financing to cover acute and chronic illnesses as well.

Biopsychosocial Theories of Aging

Defining mental health in later life is a difficult task. Many variables affect mental health as a person ages. Researchers focusing on the elderly look at a variety of factors that explain normal aging. The theories of aging may be divided into biologic and psychosocial. At this time the research continues to be theoretic, and in the case of the disengagement theory, controversial.

Biologic Theories

GENETIC THEORY According to genetic theory, aging is an involuntary process that operates over time to alter cellular structures. Genetic theories (gene theory, error theory, somatic mutation theory, and programmed theory) suggest that there is deliberate programming and that the life span is predetermined. Evidence that supports these theories provides clues, but at the same time raises questions, such as: Are the symptoms due to decreased circulation or cells that no longer divide? (Ebersole and Hess 1994).

WEAR-AND-TEAR THEORY The wear-and-tear theory proposes that the accumulation of waste products from metabolism damages DNA synthesis, leading eventually to organ malfunction. This theory allows for individual rates of system degradation, but the theory emphasizes loss and decline (Stanley and Beare 1995).

IMMUNITY THEORY This theory describes the age-related decline in an individual's immune system. The theory suggests that as a person ages, his or her ability to defend against foreign organisms declines, with a corresponding increase in susceptibility to such diseases as cancer and serious infections. Theorists suggest that the cellular changes with aging allow the body to misidentify old, irregular cells as foreign bodies, and the body then attacks these cells as if they were foreign bodies. Multiple neurochemical and viral theories are being developed as cellular research increases (Stanley and Beare 1995).

NUTRITION The importance of good nutrition pertains to people of all age groups. The belief is that how we eat has an influence on how we age. The quality of the diet is as important as the quantity, because vitamin and nutrient deficiencies or excesses have an influence on disease processes. The relationship between diet and aging is not clearly understood, but enough is known to indicate that a good diet helps minimize some of the ill effects of aging (Eliopoulos 1993).

ENVIRONMENT A number of environmental factors are known to threaten health and may be associated with aging. The ingestion of lead, arsenic, pesticides, and other substances can seriously harm the body, as can smoking and air pollution. Environmental factors such as crowded living conditions and high levels of noise are also stressful. While these factors are too complex for us to fully understand how they affect the aging process, it is helpful for nurses to have an awarness of them (Eliopoulos 1993).

Psychosocial Theories

DISENGAGEMENT THEORY First developed in the 1960s, the **disengagement theory** described the process of older adults withdrawing from society. This withdrawal process was considered to be inevitable for the proper functioning of a growing society. The theory indicated that elders were happy to reduce their social contacts and turn over their responsibilities to the younger generation. This theory is controversial because many older adults continue to be engaged and responsible well into old age. More recent research emphasizes the need for continued mental activity in order to maintain health throughout the life span. This is demonstrated by the number of elders who continue to be productive into their 80s and 90s (Stanley and Beare 1995).

ACTIVITY THEORY The activity theory is the direct opposite of the disengagement theory. The theory proposes that the way to successfully age is to stay active. According to this theory, older adults stay active and involved in order to maintain the satisfactions of life.

CONTINUITY THEORY The continuity theory was proposed as a reaction to the disengagement theory. The theory focuses on the relationship between life satisfaction and activity. The personality is considered an important factor in the determination of the relationship between life satisfaction and role activity. The theory indicates that the personality becomes more pronounced as one ages. The continuity theory relies on self-report to identify life satisfaction (Ebersole and Hess 1994).

Psychiatric Disorders in the Elderly

The ageist attitudes in our culture are responsible for many misperceptions about mental disorders in the elderly. Older people are believed to be more prone to mental disorders than the young. For several reasons, it is difficult to obtain exact incidence and prevalence rates of mental disorders in later life. The elderly are often difficult to reach with communitywide surveys. Researchers have noted that older adults are reluctant to respond to research questions dealing with emotions. As mentioned earlier, elderly people often do not seek treatment, or they consult their primary care providers rather than mental health care professionals (Callahan et al. 1994). As a result, they are underrepresented in clinical samples.

Different researchers diagnose mental problems differently, making comparisons between communitywide surveys difficult. Symptoms of mental illness in the elderly often differ from those of other age groups. While the *DSM-IV* has greatly enhanced our ability to make reliable and valid diagnoses of mental disorders, there are few age-specific categories for mental disorders in later life. Thus, in spite of the *DSM-IV's* extensive, detailed description of each problem category, clinicians and researchers continue to have difficulty applying the written descriptions to symptoms in later life.

The epidemiologic studies to date indicate that the elderly suffer no more than other groups from disorders, such as adjustment disorders, personality disorders, and grief reactions. Older adults do have a disproportionately high incidence of depression and are somewhat more likely to become paranoid. They also frequently have sleep disturbances. Two recent areas of exploration, for which there is very little epidemiologic information at present, are substance abuse in later life and the severely and persistently mentally ill elderly.

Mood Disorders

Mood disorders are primarily characterized by disturbed affect or emotional experience. Mood disturbances in the elderly, as in other age groups, may present as:

- Sustained elation and hyperactivity, as seen in a manic episode.
- Changes from elation to depression, as seen in a bipolar disorder.
- Pervasive depressed mood not accompanied by mania, as seen in major depression.

Depression is the most prevalent and most treatable mental disorder in later life (Eliopoulos 1993).

A 79-year-old male, Mr G, came to his physician's office complaining of "not feeling well." After a physical examination the doctor told Mr G he had a weight loss of 10 pounds, mild COPD, and slight hypertension, but otherwise was in good health for his age. Mr G responded angrily, "I know I am dying, but it doesn't matter because I have nothing to live for now that my wife has died. She has been gone for six months and everyone says I should be feeling better, but I feel worse! I can't eat, can't sleep, I don't even have enough energy to work in my shop!" Mr G says he is tired all day, but cannot sleep at night, "I am up at 4:00 AM every morning and can't go back to sleep." He tries to eat, but he does not cook well and "the food just does not taste right."

DEPRESSION IN THE ELDERLY Depression robs the person of later life satisfaction, inhibits ego integrity, and may substantially decrease life expectancy, since symptoms may precipitate or aggravate physical deterioration. The rate of completed suicide is highest among the elderly (Meehan, Saltzman, and Sattin 1991).

Although the signs and symptoms of depression are relatively consistent throughout the life span, certain characteristics of depression are particular to the elderly. It is crucial for clinicians to note that depression in older adults, which responds well to treatment, may present with cognitive changes similar to those that accompany other organically based, irreversible disorders (Alexopoulos et al. 1993). Lachner and Engel (1994) suggest that many elderly clients thought to be demented actually have a depressive disorder with misleading cognitive symptoms such as disorientation, agitation, and memory loss. See this chapter's Research Note concerning a study to identify clinical characteristics of depression in older adults.

In addition to cognitive changes, another sign of depression in older adults is an excessive preoccupation with physical symptoms, which is known as **somatization.** Expressing discomfort through the body may be more familiar to an older person than recognizing symptoms of psychic pain. Chronic complaints of constipation, headaches, musculoskeletal pain, chest tightness and dyspnea with no physical basis, and chronic gastrointestinal upset may be the result of a depressed elder's unconscious shifting of attention away from distressing emotions to more "acceptable," familiar, and less-stigmatized physical complaints. Clinicians have noted that because of the stigma associated with mental illness, depressed elderly clients sometimes cover up a dysphoric mood by maintaining meticulous grooming and feigning a cheerful affect (Love and Buckwalter 1991; Kennedy 1995). Nurses must be persistent and perceptive in looking for signs of depression. Depressed apathetic elders

RESEARCH NOTE

Citation

Callahan CM, Hendrie HC, Dittus RS, Brater DC, Hui SL, Tierney WM: Depression in late life: The use of clinical characteristics to focus screening efforts. *J Gerontology* 1994;49(1):M9–M14.

Study Problem/Purpose

The purpose of this study was to identify clinical characteristics associated with depressive symptoms late in life so that screening could focus on the elderly clients most likely to benefit from further evaluation.

Findings

There were 251 older clients (15%) with significant symptoms of depression. One-seventh of the clients with symptoms of depression received antidepressants. The client population most likely to have symptoms of depression were white, female, without health insurance, and may also demonstrate alcoholism, with mild cognitive loss, and be medicated with benzodiazepines, narcotics, or histamine H2 antagonists (cimetidine). Factors not significantly correlated with depressive symptoms included age, education, income, and chronic medical conditions such as hypertension, pain, arthritis, diabetes, obstructive lung disease, and coronary artery disease.

Implications

The results of this study indicate that while there are several clinical variables associated with depression in later life, there was no predictive model for identification of clients who are more likely to have significant symptoms of depression. The clinical characteristics that were significantly correlated with depressive symptoms, including cognitive loss, alcoholism, and poor access to health care, are all problems amenable to intervention. These conditions are screenable through a variety of assessment and data-collection models. The determination or identification of the predisposition toward depression, especially when there are concurrent variables, help nurses in the identification of individuals who have the potential for developing depression. Formal teaching programs as well as informational sessions can help predisposed individuals have a better understanding of their illness and possible accompanying pathology.

may believe they are supposed to feel blue and "down in the dumps" as they age. Nurses need to inform them and their families that depression is a pathologic condition often caused by biochemical imbalances. Interventions should be instituted to correct depressive states in the elderly as aggressively and comprehensively as in any other age group. Kennedy (1995) suggests that while depression in the elderly may result from the psychiatric syndrome of depression, it may also be the result of sociodemographic situations such as social isolation or neglect, or the result of a medical condition that results in a disability such as stroke, Parkinson's disease, or even a hip fracture. An individual's response to these traumatic events may result in a depressive reaction that must be treated as a syndrome with multiple areas for intervention. Treatment of only the depression may result in delayed rehabilitation of underlying treatable conditions. Because late-life depression may be intimately tied to a functional disability it is imperative to have a comprehensive geriatric assessment of the client before beginning a treatment regime.

Suicide The depressed elderly are more prone to completing suicide than any other age group in the United States (Zweig and Hinrichsen 1993). This fact does not even begin to tap the passive, indirect suicides accomplished by starvation and "accidental" overmedication. Older adults make up 12.4% of the population but account for 21% of reported suicides (McBride and Burgener 1994). The high rates clearly indicate that suicide is a significant problem in later life (Eliopoulos 1993).

Older adults who present a greater suicide risk include (Ebersole and Hess 1994):

- Males.
- Widowed or divorced people.
- Caucasians.
- Those of lower socioeconomic status.
- Those with chronic pain and terminal illness.
- Alcoholics.
- Those with mental illnesses.

Suicidal elderly people have been known to seek help (often for a vague or nonspecific physical problem) from physicians, clergy, and nurses within 1 month prior to their self-destructive act (Ebersole and Hess 1994). Thus, accurate assessment of suicide potential is crucial and requires perception, active listening, and direct questioning. A suicidal older client may present with:

- Verbal cues ("I'm going to end it all; life is not worth living; I won't be around much longer").
- Behavioral cues (completing a will, making funeral plans, acting-out, withdrawing, somatic complaints).

- Situational cues (a recent move, loss of a loved one, the diagnosis of a terminal illness).

For information on suicide and the assessment of suicide potential including a lethality index, see Chapter 24.

Schizophrenia

Older adult clients with schizophrenia present a challenge to the caregiver. These clients are often survivors of the institutional care of the past and now reside in a nursing home or residential care setting. They probably have been taking neuroleptics for years and are at high risk for tardive dyskinesia (Krach 1993).

The symptoms of an elderly client with schizophrenia diminish in intensity with a concurrent improvement in social adaptability (Ebersole and Hess 1994). Those who take their medications can maintain an adequate lifestyle in the community (Ebersole and Hess 1994).

The older person with schizophrenia will seldom verbalize pain or discomfort, but instead will demonstrate an exacerbation of psychiatric symptoms (Krach 1993). This information is important for nurses providing care. Understanding that changes in performing activities of daily living may be the first sign of a medical illness and not an exacerbation of the schizophrenia enables the nurse to intervene appropriately (Krach 1993).

Adjustment Disorders

Older adults often experience dramatic life changes because of losses through death, relocation, dependence (loss of autonomy), retirement, illness, and financial stress. One or a combination of life changes and losses may contribute to the development of an **adjustment disorder**, the essential feature of which is a maladaptive reaction to an identifiable psychosocial stressor (or stressors) that occurs within 3 months after the onset of the stressor and has persisted for no longer than 6 months (American Psychiatric Association 1994). Adjustment disorders in the elderly may have a variety of psychiatric symptoms including:

- Anxious mood.
- Depressed mood.
- Mixed emotional features.
- Physical complaints.
- Withdrawal.

Anxiety Disorders

Anxiety is very common across age groups and increases in frequency with advancing age. Adjustments to physical, emotional, and socioeconomic changes as one ages add to the variety of causes for anxiety. Anxiety reactions in the elderly may manifest themselves as somatic complaints, rigid thinking and behavior, insomnia, fatigue, hostility, restlessness, confusion, and increased dependence. Physiologic indicators of anxiety include increased blood pressure, pulse, respirations, psychomotor restlessness, and increased voiding (Eliopoulos 1993).

Mrs S, 82, is rushed to the emergency room by her bridge group with what they think may be a "heart attack." Mrs S is short of breath, diaphoretic, her pulse is rapid, her hands are shaking, and she is having difficulty sitting still during her assessment. She is tearful, but cannot tell the advice nurse what is wrong. "I don't know why I feel this way, something bad is going to happen. I have to leave and get home. Why are you asking me all these questions? No, I don't have chest pain, I tried to tell them I was just nervous. I just get this way sometimes." Mrs S was diagnosed with an anxiety disorder.

Unfortunately, anxiety disorders are often missed in older clients because, as with depression, they often present with a predominance of physical complaints that mask the underlying disorder. In addition, anxiety in elderly people is often the main feature a depressive disorder, and too often the anxiety is treated but the depression persists, leading to a cycle of anxiety-depression and physical illness.

Anxiety disorders in the elderly must be differentiated from agitation secondary to adverse drug reactions (such as akathisia from neuroleptics), delirium, dementia, parkinsonism, paranoid disorders, hypoxia, and pain (Smith, Sherril, and Colenda 1995). Anxiety may also have predominant psychologic features, as seen in anxiety stemming from perceived powerlessness, fear, perceived loss of control and mastery, anticipated loss, despair, and grief reactions. The etiology of the anxiety state determines the appropriate treatment, which most often involves a combination of psychotherapy, relaxation training, behavior modification, systematic desensitization, social support, and judicious use of the appropriate class of psychoactive medication. Low-dose medication should be initiated when symptoms interfere with the person's ability to benefit from the other psychoeducative and psychosocial therapies.

Delusional Disorders

Delusions in older adults are a cognitive mechanism for maintaining a sense of power and control. The delusions may be comforting or threatening, but they always form a structure for understanding a situation that otherwise seems unmanageable (Ebersole and Hess 1994). Persecutory delusions involve the belief that the person is under investigation, being harassed, or at the mercy of some powerful force. With somatic delusions, the predominant theme is an imagined physical disorder or abnormality of appearance. Somatic delusions in older people are frequently characterized by extremely morbid content.

Delusion processes in the elderly are often associated with delirium, depression, dementia, or anxiety disorders. Persecutory delusions may be a response to an older person's diminishing sense of self-mastery. Among the various symptoms exhibited by elderly people with psychiatric problems, delusions involving suspiciousness and persecutory ideation are among the most disturbing and unsettling for their families and caregivers. As older adults gradually give up important areas of function, such as financial management, cooking, and shopping, they may begin to develop delusions that people are robbing them or poisoning their food. They respond to these delusional processes by "dismissing" or rejecting their caregivers in an effort to regain control over these areas of life. Delusions may also result from internalized ageist attitudes, sensory losses (particularly hearing impairment), and social isolation.

Caregivers must work to establish trust and consistency with delusional elders. It is important to assess the situation to validate that the persecutory and somatic content is not reality-based. Clients need consistent social interaction, with caring people and consistent reality orientation. Relieving social isolation and correcting sensory losses may solve the problem. Delusional processes associated with delirium often abate when the cause of the delirium is treated. Medication in small doses, geared toward relieving an underlying anxiety or depressive disorder, may be helpful, although compliance is often a problem because of the client's suspiciousness.

Substance-Related Disorders

The actual extent of alcoholism and drug- and alcohol-related problems among older adults is not known. It is generally reported that the elderly constitute the age group with the lowest rate of alcohol and illegal drug use, which may be attributed to certain sociocultural influences earlier in life: prohibition and a historical disapproval of drinking by women (McMahon 1993). Older adults are more vulnerable than younger people to the effects of alcohol and other substances. They are also the largest consumers of OTC preparations and prescribed medications. Nurses caring for the elderly are in the unique position of being able to screen for the use and misuse of alcohol, OTC drugs, and prescription drugs (McMahon 1993). Refer to the color plates to identify commonly prescribed drugs.

It is estimated that 10–15% of the over-65 population have an alcohol-related problem. Many abstain or are infrequent drinkers because drinking would complicate preexisting medical problems (McMahon 1993). The typical signs of alcoholism, such as absence from work, difficulties in the family, and driving when intoxicated, may not be apparent in older people because often they are retired, live alone, and do not drive.

Data on the prevalence of illegal drug use in the older population are sparse. Early studies of addiction suggest that drug abuse diminishes in users after age 45. Presently the elderly consume 25–30% of all prescription drugs and 35–45% of all OTC drugs (McMahon 1993). Older adults also often take a variety of medications for one or more chronic medical conditions. **Polypharmacy**, the mixing of medications, with or without alcohol use, is potentially dangerous and adds to the chance of harmful drug interactions in elderly clients (McMahon 1993).

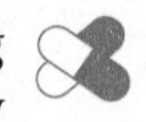

Alcohol abuse and dependence among older adults is a serious mental health problem. It affects an estimated 2.5 million people, but the true extent is unknown because many problem drinkers go undetected. Alcohol abuse can predispose elderly people to accidents, nutritional deficiencies, and diseases that may ultimately lead to the loss of autonomy (Mackel, Sheehy, and Badger 1994).

Alcoholism increases the likelihood of falls and other accidents that may lead to the inability to live at home. When older drinkers seek medical help for alcohol-related problems (such as malnutrition, injuries from falling, and sleep problems), the alcoholism is rarely the presenting problem. The presenting symptoms may be treated and other symptoms simply attributed to the aging process.

Clinical manifestations of alcohol dependence in the elderly include tolerance, a physiologic dependence on alcohol, multiple social complications, frequent behavioral problems such as aggression and traffic accidents, and alcohol-related physical health problems. The elderly individual who became a drinker early in life may have an established pattern of problematic relationships. Late-onset alcoholics manifest fewer alcohol-related problems, are less aggressive, and are believed to have turned to drinking in response to stressful life events such as bereavement, health problems, changes in their financial situation after retirement, marital stress, or depression (Hoffman 1995).

The clinical manifestations of substance-related disorders in the elderly frequently mimic the aging process or are nonspecific and include such signs as malnutrition, falls and other accidents, incontinence, mood swings, depression, confusion, self-neglect, and unexpected reactions to prescribed medications (McMahon 1993). Assessment for drug and alcohol abuse in elderly clients, especially socially isolated elders who have suffered recent losses, should be approached with care. All older clients must be educated about the danger of mixing and altering medications. Approach them nonjudgmentally, and teach them and their families about the risks of mixing medications and alcohol. Preventing reactive drinking may be accomplished by providing social support and mental health services for elders at risk for social isolation and depression.

Disorders of Arousal and Sleep

The quantity and quality of sleep change with the aging process. In a comprehensive review of research on sleep and aging, the elderly demonstrated more frequent awakening during the night than younger adults, increased total time awake, and longer time spent in bed before finally falling asleep (Bahr 1995). Changes in sleep patterns are believed to be related to changes in internal body rhythm (circadian asynchrony), emotional stress, physical illness, and medication or drugs (Ebersole and Hess 1994). Over one-third of people over 60 complain of sleep disturbances. The elderly nap more during the day and use a disproportionately high amount of OTC and prescription sleeping aids: approximately 40% of all sold (Ebersole and Hess 1994).

Problems Using Sleep Medication The chronic use of sedatives and hypnotics by elderly people has *not* been shown to improve the quality of sleep and can lead to many undesirable and dangerous side effects (Table 38–1). Older people excrete these drugs more slowly than the young and thus are prone to develop toxic effects, including delirium, daytime drowsiness, and loss of equilibrium. Respiration can be significantly disturbed with the use of sleeping medication, which may lead to a physiologically adaptive response of frequent arousal to stimulate respiration (Bahr 1995).

Guidelines for Improving Sleep The following guidelines can be used to improve sleep in the elderly (Bahr 1995):

- Steady daily physical activity.
- A cool room.
- A light bedtime snack.
- Stress reduction to promote relaxation.
- Regular arousal time.
- Avoiding napping during the day.
- Clean bed linen every day.
- Avoiding caffeine and tobacco.

The Nursing Process and the Elderly

Assessment

The Nursing Assessment Interview The variety of theories on aging and the complex interrelationship of physical, emotional, and environmental factors point to the importance of an individualized, multifactorial approach to assessment. The assessment information must be comprehensive and multidimensional. If available, a multidisciplinary team approach is usually most effective in securing comprehensiveness and providing validation of assessment impressions, leading to accurate diagnoses and effective intervention strategies.

The interview is the initial step in the assessment process and the most important procedure in differentiating between psychiatric disorders in elderly clients. Interviewing requires skill and heightened sensitivity and typically takes more time with older adults than with members of other age groups. Try to make the interview pleasant for the client, conveying a sense of respect and caring. Be close to the client, use touch when appropriate to relieve anxiety, and be clear in stating the purpose of the interview and length of time it will take. A skilled diagnostician attends to verbal, nonverbal, and environ-

Table 38–1 Examples of Medications Used as Hypnotics in the Elderly

Medication	*Class*	*Hypnotic Efficacy*	*Risk of Hangover*	*Risk of Tolerance or Dependence*	*Other Complications*
Diphenhydramine	Antihistamine	Unpredictable	High	Low	Anticholinergic
Amitriptyline	Tricyclic	Unpredictable	High	Low	Anticholinergic
Trazodone	Triazolopyridine	High	High	Low	Priapism
Flurazepam	Benzodiazepine	Very high	High	High	Falls, worsens sleep apnea
Temazepam	Benzodiazepine	Very high	Low	High	Falls, worsens sleep apnea
Triazolam	Benzodiazepine	Very high	Low	High	Memory disturbance

Source: McCall 1995.

Instructions: Ask questions 1–10 in this list and record all answers. Ask question 4A only if patient does not have a telephone. Record total number of errors based on ten questions.

\+ −

_____ 1. What is the date today? _____ (month/day/year)

_____ 2. What day of the week is it? _____

_____ 3. What is the name of this place? _____

_____ 4. What is your telephone number? _____

_____ 4A. What is your street address? _____

_____ 5. How old are you? _____

_____ 6. When were you born? _____

_____ 7. Who is the president of the U.S. now? _____

_____ 8. Who was the president before him? _____

_____ 9. What was your mother's maiden name? _____

_____ 10. Subtract 3 from 20 and keep subtracting 3 from each new number, all the way down.

_____ Total Errors

To be completed by interviewer

Patient Name: _____

Sex: 1. Male 2. Female Race: 1. White 2. Black 3. Other

Years of Education: _____

1. Grade School 2. High School 3. Beyond High School

Interviewer's Name: _____

The total number of errors constitutes the score in the SPMSQ. The test is sensitive to educational attainment.

For persons with 9–12 years of education, the following scoring applies:

0–2 Errors:	Intact intellectual functioning
3–4 Errors:	Mild intellectual impairment
5–7 Errors:	Moderate intellectual impairment
8–10 Errors:	Severe intellectual impairment

For persons with 8 or fewer years of education, one additional error is allowed for each scoring category. Persons with more than 12 years of education, one less error is allowed for each category.

Figure 38–1 Short Portable Mental Status Questionnaire (SPMSQ). *Source: From Pfeiffer E: The psychosocial evaluation of the elderly client, in Busse EW, Blazer DG (eds):* Handbook of Geriatric Psychiatry. *Van Nostrand Reinhold, 1980. Copyright © E. Pfeiffer, 1974.*

mental cues, as well as the cognitive and behavioral aspects of the client. It may become necessary to repeat the purpose and time frame of the interview because the client may forget.

Sensory loss, confusion, communication disorders, cultural influences, shame, and the fear of stigmatization may inhibit the expression of feelings in older people. They may be unaware of changes in their behavior or expect negative changes as a "normal" part of aging. It is important to solicit interpretations from family and staff members to help fill in aspects of the clinical picture and validate the information the client has provided.

The assessment information should include objective and subjective data regarding the client's physiologic status, psychologic status, cognitive status, and social and financial status. There are a variety of self-report screening tools designed for use specifically with elderly clients. These require minimal special training to administer and help the nurse obtain subjective assessment information. These tools may also be used as objective evaluation instruments to measure the effectiveness of interventions. The **Iowa Self-Assessment Inventory** (Morris and Buckwalter 1988) is useful for obtaining a subjective functional assessment from elderly clients in a variety of settings. The **Geriatric Depression Scale** (Yesavage et al. 1982–1983) and the **Short Portable Mental Status Questionnaire (SPMSQ)** (Pfeiffer 1975) are other useful tools for collecting information about depressive symptoms and mental status, respectively (Figure 38–1).

The following section provides guidelines for obtaining subjective and objective assessment information about the client's physiologic, cognitive, emotional, and psychosocial status.

BIOLOGIC ASSESSMENT Before a definitive psychiatric diagnosis can be made, all medically based illnesses that may present with psychiatric symptoms (depression, confusion, restlessness, and anxiety) must be ruled out. In addition, a complete medical and neurologic workup is necessary to differentiate irreversible, untreatable dementing illnesses from reversible, treatable conditions (pseudodementia). Emergency room admissions for "psychiatric" problems in the elderly often prove to have an underlying medical (organic) etiology, such as infection. As previously noted, older adults tend to go to their primary care provider, not to mental health care professionals (Callahan et al. 1994). Therefore, all medical and nursing personnel must maintain a high degree of alertness whenever an elderly client presents with apparent psychiatric symptoms.

Objective assessment information includes lab results, a complete history and physical including weight, vital signs, and a description of the physical appearance of the client. Standard diagnostic laboratory analysis should include complete blood chemistry, electrolytes, glucose, CBC, urinalysis, thyroid studies, BUN, creatinine, and liver function tests. The dexamethasone suppression test (DST) may be useful in identifying major depression in clients with early and/or mild-to-moderate dementia (Haggerty et al. 1988). Other procedures important for ruling out infectious processes, space-occupying lesions, drug toxicities, and cancers include chest radiography, drug toxicology screening, CT scanning, PET scanning, EKG, EEG, and lumbar puncture. In cases where normal-pressure hydrocephalus is suspected, a cysternogram is diagnostic. Dementia workup should include serologic tests for syphilis, folate, B_{12} levels, and trace minerals. See the color plates of brain scan images for an example of test findings.

Subjective assessment information includes clients' perceptions of their physical health and a description of their chronic illnesses, symptoms, and self-care activities.

COGNITIVE STATUS A thorough mental status examination is essential. Objective information includes the *presence* and *extent* of cognitive impairment. Include the family and caregivers to determine the course of the mental changes. Did the changes happen gradually (AD, drug toxicity, metabolic imbalances), suddenly (depression, CVA, drug toxicity), or in a graduated, stepwise fashion (multiinfarct dementia)? The SPMSQ is a simple, reliable, and valid ten-item cognitive performance evaluation tool. It was designed to assess and monitor cognitive changes in an elderly client. Remember that older people are sensitive to fatigue, boredom, medication, and environmental influences, which can affect their mental status. The SPMSQ cannot distinguish delirium from dementia, however. Keep in mind that assessment tools designed for use with other age groups may not be accurate or complete for use with older adults.

Subjective information regarding cognitive status includes clients' own perceptions of their mental status. Questions to ask include: "How has your thinking been lately?" "Is your memory as good as it used to be?" "Have you been able to keep track of your medicines (days of the week, meals, time)?"

PSYCHOLOGIC/EMOTIONAL STATUS Objective data regarding the client's psychologic and emotional status include your impressions taken from both content and process aspects of the interview. This information overlaps significantly with the mental status exam information. Several aspects of this assessment require synthesis and inferences made from the history and subjective information provided by the client. Therefore, this assessment cannot be made with the same objectivity as an examination of the client's skin for example. The assessment summary should include descriptions, not labels. The overuse of psychiatric terminology does not give an adequate picture of the client or the illness. Give examples of the client's behavior and, when appropriate, direct quotations to substantiate inferences and to present a vivid picture. Describe the following:

- The client's overall mood, affect, and response to you.
- Impressions from observing the client's interactions with family and others.
- Coping skills and defenses used by the client.
- The client's educational level and insight into the illness, and pertinent cultural factors.
- Components such as psychomotor activity, somatization, anxiety, judgment, substance abuse (past and present), obsessive-compulsive symptoms, irrational guilt, aggressive behavior, and impairment in concentration.
- The client's speech, production and continuity of thought, emotional regulation, impulse control, suicidal ideation, and frustration tolerance.

Be sure to include significant negative findings, such as the absence of delusional thought processes, the absence

ASSESSMENT

Guidelines for Assessing Psychologic Strengths

- What are some things you like about yourself?
- What are some of the upsetting (stressful, difficult) times you can remember?
- What did you do to comfort yourself when your husband (wife) died?
- How did you make it through the death of your son?
- What kinds of things do you do to cheer yourself up?
- What things make you happy? Content?
- What do you do to nurture yourself?
- What do you do to relax? To have fun?
- What things do you think you can do to get you through these rough times?
- How have the passing years affected your sexuality?
- Do you enjoy sex as much as you used to?
- Are you happily married/partnered?
- What are you most concerned about right now?
- How can I (we) help you through this difficult time?

of suicidal ideation, and the absence of hallucinations. The assessment should include not only pathology and problems but also health, adaptive strengths, and personal assets (ego strengths).

Strengths and Coping Strategies Aging is a continuous process, punctuated by positive and negative stress-producing life events. The elderly are individuals who have learned to cope with stress. Information regarding an older adult's coping strategies and strengths is as important as his or her psychologic symptoms. Bringing up the subject of adaptive strengths, you might begin by asking, "You have certainly lived a long, full life. Would you be willing to share some of your survival secrets with me?" Sample questions to gather information regarding the psychologic strengths of the elderly client are listed in the accompanying Assessment box.

Having gained an understanding of an elderly client's strengths and coping strategies (such as spiritual expression, listening to music, reading, reaching out to others), foster these strengths and adaptive strategies by including them in the care plan and encouraging significant others and the client to mobilize them to deal with the situation at hand.

Sexuality Sexuality is an important assessment area often overlooked by health care professionals. Sexual activity can and does continue into later life. Remember that sexuality does not refer only to sexual activity, it includes a broad multidimensional component of personhood and identity. Sexual expression includes body image, affection and love, flirtation, and social roles and interaction. Older people may abstain from sexual activity because they are denied the opportunity or they perceive negative social pressure and social norms regarding sexuality among people their age. They may abstain out of fear of HIV/AIDS or other sexually transmitted infections. Broaching the subject of sexuality with older clients may be just what they need to allay fears and give them permission to explore an untapped source of pleasure they may have long since forgotten. Approach the topic in a tactful, caring, nonjudgmental manner. An elderly client who does not wish to discuss sexual issues most likely will make that clear, by stating it directly, not answering the question, or changing the subject. An older person who was socialized in a different, more conservative time may not feel comfortable discussing sex. However, bringing up the subject may give an elderly client the opportunity to explore his or her sexuality privately or with a significant other.

SOCIAL AND FINANCIAL STATUS The quality and quantity of social support (past and present) available to the elderly person must be assessed. Quantity does not guarantee quality. Social support has important implications for recovery from psychologic disturbances. The more social support available, the better equipped an elderly person will be to overcome a stressful life event (Thompson et al. 1993). Maintaining an abundant, meaningful social network suggests strong interpersonal skills that can be mobilized to help negotiate stresses and losses later in life. The formation of a new social network, when others have dissolved, is easier for an elderly person with social skills and personal resources—assertiveness, friendliness, and warmth. Older adults who have been unsuccessful or disinclined to develop strong ties and friendships may benefit from exploring the interpersonal factors that prevented them from reaching out to others in the past.

The elderly, who often survive on a low fixed income, may be plagued by financial problems that affect their mental and physical health. Some communities have services for helping older people manage their finances and learn about financial aid and assistance programs. The removal of financial strain may dramatically improve the health of an aging person who is pressured by inadequate funds and inexperience with financial management. Sample questions for obtaining information about a client's social and financial status are listed in the accompanying Assessment box.

ELDER ABUSE The abuse of elders has generated interest because the prevalence of the problem has been increasing (Ebersole and Hess 1994). The mistreatment of elderly people is a serious, underreported, underdetected phenomenon. It is estimated that as many as a million elders are victims of mistreatment each year (Fulmer 1995). Elder mistreatment or abuse may take many forms, including physical abuse, neglect, exploitation, abandonment, and psychologic abuse.

Signs and symptoms of physical abuse may reflect direct beatings, the infliction of pain, or signs of coercion like abrasions, sprains, or dislocations. Signs of neglect may include the withholding of food, fluids, basic physical care, or medical attention. Exploitation includes the taking of social security or other pension checks, as well as the taking of other possessions against the person's will. Abandonment may occur when the caregiver drops the elder off in a local emergency room with no intention of returning to get the individual, or, for the elder who is incapacitated but living at home, the failure of the caregiver to show up to provide basic services. Finally, psychologic abuse includes continuous degrading, threatening, or scare tactics used against an older person unable to provide his or her own care (Fulmer 1995).

Elders who are at the greatest risk for abuse and neglect are those who are dependent on others for care. The degree of dependence may overwhelm the caregiver, and the resultant expression may harm the elder. Stressors related to caregiving can overwhelm any caregiver, but the caregiver of a frail elderly person is usually an adult child of the elder or the elder's spouse. In both instances, the daily pressures of care plus the exhaustion and frustration felt by the caregiver about his or her situation may be enough to cause the problems to occur (Ebersole and Hess 1994).

AMA guidelines suggest that during the assessment interview, nurses directly question older clients about the presence and nature of abuse. However, elders fearful of reprisal may not provide an accurate picture of the situation. Ebersole and Hess (1994) report that caregivers were often willing to talk about caregiving difficulties, but the elders themselves rarely did so.

An increasing number of states provide legal alternatives for the removal of an older adult to a protective situation. Nursing home placement may be necessary, but elders in this situation may react negatively and wish to return to the potentially harmful situation. Nurses must be aware of this reaction and prepare the elderly client as well as the caregiver for this type of response. In-home assistance may decrease the burden for caregivers who keep elders at home, but it is necessary for health care professionals to maintain regular contact with the elders to ascertain their health and safety in the situation (Fulmer 1995).

ASSESSMENT

Guidelines for Assessing Social and Financial Status

- How many phone calls do you get in a week?
- How frequently do you receive visitors?
- How frequently do you go visiting?
- Are you happily married/partnered?
- How would you describe your relationship with your (family, daughter, husband, wife, etc.)?
- Who do you know well enough to go visiting at their home (room, if in nursing home)?
- Do you have someone you can trust and confide in?
- Do you find yourself feeling lonely?
- Do you have someone who can drive you to the doctor or the hospital if you need it?
- How is your financial situation? Do you worry about money?

Nursing Diagnosis

The following nursing diagnoses are integral to any nursing care plan for elderly clients with the DSM-IV diagnoses given below.

MAJOR DEPRESSION

Low Self-Esteem Low self-esteem is a hallmark feature of depression. Not only do the elderly internalize social ageist biases, but they often are plagued with irrational guilt in the form of intrusive, obsessional, self-deprecating thoughts.

Risk for Violence: Self-Directed Feelings of hopelessness, low self-esteem, obsessive-compulsive symptoms, apathy, and powerlessness often contribute to suicidal ideation and attempts in the depressed elderly.

Activity Intolerance Psychomotor agitation and/or psychomotor retardation are both symptoms of depression. Psychomotor agitation in individuals with agitated depression affects social interaction, self-care abilities, and the sleep-wake cycle. Psychomotor retardation is a common vegetative sign of depression in the elderly. These individuals also experience compromised self-care abilities, lack physical exercise, and are at risk for developing complications of decreased mobility.

Self-Care Deficit: Feeding Many depressed older clients have dramatic weight losses, which in some cases indicate a passive suicide attempt. Less frequently, elderly individuals may experience a weight gain secondary to overeating and the decreased activity accompanying vegetative signs.

Altered Health Maintenance The depressed elderly are at risk for developing physical health complications secondary to poor self-care and poor health-maintenance habits.

Sleep Pattern Disturbance Often, older clients with depression experience sleep pattern disturbance, particularly early morning awakening. Occasionally, depressed elders report excessive sleeping.

Altered Thought Processes Often the elderly present with cognitive changes, such as short-term memory loss, accompanying the depression. These changes are not often seen in younger clients with depression. Concentration is often impaired, and lack of motivation hinders ability to learn new information.

Adjustment Disorder with Depressed Mood

Dysfunctional Grieving The client becomes immobilized with the stress of the loss. Often depression ensues to the point that the only factor differentiating an adjustment disorder from major depression is the identified stressor that precipitated the loss.

Self-Care Deficits Because of depression, individuals lose interest in and motivation to perform self-care activities. Grooming, hygiene, and activities of daily living are neglected. In extreme cases, the elderly person is at risk for developing other physical illnesses as a result of not taking medication and refusing to eat or engage in health-care practices.

Altered Role Performance The loss often leads to changes in social interaction and role performance, with potential for social withdrawal and loneliness and mental status changes due to lack of social stimulation and validation.

Hopelessness Hopelessness is a symptom of depression. The loss, coupled with the pervasive dysphoria, places the individual at risk for developing dependence and loss of function, as self-concept and motivation wane.

Anxiety Disorders

Ineffective Individual Coping Anxiety symptoms often impair an individual's ability to concentrate and think clearly, thus affecting judgment and often causing the client to decrease activities and avoid potentially stressful situations.

Activity Intolerance Often the anxiety is accompanied by psychomotor agitation and restlessness.

Anxiety Individuals with anxiety disorders experience fear, anxiety, and irritability to the point that they inhibit their usual pastimes and activities.

Delusional Disorders

Altered Thought Processes Elderly individuals with delusional disorders often become paranoid and suspect others of trying to rob them, cheat them, or harm them in some way. They also often have delusions about their body or bodily functions. The delusion is often accompanied by feelings of fear, paranoia, anger, and anxiety. Behavioral manifestations of these feelings may include suspiciousness, aggression, lashing out, social isolation, and unusual eating behaviors and "health" practices. Caregivers must sometimes go to great lengths to validate that the client's claims are not reality-based.

Impaired Social Interaction Often the delusions are centered around family members and caregivers, making relationships strained—if not impossible to maintain.

Planning and Implementing Interventions

The method is much less important than the process of what happens between the nurse and the elderly client (Hall et al. 1995).

Reminiscence and Life Review Reminiscence and life review are useful interventions for elderly clients experiencing self-esteem disturbance, grief, hopelessness, powerlessness, altered role performance, and social isolation. **Reminiscence** normally occurs to some degree throughout the life span but is of special significance for the elderly. During periods of crisis and transition, the process of reminiscence occurs quite naturally for many individuals (Ebersole and Hess 1994). The goals of **life review** include (Hall et al. 1995):

- Reexamining one's life.
- Resolution of old problems.
- Restoration of harmony with friends and family.
- Taking responsibility for one's own actions.
- Identifying with past accomplishments.
- Reviving happy memories to relieve depression.
- Improving interaction to decrease withdrawal.
- Reducing the fear of death.

Reminiscing can and should be encouraged for elders, individually and in groups. Creative uses of food, music, pets, and special events can facilitate the process and make it fun. Materials such as photo albums, journals, and tape and video recorders provide a means for clients to establish a permanent record of their life review, creating a legacy for those who follow.

REALITY ORIENTATION **Reality orientation** is a structured program for older adult clients that places an emphasis on orientation to time, place, and person. The approach provides consistency and a constant reminder to the client of where he or she is, why he or she is there, and what is expected. The use of periodic reality orientation tests the elder's level of confusion and disorientation. The rationale for reality orientation is the need to use a portion of the person's mind that is still intact (Ebersole and Hess 1994).

RESOCIALIZATION **Resocialization groups** are often unstructured and help meet the needs of the elderly for socializing activities within the nursing home or senior center. Group discussion focuses on topics chosen by the individual members of the group and may include reliving happy experiences, world affairs, or current local activities. Meetings usually occur weekly or several times a week, as opposed to the daily meetings of those in reality orientation groups (Ebersole and Hess 1994).

REMOTIVATION THERAPY **Remotivation therapy** is designed to renew interest in the individual's surroundings through stimulating discussion topics related to the real world. The group helps older people sense a feeling of belonging and encourages them to view themselves in terms of relationships with others. The group encourages active participation and attentiveness to others when discussions are not directly focused on an individual. Topics of discussion help group members pool knowledge and develop stimulating discussions related to the particular topic at hand (Buckwalter 1995).

PET THERAPY **Pet therapy** is used with elderly clients to decrease depression and fulfill the need to love and be loved (Buckwalter 1995). The animals, often provided by local SPCA groups, are trained to respond to elders in a calm, nonthreatening manner. The use of a certain type of animal is not as great a concern as the animal's and person's responses. Small animals are used for older clients who need to hold something on their lap, while larger animals are trained to stand next to a wheelchair and allow the client to pet or stroke without having to actually hold the animal.

MOVEMENT THERAPY **Movement therapy** helps provide a sense of relatedness to others while increasing sensory input through touch, vision, and hearing. Movement therapy has an additional benefit of increasing the elder's circulation, thereby enhancing cardiovascular capacity. It may include stretching and reaching exercises, hand-holding exercises, and/or mirroring the leader of the particular exercise (Buckwalter 1995). Movement therapy may include complex exercises for those who are able to participate, or it may have very simple, concrete exercises for those who are incapacitated either physically or cognitively.

SOCIAL SUPPORT AND GROUP INTERVENTIONS Social support and group interventions are useful when working with clients who experience altered family processes, knowledge deficit, ineffective individual coping, anticipatory and dysfunctional grieving, powerlessness, social isolation, and spiritual distress. Loss of affiliation with significant groups (family, professional and work group, bridge club) and social support can lead to identity dissolution, isolation, loneliness, and despair in the elderly.

Group therapy is considered by many to be the treatment of choice for older adult clients. It is efficient, because 8–10 people can benefit at one time. Long-term care facilities are ideally suited for group work because the members are easily accessible and transportation is not a problem.

INPATIENT AND OUTPATIENT THERAPY The care of elderly psychiatric clients and their families may extend over settings from homes to institutions. There are new models for home care, outpatient services, and long-term care. There are even special care units for elderly clients with dementia. The diversity of mental health problems requires a therapeutic environment that focuses on meeting the needs of the population in each special institution or outpatient setting.

The development of psychiatric units for elderly clients is a relatively new phenomenon. The difficulty with the mixture of clients was the great diversity of needs. A geropsychiatric facility, on the other hand, can provide for the unique needs of the elderly individual who has a long-term history of psychiatric illness (Abraham and Buckwalter 1994).

The mental health problems of older adults are biopsychosocial in nature. Nurses must avoid the error of focusing on psychologic and social dimensions at the expense of the biologic aspects (Abraham, Fox, and Cohen 1992). According to Abraham and Buckwalter (1994), the goals of care for the elderly mentally ill should include:

- Maintaining optimal functional independence.
- Supporting clients and families in homes, communities, and institutions.
- Delaying institutionalization.
- Enhancing self-esteem and personal integrity.
- Optimizing the role of the family and other informal caregivers in treatment strategies.
- Ensuring coordinated and supportive daily life activities that enhance the client's and family's capacity to cope.

These goals emphasize the areas of dysfunction and related problems that may evolve. Basic care includes keeping the client as independent as possible and encouraging client functioning at the highest physical, emotional, and social levels possible. Interventions depend on the thorough assessment of the client's abilities and limitations, and they build on the remaining capacity of the individual and attempt to compensate for the deficits.

Biologic Therapies

Medications Used judiciously, medication can be an effective adjunct to psychotherapy for mental disorders in later life. The high incidence of adverse drug reactions in older clients underscores the need for careful monitoring and conservative dosages. Medical and nursing personnel caring for elderly clients taking psychoactive medication require special training and for ongoing staff development.

Dosages of medication should be divided over the course of the day. The action of drugs in elderly clients is affected by the following factors:

- Biochemical and biologic changes.
- Stress.
- Nutritional status.
- Drug and alcohol use.
- Genetics.
- Changes in metabolism, absorption, distribution, and excretion.

The elderly are more susceptible to the side effects of psychotropic medications, such as:

- Constipation.
- EPS (dystonias, akathisia, perioral tremor, pseudoparkinsonism).
- Anticholinergic effects (urinary retention, blurred vision, dry mouth, sexual dysfunction, anticholinergic psychosis).
- Cardiovascular effects (postural hypotension, arrhythmias).
- Drug interactions (delirium, confusion, disorientation).
- Sedation.

Medications within each psychotropic class vary widely in the intensity of hypotension (postural blood pressure changes), anticholinergic effects, sedation, and extrapyramidal responses.

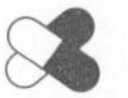

The choice of psychoactive medication in the elderly should be partially guided by a consideration of relative lack of side effects (Ebersole and Hess 1994). See Tables 38–2 and 38–3. Usually the desired effects have to be weighed against negative side effects in determining the course of treatment. It is generally recommended that the elderly client be started on dosages 30–50% of the recommended starting dosage for younger clients of similar size. The medication should be titrated until the desired therapeutic effect is established. See Table 38–4 on page 919 showing how aging affects medication absorption.

Ideally, psychotropic drug therapy should be supervised by a geropsychiatrist. General medical practitioners unfamiliar with pharmacology in the elderly often unknowingly overmedicate older clients. Among the elderly, psychotropic drugs are often prescribed inappropriately and the best drug within each class is often not selected. Medication should never take the place of psychotherapeutic modalities. Psychotherapy should always be continued along with medications.

Electroconvulsant Therapy The 2- to 3-week lag time between onset of antidepressant drug therapy and symptom relief is significant for severely depressed older clients whose health is in danger. When suicide or starvation is a real threat, or when antidepressants are ineffective or contraindicated, electroconvulsant therapy (ECT) should be considered. The main criteria for selecting ECT as the treatment of choice in the elderly are severity of depression and the need for immediate results (Zung 1980).

ECT is rapidly effective and safe, with judicious screening and advances in the use of muscle relaxants and anesthesia. The unilateral method has been shown to decrease the confusion and recent memory loss associated with ECT. Essentially, ECT may serve as a lifesaving measure in the elderly. Ignorance and negative emotions associated with early, less-sophisticated use of ECT should not enter into decisions regarding the appropriateness of this intervention with the severely depressed elderly client.

Table 38–2 Antidepressant Medications for the Elderly

Agent	*Geriatric Dose/Day (mg)*	*Sedation*	*Anticholinergic*	*Cardiac Toxicity*	*Hypertension*
Cyclic Agents					
Amitriptyline (Amitril, Elavil)	10–75	high	very high	high	medium
Imipramine (SK-Pramine, Tofranil)	10–75	medium	medium/high	medium	medium
Doxepin (Adapin, Sinequan)	10–75	high	medium	medium	medium
Desipramine (Norpramin, Pertofrane)	10–75	low	low	low	low
Nortriptyline (Aventyl, Pamelor)	10–50	low	medium	low	low
Trimipramine (Surmontil)	10–75	high	medium/high	high	medium
Protriptyline (Vivactil)	5–20	low	high	medium	medium
Maprotiline (Ludiomil)	10–75	medium	low/medium	low	medium
Amoxapine (Asendin)	10–100	medium	low	medium	medium
Fluoxetine (Prozac)	10–20 daily or every other day	unusual	none	none	none
Sertraline (Zoloft)	25–50	unusual	none	none	none
Paroxetine (Paxil)	10–20	unusual	none	none	none
Atypical Agents					
Trazodone (Desyrel)	75–150	high	none	low	medium
MAOIs					
Phenelzine (Nardil)	15–45	medium	low	none	medium/high
Tranylcypromine (Parnate)	10–40	medium	low	none	medium/high
Isocarboxazid (Marplan)	10–40	medium	low	none	medium/high

Source: Hogstel 1995.

Evaluation and Outcome Criteria

As with assessment and diagnosis, evaluation in psychosocial nursing is based primarily on the client's appearance, behavior, and self-report. Realistic expectations and stated objectives should guide the evaluation process. Key parameters of evaluation include mood, affect, and mental status. Whenever possible, involve the client in the evaluation process.

Altered Mood Subjective evidence of improved mood includes clients stating that they feel better, with increased sources of pleasure in daily activities and relationships. Objective signs of improved mood include expressive affect with more appropriate smiling and laughing. The range of affect is fuller and accompanied by less self-deprecating reference. Scores on depression and anxiety inventories show marked improvement over initial assessment scores, and a decrease in somatization and obsessive signs.

Altered Thought Processes Subjective indications of improvement include client reports that they are thinking more clearly and are better able to concentrate and remember recent and remote events. Individuals who pre-

Table 38–3 Antipsychotic Medications for the Elderly

Agent	Dose Equivalent	Sedation	Hypotension	Anticholinergic	Extrapyramidal Problems
Phenothiazines					
Chlorpromazine (Thorazine)	100	high	high	medium	low
Mesoridazine (Serentil)	50	medium	medium	medium	medium
Thioridazine (Mellaril)	95	high	high	high	low
Acetophenazine (Tindal)	15	low	low	low	medium
Fluphenazine (Prolixin)	2	medium	low	low	high
Perphenazine (Trilafon)	8	low	low	low	high
Trifluoperazine (Stelazine)	5	medium	low	low	high
Thioxanthenes					
Chlorprothixene (Taractan)	75	high	high	high	low
Thiothixene (Navane)	5	low	low	low	high
Dibenzoxazepine					
Loxapine (Loxitane)	10	medium	medium	medium	high
Butyrophenone					
Haloperidol (Haldol)	2	low	low	low	high
Indolone					
Molindone (Moban)	10	medium	low	medium	high

SOURCE: *Hogstel 1995.*

sented with delusions and other signs of psychosis will note they feel more like themselves and will be able to make more accurate, reality-based interpretations. In clients with symptoms of mania, the euphoria, grandiosity, and expansiveness of mood will resolve into a more contained reality-based affect.

Objective indications of improved mental status and cognition include orientation to person, place, and time; improved mental status exam scores; and appropriate dress, behavior, and interpersonal interactions. Tests of judgment, abstract thinking, and recent and remote memory improve over initial presentation. Communication will improve, and thought processes and content of speech will return to premorbid abilities. Clients will demonstrate tighter associations, and an improved ability to concentrate and to take in, process, and retain new information. It should be noted that improvement in thought process alteration is not a realistic goal for clients with an irreversible form of dementia.

HOPELESSNESS Expressions of hope and self-acceptance, renewed involvement and motivation in activities, and planning for the future indicate improvement and replace dependence, apathy, and negative self-talk.

SELF-CARE DEFICIT Clients will resume their premorbid level of self-care and health-maintenance behaviors.

ACTIVITY/REST DISTURBANCES: ALTERED PSYCHOMOTOR ACTIVITY Vegetative signs will be replaced with more appropriately paced activities, movement, gait, speech, appetite, and sleep-wake cycle. Anxiety and fear will be replaced with subjective feelings of calmness, restfulness, and well-being.

ALTERED NUTRITION: LESS THAN BODY REQUIREMENTS Clients will report that their appetites are returning to premorbid level, with increased pleasure associated with eating. Weight will return to normal range.

RISK FOR VIOLENCE: SELF-DIRECTED Clients will report that suicidal ideation has markedly decreased if not resolved, and there will be less morbid preoccupation with death and dying.

Table 38–4 Normal Changes in Aging That Affect Medication Absorption

Physical Change	*Pharmocologic Result*
Increase in gastric pH	Decrease in drug absorption
Increase in body fat	Decrease in concentration of fat-soluble drug
Decreased cardiac output	Delayed availability of drug at receptor sites and delayed excretion of drug
Decrease in total body water	Altered cellular distribution of drugs
Decrease in intestinal motility	Increase contact time and absorption
Decrease in plasma albumin	Decreased ability of drug to bind with protein
Decrease in hepatic blood flow	Decreased drug clearance and increased drug half-life

SOURCE: *Ebersole and Hess 1994.*

Chapter Highlights

- The aging population is increasing at a faster rate than the general population.
- Most elderly people remain relatively healthy, active, and vital well into later life.
- Older adults are the most underserved population in need of mental health care because of ageist biases, stigmatization, myths regarding normal aging, and inaccessibility of care.
- Mental health in later life is linked closely to intrapersonal, environmental, and interpersonal interactive processes.
- Depression is the most prevalent, most treatable mental disorder in later life.
- Somatization, or excessive preoccupation with bodily functions, may be a sign of depression in an older adult.
- The suicide rate for elderly people is nearly three times the rate of the general population.
- Electroconvulsant therapy may be a lifesaving intervention for severely depressed, suicidal older adults.
- Comprehensive, accurate, ongoing assessment is essential for differentiating treatable mental disorders from irreversible states.
- The elderly metabolize and excrete medication less efficiently, and are at risk for drug toxicity, which can mimic different mental disorders.
- Medication is not a substitute for psychotherapy. Medication should be prescribed primarily to enhance the effectiveness of psychotherapeutic interventions by reducing disabling symptoms.
- When the elderly are given psychotropic medication, they require only one-half to one-third the amount prescribed for younger adults of comparable weight, in doses divided over the course of the day.
- Family members caring for a dependent older adult need much emotional support and psychoeducative interventions.
- The elderly respond best to therapy that is goal-oriented and practical and has built-in short-term goals that enable them to monitor their accomplishments and progress over time.
- For the older adult, social support and group affiliation are important means for maintaining orientation, self-esteem, and a sense of identity and belonging.
- Reminiscing can be a significant therapeutic tool for enhancing self-esteem and maintaining a sense of identity in the older adult.

References

Abraham IL, Buckwalter KC: Geropsychiatric nursing: Clinical knowledge base in community and institutional settings. *J Psychosoc Nurs Ment Health Serv* 1994;32(4):20–26.

Abraham IL, Fox JC, Cohen BT: Integrating the bio into the biopsychosocial: Understanding and treating biological phenomena in psychiatric–mental health nursing. *Arch Psychiatr Nurs* 1992;5:296–305.

Alexopoulos GS, Meyers BS, Young RC, Mattis S, Kakuma T: The course of geriatric depression with "reversible dementia": A controlled study. *Am J Psychiatr* 1993;150:1693–1699.

American Psychiatric Association: *Diagnostic and Statistical Manual of Mental Disorders,* ed 4. American Psychiatric Association, 1994.

Bahr RT: Sleep disturbances, in Stanley M, Beare PG: *Gerontological Nursing.* F. A. Davis, 1995.

Buckwalter KC, Light E: New directions for psychiatric mental health nurses: The chronically mentally ill elderly. *Arch Psychiatr Nurs* 1989;3(1):53–54.

Callahan CM, Hendrie HC, Dittus RS, Brater DC, Hui SL, Tierney WM: Depression in late life: The use of clinical characteristics to focus screening efforts. *J Gerontology* 1994; 49(1):M9–M14.

Ebersole PE, Hess PA: *Toward Healthy Aging: Human Needs and Nursing Response,* ed 4. Mosby, 1994.

Eliopoulos C: *Gerontological Nursing,* ed 3. Lippincott, 1993.

Fulmer T: Elder mistreatment, in Stanley M, Beare PG: *Gerontological Nursing.* F. A. Davis, 1995.

Haggerty JJ, Golden RN, Evens DL, Janowsky DS: Differential diagnosis of pseudodementia in the elderly. *Geriatrics* 1988;43(3):61–74.

Hall, JR et al.: Standardized Care Plan: Managing Alzheimer's Patients at Home. *Gerontological Nursing.* 1995;21(1):37–47.

Harper M, Grau L: State of the art in geropsychiatric nursing. *J Psychosoc Nurs Ment Health Serv* 1994;32(4):7–12.

Hoffman AL: Alcohol problems in elder persons, in Stanley M, Beare PG: *Gerontological Nursing.* F. A. Davis, 1995.

Hogstel M: *Geropsychiatric Nursing,* ed 2. Mosby, 1995.

Kennedy G: The geriatric syndrome of late-life depression. *Psychiatr Services* 1995;46(1):43–48.

Krach P: Nursing implications: functional status of older persons with schizophrenia. *J Gerontological Nurs* 1993;19(8): 21–27.

Lachner G, Engel RR: Differentiation of dementia and depression by memory tests: A meta-analysis. *J Nervous Ment Disease* 1994;182(1):34–39.

Love CC, Buckwalter KC: Reactive depression, in Mass M, Buckwalter KC (eds): *Nursing Diagnosis and Interventions for the Institutionalized Elderly.* Addison-Wesley, 1991.

Mackel CL, Sheehy CM, Badger TA: The challenge of detection and management of alcohol abuse among elders. *Clini Nurse Specialist* 1994;8(3):129–135.

McBride AB, Burgener S: Strategies to implement geropsychiatric nursing curricula content. *J Psychosoc Nurs Ment Health Services* 1994;32(4):13–18.

McCall WV: Management of primary sleep disorders among elderly persons. *Psychiatr Services* 1995;46(1):49–54.

McMahon AL: Substance abuse among the elderly. *Nurse Practitioner Forum* 1993;4(4):231–238.

Meehan PJ, Saltzman LE, Sattin RW: Suicides among older United States residents: Epidemiologic characteristics and trends. *Am J Public Health* 1991;81:1198–1200.

Morris R, Buckwalter KC: Iowa Self-Assessment Inventory, in Busse EW, Blazer DG (eds): Handbook of Geriatric Psychiatry. Van Nostrand Reinhold, 1980.

Pfeiffer E: A Short Portable Mental Status Questionnaire for the assessment of organic brain deficit in elderly patients. *J Am Geriatr Soc* 1975;23:441–443.

Rabin DL: Characteristics of the elderly population, in Reichel W (ed): *Clinical Aspects of Aging.* Williams & Wilkins, 1989.

Smith SL, Sherril KA, Colenda CC: Assessing and treating anxiety in elder persons. *Psychiatr Services* 1995;46(1): 36–42.

Stanley M, Beare PG: *Gerontological Nursing.* F. A. Davis, 1995.

Thompson EH, Futterman AM, Gallagher-Thompson D, Rose JM, Lovett SB: Social support and caregiving burden in family caregivers of frail elders. *J Gerontology* 1993;48(3): S245–S254.

Yesavage JA, Brink TL, Lum O, Huang V, Adley MB, Leirer VO: Development and validation of a geriatric depression rating scale: A preliminary report. *J Psychiatr Res* 1982–1983; 17:37.

Zung, WK: Affective disorders, in Busse EW, Blazer DG (eds): *Handbook of Geriatric Psychiatry.* Van Nostrand Reinhold, 1980.

Zweig RA, Hinrichsen GA: Factors associated with suicide attempts by depressed older adults: A prospective study. *Am J Psychiatry* 1993;150:1687–1692.

APPENDICES

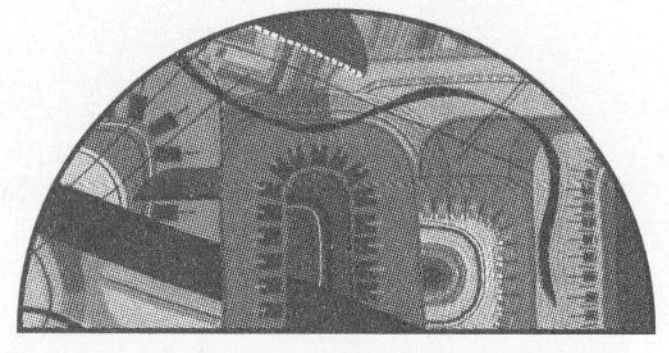

APPENDIX A

PSYCHOTROPIC DRUGS IN COMMON USAGE

Eileen Trigoboff

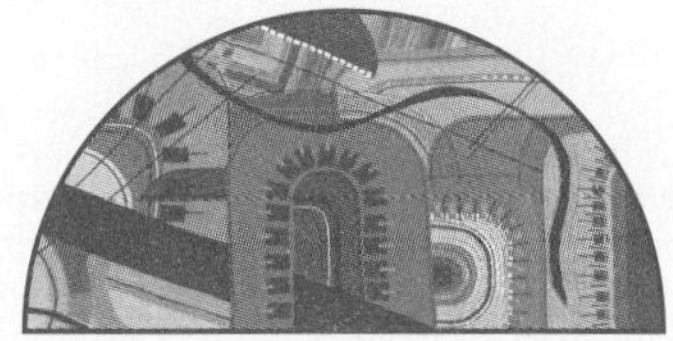

Index of Drugs

Product Information

Note: The information that follows has been selectively abstracted from the sources listed under "References" for use as an educational aid and does not cover all possible uses, actions, precautions, side effects, or interactions of this medicine. It is not intended as medical advice for individual problems.

Generic name: alprazolam
Brand name: Xanax
Classification: Antianxiety; benzodiazepine; skeletal muscle relaxant
Common uses: Anxiety disorders; relief of anxiety associated with depression; panic disorder
Should not be used if: Client is pregnant or nursing; client has narrow-angle glaucoma, hepatic, or renal disease.
Possible side effects: Drowsiness; fatigue; ataxia; dizziness; orthostatic hypotension; ECG changes; tachycardia; blurred vision; tolerance; physical and psychologic dependence; may aggravate symptoms in some depressed patients.
Possible drug interactions: Increases central nervous system depression from other drugs, including alcohol, antipsychotics, antihistamines, antidepressants, anticonvulsants, barbiturates, and narcotics. Nicotine, caffeine, valproic acid, and rifampin decrease alprazolam's effectiveness.
Nursing considerations: Assess anxiety level; potential for addiction; history of allergies and or medical problems; watch for symptoms of overdose, such as intoxication, disinhibition, impairment in judgment and memory, depressed vital signs; evaluate blood pressure reclining and standing, blood studies, hepatic studies, I&O. Educate client about potential for injury from operating cars or machinery, abrupt withdrawal, and combining with CNS depressants. Refer to Client/Family Teaching: Benzodiazepines, Chapter 33.

Usual dosage: 1.5–4 mg/day, should be gradually increased from 0.25–0.5 mg/day in 2–3 divided doses. Take with food to reduce GI symptoms.
Onset: 30–60 minutes, peaks in about 1 hour.

Generic name: amantadine HCl
Brand name: Symmetrel
Classification: Antiparkinsonian; cyclic primary amine
Common uses: Prophylaxis and/or treatment of extrapyramidal reactions; parkinsonism; symptomatic treatment of influenza caused by A influenza virus strains.
Possible side effects: Headache; dizziness; drowsiness; fatigue; orthostatic hypotension; CHF; blurred vision; leukopenia; nausea and vomiting; dry mouth; urinary frequency or retention; peripheral edema; skin mottling; photosensitivity; depression; psychosis; hallucinations.
Possible drug interactions: Additive with other anticholinergic drugs and CNS stimulants; thiazide-type diuretics may decrease excretion and lead to toxic buildup of amantadine.
Nursing considerations: Assess I&O; give after meals for better absorption; evaluate therapeutic response, skin problems, respiratory status or allergic reactions; advise gradual changes in body position to avoid orthostatic hypotension, avoidance of abrupt discontinuation of drug and caution in activities that require concentration.
Usual dosage: PO (adults 13–64)—100 mg BID or 200 mg as a single daily dose; reduced dose for children, elders, and patients with renal impairment.
Onset: For therapeutic effect, two weeks is required, then it takes effect in 4–48 hours, peaks in 1–4 hours, and will last 12–24 hours.

Generic name: amitriptyline
Brand names: Amitril; Elavil; Emitrip; Endep; Enovil; Levate; Meravil; Novotriptyn; Rotavil
Classification: Tricylic antidepressant; tertiary amine
Common uses: Major depression; depressive phase of bipolar disorder; chronic pain; and various types of headaches.
Should not be used if: Client is taking MAO inhibitors; pregnant or lactating; under 12 years of age; has a history of hypersensitivity to tricyclics; is in recovery phase of myocardial infarction; has untreated angle-closure glaucoma.
Possible side effects: Drowsiness; dizziness; orthostatic hypotension; tachycardia; hypertension; heart block; CHF; cardiovascular collapse; ECG changes; agranulocytosis; thombocytopenia; leukopenia; dry mouth; constipation; weight gain; and urinary retention. Other less common effects are noted.
Possible drug interactions: Potentiates CNS depressants, including alcohol, barbiturates, and benzodiazepines; severe systemic reactions with MAO inhibitors; nicotine increases amitriptyline metabolism; thyroid medications may interact to produce arrhythmias and tachycardia.
Nursing considerations: Assess initial vital signs and weight, monitor throughout therapy; be aware of sudden changes in mood, which may indicate lethality. Evaluate for symptoms of blood dyscrasias, including sore throat, fever, malaise, unusual bleeding or bruising; and symptoms of overdose, such as confusion, agitation, irritability. Caution client to be careful when operating machinery, standing up, and in exposure to the sun. Refer to Client/Family Teaching: Tricyclic Antidepressants, Chapter 33.
Usual dosage: Initially 75–100 mg/day for adults, less for elders and adolescents; increasing to 150–200 mg/day. Maintenance doses may be as low as 25–40 mg/day.
Onset: May take 2–4 weeks to see therapeutic results, will peak 2–12 hours after administration, and lasts for weeks.

Generic name: amoxapine
Brand name: Asendin
Classification: Tricyclic antidepressant; dibenzoxazepine derivative-secondary amine
Common uses: Major depression with psychotic symptoms; depression associated with organic causes; depressive phase of bipolar disorder; and mixed symptoms of depression, anxiety.
Should not be used if: Client is hypersensitive to tricyclics; pregnant or lactating; under 14 years of age; taking MAO inhibitor; in an acute recovery period following a myocardial infarction. Use caution with patients having history of seizures, prostatic hypertrophy, cardiovascular, hepatic, renal, or respiratory difficulties, or who are elderly, debilitated, or psychotic.
Possible side effects: Drowsiness; dizziness; orthostatic hypotension; blurred vision; nasal congestion; tachycardia; myocardial infarction; ECG changes; dry mouth; constipation; urinary retention; and many other less common problems.
Possible drug interactions: Potentiates CNS depressants, including alcohol, barbiturates and benzodiazepines; severe systemic reactions with MAO inhibitors; nicotine increases amoxapine metabolism; thyroid medications may interact to produce arrhythmias and tachycardia.
Nursing considerations: Assess initial vital signs and weight, monitor throughout therapy; be aware of sudden changes in mood, which may indicate lethality. Evaluate for symptoms of blood dyscrasias, including sore throat, fever, malaise, unusual bleeding or bruising; and symptoms of overdose, such as confusion, agitation, irritability, and physical signs. Caution client to be careful when operating machinery, standing up, and in exposure to the sun. Refer to Client/Family Teaching: Tricyclic Antidepressants, Chapter 33.
Usual dosage: Initially, 50 mg two or three times daily. Increase to 300 mg/day. NTE 400–600 mg/day, depending on available supervision.
Onset: Therapeutic effect in 2–4 weeks, thereafter blood level peaks 90 minutes after ingestion.

Generic name: benztropine mesylate
Brand name: Cogentin
Classification: Antiparkinsonian; anticholinergic
Common uses: Parkinsonism; extrapyramidal symptoms associated with antipsychotic drugs (not including tardive dyskinesia); prevention of extrapyramidal side effects.
Possible side effects: Drowsiness; dizziness; blurred vision; dry mouth; constipation; paralytic ileus; and other physical problems.
Possible drug interactions: May increase CNS depression with alcohol, barbiturates, narcotics, and benzodiazepines. May decrease antipsychotic effects of the phenothiazines or haloperidol. May increase anticholinergic effects of any other drug with anticholinergic properties.
Should not be used if: Client is hypersensitive; pregnant or lactating; under 3 years of age; routinely exposed to elevated external temperatures; has cardiac or GI problems; has glaucoma or urinary obstructions; has hypertension or hyperthyroidism.
Nursing considerations: Assess for symptoms of Parkinson's disease, such as tremors, muscular weakness and rigidity, drooling, shuffling, flat affect, and disturbance in balance or posture; extrapyramidal symptoms are similar with the addition of akinesia (muscular weakness), akathisia (restlessness), dystonia (involuntary muscular movements), oculogyric crisis (rolling back of the eyes), and tardive dyskinesia (bizarre facial and tongue and/or body movements). Evaluate for constipation, GI disturbance, or paralytic ileus, which may be life threatening. Educate client to avoid OTC medications until physician agrees, to avoid driving or other activities that require intense concentration, and not to stop medication abruptly.
Usual dosage: May be given PO or IM. For Parkinsonism, begin at 0.5–1.0 mg and increase gradually to smallest effective dose. Maximum daily dose is 6 mg/day. For extrapyramidal symptoms, give 1–4 mg daily or BID.
Onset: PO—onset, 1–2 hours; duration 24 hours. IM—15 minutes; duration 6–10 hours.

Generic name: bupropion
Brand name: Wellbutrin
Classification: Monocyclic antidepressant; amino ketone type

Common uses: Clients with depression who fail to respond or who cannot tolerate alternative antidepressant treatments. Not recommended as a first choice.
Should not be used if: Client is hypersensitive; taking MAO inhibitors; pregnant or lactating; under 18 years of age; has a history of seizure disorder, cranial trauma, bulimia, or anorexia nervosa. Use caution if client has cardiovascular, hepatic, or renal problems or if client is suicidal, psychotic, elderly, or debilitated.
Possible side effects: Agitation; insomia; headache; migraine; tremors; seizures; blurred vision; sedation; dizziness; tachycardia; dry mouth; constipation; nausea; vomiting; weight loss; anorexia; leukopenia; and other not so common physical problems. Slight increase in BP; orthostatic hypotension; slight weight loss.
Possible drug interactions: Drugs that alter hepatic enzyme activity may decrease metabolism of bupropion; levodopa may increase incidence of adverse effects; MAO inhibitors enhance toxicity of bupropion; drugs that lower seizure threshold may increase risk of seizures.
Nursing considerations: Assess for lethality and sudden mood elevation that may precede suicide attempt; vital signs and weight; malaise. Evaluate history of seizures, allergies, glaucoma, alcohol/drug consumption, contraceptive use. Educate client to understand precautions about illness, medications, and precautions that must be taken in regard to driving and operation of machinery.
Usual dosage: PO (adults)—initially 200 mg/day given as 100 mg BID, increased to a maximum of 450 mg over several weeks of treatment.
Onset: May take up to 4 weeks for clinical efficacy, peaks in 1–3 hours and stays in the system for 1–2 weeks.

Generic name: buspirone
Brand name: Buspar
Classification: Antianxiety agent
Common uses: Generalized anxiety states
Should not be used if: Client is hypersensitive; using MAO inhibitors; elderly or debilitated; pregnant or lactating; under 18 years of age. Use caution with clients who have hepatic or renal dysfunction. Clients should be withdrawn from benzodiazepines or sedative/hypnotics before therapy with buspirone.
Possible side effects: Drowsiness; dizziness; headache; nervousness; nausea; and several other less common problems.
Possible drug interactions: Use with MAO inhibitors may elevate blood pressure.
Nursing considerations: Assess extent of anxiety, lethality, presence of side effects. Evaluate history for allergies, contraceptive use, childbearing status, alcohol/drug abuse. Educate client to take care in activities that require concentration and to avoid potential hazards. This medication is less sedating than benzodiazepines.
Usual dosage: PO (adults)—5 mg TID, to be increased at intervals of 2–3 days, NTE 60 mg/day, usually effective dose: 20–30 mg/day.
Onset: Therapeutic levels may be reached in 7–10 days; it peaks in 40–90 minutes; its duration in the body is unknown.

Generic name: carbamazepine
Brand name: Tegretol
Classification: Anticonvulsant
Common uses: Seizure disorders; trigeminal neuralgia
Should not be used if: Sensitivity to tricyclic antidepressants; baseline hematologic abnormalities or receiving other myelotoxic drugs; history of bone marrow depression. Use caution if client has history of cardiac damage, liver disease, increased intraocular pressure.
Possible side effects: Sedation; anticholinergic effects; dizziness; drowsiness; blurred vision; speech disturbances; abnormal involuntary movements; GI distress; muscle relaxation; antiarrhythmic action; antidiuretic effects; nystagmus; minor hematologic changes; hypotension; aggravation of hypertension; pruritus; photosensitivity; diaphoresis; chills.
Possible drug interactions: Serum concentrations of anticonvulsants may be decreased; calcium-channel blocking, agents (verapamil) may be increased to toxic level; erythromycin decreases clearance of carbamazepine; doxycycline should not be given concomitantly; serum concentration of warfarin decreased; MAO inhibitors not recommended; reliability of oral contraceptives may be adversely affected.
Nursing considerations: Tasks requiring mental alertness or physical coordination may become difficult; assess for carbamazepine toxicity if erythromycin is also utilized; discuss contraception; assess elimination patterns; assure proper hydration.
Usual dosage: Oral suspensions produce higher peak concentrations. Children 6–12 years: 50 mg 4 times/day; over 12 and adults: 400 mg/day to 1.2 grams/day.
Onset: Peak plasma concentration within 2–8 hours.

Generic name: chloral hydrate
Brand name: Notec; Aquachloral Supprettes; Cohidrate; Novochlorhydrate
Classification: Sedative-hypnotic; CNS depressant; chloral derivative
Common uses: Insomnia; moderate anxiety; preoperative sedation; anxiety associated with drug withdrawal.
Should not be used if: Client is hypersensitive; pregnant or lactating; elderly or debilitated; has severe hepatic, renal, or cardiac disease, gastritis, esophagitis, peptic or oral ulcers, history of porphyria or drug abuse.
Possible side effects: Drowsiness; dizziness; skin rashes; nausea and vomiting; diarrhea; leukopenia; physical and psychologic dependence.
Possible drug interactions: Potentiates action of other CNS depressants such as alcohol and opiates; increases effects of anticoagulants; in combination with furosemide, may produce blood pressure changes; flushing and diaphoresis.
Nursing considerations: Assess level of anxiety/agitation, sleep patterns, lethality, presence of side effects. Evaluate history of allergies, use of contraceptives, childbearing status, use of drugs/alcohol. Educate about need for medication, caution in operation of cars and machinery.
Usual dosage: PO (adults)—insomnia, 500–1000 mg at bedtime.
Onset: Effective in 30–60 minutes, lasts 4–8 hours.

Generic name: chlordiazepoxide
Brand name: Librium
Classification: Antianxiety; benzodiazepine
Common uses: Temporary relief of anxiety; acute alcohol withdrawal
Should not be used if: Client is hypersensitive to benzodiazepines; using other CNS depressants; pregnant or lactating; an infant; in shock or coma; elderly; or debilitated. Use caution with clients with narrow-angle glaucoma, hepatic or renal dysfunction, a history of drug abuse/addiction, or lethality.
Possible side effects: Drowsiness; fatigue; ataxia; dizziness; shock; cardiovascular collapse; and many other less common physical effects.
Possible drug interactions: Other CNS depressants produce additive CNS depression; effects of chlordiazepoxide are increased by cimetidine and decreased by valproic acid; oral contraceptives are contraindicated; phenytoin is increased in the system; the effects of levodopa are increased; digoxin's excretion is decreased; antitubercular drugs have contradictory effects; disulfiram decreases clearance of chlordiazepoxide.
Nursing considerations: Assess vital signs, reclining and standing; lab values; level of anxiety; lethality; presence of side effects; childbearing status; contraceptive use. Evaluate for history of allergies, drug/alcohol abuse, glaucoma. Educate client to understand the problems of the disease and use of medication, take drug with food, use caution in operation of automobiles and other machinery. Refer to Client/Family Teaching: Benzodiazepines, Chapter 33.

Usual dosage: PO (adults)—5–25 mg TID or QID for anxiety; PO (adults)—50–100 mg for acute alcohol withdrawal; maximum daily dose 300 mg/day.
Onset: Is effective in 15–30 minutes and peaks in 2–4 hours.

Generic name: chlorpromazine
Brand name: Thorazine; Chlorazine; Klorazine; Ormazine; Promapar; Promaz; Thor-Prom
Classification: Antipsychotic/neuroleptic; antiemetic; phenothiazine
Common uses: Management of psychotic disorders such as schizophrenia; manic phase of bipolar disorder (until lithium takes effect); brief reactive psychosis; intractable hiccups; severe behavior problems in children; nausea and vomiting; pre- and postoperative sedation.
Should not be used if: Client is hypersensitive to phenothiazines; comatose or CNS-depressed; taking CNS depressants; pregnant or lactating; under 2 years of age; has bone marrow depression, blood dyscrasias, subcortical brain damage, Parkinson's disease, liver, renal, or cardiac insufficiency, severe hypo- or hypertension. Use caution for clients with a history of seizures, prostatic hypertrophy, diabetes, hypocalcemia, severe reactions to insulin or ECT; who may be exposed to extreme temperatures or organophosphate insecticides; if client is withdrawing from alcohol or barbiturates.
Possible side effects: Sedation; headache; extrapyramidal symptoms; tardive dyskinesia; blurred vision; neuroleptic malignant syndrome, orthostatic hypotension; skin rashes; photosensitivity; dry mouth; nausea; vomiting; increased or decreased appetite; constipation; agranulocytosis; leukopenia; anemia; thrombocytopenia; pancytopenia; laryngeal edema; laryngospasm; bronchospasm; suppression of cough reflex.
Possible drug interactions: Additive effects with CNS depressants and anticholinergic drugs; with epinephrine, may reverse action and lead to decreased blood pressure and tachycardia; aluminum or magnesium hydroxide may decrease absorption; the effects of lithium and levodopa may be decreased; may be neurotoxic in combination with lithium; may increase plasma levels of propranolol and metoprolol; cimetidine may decrease the effectiveness of phenothiazines; clonidine may produce severe hypotension; caffeine may counteract antipsychotic effects.
Nursing considerations: Assess therapeutic effects of medication; level of sedation; vital signs; childbearing status; ability to carry out activities of daily living. Evaluate lab values for symptoms of blood dyscrasias, extrapyramidal symptoms, tardive dyskinesia, symptoms of neuroleptic malignant syndrome, history of allergies and drug/alcohol consumption. Educate about nature of illness and use of medications; caution client to be careful when operating vehicles and machinery, and in processes that involve concentration. Refer to Client/Family Teaching: Antipyschotics, Chapter 33.
Usual dosage: PO (adults)—10 mg TID or QID, or 25 mg BID or TID; increased by 20–50 mg until symptoms are controlled; maximum daily dose of 200 mg.
Onset: 30–60 minutes, peaking in 2–4 hours and lasting 4–5 hours.

Generic name: clomipramine
Brand name: Anafranil
Classification: Tricyclic antidepressant
Common uses: Severe obsessive-compulsive disorder; depressive symptoms; panic disorder, or phobic disorder, but only if OCD is the primary diagnosis and strongly dominates the clinical picture.
Should not be used if: Client is hypersensitive to tricyclic antidepressants; using MAO inhibitors; in acute recovery from myocardial infarction; pregnant or lactating; under 18 years of age. Use with caution for clients with a history of seizures; urinary retention, glaucoma, cardiovascular disorders, hepatic or renal insufficiency, psychosis, acute intermittent porphyria, or who are elderly or debilitated.
Possible side effects: Drowsiness; dizziness; mania; tremors; lowered seizure threshold; blurred vision; orthostatic hypotension; delayed ejaculation; anorgasmia; cardiac arrest; dry mouth; constipation; agranulocytosis; neutropenia; pancytopenia; and many other less common physical symptoms.
Possible drug interactions: Potentiates CNS depressants, including alcohol, barbiturates, and benzodiazepines; severe systemic reactions with MAO inhibitors; methylphenidate, phenothiazines, haloperidol, and cimetidine increase clomipramine serum levels; quinidine, procainamide, disopyramide potentiate adverse cardiovascular effects of clomipramine; smoking increases clomipramine metabolism; disulfiram decreases clomipramine metabolism; the absorption of levodopa and phenylbutazone is delayed; warfarin increases prothrombin time; dicumarol increases in the plasma; thyroid medications may interact to produce arrhythmias and tachycardia.
Nursing considerations: Assess initial vital signs (BP, lying down and standing) and weight, monitor throughout therapy; be aware of sudden changes in mood that may indicate lethality, note presence of obsessions and compulsions. Evaluate for symptoms of blood dyscrasias, including sore throat, fever, malaise, unusual bleeding or bruising, and symptoms of overdose, such as confusion, agitation, irritability, and physical signs. Educate client as to nature of disease, need for medication as withdrawal from medication may cause recurrence, properties of medication, including length of time drug takes to reach effective levels, to be careful when operating machinery and motor vehicles, standing up, and in exposure to the sun. Refer to Client/Family Teaching: Tricyclic Antidepressants, Chapter 33.
Usual dosage: OCD PO (adults)—75–150 mg/day in three divided doses.
Onset: Peak plasma in under 2 hours, takes effect in 5–10 weeks.

Generic name: clonazepam
Brand name: Klonopin; Rivotril
Classification: Anticonvulsant; benzodiazepine derivative
Common uses: Prophylactic treatment of seizures; panic attacks; mild sedation
Should not be used if: Client is hypersensitive to benzodiazepines; lactating, has acute angle-closure glaucoma, chronic respiratory or severe liver disease. Use caution if client is pregnant, elderly, or debilitated; depressed or suicidal; has a history of drug abuse/addiction.
Possible side effects: Drowsiness; ataxia; behavior problems; nausea/vomiting; constipation; blood dyscrasias; increased salivation; nystagmus; diplopia; respiratory depression; and several other less common physical effects.
Possible drug interactions: Additive with other CNS depressants; may increase absence seizures with valproic acid; phenobarbital, phenytoin, and carbamazepine decrease the effect of clonazepam; disulfiram increases its effect but may also lead to toxic reactions.
Nursing considerations: Assess vital signs; lab values; lethality; presence of side effects. Evaluate history of allergies, glaucoma, drug and alcohol consumption, childbearing status. Educate about usefulness of medication and disease process, caution needed in operation of vehicles and machinery. Refer to Client/Family Teaching: Benzodiazepines, Chapter 33.
Usual dosage: PO (adults)—initially 15 mg/day in three divided doses; may be increased to 20 mg/day.
Onset: Takes effect in 20–60 minutes; peaks in 1–2 hours; lasts from 6–12 hours.

Generic name: clorazepate
Brand name: Tranxene
Classification: Antianxiety; benzodiazepine
Common uses: Anxiety disorders and anxiety symptoms; partial seizures (adjunctive management); acute alcohol withdrawal
Should not be used if: Client is hypersensitive to benzodiazepines; taking other CNS depressants; pregnant or lactating; under 9 years of age. Use caution with elderly or debilitated

patients; those with hepatic or renal dysfunction; a history of drug abuse/addiction; depression or lethality.

Possible side effects: Drowsiness; fatigue; ataxia; dizziness; and many other less common effects.

Possible drug interactions: Additive with other CNS depressants; effects increased by cimetidine; nicotine and caffeine decrease effects; neuromuscular blocking agents increase respiratory depression; reduces excretion of digoxin, increasing potential for toxicity; antacids reduce effectiveness.

Nursing considerations: Assess anxiety level; potential for addiction; history of allergies and/or medical problems; watch for symptoms of overdose, such as intoxication, disinhibition, impairment in judgment and memory, depressed vital signs. Evaluate blood pressure reclining and standing, blood studies, hepatic studies, I&O. Educate client about potential for injury from operating cars or machinery, abrupt withdrawal, and combining with CNS depressants. Refer to Client/Family Teaching: Benzodiazepines, Chapter 33.

Usual dosage: For anxiety, PO (adults)—15–60mg/day in divided doses.

Onset: Takes effect in 30–60 minutes and peaks in 1–2 hours.

Generic name: clozapine
Brand name: Clozaril
Classification: Antipsychotic; tricyclic dibenzodiazepine derivative

Common uses: Management of psychotic symptoms in schizophrenic patients for whom other antipsychotics have failed.

Should not be used if: Client is hypersensitive to tricyclics; CNS-depressed or comatose; has myeloproliferative disorders, severe granulocytopenia.

Possible side effects: Agranulocytosis; sedation; salivation; dizziness; headache; tremors; sleep problems; akinesia; fever; seizures; sweating; akathisia; confusion; fatigue; insomnia; dry mouth; constipation, nausea; abdominal discomfort; vomiting; diarrhea; tachycardia; hypotension; hypertension; urinary abnormalities; leukopenia, neutropenia, eosinophilia.

Possible drug interactions: Anticholinergic effects increased with other anticholinergic drugs, in combination with antihypertensive drugs produces increased hypotension; potentiates CNS depressive drugs; bone marrow suppression is increased with antineoplastic medications; plasma concentration of warfarin, digoxin and other protein-bound drugs.

Nursing considerations: Evaluate for symptoms of blood dyscrasias, including sore throat, fever, malaise, unusual bleeding or bruising. Assess initial vital signs and weight, monitor throughout therapy; be aware of sudden changes in mood, which may indicate lethality; skin turgor, presence of side effects including pseudoparkinsonism, constipation and/or urinary retention. Educate about disease process, uses of medication and side effects. Caution client to be careful when operating machinery and motor vehicles, standing up and walking slowly until stabilized, and in exposure to excessive external or environmental temperatures including hot tubs and showers; avoid use of OTC medications, alcohol or CNS depressant medications until cleared by doctor; observe when use in combination with other medications that lower seizure threshold. Refer to Client/Family Teaching: Antipsychotics, Chapter 33.

Usual dosage: PO (adult)—initially 25 mg/day QD or BID; may increase to 300–450 mg/day gradually over 2 weeks, NTE 900 mg/day.

Onset: May take 2–4 weeks for therapeutic effect.

Generic name: diazepam
Brand name: Valium, Valrelease
Classification: Antianxiety; benzodiazepine

Common uses: Anxiety disorders; acute alcohol withdrawal; skeletal muscle spasms; convulsive disorders (adjunctive therapy); status epilepticus; preoperative sedation and relief or anxiety; anterograde amnesia.

Should not be used if: Client is hypersensitive to benzodiazepines; using other CNS depressants; pregnant or lactating; an infant; in shock or coma; elderly or debilitated. Use with caution if client has narrow-angle glaucoma, hepatic or renal dysfunction, a history of drug abuse/addiction or lethality.

Possible side effects: Drowsiness; fatigue; ataxia; dizziness; shock; cardiovascular collapse; agranulocytosis; and many other less common physical effects.

Possible drug interactions: Other CNS depressants have additive depressant effects; cimetidine and valproic acid increase effects of diazepam; oral contraceptives and antitubercular drugs have contradictory effects; nicotine and caffeine decrease effects of diazepam; serum levels of phenytoin may be increased; the effects of levodopa are decreased; excretion of digoxin may increase potential for toxicity.

Nursing considerations: Assess vital signs reclining and standing; lab values; level of anxiety; lethality; presence of side effects; childbearing status; contraceptive use. Evaluate for history of allergies, drug/alcohol abuse, glaucoma. Caution client that drug may become habit forming, to take drug with food, to use caution in operation of automobiles and other machinery; drug should not be used longer than four months unless directed by a physician; consult with physician before taking any OTC preparations in conjunction with diazepam. Refer to Client/Family Teaching: Benzodiazepines, Chapter 33.

Usual dosage: PO (adults)—2–10 mg BID or QID.

Onset: Takes effect in 30–60 minutes; peaks in 1–2 hours.

Generic name: diphenhydramine
Brand name: Benadryl; Bendylate; Benylin; Compoz; Fenylhist; Surfadil
Classification: Antihistamine with anticholinergic and sedative side effects

Common uses: Relief from allergies, cold symptoms, extrapyramidal side effects, Parkinson's disease, motion sickness, nausea and vomiting, dizziness; for mild sedation.

Should not be used if: MAO inhibitors have been used in previous 2 weeks. Use caution with clients with pregnancy, lactation, asthma, heart or lung disease, glaucoma, ulcers, difficulty urinating, high BP, seizures, hyperthyroidism; under 6 years of age.

Possible side effects: Sedation; dry mouth and mucous membranes; vision problems; difficulty urinating; muscle weakness; excitement (especially in children); nervousness.

Possible drug interactions: Potentiates alcohol and other CNS depressants; MAO inhibitors prolong and intensify anticholinergic effects.

Nursing considerations: If a dose is missed, do not double dose; caution advised in tasks requiring alertness, I&O.

Usual dosage: Usual daily dose range 75–200 mg, nighttime sleep aid dosage 50 mg.

Onset: Takes effect and peaks in 1 hour, lasts for 4–6 hours.

Generic name: disulfiram
Brand name: Antabuse
Classification: Alcohol deterrent; aldehyde dehydrogenase inhibitor

Common uses: Chronic alcoholism (aversion therapy)

Should not be used if: Client is hypersensitive to thiuram derivatives; has severe myocardial disease, coronary occlusion, psychoses; has recently received or is receiving metronidazole, paraldehyde, alcohol or alcohol-containing preparations; use caution with clients who have hepatic or renal insufficiency, diabetes mellitus, seizure disorders, cerebral damage, history of rubber-contact dermatitis, chronic or acute nephritis, hepatic cirrhosis, abnormal EEG results, multiple drug dependence, hypothyroidism; or who are pregnant.

Possible side effects: Drowsiness; headache; metallic or garlic-like aftertaste; hepatotoxicity; blood dyscrasias; disulfiram-alcohol reaction, which includes tachycardia, hypotension, flushing, dyspnea, headache, nausea and vomiting.

Possible drug interactions: Mild to severe life-threatening reactions with alcohol-containing preparations (including topical), increased effects of diazepam and chlordiazepoxide;

phenytoin intoxication, prolonged prothrombin time with oral anticoagulants; unsteady gait or marked changes in behavior with isoniazid; acute toxic psychosis with metronidazole; additive CNS stimulation with marijuana; with barbiturates and paraldehyde, increased serum concentration and posssible toxicity; combination with tricyclic antidepressants may produce acute organic brain syndrome and enhance the disulfiram-alcohol reaction; decreased clearance of caffeine.

Nursing considerations: Assess baseline vital signs and weight; mood, appearance, orientation, and behavior; assess for symptoms of alcohol withdrawal, oral contraceptive use, childbearing status. Evaluate alcohol and drug use, history of allergies, diabetes, cardiac disease, epilepsy, hypothyroidism, liver disease, psychosis, adverse side effects (symptoms can occur within 5–10 minutes after ingestion of alcohol). Educate about condition and need for therapy, medication effects and contraindications. Refer to Chapter 13.

Usual dosage: PO (adults)—initial dosage 250–500 mg/day in a single dose for 1–2 weeks. Not to exceed 500 mg/day.

Onset: Takes effect in 3–12 hours, lasts up to 14 days.

Generic name: doxepin HCl

Brand name: Adaptin; Sinequan

Classification: Tricyclic antidepressant; debenzoxepin; tertiary amine

Common uses: Major depression with melancholia or psychotic symptoms; depression associated with organic disease and alcoholism; depressive phase of bipolar disorder; psychoneurotic anxiety; mixed symptoms of anxiety and depression.

Should not be used if: Client is hypersensitive to tricyclic antidepressants; taking a MAO inhibitor; in acute recovery phase after myocardial infarction; pregnant or lactating; under 12 years of age; has untreated angle-closure glaucoma, a history of urinary retention. Use caution if client has cardiovascular, hepatic, or renal problems or if client is suicidal, psychotic, elderly, or debilitated.

Possible side effects: Drowsiness; dizziness; orthostatic hypotension; tachycardia; myocardial infarction; heart block; CHF; ECG changes; cardiovascular collapse; dry mouth; constipation; urinary retention; agranulocytosis; thrombocytopenia; leukopenia; and several less common problems.

Possible drug interactions: Potentiates CNS depressants, including alcohol, barbiturates, and benzodiazepines; severe systemic reactions with MAO inhibitors; nicotine increases doxepin metabolism; thyroid medications may interact to produce arrhythmias and tachycardia; cimetidine, phenothiazines, and haloperidol increase doxepin serum levels; oral contraceptives decrease effects of doxepin; disulfiram decreases doxepin metabolism, absorption of levodopa, and phenylbutazone is decreased; plasma concentration of dicumarol is increased.

Nursing considerations: Assess for lethality and sudden mood elevation that may precede suicide attempt, vital signs, weight, malaise. Evaluate history of seizures, allergies, glaucoma, alcohol/drug consumption, contraceptive use. Educate client to understand precautions about illness, medications, and precautions that must be taken in regard to driving and operation of machinery. Refer to Client/Family Teaching: Tricyclic Antidepressants, Chapter 33.

Usual dosage: PO (adults)—initial dosage 10–25 mg TID; usual optimal dose 75–150 mg/day; entire dose may be taken at bedtime.

Onset: May take from 2–4 weeks, peaks in less than 2 hours and lasts for weeks in the system.

Generic name: fluoxetine

Brand name: Prozac

Classification: Bicyclic antidepressant

Common uses: Major depressive disorder

Should not be used if: Client is hypersensitive; pregnant or lactating. Use caution if client has a history of seizures, lethality, being underweight, hepatic or renal insufficiency, drug abuse, a recent MI; if client is elderly or debilitated.

Possible side effects: Headache; nervousness; insomnia; drowsiness; anxiety, tremors; dizziness; fatigue; rash; nausea; diarrhea; dry mouth, anorexia; weight loss; anemia; thrombocytopenia; leukopenia; thrombocythemia; excessive sweating.

Possible drug interactions: Prolongs half-life of diazepam; potential for hypertensive crisis with MAO inhibitors; with tryptophan, there may be increased central and peripheral toxicity, agitation, restlessness, GI distress; fluoxetine increases activity of warfarin.

Nursing considerations: Assess for suicidal ideation, sudden elevation in mood, mental status, symptoms of blood dyscrasias. Evaluate vital signs, weight, history for drug/alcohol abuse, glaucoma, childbearing status. Educate client about disease process and value of medication therapy, possible side effects, when to expect results, to be cautious with machinery or motor vehicles.

Usual dosage: PO (adults)—initial dose 20 mg/day given in the morning, may be increased after several weeks if no improvement is noted; doses above 20 mg/day should be administered BID (morning and noon); maximum daily dose of 80 mg/day.

Onset: Takes effect in 3–5 weeks, will peak in 6–8 hours and remains in system for weeks.

Generic name: fluphenazine

Brand name: Prolixin HCl; prolixin decanoate

Classification: Antipsychotic/neuroleptic; phenothiazine; piperazine

Common uses: Acute and chronic psychotic disorders; schizophrenia

Should not be used if: Client is hypersensitive to phenothiazines, sulfites, or tartrazine; comatose or CNS depressed; taking large amounts of CNS depressants; hyper/hypotensive, under 12 years of age; pregnant or lactating; client has bone marrow depression, subcortical brain damage, Parkinson's disease, hepatic, renal or cardiac insufficiency. Use caution with clients who have a history of seizures, respiratory, renal, hepatic, thyroid, or cardiovascular disorders, prostatic hypertrophy, glaucoma, diabetes, hypocalcemia, a history of severe reactions to insulin or ECT; clients who are exposed to extremes of temperatures or organophosphate insecticides or who are elderly or debilitated.

Possible side effects: Sedation; headache; extrapyramidal symptoms; tardive dyskinesia; blurred vision; neuroleptic malignant syndrome, orthostatic hypotension; skin rashes; photosensitivity; dry mouth, nausea; vomiting; increased or decreased appetite; constipation; agranulocytosis; leukopenia; anemia; thrombocytopenia; pancytopenia; laryngeal edema; laryngospasm; bronchospasm; suppression of cough reflex.

Possible drug interactions: Cumulative effects with other CNS depressants; decreases effects of levodopa; additive anticholinergic effects; decreased antipsychotic effects with anticholinergic agents; barbiturates may decrease effects of fluphenazine; may be toxic with epinephrine; clonidine may produce acute brain syndrome; magnesium/aluminum containing antacids reduce absorption/effectiveness; lithium decreases plasma levels and effectiveness, may be neurotoxic; decreased phenytoin metabolism; increased risk of toxicity; cimetidine decreases effectiveness of fluphenazine; possibility of severe hypotension with clonidine; increased seizure potential with piperazine.

Nursing considerations: Assess therapeutic effects of medication; level of sedation; vital signs; childbearing status; ability to carry out activities of daily living. Evaluate lab values for symptoms of blood dyscrasias; evaluate for extrapyramidal symptoms, tardive dyskenisia, symptoms of neuroleptic malignant syndrome, history of allergies and drug/alcohol consumption. Educate about nature of illness and use of medications; caution in operation of vehicles and machinery, and in processes that involve concentration. Refer to Client/Family Teaching: Antipsychotics, Chapter 33.

Usual dosage: Fluphenazine HCl, PO (adults)—initial dose 0.5–10 mg/day in divided doses Q 6–8 hours. Optimal effect usually under 20 mg/day, occasionally 40 mg/day is required. Fluphenazine decanoate (adults), 12.5–25 mg IM every 1–3 weeks. Conversion approximately 12.5 mg of fluphenazine decanoate every 3 weeks for every 10 mg fluphenazine HCl daily.

Onset: PO (HCl)—takes effect in 60 minutes, peaks in 1.5–2 hours, lasts for 6–8 hours; IM (HCl)—takes effect in 60 minutes, peaks in 0.5 hour, lasts 6–8 hours; IM (decanoate)—takes effect in 1–3 days, peaks in 1–2 days, lasts for 1–3 weeks.

Generic name: flurazepam
Brand name: Dalmane
Classification: Sedative-hypnotic; benzodiazepine derivative
Common uses: Short-term use for insomnia, characterized by difficulty falling asleep, frequent nocturnal awakening, and/or early morning awakening.
Should not be used if: Client is hypersensitive to benzodiazepines; pregnant or lactating; under 15 years of age. Use caution with elderly or debilitated patients, those with anemia, hepatic or renal dysfunctions, a history of drug abuse/addiction, or who are depressed/suicidal, are using other CNS depressants, or have low serum albumin.
Possible side effects: Residual sedation, dizziness; confusion; headache; lethargy; weakness; paradoxical excitement; blurred vision; encephalopathy; rashes; nausea and vomiting; diarrhea; constipation; agranulocytosis; tolerance; physical and psychologic dependence.
Possible drug interactions: Other CNS depressants, antipsychotics, antidepressants, antihistamines, anticonvulsants, and cimetidine are all cumulative in effect with flurazepam; neuromuscular blocking agents may increase respiratory depression; disulfiram may increase the duration of action.
Nursing considerations: Assess lab values and baseline vital signs, sleep patterns, suicidal ideation, childbearing status, presence of side effects. Evaluate history of allergies or glaucoma, current and past history of alcohol/drug use, oral contraceptive use, mental status, blood dyscrasias. Educate about illness and need for medication, about other techniques for sleep induction, to avoid driving, operation of hazardous machinery or other functions that require concentration until drug is stabilized, other safety precautions such as raised side rails on the beds. Active metabolites are retained in the body for several days.
Usual dosage: PO (adults)—15–30 mg at bedtime.
Onset: Takes effect in 15–45 minutes; peaks in 30–60 minutes and stays in the system for days.

Generic name: haloperidol
Brand name: Haldol; Haldol Enthante; Peridol/Haloperidol Decanoate
Classification: Antipsychotic/neuroleptic; butyrophenone
Common uses: Management of acute and chronic psychosis; control of Tourette syndrome; symptoms of dementia in the elderly; short-term treatment of hyperactive children; prolonged treatment of chronic schizophrenia.
Should not be used if: Client is hypersensitive to haloperidol or tartrazine, comatose or severely CNS depressed, taking other CNS depressants; pregnant or lactating; under 3 years of age; has bone marrow depression, blood dyscrasias, subcortical brain damage, Parkinson's disease, respiratory, hepatic, renal, thyroid or cardiovascular disorders, severe hypo/hypertension. Use caution with clients with history of seizures, prostatic hypertrophy, glaucoma, diabetes, hypocalcemia, acute illness or dehydration; clients who are elderly or debilitated, exposed to extreme environmental temperatures, or have severe reactons to insulin or ECT.
Possible side effects: Sedation; headache; extrapyramidal symptoms; tardive dyskinesia; blurred vision; neuroleptic malignant syndrome; orthostatic hypotension; photosensitivity; dry mouth; anorexia; constipation; paralytic ileus; impaired liver function; hypersalivation; agranulocytosis; leukopenia; anemia; laryngeal edema; laryngospasm; bronchospasm; suppression of cough reflex; diaphoresis; and many other less common physical symptoms.
Possible drug interactions: CNS depressants have an additive effect; anticholinergic agents have additive anticholinergic and decreased antipsychotic effects; barbiturate anesthetics have increased incidence of excitatory effects and hypotension; barbiturates may decrease antipsychotic effects; metyrosine potentiates extrapyramidal side effects; the efficacy of levodopa is decreased; additive cardiac depressive effects with quinidine; the antihypertensive action of guanethidine is decreased; the hypotensive action of propranolol and metoprolol is increased; lithium may produce neurologic toxicity or encephalopathy; carbamazepine decreases the effects of haloperidol; with epinephrine may decrease blood pressure; phenytoin may decrease the effects of haloperidol; methyldopa leads to increased sedation and abnormal mental symptoms; caffeine may counteract antipsychotic effect.
Nursing considerations: Assess mental status, ability to carry out activities of daily living, presence of spastic facial movements or unusual vocal utterances, symtoms of blood dyscrasias, extrapyramidal symptoms, symptoms of neuroleptic malignant syndrome, baseline vital signs and weight. Evaluate history for allergies, childbearing status, oral contraceptive use, drug/alcohol use, signs and symptoms of cholestatic jaundice. Educate about nature of illness and effective use of medication, to avoid hot tubs and showers and to get up slowly to avoid orthostatic hypotension, to use a sunscreen during exposure. Educate about nature of side effects and to report problems, to avoid driving or operation of machinery that requires concentration until more stable, that constipation may occur and should be reported, to avoid OTC preparations until physician is consulted. Refer to Client/Family Teaching: Antipsychotics, Chapter 33.
Usual dosage: PO (adults)—tablets or concentrate 3–5 mg BID or TID; daily dosages of up to 100 mg may be necessary for severely resistant patients. IM (adults)—2–5 mg Q 4–8 hours, may be administered as often as Q 60 minutes if client is severely agitated. Maintenance with IM decanoate is initially 10–15 times the daily oral dosage, to a maximum of 100 mg per dose every 4 weeks.
Onset: PO—erratic in length of time to effective therapy, peaks in 2–6 hours, full therapeutic effects may not be observed for 4–8 weeks; IM—takes effect in 30–60 minutes, peaks in 10–20 minutes, and stays in the system for 4–8 hours. IM decanoate—peaks in 6–7 days and will remain effective for 3–4 weeks.

Generic name: hydroxyzine
Brand name: Vistaril; Atarax; Atozine; Durrax; Vamate
Classification: Antihistamine; antianxiety; piperazine derivative
Common uses: Anxiety; relief from allergies; pruritus; nausea and vomiting; motion sickness
Should not be used if: Caution should be exercised in clients with pregnancy or lactation; asthma; heart disease; glaucoma; ulcers; difficulty urinating; high BP; seizures; hyperthyroidism.
Possible side effects: Sedation; decreases mental alertness and physical coordination; dry mouth; headache; increased anxiety; ischemia.
Possible drug interactions: Enhances alcohol and other CNS depressants; epinephrine should not be used to administer vasopressor effects; MAO inhibitors prolong and intensify anticholinergic effects.
Nursing considerations: Caution client to be careful when doing tasks requiring alertness; falsely elevated urine hydroxycorticosteroids. Evaluate for vital signs, assure proper hydration, I&O.
Usual dosage: 75–100 mg/day to 200–400 mg/day.
Onset: 15–30 minutes, effects for 4–6 hours.

Generic name: lithium carbonate
Brand name: Lithane; Eskalith; Lithonate; Lithotabs; Lithobid; Lithium Citrate; Lithonate-S

Classification: Antimanic; alkali metal ion salt
Common uses: Manic phase of bipolar disorder; maintenance therapy to prevent or diminish intensity of subsequent manic episodes; depression associated with bipolar disorder.
Should not be used if: Client has severe renal or cardiovascular disease, dehydration, sodium depletion, brain damage, or is pregnant or lactating. Use caution with elderly clients, those having thyroid disorders, diabetes mellitus, urinary retention, a history of seizure disorder.
Possible side effects: Fine hand tremors; fatigue; dizziness; confusion; restlessness; headache; lethargy; drowsiness; ECG changes; acne; rash; hypothyroidism; excessive weight gain; anorexia; nausea and vomiting; diarrhea; dry mouth; thirst; polyuria; glycosuria; diabetes insipidus; reversible leukocytosis (WBC 10,000–15,000).
Possible drug interactions: Aminophylline; mannitol; acetazolamide; sodium bicarbonate; drugs high in sodium content may increase renal elimination and decrease effectiveness of lithium; haloperidol may cause encephalopathic syndrome and result in brain damage; neuromuscular blocking agents prolong effects of skeletal muscle relaxation; paroxicam, indomethacin, and nonsteroidal anti-inflammatory drugs produce significant increases in plasma lithium levels thereby increasing potential for toxicity; thiazide diuretics decrease renal clearance of lithium, thus increasing risk of toxicity; phenothiazines produce decreased antipsychotic effect and/or increased lithium excretion; phenytoin and carbamazepine may have adverse neurological effects; iodides have additive hypothyroid effects; increased dietary sodium increases renal elimination of lithium while decreased dietary sodium decreases renal excretion of lithium, thus increasing risk of toxicity.
Nursing considerations: Assess mood and behavior, baseline vital signs and weight, lab values, lethality. Evaluate renal and thyroid function tests and baseline ECG in collaboration with physician, any physical symptoms that the client displays; wrists and ankles for edema; hydration; neurologic state. Educate client and family about the disease and the effective use of medication, including side effects and when to notify physician; about taking medication with meals to avoid GI upset; to use contraception; not to operate machinery until lithium levels are stable; to avoid increasing normal fluid intake. Refer to Client/Family Teaching: Lithium Carbonate, Chapter 33.
Usual dosage: Acute mania—PO (adults): 600 mg TID or QID. Maintenance therapy—PO (adults): 300–1200 mg/day in divided doses.
Onset: Normalization of symptoms is usually apparent after 1–3 weeks. Takes effect rapidly after stabilization, peaks in 0.5–3 hours, duration is variable.

Generic name: lorazepam
Brand name: Ativan
Classification: Antianxiety agent; benzodiazepine
Common uses: Anxiety; irritability in psychiatric or organic disorders; insomnia
Should not be used if: Client is hypersensitive to benzodiazepines; using other CNS depressants; pregnant or lactating; under 12 years of age; in shock or coma; elderly or debilitated. Use with caution if client has narrow-angle glaucoma, hepatic or renal dysfunction, a history of drug use, or lethality.
Possible side effects: Drowsiness; fatigue; ataxia; dizziness; constipation; dry mouth; ECG changes; tachycardia; orthostatic hypotension; blurred vision; and many other less common physical effects.
Possible drug interactions: Other CNS depressants produce additive CNS depression; effects of lorazepam are decreased by nicotine and caffeine; neuromuscular blocking agents increase respiratory depression; digoxin excretion is reduced, thus increasing potential for toxicity.
Nursing considerations: Assess vital signs, lying and standing; lab values; level of anxiety; lethality; presence of side effects; childbearing status; contraceptive use. Evaluate for history of allergies, drug/alcohol abuse, glaucoma. Educate client to understand the problems of the disease and use of medication, not to take drug for everyday stressors, to take drug with food, to use caution in operation of automobiles and other machinery, to avoid use of alcohol and OTC medications until physician is consulted, not to discontinue medication abruptly. Refer to Client/Family Teaching: Benzodiazepines, Chapter 33.
Usual dosage: PO (adults)—2–3 mg BID or TID. IM form available.
Onset: Takes effect in 15–45 minutes, peaks in 2 hours, duration is variable.

Generic name: molindone HCl
Brand name: Moban
Classification: Tranquilizer; antipsychotic; dihydroindolone
Common uses: Management of psychosis
Should not be used if: Severe CNS depression; known sensitivity to drug; pregnant or lactating; under 12 years of age.
Possible side effects: Blurred vision; glaucoma; constipation; akathisia; akinesia; dry mouth; decreased sweating; headache; drowsiness; orthostatic hypotension; tachycardia; difficulty talking; mask-like face; restlessness; stiff extremities; trembling; tardive dyskinesia; muscle spasms; neuroleptic malignant syndrome; agranulocytosis.
Possible drug interactions: Antacids and diarrhea medication decrease absorption; potentiates alcohol and other CNS depressants; may decrease absorption of phenytoin or tetracyclines.
Nursing considerations: Assess for neuroleptic malignant syndrome; allergic reaction to sulfite. Caution client to be careful when doing tasks requiring alertness. Educate about use of care to avoid becoming overheated. Assure good hydration, I&O. Refer to Client/Family Teaching: Antipsychotics, Chapter 33.
Usual dosage: Initially 50 mg/day to 225 mg/day; maintenance doses 15–150 mg day.
Onset: Peak within 1 hour, duration of action 36 hours.

Generic name: oxazepam
Brand name: Serax
Classification: Sedative-hypnotic; benzodiazepine
Common uses: Anxiety; agitation during alcohol withdrawal
Should not be used if: Caution in prescribing for clients who are pregnant or lactating, have kidney or liver disease, allergy to aspirin or tartrazine (yellow dye).
Possible side effects: Drowsiness; muscle incoordination; fatigue; dizziness; confusion; restlessness; excitement; muscle spasms; nightmares; dose dependent CNS adverse effects.
Possible drug interactions: Nicotine decreases effectiveness; alcohol potentiates sedation and dizziness; levodopa-treated patients may experience decreased control of parkinsonian symptoms. Closely observe patients on anticonvulsants.
Nursing considerations: Caution client to be careful when doing tasks requiring alertness; this medication may become habit forming; if a dose is missed do not double dose; some evidence that ataxia and risk of falls is increased in geriatrics; gradual tapering off medication; the need for continued use should be reassessed regularly. Refer to Client/Family Teaching: Benzodiazepines, Chapter 33.
Usual dosage: 30–60 mg/day, for severe anxiety or agitation associated with ETOH withdrawal 45–120 mg/day in divided doses.
Onset: 15–45 minutes, duration 7–8 hours.

Generic name: paroxetine
Brand name: Paxil
Classification: Antidepressant, selective serotonin reuptake inhibitor
Common uses: Depressive mood disorders (e.g., major depression)
Should not be used if: Patient taking monoamine oxidase inhibitors (at least 14 days should elapse between end of one

medication and the start of the other). Patient has a history of hypomania or mania.
Possible side effects: Dry mouth, nausea, headache, somnolence, weakness, dizziness, insomnia, sexual dysfunction, sweating, diarrhea, constipation, tremor, decreased appetite, nervousness.
Possible drug interactions: Caution with oral anticoagulants; do not mix with MAO inhibitors.
Nursing considerations: Unaffected by food or antacids; does not potentiate the effects of alcohol, barbiturates, antipsychotics, or benzodiazepines. Used as maintenance treatment for preventing relapse in depressions.
Usual dosage: Usual initial dose 20 mg/day with upper limit dose of 50 mg daily; renal impairment patients: initial dose 10 mg/day and doses increased as clinically warranted.
Onset: 4–14 days.

Generic name: perphenazine
Brand name: Trilafon
Classification: Antipsychotic; phenothiazine
Common uses: Symptomatic management of psychotic disorders; severe nausea and vomiting in adults.
Should not be used if: Sulfite sensitivity, under 12 years of age.
Possible side effects: Dizziness; orthostatic hypotension; dry mouth; muscle spasms; slow or difficult speech; tremors; shuffling gait; drooling; restlessness; weakness; blurred vision; constipation; difficulty urinating; tardive dyskinesia; photosensitivity; decreased body temperature regulation; drowsiness; tachycardia; agranulocytosis, pruritus; depositions of pigment in body tissues and fine particulate matter in lens and cornea; GI distress.
Possible drug interactions: Potentiating effects of alcohol and other CNS depressants; lowered seizure threshold therefore dosage adjustment on anticonvulsants; lithium used concurrently may cause unusual adverse neurologic effects; do not use with metrizamide.
Nursing considerations: Caution client to be careful when doing tasks requiring alertness; avoid overheating. Assess for extrapryamidal reactions; track elimination patterns; observe for unusual hematologic occurrences. Due to enhanced response, CNS depressants (alcohol, etc.) cannot be used; with hypocalcemia increased dystonia occurs; assure proper hydration; may be necessary to continue antiparkinsonian medication after discontinuance of drug; protect medication from light. Educate about tardive dyskinesia. Refer to Client/Family Teaching: Antipsychotics, Chapter 33.
Usual dosage: 12–24 mg/day to 16–64 mg/day.
Onset: For prompt control of severe symptoms, IM administration recommended; specific onset information not available.

Generic name: phenelzine sulfate
Brand name: Nardil
Classification: Antidepressant; monoamine oxidase inhibitor
Common uses: Atypical, nonendogenous, or neurotic depression; depression accompanied by anxiety; clients unresponsive to other antidepressants (usually not drug of choice).
Should not be used if: Client is hypersensitive to MAO inhibitors; a paranoid schizophrenic; pregnant or lactating; over 60/under 16 years of age; has pheochromocytoma, CHF, diseases of cardiovascular, renal, or hepatic systems, hypertension, a history of severe headaches. Use caution with clients with history of seizures, lethality, schizophrenia, diabetes mellitus, angina pectoris, hyperthyroidism or who are agitated/hypomanic, suicidal, sensitive to tartrazine (FD&C yellow No. 5).
Possible side effects: Hypertensive crisis; dizziness; headache; drowsiness; blurred vision; orthostatic hypotension; hypertension; cardiac dysrhythmias; dry mouth; constipation; weight gain; photosensitivity; flushing; increased perspiration; urinary frequency; anorexia.
Possible drug interactions: Specific food (containing tyramine, tryptophan); drink and other medications may cause severe reactions; alcohol is to be avoided; OTC or prescription cold, hay fever or weight-reducing medication, other MAO inhibitor or tricyclic antidepressant; fluoxetine may result in severe adverse effects; amphetamines; may be additive with CNS depressants; elevated BP with buspirone; exaggerated effects of general anesthetics; caution with disulfiram.
Nursing considerations: Diet must be regulated to prevent dangerous reactions (e.g., sudden hypertension); know and teach symtoms of hypertensive crisis (severe headache, palpitation, neck stiffness, nausea, sweating, visual disturbances); closely monitor blood pressure; assess lethality; assure proper hydration; medication may take several weeks to begin effect; caution advised in tasks requiring alertness; evaluate for lethality; protect medication from excessive exposure to heat and light; medication must be discontinued 7–14 days prior to elective surgery. Refer to Client/Family Teaching: MAO Inhibitors, Chapter 33.
Usual dosage: 45 mg/day–90 mg/day, maintenance therapy as low as 15 mg/day.
Onset: Maximum benefit 2–6 weeks.

Generic name: phenobarbital
Brand name: Bar; Barbita; Eskabarb; Floramine; Luminal; Orpine; Solubarb; Stental; Luminal sodium
Classification: Sedative-hypnotic; anticonvulsant; barbiturate; CNS depressant
Common uses: Moderate anxiety states; insomnia; seizures (long term); status epilepticus; pre- or postoperative sedation.
Should not be used if: Client is hypersensitive to barbiturates; has hepatic, renal, cardiac, or respiratory disease; a history of previous drug addiction or of porphyria; use caution with clients who are anemic, elderly, or debilitated, depressed/suicidal, pregnant, lactating, or have ammonia intoxication.
Possible side effects: Drowsiness; dizziness; lethargy; residual sedation; agranulocytosis; thrombocytopenia; respiratory depression; laryngospasm; bronchospasm; tolerance; nausea and vomiting; and other less common physical and psychologic problems.
Possible drug interactions: Additive with other CNS depressants, chloramphenicol, MAO inhibitors, valproic acid, cimetidine, disulfuram all increase effects of phenobarbital; with phenytoin the effects of either drug may be increased or decreased; the effectiveness of oral contraceptives, oral anticoagulants, corticosteroids, digitoxin, and doxycycline are decreased; with furosemide there is a risk of orthostatic hypotension; phenobarbital decreases levels of griseofulvin.
Nursing considerations: Assess sleep patterns, seizure activity, suicidal ideations, baseline vital signs, laboratory tests; evaluate effectiveness of therapy, history of alcohol and drug use, childbearing status/contraceptive use, presence of adverse reactions, client and family's response to diagnosis. Educate family and client concerning diagnosis, need for medication, possible effects of medication, dangers of operating vehicles or machinery while medication is effective.
Usual dosage: PO (adults)—15–30 mg BID or TID. PO (children)—2 mg/kg TID.
Onset: PO—takes effect in 20–60 minutes; peaks in 8–12 hours and lasts from 6–10 hours.

Generic name: phenytoin, phenytoin sodium
Brand name: Dilantin; Di-Phen; Diphenylan
Classification: Anticonvulsant; hydantoin; antiarrhythmic
Common uses: Tonic-clonic (grand mal) and partial seizures with complex symptomatology; grand mal seizures associated with status epilepticus or occurring during or following neurosurgery; autonomic seizures; cardiac arrhythmias.
Should not be used if: Client is hypersensitive to phenytoin; lactating; has sinus bradycardia; heart block; absence (petit mal) seizures and seizures related to hypoglycemia. Use with caution for clients with hepatic or renal dysfunction, diabetes mellitus, hypotension, myocardial insufficiency, or who are elderly, pregnant or debilitated.
Possible side effects: Nystagmus; ataxia; drowsiness; decreased alertness; hypotension; arrhythmias; circulatory collapse; car-

diac arrest; skin rashes; hypertrichosis; exfoliative dermatitis; nausea and vomiting; blood dyscrasias; gingival hyperplasia.

Possible drug interactions: Trimethoprim, amiodarone, benzodiazepines, disulfiram, isoniazid, phenylbutazone, chloramphenicol, cimetidine, sulfonamides, salicylates, acute alcohol intake, phenothiazines all increase the effects of phenytoin, thus increasing the risk of toxicity; barbiturates, diazoxide, rifampin, antineoplastic agents, chronic alcohol abuse, antacids, calcium gluconate, carbamazepine decrease the effects of phenytoin; effects may increase or decrease with phenobarbital, valproic acid, sodium valproate; phenytoin decreases effects of corticosteroids, oral contraceptives, digoxin, furosemide, doxycycline, dopamine, and levodopa; phenytoin increases effects of primidone.

Nursing considerations: Assess baseline vital signs, seizure activity, laboratory values, for presence of skin rashes, adverse reactions and side effects. Evalute history of past and present disease states, drug/alcohol use, allergies, contraceptive use and childbearing status. Educate family and client about the disease process, need for and properties of medication, dangers of operating motor vehicles and machinery while drug is active in the system.

Usual dosage: PO (adults)—100 mg TID or QID (MDD 600 mg).

Onset: PO—Takes effect in 0.5–2 hours; peaks in 1.5–3 hours and lasts from 6–12 hours.

Generic name: propranolol HCl

Brand name: Inderal

Classification: Antihypertensive; antianginal; anti-arrhythmic; beta-adrenergic blocker

Common uses: Hypertension; angina pectoris; cardiac arrhythmias; migraine headaches; essential tremor; acute exacerbation of schizophrenic disorder and anxiety states; action tremors (drug-induced), tardive dyskinesia; acute panic symptoms; intermittent explosive disorder.

Should not be used if: Client is hypersensitive to beta-adrenergic blocking agents; pregnant or lactating; has heart block greater than first degree, cardiogenic shock, CHF, overt cardiac failure, bronchial asthma, bronchospasm, severe COPD, allergic rhinitis during the pollen season, Raynaud's syndrome, malignant hypertension, sinus bradycardia. Use with caution if client has diabetes mellitus, myasthenia gravis, Wolff-Parkinson-White syndrome, thyrotoxicosis, impaired hepatic or renal function, inadequate cardiac function, sinus node dysfunction, or is undergoing surgery.

Possible side effects: Dizziness; fatigue; insomnia; weakness; bradycardia; peripheral arterial insufficiency; hypotension; first and third degree heart block; intensification of AV block; nausea; diarrhea; agranulocytosis; depression; bronchial obstruction; bronchospasm; laryngospasm; and many other less common problems.

Possible drug interactions: Catecholamine depleting drugs produce additive reduction in sympathetic tone, resulting in hypotension, bradycardia, vertigo, syncope; digitalis glycosides produce additive depression of AV conduction, potentiation of bradycardia; the effects of sympathomimetics are decreased; antimuscarinics and tricyclic antidepressants antagonize propranolol's cardiac effects; smoking increases clearance of propranolol; diuretics and other antihypertensives increase hypotensive effects; prolongs hypoglycemic effects of insulin; severe rebound hypertension when propranolol is discontinued abruptly; increased effects of chlorpromazine, cimetidine, oral contraceptives, furosemide, hydralazine, succinylcholine and tubocurarine; phenytoin, rifampin, phenobarbital, and other barbiturates decrease levels of propranolol; thyroid hormones decrease its effects; isoproterenol, norepinephrine, dopamine, dobutamine reverse its effects; aluminum hydroxide gel reduces its absorption; ethanol slows its absorption; phenothiazines are additive pharmacologically.

Nursing considerations: Assess baseline vital signs, including weight, orthostatic blood pressure, extremities for coldness and paresthesia. Evaluate blood pressure and pulse before administration of drug, history of allergies, drug/alcohol use, use of oral contraceptives/childbearing status, presence of adverse reactions (including symptoms of CHF). Educate client and family about illness, need for medication, and side effects, caution in operation of motor vehicles and other machinery.

Usual dosage: PO (adults)—wide range of dosages from 10–30 mg/day TID/QID for cardiac arrhythmias to 80–120 mg/day TID for exacerbation of schizophrenia or anxiety states.

Onset: Takes effect in 30 minutes, peaks in 60–90 minutes and lasts for 4–6 hours.

Generic name: risperidone

Brand name: Risperdal

Classification: Antipsychotic

Common uses: Symptomatic management of psychotic disorders, treatment of positive, negative, and affective symptoms of schizophrenia.

Should not be used if: Known sensitivity to risperidone, suffering intolerable side effects.

Possible side effects: Sedation, nausea, vomiting, agitation, dizziness, increased salivation, weight gain, induces few extrapyramidal reactions, orthostatic hypotension, neuroleptic malignant syndrome is possible with all antipsychotic drugs, can lengthen the QT interval leading to arrhythmia, muscle spasms, priapism, seizures.

Possible drug interactions: Caution suggested with other centrally acting agents or alcohol, may enhance effects of certain antihypertensive agents, may antagonize effects of levodopa, clearance of risperidone may increase with carbamazepine or decrease with clozapine.

Nursing considerations: Slower titration leads to fewer side effects, can overlap with other antipsychotics at least 3 weeks (while tapering down on other antipsychotic can be introducing risperidone), tardive dyskinesia has decreased or resolved with drug use without increasing parkinsonism, does activate/motivate patients, if nausea or vomiting occurs take medication with food, patients who were nonresponders to other antipsychotics may have difficult coping without psychotic symptoms, help patients cope if they are nonresponding to risperidone, orthostatic hypotension.

Usual dosage: Initial dosing titrated over 3 days—first day 1 mg BID, second day 2 mg BID, third day 3 mg BID. Therapeutic window is 4–8 mg/day. A minimum of 1–2 weeks necessary for dose evaluation. Maximum dose 16 mg/day. Comes as 1, 2, 3, or 4 mg tablets. The 1 mg tablet is scored. Geriatric, renal and hepatic impaired dosing: start with .5 mg BID, increase dose .5 mg BID once weekly and evaluate, maximum dose 1.5 mg BID.

Onset: Often within first treatment week, usually by the second treatment week, maximum treatment effect seen by 10th week.

Generic name: sertraline

Brand name: Zoloft

Classification: Antidepressant, selective serotonin reuptake inhibitor

Common uses: Depression including depressed mood, difficulty concentrating, decreased activity

Should not be used if: Patient taking momoamine oxidase inhibitors (at least 14 days should elapse between end of one medication and the start of the other). Binds tightly to plasma proteins and may interact with other medications that are also highly protein-bound and produce adverse effects. Caution with other CNS-active medications.

Possible side effects: nausea, sedation, dizzinesss, insomnia, sweating, tremor, decreased appetite, nervousness, ejaculatory disturbance, aggravated depression, hypervigilance, suicidal thoughts.

Possible drug interactions: MAO inhibitors (see above).

Nursing considerations: Far safer in overdose situations than tricyclic antidepressants, supplied as 20 mg tablet scored and 30 mg tablet. Drug should be administered with food, does not potentiate alcohol or other recreational drugs.

Usual dosage: Starting single daily dose 50–200 mg/day, usual initial dose 50 mg/day.
Onset: Early improvement seen within 3 weeks, maximum difference occurs in 6 weeks.

Generic name: temazepam
Brand name: Restoril
Classification: Sedative-hypnotic; benzodiazepine
Common uses: Relief of anxiety; short-term treatment of insomnia; acute alcohol withdrawal; adjunct with anticonvulsants for seizure control.
Should not be used if: Client is pregnant or lactating. Use caution with geriatric, liver disease patients.
Possible side effects: Drowsiness; ataxia; weakness; confusion; agitation; GI complaints; urinary retention; dry mouth; increased appetite; increased salivation; constipation; menstrual irregularities.
Possible drug interactions: Alcohol, psychotropic drugs, anticonvulsants, antihistaminics and other CNS depressants are enhanced; levodopa-treated patients may experience decreased control of parkinsonian symptoms; closely observe patients on anticonvulsants.
Nursing considerations: Relatively slow GI absorption, therefore may be more effective 1–2 hours before bed. Caution client to be careful when doing tasks requiring alertness, this medication may become habit forming, if a dose is missed do not double dose, some evidence that ataxia and risk of falls is increased in geriatrics. Assess for contraceptive use, gradual tapering off medication, sleep pattern; the need for continued use should be reassessed regularly. Refer to Client/Family Teaching: Benzodiazepines, Chapter 33.
Usual dosage: 15–30 mg/day
Onset: 15–45 minutes, duration of action 7–8 hours.

Generic name: thioridazine HCl
Brand name: Mellaril; Millazine; SK Thioridazine
Classification: Antipsychotic/neuroleptic; phenothiazine; piperidine
Common uses: Psychotic disorders; moderate to marked depression with variable degrees of anxiety (short term); multiple symptoms such as agitation, anxiety, depression, sleep disturbances, tension, and fears in geriatric patients; hyperkinesis, combativeness, and severe behavioral problems in children.
Should not be used if: Client is hypersensitive to phenothiazines, sulfites, or tartrazine; comatose or severely CNS depressed; pregnant or lactating; under 2 years of age; has bone marrow depression, blood dyscrasias, subcortical brain damage, Parkinson's disease, liver, renal, and/or cardiac insufficiency, severe hypotension or hypertension. Use caution with clients who have a history of seizures, respiratory, renal, hepatic, thyroid and cardiac disorders, prostatic hypertrophy, glaucoma, diabetes, or if exposed to extreme environmental temperatures, have a history of severe reactions to insulin or ECT, or who are elderly or debilitated.
Possible side effects: Sedation; headache; extrapyramidal symptoms; blurred vision; neuroleptic malignant syndrome; orthostatic hypotension; cardiac arrest; ECG changes; arrhythmias, pulmonary edema; circulatory collapse; skin rashes; photosensitivity; exfoliative dermatitis; dry mouth; nausea and vomiting; constipation; paralytic ileus; agranulocytosis; leukopenia; anemia; thrombocytopenia; pancytopenia; laryngeal edema; laryngospasm; bronchospasm; suppression of cough reflex; and other less common symptoms.
Possible drug interactions: Cumulative effects with other CNS depressants; decreases effects of levodopa; additive anticholinergic effects, decreased antipsychotic effects with anticholinergic agents; barbiturates may decrease effects of thioridazine; may be toxic with epinephrine; clonidine may produce acute brain syndrome; magnesium/aluminum containing antacids reduce absorption/effectiveness; lithium decreases plasma levels and effectiveness, may be neurotoxic; decreased phenytoin metabolism, increased risk of toxicity, cimetidine decreases effectiveness of thioridazine; possibility of severe hypotension with clonidine; increased seizure potential with piperazine.
Nursing considerations: Assess therapeutic effects of medication; level of sedation; vital signs; childbearing status; ability to carry out activities of daily living. Evaluate lab values for symptoms of blood dyscrasias, extrapyramidal symptoms, tardive dyskinesia, symptoms of neuroleptic malignant syndrome, history of allergies and drug/alcohol consumption. Educate about nature of illness and use of medications; caution in operation of vehicles and machinery, and in processes that involve concentration. Refer to Client/Family Teaching: Antipsychotics, Chapter 33.
Usual dosage: PO (adults)—50–100 mg TID initially; may be gradually increased to maximum daily dose of 800 mg, then reduced gradually to maintenance dose.
Onset: Takes effect in 30–60 minutes; peaks in 2–4 hours; lasts for 4–6 hours.

Generic name: thiothixene
Brand name: Navane
Classification: Antipsychotic/neuroleptic; thioxanthene
Common uses: Psychotic disorders; schizophrenia; acute agitation
Should not be used if: Client is hypersensitive to thioxanthenes or phenothiazines, comatose or severely CNS-depressed, taking large amounts of CNS depressants, hyper/hypotensive; under 12 years of age; pregnant or lactating; has bone marrow depression, subcortical brain damage, Parkinson's disease, hepatic, renal or cardiac insufficiency. Use caution with clients who have a history of seizures, respiratory, renal, hepatic, thyroid, or cardiovascular disorders, prostatic hypertrophy, glaucoma, diabetes, hypocalcemia, a history of severe reactions to insulin or ECT; clients who are exposed to extremes of temperatures or organophosphate insecticides or who are elderly or debilitated.
Possible side effects: Sedation; headache; extrapyramidal symptoms; tardive dyskinesia; blurred vision; neuroleptic malignant syndrome; glaucoma; orthostatic hypotension; skin rashes; photosensitivity; contact dermatitis; dry mouth; nausea and vomiting; anorexia; constipation; agranulocytosis; leukopenia; anemia; thrombocytopenia; pancytopenia; laryngeal edema; laryngospasm; bronchospasm; suppression of cough reflex; and other less common symptoms.
Possible drug interactions: Cumulative effects with other CNS depressants; decreases effects of levodopa; additive anticholinergic effects, decreased antipsychotic effects with anticholinergic agents; barbiturates may decrease effects of thiothixene; may be toxic with epinephrine; clonidine may produce severe hypotension; magnesium/aluminum containing antacids reduce absorption/effectiveness; lithium decreases plasma levels and effectiveness, may be neurotoxic; decreased phenytoin metabolism, increased risk of toxicity; cimetidine decreases effectiveness of thiothixene; increased seizure potential with piperazine; caffeine counteracts antipsychotic effects.
Nursing considerations: Assess mental status, therapeutic effects of medication, level of sedation, vital signs and weight, childbearing status, ability to carry out activities of daily living. Evaluate lab values for symptoms of blood dyscrasias and cholestatic jaundice; extrapyramidal symptoms; tardive dyskinesia; symptoms of neuroleptic malignant syndrome; history of allergies and drug/alcohol consumption. Educate about nature of illness and use of medications, caution in operation of vehicles and machinery, and in processes that involve concentration. Refer to Client/Family Teaching: Antipsychotics, Chapter 33.
Usual dosage: PO (adults)—initial dose 2–5 mg/day; increased to maximum daily dose of 60 mg; usual optimal dose 20–30 mg/day.
Onset: Takes effect slowly, peaks in 2–8 hours, lasts for 12–24 hours.

Generic name: trazodone HCl
Brand name: Desyrel
Classification: Antidepressant
Common uses: Depression; anxiety; sleep disturbances; alcohol dependence
Should not be used if: Initial phase of MI recovery; pregnant or lactating; under 18 years of age.
Possible side effects: Drowsiness; dry mouth; dizziness; orthostatic hypotension; muscle aches; sinus bradycardia; akathisia; anemia; early menses; delayed urine flow; hypersalivation; impotence; impaired speech; increased appetite; increased libido; nausea and vomiting; rash; priapism.
Possible drug interactions: Alcohol, barbiturates and other CNS depressants may be enhanced; antihypertensive medication may require dose reduction; digoxin and phenytoin levels may increase.
Nursing considerations: Caution client to be careful when doing tasks requiring alertness; medication has been associated with incidence of priapism; should be taken shortly after food. Assess lethality, depression, side effects, alcohol/drug abuse. Evaluate history of allergies.
Usual dosage: Initially 150 mg/day, increased to 400 mg/day (to 600 mg/day for inpatients)
Onset: Therapeutic levels reached in 7–14 days, peak after 1 hour (if taken on empty stomach); 2 hours (if taken with food).

Generic name: triazolam
Brand name: Halcion
Classification: Hypnotic; benzodiazepine
Common uses: Relief of anxiety; short-term management of initial insomnia; muscle spasm; epilepsy.
Should not be used if: Client is pregnant or lactating; depressed. Use caution with clients with impaired renal or hepatic function or chronic pulmonary insufficiency; under 18 years of age.
Possible side effects: Sedation; dizzinesss; lightheadedness; headache; nervousness; ataxia; nausea and vomiting; confusion.
Possible drug interactions: Alcohol, psychotropic drugs, anticonvulsants, antihistaminics and other CNS depressants are enhanced; may interact with disulfiram; cimetidine reduces plasma clearance; levodopa-treated patients may experience decreased control of parkinsonian symptoms; closely observe patients on anticonvulsants.
Nursing considerations: This medication may become habit forming; if a dose is missed do not double dose. Caution client to be careful when doing tasks requiring alertness. Evaluate for signs of OD (slurred speech, confusion, shakiness, SOB or trouble breathing, severe drowsiness, severe weakness, staggering), which may occur at 4 times maximum therapeutic dose; sedative effect may decrease over time; contraceptive use. Assess lethality, rebound insomnia after discontinuance; abrupt discontinuance should be avoided. Refer to Client/Family Teaching: Benzodiazepines, Chapter 32.
Usual dosage: 0.125–0.25 mg for elderly, debilitated; 0.25–0.5 mg HS
Onset: Peak in 1.3 hours, duration in body under 5.5 hours.

Generic name: trifluoperazine
Brand name: Stelazine; Suprazine
Classification: Antipsychotic; phenothiazine
Common uses: Management of psychotic disorders; short-term treatment of nonpsychotic anxiety.
Should not be used if: Sulfite sensitivity; metrizamide being administered. Use caution with clients with severe cardiovascular disorders, seizure history, lactating mothers, children with acute illnesses or dehydration, geriatric, debilitated, renal or hepatic disease, glaucoma, prostatic hypertrophy, hypocalcemia; safety during pregnancy has not been established.
Possible side effects: Akathisia; blurred vision; decreased alertness; dizziness; dry mouth; muscle spasms; slow or difficult speech; tremors; shuffling gait; drooling; restlessness; weakness; blurred vision; constipation; difficulty urinating; tardive dyskinesia; photosensitivity; decreased body temperature regulation; orthostatic hypotension; tachycardia; agranulocytosis; pruritus; pigment depositions in various body tissues; deposits of fine particulate matter in lens and cornea; breast engorgement with lactation.
Possible drug interactions: Additive or potentiating with other CNS depressants; lowered seizure threshold therefore dosage adjustment on anticonvulsants; lithium used concurrently may cause unusual adverse neurologic effects; do not use with metrizamide.
Nursing considerations: Geriatric clients may be more susceptible to hypotension and neuromuscular reactions; monitor for phenytoin toxicity (this medication lowers the seizure threshold). Caution client to be careful when doing tasks requiring alertness. Assess elimination patterns, avoid overheating; protect liquid medication from light. Assess for extrapyramidal reactions. Educate about tardive dyskinesia and photosensitivity. Refer to Client/Family Teaching: Antipsychotics, Chapter 33.
Usual dosage: Psychotic disorders—Adults 2–4 mg/day up to 40 mg/day, children 6–12 years 1–2 mg/day. Nonpsychotic anxiety: Adult—2–4 mg/day not to exceed 6 mg/day, 12 weeks.
Onset: Optimum therapeutic response usually within 2–3 weeks.

Generic name: trihexyphenidyl HCl
Brand name: Aphen; Artane; Hexaphen; Trihexane; Trihexidyl
Classification: Antiparkinsonian agent; anticholinergic; synthetic tertiary amine
Common uses: All forms of parkinsonism (adjunctive therapy); extrapyramidal symptoms (except tardive dyskinesia) associated with antipsychotic drugs.
Should not be used if: Client is hypersensitive to anticholinergics; under 3 years of age; has angle-closure glaucoma, pyloric or duodenal obstruction, stenosing peptic ulcers, prostatic hypertrophy or bladder neck obstructions, achalasia, myasthenia gravis, ulcerative colitis, toxic megacolon, tachycardia secondary to cardiac insufficiency or thyrotoxicosis. Use with caution if client is elderly or debilitated, pregnant or lactating, exposed to extreme environmental temperatures, has narrow-angle glaucoma, hepatic, renal, or cardiac insufficiency, hyperthyroidism, hyptertension, autonomic neuropathy, or a tendency toward urinary retention.
Possible side effects: Drowsiness; dizziness; blurred vision; nervousness; dry mouth; nausea; constipation; paralytic ileus; and numerous other less common problems.
Possible drug interactions: Other drugs with anticholinergic properties increase anticholinergic effects, which may produce anticholinergic toxicity manifested by confusion, overt psychosis, visual hallucinations, hot dry skin, dilated pupils; decreases absorption of levodopa and digoxin; increased CNS depressant effects; decreases therapeutic effect of chlorpromazine, phenothiazines, and haloperidol; MAO inhibitors increase effects of trihexyphenidyl; antacids decrease its absorption; decreased antipsychotic effect with phenothiazines and haloperidol.
Nursing considerations: Assess baseline vital signs and weight, oral contraceptive use and childbearing status, symptoms of Parkinson's disease, such as tremors, muscular weakness and rigidity, drooling, shuffling, flat affect and disturbance in balance or posture; extrapyramidal symptoms are similar with the addition of akinesia (muscular weakness), akathisia (restlessness), dystonia (involuntary muscular movements), oculogyric crisis (rolling back of the eyes), and tardive dyskinesia (bizarre facial and tongue movements with stiff neck and difficulty in swallowing). Evaluate for constipation, GI disturbance, or paralytic ileus which may be life-threatening. Educate patient to avoid OTC medications until physician agrees, to avoid driving or other activities that require intense concentration and not to stop medication abruptly.
Usual dosage: For drug-induced side effects, usual daily dose range 5–15 mg.
Onset: Takes effect in 1 hour, peaks in 1.5 hours, lasts for 6–12 hours.

Generic name: valproic acid
Brand name: Depakote
Classification: Anticonvulsant
Common uses: Management of simple and complex absence seizures (petit mal); adjunct to other anticonvulsants
Should not be used if: Safe use during pregnancy has not been established; caution in lactating women.
Possible side effects: Nausea and vomiting; sedation; drowsiness; ataxia; headache; hepatic effects including hepatotoxicity, hyperammonemia, hyperglycinemia, prolonged bleeding time; transient alopecia, generalized pruritus.
Possible drug interactions: Additive with CNS depressants including other anticonvulsants; increased phenobarbital plasma concentrations with possible severe CNS depression; barbiturates require observation for neurologic toxicity; clonazepam produces petit mal; potentiates MAO inhibitors; aspirin and warfarin also decrease bleeding time.
Nursing considerations: May impair ability to perform hazardous activities requiring mental alertness or physical coordination; overdosage may cause somnolence or coma. Evaluate seizure activity.
Usual dosage: Initially 15 mg/kg daily, maximum 60 mg/kg daily
Onset: Therapeutic effects in several days to more than one week.

Generic name: venlafaxine
Brand name: Effexor
Classification: Antidepressant, inhibits both norepinephrine and serotonin reuptake
Common uses: Treatment of depression
Should not be used if: Patient is taking MAO inhibitos, monamine oxidase inhibitors (at least 14 days should elapse between end of MAO inhibitor treatment and the start of venlafaxine, at least 7 days between end of venlafaxine treatment and the start of MAO inhibitor).
Possible side effects: Dose dependent weight loss, activation of mania/hypomania in patients with major affective disorder, anxiety, nervousness, insomnia, dose related seizures, nausea, somnolence, dizziness, abnormal ejaculation, headache, dry mouth, constipation, sweating. With doses higher than 300 mg/day an increase in systolic blood pressure.
Possible drug interactions: MAOIs (see above). Any drug that would reduce the metabolism of venlafaxine would increase the plasma concentration of venlafaxine (such as quinidine).
Nursing considerations: This is a new compound and there may be interactions with OTC drugs, advise patients to avoid alcohol when taking venlafaxine, 25, 37.5, 50, 75, and 100 mg tablets, all scored.
Usual dosage: Initial dose 75 mg/day in 2 or 3 divided doses, taken with food. Dose may be increased to 150 mg/day to 225 mg/day in increments of 75 mg/day every 4 or more days. More severely depressed patients may benefit from 350–375 mg/day in 3 divided doses. Taper to discontinue. Hepatic/renal impairment dosing: individualization of dosing to more than 50% reduction of dose.
Onset: 2–4 weeks.

References

American Hospital Formulary Service, American Society of Hospital Pharmacists, Bethesda, MD, 1994.

Computerized Clinical Information System, Micromedex Inc., Denver, 1994.

Guze BH, Gitlin M: "New Antidepressants and the Treatment of Depression," *The Journal of Family Practice* 38(1), 1994: 49–57.

The Medical Letter on Drugs and Therapeutics, Vol. 36 (924), June 10, 1994.

Nursing93 Drug Handbook, Springhouse, Springhouse PA, 1993.

Physician's Desk Reference, 48th Edition, Medical Economics Company, Oradell, NJ, 1994.

Zito, Julie Magno: *Psychotherapeutic Drug Manual* ed 3, revised, Wiley, 1994.

APPENDIX B

DSM-IV CLASSIFICATION AND CODES

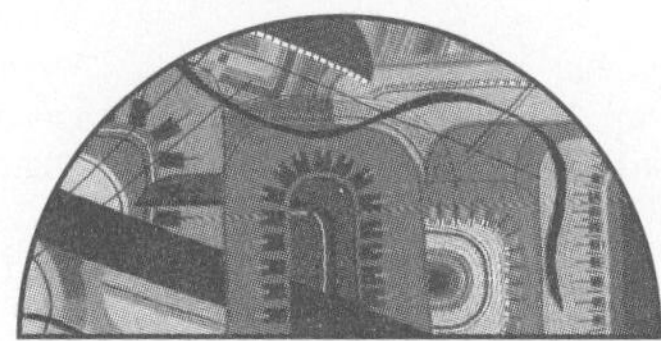

NOS = Not Otherwise Specified.

An *x* appearing in a diagnostic code indicates that a specific code number is required.

An ellipsis (. . .) is used in the names of certain disorders to indicate that the name of a specific mental disorder or general medical condition should be inserted when recording the name (e.g., 293.0 Delirium Due to Hypothyroidism).

If criteria are currently met, one of the following severity specifiers may be noted after the diagnosis:

Mild
Moderate
Severe

If criteria are no longer met, one of the following specifiers may be noted:

In Partial Remission
In Full Remission
Prior History

Source: American Psychiatric Association: *Diagnostic and Statistical Manual of Mental Disorders,* ed 4, APA, 1994.

Disorders Usually First Diagnosed in Infancy, Childhood, or Adolescence

MENTAL RETARDATION

Note: These are coded on Axis II.

317 Mild Mental Retardation
318.0 Moderate Mental Retardation
318.1 Severe Mental Retardation
318.2 Profound Mental Retardation
319 Mental Retardation, Severity Unspecified

LEARNING DISORDERS

315.00 Reading Disorder
315.1 Mathematics Disorder
315.2 Disorder of Written Expression
315.9 Learning Disorder NOS

MOTOR SKILLS DISORDER

315.4 Developmental Coordination Disorder

COMMUNICATION DISORDERS

315.31 Expressive Language Disorder
315.31 Mixed Receptive-Expressive Language Disorder
315.39 Phonological Disorder
307.0 Stuttering
307.9 Communication Disorder NOS

PERVASIVE DEVELOPMENTAL DISORDERS

299.00 Autistic Disorder
299.80 Rett's Disorder
299.10 Childhood Disintegrative Disorder
299.80 Asperger's Disorder
299.80 Pervasive Developmental Disorder NOS

ATTENTION-DEFICIT AND DISRUPTIVE BEHAVIOR DISORDERS

314.xx Attention-Deficit/Hyperactivity Disorder
.01 Combined Type
.00 Predominantly Inattentive Type
.01 Predominantly Hyperactive-Impulsive Type
314.9 Attention-Deficit/Hyperactivity/Disorder NOS
312.8 Conduct Disorder
Specify type: Childhood-Onset Type/Adolescent-Onset Type
313.81 Oppositional Defiant Disorder
312.9 Disruptive Behavior Disorder NOS

FEEDING AND EATING DISORDERS OF INFANCY OR EARLY CHILDHOOD

307.52 Pica
307.53 Rumination Disorder
307.59 Feeding Disorder of Infancy or Early Childhood

TIC DISORDERS

307.23 Tourette's Disorder
307.22 Chronic Motor or Vocal Tic Disorder
307.21 Transient Tic Disorder
Specify if: Single Episode/Recurrent
307.20 Tic Disorder NOS

ELIMINATION DISORDERS

___._ Encopresis
787.6 With Constipation and Overflow Incontinence
307.7 Without Constipation and Overflow Incontinence
307.6 Enuresis (Not Due to a General Medical Condition)
Specify type: Nocturnal Only/Diurnal Only/Nocturnal and Diurnal

OTHER DISORDERS OF INFANCY, CHILDHOOD, OR ADOLESCENCE

309.21 Separation Anxiety Disorder
Specify if: Early Onset
313.23 Selective Mutism
313.89 Reactive Attachment Disorder of Infancy or Early Childhood
Specify type: Inhibited Type/Disinhibited Type
307.3 Stereotypic Movement Disorder
Specify if: With Self-Injurious Behavior
313.9 Disorder of Infancy, Childhood, or Adolescence NOS

Delirium, Dementia, and Amnestic and Other Cognitive Disorders

DELIRIUM

293.0 Delirium Due to . . . *[Indicate the General Medical Condition]*
___._ Substance Intoxication Delirium *(refer to Substance-Related Disorders for substance-specific codes)*
___._ Substance Withdrawal Delirium *(refer to Substance-Related Disorders for substance-specific codes)*
___._ Delirium Due to Multiple Etiologies *(code each of the specific etiologies)*
780.09 Delirium NOS

DEMENTIA

290.xx Dementia of the Alzheimer's Type, With Early Onset *(also code 331.0 Alzheimer's disease on Axis III)*
.10 Uncomplicated
.11 With Delirium
.12 With Delusions
.13 With Depressed Mood
Specify if: With Behavioral Disturbance
290.xx Dementia of the Alzheimer's Type, With Late Onset *(also code 331.0 Alzheimer's disease on Axis III)*
.0 Uncomplicated
.3 With Delirium
.20 With Delusions
.21 With Depressed Mood
Specify if: With Behavioral Disturbance
290.xx Vascular Dementia
.40 Uncomplicated
.41 With Delirium
.42 With Delusions
.43 With Depressed Mood
Specify if: With Behavioral Disturbance
294.9 Dementia Due to HIV Disease *(also code 043.1 HIV infection affecting central nervous system on Axis III)*
294.1 Dementia Due to Head Trauma *(also code 854.00 head injury on Axis III)*
294.1 Dementia Due to Parkinson's Disease *(also code 332.0 Parkinson's disease on Axis III)*
294.1 Dementia Due to Huntington's Disease *(also code 333.4 Huntington's Disease on Axis III)*
290.10 Dementia Due to Pick's Disease *(also code 331.1 Pick's Disease on Axis III)*
290.10 Dementia Due to Creutzfeldt-Jakob Disease *(also code 046.1 Creutzfeldt-Jakob Disease on Axis III)*
294.1 Dementia Due to . . . *[Indicate the General Medical Condition not listed above] (also code the general medical condition on Axis III)*
___._ Substance-Induced Persisting Dementia *(refer to Substance-Related Disorders for substance-specific codes)*
___._ Dementia Due to Multiple Etiologies *(code each of the specific etiologies)*
294.8 Dementia NOS

AMNESTIC DISORDERS

294.0 Amnestic Disorder Due to . . . *[Indicate the General Medical Condition]*
Specify if: Transient/Chronic
___._ Substance-Induced Persisting Amnestic Disorder *(refer to Substance-Related Disorders for substance-specific codes)*
294.8 Amnestic Disorder NOS

OTHER COGNITIVE DISORDERS

294.9 Cognitive Disorder NOS

Mental Disorders Due to a General Medical Condition Not Elsewhere Classified

293.89 Catatonic Disorder Due to . . . *[Indicate the General Medical Condition]*
310.1 Personality Change Due to . . . *[Indicate the General Medical Condition]*
Specify type: Labile Type/Disinhibited Type/Aggressive Type/Apathetic Type/Paranoid Type/Other Type/Combined Type/Unspecified Type
293.9 Mental Disorder NOS Due to . . . *[Indicate the General Medical Condition]*

Substance-Related Disorders

[a]The following specifiers may be applied to Substance Dependence:
With Physiological Dependence/Without Physiological Dependence
Early Full Remission/Early Partial Remission
Sustained Full Remission/ Sustained Partial Remission
On Agonist Therapy/In a Controlled Environment

The following specifiers apply to Substance-Induced Disorders as noted:
[I]With Onset During Intoxication/[W]With Onset During Withdrawal

ALCOHOL-RELATED DISORDERS

Alcohol Use Disorders

303.90 Alcohol Dependence[a]
305.00 Alcohol Abuse

Alcohol-Induced Disorders

303.00 Alcohol Intoxication
291.8 Alcohol Withdrawal
Specify if: With Perceptual Disturbances
291.0 Alcohol Intoxication Delirium

291.0 Alcohol Withdrawal Delirium
291.2 Alcohol-Induced Persisting Dementia
291.1 Alcohol-Induced Persisting Amnestic Disorder
291.x Alcohol-Induced Psychotic Disorder
.5 With Delusions[I,W]
.3 With Hallucinations[I,W]
291.8 Alcohol-Induced Mood Disorder[I,W]
291.8 Alcohol-Induced Anxiety Disorder [I,W]
291.8 Alcohol-Induced Sexual Dysfunction[I]
291.8 Alcohol-Induced Sleep Disorder [I,W]
291.9 Alcohol-Related Disorder NOS

AMPHETAMINE (OR AMPHETAMINE-LIKE) RELATED DISORDERS

Amphetamine Use Disorders
304.40 Amphetamine Dependence[a]
305.70 Amphetamine Abuse

Amphetamine-Induced Disorders
292.89 Amphetamine Intoxication
Specify if: With Perceptual Disturbances
292.0 Amphetamine Withdrawal
292.81 Amphetamine Intoxication Delirium
292.xx Amphetamine-Induced Psychotic Disorder
.11 With Delusions[I]
.12 With Hallucinations[I]
292.84 Amphetamine-Induced Mood Disorder[I,W]
292.89 Amphetamine-Induced Anxiety Disorder[I]
292.89 Amphetamine-Induced Sexual Dysfunction[I]
292.89 Amphetamine-Induced Sleep Disorder[I,W]
292.9 Amphetamine-Related Disorder NOS

CAFFEINE-RELATED DISORDERS

Caffeine-Induced Disorders
305.90 Caffeine Intoxication
292.89 Caffeine-Induced Anxiety Disorder [I]
292.89 Caffeine-Induced Sleep Disorder [I]
292.9 Caffeine-Related Disorder NOS

CANNABIS-RELATED DISORDERS

Cannabis Use Disorders
304.30 Cannabis Dependence[a]
305.20 Cannabis Abuse

Cannabis-Induced Disorders
292.89 Cannabis Intoxication
Specify if: With Perceptual Disturbances
292.81 Cannabis Intoxication Delirium
292.xx Cannabis-Induced Psychotic Disorder
.11 With Delusions[I]
.12 With Hallucinations[I]
292.89 Cannabis-Induced Anxiety Disorder[I]
292.9 Cannabis-Related Disorder NOS

COCAINE-RELATED DISORDERS

Cocaine Use Disorders
304.20 Cocaine Dependence[a]
305.60 Cocaine Abuse

Cocaine-Induced Disorders
292.89 Cocaine Intoxication
Specify if: With Perceptual Disturbances
292.0 Cocaine Withdrawal
292.81 Cocaine Intoxication Delirium
292.xx Cocaine-Induced Psychotic Disorder
.11 With Delusions[I]
.12 With Hallucinations[I]
292.84 Cocaine-Induced Mood Disorder[I,W]
292.89 Cocaine-Induced Anxiety Disorder[I,W]
292.89 Cocaine-Induced Sexual Dysfunction[I]
292.89 Cocaine-Induced Sleep Disorder[I,W]
292.9 Cocaine-Related Disorder NOS

HALLUCINOGEN-RELATED DISORDERS

Hallucinogen Use Disorders
304.50 Hallucinogen Dependence[a]
305.30 Hallucinogen Abuse

Hallucinogen-Induced Disorders
292.89 Hallucinogen Intoxication
292.89 Hallucinogen Persisting Perception Disorder (Flashbacks)
292.81 Hallucinogen Intoxication Delirium
292.xx Hallucinogen-Induced Psychotic Disorder
.11 With Delusions[I]
.12 With Hallucinations[I]
292.84 Hallucinogen-Induced Mood Disorder[I]
292.89 Hallucinogen-Induced Anxiety Disorder[I]
292.9 Hallucinogen-Related Disorder NOS

INHALANT-RELATED DISORDERS

Inhalant Use Disorders
304.60 Inhalant Dependence[a]
305.90 Inhalant Abuse

Inhalant-Induced Disorders
292.89 Inhalant Intoxication
292.81 Inhalant Intoxication Delirium
292.82 Inhalant-Induced Persisting Dementia
292.xx Inhalant-Induced Psychotic Disorder
.11 With Delusions[I]
.12 With Hallucinations[I]
292.84 Inhalant-Induced Mood Disorder[I]
292.89 Inhalant-Induced Anxiety Disorder[I]
292.9 Inhalant-Related Disorder NOS

NICOTINE-RELATED DISORDERS

Nicotine Use Disorder
305.10 Nicotine Dependence[a]

Nicotine-Induced Disorder
292.0 Nicotine Withdrawal
292.9 Nicotine-Related Disorder NOS

OPIOID-RELATED DISORDERS

Opioid Use Disorders
304.00 Opioid Dependence[a]
305.50 Opioid Abuse

Opioid-Induced Disorders
292.89 Opioid Intoxication
Specify if: With Perceptual Disturbances
292.0 Opioid Withdrawal
292.81 Opioid Intoxication Delirium
292.xx Opioid-Induced Psychotic Disorder
.11 With Delusions[I]
.12 With Hallucinations[I]

292.84 Opioid-Induced Mood Disorder[I]
292.89 Opioid-Induced Sexual Dysfunction[I]
292.89 Opioid-Induced Sleep Disorder[I,W]
292.9 Opioid-Related Disorder NOS

PHENCYCLIDINE (OR PHENCYCLIDINE-LIKE) RELATED DISORDERS

Phencyclidine Use Disorders
304.90 Phencyclidine Dependence[a]
305.90 Phencyclidine Abuse

Phencyclidine-Induced Disorders
292.89 Phencyclidine Intoxication
Specify if: With Perceptual Disturbances
292.81 Phencyclidine Intoxication Delirium
292.xx Phencyclidine-Induced Psychotic Disorder
.11 With Delusions[I]
.12 With Hallucinations[I]
292.84 Phencyclidine-Induced Mood Disorder[I]
292.89 Phencyclidine-Induced Anxiety Disorder[I]
292.9 Phencyclidine-Related Disorder NOS

SEDATIVE-, HYPNOTIC-, OR ANXIOLYTIC-RELATED DISORDERS

Sedative, Hypnotic, or Anxiolytic Use Disorders
304.10 Sedative, Hypnotic, or Anxiolytic Dependence[a]
305.40 Sedative, Hypnotic, or Anxiolytic Abuse

Sedative-, Hypnotic-, or Anxiolytic-Induced Disorders
292.89 Sedative, Hypnotic, or Anxiolytic Intoxication
292.0 Sedative, Hypnotic, or Anxiolytic Withdrawal
Specify if: With Perceptual Disturbances
292.81 Sedative, Hypnotic, or Anxiolytic Intoxication Delirium
292.81 Sedative, Hypnotic, or Anxiolytic Withdrawal Delirium
292.82 Sedative-, Hypnotic-, or Anxiolytic-Induced Persisting Dementia
292.83 Sedative-, Hypnotic-, or Anxiolytic-Induced Persisting Amnestic Disorder
292.xx Sedative-, Hypnotic-, or Anxiolytic-Induced Psychotic Disorder
.11 With Delusions[I,W]
.12 With Hallucinations[I,W]
292.84 Sedative-, Hypnotic-, or Anxiolytic-Induced Mood Disorder[I,W]
292.89 Sedative-, Hypnotic-, or Anxiolytic-Induced Anxiety Disorder[W]
292.89 Sedative-, Hypnotic-, or Anxiolytic-Induced Sexual Dysfunction[I]
292.89 Sedative-, Hypnotic-, or Anxiolytic-Induced Sleep Disorder[I,W]
292.9 Sedative-, Hypnotic-, or Anxiolytic-Related Disorder NOS

POLYSUBSTANCE-RELATED DISORDER
304.80 Polysubstance Dependence[a]

OTHER (OR UNKNOWN) SUBSTANCE-RELATED DISORDERS

Other (or Unknown) Substance Use Disorders
304.90 Other (or Unknown) Substance Dependence[a]
305.90 Other (or Unknown) Substance Abuse

Other (or Unknown) Substance-Induced Disorders
292.89 Other (or Unknown) Substance Intoxication
Specify if: With Perceptual Disturbances
292.0 Other (or Unknown) Substance Withdrawal
Specify if: With Perceptual Disturbances
292.81 Other (or Unknown) Substance-Induced Delirium
292.82 Other (or Unknown) Substance-Induced Persisting Dementia
292.83 Other (or Unknown) Substance-Induced Persisting Amnestic Disorder
292.xx Other (or Unknown) Substance-Induced Psychotic Disorder
.11 With Delusions[I,W]
.12 With Hallucinations[I,W]
292.84 Other (or Unknown) Substance-Induced Mood Disorder[I,W]
292.89 Other (or Unknown) Substance-Induced Anxiety Disorder[I,W]
292.89 Other (or Unknown) Substance-Induced Sexual Dysfunction[I]
292.89 Other (or Unknown) Substance-Induced Sleep Disorder[I,W]
292.9 Other (or Unknown) Substance-Related Disorder NOS

Schizophrenia and Other Psychotic Disorders

295.xx Schizophrenia

The following Classification of Longitudinal Course applies to all subtypes of Schizophrenia:

Episodic With Interepisode Residual Symptoms (*specify if:* With Prominent Negative Symptoms)/Episodic With No Interepisode Residual Symptoms/Continuous (*specify if:* With Prominent Negative Symptoms)
Single Episode In Partial Remission (*specify if:* With Prominent Negative Symptoms)/Single Episode In Full Remission
Other or Unspecified Pattern

.30 Paranoid Type
.10 Disorganized Type
.20 Catatonic Type
.90 Undifferentiated Type
.60 Residual Type

295.40 Schizophreniform Disorder
Specify if: Without Good Prognostic Features/With Good Prognostic Features
295.70 Schizoaffective Disorder
Specify type: Bipolar Type/Depressive Type
297.1 Delusional Disorder
Specify type: Erotomanic Type/Grandiose Type/Jealous Type/Persecutory Type/Somatic Type/Mixed Type/Unspecified Type
298.8 Brief Psychotic Disorder
Specify if: With Marked Stressor(s)/Without Marked Stressor(s)/With Postpartum Onset
297.3 Shared Psychotic Disorder
293.xx Psychotic Disorder Due to . . . *[Indicate the General Medical Condition]*
.81 With Delusions
.82 With Hallucinations
___._ Substance-Induced Psychotic Disorder (refer to Substance-Related Disorders for substance-specific codes)
Specify if: With Onset During Intoxication/With Onset During Withdrawal
298.9 Psychotic Disorder NOS

Mood Disorders

Code current state of Major Depressive Disorder or Bipolar I Disorder in fifth digit:

1 = Mild
2 = Moderate
3 = Severe Without Psychotic Features
4 = Severe With Psychotic Features
Specify: Mood-Congruent Psychotic Features/Mood-Incongruent Psychotic Features
5 = In Partial Remission
6 = In Full Remission
0 = Unspecified

The following specifiers apply (for current or most recent episode) to Mood Disorders as noted:

[a]Severity/Psychotic/Remission Specifiers/[b]Chronic/[c]With Catatonic Features/[d]With Melancholic Features/[e]With Atypical Features/[f]With Postpartum Onset

The following specifiers apply to Mood Disorders as noted:

[g]With or Without Full Interepisode Recovery/[h]With Seasonal Pattern/[i]With Rapid Cycling

DEPRESSIVE DISORDERS

296.xx Major Depressive Disorder,
.2x Single Episode[a,b,c,d,e,f]
.3x Recurrent[a,b,c,d,e,f,g,h]
300.4 Dysthymic Disorder
Specify if: Early Onset/Late Onset
Specify: With Atypical Features
311 Depressive Disorder NOS

BIPOLAR DISORDERS

296.xx Bipolar I Disorder,
.0x Single Manic Episode[a,c,f]
Specify if: Mixed
.40 Most Recent Episode Hypomanic[g,h,i]
.4x Most Recent Episode Manic[a,c,f,g,h,i]
.6x Most Recent Episode Mixed[a,c,f,g,h,i]
.5x Most Recent Episode Depressed[a,b,c,d,e,f,g,h,i]
.7 Most Recent Episode Unspecified[g,h,i]
296.89 Bipolar II Disorder[a,b,c,d,e,f,g,h,i]
Specify (current or most recent episode): Hypomanic/Depressed
301.13 Cyclothymic Disorder
296.80 Bipolar Disorder NOS
293.83 Mood Disorder Due to . . . *[Indicate the General Medical Condition]*
Specify type: With Depressive Features/With Major Depressive-Like Episode/With Manic Features/With Mixed Features
___._ Substance-Induced Mood Disorder *(refer to Substance-Related Disorders for substance-specific codes)*
Specify type: With Depressive Features/With Manic Features/With Mixed Features
Specify if: With Onset During Intoxication/With Onset During Withdrawal
296.90 Mood Disorder NOS

Anxiety Disorders

300.01 Panic Disorder Without Agoraphobia
300.21 Panic Disorder With Agoraphobia
300.22 Agoraphobia Without History of Panic Disorder
300.29 Specific Phobia
Specify type: Animal Type/Natural Environment Type/Blood-Injection-Injury Type/Situational Type/Other Type
300.23 Social Phobia
Specify if: Generalized
300.3 Obsessive-Compulsive Disorder
Specify if: With Poor Insight
309.81 Posttraumatic Stress Disorder
Specify if: Acute/Chronic
Specify if: With Delayed Onset
308.3 Acute Stress Disorder
300.02 Generalized Anxiety Disorder
293.89 Anxiety Disorder Due to . . . *[Indicate the General Medical Condition]*
Specify if: With Generalized Anxiety/With Panic Attacks/With Obsessive-Compulsive Symptoms
___._ Substance-Induced Anxiety Disorder *(refer to Substance-Related Disorders for substance-specific codes)*
Specify if: With Generalized Anxiety/With Panic Attacks/With Obsessive-Compulsive Symptoms/With Phobic Symptoms
Specify if: With Onset During Intoxication/With Onset During Withdrawal
300.00 Anxiety Disorder NOS

Somatoform Disorders

300.81 Somatization Disorder
300.81 Undifferentiated Somatoform Disorder
300.11 Conversion Disorder
Specify type: With Motor Symptom or Deficit/With Sensory Symptom or Deficit/With Seizures or Convulsions/With Mixed Presentation
307.xx Pain Disorder
.80 Associated With Psychological Factors
.89 Associated With Both Psychological Factors and a General Medical Condition
Specify if: Acute/Chronic
300.7 Hypochondriasis
Specify if: With Poor Insight
300.7 Body Dysmorphic Disorder
300.81 Somatoform Disorder NOS

Factitious Disorders

300.xx Factitious Disorder
.16 With Predominantly Psychological Signs and Symptoms
.19 With Predominantly Physical Signs and Symptoms
.19 With Combined Psychological and Physical Signs and Symptoms
300.19 Factitious Disorder NOS

Dissociative Disorders

300.12 Dissociative Amnesia
300.13 Dissociative Fugue
300.14 Dissociative Identity Diusorder
300.6 Depersonalization Disorder
300.15 Dissociative Disorder NOS

Sexual and Gender Identity Disorders

SEXUAL DYSFUNCTIONS

The following specifiers apply to all primary Sexual Dysfunctions:
Lifelong Type/Acquired Type
Generalized Type/Situational Type
Due to Psychological Factors/Due to Combined Factors

Sexual Desire Disorders

302.71 Hypoactive Sexual Desire Disorder
302.79 Sexual Aversion Disorder

Sexual Arousal Disorders

302.72 Female Sexual Arousal Disorder
302.72 Male Erectile Disorder

Orgasmic Disorders

302.73 Female Orgasmic Disorder
302.74 Male Orgasmic Disorder
302.75 Premature Ejaculation

Sexual Pain Disorders

302.76 Dyspareunia (Not Due to a General Medical Condition)
306.51 Vaginismus (Not Due to a General Medical Condition)

Sexual Dysfunction Due to a General Medical Condition

625.8 Female Hypoactive Sexual Desire Disorder Due to . . . *[Indicate the General Medical Condition]*
608.89 Male Hypoactive Sexual Desire Disorder Due to . . . *[Indicate the General Medical Condition]*
607.84 Male Erectile Disorder Due to . . . *[Indicate the General Medical Condition]*
625.0 Female Dyspareunia Due to . . . *[Indicate the General Medical Condition]*
608.89 Male Dyspareunia Due to . . . *[Indicate the General Medical Condition]*
625.8 Other Female Sexual Dysfunction Due to . . . *[Indicate the General Medical Condition]*
608.89 Other Male Sexual Dysfunction Due to . . . *[Indicate the General Medical Condition]*
___._ Substance-Induced Sexual Dysfunction *(refer to Substance-Related Disorders for substance-specific codes)*
Specify if: With Impaired Desire/With Impaired Arousal/With Impaired Orgasm/With Sexual Pain
Specify if: With Onset During Intoxication
302.70 Sexual Dysfunction NOS

PARAPHILIAS

302.4 Exhibitionism
302.81 Fetishism
302.89 Frotteurism
302.2 Pedophilia
Specify if: Sexually Attracted to Males/Sexually Attracted to Females/Sexually Attracted to Both
Specify if: Limited to Incest
Specify type: Exclusive Type/Nonexclusive Type
302.83 Sexual Masochism
302.84 Sexual Sadism
302.3 Transvestic Fetishism
Specify if: With Gender Dysphoria
302.82 Voyeurism
302.9 Paraphilia NOS

GENDER IDENTITY DISORDERS

302.xx Gender Identity Disorder
.6 in Children
.85 in Adolescents or Adults
Specify if: Sexually Attracted to Males/Sexually Attracted to Females/Sexually Attracted to Both/Sexually Attracted to Neither
302.6 Gender Identity Disorder NOS
302.9 Sexual Disorder NOS

Eating Disorders

307.1 Anorexia Nervosa
Specify type: Restricting Type; Binge-Eating/Purging Type
307.51 Bulimia Nervosa
Specify type: Purging Type/Nonpurging Type
307.50 Eating Disorder NOS

Sleep Disorders

PRIMARY SLEEP DISORDERS

Dyssomnias

307.42 Primary Insomnia
307.44 Primary Hypersomnia
Specify if: Recurrent
347 Narcolepsy
780.59 Breathing-Related Sleep Disorder
307.45 Circadian Rhythm Sleep Disorder
Specify type: Delayed Sleep Phase Type/Jet Lag Type/Shift Work Type/Unspecified Type
307.47 Dyssomnia NOS

Parasomnias

307.47 Nightmare Disorder
307.46 Sleep Terror Disorder
307.46 Sleepwalking Disorder
307.47 Parasomnia NOS

SLEEP DISORDERS RELATED TO ANOTHER MENTAL DISORDER

307.42 Insomnia Related to . . . *[Indicate the Axis I or Axis II Disorder]*
307.44 Hypersomnia Related to . . . *[Indicate the Axis I or Axis II Disorder]*

OTHER SLEEP DISORDERS

780.xx Sleep Disorder Due to . . . *[Indicate the General Medical Condition]*
.52 Insomnia Type
.54 Hypersomnia Type
.59 Parasomnia Type
.59 Mixed Type
___._ Substance-Induced Sleep Disorder *(refer to Substance-Related Disorders for substance-specific codes)*
Specify type: Insomnia Type/Hypersomnia Type/Parasomnia Type/Mixed Type
Specify if: With Onset During Intoxication/With Onset During Withdrawal

Impulse-Control Disorders Not Elsewhere Classified

312.34 Intermitten Explosive Disorder
312.32 Kleptomania
312.33 Pyromania
312.31 Pathological Gambling
312.39 Trichotillomania
312.30 Impulse-Control Disorder NOS

Adjustment Disorders

309.xx Adjustment Disorder
.0 With Depressed Mood
.24 With Anxiety
.28 With Mixed Anxiety and Depressed Mood
.3 With Disturbance of Conduct
.4 With Mixed Disturbance of Emotions and Conduct
.9 Unspecified
Specify if: Acute/Chronic

Personality Disorders

Note: *These are coded on Axis II.*

301.0 Paranoid Personality Disorder
301.20 Schizoid Personality Disorder
301.22 Schizotypal Personality Disorder
301.7 Antisocial Personality Disorder
301.83 Borderline Personality Disorder
301.50 Histrionic Personality Disorder
301.81 Narcissistic Personality Disorder
301.82 Avoidant Personality Disorder
301.6 Dependent Personality Disorder
301.4 Obsessive-Compulsive Personality Disorder
301.9 Personality Disorder NOS

Other Conditions That May Be a Focus of Clinical Attention

PSYCHOLOGICAL FACTORS AFFECTING MEDICAL CONDITION
316 . . . *[Specified Psychological Factor]* Affecting . . . *[Indicate the General Medical Condition]*
Choose name based on nature of factors:
Mental Disorder Affecting Medical Condition
Psychological Symptoms Affecting Medical Condition
Personality Traits or Coping Style Affecting Medical Condition
Maladaptive Health Behaviors Affecting Medical Condition
Stress-Related Physiological Response Affecting Medical Condition
Other or Unspecified Psychological Factors Affecting Medical Condition

MEDICATION-INDUCED MOVEMENT DISORDERS
332.1 Neuroleptic-Induced Parkinsonism
333.92 Neuroleptic Malignant Syndrome
333.7 Neuroleptic-Induced Acute Dystonia
333.99 Neuroleptic-Induced Acute Akathisia
333.82 Neuroleptic-Induced Tardive Dyskinesia
333.1 Medication-Induced Postural Tremor
333.90 Medication-Induced Movement Disorder NOS

OTHER MEDICATION-INDUCED DISORD
995.2 Ad se Effects of Me n NOS

RELATION LEMS
V61.9 Rela blem Re o a Me sorder or General Medica n
V61.20 Parent-Ch tiona em
V61.1 Partner Relat al Prob
V61.8 Sibling Relational Probl
V62.81 Relational Problem NO

PROBLEMS RELATED TO ABU NEG
V61.21 Physical Abuse of Child
(code 995.5 if focus of atte s on vi
V61.21 Sexual Abuse of Child
(code 995.5 if focus of att s on vi
V61.21 Neglect of Child
(code 995.5 if focus of atten on vi
V61.1 Physical Abuse of Adult
(code 995.81 if focus of atte s on v
V61.1 Sexual Abuse of Adult
(code 995.81 if focus of atte s on v

ADDITIONAL CONDITIONS THA BE S OF CLINICAL ATTENTION
V15.81 Noncompliance With Treat
V65.2 Malingering
V71.01 Adult Antisocial Behavior
V71.02 Child or Adolescent Antisoc hav
V62.89 Borderline Intellectual Funct g
Note: *This is coded on Axis II.*
780.9 Age-Related Cognitive Declin
V62.82 Bereavement
V62.3 Academic Problem
V62.2 Occupational Problem
313.82 Identity Problem
V62.89 Religious or Spiritual Problem
V62.4 Acculturation Problem
V62.89 Phase of Life Problem

Additional Codes

300.9 Unspecified Mental Disorder otic)
V71.09 No Diagnosis or Condition
799.9 Diagnosis or Condition Def red is I
V71.09 No Diagnosis on Axis I
799.9 Diagnosis Deferred xis II

Multiaxial System

Axis I Clinical Disor
Other Condi That M cus of Clinical Attention
Axis II Personality ders
Mental Re ion
Axis III General al Co
Axis IV Psychos and E Problems
Axis V Globa ssme g

AXIS II

Personality Disorders, Mental Retardation

Paranoid Personality Disorder
Schizoid Personality Disorder
Schizotypal Personality Disorder
Antisocial Personality Disorder
Borderline Personality Disorder
Histrionic Personality Disorder
Narcissistic Personality Disorder
Avoidant Personality Disorder
Dependent Personality Disorder
Obsessive-Compulsive Personality Disorder
Personality Disorder Not Otherwise Specified

Mental Retardation

AXIS III

General Medical Conditions

Infectious and Parasitic Diseases
Neoplasms
Endocrine, Nutritional, and Metabolic Diseases and Immunity Disorders
Diseases of the Blood and Blood-Forming Organs
Diseases of the Nervous System and Sense Organs
Diseases of the Circulatory System
Diseases of the Respiratory System
Diseases of the Digestive System
Diseases of the Genitourinary System
Complications of Pregnancy, Childbirth, and the Puerperium
Diseases of the Skin and Subcutaneous Tissue
Diseases of the Musculoskeletal System and Connective Tissue
Congenital Anomalies
Certain Conditions Originating in the Perinatal Period
Symptoms, Signs, and Ill-Defined Conditions
Injury and Poisoning

AXIS IV

Psychosocial and Environmental Problems

Problems with primary support group
Problems related to the social environment
Educational problems
Occupational problems
Housing problems
Economic problems
Problems with access to health care services
Problems related to interaction with the legal system/crime
Other psychosocial and environmental problems

Global Assessment of Functioning (GAF) Scale

Consider psychological, social, and occupational functioning on a hypothetical continuum of mental health–illness. Do not include impairment in functioning due to physical (or environmental) limitations.

Code (**Note:** Use intermediate codes when appropriate, e.g., 45, 68, 72.)

100 **Superior functioning in a wide range of activities, life's problems never seem to get out of hand, is sought out by others because of his or her many positive qualities.**
91 **No symptoms.**

90 **Absent or minimal symptoms** (e.g., mild anxiety before an exam), **good functioning in all areas, interested and involved in a wide range of activities, socially effective, generally satisfied with life, no more than everyday problems or concerns** (e.g., an occasional argument with fam-
81 ily members).

80 **If symptoms are present, they are transient and expectable reactions to psychosocial stressors** (e.g., difficulty concentrating after family argument); **no more than slight impairment in social, occupational, or school**
71 **functioning** (e.g., temporarily falling behind in schoolwork).

70 **Some mild symptoms** (e.g., depressed mood and mild insomnia) **OR some difficulty in social, occupational, or school functioning** (e.g., occasional truancy, or theft within the household), **but generally functioning pretty well, has**
61 **some meaningful interpersonal relationships.**

60 **Moderate symptoms** (e.g., flat affect and circumstantial speech, occasional panic attacks) **OR moderate difficulty in social, occupational, or school functioning**
51 (e.g., few friends, conflicts with peers or coworkers).

50 **Serious symptoms** (e.g., suicidal ideation, severe obsessional rituals, frequent shoplifting) **OR any serious impairment in social, occupational, or school functioning** (e.g., no
41 friends, unable to keep a job).

40 **Some impairment in reality testing or communication** (e.g., speech is at times illogical, obscure, or irrelevant) **OR major impairment in several areas, such as work or school, family relations, judgment, thinking, or mood** (e.g., depressed man avoids friends, neglects family, and is unable to work; child frequently beats up younger children, is defiant at
31 home, and is failing at school).

30 **Behavior is considerably influenced by delusions or hallucinations OR serious impairment in communication or judgment** (e.g., sometimes incoherent, acts grossly inappropriately, suicidal preoccupation) **OR inability to function in almost all areas** (e.g., stays in bed all day; no job, home, or
21 friends).

20 **Some danger of hurting self or others** (e.g., suicide attempts without clear expectation of death; frequently violent; manic excitement) **OR occasionally fails to maintain minimal personal hygiene** (e.g., smears feces) **OR gross impair-**
11 **ment in communication** (e.g., largely incoherent or mute).

10 **Persistent danger of severely hurting self or others** (e.g., recurrent violence) **OR persistent inability to maintain minimal personal hygiene OR serious suicidal act with**
1 **clear expectation of death.**

0 Inadequate information

The rating of overall psychological functioning on a scale of 0–100 was operationalized by Luborsky in the Health-Sickness Rating Scale (Luborsky L: "Clinicians' Judgments of Mental Health." *Archives of General Psychiatry* 7:407–417, 1962). Spitzer and colleagues developed a revision of the Health-Sickness Rating Scale called the Global Assessment Scale (GAS) (Endicott J, Spitzer RL, Fleiss JL, Cohen J: "The Global Assessment Scale: A Procedure for Measuring Overall Severity of Psychiatric Disturbance." *Archives of General Psychiatry* 33:766–771, 1976). A modified version of the GAS was included in *DSM-III-R* as the Global Assessment of Functioning (GAF) Scale.

APPENDIX C

OUTLINE FOR CULTURAL FORMULATION AND GLOSSARY OF CULTURE-BOUND SYNDROMES

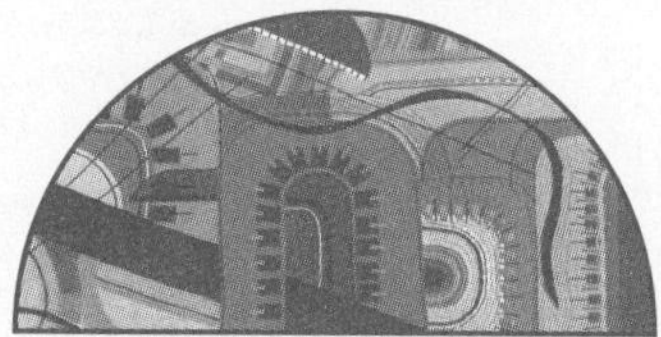

This appendix is divided into two sections. The first section provides an outline for cultural formulation designed to assist the clinician in systematically evaluating and reporting the impact of the individual's cultural context. The second is a glossary of culture-bound syndromes.

Outline for Cultural Formulation

The following outline for cultural formulation is meant to supplement the multiaxial diagnostic assessment and to address difficulties that may be encountered in applying DSM-IV criteria in a multicultural environment. The cultural formulation provides a systematic review of the individual's cultural background, the role of the cultural context in the expression and evaluation of symptoms and dysfunction, and the effect that cultural differences may have on the relationship between the individual and the clinician.

As indicated in the introduction to the *DSM-IV* manual it is important that the clinician take into account the individual's ethnic and cultural context in the evaluation of each of the DSM-IV axes. In addition, the cultural formulation suggested below provides an opportunity to describe systematically the individual's cultural and social reference group and ways in which the cultural context is relevant to clinical care. The clinician may provide a narrative summary for each of the following categories:

Cultural identity of the individual. Note the individual's ethnic or cultural reference groups. For immigrants and ethnic minorities, note separately the degree of involvement with both the culture of origin and the host culture (where applicable). Also note language abilities, use, and preference (including multilingualism).

Cultural explanations of the individual's illness. The following may be identified: the predominant idioms of distress through which symptoms or the need for social support are communicated (e.g., "nerves," possessing spirits, somatic complaints, inexplicable misfortune), the meaning and perceived severity of the individual's symptoms in relation to norms of the cultural reference group, any local illness category used by the individual's family and community to identify the condition (see "Glossary of Culture-Bound Syndromes" below), the perceived causes or explanatory models that the individual and the reference group use to explain the illness, and current preferences for and past experiences with professional and popular sources of care.

Source: American Psychiatric Association: *Diagnostic and Statistical Manual of Mental Disorders,* ed 4, APA, 1994.

Cultural factors related to psychosocial environment and levels of functioning. Note culturally relevant interpretations of social stressors, available social supports, and levels of functioning and disability. This would include stresses in the local social environment and the role of religion and kin networks in providing emotional, instrumental, and informational support.

Cultural elements of the relationship between the individual and the clinician. Indicate differences in culture and social status between the individual and the clinician and problems that these differences may cause in diagnosis and treatment (e.g., difficulty in communicating in the individual's first language, in eliciting symptoms or understanding their cultural significance, in negotiating an appropriate relationship or level of intimacy, in determining whether a behavior is normative or pathological).

Overall cultural assessment for diagnosis and care. The formulation concludes with a discussion of how cultural considerations specifically influence comprehensive diagnosis and care.

Glossary of Culture-Bound Syndromes

The term *culture-bound syndrome* denotes recurrent, locality-specific patterns of aberrant behavior and troubling experience that may or may not be linked to a particular DSM-IV diagnostic category. Many of these patterns are indigenously considered to be "illnesses," or at least afflictions, and most have local names. Although presentations conforming to the major DSM-IV categories can be found throughout the world, the particular symptoms, course, and social response are very often influenced by local cultural factors. In contrast, culture-bound syndromes are generally limited to specific societies or culture areas and are localized, folk, diagnostic categories that frame coherent meanings for certain repetitive, patterned, and troubling sets of experiences and observations.

There is seldom a one-to-one equivalence of any culture-bound syndrome with a DSM diagnostic entity. Aberrant behavior that might be sorted by a diagnostician using DSM-IV into several categories may be included in a single folk category, and presentations that might be considered by a diagnostician using DSM-IV as belonging to a single category may be sorted into several by an indigenous clinician. Moreover, some conditions and disorders have been conceptualized as culture-bound syndromes specific to industrialized culture (e.g., Anorexia Nervosa, Dissociative Identity Disorder) given their apparent rarity or absence in other cultures. It should also be noted that all industrialized societies include distinctive subcultures and widely diverse immigrant groups who may present with culture-bound syndromes.

This glossary lists some of the best-studied culture-bound syndromes and idioms of distress that may be encountered in clinical practice in North America and includes relevant DSM-IV categories when data suggest that they should be considered in a diagnostic formulation.

amok A dissociative episode characterized by a period of brooding followed by an outburst of violent, aggressive, or homicidal behavior directed at people and objects. The episode tends to be precipitated by a perceived slight or insult and seems to be prevalent only among males. The episode is often accompanied by persecutory ideas, automatism, amnesia, exhaustion, and a return to premorbid state following the episode. Some instances of amok may occur during a brief psychotic episode or constitute the onset or an exacerbation of a chronic psychotic process. The original reports that used this term were from Malaysia. A similar behavior pattern is found in Laos, Philippines, Polynesia *(cafard* or *cathard),* Papua New Guinea, and Puerto Rico *(mal de pelea),* and among the Navajo *(iich'aa).*

ataque de nervios An idiom of distress principally reported among Latinos from the Caribbean, but recognized among many Latin American and Latin Mediterranean groups. Commonly reported symptoms include uncontrollable shouting, attacks of crying, trembling, heat in the chest rising into the head, and verbal or physical aggression. Dissociative experiences, seizurelike or fainting episodes, and suicidal gestures are prominent in some attacks but absent in others. A general feature of an ataque de nervios is a sense of being out of control. Ataques de nervios frequently occur as a direct result of a stressful event relating to the family (e.g., news of the death of a close relative, a separation or divorce from a spouse, conflicts with a spouse or children, or witnessing an accident involving a family member). People may experience amnesia for what occurred during the ataque de nervios, but they otherwise return rapidly to their usual level of functioning. Although descriptions of some ataques de nervios most closely fit with the DSM-IV description of Panic Attacks, the association of most ataques with a precipitating event and the frequent absence of the hallmark symptoms of acute fear or apprehension distinguish them from Panic Disorder. Ataques span the range from normal expressions of distress not associated with having a mental disorder to symptom presentations associated with the diagnoses of Anxiety, Mood, Dissociative, or Somatoform Disorders.

bilis and **colera** (also referred to as *muina*) The underlying cause of these syndromes is thought to be strongly experienced anger or rage. Anger is viewed among many Latino groups as a particularly powerful emotion that can have direct effects on the body and can exacerbate existing symptoms. The major effect of anger is to disturb core body balances (which are understood as a balance between hot and cold valences in the body and between the material and spiritual aspects of the body). Symptoms can include acute nervous tension, headache, trembling, screaming, stomach disturbances, and, in more severe cases, loss of consciousness. Chronic fatigue may result from the acute episode.

boufée delirante A syndrome observed in West Africa and Haiti. This French term refers to a sudden outburst of agitated and aggressive behavior, marked confusion, and psychomotor excitement. It may sometimes be accompanied by visual and auditory hallucinations or paranoid ideation. These episodes may resemble an episode of Brief Psychotic Disorder.

brain fag A term initially used in West Africa to refer to a condition experienced by high school or university students in response to the challenges of schooling. Symptoms include difficulties in concentrating, remembering, and thinking. Students often state that their brains are "fatigued." Additional somatic symptoms are usually centered around the head and neck and include pain, pressure or tightness, blurring of vision, heat, or burning. "Brain tiredness" or fatigue from "too much thinking" is an idiom of distress in many cultures, and resulting syndromes can resemble certain Anxiety, Depressive, and Somatoform Disorders.

dhat A folk diagnostic term used in India to refer to severe anxiety and hypochondriacal concerns associated with the discharge of semen, whitish discoloration of the urine, and feelings of weakness and exhaustion. Similar to *jiryan* (India), *sukra prameha* (Sri Lanka), and *shen-k'uei* (China).

falling-out or **blacking out** These episodes occur primarily in southern United States and Caribbean groups. They are characterized by a sudden collapse, which sometimes occurs without warning but sometimes is preceded by feelings of dizziness or "swimming" in the head. The individual's eyes are usually open but the person claims an inability to see. The person usually hears and understands what is occurring around him or her but feels powerless to move. This may correspond to a diagnosis of Conversion Disorder or a Dissociative Disorder.

ghost sickness A preoccupation with death and the deceased (sometimes associated with witchcraft) frequently observed among members of many American Indian tribes. Various symptoms can be attributed to ghost sickness, including bad dreams, weakness, feelings of danger, loss of appetite, fainting, dizziness, fear, anxiety, hallucinations, loss of consciousness, confusion, feelings of futility, and a sense of suffocation.

hwa-byung (also known as **woll-hwa-byung**) A Korean folk syndrome literally translated into English as "anger syndrome" and attributed to the suppression of anger. The symptoms include insomnia, fatigue, panic, fear of impending death, dysphoric affect, indigestion, anorexia, dyspnea, palpitations, generalized aches and pains, and a feeling of a mass in the epigastrium.

koro A term, probably of Malaysian origin, that refers to an episode of sudden and intense anxiety that the penis (or , in females, the vulva and nipples) will recede into the body and possibly cause death. The syndrome is reported in south and east Asia, where it is known by a variety of local terms, such as *shuk yang, shook yong,* and *suo yang* (Chinese); *jinjinia bemar* (Assam); or *rok-joo* (Thailand). It is occasionally found in the West. Koro at times occurs in localized epidemic form in east Asian areas. This diagnosis is included in the *Chinese Classification of Mental Disorders,* Second Edition (CCMD-2).

latah Hypersensitivity to sudden fright, often with echopraxia, echolalia, command obedience, and dissociative or trancelike behavior. The term *latah* is of Malaysian or Indonesian origin, but the syndrome has been found in many parts of the world. Other terms for this condition are *amurakh, irkunii, ikota, olan, myriachit,* and *menkeiti* (Siberian groups); *bah tschi, bah-tsi, baah-ji* (Thailand); *imu* (Ainu, Sakhalin, Japan); and *mali-mali* and *silok* (Philippines). In Malaysia it is more frequent in middle-aged women.

locura A term used by Latinos in the United States and Latin America to refer to a severe form of chronic psychosis. The condition is attributed to an inherited vulnerability, to the effect of multiple life difficulties, or to a combination of both factors. Symptoms exhibited by persons with locura include incoherence, agitation, auditory and visual hallucinations, inability to follow rules of social interaction, unpredictability, and possible violence.

mal de ojo A concept widely found in Mediterranean cultures and elsewhere in the world. *Mal de ojo* is a Spanish phrase translated into English as "evil eye." Children are especially at risk. Symptoms include fitful sleep, crying without apparent cause, diarrhea, vomiting, and fever in a child or infant. Sometimes adults (especially females) have the condition.

nervios A common idiom of distress among Latinos in the United States and Latin America. A number of other ethnic groups have related, though often somewhat distinctive, ideas of "nerves" (such as *nevra* among Greeks in North America).

Nervios refers both to a general state of vulnerability to stressful life experiences and to a syndrome brought on by difficult life circumstances. The term *nervios* includes a wide range of symptoms of emotional distress, somatic disturbance, and inability to function. Common symptoms include headaches and "brain aches," irritability, stomach disturbances, sleep difficulties, nervousness, easy tearfulness, inability to concentrate, trembling, tingling sensations, and *mareos* (dizziness with occasional vertigo-like exacerbations). Nervios tends to be an ongoing problem, although variable in the degree of disability manifested. Nervios is a very broad syndrome that spans the range from cases free of a mental disorder to presentations resembling Adjustment, Anxiety, Depressive, Dissociative, Somatoform, or Psychotic Disorders. Differential diagnosis will depend on the constellation of symptoms experienced, the kind of social events that are associated with the onset and progress of nervios, and the level of disability experienced.

pibloktoq An abrupt dissociative episode accompanied by extreme excitement of up to 30 minutes' duration and frequently followed by convulsive seizures and coma lasting up to 12 hours. This is observed primarily in arctic and subarctic Eskimo communities, although regional variations in name exist. The individual may be withdrawn or mildly irritable for a period of hours or days before the attack and will typically report complete amnesia for the attack. During the attack, the individual may tear off his or her clothing, break furniture, shout obscenities, eat feces, flee from protective shelters, or perform other irrational or dangerous acts.

qi-gong psychotic reaction A term describing an acute, time-limited episode characterized by dissociative, paranoid, or other psychotic or nonpsychotic symptoms that may occur after participation in the Chinese folk health-enhancing practice of qi-gong ("exercise of vital energy"). Especially vulnerable are individuals who become overly involved in the practice. This diagnosis is included in the *Chinese Classification of Mental Disorders,* Second Edition (CCMD-2).

rootwork A set of cultural interpretations that ascribe illness to hexing, witchcraft, sorcery, or the evil influence of another person. Symptoms may include generalized anxiety and gastrointestinal complaints (e.g., nausea, vomiting, diarrhea), weakness, dizziness, the fear or being poisoned, and sometimes fear of being killed ("voodoo death"). "Roots," "spells," or "hexes" can be "put" or placed on other persons, causing a variety of emotional and psychological problems. The "hexed" person may even fear death until the "root" has been "taken off" (eliminated), usually through the work of a "root doctor" (a healer in this tradition), who can also be called on to bewitch an enemy. "Rootwork" is found in the southern United States among both African American and European American populations and in Caribbean societies. It is also known as *mal puesto* or *brujeria* in Latino societies.

sangue dormido ("sleeping blood") This syndrome is found among Portuguese Cape Verde Islanders (and immigrants from there to the United States) and includes pain, numbness, tremor, paralysis, convulsions, stroke, blindness, heart attack, infection, and miscarriage.

shenjing shuairuo ("neurasthenia") In China, a condition characterized by physical and mental fatigue, dizziness, headaches, other pains, concentration difficulties, sleep disturbance, and memory loss. Other symptoms include gastrointestinal problems, sexual dysfunction, irritability, excitability, and various signs suggesting disturbance of the autonomic nervous system. In many cases, the symptoms would meet the criteria for a DSM-IV Mood or Anxiety Disorder. This diagnosis is included in the *Chinese Classification of Mental Disorders,* Second Edition (CCMD-2).

shen-k'uei (Taiwan); **shenkui** (China) A Chinese folk label describing marked anxiety or panic symptoms with accompanying somatic complaints for which no physical cause can be demonstrated. Symptoms include dizziness, backache, fatigability, general weakness, insomnia, frequent dreams, and complaints of sexual dysfunction (such as premature ejaculation and impotence). Symptoms are attributed to excessive semen loss from frequent intercourse, masturbation, nocturnal emission, or passing of "white turbid urine" believed to contain semen. Excessive semen loss is feared because of the belief that it represents the loss of one's vital essence and can thereby be life threatening.

shin-byung A Korean folk label for a syndrome in which initial phases are characterized by anxiety and somatic complaints (general weakness, dizziness, fear, anorexia, insomnia, gastrointestinal problems), with subsequent dissociation and possession by ancestral spirits.

spell A trance state in which individuals "communicate" with deceased relatives or with spirits. At times this state is associated with brief periods of personality change. This culture-specific syndrome is seen among African Americans and European Americans from the southern United States. Spells are not considered to be medical events in the folk tradition, but may be misconstrued as psychotic episodes in clinical settings.

susto ("fright," or "soul loss") A folk illness prevalent among some Latinos in the United States and among people in Mexico, Central America, and South America. Susto is also referred to as *espanto, pasmo, tripa ida, perdida del alma,* or *chibih.* Susto is an illness attributed to a frightening event that causes the soul to leave the body and results in unhappiness and sickness. Individuals with susto also experience significant strains in key social roles. Symptoms may appear any time from days to years after the fright is experienced. It is believed that in extreme cases, susto may result in death. Typical symptoms include appetite disturbances, inadequate or excessive sleep, troubled sleep or dreams, feeling of sadness, lack of motivation to do anything, and feelings of low self-worth or dirtiness. Somatic symptoms accompanying susto include muscle aches and pains, headache, stomachache, and diarrhea. Ritual healings are focused on calling the soul back to the body and cleansing the person to restore bodily and spiritual balance. Different experiences of susto may be related to Major Depressive Disorder, Posttraumatic Stress Disorder, and Somatoform Disorders. Similar etiological beliefs and symptom configurations are found in many parts of the world.

taijin kyofusho A culturally distinctive phobia in Japan, in some ways resembling Social Phobia in DSM-IV. This syndrome refers to an individual's intense fear that his or her body, its parts or its functions, displease, embarrass, or are offensive to other people in appearance, odor, facial expressions, or movements. This syndrome is included in the official Japanese diagnostic system for mental disorders.

zar A general term applied in Ethiopia, Somalia, Egypt, Sudan, Iran, and other North African and Middle Eastern societies to the experience of spirits possessing an individual. Persons possessed by a spirit may experience dissociative episodes that may include shouting, laughing, hitting the head against a wall, singing, or weeping. Individuals may show apathy and withdrawal, refusing to eat or carry out daily tasks, or may develop a long-term relationship with the possessing spirit. Such behavior is not considered pathological locally.

APPENDIX D

NANDA-APPROVED NURSING DIAGNOSES FOR CLINICAL USE AND TESTING

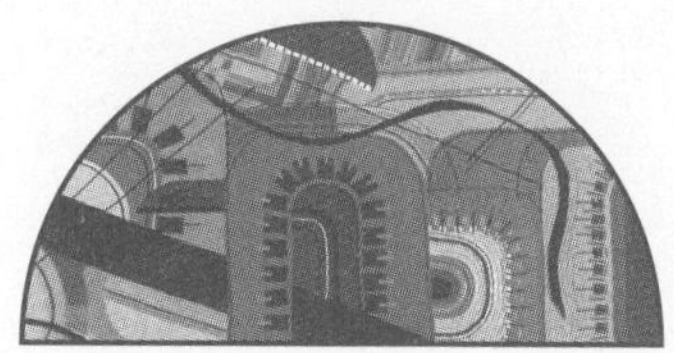

PATTERN 1: EXCHANGING

	1.1.2.1	Altered Nutrition: More than Body Requirements
	1.1.2.2	Altered Nutrition: Less than Body Requirements
	1.1.2.3	Altered Nutrition: Potential for More than Body Requirements
*	1.2.1.1	Risk for Infection
*	1.2.2.1	Risk for Altered Body Temperature
	1.2.2.2	Hypothermia
	1.2.2.3	Hyperthermia
	1.2.2.4	Ineffective Thermoregulation
	1.2.3.1	Dysreflexia
	1.3.1.1	Constipation
	1.3.1.1.1	Perceived Constipation
	1.3.1.1.2	Colonic Constipation
	1.3.1.2	Diarrhea
	1.3.1.3	Bowel Incontinence
	1.3.2	Altered Urinary Elimination
	1.3.2.1.1	Stress Incontinence
	1.3.2.1.2	Reflex Incontinence
	1.3.2.1.3	Urge Incontinence
	1.3.2.1.4	Functional Incontinence
	1.3.2.1.5	Total Incontinence
	1.3.2.2	Urinary Retention
	1.4.1.1	Altered (Specify Type) Tissue Perfusion (Renal, cerebral, cardiopulmonary, gastrointestinal, peripheral)
	1.4.1.2.1	Fluid Volume Excess
	1.4.1.2.2.1	Fluid Volume Deficit
*	1.4.1.2.2.2	Risk for Fluid Volume Deficit
	1.4.2.1	Decreased Cardiac Output
	1.5.1.1	Impaired Gas Exchange
	1.5.1.2	Ineffective Airway Clearance
	1.5.1.3	Ineffective Breathing Pattern
	1.5.1.3.1	Inability to Sustain Spontaneous Ventilation
	1.5.1.3.2	Dysfunctional Ventilatory Weaning Response (DVWR)
*	1.6.1	Risk for Injury
	1.6.1.1	Risk for Suffocation
*	1.6.1.2	Risk for Poisoning
*	1.6.1.3	Risk for Trauma
*	1.6.1.4	Risk for Aspiration
*	1.6.1.5	Risk for Disuse Syndrome
	1.6.2	Altered Protection
	1.6.2.1	Impaired Tissue Integrity
	1.6.2.1.1	Altered Oral Mucous Membrane
	1.6.2.1.2.1	Impaired Skin Integrity
*	1.6.2.1.2.2	Risk for Impaired Skin Integrity
#	1.7.1	Decreased Adaptive Capacity: Intracranial
#	1.8	Energy Field Disturbance

PATTERN 2: COMMUNICATING

	2.1.1.1	Impaired Verbal Communication

PATTERN 3: RELATING

	3.1.1	Impaired Social Interaction
	3.1.2	Social Isolation
#	3.1.3	Risk for Loneliness
	3.2.1	Altered Role Performance
	3.2.1.1.1	Altered Parenting
*	3.2.1.1.2	Risk for Altered Parenting
#	3.2.1.1.2.1	Risk for Altered Parent/Infant/Child Attachment
	3.2.1.2.1	Sexual Dysfunction
	3.2.2	Altered Family Processes
	3.2.2.1	Caregiver Role Strain
*	3.2.2.2	Risk for Caregiver Role Strain
#	3.2.2.3.1	Altered Family Process: Alcoholism
	3.2.3.1	Parental Role Conflict
	3.3	Altered Sexuality Patterns

PATTERN 4: VALUING

	4.1.1	Spiritual Distress (Distress of the Human Spirit)
#	4.2	Potential for Enhanced Spiritual Well-Being

PATTERN 5: CHOOSING

	5.1.1.1	Ineffective Individual Coping
	5.1.1.1.1	Impaired Adjustment
	5.1.1.1.2	Defensive Coping
	5.1.1.1.3	Ineffective Denial
	5.1.2.1.1	Ineffective Family Copying: Disabling
	5.1.2.1.2	Ineffective Family Coping: Compromised
	5.1.2.2	Family Coping: Potential for Growth
#	5.1.3.1	Potential for Enhanced Community Coping
#	5.1.3.2	Ineffective Community Coping

#New diagnoses added in 1994 classified at level 1.4 using new Criteria for Staging (see reference later in this book).
*Diagnoses with modified label terminology in 1994 (This change was recommended by the NANDA Taxonomy Committee and adopted to remain consistent with the ICD.)

Source: North American Nursing Diagnosis Association, *Nursing Diagnoses, Definitions and Classification 1995–1996*. 1994.

	5.2.1	Ineffective Management of Therapeutic Regimen (Individuals)
	5.2.1.1	Noncompliance (Specify)
#	5.2.2	Ineffective Management of Therapeutic Regimen: Families
#	5.2.3	Ineffective Management of Therapeutic Regimen: Community
#	5.2.4	Ineffective Management of Therapeutic Regimen: Individual
	5.3.1.1	Decisional Conflict (Specify)
	5.4	Health Seeking Behaviors (Specify)

PATTERN 6: MOVING

	6.1.1.1	Impaired Physical Mobility
*	6.1.1.1.1	Risk for Peripheral Neurovascular Dysfunction
#	6.1.1.1.2	Risk for Perioperative Positioning Injury
	6.1.1.2	Activity Intolerance
	6.1.1.2.1	Fatigue
*	6.1.1.3	Risk for Activity Intolerance
	6.2.1	Sleep Pattern Disturbance
	6.3.1.1	Diversional Activity Deficit
	6.4.1.1	Impaired Home Maintenance Management
	6.4.2	Altered Health Maintenance
	6.5.1	Feeding Self Care Deficit
	6.5.1.1	Impaired Swallowing
	6.5.1.2	Ineffective Breastfeeding
	6.5.1.2.1	Interrupted Breastfeeding
	6.5.1.3	Effective Breastfeeding
	6.5.1.4	Ineffective Infant Feeding Pattern
	6.5.2	Bathing/Hygiene Self Care Deficit
	6.5.3	Dressing/Grooming Self Care Deficit
	6.5.4	Toileting Self Care Deficit
	6.6	Altered Growth and Development
	6.7	Relocation Stress Syndrome
#	6.8.1	Risk for Disorganized Infant Behavior
#	6.8.2	Disorganized Infant Behavior
#	6.8.3	Potential for Enhanced Organized Infant Behavior

PATTERN 7: PERCEIVING

	7.1.1	Body Image Disturbance
	7.1.2	Self Esteem Disturbance
	7.1.2.1	Chronic Low Self Esteem
	7.1.2.2	Situational Low Self Esteem
	7.1.3	Personal Identity Disturbance
	7.2	Sensory/Perceptual Alterations (Specify) (Visual, Auditory, Kinesthetic, Gustatory, Tactile, Olfactory)
	7.2.1.1	Unilateral Neglect
	7.3.1	Hopelessness
	7.3.2	Powerlessness

PATTERN 8: KNOWING

	8.1.1	Knowledge Deficit (Specify)
#	8.2.1	Impaired Environmental Interpretation Syndrome
#	8.2.2	Acute Confusion
#	8.2.3	Chronic Confusion
	8.3	Altered Thought Processes
#	8.3.1	Impaired Memory

PATTERN 9: FEELING

	9.1.1	Pain
	9.1.1.1	Chronic Pain
	9.2.1.1	Dysfunctional Grieving
	9.2.1.2	Anticipatory Grieving
*	9.2.2	Risk for Violence: Self-Directed or Directed at Others
*	9.2.2.1	Risk for Self-Mutilation
	9.2.3	Post-Trauma Response
	9.2.3.1	Rape-Trauma Syndrome
	9.2.3.1.1	Rape-Trauma Syndrome: Compound Reaction
	9.2.3.1.2	Rape-Trauma Syndrome: Silent Reaction
	9.3.1	Anxiety
	9.3.2	Fear

APPENDIX E

DISCUSSION AND ANALYSIS POINTS FOR CRITICAL THINKING CHALLENGES

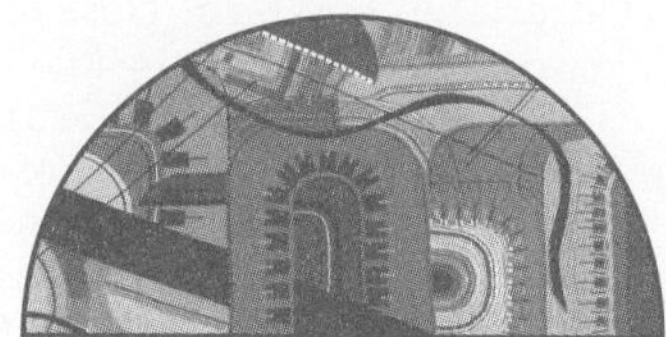

Chapter 1

Although well-intentioned, your classmate, your neighbor, and your family physician are all speaking from limited frames of reference. Today's psychiatric population has more complex problems than in the past, requiring today's psychiatric nurses to integrate the growing biologic base into their psychophysiologic clinical nursing practice. New medications have been developed, existing medications are being used in new ways, and new biologic therapies for psychiatric nurses have been introduced. What we know as traditional medical-surgical nursing skills are essential components of today's psychiatric nursing practice.

Although new medications and new biologic therapies may reduce or alleviate symptoms, it is important to remember that the maladaptive behavior of clients (because of their psychopathology) has negatively altered their relationships with others. Our ability to use ourselves therapeutically will help our clients repair these damaged relationships or form new meaningful ones.

Your classmate, your neighbor, and your family physician do not recognize the unparalled opportunities for your self-fulfillment in psychiatric–mental health nursing.

Chapter 2

This critical thinking challenge is an exercise in divergent thinking. Among the factors that contribute to the research-practice gap in psychiatric nursing are the following (you may think of additional ones that do not appear below):

- Most nursing theorists have developed grand theories with broad concepts like "self-care" and "health." Such theories do include issues relevant to psychiatric nursing practice but are so general that they do not specify researchable prescriptions for interventions.
- Most psychiatric theories have been generated based on case studies and have not been subjected to rigorous clinical trials for the effectiveness of specific treatment approaches.
- Only minimal research has been conducted, replicated, and reported on the client outcomes for one psychiatric intervention strategy versus another. Thus, with the exception of medications, clinicians have little basis for choosing one therapy over another (such as group or family therapy instead of individual therapy).
- Insurance coverage for psychiatric care has been so severely cut back that any approach requiring long-term residential care is generally impossible. Symptom management (usually through psychiatric medications) and crisis intervention have become the only economically feasible options for the majority of the population.

Directions for the future to bridge the theory-practice gap include:

- The need for "middle-range" psychiatric nursing clinical studies to evaluate the therapeutic and cost-effectiveness of alternative psychiatric nursing interventions in terms of client outcomes.
- The translation of theories of psychiatric disorders into treatment prescriptions.
- Clinical studies of innovative service delivery alternatives.
- Acceptance of an established nomenclature by psychiatric nursing for identifying psychiatric problems that fosters communication with the rest of the interdisciplinary mental health team as well as with third-party payers.
- Updating of psychiatric nurses' knowledge in the complex area of the psychobiology underlying major psychiatric disorders.

Chapter 3

Thinking critically about this challenge requires you to sort facts from opinion. Facts characterizing contemporary psychiatric care indeed include short hospital stays, cost containment, quick assessments, and cost effective interventions that focus on symptom management often in the form of biologic treatment (medications). Another fact is the explosion of new research-based knowledge about the biology of psychiatric disorders after decades of emphasis on psychodynamic and interpersonal explanations. However, to neatly equate psychobiologic variables such as family history/heritability, chronobiologic rhythms, neurotransmitter disturbances, and brain structure abnormalities with a packaged care plan based on a medical model is shortsighted at best. Contemporary conditions require competence in clinicians and effectiveness in interventions. Both can be achieved when psychiatric nurses conduct thorough biopsychosocial assessments and plan individualized care. When psychobiology synthesizes traditional psychologic knowledge and holistic psychiatric nursing care it is better able to meet the unique needs of each client. To argue otherwise is a matter of opinion reflecting the response to a paradigm shift that challenges psychiatric nurses to become comfortable with a new, complex, and possibly unfamiliar body of research knowledge. Client assessments that include psychobiologic factors will lead to improved communication, more astute diagnoses, better suited treatment plans, and improved client outcomes.

Chapter 4

Both the man and the woman were in the state of anxiety known as panic. Not all those in panic behave alike. The man's behavior put him in danger of injury in case the car exploded. The woman's behavior caused her physical injury. Neither person was able to think logically or make effective decisions.

Be cautious also about gender stereotyping. Control behaviors may be seen as masculine and appropriate. Loss of control, as in the hysteria the woman demonstrated, is often perceived as a feminine, helpless, inappropriate behavior. The truth is, both people experienced intense terror. Neither behavior was purposeful.

Chapter 5

Clients in clinical settings reflect a subgroup that may not represent all individuals with mental disorders in the general population. Those seeking treatment tend to have more chronic, more severe, and a greater number of mental disorders. The majority of individuals with mental disorders never seek treatment. Three levels of prevention (primary, secondary, and tertiary) may serve as a framework as you learn to develop mental health prevention strategies. Nursing assessment needs to address a client's cultural and ethnic background which may influence the experience, expression, reporting, and evaluation of psychiatric disorders.

Chapter 6

At issue here is one of the most perplexing of all clinical psychiatric nursing dilemmas: how to predict the potential for dangerousness in a client. Despite the lack of accepted research indicators in this area, clinical reasoning mandates that the psychiatric nurse report and document evidence of dangerousness, put into effect all measures that are feasible, and communicate problems such as insufficient staff to supervisors and the client's physician. Sometimes clients can be transferred to locked units where higher levels of observation are possible. Sometimes family members can be recruited to "sit with and monitor" the client. Sometimes hospitals refer to or provide "sitters" when "eyes-on" (a staff member can see the client at all times) and "hands-reach" (a staff member can physically restrain a client at all times) levels of observation are indicated. Be aware of the options.

Chapter 7

It is important to recognize that the facilitative communication skills described in this chapter are given as guidelines. You can make them your own by translating them into language you are more comfortable with, so that the "fit" with your personal style is more congruent. Some students find that role playing with classmates helps. You may do this independently or suggest to your instructor that time for role playing be included in preparation for this clinical experience. Discussing your fears and concerns with others, including your instructor, will help minimize your fears, bringing them to a more manageable level.

Chapter 8

A thorough suicide assessment must include the self-report of the client *and* consider the background and demographic data from the client's history that research has linked to higher suicide risks. This is particularly crucial when the client has psychotic symptoms. Motivations for suicide are far-ranging and not limited to despair. This particular client denies suicide ideation and intent but presents with a classic background from demographics to diagnosis associated with suicide in retrospective studies.

Among recommendations for "admission orders" for any client who may be depressed, anxious, and psychotic; who has a history of past lethal suicidal attempts; and who meets the demographic profile include locked unit, if possible; room assignment close to nurses' station; close level of observation for at least the first 72 hours, with careful charting to note any changes in client behavior that suggest the wisdom of eyes-on or arm's-reach level of observation, and customary hospital policy regarding removal of dangerous possessions. There is a fine line to be drawn between stripping a client of all personal possessions that could be dangerous (belts, shoelaces, bras, etc.) and making client safety a first priority. Only rigorous assessment and responsible observation can inform the psychiatric nurse's judgment on these issues.

Chapter 9

Moral therapy values and milieu therapy techniques have influenced current thinking about the therapeutic capacity of the treatment environment. Yet these values and interventions reflect an era when clients were maintained, sometimes for years, in institutional settings and few pharmacologic agents were available. Efforts to control the spiraling costs of mental health inpatient care and the availability of symptom-specific psychotropic agents have drastically reduced the length of inpatient treatment. In turn, the therapeutic nature of the inpatient treatment environment has evolved to emphasize its importance in promoting safety and security, achieving the rapid reduction of acute symptoms, and enhancing client functioning in order to return to the community. While long-term maintenance and intervention based solely on interpersonal relationships contrast with current brief hospitalizations and the use of psychotropic medications, the therapeutic capacity of the environment and value for the humanity of the client transcend the changes in setting and medical intervention.

Chapter 10

Managed care for psychiatric clients raises main ethical concerns: client autonomy, encroachment on the therapeutic relationship between clinician and client, and client responsibility.

At issue with respect to client autonomy is that managed care denies clients the right to choose treatment (for example, inpatient versus outpatient treatment for substance abuse rehabilitation). Ethical reasoning requires that the following question be considered: What restrictions on client autonomy of choice are proper, and with what justification? One example of an ethically valid reason for limiting autonomy is if a client's mental competence is sufficiently impaired. Another is if a client is dangerous to self or others.

At issue in the clinician-client relationship dilemma is that financial considerations inherent in the purpose of managed care will contaminate the judgment of the person making treatment decisions. Ethical reasoning requires that the following question be asked: What is the proper relationship between the psychiatric nurse, the managed care agent, and the client? Some authorities have addressed this ethical dilemma by reaffirming the obligations inherent in the therapeutic nurse-client relationship, emphasizing that some balance must be sought with the fiscal concerns of managed care (see Olsen 1994 for a complete discussion).

With respect to client responsibility, ethical reasoning requires that the following question be asked: Is it ever proper to deny, curtail, or alter access to treatment based on client noncompliance? Experts suggest that resolution of this dilemma rests not with a *blaming the victim* approach but rather with reframing the question to this one: Who has been unable to benefit from treatment?

Clearly, mental health professionals must continue to examine managed care in view of complex client circumstances and bioethical principles.

Chapter 11

The core of this question relates to the dignity of each client, even if the client does not want to cooperate. The nurse must make every attempt to listen to the client in order to understand the client's view. The nurse must be honest in sharing the choices that are within the law. The nurse must not mislead the client.

A second issue is the determination of competency. Each state varies in the specific guidelines used to determine competency. The nurse, in cooperation with the mental health team, must determine if the assessment of the client suggests that the client is sufficiently competent to refuse treatment. If so, the nurse must act to inform the client of the potential effects of the choices and what the professional staff can and cannot do in the light of the client's refusal. It is preferable that this information be given verbally and in writing. Conversely, if the assessment suggests that the client is not competent to make decisions, all reasonable means must be taken in order to protect the client. This might begin with actions aimed at forcing the client to be in treatment. However, ongoing assessment must occur. The right to freedom can only be lost while the client is not competent.

A third issue is the nurse's ability to balance the desire to help, the duty to act, and the right of client refusal and remain able to work in the field. Supervision may be required to help nurses know when to let go of certain issues.

Chapter 12

The relevant ethical principle in this challenge is respect for people. The principle concerns autonomy and affirms that individuals have the right to determine a course of action. Families report that physicians are quick to suggest institutionalization when they describe their fatigue or difficulties with AD symptoms and behaviors. Such a pat recommendation without *listening* carefully to the family—assessing their strengths and weaknesses, successes and failures in caregiving—does not work. Instead, family members become angry at the physician; communication is closed down rather than opened up. Institutionalizing a family member is a huge decision that is accompanied by much grief and, at times, family discord. Sensitivity to the salient issues, *listening* to families and *supporting* them to do *what is best for them,* is critical to a successful decision.

Chapter 13

Crack mothers present professionals with what Kearney et al. (1994) have called a moral ambiguity. For many, it is never justified to risk damaging a child to satisfy a selfish need. Yet in Kearney's research, she found that the world of the addicted mothers she interviewed was neither amoral nor asocial. They had, instead, a deep sense of duty regarding the care of their children, a strong mothering ethic, and described their children as the center of their world. The first step in offering effective treatment for Billie and mothers like her is to conquer our own prejudicial attitudes. Addicts who continue to use often have lost control and cannot quit without help even when they desire to do so. A critical thinking approach to treatment would address several other considerations in this story:

- Give the client clear and full assurance that to the extent possible, withdrawal and craving suffering will be medically managed.
- Look for strategies to avoid punitive removal of children from mothers during drug treatment and instead develop ways to support and enhance the woman's mothering role. Kearney urges the establishment of treatment settings for addicted women where they could be with their children.
- Become a resource for locating 12-step self-help groups (AA, NA, CA) that deviate from the norm of "white men who pray the Our Father." Look for women's groups. Let clients know that while certain traditions from AA are consistent across groups, there are many variations, including prayers to "Our Mother."
- Address social problems such as homelessness, joblessness, and poverty. Often drugs have been the only solace or escape from a dead-end life situation.
- Deal empathically with the guilt, shame, and stigma that go along with being a "crack mother."
- Educate your team members about research such as the study by nurse scientist Kearney from which these guidelines emerged.

Chapter 14

Historically, people with schizophrenia were treated for long periods of time in the protected environments of large state psychiatric hospitals. Unfortunately, these environments often caused problems that paralleled and even surpassed the illness difficulties. Decline in social skills, interest in life activities, and the basic capacity to care for oneself were common. Currently, the optimal environment is thought to be one that is stimulating but not overly stressful, where the person with schizophrenia self-determines activities and involvements, but has access to support for managing the illness.

Chapter 15

If clients are committed and are legal wards of relatives or the state, they lose many of their rights. Others, however, are voluntarily admitted, and the level to which they are allowed to make decisions regarding their own care becomes an ethical decision rather than a legal one. The extent to which severely ill psychiatric clients should be allowed or encouraged to collaborate as equal members of the health care team in planning their own care is a highly charged issue. There are not right or wrong answers. Identify the steps of the ethical decision-making process you are using as you debate this critical thinking challenge. This will prevent the debate from deteriorating into a mere sharing of opinions and emotionally based arguments. Explore how a philosophy of care can be translated into hospital policy.

Chapter 16

Imagine a person who has so much anxiety or so much pain that he or she develops strange or bizarre symptoms. For example, some individuals who were abused as children develop separate identities as a mechanism for survival. As you meet people with these disorders during your professional career, maintain a nonjudgmental attitude. Keep in mind that psychogenic pain is just as real as pain with organic etiologies. Caregivers' skepticism and doubt interfere with the healing process.

Chapter 17

The issue is one of power and control. Professional staff members often believe that they "know what is best" for clients without consulting with them. The United States is a sex-negative culture, and it is difficult to discuss sexual matters with our own partners, let alone with our clients. When people are in need of mental health care, we often consider them to be asexual throughout the treatment time. We often label them as "perverted" if they express the need for sexual interaction with their partner.

Chapter 18

This issue involves the ethical responsibility of nurses to educate the public about a significant health problem. It also addresses nursing's scope of practice. Parents and teachers should be taught about the relationship between eating and feeding patterns and stages of growth and development, and what to expect in each stage. Gymnastic and wrestling coaches and ballet teachers should engage in discussions with parents about the "winning at any cost" philosophy and the negative impact this has on the self-esteem of young people. As you reflect on your own eating attitudes and behaviors, realize that studying this content will probably cause you to question your own attitudes. Doubts you have about your own body size and shape may emerge, and this is expected.

Chapter 19

The issue is one of dealing with apparently conflicting subjective and objective data. Students may initially frame this issue in black-and-white terms; either what the client says is most important, or the client's view cannot be trusted when there is objective evidence to the contrary. The challenge is to help broaden your thinking about possibilities. Interpretations may include but are not limited to these: quantity of sleep and quality of sleep are not the same; perceptions of whether or not one is sleeping vary and are essentially learned second-hand because sleep is a subjective experience; there is debate even among sleep specialists as to whether stage 1 sleep as measured in polysomnography is really sleep or not.

Chapter 20

The issues are manipulation, the desire for special consideration, implied threats, and splitting of work staff. The request of the client involves dishonesty and noncompliance with unit policy. This behavior has the potential for diminishing morale on a nursing unit and ultimately compromising care. The anger of the client and her implied threats may be intimidating to the new employee. The request places you in an ethical dilemma. If you agree to the request, your integrity is also compromised. A suitable solution to this incident would be the use of the SET (support, empathy, truth) system of assertive communication, stating your understanding of the client's request while setting limits with kind firmness. An example of the "S" or support statement would be, "I am concerned about how you are feeling." The "E" or empathy segment acknowledges her desire to be with her boyfriend. An example of an empathy statement would be, "It is a difficult feeling to imagine not being with him when you want to be." The "T" or truth statement represents reality and responsibility. An example would be, "This is what I can do to get you in touch with the team. What do you plan to do to work this out?" All three stages of the SET communication system should be used, even though the client may not hear or integrate all of them (Kreisman, Strauss, 1989).

Chapter 21

The relative value that a nurse places on independence or on long-term support may be a question of individual moral beliefs. However, the goal of professional nursing care is to allow the client to achieve his or her own desired level of self-care and autonomy. It becomes a matter of clinical practice and not of individual belief when the nurse develops a plan of care that helps the client to achieve goals for some level of autonomous or independent functioning. This plan may involve extensive commitment and support since the nurse provides the kinds of environmental resources that make more independent living a possibility. Frequently the goal of increased autonomy and the goal of providing supports are compatible rather than in opposition. Environmental resources and interpersonal assistance enhance individual function. Further, from a rehabilitation perspective, these resources are not withdrawn when function improves, but rather maintained to continue to maintain that level of function.

Chapter 22

Nurses have traditionally viewed disease as caused by many factors: biologic, psychologic, social, and environmental. An individual's susceptibility to illness is mediated by these and other factors that are not always fully understood by the client or the clinician. Moreover, all the factors that contribute to disease are perceived and given meaning by the client (and the clinician) in ways that affect the diagnosis, progression, and treatment of the disease. For example, a client with chronic fatigue may believe that her illness is biologically based and seek biologic interventions to relieve her symptoms. The clinician she consults, however, may view her condition as stemming from depression and recommend an antidepressant and psychotherapy. Unless both client and clinician reach consensus on the meaning of the condition, its diagnosis, treatment, and outcome may be negatively affected.

Very often clients resist considering the possibility that psychologic factors may have contributed to their physical illness. However, psychologic factors contribute in some way to almost all physical illness and disease causation. Nurses must assess clients' perceptions about illness and, applying knowledge from the biopsychosocial sciences, help them understand their condition, identify and strengthen coping skills, and engage in self-care.

Chapter 23

The issue is whether you believe that men are dominant by nature and women are subordinate by nature. The argument is one of biology versus social learning and cultural values. Ask yourself: Why is it that men, in American culture, are very resistant to giving up their birth name and adopting their wife's name? In other cultures, women keep their own name after marriage, and there is a cultural system for naming the children. What is the message when women earn significantly more than their male partners?

Under what conditions is violence tolerable and even appropriate? Our institutions cannot intervene to protect people from beatings, imprisonment, starvation, rape, and murder within the home, unless these acts are explicitly prohibited by law.

Chapter 24

The practice of controlling clothing only gives staff members a false sense of security and may in fact keep them from determining the appropriate level of observation or containment for the client. Besides being of little clinical value, the practice is dehumanizing. When one client was asked about the practice, he stated "Do you think if I'm going to go kill myself I would worry if I had shoes on?"

This issue also speaks to the staff's need to control a client whose behavior is making them anxious. It is important for staff members and students to understand that some of the behaviors they use to control clients relieve the staff's own anxiety and have little to do with helping clients manage their suicidal impulses or ideas. Clients have often stated that the staff members who have been most helpful to them are those who have encouraged them to find ways to assume greater control and more responsibility over their own lives.

Chapter 25

Such a policy is unlikely to be an incentive to substance-abusing clients to stop using, and is more likely to be a barrier to their seeking necessary mental health care. As well as having many of the same reasons for using drugs or alcohol as anyone else, people with mental disorders may also use substances to self-medicate such symptoms as anxiety, sleeplessness, and auditory hallucinations. Thus, mental health care that addresses some of these special needs is a particularly important component of any plan to treat substance abuse.

Although abstinence may be a desirable goal of treatment, research and clinical experience indicate that achieving stable abstinence may be a long-term process, with many relapses along the way. Even if mentally ill clients are still using, helping them find less harmful patterns of substance use is an important nursing intervention.

Staff in mental health clinics may have reasons to be reluctant to work with dual diagnosis clients. Educational programs for mental health care professionals often fail to include content on substance abuse, and the placement of substance abuse treatment outside the mainstream of mental health care means that many caregivers have had little exposure to methods of working with substance-abusing clients.

In addition, clients with psychiatric/substance abuse comorbidity can be difficult to work with. Research indicates that such clients are more likely to manifest problematic behaviors, such as assaultiveness and hostility, and are less likely to comply with treatment. Since relapses are common in recovery from substance abuse, and because homelessness, legal problems, and poor self-care are also common sequelae of substance abuse in mentally ill clients, the enormity of their problems can make them frustrating for clinicians who hope to see immediate improvement.

Chapter 26

Codependence is very active in this colleague. She takes control by stepping in to do others' work. She expects others to be perfect and denies the problems that are apparent to a new staff member by describing the ward as "well run." Martyr behavior is exhibited by the "I don't get credit but I'll still do it" comments.

Healthy responses to codependence are imperative. When something happens that does not allow you to be an adult and take care of circumstances occurring in your career, certain steps must be taken. It takes two dysfunctional people to keep a codependent relationship alive. If one refuses to allow it and defines more functional approaches, the relationship can be turned into a healthier one.

In deciding to be healthy in this relationship, first recognize that your goal is not to remove codependence from your colleague's interactions. Having that as your goal is taking responsibility for another adult, which is also codependent. Your goal is to communicate clearly that adult interactions between you and your colleague are to occur. Use statements such as, "I know I have to learn how to do this efficiently. Why don't you tell me what you would do, and I'll incorporate my own methods and see if the result suits me," or "Once I do a few of these on my own, I'll be pretty good at it," or "I appreciate your interest in how I'm doing, but I like to do things on my own once I have the information necessary to do it." These statements will define your personal boundaries, help you anticipate situations, and respond without criticism.

Chapter 27

Approximately 25% of the AIDS cases in the United States occur among heterosexual injection drug users (IDUs). In addition, HIV occurs in those whose sole risk factor is having an IDU sex partner. More than half of pediatric AIDS cases are attributed to HIV transmission from mothers who were IDUs themselves or who engaged in sexual activity with IDUs. Successful prevention of the further spread of HIV in this population is crucial.

Review the information on needle and syringe programs earlier in the chapter. Share the results of the research studies with others. Above all, remember that studies have not shown that needle and syringe exchange programs stimulate illicit drug injection. Needle and syringe exchange programs keep infected drug paraphernalia off the streets, thus promoting community safety.

Communities should not view needle and syringe exchange programs as a substitute for a comprehensive approach to drug abuse treatment and prevention or as the ultimate HIV prevention strategy. The process of ethical reasoning in Chapter 10 will help you sort out your feelings about this issue.

Chapter 28

The primary issue involves how you as a nursing student perceive and react to initial client behaviors. Feelings of confusion, anger, discouragement, and failure may accompany work with a difficult client, especially when this is the first such experience. Use your instructor as a clinical supervisor to explore your personal feelings and perceptions, understand how the client's offensive behaviors may serve the client, and continue to focus on the goals, tasks, and interventions in the orientation phase of one-to-one relationships, as discussed in the chapter.

Chapter 29

Learning how to manage your stress will facilitate your personal and professional renewal. The stress-management exercises in this chapter, especially the breathing, meditation, and visualization exercises, will help you connect with your spirit. Try them out, one at a time, and incorporate them into your life. Find those that you enjoy, and use them to maintain balance in body, mind, and spirit.

Chapter 30

The issues are: how to accurately assess and effectively intervene with this man in crisis; what cultural factors may be involved in the assessment and treatment of this client; and how cultural and personal factors of the nurse will affect the client's care. The nurse has difficulty with her client's expression of his own distress, including crying. It is likely that her reluctance to accept his crying will render her ineffective in being able to help him learn new coping mechanisms and will make it difficult for her to understand his current problems.

The fact that the man has returned several times may indicate either an unmet need or a maladaptive response to prior crisis or trauma. A complete assessment will be needed to understand exactly what the situation is and who is in the best position to work with him. Distancing oneself from the individual may result in incomplete or inaccurate assessment and lead to inaccurate attention to his problems and perpetuation of the cycle. In addition, the nurse's behavior is intended to distance herself from the client as a means of managing her own anxiety. While this may help her feel less threatened, it could have a disastrous effect on the client.

Clients are generally very attuned to the attitudes and feelings of those who provide assistance. Asking for help is often difficult for most adults who pride themselves on being accomplished at self-care. Clients are often sensitive to the nurse's condescension or disgust and may feel rejected, all of which could lead to an ineffective, nonsupportive interaction between nurse and client. Self-awareness of your own biases and cultural values (men should be strong; men should not cry) will help avoid errors that may harm the client. Clients need to be able to have someone who can understand their point of view and help them find some ways to assume more responsibility and control over their own lives.

Chapter 31

Group therapy can be helpful to Mark for several reasons, but perhaps the primary reason is that one of the curative factors in interactional group therapy is the corrective recapitulation of the primary family group. Group members are influenced by their history. They usually perceive the behavior of other members and the leader as like that of their siblings and parents. The responses of group members and the leader offer the client the opportunity to review and correctively relive early family conflicts and growth-inhibiting relationships. The client has the opportunity to test out other ways of being in a safe setting. It is possible for Mark to transfer these new learnings to future interactions with his siblings and his parents, and other people important to him.

Chapter 32

Anger, embarrassment, reluctance, and feeling overwhelmed are common experiences for family members. Families often don't have the skills, resources, or training to deal with the behavioral problems, role changes, financial obligations, and social stigma that accompany mental illness.

You can be helpful by assisting the family in accessing available community services such as day care programs, respite care, and organizations such as the National Alliance for the Mentally Ill (NAMI). Support groups and short-term therapy may be needed.

Providing the family with factual, honest information about Mark's diagnosis, medications, treatment plan, and prognosis will help them understand Mark's illness. Don't be reluctant to give practical advice and provide emotional support. Families dealing with the burden of mental illness need information and support from mental health care professionals.

Remember that the family is a system. Respect the ability of family members to share their experience and information with you and with other staff. Incorporate them into the discharge planning and treatment team. Provide for regular communication with the family.

Become politically active and lobby for changes in the mental health system. Join NAMI and learn how families help each other. And then, reach out to your clients' families.

Chapter 33

There are legitimate concerns when a client with a violent history and new (if any) coping mechanisms starts to show strong feelings. In this circumstance, the nurse was trying to anticipate the client's behavior. She had special contact with his past problems and wanted to head off an escalation. However, the timing is very important when you are evaluating a client's coping. The client had not shown undue anger. It is OK to become angry and to want to express it. One of the goals for this client may very well be learning how to express his anger in a variety of ways. The nurse acted too soon and may have used the anxiolytic as a restraining device to rein in strong feelings. Medication is an adjunct to learning; it does not teach people how to handle stress and anger. It helps reduce the power and intensity of feelings. Using medication in this circumstance may have only served to show the client that he is distrusted and that he cannot, and likely will not be able to, control himself. This is not the best message to send to a struggling psychiatric client.

Chapter 34

The issue here is one of social control in psychiatry. Use of the dangerousness criterion as the basis for treatment decisions pits the rights of individual clients against the rights of the group to safety. The inaccuracy of a dangerousness decision makes it particularly difficult to justify its use, yet when we try to think of other standards as the basis for treatment decisions, they, too, are complex. As a group, the violent mentally ill represent a particularly vulnerable population who are easily stigmatized. Those who care for them must pay special attention to the moral-ethical questions raised by the tension between an individual's right to liberty and the right of the group to safety.

Chapter 35

Many parties have a stake in changing the health care system or keeping it the same. The issue confronted in this critical thinking challenge is to comprehend all of the various interests and how changing the system might affect them. Change in any system involves risk, and in changing the health care delivery system we are talking about redistributing economic risk—that is, who pays for those who cannot pay and what services insured clients may expect when someone else pays all or part of the premium.

Nursing is directly confronted by virtually every change to the system that is proposed or implemented. As positions are redefined and move from inpatient to outpatient settings, nurses will gain or lose employment and scope of professional responsibility. As a profession, nursing will be better off if it can foresee new roles and occupy them.

Chapter 36

There are a number of important factors for consideration here. In general, mental health problems in children should no longer be viewed as resulting from *either* nature *or* nurture deficits. For most conditions, it is the delicate interaction between the two that we must address. However, the relative influence of the environment versus genetic or biologic factors depends on the specific disorder. For example, there is little evidence to suggest that reactive attachment disorder has any biologic basis, but the child's biologic vulnerability can put her at greater risk from the gross pathologic care that is thought to cause an attachment disorder. In contrast, pervasive developmental disorders appear to be strongly influenced by biologic dysfunction in the child, but an intrusive, overstimulating parent can increase symptoms experienced by a child with autism.

The family's role in a child's mental illness should never be assumed. A combination of careful observation of family interaction, medical and psychologic testing of the child, and interviews of all family members will eventually produce a better understanding of the etiology of each child's unique constellation of problems. If we make assumptions that either biology or the family are the sole or primary cause without a careful assessment, we may target our interventions inappropriately and actually increase the problems that a child and family are facing.

Chapter 37

Of the more than 300 clinics associated with elementary, junior high, and senior high schools, only 12% of them provide reproductive health services, and only a small proportion actually dispense contraceptive devices on site. Moreover, surveys indicate that providing such services does not lead to an increase in sexual activity. However, these services do provide strong programs that emphasize the prevention of pregnancy and HIV/AIDS. In addition, these clinics offer a wider variety of services, including well-child care, immunizations, treatment of acute illness and accidents, management of mental health counseling, nutrition counseling, substance abuse programs, and general health education. Moreover, school clinics are an ideal place in which to reach disadvantaged families who may not avail themselves of other community programs or have the financial means for health maintenance. Nurses in these clinics should get to know the adolescents in the school, identify those at risk, and intervene early with potentially self-destructive behaviors. Comprehensive health care for adolescents is a basic element for the social development of young people into adults. This goal affects not only the ultimate well-being of a generation of individuals but the future of the larger society.

Chapter 38

Your client has some difficulty with his memory, but has additional symptoms that should be addressed through a thorough physical examination. The areas that should be assessed include:

- Changes in physical status—what other physical complaints may he have? He already has revealed that he has an appetite loss and is tired.
- Changes in cognition—is his memory decreased or is he simply not interested in his surroundings, so that he appears unable to concentrate?
- Recent losses—the loss of his brother and his retirement within the last year provide a beginning for the assessment of any other losses in his life. Remember that this loss in itself may be very significant since he lost both so recently.
- Medications—there have been no questions related to any medications that he might be taking. Is he taking anything over-the-counter? Something for sleep? Has he had a cold and taken antihistamines? Prescription medications—either his own or from his wife? Elders often share their medications, so he may have taken someone else's prescriptions. Does he have any chronic illnesses for which he is receiving medication?
- Chronic diseases—does he have any illnesses related to his work? Chronic back pain? Joint difficulties? Other chronic ailments related to lifting and stooping? What are his fluid and electrolytes like if he has not been eating?

Deal directly with your client and get a thorough history. Encourage him to talk about what it was like to work and compare that to how he feels now. Once you have obtained a history and physical from him, with his permission interview his wife for additional information.

GLOSSARY

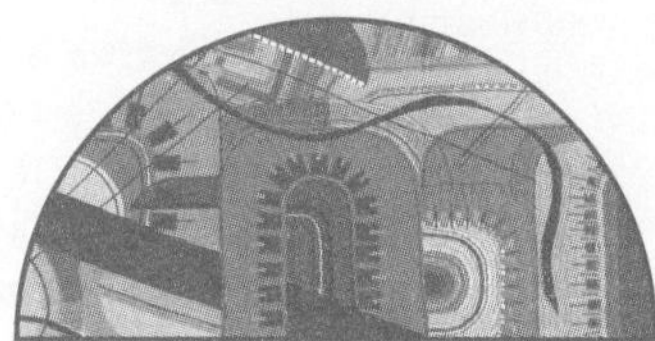

Abreaction The reliving of past events and their related feelings through play or imagery.

Abstinence Cessation of any use of non-prescribed psychoactive substances.

Abuse Misuse of a drug that can be discontinued at will.

Acquaintance (or date) rape Rape by an acquaintance, friend, lover, boyfriend, or husband.

Acquired immune deficiency syndrome (AIDS) A contagious and fatal condition of immune system depression for which there is no known cure.

Acting out Term used to describe a recreation of the client's life experiences and relationships with significant others with resultant unresolved conflicts. Acting out may include, but is not limited to, destructive actions.

Action potential The electrical activity developed in a nerve or muscle cell during activity. The electrical activity signals the vesicles to release neurotransmitters.

Active euthanasia *See Euthanasia*

Active listening Paying undivided attention to what the client says and does.

Active progressive relaxation Purposeful muscle tensing followed by a conscious relaxing of the muscles.

Acute stress disorder An anxiety disorder characterized by development of anxiety, dissociative, or other symptoms within one month after exposure to a traumatic event.

Addiction Term synonymous with substance dependence.

Adjustment disorder Maladaptive reaction to an identifiable psychological stressor.

Adult children of alcoholics (ACoA) Adults who suffer difficulties and problems in their adult life as a result of having an alcoholic parent, parents, or guardian. Adult children of alcoholics were often deprived of a nurturing parent in their formative years. They are at increased risk for developing alcoholism themselves.

Adult ego state In transactional analysis theory, the ego state responsible for the objective appraisal of reality and the capacity to process data.

Advocacy The component of community mental health practice that focuses on generating and maintaining resources for mental health consumers.

Affect An outward manifestation of a person's feelings or emotions in response to persons or events, sometimes referred to as emotional "climate."

Affection need The interpersonal need to establish and maintain a satisfactory relation between self and other people.

Aggression Refers to a broad range of behaviors, including conduct necessary for success and creativity, as well as destructive behaviors characterized, in the extreme, by violence.

Agnosia Loss of sensory ability to recognize objects.

Agoraphobia A type of anxiety disorder characterized by extreme anxiety about, or avoidance of, places or situations from which escape might be difficult or embarrassing, or in which help may not be available if panic symptoms should occur.

Agraphia Inability to express thoughts in writing.

Akathisia One of the classes of side effects caused by neuroleptic drugs. Signs of this condition include motor restlessness, an urge to pace, a need to shift weight, or an inability to stand or sit still.

Akinesia Partial or complete loss of muscle movement; characterized by slowed movement, shuffling gait, absence of spontaneous muscle movement, and lifeless appearance; responds to antiparkinsonian agents.

Al-Anon A support group for spouses and parents of alcoholics.

Al-Ateen A support group for teenage children of alcoholics.

Alcohol withdrawal syndrome The constellation of physiologic and behavioral symptoms that occurs when an addicted individual stops drinking.

Alcoholics Anonymous (AA) A self-help organization that uses a twelve-step program to assist alcoholics in achieving and maintaining sobriety.

Alexia Inability to understand written language.

Alter An occurrence in dissociative identity disorder; an alter is a separate identity completely distinct from the host personality. Each alter performs different functions and stores different memories and feelings.

Alternate nostril breathing A general relaxation exercise that helps a person reduce tension and sinus headaches by inhaling and exhaling through alternate nostrils one at a time.

Alzheimer's disease A chronic progressive disorder that is the major cause of degenerative dementia in the United States. With the progression of the condition, there is often memory and judgment loss, loss of interest, and carelessness. The cause of the disease is unknown, and there is no known cure. Diagnosis is based on changes in the brain plaques and neurofibrillary tangles on autopsy.

Ambivalence Simultaneous conflicting feelings or attitudes towards a person, object, conflict or desire.

Amnestic disorder A category of cognitive disorders in which relatively selected areas of cognition (short- and long-term memory) are impaired.

Amotivation syndrome Confusion, declining performance, and difficulty finishing tasks associated with frequent marijuana use.

Anergdola Brain structure associated with strong emotions—rage, fear, elation, which helps pattern behavioral responses appropriate to the occasion.

Anergy Decrease in or absence of energy; profound fatigue.

Anger rape Rape distinguished by physical violence and cruelty to the victim. The ability to injure, traumatize, and shame the victim provides the rapist with an outlet for rage and temporary relief from turmoil.

Anhedonia The absence of pleasure normally derived from participation in activities, sports, and interpersonal relationships.

Anomia Difficulty in finding words.

Anorexia nervosa Refusal to maintain a minimally normal body weight, intense fear of gaining weight, and significant disturbance of perception of body shape or size.

Anterograde amnesia Amnesia for short-term memories; remote memories remain intact. Present in blackouts, a symptom of alcoholism.

Anticholinergic side effects Side effects caused by the use of neuroleptic medications, including symptoms such as dry mouth, constipation, urinary retention, blurred vision, and dry mucous membranes.

Antidepressant medications Psychopharmacologic preparations used to treat symptoms of depression and depressive equivalents.

Antimanic medications Medications used in the treatment of mania or a cluster of symptoms such as exalted feelings, delusions of grandeur, elevation of mood, psychomotor overactivity, and an overproduction of ideas. The main antimania medication is lithium carbonate; however, other medications have been used as alternatives, or adjunct therapy such as haloperidol and carbamazepine.

Antipsychotic medications Psychopharmacologic preparations used to treat symptoms of disintegrated thought, perception, and affect; also called neuroleptics, they include the following classes: phenothiazine, thioxanthene, butyrophenone, dihydroindolene, dibenzoxazepine.

Antisocial personality disorder A personality disorder with the essential feature of a pattern of disregard for and violation of the rights of others beginning at 15 years of age.

Anxiety Nonspecific, unpleasant feeling of apprehension and discomfort that can be communicated interpersonally and that prompts the person to take some action to seek relief.

Anxiety disorder A maladaptive coping pattern in which anxiety is the predominant characteristic.

Anxiolytic medications Psychopharmacologic preparations used in the abatement of anxiety-related symptoms. Drug classes in this group include benzodiazepines, beta-blockers, antihistamines, sedatives with hypnotic effects, and propanedides.

Anxious-fearful A category of personality disorders that includes avoidant, dependent and compulsive disorders.

Aphasia Loss of language ability.

Apraxia Loss of purposeful movement without loss of muscle power or coordination in general.

Asperger's disease A pervasive developmental disorder involving severe problems in the quality of a child's social interaction, as well as restricted, repetitive behavior.

Assault A legal (rather than clinical) term, applying to behavior categorized as simple assault, assault and battery, or aggravated assault.

Assertive behavior Asking for what one wants or acting to get what one wants in a way that respects the other person.

Athetoid Involuntary movements that are slow, writhing, snakelike, and irregular.

Attention deficit hyperactivity disorder A disorder involving inattention to the surrounding environment and/or hyperactivity/impulsiveness.

Autistic disorder A pervasive developmental disorder which involves severe problems in the quality of social interaction, delays in language and cognitive development, and a restricted repertoire of interests or behaviors.

Autogenic training A systematic training program of structured exercises to reduce stress-related conditions, modify the reaction to pain, and reduce or eliminate stress disorders.

Autonomic nervous system The system of nerves that regulates involuntary bodily processes, i.e. blood pressure, heartbeat, breathing.

Avoidant personality disorder A personality disorder with the essential feature of a pervasive pattern of social inhibition, feelings of inadequacy, and hypersensitivity to negative evaluation that begins in early adulthood.

Axon The long fiber in a nerve cell that transmits chemical impulses.

Basal ganglia Group of structures involved in starting and stopping movement, planning motor activities, and processing of emotions and memories.

Behavior modification Aims to bring about behavior change through use of the environment; however, emphasizes consequences for actions rather than group pressure. Based on the following principles:

–frequency of behavior depends on positive or negative consequences

–events that occur together will become associated

–new behaviors are developed through others' teaching and role modeling

Bender-Gestalt test A psychological test that asks clients to reproduce, as best they can, nine geometric designs that are printed on separate cards. Believed useful in identifying organic brain damage.

Binge eating The act of ingesting large amounts of food in a short time, usually two hours or less. Easily ingested foods such as snack foods, doughnuts, or ice cream are usually selected.

Bioenergetics Techniques for reducing muscular tension by releasing feelings, consisting of physical exercises and verbal techniques.

Biofeedback A technique for gaining conscious control over unconscious body functions such as blood pressure and heartbeat to achieve relaxation or the relief of stress-related physical symptoms; involves the use of self-monitoring equipment.

Biparental failure A family situation in which the male parent fails to offset the child's troubled relationship with the mother by providing positive experiences for the child.

Bipolar disorders Major mood disorders characterized by episodes of mania and depression.

Blackout See Anterograde Amnesia

Blended family A family in which one or both marital partners have previously been divorced or widowed and bring with them their children from the former relationship.

Blunted affect An extreme restriction in emotional expression; only minor degrees of emotional intensity are evident.

Body dysmorphic disorder A somatoform disorder characterized by preoccupation with an imagined or exaggerated defect in physical appearance.

Body scanning Focusing separately on all parts of the body to note the location of any tension or tightness.

Borderline personality disorder A personality disorder with the essential feature of a pervasive pattern of unstable interpersonal relationships, self-image, and moods along with impulsive behavior beginning in early adulthood.

Boundary The personal limits one uses to differentiate between one event and another; for example, one's boundaries keep one from experiencing another person's pain.

Brain imaging A variety of technologic techniques for looking into the living human brain.

Bulimia nervosa Recurrent episodes of binge eating accompanied by purging and persistent overconcern with body shape and weight.

Burnout A condition in which health professionals lose their concern and feeling for the clients with whom they work and begin to treat them in detached or dehumanizing ways. An attempt to cope with the intense stress of interpersonal work by distancing.

Capitation An insurance term referring to a set amount of money received or paid out (slang: "cap"). It is based on membership enrollment requirements rather than on services delivered and is usually expressed in units of PMPM or per member per month. May vary by factors such as age and sex of enrolled member.

Cardiac neurosis A "disorder" in which the individual is overly concerned about the heart and its functioning. May occur following a cardiac illness and may lead individual to restrict behavior. A term of historical rather than diagnostic interest.

Case management A method of managing the provision of health care or high-cost medical conditions. The goal is to coordinate the care so as to both improve continuity and quality of care, as well as lower cost. Usually a dedicated function in the utilization management department of a managed care organization.

Catalysts Unconflicted members of a group who are able to move the group on to the next phase of group work.

Cataplexy Episodes of sudden collapse of muscle tone, usually associated with intense emotion, observed most often in narcolepsy, thought to be related to REM sleep breakthrough into daytime functioning.

Catatonia A disturbance in psychomotor behavior that can either take the form of stupor, in which the client appears unaware of the environment, or rigidity, in which the client may maintain a rigid posture and resist efforts to be moved.

Catharsis The release of strong emotions, with a resulting relief from inner tension and distress caused by the feelings.

Cathexis In psychoanalysis, the attachment of emotion to an object, person, or idea. It may be positive or negative emotion (love or hate).

Checking perceptions A communication skill in which the therapist shares how he or she perceives and hears the client and asks the client to verify these perceptions. Perception checks are used to make sure that one person understands the other.

Chemical dependence Term synonymous with substance dependence.

Chief complaint A client's own words for explaining why he/she has come to the attention of psychiatric services.

Child ego state In transactional analysis theory, the ego state that represents the archaic relics of early childhood.

Child neglect The compromise of a child's health or welfare by negligence from the person or persons who are responsible for the care.

Child within A phrase from inner child theorists that represents the thoughts, needs, and feelings of a child who exists within an adult.

Childhood disintegrative disorder A pervasive developmental disorder involving multiple losses during early or middle childhood of previously acquired social, language and play skills, as well as bladder and bowel control.

Childhood onset schizophrenia A disorder involving delusions, hallucinations, disorganized speech and behavior, affective blunting and social withdrawal.

Chorea Quick, jerky, purposeless, involuntary movements associated with Huntington's disease.

Choreiform movements Involuntary muscle movements, especially of face and extremities, involving twitching or sudden contractions of muscle groups.

Chronic motor or vocal tic disorder Rapid, recurring, nonrhythmic, stereotyped movements or vocalizations which occur suddenly and without voluntary control.

Circadian rhythms Automatic internal physiologic rhythms such as body temperature, sleep, and appetite that occur every 24 hours.

Clarifying Asking the client to give an example to clarify a meaning in order to understand the basic nature of the client's statement.

Clinical case management A service approach that blends the service broker function with the role of out-patient clinician.

Clinical specialist in psychiatric-mental health nursing A graduate of a master's program providing specialization in the clinical area of psychiatric/mental health nursing.

Closed panel A managed care plan that contracts with physicians on an exclusive basis for service and does not allow those physicians to see patients for other managed care organizations.

Cluster suicide Any excessive number of suicides occurring in close temporal or geographic proximity to each other.

Co-alcoholic A term coined by Al-Anon referring to the spouses and families of alcoholics.

Cocaine crash *See Crashing*

Codependence A group of learned behaviors that includes denial, urges to control others, and a preoccupation with the thoughts and feelings and circumstances of other adults who are often addicts. May interfere with an individual's ability to take care of personal needs.

Cognitive restructuring A technique of cognitive therapy that attempts to modify inaccurate or biased ways of processing information that cause the child to misperceive or distort what is experienced.

Cogwheeling An extrapyramidal side effect of antipsychotic medications where tremor and rigidity combine to create a cogging motion of a limb when it is manipulated. External movement of, for example, the arm would feel like the arm was slipping into a notched position when moved.

Commitment The legal process by which a person is confined to a mental hospital, usually associated with involuntary hospitalization. Also a sense of dedication and responsibility.

Communication disorders Severe impairments in language expression, understanding of language, stuttering or failure to use speech sounds appropriate for a child's age and dialect.

Community support program Programs providing a full range of treatment, rehabilitative, and support services to promote quality of life for the severely and persistently mentally ill in the community.

Comorbidity Simultaneous experience of more than one pathological condition. In this text, refers to concurrent mental illness and substance use disorder.

Competency Having the mental capacity to understand the nature of an act.

Complementary relationships Relationships based on the enjoyment of differences and interdependence. They may deteriorate when one partner controls what the complementarity is and how it is maintained.

Complementary transactions Transactions in which the transactional stimulus and the transactional response occur on identical ego levels.

Compulsion An uncontrollable, persistent urge to perform an act repetitively in an attempt to relieve anxiety; performed in response to an obsession, according to certain rules, or in a stereotyped fashion.

Compulsive overeating A pattern of consistent, irresistible urges to ingest larger amounts of food than the body requires, even when not physically hungry.

Compulsive use The need for larger amounts of the substance than intended.

Conditioned response Behavior that occurs as a consequence of rewarding conditions that act as a stimulus.

Condom A barrier protection placed on the penis to prevent the transmission of body fluids during sexual activity.

Conduct disorder Repetitive and persistent behavior in which the basic rights of others or major societal norms as rules are violated.

Confabulations Invented memories to take the place of those the client cannot recall.

Confidentiality Treating as private the information clients provide about themselves so that no harm will befall the client for having disclosed the information; includes releasing information about clients only with their permission.

Conflict A clash between opposing forces. It may be conscious or unconscious, intrapersonal or interpersonal.

Conflicted member A member of a group whose posture toward authority or intimacy is inflexible, rigid, or compulsive.

Confrontation A communication that deliberately invites another to self-examine some aspect of behavior in which there is a discrepancy between what the person says and does.

Continuous treatment teams An intensive case management approach that relies on teams rather than creating dependence on one case manager.

Contract A set of expectations agreed on by two or more people about what each will contribute to the relationship.

Control need The interpersonal need to establish and maintain a satisfactory relation between self and others with regard to power and influence.

Copayment A portion of claim or medical expense that a member must pay out of pocket. Usually a fixed amount.

Coping behavior The behaviors people under stress use in struggling to improve their situations.

Coprolalia A type of vocal tic in which obscenities are uttered suddenly and without voluntary control.

Countertransference The term used to denote transference feelings experienced by the therapist or mental health professional toward the client. The term is commonly employed in referring to feelings or attitudes of the professional that compromise the therapeutic work with the client. The concept originated in psychoanalytic theory in describing feelings/attitudes of the analyst toward the patient. It is important to seek supervision to deal with this.

Crashing A terrible letdown called the "postcoke blues" or cocaine abstinence syndrome.

Credentialing Obtaining and reviewing the documentation of professional providers. Includes: licensure, certification, insurance, evidence of malpractice insurance and history of malpractice incidents. The information is reviewed and verified when a provider is credentialed.

Creutzfeld-Jakob disease A transmissible degenerative dementia with rapid onset affecting the cerebral cortex through cell destruction and overgrowth.

Crisis A situation in which usual problem-solving or adapting methods are inadequate to resolve a problem or conflict, causing a state of disequilibrium; this is the crisis. A crisis may be a time of great personal growth for an individual.

Crisis intervention A conceptual framework for intervention that calls for short-term, action-oriented assistance to be focused on problem-solving with a goal of restoring the individual's equilibrium (to be given to the person in crisis).

Critical path A standard written plan and timetable for care that identifies routine treatments, activities, medications, expected length of stay, and discharge planning.

Cross-sectional study A survey of a group of individuals (some with and some without a disorder) conducted at one point in time. This type of study is often called a prevalence study.

Crossed transaction A transaction in which a change in ego state occurs, terminating a complementary relationship.

Cultural diversity A sensitivity to cultural and ethnic background which may influence the expression, reporting, and evaluation of mental disorder.

Cultural relativism The belief that all cultures are equally valued and that they can be evaluated based on their own values.

Cyclothymia A chronic, fluctuating mood disturbance characterized by numerous periods of hypomania alternating with numerous periods of depression during a two-year period.

Dangerousness The prediction of who poses a risk for violence and the perception that someone is more likely to be violent.

Defense mechanisms Operations outside of a person's awareness that the ego calls into play to protect against anxiety; the psychoanalytic term for coping mechanisms; also called mental mechanism.

Deinstitutionalization A humanitarian philosophy committed to community-based care for the mentally ill which has resulted in decreased census for the state mental hospitals and emergence of community-based treatment facilities as well as unanticipated consequences including the homeless mentally ill.

Delirium An acute disturbance of consciousness that involves problems with attention, perception, thinking, memory, psychomotor behavior and sleep-wake cycle.

Delusions An important personal belief that is almost certainly not true and resists modification.

Dementia Impairment in short- and long-term memory due to varied etiologies, including vascular disease, HIV, head trauma, Parkinson's disease, substance abuse, among others. Dementia is considered a cognitive disorder in the DSM-IV.

Dendrites Filaments that branch out from the body of a neuron to receive information transmitted by the axons of other neurons.

Denial A defense mechanism, or coping mechanism, by which the mind refuses to acknowledge a thought, feeling, wish, need or reality factor.

Dependent personality disorder A personality disorder with the essential feature of a pervasive and excessive need to be taken care of that leads to submissive and clinging behavior and fears of separation that begins by early adulthood.

Depersonalization disorder A dissociative disorder characterized by persistent or recurrent feeling of being detached from one's body or thoughts; reality testing remains intact.

Depot medications A term used to describe the slow release of long-term medications given by injection (either intramuscularly or subcutaneously), using the body as a temporary storage of the entire dose. Antipsychotic medications such as fluphenazine decanoate and haloperidol decanoate are depot medications.

Descriptive study Study that identifies the amount and distribution of disorder within a population by answering questions related to "who," "where," and "when."

Desensitization A counterconditioning technique used by behaviorists to overcome fears by gradually increasing exposure to the fearful stimuli.

Devaluation Sustained criticism used to defend against feelings of inadequacy.

Deviance Behavior outside the social norm of a specific group; should not be construed to mean negative behavior.

Disengagement A family pattern characterized by unresponsive and unconnected interactions between members. Structure, order, and authority may be absent or weak.

Displacement A defense or coping mechanism in which a person discharges pent-up feelings on persons less threatening than those who initially aroused the emotion.

Dissociation A defense or coping mechanism that protects the self from a threatening awareness of uncomfortable feelings by denying their existence in awareness.

Dissociative amnesia An inability to recall significant personal information; the forgotten information is usually traumatic; the memory loss is not due to "usual" forgetfulness or organic factors.

Dissociative disorders A group of altered coping patterns in which the usually integrated functions of memory, consciousness, identity, or perception of the environment are disrupted.

Dissociative fugue A state in which the individual is unable to recall one's past and often has sudden, unexpected travel away from routine surroundings; may be accompanied by identity confusion or assumption of a new identity.

Dissociative identity disorder A condition characterized by the presence of two or more distinct identities or personality states; formerly called multiple personality disorder.

DNA The complex molecule (deoxyribonucleic acid) that, along with structural proteins, makes up chromosomes. It consists of two twisted strands, made up of sugars and phosphates, to which are attached four types of bases.

Double bind A complex series of paradoxical interactions in which one person demands a response to a message containing mutually contradictory signals, while the other person is not able to comment on the incongruity or to escape from the situation.

Dramatic-erratic A category of personality disorders that includes histrionic, narcissistic, antisocial, and borderline disorders.

Drives The source of psychic energy, according to Freud.

DSM-IV The diagnostic and statistical manual published in its fourth edition by the American Psychiatric Association; the nomenclature for mental disorders.

Dual diagnosis Term commonly used by clinicians to refer to persons manifesting problems with both mental illness and substance use disorder.

Duty to intervene A professional obligation to take reasonable, prudent action.

Dysarthria Difficulty in speaking.

Dysomnia A disorder of either difficulty initiating or maintaining sleep, or excessive sleepiness.

Dyspareunia Pain during, or immediately after, intercourse.

Dysthymia A chronically depressed mood that occurs on a nearly daily basis for most of the day for at least 2 years.

Dystonia Impaired or disordered muscle tone occurring with antipsychotic medications as an extrapyramidal side effect. This is a painful side effect and is usually treated with anticholinergic medications.

Eccentric A category of personality disorders that includes paranoid, schizoid, and schizotypal disorders.

Ego A concept of the organized part of personality that screens stimuli from the outside world and controls internal demands. As intermediary between the unconscious and the world, it includes defensive, cognitive, and executive functions. Consciousness resides in the ego, but some of its operations are out of the person's awareness.

Ego-dystonic A perspective on oneself that may motivate change due to symptoms that are not compatible or harmonious with the person's view of himself or herself.

Ego-syntonic A perspective on oneself that does not motivate seeking change.

Electroconvulsive therapy (ECT) A treatment procedure that involves inducing a brief convulsion by passing an electric current through the brain; used in the treatment of mood disorders in persons resistant to psychoactive drug therapy.

Elopement The departure or flight of a client from a psychiatric hospital.

Empathy The ability to feel the feelings of other people so that one can respond to and understand their experiences on their terms. It is distinguished from sympathy by lack of condolence, agreement, or pity.

Enabler Family member in an alcoholic's or addict's life whose behavior contributes to the continuation of chemical use.

Encopresis The repeated passing of feces by the child into inappropriate places such as clothing or a corner of the room.

Endocrine system A network of endocrine glands in the body, as well as organs, that secretes hormones.

Enmeshment A family pattern characterized by a fast tempo of interpersonal exchange, overcontrol, and intrusiveness, usually from parent to child.

Enuresis The repeated voiding of urine into the bed or clothes during the day or at night.

Ethnocentrism People's beliefs that their cultural values and behaviors are superior and preferable to any other culture.

Euthanasia The intentional termination of a life of such poor quality that it is considered not worth living; can be active or passive.

Exhibitionism Intentional exposure of the genitals to a stranger or unsuspecting person; may be accompanied by arousal and masturbation, either during or after the exposure.

Expressed emotion A characteristic of families of schizophrenics who are highly critical, hostile or overinvolved with their ill relative. High EE is associated with more frequent relapse.

Extended family All persons related by birth, marriage, or adoption to the nuclear family.

Extrapyramidal side-effects (EPS) Side-effects caused by the use of neuroleptic medications, including three separate classes: parkinsonism, dystonias, and akathisia.

Extrapyramidal system A system of descending motor tracts that originate from various regions of the cerebral cortex and subcortical areas. Because these tracts do not travel through the pyramids of the medulla, they are called extrapyramidal.

Factitious disorder A state characterized by symptoms (psychological or physical) that are intentionally produced or feigned in order to assume the sick role and experience its benefits.

False memory Incomplete or inaccurate memories that are the result of faulty recollection or the result of suggestion from another person.

Family burden A term that refers to the difficulties and responsibilities of family members who assume a caregiving function for relatives with psychiatric disabilities.

Family lifestyle A family's biased perception of the outside world and its automatic means of coping with this world. It is the front or facade the family presents to others.

Family myths Well-integrated unchallenged beliefs, shared by all family members, about each other and their positions in family life.

Family of origin The family in which an individual grew up.

Family theme A family's perception of its development and history.

Fantasy A defense mechanism that is a sequence of mental images, like a daydream. It may be conscious or unconscious. It is considered by some to be an individual's attempt to resolve an emotional conflict.

Feedback The process by which performance is checked and malfunctions corrected; a regulatory function in the communication process, requiring two persons—one to give and one to receive it.

Feeding disorder of infancy or early childhood The persistent failure of a child to eat adequately, accompanied by a failure to gain weight, or significant weight loss.

Female orgasmic disorder Cessation of sexual response before orgasm occurs.

Female sexual arousal disorder Persistent and recurring lack of subjective sexual excitement or pleasure.

Feminism A viewpoint that examines the impact of being female and exhorts the rights of females.

Fetal alcohol syndrome (FAS) Physical and mental defects found in babies of alcoholic women.

Fetishism An association with or stimulus for sexual arousal elicited by inanimate objects (shoes, leather, rubber) or specific body parts (feet, hair) that is not typical for the culture.

Fight-flight Aggression (fight)–withdrawal (flight) response to stress.

Flashbacks A spontaneous reliving of the experiences the person felt while under the influence of the drug, although the person is drug-free.

Flat affect (shallowness) A lack of emotional expression; an insufficiently intense emotional display in association with ideas or situations that ordinarily would call for a stronger response.

Flight of ideas The rapid and continuous succession of accelerated, fragmentary thoughts in which content changes abruptly. Manifested in pressured speech which, when severe, may be incoherent.

Frail elderly Dependent, chronically ill older people.

Freebase A purified form of cocaine made by applying solvents to ordinary cocaine to produce a more intense "high."

Frotteurism Intense sexual arousal elicited by rubbing the genitals against a nonconsenting person.

G protein Large family of receptors which are the links in second messenger transactions.

Games In transactional analysis theory, a series of ulterior transactions with a concealed motivation.

Gatekeeper An informal term that refers to a primary care case management model health plan. In this model, all care from providers other than primary care, except true emergencies, must be authorized by primary care providers before care is rendered.

Gender identity An individual's personal or private sense of identity as female or male.

Gender identity disorder Feeling persistent and intense distress about one's biologic gender and desiring to be of the other sex.

Gender role The role a person is expected to perform as a result of being male or female in a particular culture.

General adaptation syndrome (GAS) The objectively measurable structural and chemical changes produced in the body when stress affects the whole body. The GAS occurs in three stages: (1) alarm, (2) resistance, and (3) exhaustion.

General systems theory A conceptual framework that can be applied to living systems or people and that integrates the biologic and social sciences logically with the physical sciences.

Generalized anxiety disorder A coping pattern in which anxiety is the predominant feature; there is a history of at least six months of persistent and excessive anxiety.

Genes Units of functional information of the chromosome; a length of DNA that codes for the production of a specific protein.

Geriatric depression scale A tool for assessing depressive symptoms in elderly clients.

Geropsychiatry A clinical specialty within psychiatry that focuses on the psychosocial aspects of the care of the aged.

Global Assessment of Functioning Scale (GAF) Axis V of DSM-IV that consists of a rating scale from 0–100. Often associated with prognosis.

Grandiosity An exaggerated appraisal of one's worth, importance, power, knowledge, or identity. Sometimes assumes delusional proportions.

Group model An HMO that contracts with a medical group for provision of health care services. A form of closed panel health plan.

Hallucination A false perception, the most common of which is auditory and involves hearing voices; other types of hallucinations are tactile, somatic, visual, gustatory, and olfactory. A sensory impression in the absence of external stimuli that occurs during the waking state.

Health maintenance organization (HMO) An entity that provides, offers, or arranges for coverage of designated health services needed by plan members for a fixed, prepaid premium. There are four basic models of HMOs: group model, individual practice association, network model, and staff model.

Hippocampus Limbic structure involved in emotional reactions and short- and long-term memory drive.

Histrionic personality disorder A personality disorder with the essential feature of a pervasive and excessive emotionality and attention-seeking behavior beginning in early adulthood.

HIV-related dementia A progressive dementia caused by direct HIV infection of the CNS.

Holism A philosophic perspective that views the person as an integrated whole whose parts share an organic and functional relationship.

Homeostasis The principle that all organisms react to changing conditions in an effort to maintain a relatively constant internal environment; in general systems theory, the characteristics of systems to strive to maintain a dynamic equilibrium, or balance, among various forces that operate within and on it.

Homophobia The unrealistic fear of homosexuality and homosexuals that stems from myths and stereotypes associated with homosexuality.

Hormone A chemical, released by glands and other organs, that travels through the bloodstream and regulates the activities of specific tissue, organs, and other glands.

Hostility A type of aggression that is oriented to do purposeful harm because of anger or provocation.

Human immunodeficiency virus (HIV) The tiny but virulent retrovirus that causes AIDS. It consists of a double-layered shell or envelope full of proteins surrounding a bit of ribonucleic acid (RNA).

Humanism A view of human beings that values the individual's freedom of choice. In psychiatric nursing practice, a philosophy of devotion to the interests of human beings wherever they live and whatever their status. It reaffirms the spirit of compassion and caring for others, and constructively and wholeheartedly affirms the joys, beauties, and value of human living.

Huntington's disease A progressive, degenerative genetic disorder characterized by both motor and cognitive changes. This is one of the more frequently observed types of hereditary nervous system diseases.

Hypersomnia Excessive sleepiness, sleep of abnormal depth or duration.

Hypervigilance An increased state of guardedness or watchfulness.

Hypnagogic hallucinations Vivid dreamlike images which may appear just before sleep onset.

Hypoactive sexual desire disorder A deficiency in or absence of sexual fantasies, and persistently low interest or a total lack of interest in sexual activity.

Hypochondriasis A somatoform disorder characterized by the persistent belief or fear that one is ill with no evidence of organic pathology.

Hypomania A distinct period during which there is an abnormally and persistently elevated, expansive, or irritable mood lasting at least 4 days, but somewhat less intense than in mania.

Hypothalamus Neuroanatomic structure that regulates hormone levels, circadian rhythms, pleasure and pain, and control in the autonomic nervous system.

Id In psychoanalytic theory, all inherited psychic properties of the person, most notably the instincts and drives.

Identification A defense mechanism; the wish to be like another person and to assume the characteristics of that person's personality.

Identity diffusion The failure to integrate various childhood identifications into a harmonious adult, psychosocial identity; the "as if" personality.

Illusions Misperceptions and misinterpretations of externally real stimuli. Visual and auditory illusions are much more common than tactile, olfactory, and gustatory illlusions.

Imparting information A communication skill in which the nurse makes statements that give needed data to the client.

Incidence rate A measure of the number of *new* cases of a disease or disorder in a population over a period of time.

Inclusion need The interpersonal need to establish and maintain relationships with others.

Incompetence Lack of ability or legal qualification to perform a specified act.

Informational confrontation Describing the visible behavior of another person.

Informed consent A client's right to have treatment explained in order to agree with it or to refuse it.

Insanity An obsolete medical term for psychosis or mental illness. Continues to be used in legal terminology.

Insomnia The chronic inability to get to sleep or to remain asleep during the usual sleep period.

Institutionalization The process of decline in functioning characterized by dependence, apathy, resignation, and inability to manage daily living outside an institution and created by an environment that controls all individual decision making, negates independence and autonomy, and segregates inmates from the mainstream community.

Intellectualization A defense mechanism in which intellectual processes are overused to avoid closeness or affective experience and expression and for a standardized intelligence assessment.

Intelligence test Method to evaluate the presence and degree of mental retardation and for a standardized intelligence assessment.

Intensive case management Case management models for high-risk subgroups of the mentally ill who require assertive outreach and skilled service providers.

Interpretative confrontation Expressing thoughts and feelings about another's behavior and drawing inferences about the meaning of the behavior.

Intoxication Reversible substance-specific syndrome caused by recent ingestion. May include such behavioral changes as mood lability, motor dysfunction, and cognitive impairment.

Introjection A defense mechanism closely related to identification; the process of accepting another's values and opinions as one's own.

Involuntary commitment The legal process by which a person is confined without consent to a mental hospital. There are three categories: (1) emergency, (2) temporary, and (3) extended. Criteria vary from state to state.

Ion channels Water-filled molecular tunnels that pass through the cell membrane and allow charged atoms or small molecules to enter or leave the cell.

Iowa self-assessment inventory A tool for obtaining a subjective functional assessment from elderly clients.

Irrational self-talk In rational-emotive therapy, the untrue thoughts with which one describes and interprets the world to oneself; usually catastrophic interpretations of an event or the need to live up to an absolute standard.

Kindling Repeated administration of a stimulus to the neuron.

Korsakoff's psychosis (alcohol amnestic disorder) A chronic neurological condition associated with alcoholism that may follow an acute phase called Wernicke's encephalopathy. Retrograde and anterograde amnesia are present.

La belle indifference The lack of concern about one's physical symptom; is typically seen in clients experiencing conversion disorder.

Learned helplessness (excessive dependence) A condition in which a person attempts to establish and maintain contact with another by adopting a helpless, powerless stance.

Learning disorders Achievement significantly below age-appropriate expectations on standardized tests of reading, mathematics, or written expression.

Least restrictive alternative Imposition of the least amount of limitation or interference on an individual's thought and decision-making, physical activity, and sense of self as necessary to provide for safety.

Lethality assessment A systematic method of assessing a client's suicide potential.

Life review The process of reexamination of one's own life to resolve old problems, restore harmony within the family unit, identify past accomplishments, and take responsibility for one's own actions.

Life script Life expectations that have evolved over time due to the client's life experiences and relationships with significant others. The life script can affect numerous areas of living, such as the client's choices for career, life mate (to have or not to have), and patterns of behavior.

Limbic system A group of structures within the brain thought to play a major role in emotions and memory.

Limit-setting The reasonable and rational setting of parameters for client behavior that provide for control and safety.

Linking A communication skill in which the nurse responds to the client in a way that ties together two events, experiences, feelings, or people. It may be useful in connecting the past with current behaviors.

Lithium carbonate A lithium salt effective in the treatment of bipolar disorder, particularly during acute mania.

Locus ceruleus A cluster of nuclei in the pons, brainstem, that produce the neurotransmitter norepinephrine. Comes from Latin for "blue area," for the color of its cells.

Major depressive disorder A period of at least 2 weeks during which there is either depressed mood or the loss of interest or pleasure in nearly all activities.

Male erectile disorder Inability to attain a full erection or losing the erection prior to orgasm.

Male orgasmic disorder Extreme difficulty ejaculating.

Malingering A conscious, deliberate feigning of an illness used to avoid a painful situation or for personal gain.

Malpractice Negligent act of professionals when they fail to act in a responsible and prudent manner in carrying out their professional duties.

Managed care Cost-containment systems in which a population at risk receives care that is constrained by a specified budget and is held accountable for defined client outcomes or results.

Managed care organization (MCO) A system of health care delivery that influences utilization of services, cost of services, and measures performance. The goal is a system that delivers value by giving people access to quality, cost-effective health care.

Mania A period of abnormal mood lasting at least 1 week characterized by abnormally and persistently elevated, expansive, or irritable mood accompanied by at least 3 additional symptoms, such as inflated self-esteem or grandiosity, decreased need for sleep, pressured speech, flight of ideas, and others.

Mantra A syllable, word, or name that is chanted over and over during meditation.

Meditation A method of achieving a state of deep rest and increasing alpha wave brain activity enabling one to focus on one thing at a time in order to achieve inner peace and harmony.

Mental disorder A clinically significant behavioral or psychologic syndrome or pattern that occurs in a person and is associated with distress or disability or with an increased risk of suffering, death, pain, disability, or an important loss of freedom; is not an expected response to a particular event or experience.

Mental health The relationship between the individual's optimal psychobiologic health and feelings of self-worth, personal integrity, self-fulfillment, creative expression, the satisfying of basic living needs, comfortable relationships with others and the recognition of human rights.

Mental retardation A disorder involving subaverage intellectual functioning (IQ below 70) and impairments in either communication, social skills, or safety.

Mental Status Examination A customary part of psychiatric assessment that addresses orientation, thinking, mood, judgment and the like through structured questions.

Metabolites Product or substance produced from the breakdown or metabolic process of neurochemicals.

Methadone A synthetic narcotic.

Milieu therapy/therapeutic environment A type of psychotherapy using the total environment (such as physical surroundings, stable social structure, structured activities) to promote therapeutic interactions and personal growth.

Mixed message Communication in which the verbal and the nonverbal aspects contradict one another.

MMPI A lengthy written psychometric test.

Mnemonic disturbances Memory loss.

Monoamine oxidase (MAO) inhibitors A group of drugs used primarily in the treatment of depression; also used in treating phobias, migraine headache, and hypertension.

Mood disorders A group of psychiatric diagnoses characterized by disturbances in physical, emotional, and behavioral response patterns.

Moral claims Conflicting claims to the truth that require ethical reasoning.

Motor skills disorder Marked impairment in the development of motor coordination which significantly interferes with the child's academic achievement or activities of daily living.

Movement therapy A therapeutic technique that provides elderly clients a sense of relatedness to others, while increasing sensory input (touch, vision, and hearing) through a series of exercises ranging from simple to complex, depending on the individual's physical and cognitive ability.

Multifactorial causation A term used to describe the requirement that a combination of causes or factors may be required to produce a disorder.

Mutism The absence of verbal response.

Narcissism Self-love or extreme self-centeredness.

Narcissistic personality disorder A personality disorder characterized by a pervasive pattern of grandiosity, need for admiration of others, and a lack of empathy; onset beginning in early adulthood.

Narcotics Anonymous (NA) A 12-step self-help program for addicts.

National Committee on Quality Assurance (NCQA) A not-for-profit organization that performs quality-oriented accreditation reviews on health maintenance organizations and similar managed care plans.

Natural history of disorder The course of disorder over time in the absence of intervention.

Negative reinforcement In behaviorist/learning theory, alteration of an adversive stimulus to increase the probability that a behavioral response will occur.

Negative symptoms Schizophrenic symptoms, including flattening of affect, loss of motivation, and poverty of speech.

Negative transference Client reactions in therapeutic work based on negative feelings (such as hate, bitterness, contempt, annoyance) left over from unsatisfying past relationships.

Negligence Failure to exercise the standard of care that a reasonable person would exercise under the same or similar circumstances.

Negotiated reality The creation of a mutually understood common ground.

Neologism A private, unshared meaning of a word or term. Neologisms are frequently characteristic of the language of schizophrenic individuals.

Neurofibrillary tangles Characteristic in Alzheimer's disease, the tangle is composed of interneurons that have increased in thickness and twisted into tangled masses of fibrous strands or bundles in the temporal lobe.

Neuroleptic malignant syndrome (NMS) An infrequent, yet extreme, condition that occurs in clients who are severely ill and is believed to be the result of dopamine blockade. Symptoms of this syndrome include diaphoresis, muscle rigidity, and hyperpyrexia.

Neurolinguistic programming (NLP) A communication model derived from theory in linguistics, neurophysiology, psychology, cybernetics, and psychiatry.

Neuron A nerve cell consisting of a central body, or soma, from which extend a number of dendrites and a single axon.

Neurosyphilis A dementia that is the direct result of untreated primary syphilis.

Neurotic conflict In psychoanalytic theory, the consequence of a traumatic experience in which client experiences ideas or feelings that are incompatible with his or her ego; believed to generate anxiety and use of defense mechanisms.

Neurotransmitter A highly specialized neurochemical that allows transmission of an electrical impulse from one neuron to the next across the synapse.

No self-harm/no suicide contract An agreement between two people that sets as an expectation that the first individual will not harm him/herself, and the second individual agrees to be available to assist the other.

Nonassertive behavior Timid holding back.

Nonverbal communication Communication between two or more people without the use of words. Facial expressions, gestures, and body postures are examples.

Normal pressure hydrocephalus A relatively uncommon cause of dementia correctable by a shunt placed in the brain that drains cerebral spinal fluid to the abdomen.

Normal weight bulimic An individual who, in spite of engaging in bulimic behaviors of binge eating and purging, maintains near-normal body weight.

Norms The set of unwritten rules of conduct or prescriptions of behavior established by members of a group.

North American Nursing Diagnosis Association (NANDA) The organization that publishes the approved lists of nursing diagnoses.

Nuclear family The "traditional" family consisting of two parents in a time-limited, two-generational relationship.

Nucleotides A fundamental unit of DNA and RNA, consisting of a sugar and phosphate unit/compound joined.

Nucleus A specialized component of all cells, except erythrocytes, that contains the cell's chromosomes.

Nursing process The conscious, systematic set of cognitive and behavioral steps that make up the clinical act of nursing practice.

Obesity Body weight 20 percent or more higher than the ideal weight for age, gender, and height.

Object loss The forced, often traumatic, separation of a person from a significant object of attachment.

Objective data Data collected and verified from sources other than the client and family.

Obsession A persistent unwanted intrusive thought which cannot be eliminated from conscious thought by logic; leads to intense anxiety which is responded to by compulsive behaviors.

Obsessive-compulsive disorder An anxiety disorder characterized by unwanted intrusive thoughts (obsessions) and/or compulsions, behaviors which seek to alleviate the anxiety caused by obsessions.

Obsessive-compulsive personality disorder A personality disorder with the essential feature of preoccupation with orderliness, perfectionism, and mental and interpersonal control, at the expense of flexibility, openness and efficiency that begins by early adulthood.

Oculogyric crisis An involuntary deviation and fixation of the eyeballs, usually upward and to one side. Side effect of antipsychotic medications. An extrapyramidal side effect.

Omnipotence Fantasies of greatness or power.

One-to-one relationship A mutually defined, collaborative, goal-directed client-therapist relationship for the purpose of crisis intervention, counseling, or individual psychotherapy.

Open panel A managed care plan that contracts with private physicians to deliver care in their own offices. Examples are direct contract HMOs and PPOs.

Operant conditioning *See Positive Reinforcement*

Opisthotonos A manifestation of an acute dystonic reaction in which the affected person demonstrates spasms of the neck and back, forcing the back to arch and the neck to bend backward.

Oppositional defiant disorder A recurrent and hostile pattern of behavior toward authority figures, but without violating the rights of other or major rules.

Orientation A part of the mental status exam to determine the presence of confusion or clouding of consciousness.

Orientation phase The beginning phase of a one-to-one relationship characterized by the establishment of contact with the client.

Overload In communication theory, sensory input that exceeds a person's tolerance level or capacity.

Pain disorder A somatoform disorder with pain as the predominant feature. Psychological factors have great influence on the onset, severity, and exacerbation of the pain.

Panic disorder A type of anxiety disorder in which the fear of an impending panic attack causes severe restrictions in lifestyle.

Paradox A self-contradictory communication; for example, the demand "Stand up for yourself!"

Parallel process The unconscious process of mutual influencing that occurs during social interactions.

Paranoid personality disorder A personality disorder with the essential feature of a pervasive distrust and suspiciousness of others interpreted as being deliberately demeaning, threatening, or malevolent.

Paraphilia A group of psychosexual disorders characterized by unconventional sexual behaviors.

Paraphrasing An activity or communication skill in which the nurse restates what she or he has heard the client communicating. Paraphrasing offers an opportunity to test the nurse's understanding of what the client is attempting to communicate.

Parasomnia A disorder of arousal, partial arousal, or sleep stage transition.

Parent ego state In transactional analysis theory, the ego state that incorporates the feelings and behaviors learned from parents or authority figures.

Parens patriae Enables the state to take the role of protector and involuntarily hospitalize individuals "for their own good."

Parkinsonian syndrome An adverse reaction that resembles Parkinson's disease resulting from the effects of antipsychotics on the extrapyramidal tracts of the CNS.

Parkinson's disease A cognitive disorder occasionally associated with Alzheimer's dementia, thus confusing the diagnosis. Several varieties of Parkinson's disease exist; the cause is unknown.

Passive progressive relaxation Relaxing the muscles without first tightening them.

Pedophile An adult who is sexually aroused by, and engages in sexual activity with, children.

Peptides Member of a class of compounds which yield amino acids. Peptides form the constituent parts of proteins.

Perception The experience of sensing, interpreting, and comprehending the world; a highly personal and internal act.

Perseveration A communication disturbance in which the client repeats the same words or phrase over and over.

Personal space The "invisible bubble" of territory around a person's body into which intruders may not come.

Personality disorder NOS A category of personality disorders used when a personality pattern meets general criteria, but criteria for a specific personality disorder are not met or the individual's personality disorder is not included in the DSM-IV classification (such as passive-aggressive personality disorder)

Personality disorders Enduring patterns of perceiving, relating to, and thinking about the environment and oneself that become inflexible and maladaptive and cause either functional impairment or subjective distress; coded on Axis II of DSM-IV.

Personality traits Lifelong personality patterns that do not significantly interfere with one's life but may charm, annoy, or frustrate others.

Pervasive developmental disorders A group of 4 disorders which arise in the first years of life, each involving severe developmental impairment in several areas.

Pet therapy A therapeutic activity often utilized with elderly clients to decrease depression and fulfill the need to be loved through the use of animals that respond to the clients in a calm, nonthreatening manner.

Pica A disorder in which a child persistently eats nonnutritive substances such as paint or hair.

Pinpointing Calling attention to statements, inconsistencies among statements, or similarities or differences in points of view, feelings, or actions.

Pituitary Gland, under the direction of the hypothalamus, which secretes hormones into the bloodstream and triggers other glands.

Pleasure principle In psychoanalytic theory, the tendency for the id to seek pleasure and avoid pain. The demands of the pleasure principle become modified by the reality principle, and the individual thereby develops the capacity to delay immediate release of tension or achievement of pleasure.

Point-of-service plan A type of health plan allowing the covered person to choose to receive a service from a participating or a non-participating provider, with different benefit levels associated with the use of participating providers. Points of service can be provided in several ways:

–an HMO may allow members to obtain limited services from non-participating providers

–an HMO may provide non-participating benefits through a supplemental major medical policy

–a PPO may be used to provide both participating and non-participating levels of coverage and access

–various combinations of the above may be used

Polypharmacy Mixing of multiple medications.

Polysomnography The electrophysiological recording of parameters such as electroencephalogram (EEG), electromylogram (EMG) and electro-oculargram (EOG) which, taken together, permit the identification of discrete sleep stages.

Pons The middle segment of the brain stem linking the cerebral cortex and the cerebellum.

Positive reinforcement In behavioral theory and operant conditioning, an environmental event that rewards, and thus increases the probability of, a behavioral response.

Positive symptoms Schizophrenic symptoms, including hallucinations, delusions, and thought disorders.

Positive transference Client reactions in therapeutic work based on positive feelings (love, affection, respect, trust) from satisfying past relationships.

Posttraumatic stress disorder An anxiety disorder in which an extremely traumatic event is reexperienced and accompanied by symptoms of autonomic arousal and avoidance of stimuli associated with the trauma.

Power rape Rape distinguished by the rapist's intent to command and master another person sexually, not to injure the victim.

Preconscious Mental events that could be brought into conscious awareness through an act of attention.

Preferred provider organization (PPO) A program in which contracts are established with providers of medical care. Providers under such contracts are referred to as preferred providers. Usually, the benefit contract provides significantly better benefits (fewer co-payments) for services received from preferred providers, thus encouraging members to use these providers. Members are generally allowed benefits for non-participating providers' services, usually on an indemnity basis with significant co-payments. Providers may be, but are not necessarily, paid on a discounted fee-for-service basis.

Premature ejaculation The absence of voluntary control of ejaculation.

Prescription authority The authority granted by state law for advanced practice nurses to prescribe some types of drugs and devices as a component of a professional's scope of practice.

Prevalence rate Measures the number of people in a population who have a disease or disorder at a given time.

Primary care provider The physician who is assigned or chosen by the member when they enroll in a managed care plan. Usually a family practice or internal medicine specialist; may also be a nurse practitioner or physician assistant.

Primary data source The client himself or herself as the provider of assessment information.

Primary gain A decrease in anxiety as a result of an individual's coping mechanisms.

Primary prevention The first level of prevention which involves prevention of the occurrence of disorder by removal of risk factors.

Primitive idealization Assigning unrealistic powers to an individual on whom one is dependent.

Prior authorization The process of obtaining coverage approval for a service or medication; without such prior authorization, the service or medication is not covered.

Problem-solving strategies Specific forms of intellectual activity used when an individual faces a situation he or she is unable to handle in terms of past learning. Problem-solving strategies are considered crucial in any psychotherapeutic endeavor. Strategies consist of the following essential steps: observation, definition, preparation, analysis, ideation, incubation, synthesis, evaluation, and development.

Process recording A verbatim and progressive recording of the verbal and non-verbal interactions between client and nurse within a given period of time.

Processing A complex and sophisticated communication skill in which direct attention is given to the interpersonal dynamics of the nurse-client experience. Process comments focus on the content, feelings, and behavior experienced within the nurse-client relationship.

Program structure Organization of the daily schedule of activities and communication to clients of the expectations for participation.

Progressive supranuclear palsy A disorder similar to Parkinson's disease that occurs when the patient is in his/her 60s. Symptoms include difficulties in balance, visual disturbances, slurred speech, and personality changes.

Projection An unconscious defense mechanism in which what is emotionally unacceptable to the individual is rejected and attributed to others.

Projective identification The placement of one's aggressive feelings onto another, thereby justifying expression of anger and self-protection.

Projective tests A personality test that evokes projection in the response of the person tested.

Pseudodelirium A delirium that does not have all the hallmarks of delirium. Inconsistencies in cognitive functioning are present; a history of psychiatric illness is common.

Pseudodementia Affective disorders, especially depression, can be marked by symptoms of dementia. Accurate diagnosis is critical because these patients can recover with treatment.

Pseudohostility Chronic conflict, alienation, tension, and inappropriate remoteness among members of a family. The problems of family life are denied in an attempt to negate the hostility among the members.

Pseudomutuality A method of family functioning in which the members act "as if" it is a close, happy family, when in fact it is not.

Pseudo-Parkinsonian syndrome Side effect of neuroleptic medications mimicking Parkinson's disease, including masked facies, muscle weakness, and rigidity.

Psychiatric audit A means of evaluation in which criteria for quality care are compared with actual practice as recorded on the client's chart.

Psychiatric epidemiology The study of the distribution and determinants of mental disorders (or other health-related conditions or events) in human populations. Purposes include the prevention, surveillance (monitoring), and control of mental disorders.

Psychiatric history A set of interview questions oriented to the medical model, designed to elicit information about an individual's present and previous psychiatric experiences. Information may be provided by family, friends, and others about the client, resulting in a variety of perceptions.

Psychiatric home care Services delivered by psychiatric nurses to the homebound severely mentally ill, including the elderly and persons with severe medical problems such as HIV. Psychiatric home care nurses provide a form of case management adapted to the needs of the medically ill.

Psychiatric nursing A specialty within the nursing profession in which the nurse directs efforts toward the promotion of mental health, the prevention of mental disturbance, early identification of an intervention in emotional problems, and follow-up care to minimize long-term effects of mental disturbance.

Psychiatric rehabilitation A treatment philosophy and a set of strategies and interventions that minimize a client's impairment and emphasizes function in a normalized milieu.

Psychiatric violence Behavior by a psychiatric inpatient that threatens or actually harms or injures people or destroys property.

Psychic determinism In psychoanalytic theory, the tenet that none of human behavior is accidental, that emotional and behavioral events do not happen randomly or by chance. Each psychic event is believed to be determined by the ones that preceded it.

Psychoactive substance Chemical substance that, when ingested, causes physiologic effects on the nervous system that produce changes in consciousness, cognition, mood, and other mental functions.

Psychoanalysis A theory of human development and behavior and a form of psychotherapy developed by Sigmund Freud and his followers. Psychoanalysis is a form of insight therapy that relies on the technique of free association to explore the dynamic, psychogenic, and transference aspects of a client's personality.

Psychobiologic revolution A major advance in knowledge about the brain, the mind, the spirit, and behavior.

Psychobiology The study of biochemical foundations, molecular and genetic, and the interactions among cognition, mood, emotion, affect and behavior.

Psychoeducation An intervention often used with clients and their families based on information-giving and support.

Psychogerontology A clinical specialty within gerontology that focuses on the psychosocial aspects of the care of the aged.

Psychoimmunology The study of the links between thoughts, emotions, the nervous system and brain, and the immune system.

Psychological factors affecting mental condition (PFAMC) One or more specific or behavioral factors that adversely affect a medical condition, such as depression or anxiety causing or aggravating a medical condition.

Psychomotor retardation Noticeable slowing of thinking, speech, and body movements seen in depression.

Psychoneuroimmunology An exploration of relationships between the central nervous system, the immune system, behavior, and human biology.

Psychophysiologic disorder A large group of disorders characterized by dysfunction of an organ or organ system controlled by the autonomic nervous system that may be caused or aggravated by emotional factors. Also called psychosomatic illness. Deleted from DSM IV.

Psychosomatic disorder *Same as Psychophysiologic disorder*

Psychosurgery The surgical removal or destruction of brain tissue with the intent of altering behavior.

Psychotherapy A process in which a client enters into an implicit or explicit contract to interact in a prescribed way with a psychotherapist. Goals of psychotherapy may include seeking personal growth, resolving problems in living, and relieving symptoms.

Purging The act of evacuating the gastrointestinal tract by self-induced vomiting or use of emetics, laxatives, or enemas.

Questioning A very direct communication activity that may be useful when the nurse needs specific information from the client. There are two types: (1) open-ended questioning focuses on the topic but at least allows freedom of response; and (2) closed-ended questioning limits the client's responses to yes or no. When used to excess, questioning acts to control the nature and extent of the client's responses.

Rape Any forced sexual activity; the key factor is the absence of consent.

Rape trauma syndrome A syndrome of specific responses to the experience of being raped; also a nursing diagnosis.

Rational Recovery (RR) A secular rather than spiritual program for alcohol or drug recovery.

Rationalization A defense or coping mechanism in which a person falsifies experience by constructing logical or socially approved explanations of behavior.

Reaction formation A defense or coping mechanism in which unacceptable feelings are disguised by repression of the real feeling and reinforcement of the opposite feeling.

Reactive attachment disorder A disorder resulting from gross pathological care that can take one of two forms: failure to initiate and respond to social interactions or indiscriminate sociability and lack of selectivity in the choice of attachment figures.

Reality orientation A structured program for older adult clients that places an emphasis on orientation to time, place, and person.

Reality orientation resources Use of normal resources in the daily environment, such as clocks, calendars, and newspapers, as well as more specialized accommodations such as ramps or telecommunication devices for the hearing impaired, that promote functioning and involvement within the current environment.

Reality principle In psychoanalytic theory, largely a learned ego function whereby people develop the capacity to delay immediate release of tension or achievement of pleasure. This is Sigmund Freud's term for the practical demands of society, which are often in conflict with the individual's own wishes.

Receptors Highly socialized proteins in the neuronal cell membrane.

Recovered memory Memories that emerge into consciousness after being repressed for a period of time, sometimes years.

Reflected appraisals In Harry Stack Sullivan's interpersonal theory of psychiatry, the means by which one's self-view is learned through interaction with significant others.

Reflecting A communication skill in which the nurse reiterates either the content or the feeling message of the client. In "content" reflection, the nurse repeats basically the same statement as the client. In "feeling" reflection, the nurse verbalizes what seems to be implied about feelings in the client's comment.

Rehash A small, spontaneous group led by staff members that discusses what happened just after a violent incident. Also included is a discussion of the outcome and feelings of the community about the event.

Reinforcement Term from behaviorist or learning theory that refers to altering environmental stimuli to increase the probability that a behavioral response will occur; can be positive as a reward or negative as a removal of adversive stimuli.

Reminiscence A therapeutic modality that allows the elderly client to share memories of the past while increasing self-esteem, enhancing socialization, and decreasing depression.

Remotivation therapy Structured groups designed to increase the participant's sense of reality through resocialization of regressed and apathetic elderly clients.

Repression A coping mechanism in which unacceptable feelings are kept out of awareness.

Resistance All the phenomena that interfere with and disrupt the smooth flow of feelings, memories, and thoughts. In the traditional psychoanalytic sense, anything that inhibits the client from producing material from the unconscious. Resistance is often cited by psychotherapists to "explain" unsuccessful treatment of a client.

Resocialization group Unstructured groups, usually within nursing homes, that help meet the socialization needs of elderly clients.

Restraint The application of devices (locked leather, cloth camisoles) to contain and restrict clients who do not respond to seclusion.

Restricting A type of anorexia nervosa in which weight loss is accomplished through dieting, fasting, or excessive exercise in the absence of binge eating or purging.

Restrictiveness The degree to which the physical setting, psychological, or social aspects of the treatment environment interfere with the client's personal autonomy and self-determination. The concept of the "least restrictive alternative" has affected legal, clinical, and regulatory standards.

Reticular activating system Nerve pathways of the reticular formation of the medulla oblongata. These cells control the overall degree of central nervous system activity such as wakefulness, attentiveness, and sleep.

Rett's disorder A pervasive development disorder involving multiple losses during the first 5 months of life of previously acquired motor, social and language skills, as well as deceleration in head growth.

Risk factor A factor whose presence is associated with an increased chance or probability of mental disorder.

RNA Ribonucleic acid—a complex molecule like DNA; composed of a single strand, and plays a major role in the translation of DNA's coding instructions for making protein.

Role taking A process through which individuals can sense the feelings of another, having internally aroused the attitude of the person to whom they are relating.

Rolfing Structural realignment of the body in proper relationship to the field of gravity; a body-mind therapy.

Rorschach test (inkblot test) A personality test in which a person says whatever comes to mind while looking at a series of ten standardized cards with inkblots on them. It is believed to reveal many aspects of the individual's personality structure and emotional functioning.

Rumination A disorder involving the repeated regurgitation and rechewing of food by a child after a period of normal eating behavior has developed.

Sadistic rape Rape distinguished by brutality as a necessary ingredient for the rapist to become sexually excited.

Safer sex practices Sexual behaviors that avoid the risk of HIV infection by preventing the transmission of body fluids during sexual activity.

Satiety The sensation of having eaten enough; satisfaction of hunger.

Scapegoating A process by which an individual or group of individuals is identified as different from others and becomes the object of the group's fears, frustration, or anger.

Schismatic family A family in which the children are forced to join one or the other camp of two warring spouses.

Schizoid personality disorder A personality disorder with the essential features of the lack of enjoyment of close relationships and lack of desire for social or sexual involvement.

Schizophrenia A disturbance that lasts for at least six months and includes at least one month of active phase symptoms (delusions, hallucinations, disorganized speech, grossly disorganized or catatonic behavior, negative symptoms).

Schizotypal personality disorder A personality disorder with the essential feature of a pervasive pattern of peculiarities of ideas, appearance, and behavior and deficits in interpersonal relatedness accompanied by acute discomfort.

Seasonal affective disorder (SAD) A major depressive episode with a seasonal pattern.

Seclusion A type of limit-setting that provides safety, containment, security, and boundaries for a patient.

Second messenger transmission Complex intracellular cell membrane proteins that relay the message from the neurotransmitter complex through a cascade of chemical reactions to the cell neoplasm.

Secondary data sources Sources other than the client, including laboratory findings, psychologic test results, brain scan results, and reports from family and other mental health care professionals.

Secondary gain Outcomes of the sick role, other than the alleviation of anxiety; examples include financial rewards, gaining sympathy and attention, avoidance of responsibilities.

Secondary prevention The second level of prevention involving the early detection and prompt treatment of disorder.

Selective inattention A filtering out of stimuli under conditions of moderate and severe anxiety.

Selective mutism The persistent failure to speak in specific social situations, even though the child can speak in other situations.

Selective serotonin reuptake inhibitors (SSRIs) A new class of antidepressant drugs that reportedly have fewer disturbing side effects than tricyclic antidepressants.

Self actualization According to Maslow, the state achieved by people who make full use of their talents and potentialities. Those doing the best they can understand themselves better than other people, and do not allow their own desires to distort their judgment.

Self-awareness A sense of knowing what one is experiencing, a major goal of all therapy.

Self-destructive behavior Action by which people emotionally, socially, and physically either damage themselves or end their life.

Self-disclosure Being open to personal feelings and experiences; sharing information and feelings with others.

Self-fulfilling prophecy An idea or expectation that is acted out, largely unconsciously, thus "proving" itself.

Self-hypnosis Putting oneself into a hypnotic state, often used to achieve significant relaxation, to make positive suggestions for changes in one's life, or to uncover forgotten events that continue to influence oneself.

Self-medication In this context, self-directed use of psychoactive substances to achieve relief from unpleasant feelings, symptoms of mental illness, or medication side effects. Includes use of prescribed medications in ways other than those specified by the physician, and OTC drugs, as well as alcohol and street drugs.

Self-mutilation The deliberate destruction of body tissue without conscious intent to commit suicide.

Self-system (self dynamism) One of Harry Stack Sullivan's central concepts—that the self is a construct built out of the child's experience. It is made up of "reflected appraisals" learned in contacts with other significant people.

Senile plaques Starch-like protein materials deposited in brain tissues in Alzheimer's clients. The extracellular plaques are comprised of a cluster of degenerating nerve terminals.

Separation anxiety disorder A disorder involving developmentally inappropriate and excessive anxiety over separation from home or from attachment figures.

Separation–individuation The process of identifying oneself as different from the primary caretaker, while maintaining an emotional attachment to that person.

Severely and persistently mentally ill Individuals with psychiatric disorders that impinge on major role functioning over time, involving some level of disability, or otherwise disabling in the absence of appropriate services and treatment.

Sexual abuse Inappropriate sexual behavior, instigated by an adult.

Sexual aversion disorder A severe distaste for sexual activity or the thought of sexual activity, which then leads to a phobic avoidance of sex.

Sexual dysfunction Problems or difficulties with sexual expression.

Sexual masochism Being sexually aroused by receiving emotional or physical pain.

Sexual sadism Being sexually aroused by inflicting emotional or physical pain.

Shallow affect *See Flat affect*

Shaping An intervention procedure in behaviorist/learning theory in which reinforcement is manipulated to bring the client closer and closer to a desired behavior.

Short Portable Mental Status Questionnaire (SPMSQ) A tool for assessing the mental status of elderly clients.

Show of force The gathering of support staff with a leader to approach an out-of-control patient.

Skewed family A family in which one partner is severely dysfunctional; the other partner, usually aware of the dysfunction, assumes a passive, peacemaking stance to preserve the relationship.

Sleep apnea Repetitive episodes of disrupted breathing during sleep; may be of the obstructive or central type.

Sleep bruxism A parasomnia in which there is grinding or clenching of the teeth during sleep.

Sleep enuresis A parasomnia in which there is inability to maintain urinary control during sleep.

Sleep latency The length of time it takes to fall asleep after deciding to go to sleep.

Sleep paralysis A sense of being totally unable to move for a brief period after wakening or at sleep onset.

Sobriety A state of purposeful abstention from the use of nonprescribed psychoactive substances.

Social interaction interventions Intervention based on the following principles: expectations for behavior are clearly communicated; acquisition of new behaviors depends on the degree of personal involvement in learning new skills; membership in a group has significant influence on the occurrence of behavior.

Social phobia An anxiety disorder characterized by extreme anxiety resulting from exposure to certain types of social or performance situations; avoidance behavior usually occurs.

Somatization Excessive preoccupation with physical symptoms.

Somatization disorder A somatoform disorder characterized by multiple physical complaints, including gastrointestinal, sexual, and pain, with no evidence of physiologic impairment.

Somatoform disorder Group of disorders characterized by physical symptoms for which there is no evidence of physiologic disorder.

Somnambulism The parasomnia commonly known as sleepwalking.

Specific phobia A disorder in which severe anxiety occurs with exposure to a specific feared object, event, or situation; often accompanied by avoidance behavior.

Splitting A defense mechanism that prevents one from uniting the good (love) and bad (hate) aspects of oneself or of one's image of another person. The person views the self as all good or all bad, failing to integrate the positive and negative qualities of the self and others into a cohesive image.

Stanford-Binet scale A commonly used intelligence test for children, consisting of a series of tasks of increasing difficulty.

Stereotypic movement disorder A pattern of repetitive, nonfunctional motor behavior which the child appears driven to do, such as head banging or twirling objects.

Stress A broad class of experiences in which a demanding situation taxes a person's resources or capabilities, causing a negative effect.

Stressor The source of stress; the demanding situation.

Structuring An attempt to create order or evolve guidelines.

Subjective data Data reported by the client and significant others in their own words.

Substance abuse Repeated use of a substance despite significant and repeated substance-related consequences.

Substance dependence A pattern of compulsive substance use that is continued despite significant consequences. For most substances, tolerance will result, as will withdrawal if substance use is stopped.

Substance intoxication *See Intoxication*

Substance-related disorder Mental disorder caused by use of a psychoactive substance; includes acute syndromes, such as intoxication and withdrawal, as well as habitual substance misuse.

Substance use disorder Substance abuse or dependence, as in DSM-IV.

Substance withdrawal *See Withdrawal*

Suicide The willful act of ending one's own life. Suicide is purposeful self-destruction and arouses intense and complicated emotions in others.

Suicide attempt A strong and often desperate call for help. This is behavior, direct or indirect, that is intended to kill oneself.

Suicide precautions A set of protocols or guidelines for observing and monitoring client behavior.

Suicide threat A statement of suicidal intent from an individual. All threats should be taken seriously.

Summarizing A communication skill in which main ideas are highlighted. Summarizing reviews for client and nurse the main themes of a conversation; useful in helping the client to focus thinking.

Sundowning Increased restlessness and agitation during the evening and night hours; a phenomenon observed in Alzheimer's disease and other dementias.

Superego In psychoanalytic theory, a special agency of the ego that embodies rules (conscience) and values (ego ideal) resulting from influences of parental figures.

Supported employment Models of vocational rehabilitation that train and support the mentally ill at the worksite and in a normal job environment.

Suppression A defense or coping mechanism in which unacceptable feelings and thoughts are consciously kept out of awareness.

Suprachiasmatic nuclei A group of neurons located in the hypothalamus, which is the body's internal synchronizer for temperature and sleep.

Suspiciousness Behaviors that include hypervigilence and hyperalertness to the environment.

Symbolic interactionism A distinctive approach to the study of human conduct based on the premises that (1) human beings act toward things on the basis of the meaning that the things have for them, (2) the meaning of things in life is derived from the social interactions a person has with others, and (3) people handle and modify the meanings of the things they encounter through an interpretive process.

Symmetrical relationships Relationships based on maintaining equality between members allowing for respect and trust, but which may deteriorate into competition.

Synapse A narrow gap between the axon terminal of a presynaptic neuron and the dendrites or cell body of the post-synaptic neuron.

Synaptic vesicles A structure located in the axon terminal that contains molecules of neurotransmitters.

Systematic desensitization A behavior modification technique in which an individual is gradually introduced to the phobic object until contact can be made without resulting debilitating anxiety.

Tangential response An inappropriate response to a statement in which the content of the statement is disregarded. The reply is directed toward an incidental aspect of the initial statement, the type of language used, the emotions of the sender, or another facet of the same topic.

Tardive dyskinesia Usually a nonreversible and late-onset complication of antipsychotic medications. Characteristically, this condition is evidenced by the presence of abnormal, involuntary movements of the face, jaw and tongue that produce bizarre grimaces, lip smacking, and protrusion of the tongue.

Termination phase The end phase of the one-to-one relationship characterized by the termination of contact with the client.

Territoriality The assumption of a proprietary attitude toward a geographic area by a person or a group.

Tertiary prevention The third level of prevention which involves limitation of disability and rehabilitation when disorder has occurred.

Tetrahydroisoquinolones (TIQs) Opiatelike compounds that affect nerve receptors much like morphine and endorphins.

Thematic apperception test (TAT) A projective psychological test.

Therapeutic alliance A conscious relationship between a facilitative person and a client in which each implicitly agrees to work together to help the client address personal problems and concerns.

Therapeutic community Creation of a milieu in which the hospitalized client can have a corrective interpersonal experience by recreating and resolving obstacles to social relationships; traditional hierarchical roles and authority structures are minimized; originally attributed to Maxwell Jones.

Therapeutic contract The client's definition of personal goals for treatment, plus the nurse's professional responsibilities.

Therapeutic environment The therapeutic potential of people, resources, and events in the client's immediate environment to promote optimal functioning in the activities of daily living, development or improvement of interpersonal skills, and ability to manage outside the institutional setting.

Therapeutic touch The specific transfer of energy in a therapeutic manner in which some of the excess energies of the healer are directed to the client, or energy is transferred from one place to another in the client's body.

Therapeutic use of the self The ability of the psychiatric nurse to use theory and experiential knowledge, along with self-awareness and the ability to evaluate one's personal impact on others, in assessments and interventions with the client.

Thought blocking Stopping the expression of a thought midway.

Thought stopping A method of overcoming obsessive and phobic thoughts by first concentrating on the unwanted thoughts and, after a short time, stopping or interrupting the unwanted thoughts.

Token economy A behavioral approach that rewards clients for desired behavior using token reinforcers, such as food, candy, and verbal approval.

Tolerance Physiologic habituation to a substance, resulting in need for progressively greater amounts to achieve intoxication, or a diminished effect from continued use of the same amount of the substance.

Tort Any private or civil wrong by act or omission, but not including breach of contract.

Torticollis Contraction of the neck muscles, drawing the head to one side with chin pointing in other direction. Extrapyramidal side effect of antipsychotic medications.

Tourette's syndrome A disorder involving multiple motor tics and one or more vocal tics which occur simultaneously or at different periods during the illness.

Toxic shame John Bradshaw's phrase describing the codependent individual's tremendous amount of shame that interferes with the individual's ability to seek happiness.

Transactional analysis (TA) A system introduced by Eric Berne that has four components: (1) structural analysis of intrapsychic phenomena, (2) transactional analysis proper, (3) game analysis, and (4) script analysis—used in both individual and group psychotherapy.

Transference An unconscious phenomenon in which feelings, attitudes, and wishes originally linked with significant figures in one's early life are projected onto others in one's current life. The concept originated in psychoanalytic theory in describing the therapeutic work between the patient and analyst.

Transient tic disorder A disorder involving one or more tics of any type which do not last longer than a 12-month period.

Transsexualism Consistently strong feelings of being trapped in the body of the wrong sex.

Transvestic fetishist A man who becomes sexually aroused by dressing in women's clothing.

Triage The classification of sick or injured persons according to severity in order to direct care and ensure the efficient use of medical and nursing staff and facilities.

Triangulation In family systems theory, the process of forming a triad. Dysfunctional triangulation is a major concept in the Bowen approach to family therapy.

Tricyclic antidepressants (TCAs) A group of antidepressant drugs, named for their three-ringed structure, widely used in the treatment of depression.

Type A personality A behavioral pattern associated with persons who are highly competitive and compulsive in their work habits. Associated with coronary artery disease.

Ulterior transaction A transaction that occurs on both overt (social) and covert (psychologic) levels.

Unconflicted member (*also* independent member) A group member who is able to assess situations and alter roles or behavior.

Unconscious In psychoanalytic theory, the part of the mind that is out of awareness and helps to determine personality.

Underload A situation that occurs when delay or lack of information interferes with one person's ability to comprehend the message of another.

Undifferentiated somatoform disorder A condition characterized by unexplained physical complaints of at least six months' duration.

Universality Ethical principle that one will make the moral decision regardless of the people or place involved.

Using silence Purposeful silence that allows the client time to ponder what has been said, to make a connection, to collect his or her thoughts, or to consider alternatives.

Vaginismus Involuntary spasm of the outer one-third of the vaginal muscles, making penetration of the vagina painful and sometimes impossible.

Vascular dementia A dementia that is abrupt in onset and episodic, with multiple remissions. Brain tissue is destroyed by intermittent emboli.

V-codes Conditions such as marital problems, occupational problems, and parent-child problems that may be a focus of clinical attention but are not a mental disorder.

Vegetative symptoms Changes in physiological functioning, such as appetite, sleep patterns, and elimination patterns, experienced during depression.

Verbal de-escalation Redirection of patient to a calmer state through verbal interventions by staff members.

Visualization Using a person's own imagination and positive thinking to reduce stress or promote healing.

Voluntary admission A legal process by which a person chooses to be admitted to a mental hospital; requires written application by the person or someone acting in his or her behalf, such as a partner or guardian.

Voyeurism Secret observation of an unsuspecting person (usually a woman) engaged in a private act such as undressing or having sex. The voyeur often masturbates during or after the viewing.

Water intoxication A physiologic state brought on by excessive drinking, characterized by hyponatremia, confusion, disorientation, apathy and lethargy. In severe cases, seizures and death may result.

Wechsler Intelligence Scale A commonly used intelligence test.

Wernicke's encephalopathy (*also* **alcoholic encephalopathy)** A neurological syndrome due to thiamine deficiency that may result in delirium, often associated with alcoholism. Symptoms include mental confusion, oculomotor disturbances, and cerebellar ataxia.

Withdrawal Uncomfortable and maladaptive physiologic and cognitive behavioral changes associated with lowered blood or tissue concentrations of a substance after an individual has been engaged in heavy use.

Working phase The middle phase of the one-to-one relationship characterized by the maintenance and analysis of contact.

World view Refers to how a group of people (culture or subculture) see their social world, symbolic system, and physical environment, and their own place in each of them.

Writ of habeas corpus A means by which a person can challenge the legality of his or her detention.

CREDITS

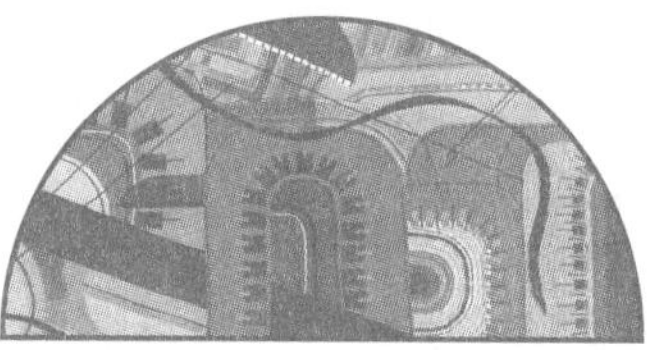

Table 1.1 Comparison of Nonassertive, Aggressive, and Assertive Behaviors. Emily E M Smythe, *Surviving Nursing,* Addison-Wesley, 1984. Copyright © 1984 Emily E M Smythe.

Box p 16 1994 ANA Standards of Psychiatric–Mental Health Clinical Nursing Practice. American Nurses Association, *A Statement on Psychiatric–Mental Health Clinical Nursing Practice.* American Nurses Publishing, 1994.

Table 2.1 Adapted from Karen S Danley and William A Anthony, The choose-get-keep model: Serving severely psychiatrically disabled people, *American Rehabilitation,* 1987; 13(4):6–9.

Table 2.2 Erikson's Eight Stages. From *Childhood and Society,* 2nd Ed, adapted from Erik H Erikson, *Childhood and Society,* W W Norton & Company, Inc ©1950, 1963 W W Norton & Company, Inc, Renewed 1978, 1991 by Erik H Erikson; by permission of the estate and Chatto & Windus, Ltd, The Hogarth Press Ltd.

Fig. 2.2 Maslow's Hierarchy of Needs. H Maslow, *Toward a Psychology of Being,* NY: Van Nostrand Reinhold, 1962. © 1962 H Maslow.

Box p 104 NANDA Nursing Diagnosis: Hopelessness. North American Nursing Diagnosis Association 1995. *NANDA Nursing Diagnoses: Definitions and Classification 1995–1996.* Philadelphia: NANDA.

Fig. 3.1 Delineation of the Cerebral Lobes. Alexander P Spence and Elliott B Mason, *Human Anatomy & Physiology,* 3rd Ed, p 341, Benjamin/Cummings, 1987. Illustrations ©1987 Benjamin/Cummings Publishing Co.

Fig. 3.3 Basal Ganglia. From Guyton, *Basic Neuroscience: Anatomy and Physiology,* p 234, fig 18.19, Philadelphia: W B Saunders, 1987. ©1987 W B Saunders.

Fig. 3.4 Structure of the Generalized Cell. From Marieb E, *Human Anatomy and Physiology,* 3rd Ed, Benjamin/Cummings, 1995. Copyright 1995 Benjamin/Cummings Publishing Co.

Fig. 3.8 Major Neurotransmitter Tracts. From Andreasen N C, *The Broken Brain: The Biological Revolution in Psychiatry,* NY: Harper & Row, 1984, pp 134–35.

Fig. 7.4 A Symbolic Interactionist Model of Communication. Adapted from Hulett J E, Jr, A symbolic interactionist model of human communication, *A V Communication Review* 1966 (14)14.

Fig. 7.5 The Covert Rehearsal Phase of the Symbolic Interactionist Model. Adapted from Hulett J E, Jr, A symbolic interactionist model of human communication, *A V Communication Review,* (14)18.

Fig. 8.1 Initial Contact Sheet. Erie County Department of Mental Health; Mental Health Services, Erie County, Corporation IV, South East Corporation V, and Lakeshore Corporation VI.

Text p 134 Mental Status Examination. Small, S M , Outline for Psychiatric Examination, Sandoz Pharmaceuticals, Division of Sandoz, Inc., 1980.

Fig. 8.2 Neurologic Assessment Guide. From *American Journal of Nursing,* (77)9 ©1977 American Journal of Nursing Company.

Fig. 8.3 Thematic Apperception Test. Reprinted from Murray H A, Thematic Apperception Test, Harvard University Press, 1943. ©1943 by the President and Fellows of Harvard College; 1971 by Henry A Murray.

Fig. 8.4 Examples of the Draw-A-Person Test. Spire R H, Project in partial fulfillment of MS degree, State University of New York at Buffalo, 1967, pp. 243, 248, 249, 251, 256.

Fig. 8.6 A Mental Health Supplement to the Standard Database. Veterans Administration Hospital, Buffalo, NY.

Fig. 8.7 Sample Form for Problem-oriented Progress Notes. Veterans Administration Hospital, Buffalo, NY.

Table 8.1 Differentiation of Mental Status Examination Findings. Adapted from Bates B, *A Guide to Physical Examination,* 3rd Ed, Lippincott, 1983, pp 312–313. ©1974 Lippincott/Harper & Row.

Fig. 9.1 Example of No-harm Contract. Langley Porter Psychiatric Hospital and Clinics, Nursing Staff, Behavioral Neurosciences Service.

Fig. 9.2 Contract of Basic Expectations. Adapted from Langley Porter Psychiatric Hospital and Clinics, 1985, Behavioral Neurosciences Service.

Box p 172 Incorporating Spirituality into the Therapeutic Environment. Adapted from Waldfogel and Wolpe, Using awareness of religious factors to enhance interventions in consultation-liaison psychiatry, *Hospital and Community Psychiatry,* 1993; (44)473–477. ©1993 by the American Psychiatric Association. Reprinted by permission.

Box p 175 Suggestions for Establishing a Therapeutic Environment Outside the Hospital: C C Bisbee, *Educating Patients and Families About Mental Illness,* Aspen Publishers, 1991, pp 365–380. ©1991 Aspen Publishers, Inc.

Text p 178 Dominant Ethical Perspectives. Adapted from Davis A J and Aroskar M A, *Ethical Dilemmas and Nursing Practice,* Appleton Century Crofts, 1978.

Box p 179 Principles of Bioethics. Davis A J, Ethical dilemmas in nursing. Recorded at JONA and Nurse Educator's 1981 Joint Leadership Conference.

Box p 184 Mental Patient's Bill of Rights. Mental Patients Alliance of Central New York, Inc.

Fig. 10.1 Integrated Model: Diagnostic, Therapeutic and Ethic of Reasoning. Gordon et al., Clinical judgment: An integrated model, *Advances in Nursing Science* 16(4): 55–70.

Table 12.1 Impaired Cognitive Function. Blazer D, Hughes D, George I, The epidemiology of depression in an elderly community population, *Gerontologist* 1987; 27(3):281–287.

Table 12.2 Global Deterioration Scale Stages and Functional Assessment Stages in Alzheimer's. Adapted from Reisberg et al., The stage-specific temporal course of Alzheimer's disease, Kqbal et al., eds, *Prog Clin Biol Res* 1989. ©1989 John Wiley & Sons. Reprinted by permission of Wiley-Liss, Inc, a subsidiary of John Wiley & Sons, Inc.

Table 12.3 Aids in the Evaluation of Clients with Possible Dementia. From Bennett B and Knopman D, 1994, Alzheimer's Disease, *Geriatrics,* 49(8):22. ©1994 Advanstar Communications. Reprinted with permission.

Box p 226 Physiologic, Psychologic, and Environmental Etiologies of Acute Confusional States in the Hospitalized Elderly. Foreman, M D, *Nursing Research* 1986, 35:37. Copyright © 1986 The American Journal of Nursing Co.

Fig. 13.3 Cocaine Use Cycle: Landry M, Smith D E, Crack: Anatomy of addiction. *Calif Nurs* March/April 1987:13.

Box p 255 Physical Effects of Chronic Alcoholism. Kneisl C R, Ames S A, *Adult Health Nursing: A Biopsychosocial Approach,* Addison-Wesley, 1986. Copyright © 1986 Addison-Wesley Publishing Co.

Box p 277 A Guide to Analyzing Personal Responses Toward Substance Abusers. Kneisl C R, Ames S A, *Adult Health Nursing: A Biopsychosocial Approach,* Addison-Wesley, 1986. Copyright © 1986 Addison-Wesley Publishing Co.

Box p 281 Signs and Symptoms of Liver Cirrhosis. Adapted from Meissner J E, Caring for Patients with Cirrhosis, *Nurs* 1994, 9:44–45.

Box p 282 The Twelve Steps of Alcoholics Anonymous. Twelve Steps and Twelve Traditions, reprinted with permission of Alcoholics Anonymous World Services, Inc.

Box p 308 Assessment: Hallucinations. Murphy M F, Moller M D, Relapse management in neurobiological disorders: The Moller-Murphy symptom management assessment tool, *Arch Psych Nurs* 1993: 8(4):226–235.

Fig. 14.1 A Stress-Vulnerability Model for Symptom Etiology: O'Connor F W, *Image: Journal of Nursing Scholarship,* 1994 (26)3, fig 1, p 232.

Table 14.3 Action and Side Effects of Antipsychotic Medications. Adapted from Mathewson M A and Kun M A, *Pharmacotherapeutics: A Nursing Approach,* 3rd Ed, F A Davis Co, 1994.

Box p 374 Assessment: Common Features of Anxiety. *Diagnostic and Statistical Manual of Mental Disorders,* 4th Ed, Washington, D C: American Psychiatric Association, 1994.

Box p 379 Guidelines for Working with Anxious Clients. Peplau H, Interpersonal techniques: The crux of nursing. *American Journal of Nursing,* (62)6. © 1962 American Journal of Nursing Co.

Fig. 18.1 Client Contract for Weight Gain. Patricia Worthy, Head Nurse, and the Nursing Staff of the Adolescent and Young Adult Treatment Unit, Yale-New Haven Hospital, New Haven, CT.

Box p 499 Nursing Self-Awareness. Recognizing and Working with Borderline Personalities. Wester C M, Managing the Borderline Personality, *Nurs Mngmt* 1989, 20:49–51.

Table 21.1 Phases of Supported Employment. Anthony W A, Farkas M D, Cohen M R, *Psychiatric Rehabilitation,* Boston. Boston University, Center for Psychiatric Rehabilitation, 1990.

Fig. 21.1 The WHO Parallel Sequence for Long-term Illness. World Health Organization, Internal Classification of Impairments, Disabilities and Handicaps, 1980.

Box p 563 Rape Myths Versus Rape Facts. Adapted from *Resources Against Sexual Assault,* Rape Prevention Education Program, 1987, pp 5–6, University of California, San Francisco.

Box p 594 Signs That Help Predict Suicide Risk. Lee Ann Hoff, *People in Crisis,* San Francisco, CA: Jossey-Bass, 1995, pp 207–208. ©1995 Jossey-Bass, Inc.

Box p 597 Lethality Assessment Scale. Lee Ann Hoff, *People in Crisis,* San Francisco, CA: Jossey-Bass, 1995, p 209. ©1995 Jossey-Bass, Inc.

Fig. 27.1 The HIV Mental Health Spectrum. Knox, Davis, Friedrich, The HIV mental health spectrum, *Community Mental Health Journal* 1994; 30(1): 77.

Box p 662 Counseling Plan for Clients with a Dual Diagnosis of HIV and Substance Use. Hughes, Martin, Franks, *AIDS Home Care and Hospice Manual,* Visiting Nurses Association of San Francisco, 1987, p 137.

Box p 703 Visualization for the Bath. Mason J L, *Guide to Stress Reduction,* Berkeley, CA: Celestial Arts, 1986, 1980, pp 61–63.

Box p 708 Albert Ellis' Ten Basic Irrational Ideas. Davis, Eshelman, McKay, *The Relaxation and Stress Reduction Handbook,* 2nd Ed, New Harbinger Publications, 1982, pp 106–107.

Table 30.1 Assistance During Three Stages of Natural Disaster. Lee Ann Hoff, *People in Crisis,* San Francisco, CA: Jossey-Bass, 1995, pp 316–317. ©1995 Jossey-Bass, Inc.

Fig. 30.1 The Effect of Balancing Factors in a Stressful Event. Aguilera, D C, *Crisis Intervention:* Theory and Methodology, 7th Ed, C V Mosby, 1994, p 66.

Box p 715 Myths and Realities About Crisis. Adapted from Lee Ann Hoff, *People in Crisis,* San Francisco, CA: Jossey-Bass, 1995, pp 6–8. ©1995 Jossey-Bass, Inc.

Fig. 32.1 Main Flow of a Family Life Chronology. Satir, *Conjoint Family Therapy,* Rev Ed, Science and Behavior Books, Inc, 1967.

Box p 795 Medication Teaching Plan: Antipsychotics. Adapted from Langley Porter Psychiatric Institute Hospital and Clinics, 1984. University of California, San Francisco.

Box p 797 Dexamethasone Suppression Test Information. Adapted from Langley Porter Psychiatric Institute Hospital and Clinics, 1985. University of California, San Francisco.

Box p 800 Medication Teaching Plan: TCAs. Adapted from Langley Porter Psychiatric Institute Hospital and Clinics, 1984. University of California, San Francisco.

Box p 802 Medication Teaching Plan: MAOIs. Box Ch. 33: Adapted from Langley Porter Psychiatric Institute Hospital and Clinics, 1984. University of California, San Francisco.

Fig. 33.2 The Simpson Neurological Scale. The Simpson Neurological Scale: Dept of Health and Human Services, Public Health Service, Alcohol, Drug Abuse and Mental Health Administration, NIMH Treatment Strategies in Schizophrenia Study.

Fig. 33.3 The Abnormal Involuntary Movement Scale. Dept of Health and Human Services, Public Health Service, Alcohol, Drug Abuse and Mental Health Administration, NIMH Treatment Strategies in Schizophrenia Study.

Box p 806 Medication Teaching Plan: Carbamazepine. Adapted from Langley Porter Psychiatric Institute Hospital and Clinics, 1984. University of California, San Francisco.

Box p 808 Medication Teaching Plan: Lithium Carbonate. Adapted from Langley Porter Psychiatric Institute Hospital and Clinics, 1984. University of California, San Francisco.

Box p 812 Medication Teaching Plan: Benzodiazepines. Adapted from Langley Porter Psychiatric Institute Hospital and Clinics, 1984. University of California, San Francisco.

Table 33.4 Antipsychotic Medication and Lithium Compatibility with Liquids and Other Drugs. Department of Pharmacy, Buffalo Psychiatric Center, Buffalo, New York, 1994.

Table 35.2 Four Models of Health Maintenance Organizations. Group Health Insurance Association of America, 1990.

Box p 853 Functions of the Case Manager in Managed Mental Health Care. Adapted from Bower K A, *Case Management by Nurses,* American Nurses Publishing, 1992.

Table 35.3 Comparative Dominant Values of Long-Term and Short-Term Therapists. Simon Budman, *Psychotherapy and Managed Care: The Optimal Use of Time and Resources,* American Psychiatric Press, 1991. Copyright ©1991 American Psychiatric Press.

Box p 860 ANA Standards of Child and Adolescent Psychiatric and Mental Health Nursing. American Nurses Association, 1985. Reprinted with permission of the American Nurses Association.

Table 37.1 Life Priorities by Ethnic Group. Public Health Service, 1992.

Fig. 37.1 The Continuous Chain of Prevention. Serrano, C V, Adoles J, *Health* 1993;14:613–618. ©1993 Elsevier Science Publishing.

Box p 894 National Health Objectives Measured by the Youth Risk Behavior Surveillance. Adapted from Public Health Service, 1993.

Table 38.1 Examples of Medications Used as Hypnotics in the Elderly: McCall, W V, Management of Primary Sleep Disorders Among Elderly Persons. *Psychiatric Services,* 1995; 46(1):49–54. ©1995 American Psychiatric Association.

Table 38.2 Antidepressant Medication for the Elderly: Hogstel M, ed, *Geropsychiatric Nursing,* 2nd Ed, Mosby, 1995, T5.1. ©1995 Mosby-Year Book, Inc.

Table 38.3 Antipsychotic Medication for the Elderly: Hogstel M, ed, *Geropsychiatric Nursing,* 2nd Ed, Mosby, 1995, T5.2. ©1995 Mosby-Year Book, Inc.

Fig. 38.1 Short Portable Mental Status Questionnaire. Pfeiffer E, The Psychological Evaluation of the Elderly Client, in Busse, E W, Blazer, D G, eds, *Handbook of Geriatric Psychiatry.* Van Nostrand Reinhold, 1980. ©1974 E Pfeiffer.

Table 38.4 Normal Changes in Aging that Affect Medical Absorption. Ebersole P E, and Hess P A, *Toward Healthy Aging: Human Needs and Nursing Response,* 4th Ed, Mosby, 1994. ©1994 C V Mosby.

DSM-IV Diagnostic Criteria on pages 218, 222, 223, 225, 248, 249, 250, 299, 300, 301, 326, 327, 362, 366, 367, 400, 401, 403, 421, 422, 450, 451, 452, 454, 455, 456, 457, 458, 471, 476, 485, 486, 497, 502, 504, 506, 512, 513, 517, 716: American Psychiatric Association, Diagnostic and Statistical Manual of Mental Disorders, 4th Edition. Copyright ©1994 American Psychiatric Association.

INDEX

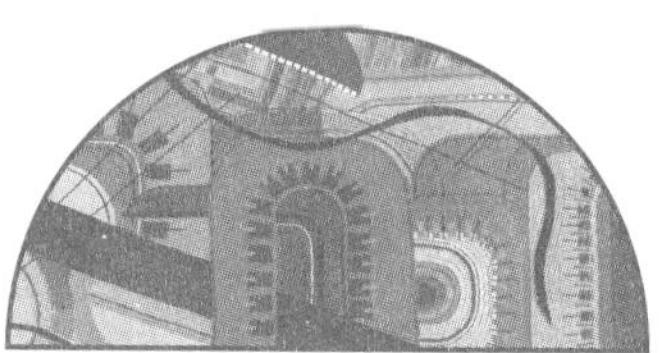

Note: *t* following a page number indicates a table, *i* following a page number indicates an illustration.

B

D

F

J

K

L

O